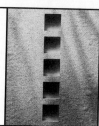

MANUAL OF
PEDIATRIC
EMERGENCY
NURSING

P9-DUC-480

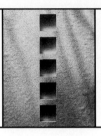

Manual of Pediatric Emergency Nursing

Treesa E. Soud, RN, BSN
Pediatric Emergency Nurse Consultant and Staff Nurse
Children's Emergency Center
Baptist Medical Center
Jacksonville, Florida

Janice Steiner Rogers, MS, RN, CS, PNP
Pediatric Nurse Practitioner
Emergency Department
University of Rochester Medical Center

Instructor of Clinical Nursing
University of Rochester
School of Nursing
Rochester, New York

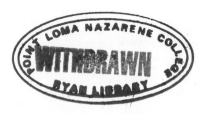
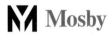

Mosby

St. Louis Baltimore Boston Carlsbad Chicago Minneapolis New York Philadelphia Portland
London Milan Sydney Tokyo Toronto

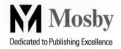
Mosby
Dedicated to Publishing Excellence

**A Times Mirror
Company**

Vice President and Publisher: Nancy L. Coon
Executive Editor: Sally Schrefer
Developmental Editor: Michele D. Hayden
Project Manager: John Rogers
Production Editor: Jeanne Genz
Designer: Yael Kats
Manufacturing Manager: Linda Ierardi

Copyright © 1998 by Mosby–Year Book, Inc.

Printed in the United States of America
Composition by Graphic World, Inc.
Printing/binding by R.R. Donnelley & Sons Company

Mosby–Year Book, Inc.
11830 Westline Industrial Drive
St. Louis, Missouri 63146

Library of Congress Cataloging in Publication Data
Soud, Treesa Etheredge.
     Manual of pediatric emergency nursing / Treesa Etheredge Soud,
   Janice S. Rogers. — 1st ed.
        p.   cm.
     Includes bibliographical references and index.
     ISBN 0-8016-7891-9
     1. Pediatric emergencies.   2. Pediatric nursing.   3. Emergency
nursing.   I. Rogers, Janice S.   II. Title.
     [DNLM: 1. Emergency Nursing.   2. Pediatric Nursing.   WY 154 S719m
1988] RJ370.S66   1998
     610.73′62—dc21
     DNLM/DLC
     for Library of Congress   97-14312
                                                                CIP

97 98 99 00 01 / 9 8 7 6 5 4 3 2 1

Contributors

Connie Toney Andry, RN
Nurse Manager, Children's Emergency Center
Baptist Medical Center
Jacksonville, Florida

Nancie Mlakar Bechtel, RN, BSN, CEN, EMT
Staff Nurse, Emergency Department
Children's Hospital
Columbus, Ohio

Valerie L. Benjamin, RN, CPNP
Pediatric Care Center
Hughes-Spalding Children's Hospital
Atlanta, Georgia

Lisa Marie Bernardo, RN, PhD, CEN
Assistant Professor
University of Pittsburgh
School of Nursing
Pittsburgh, Pennsylvania

Syvil S. Burke, RN, MSN, CCRN
Head Nurse, Intensive Care Nursery
Duke University Medical Center
Durham, North Carolina

Karen Chalanick, RN, MS, PNP
Pediatric Nurse Practitioner
Pediatric Pulmonary Division
University of Rochester Medical Center
Children's Hospital at Strong
Rochester, New York

Marianne Chiafery, RN, MSN
Nurse Educator, Department of Nursing and Career
    Development
University of Rochester Medical Center
Strong Memorial Hospital
Rochester, New York

Alice E. Conway, RN, PhD
Associate Professor
Edinboro University of Pennsylvania
Edinboro, Pennsylvania

Sandra L. Elvik, RN, MS, CPNP
Associate Professor of Pediatrics
UCLA School of Medicine;
Assistant Medical Director
Child Crisis Center
Harbor UCLA Medical Center
Torrance, California

Joanne Fioravanti, RN, MS, PNP
Assistant Professor of Clinical Nursing
University of Rochester School of Nursing
Rochester, New York

Kathy Haley, RN, BSN, CEN
Trauma Coordinator, Trauma Services
Children's Hospital
Columbus, Ohio

Mary Fran Hazinski, RN, MSN, FAAN
Clinical Specialist
Division of Trauma
Departments of Surgery and Pediatrics
Vanderbilt University Medical Center
Vanderbilt Children's Hospital
Nashville, Tennessee

Deborah Parkman Henderson, RN, PhD
Lecturer
Department of Pediatrics
UCLA School of Medicine
Harbor UCLA Medical Center
Torrance, California

Marilyn M. Robertson Horton, RN, CEN
Staff Nurse
Children's Emergency Center
Wolfson's Children's Hospital
Baptist Medical Center
Jacksonville, Florida

Connie Parnaby Inman, RN
Staff Nurse
Children's Emergency Center
Wolfson's Children's Hospital
Baptist Medical Center
Jacksonville, Florida

Jean E. Mack-Fogg, RN, MS, PNP, CS
Pediatric Nurse Practitioner
Pediatric Endocrinology
University of Rochester Medical Center
Strong Memorial Hospital
Rochester, New York

Saniyyah I. Mahmoudi, RN, MSN, CCRN, ARNP
Pediatric Nurse Practitioner
Education Coordinator
Pediatric Infectious Diseases and Immunology
University of Florida Health Science Center
Jacksonville, Florida

Linda Manley, RN, BSN, CEN, CCRN
EMS Coordinator, Children's Hospital;
Flight Nurse, Med Flight
Columbus, Ohio

Barbara S. Masiulis, RN, MS, CS, PNP
Pediatric Nurse Practitioner
Child Neurology
University of Rochester Medical Center
Rochester, New York

Bernadette Mazurek Melnyk, RN-C, PhD, PNP
Assistant Professor of Nursing
University of Rochester School of Nursing
Rochester, New York

Marcy Moag Noble, RN, BSN, CEN
Pediatric Nurse Leader
Emergency Department
University of Rochester Medical Center
Strong Memorial Hospital
Rochester, New York

Scott E. Pikulski, RN
Flight Nurse
Life Flight
Baptist Medical Center
Jacksonville, Florida

Theresa D. Pye, RN, BSN
Clinical Nurse Educator
Emergency Department
University Medical Center
Jacksonville, Florida

Sharon P. Redfearn, RN, MSN, ARNP
Pediatric Cardiology Nurse Practitioner
Division of Pediatric Cardiology
University of Florida
Wolfson's Children's Hospital
Jacksonville, Florida

Peggy D. Saum, RN, CEN, EMT-P
Chief Flight Nurse
Life Flight
Baptist Medical Center
Jacksonville, Florida

Jay L. Schauben, PharmD, ABAT
Clinical Professor and Director
Florida Poison Information Center
University Medical Center
University of Florida Health Science Center
Jacksonville, Florida

Kimberly A. Schriefer, RN, BSN
Assistant Nurse Manager
Children's Emergency Center
Baptist Medical Center
Jacksonville, Florida

Alison W. Schultz, RN, EdD
Associate Clinical Professor of Nursing
University of Rochester School of Nursing
Rochester, New York

Melinda Sciera, RN, MS, CS, PNP
Pediatric Nurse Practitioner
Emergency Department
University of Rochester Medical Center
Strong Memorial Hospital
Rochester, New York

Patricia Regina Julian Standifer, RN
Staff Nurse
East Tennessee Children's Hospital
Knoxville, Tennessee

Melissa Lawson Stimler, RN, BSN
Nurse Manager
Emergency Services
Baptist Medical Center
Jacksonville, Florida

Rita A. Dello Stritto, RN, MSN, CEN, CNS, ENP
Emergency Nurse Practitioner
Kelsey-Seybold Urgent Care Clinic
Houston, Texas

Donna Ojanen Thomas, RN, MSN, CEN
Director, Emergency Department
Primary Children's Medical Center
Salt Lake City, Utah

Cheryl A. Tucker, RN, BSN, CSPI
Education Coordinator
Florida Poison Information Center
University Medical Center
Jacksonville, Florida

Elizabeth Weld Vaczy, RN, MS, PNP, CS
Pediatric Nurse Practitioner
Pediatric Practice
University of Rochester Medical Center
Children's Hospital at Strong
Rochester, New York

Karen L. Winn, RN, MSN, CCRN, ARNP
Clinical Nurse Specialist
Exu-Dry Wound Care Products, Inc.
Atlanta, Georgia;
Formerly Clinical Nurse Specialist
University of South Alabama Burn Center
Mobile, Alabama

Reviewers

Ann M. Capelli Anderson, RN
Clinical Research Associate
Shriner's Hospital for Crippled Children
St. Louis, Missouri

Roger M. Barkin, MD, MPH, FAAP, FACEP
Vice President for Pediatric and Newborn Programs
Columbia HealthONE;
Professor of Surgery and
Clinical Professor of Pediatrics
University of Colorado Health Sciences Center
Denver, Colorado

Deborah S. Boucher, RN, MS, CEN, CCRN
Emergency Clinical Nurse Specialist
UCLA Medical Center
Emergency Medicine Center
Los Angeles, California

Cynthia Cappiello, RN, MS
Nurse Practitioner, Emergency Department
University of Rochester Medical Center
Strong Memorial Hospital
Rochester, New York

Ellen M. Chiocca, RNC, MSN
Instructor, Maternal-Child Health
Loyola University
Chicago, Illinois

Patricia Codden, RN, MSN
Clinical Specialist in Hematology/Oncology
Cardinal Glennon Children's Hospital
St. Louis, Missouri

M. Colleen O'Neil Davis, MD, FAAP
Assistant Professor
Emergency Medicine and Pediatrics
University of Rochester Medical Center
Rochester, New York

Sharon Deppe, RN, BSN
Nurse Clinician, Trauma Services
Children's Hospital
Columbus, Ohio

Brian Duggan, RN, MSN, ANP, CEN
Clinical Systems Analyst
Texas Children's Hospital
Houston, Texas

Nancy J. Eckle, RN, MSN, CEN
Clinical Nurse Specialist
Emergency Department
Children's Hospital
Columbus, Ohio

Laurie Flaherty, RN, MS, CCRN, CEN
Clinical Educator, Emergency Department
Georgetown University Hospital
Washington, D.C.

Jill P. French, RN, MSN, CCRN
Clinical Educator
Pediatric Intensive Care Unit
Wake Medical Center
Raleigh, North Carolina

Gregory G. Gaar, MD
Clinical Assistant Professor of Pediatrics
University of South Florida College of Medicine;
Co-Medical Director, Florida Poison Information
   and Toxicology Resource Center;
Medical Director
Saunders Pediatric Emergency Care Center
Tampa General Hospital
Tampa, Florida

Victor F. Garcia, MD
Director, Trauma Service
Children's Hospital Medical Center
Cincinnati, Ohio

Mary Martha Hall, RN, MSN, CEN
Clinical Nurse Specialist, Emergency Center
Ben Taub Hospital
Houston, Texas

Reneé S. Holleran, RN, PhD, CEN, CCRN, CFRN
Chief Flight Nurse, University Air Care;
Emergency Clinical Nurse Specialist
University of Cincinnati Hospital
Cincinnati, Ohio

Foreword

Your children are not your children. They are the sons and daughters of Life's longing for itself. They come through you, but not from you, and though they are with you, yet they belong not to you.

Kahil Gibran

In 1986, I was a member of the flight team that was called to transport a child a little less than 2 years of age to our Children's Hospital in Cincinnati. The child's mother reported that he had been relatively healthy up until a few hours before she had brought him to the emergency department of her community hospital. In fact, his mother had taken him trick-or-treating the night before and he still bore the remnants of his Halloween makeup on his face. Now he was gravely ill with meningitis and in profound septic shock.

During the 20-minute transport, the child's vital signs continued to deteriorate and we could only maintain his central pulse with repeated boluses of intravenous fluids and epinephrine. Unfortunately, he expired a short time after admission to the pediatric emergency department.

Our resuscitation efforts had been guided by the education provided by our pediatric colleagues at Cincinnati Children's Medical Center and the training we had received from Advanced Cardiac Life Support (ACLS). It was not until 2 years later that the Pediatric Advanced Life Support Course became available nationally and direction for pediatric resuscitation and care was widely distributed.

In 1992, *U.S. News and World Report*[1] reported cases where children had been permanently damaged or had died because hospitals (particularly emergency departments) and rescue units were not properly prepared to deal with pediatric emergencies. This article brought to light nationally what many of us were already acutely aware of—there needed to be more and better resources to provide emergency care to critically ill and injured pediatric patients.

Over the past 10 years, numerous people and organizations have devoted time and energy to assure that pediatric patients receive appropriate care during an emergency. Examples of actions directed at improving pediatric care include the following: the development and funding of the Emergency Medical Services for Children (EMS-C) supported by the Maternal and Child Health Bureau of the U.S. Department of Human Services,[2,3] which provides funding on a state level to train and educate emergency care providers; the creation of the Emergency Nursing Pediatric Course (ENPC),[4] which offers a focused course on the emergency nursing care of the pediatric patient; and the revisions of the Pediatric Advanced Life Support course, which now includes a nurse coeditor.[5]

Another major focal point of the past 10 years has been the efforts put into prevention. Teaching families and communities about restraint systems, gun safety, and immunizations, and teaching them how to recognize and prevent abuse are but a few examples of prevention strategies.

This text, the *Manual of Pediatric Emergency Nursing*, has brought together many of the pediatric nursing pioneers who have contributed to pediatric emergency care. The book provides a comprehensive approach to the emergency management of the ill or injured child and information about legal and ethical considerations, crisis management, emergency care of the child with a special need, and pediatric pain management.

One of the most frightening experiences people can endure is to have to take their children to the emergency department. As parents, they expect that the people caring for their children are educated and trained to provide competent pediatric emergency care. The *Manual of Pediatric Emergency Nursing*, authored by Soud and Rogers, offers a significant resource for those responsible for pediatric emergency care.

Reneé Semonin Holleran, RN, PhD, CEN, CCRN, CFRN
Flight Nurse/Emergency Clinical Specialist
1996 President, Emergency Nurses Association

REFERENCES

1. Buckley J: The shame of emergency care for kids, *U.S. News & World Report* 1:34-43, 1992.

2. Seidel J, Henderson D: *Emergency medical services for children: A report to the nation*, 1991, National Center for Education in Maternal and Child Health.

3. Durch J, Lohr K: *Emergency medical services for children*, Washington DC, 1993, National Academy Press.

4. Haley K, Baker P: *Emergency nursing pediatric course*, Park Ridge, Il, 1993, Emergency Nurses Association.

5. Chameides L, Hazinski M: *Textbook of pediatric advanced life support*, Dallas, 1994, American Heart Association.

Preface

Emergency nursing is one of the few specialties for which the nurse must possess skills and knowledge in a wide array of topics—from complex trauma and medical care, to caring for the elderly, to caring for children. In recent years educational programs and texts have proliferated as attempts are made to assist the emergency nurse when caring for the child. This book is meant not only to be a practical guide for the emergency nurse when providing care to children and their families, but also to include controversial and often complex issues relating to the care of children. It was written with the generalist emergency nurse in mind, but it can be used in a variety of settings where acutely ill or injured children may be cared for; among these are primary care clinics or offices and prehospital systems, both primary and secondary transport services. Nurses from throughout the country participated in writing this text, allowing for a broader view of emergency nursing care interventions.

Part one includes chapters that review general approaches to care unique to the pediatric population; for example, legal considerations and pediatric triage. Part two includes emergent conditions and interventions, as well as crisis management. Part three includes specific systems and selected pediatric emergencies. Each chapter in this section includes a system-specific overview of assessment and anatomic and physiologic differences of the child as they relate to assessment findings and interventions. Part four includes trauma-related topics—from the general approach, to pediatric multiple trauma, to specific trauma-related topics including head and neck trauma, burn care, and child maltreatment. Part five includes both specialty topics such as care of the neonate and children with special needs to sometimes controversial issues such as care of the febrile child, pediatric pain management, and pediatric ingestions.

ACKNOWLEDGMENTS

The list of people who have supported this project is endless. However, the staff of the Baptist Medical Center, Children's Emergency Center deserve special mention, as they have assisted me, reviewed material, offered constructive criticism, and put up with my erratic schedule. Others who deserve special mention are those who have been behind the scenes such as my husband, Gary, who reviewed content at the last minute when no one else was available, and who put up with my late nights and weekends at the computer when he had other plans for the family. My son Ryan, who was born during this project has brought great joy and depth to my life.

Treesa E. Soud

I am most grateful for the support of my family, colleagues, and friends while I was working on this book. In particular, I would like to thank my parents, Marg and Harry Steiner, and my sisters, Pat and Mary Ellen, for their love, guidance, and encouragement; Betsy Slavinskas, Associate Nursing Director of Ambulatory Care Services at the University of Rochester Medical Center, for helping me balance my work schedule with writing and editing; and especially my children, Karin, Brian, and Katie, for putting up with the enormous amount of time I needed to put into this project and for being the greatest joy in my life.

Janice S. Rogers

Contents

PART I   APPROACH TO THE CHILD
1 Emergency Medical Services for Children (EMSC), 1
2 Legal and Ethical Considerations, 24
3 Unique Characteristics of Children, 43
4 Pediatric History and Physical Examination, 70
5 Pediatric Triage, 89

PART II   EMERGENT CONDITIONS AND INTERVENTIONS
6 Respiratory Failure and Shock, 107
7 Life-Threatening Neurologic Emergencies, 128
8 Pediatric and Neonatal Resuscitation, 147
9 Crisis Intervention and Death, 178

PART III   SYSTEMS OVERVIEW WITH SELECTED EMERGENCIES
10 Respiratory System, 193
11 Cardiovascular System, 233
12 Neurologic System, 266
13 Musculoskeletal System, 290
14 Fluid and Electrolyte Imbalances, 313
15 Gastrointestinal System, 332
16 Genitourinary System, 364
17 Hematologic and Immune Systems, 390
18 Integumentary System, 417
19 Eye, Ear, Nose, and Throat Disorders, 452
20 Endocrine System, 472

PART IV   PEDIATRIC TRAUMA
21 Multiple Trauma Management, 487
22 Trauma—Selected Systems, 511
23 Musculoskeletal and Soft Tissue Injuries, 540
24 Burn Injuries, 564
25 Child Maltreatment, 586

PART V   SELECTED CLINICAL TOPICS
26 The Febrile Child, 606
27 Environmental and Toxicologic Emergencies, 622
28 Neonatal Topics, 660
29 Pain Assessment and Management, 686
30 Children with Special Needs, 712
31 Psychosocial and Behavioral Problems, 727

APPENDIXES

A   Comparison of EMS Data Collection Recommendations, 741

B   EMSC State Contacts—1997, 742

C   Summary of Recommendations of the Committee on Pediatric Emergency Medical Services, 747

D   Growth Charts, 749

CHAPTER 1

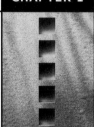

Emergency Medical Services for Children (EMSC)

Deborah P. Henderson

■ INTRODUCTION

Unquestionably, critically ill and injured children are challenging patients. Preverbal children are not able to describe their symptoms, are frightened by most aspects of physical examinations, and are often unable to indicate the location of their pain. As children mature, their needs change; each age and stage of childhood is different, and each is associated with different illnesses and injuries. To care for children effectively, emergency medical services (EMS) systems must be designed to be as responsive to their needs as to those of adults. Health care providers must have good pediatric assessment skills and be able to recognize the critically ill or injured child rapidly, plan treatment, and expedite care. Full development and integration of pediatric emergency care into EMS systems requires community commitment and creative use of national, regional, and local resources.

An EMS system is an organized system of care beginning with injury prevention and continuing through rehabilitation and reintegration of ill and injured patients into the community. Nurses play an important role in EMS systems. All across the United States, emergency nurses staff critical care ambulances, serve as flight nurses for aeromedical transports, and care for pediatric patients in many different types of settings and facilities, including community hospitals, ambulatory care centers, rural standby emergency departments, and tertiary care centers. Nurses in some areas are responsible for on-line direction of prehospital personnel, performing quality improvement and utilization review and providing tape reviews and educational programs for all levels of health care professionals in the EMS system.

■ EMERGENCY MEDICAL SERVICES SYSTEMS (EMSS)

Providing care for critically ill and injured patients before arrival at a definitive care center is a relatively new concept. The two earliest prehospital care systems in the United States (Dade County, Florida, and Los Angeles, California) are now less than 30 years old.[5] As late as the 1950s, the largest number of prehospital transport vehicles was hearses operated primarily by mortuary personnel. As ambulances became the mode of transport in emergency care, the idea of providing medical care for patients at the scene and en route to the hospital was conceived. Trained providers became a necessity; cardiac care nurses were the first prehospital providers in Los Angeles.

As the idea of prehospital care gathered impetus, EMS systems began transporting all types and all ages of patients, both ill and injured. In the late 1970s, as the number of motor vehicles and the speed of motor vehicles increased, the number of highway traffic collisions increased also, resulting in a greater number of traumatic injuries and demand for prehospital care. Care of this type of multiple trauma patient was very familiar to medics who cared for wartime casualties; the knowledge and experience gained in treatment of injured military personnel was used to develop procedures, protocols, and EMS structural components.[5] Over time, prehospital trauma and cardiac care for adult patients grew increasingly sophisticated, and more patients began to use the EMS system. Many pediatric patients were being attended to in EMS systems largely designed for adults and by personnel who were trained to care for adult illnesses and injuries.

In the last 20 years, EMS systems have taken a quantum leap forward. Some of the problems of emergency access to medical care were researched and publicized by the 1966 report by the National Research Council of the National Academy of Sciences, *Accidental Death and Disability: The Neglected Disease of Modern Society*. This report increased national awareness, stimulated discussion, and encouraged passage of legislation to support EMS system improvement. Through the EMSS Act of 1973 (PL 93-154), which was amended in 1976 and 1979, federal block grant funding for EMS systems was authorized for development of EMS systems nationally over a 5-year period. This Act identified 15 essential components for EMS systems (Box 1-1). Also in the early 1970s, the Robert Wood Johnson Foundation offered grant funding for expanding EMS systems and improving field communication in prehospital care. These two sources of funding were largely responsible for the early development of EMS systems as we now know them.

Today, many prehospital providers perform sophisticated medical interventions, with and without on-line medical direction, and are able to monitor and treat critically ill and injured patients with the latest medical procedures and equipment. Other EMS systems, however, are still staffed exclusively by volunteers who have little or no time for advanced medical training or continuing education and are provided with only the most basic equipment and supplies.[13] The term *EMS system*, therefore, is only a very basic concept; each EMS system has a different character and resources. Some very general national standards have been developed for educating, training, and equipping prehospital personnel, but these are often loosely interpreted. At present, there are many types of emergency medical technicians (EMTs) able to perform care at various levels (Box 1-2).

DEVELOPMENT OF EMERGENCY MEDICAL SERVICES FOR CHILDREN (EMSC)

With the rapid expansion of EMS systems and emergency care in the middle and late 1970s, there was growing concern among pediatricians, pediatric trauma surgeons, and others that the mortality rates for ill and injured children cared for in EMS systems were higher than in the adult population.[40] By the early 1980s, there were questions about whether EMS personnel were receiving sufficient pediatric training and whether the equipment they carried was appropriate for pediatric emergency care.[44] A study by Ramenofsky et al. was equally influential during this period. The study demonstrated that pediatric trauma patients were receiving inadequate care, and it found that there were problems in identification of critically ill and injured patients, improper care of patients, and lack of access to tertiary care centers.[40] The care given to pediatric trauma patients was divided by Ramenofsky into the following six phases:

1. Initial identification of injured patients
2. Field care: treatment and life-sustaining measures initiated and maintained until definitive care is reached
3. Triage of trauma patients to appropriate facilities
4. Transport of critically injured patients to definitive care
5. Definitive care at a level equal to the needs of the patient
6. Rehabilitation

Although Ramenofsky did not include injury prevention as a phase of trauma care, injury prevention is now included as an essential component and perhaps the most important means of reducing death and disability in pediatric patients.

Box 1-1   Components of an EMS System

1. Provision of personnel
2. Training of personnel
3. Communications
4. Transportation
5. Facilities
6. Critical care units
7. Use of public safety agencies
8. Consumer participation
9. Accessibility of care
10. Transfer of patients
11. Consumer information and education
12. Standard medical record keeping
13. Independent review and evaluation
14. Disaster linkage
15. Mutual aid agreements

From Seidel JS, Henderson DP, eds: *Emergency medical services for children: a report to the nation*, Washington, DC, 1991, National Center for Education in Maternal and Child Health.

- *First Responder*   First responder is the minimum standard for certification or licensure, with the average course running approximately 40 hours in length. Content addresses basic techniques (e.g., bandaging, splinting, simple airways). Many states do not recognize this certification.
- *EMT-Basic*   The EMT-Basic provider curriculum is a minimum of 110 hours of instruction. Skills performed are largely noninvasive, although in some states the EMT-B is allowed to apply pneumatic antishock trousers. A few states allow the EMT-B to start and maintain an IV if additional training is obtained.
- *EMT-Defibrillator*   This classification is an add-on module to the EMT-B certification. EMT-Ds are certified to use either automatic or manual defibrillators.
- *EMT-Intermediate*   This classification varies widely. The EMT-I is allowed to perform several invasive procedures under different degrees of supervision (e.g., venipuncture, administration of selected drugs). In some cases the EMT-I is allowed to provide cardiac monitoring and/or defibrillation.
- *EMT-Critical Care*   This category is similar to the EMT-I but may also include such procedures as the insertion of central lines, endotracheal intubation, and cardioversion. It is recognized in fewer than 20 states.
- *EMT-Paramedic*   The EMT-Paramedic receives an average of 749 hours of training, with a minimum curriculum of 400 hours. Skills of the EMT-P include all of the skills outlined in the above categories but may also include such skills as intracardiac injections, cricothyroidotomy, and intraosseous infusion.
- *Mobile Intensive Care Nurse (MICN)* This designation is recognized in only a few states, and the requirements vary widely. There is currently no recognized curriculum for training registered nurses to become MICNs.

Modified from Seidel JS, Henderson DP, eds: *Emergency medical services for children: a report to the nation,* Washington, DC, 1991, National Center for Education in Maternal and Child Health.

Each phase of trauma care has specific challenges, and each has the potential to affect outcomes. This study noted that the lives of some of these children might have been saved by early recognition and appropriate emergency treatment. Although Ramenofsky's research concerns trauma only, pediatric illness is of equal concern. In 1984, a study of pediatric patients cared for in the Los Angeles EMS system showed not only critically injured but also critically ill children had higher mortality rates in areas where there were no facilities with a higher level of care for pediatric patients.[44]

Pediatric patients now comprise a significant percentage of prehospital care. Data collected on over 11,000 pediatric EMS responses by the California EMSC Project in 1989 showed that 5% to 10% of prehospital responses and 20% to 35% (in some hospitals up to 50%) of emergency department visits involved pediatric patients 18 years old and under. Patients are seen for a variety of complaints, which are very similar in rural and urban areas (Table 1-1). A similar study found approximately the same percentages of pediatric patients transported by prehospital providers.[51] The number of pediatric patients documented by these studies is sufficient justification for development of a comprehensive plan for their care.

EMSC COMPONENTS

The categorization of trauma care into the six phases described by Ramenofsky is a model that is equally applicable to pediatric medical emergencies. The six components of emergency care are key factors in the development and management of an integrated approach to critically ill and injured pediatric patients. All six areas must be considered when implementing a regionalized pediatric emergency care system, and each component has the potential to affect outcomes.

PREHOSPITAL CARE

Prehospital care includes identification, dispatch, onscene treatment, and transport of patients to facilities appropriate for their care.

IDENTIFICATION

Recognition and identification of the seriously ill or injured pediatric patient, as well as injury prevention, are important components of prehospital care. EMS systems should be able to identify areas where public

4 I CHAPTER 1: Emergency Medical Services for Children (EMSC)

TABLE 1-1	Chief Complaints for Urban and Rural Pediatric Prehospital Calls			
COMPLAINT	URBAN No. (%)	RURAL No. (%)	BOTH No. (%)	P-VALUE*
Head trauma	1810 (19.6)	194 (16.3)	2004 (19.2)	0.007
Laceration/avulsion	1585 (17.1)	182 (15.3)	1767 (16.1)	0.12
Abrasion/contusion	1334 (14.4)	177 (14.9)	1511 (14.5)	0.66
Pain (knee)	1112 (12.0)	125 (10.5)	1237 (11.8)	0.14
Seizures	826 (8.9)	65 (5.5)	891 (8.5)	<0.0001
Pain—neck/back	788 (8.5)	171 (14.4)	959 (9.2)	<0.0001
Fractures	758 (8.2)	90 (7.6)	848 (8.1)	0.50
Ingestion	669 (7.2)	86 (7.2)	755 (7.2)	0.99
Respiratory distress	492 (5.3)	67 (5.6)	559 (5.4)	0.63
Abdominal pain	421 (4.6)	59 (5.0)	480 (4.6)	0.51
Full arrest	57 (0.6)	4 (0.3)	61 (0.6)	0.31
SIDS	12 (0.1)	1 (0.1)	13 (0.1)	0.99

From Seidel JS et al: Pediatric prehospital care in urban and rural areas, *Pediatr* 88(4):681-690, 1991.
*Fisher's exact test.

education and illness and injury prevention programs can be helpful. The public should be informed when to call a primary care provider, when a child should be taken to an emergency department, when to access the EMS system, and what to do until help arrives. This type of education is important in preventing overuse of limited EMS resources and ensuring appropriate care.

DISPATCH

Central dispatch using the number 9-1-1 is available in many areas of the United States, although some areas continue to use local numbers for this purpose. Dispatchers are often the first to receive emergency calls. Telephone assessment of pediatric patients requires special training to recognize the degree of severity of the illness or injury, which may appear very different from adults. Recognizing the critically ill or injured pediatric patient and providing the correct response may be lifesaving. Dispatchers should know how to give CPR instructions to caretakers and how to provide advice on the immediate care of common pediatric emergencies such as seizures and drowning.

PROVIDER EDUCATION

It is well documented that prehospital providers are particularly anxious about caring for pediatric patients;

anxiety decreases as age of the child increases.[19] This concern is apparent even when providers feel they have adequate skills and training. To decrease anxiety both in initial training and in continuing education, prehospital certification programs should include instruction about the management of pediatric patients. Sufficient time should be given for pediatric skills to become automatic, and equal attention should be given to medical illness and trauma. Important topics to be included in the program include the following:

- Approach to the pediatric patient and family
- Growth and development
- Child abuse and neglect
- Death of a child
- Sudden infant death syndrome (SIDS)

Continuing education is provided to ensure adequate performance of infrequently used pediatric skills, such as endotracheal intubation and intraosseous infusion, when these are approved field procedures. In 1993 a publication outlining the components of pediatric education for paramedics was published by the American Academy of Pediatrics (AAP) in collaboration with the American College of Emergency Physicians (ACEP)—*Guidelines for Paramedic Pediatric Education*.[11] Numerous pediatric emergency care courses for prehospital providers have also been developed, many through EMSC funding from the U.S. Department of Health and Human Services, Maternal and Child Health Bureau

(MCHB); most are public domain material.[27,33] There is no single standard of training for EMTs today, just as there are no national standards agreed upon for the licensing of these professionals; most certification is provided by individual or state EMS agencies. Currently, the Department of Transportation, National Highway Traffic Safety Administration (NHTSA), is supporting the development of national standards for EMT training curricula; training in pediatric emergency care is being included in the recommended curriculum.

In addition to education of certified prehospital providers, persons who are likely to be the first to respond to pediatric emergencies, such as school teachers, school nurses, police officers, sheriffs, lifeguards, and forest rangers, should have training in first aid and resuscitation of pediatric patients. The American Red Cross and the American Heart Association offer basic courses in first aid, as do several commercial companies such as the National Safety Council and Emergency and Safety Programs, Inc. The National Association of School Nurses has developed and disseminates an 8-hour course in pediatric emergency care that was developed in collaboration with the Emergency Nurses Association (ENA).

FIELD TREATMENT PROTOCOLS

Adult field treatment protocols for prehospital providers do not always address the special issues involved in management of the acutely ill or injured child. Guidelines for airway management of the pediatric patient, such as head positioning and appropriate use of airway adjuncts, should be included, as should protocols that provide medication dosages on a per-kilogram basis. These issues should be addressed in standard training programs and ongoing education, along with algorithms, triage protocols, and assessment guidelines for common pediatric medical and traumatic emergencies. Many examples of protocols have been developed by EMSC projects.[4,41] A list of some of the most essential pediatric protocols can be found in Box 1-3.

▌TRANSPORT SYSTEMS

Transport systems vary greatly in accessibility, availability, and personnel. Personal preference of the transferring physician or health care providers may be the deciding factor in facility destination, but it may not always represent the best choice.

Box 1-3 Pediatric Prehospital Protocols

- Abuse—suspected child abuse/sexual abuse
- Airway obstruction by foreign body
- Allergic reaction/anaphylaxis
- Altered level of consciousness
- Arrest—respiratory/cardiorespiratory
- Dysrhythmias (e.g., bradycardia, supraventricular tachycardia)
- Burns
- Cold injuries—hypothermia
- Drowning/near-drowning
- Neonatal resuscitation
- Overdose/poisonings/ingestions
- Respiratory distress
- Seizures
- Shock
- SIDS
- Inhalation injuries
- Trauma

GROUND AND AIR TRANSPORT

Regionalized care should include attention to the development of an organized approach to transport of ill and injured pediatric patients. However, the problems associated with development may be complex. For example, transports across city, county, and state lines may require agreements in advance of need, and the potential use of helicopters or other air transport must be organized in advance so that providers are well staffed and equipped and are available on a timely basis. In certain systems, air transport may be provided directly from the scene; in some of these cases, nurses provide advanced field care, and they may perform complex procedures such as endotracheal intubation, needle cricothyroidotomy, and needle thoracostomy.[18] More information about this issue may be obtained from the AAP guidebook, *Guidelines for Air and Ground Transport of Neonatal and Pediatric Patients* (available from the AAP),[1] which provides some guidance in this complex area.

TRIAGE AND TRANSPORT

Triage from the field to appropriate definitive care facilities requires planning and system development in advance of need. Triage protocols defining criteria for transport to various levels of care ensure delivery of patients to facilities capable of caring for them (Table 1-2). The levels of pediatric care available in a community or region should be mapped out, and field protocols should address destination issues. Correct triage also requires adequate pediatric assessment skills on the part of the prehospital care providers and base station personnel. In areas where radio contact is possible, it may also require radio communication and instruction by emergency physicians and nurses well versed in pediatric care issues. The definition of several levels of definitive care may be necessary for the development of transport protocols that ensure the delivery of pediatric patients to facilities able to care for them. Although there is often resistance among facilities to the concept of regionalization of care, research has shown that critically ill or injured pediatric patients can benefit from transport to appropriate facilities.[39] In regions where they are not triaged to facilities with higher levels of care, mortality increases.[44]

▍SCORING SYSTEMS

Field triage requires accurate assessment of ill and injured patients by the prehospital care provider. Most field providers have run sheets that require, at a minimum, demographics, assessment of vital signs, type of complaint, and mechanism of injury, if any. The most commonly used scoring tool in prehospital and emergency department settings is the Glasgow Coma Scale (GCS). This score was developed to assess the level of consciousness of both medical and trauma patients, and it was intended to be a means of obtaining serial assessments of alterations in mental status rather than a triage tool. It was originally intended for use by physicians and nurses in caring for hospitalized patients.[49] In its original form, it assesses three areas: motor, eye, and verbal responses. Because the assessment of verbal responses in children can be difficult, the Glasgow Coma Scale has been adapted for use in pediatric patients (see Chapter 7).[28]

Several attempts have been made to develop tools that assign numbers to the degree of criticality for field triage—there are definite advantages to using a systematic scoring system, including the following:

- Scoring tools can be used as a means of assisting in both management and triage of patients. An accurate scoring tool can provide a common language that may assist in activation of various levels of response, such as the notification of specialists and subspecialists when available.
- When there is regional system development,

scoring can help to determine the level of care needed for patients, so they can be transported directly to definitive care facilities appropriate to their needs.
- In rural or remote areas where there is only one receiving facility, scoring can be a means of assessing whether secondary transport will be necessary so that air or ground transport providers can be contacted immediately for secondary transfer.
- Comparing field scoring to the condition of the patient in the emergency department can be a means of providing objective measures of improvement or deterioration, and it can also serve as a means of reviewing assessment skills of field providers.

These compelling reasons have fueled the search for a simple method of triaging patients accurately, without excessive overtriage. Many attempts have been made to develop precise scoring systems, most often for traumatic injuries.[30] Because the first EMS systems were designed for adults, so were the first triage scoring systems. Determining the patient's level of consciousness is a requirement for most scoring systems, and this can be problematic with nonverbal pediatric patients.

FIELD SCORING INSTRUMENTS

Triage Index (TI). The TI, developed by Howard Champion in 1980, uses historical criteria, vital signs criteria, and physical examination to triage patients. It was developed to determine degree of severity of traumatic injury and to decide whether patients needed air vs. ground transport to a definitive care facility.[9] This score has been shown to relate well to the Injury Severity Score (ISS) (which uses hospital diagnoses and is only available after hospitalization), and it has been used as a tool for triaging patients.[47] This scale is rather complex for rapid assessment by field personnel, using 18 separate assessment criteria; its use for pediatric patients has not been well established.

Trauma Score (TS). The TS is a revised version of the TI; it is composed of physiologic data and does not include mechanism of injury. Using this score, a patient with a gunshot wound to the chest, who may have relatively normal vital signs on initial assessment, may be incorrectly triaged.[7] It is often used in conjunction with the ISS as a means of evaluating trauma care.

Table 1-2	Los Angeles County EDAP–PCCC* Transport Criteria

The following pediatric patients require transport to a PCCC.

Trauma criteria   **Findings**

Physical assessment   Hypotension, defined by:
    a. BP <70 systolic (6 yrs old and under)
    b. BP <90 systolic (over 6 yrs old)
Abnormal capillary refill (over 2 seconds in normothermic patient)
No spontaneous eye opening
Diffuse abdominal tenderness after blunt or penetrating trauma

Type of injury   Penetrating injury to head, neck, chest, or abdomen
Blunt injury to chest with unstable chest wall (flail chest), or obvious pneumothorax
Obvious deformity of two or more major long bones
Evidence of or presence of uncontrollable hemorrhage

Mechanism of injury   Fall from a height >15 feet
Intrusion of vehicle into passenger space
Pedestrian (walking, skateboard, bicycle) vs. auto, thrown >10 feet, run over, or hit by car going >15 mph

General criteria (other than trauma)

Assessment   Abnormal vital signs at rest, defined by:
    Pulse:
      >180 or <80 in newborns to 1 month
      >160 or <60 in over 1 month
    Respiratory rate:
      >60 or <16 in newborns to 1 month
      >50 or <8 in over 1 month
    Blood pressure:
      <70 systolic (6 yrs old and under)
      <90 systolic (over 6 yrs old)
    Skin signs:
      Cool extremities
      Mottled
      Cold
      Clammy skin
Abnormal capillary refill (>2 seconds in normothermic patient)
Severe respiratory distress, which may be defined by one or more of the following:
    • Evidence of severe supraclavicular, sternal, or intercostal retractions
    • Nasal flaring <2 yrs old
    • Grunting respirations
    • Tripod position
    • Stridor at rest
Cyanosis present or history of cyanotic event
Altered mental status, which may include one or more of the following:
    • No spontaneous eye opening
    • Unexplained combativeness

*Emergency department approved for pediatrics–pediatric critical care center.

Continued.

TABLE 1-2	Los Angeles County EDAP–PCCC Transport Criteria—cont'd
	Obvious signs of meningitis, which may include: • Purpura with fever and/or nuchal rigidity • Altered mental status, with poor eye contact and/or failure to recognize parents Monitored cardiac rhythm disturbances Status epilepticus: Defined by the occurrence of two or more generalized tonic-clonic seizures without complete recovery of full consciousness between seizures or the occurrence of continuous tonic-clonic seizure activity for more than 15 minutes Severe dehydration, which may include one or more of the following: • Dry mucous membranes • Poor skin turgor • Altered mental status • Sunken eyes
Mechanism of injury	Burns, specific signs, symptoms, or situations, such as: • Burns of greater than 10% of the body for children less than 1 year • Burns of greater than 15% of the body for children over 1 year • Singed nasal hair • Brassy sooty cough • Respiratory distress or stridor • Closed space burns • Burns involving face, ears, or perineum Submersion injuries Exposures to toxic fumes or carbon monoxide Envenomation Suspected child abuse Any other condition considered to be critical by the field provider or by the base hospital.

Prehospital Index (PHI). The PHI was specifically developed for field triage of trauma patients. It is a weighted index, using vital signs combined with level of consciousness. In field testing, it was shown to compare favorably with the CRAMS scale.[14]

Triage-Revised Trauma Score (T-RTS). The T-RTS scoring system uses the sum of coded values of the GCS, systolic blood pressure, and respiratory rate. This scoring instrument is easier to use than the TS and it has been studied in relation to sensitivity and specificity with good results. There is no research indicating that it is as accurate an instrument for children as it is for adults.[8]

CRAMS Scale. The CRAMS scale uses physiologic and anatomic parameters for assessment, forming an acronym from Circulation, Respiration, Abdomen, Motor, and Speech. It does not include mechanism of injury.[20,38]

Trauma Triage Rule (TTR). Using anatomic injury, blood pressure, and the Glasgow Coma Scale, the TTR was shown to be more specific than the CRAMS scale. It has not been tested on pediatric patients.[3,17]

Yearly, new assessment mechanisms are developed, most frequently for adult patients. Ensuring correct triage for pediatric patients is vitally important, but assessing pediatric patients by any type of scoring system is more problematic than scoring adults. Few pediatric scoring instruments are available; some have been adapted from adult models.

PEDIATRIC SCORING INSTRUMENTS

Pediatric Trauma Score (PTS). The PTS is probably the most widely used instrument for the assessment of pediatric trauma. Data from children scored with the PTS since 1985 have been entered into a common database, the National Pediatric Trauma

Registry (NPTR). This scoring system, which has six components, has been shown to have an inverse linear relationship with the ISS.[50] Some prehospital personnel may find the PTS difficult for field assessment because it uses weighted variables, some with negative values. Reliability may vary with the amount and consistency of follow-up provided (Table 1-3).

Children's Trauma Tool. Used by prehospital providers in San Diego County, the Children's Trauma Tool includes mechanism of injury and anatomic factors (Box 1-4).[31] Research regarding the use of this assessment measure has not been published.

Revised Trauma Score for Children. The Revised Trauma Score for Children alters the Revised Trauma Score so that children younger than 3 years old are not triaged solely on the basis of respiratory assessment.[15]

Severity Index for Acute Pediatric Illness. The Severity Index for Acute Pediatric Illness was developed for emergency departments rather than field triage and was devised for determination of severity of illness. The Severity Index uses a 0-1-2 rating for five variables (respiratory effort, color, activity, temperature, play).

The only scoring system that has been extensively tested for reliability and validity in triaging pediatric patients from the field is the PTS. It was found to be an effective predictor of mortality and severity of injury when used on patients entered into the NPTR. When deciding on a scoring system it is important to remember the following:

- Reliability of these instruments is dependent on the reliability of the observations of the field provider.

- Ease of use is an important factor; checklists not requiring calculation are easier to use.
- Quality improvement mechanisms should be built into EMS systems for review of scoring accuracy.
- Most scoring systems were devised for patients with traumatic injuries; these patients comprise only about one half of all pediatric patients transported by EMS.[45]

Although each new scoring method is presented as the answer to field triage of patients, clinical judgment is also an important factor.[30] Any scoring mechanism used should be reviewed on a regular basis to determine whether field providers are using it correctly; whether it is triaging patients accurately, without excessive under- or overtriage; and whether time is well spent in making the necessary assessments and calculations.

EQUIPMENT

Prehospital and interfacility transport providers should carry equipment in age-appropriate sizes. Standard lists of equipment have been recommended by the AAP, ACEP and others.[11,33,45] A sample list of pediatric equipment is presented in Box 1-5. Air transport personnel and providers of interfacility transport of pediatric patients should also have pediatric equipment available and training in pediatric emergency care. In addition, EMS transport systems must have a means of monitoring and restocking pediatric equipment and supplies.

DATA AND RESEARCH

There is virtually no documentation of the effectiveness of many prehospital procedures in reducing

TABLE 1-3	Pediatric Trauma Score		
COMPONENT	**+2**	**+1**	**−1**
Size	>20 kg	10-20 kg	<10 kg
Airway	Normal	Maintainable	Unmaintainable
CNS	Awake	Obtunded	Comatose
Systolic BP	>90 mm Hg	90-50 mm Hg	<50 mm Hg
Open wounds	None	Minor	Major or penetrating
Skeletal	None	Closed fractures	Open/multiple fractures

From Tepas JJ et al: The pediatric trauma score as a predictor of injury severity: an objective assessment, *Trauma* 28(4):425-429, 1988.

Box 1-4   Children's Trauma Tool

Pedestrian struck (significant force on the body)
_____ Damage to car or truck (fender, hood, windshield)
_____ Child thrown or found more than 5 to 6 feet from car
_____ Child dragged by moving vehicle (abrasion, road rash)
_____ Child run over (tire marks)
_____ Hit at speed of >10 mph as per witness

Motor vehicle accidents (with major vehicle damage)
_____ Rollover, unrestrained
_____ Passenger space intrusion and/or extrication
_____ Death of another passenger in same car
_____ Ejection from vehicle

Falls
_____ Greater than 15 feet (second story window)

In addition, the following *anatomic* factors should alert emergency health care providers to the pediatric victim's need for evaluation by a pediatric trauma care specialist.

Head injury
_____ Loss of consciousness for more than 1 minute
_____ Altered level of consciousness (disoriented, etc.)
_____ Seizure activity after head injury

Penetrating injuries
_____ Above the midthigh or elbow

Other anatomic injuries
_____ Pelvic tenderness (on "rocking" or "stressing")
_____ Suspected femur fracture
_____ Unequal chest expansion or lung sounds

From: *Topics in emergency medicine,* vol 9, No 3, 1987, Aspen Publisher.
Developed by IA Kaufman, MD; Joanne Stonecipher, RN, MSN; Louann Kitchen, RN, MS; Louise M. Haubner, RN, BSN; and Scott Jacobs, MD.

---

morbidity and mortality. Both outcome and epidemiologic data should be collected by EMS agencies and hospitals to provide information specific to the EMS region. Some states, such as California and Florida, are working toward making this data collection mandatory. Collaborative studies are also badly needed to answer questions about the effectiveness of many widely used procedures and treatments in improving outcomes, particularly in the prehospital arena.

Large databases of pediatric patients should be developed and maintained, such as the NPTR, but they should include illness in addition to injury. In 1993, NHTSA sponsored a data conference for EMS providers in which a panel of experts worked toward development of a set of standard data elements recommended for collection by all EMS agencies. Included in the panel's recommendations were approximately 80 data elements, including demographic elements, injury information, and assessment variables. Several elements are specific to pediatric assessment. If this information can be collected nationally, a clearer picture of the range and scope of pediatric illness and injury in the prehospital setting will be available for use in designing and refining EMS and EMSC. The Health Resources and Services Administration (HRSA), MCHB, supports a data center for EMSC, the National EMSC Data and Research Center (NEDARC), established in 1995, for the purpose of developing uniform approaches to the collection of pediatric data.

HOSPITAL CARE

EMERGENCY DEPARTMENT EDUCATION

Since approximately one third of visits to the average emergency department are pediatric patients, emergency departments must be well prepared to handle all types of pediatric emergencies. Pediatric resuscitation supplies and equipment should be readily available, preferably in one location, such as a pediatric cart (Box 1-6), and emergency personnel should receive specialized training in pediatric emergency care. Several courses have been developed for this purpose.

Physicians. Emergency department standards often include requirements for additional pediatric emergency training for physicians. The American Heart Association Advanced Cardiac Life Support Course, which has some basic information about pediatric resuscitation, is required most often. Some hospitals mandate additional pediatric training for

Box 1-5   Minimum Standards for Pediatric Equipment

BLS equipment and supplies

Essential
Oropharyngeal airways: infant, child, adult (sizes 00–5)
Self-inflating resuscitation bag: child and adult sizes
Masks for bag-valve-mask device: infant, child, and adult sizes
Oxygen masks: infant, child, and adult sizes
Nonrebreathing mask: pediatric and adult sizes
Stethoscope
Backboard
Cervical immobilization device
Blood pressure cuff: infant, child, and adult sizes
Portable suction unit with a regulator
Suction catheters: tonsil-tip and 6F–14F
Extremity splints: pediatric sizes
Bulb syringe
Obstetric pack
Thermal blanket
Water-soluble lubricant

Desirable
Infant car seat
Nasopharyngeal airways: sizes 18F–34F, or 4.5–8.5 mm
Glasgow Coma Scale reference
Pediatric Trauma Score reference
Small stuffed toy

ALS equipment and supplies
All ALS ambulances should carry everything on the BLS list, plus the following items:

Essential
Transport monitor
Defibrillator with adult and pediatric paddles
Monitoring electrodes: pediatric sizes
Laryngoscope with straight blades 0–2, curved blades 2–4
Endotracheal tube stylets: pediatric and adult sizes
Endotracheal tubes: uncuffed sizes 2.5–6.0, cuffed sizes 6.0–8.0
Magill forceps: pediatric and adult
Nasogastric tubes: 8F-16F
Nebulizer
IV catheters: 16 to 24 gauge
Intraosseous needles
Length/weight-based drug dose chart or tape
Needles: 18- to 24-gauge
Resuscitation drugs and IV fluids that meet the local standards of practice

Desirable
Blood glucose analysis system
Disposable CO_2 detection device

From Committee on Ambulance Equipment and Supplies, National EMSC Resource Alliance: Guidelines for pediatric equipment and supplies for basic and advanced life support ambulances, *Pediatric Emergency Care* 12(6):452–453, 1996.

Box 1-6   Pediatric Emergency Care Cart Equipment

Monitor-defibrillator—with infant and child paddles (4.5 cm and 8.0 cm)

Bag-valve-mask resuscitators, including reservoir
- at least 450 ml for infant/young child
- 750 ml for older child/adolescent
- masks: infant/child/adult

Blood pressure cuffs—infant, child, small adult

Back board (spinal immobilization)*

Stiff neck collars*—small, medium, large

Sand bags*

Femur splint*—pediatric

Antishock trousers—pediatric

Laryngoscope—curved and straight blades; sizes 0, 1, 2

ET Tube stylets—6F and 14F

Magill forceps—pediatric

Stethoscope—two-sided; pediatric

Pediatric emergency drug dosage book or chart—dosage by weight

Chest tube tray with pediatric-size chest tubes—8F through 16F

Cricothyrotomy and tracheostomy tray with pediatric tubes

Cutdown tray

From Wayland BW, Rowland MC: Pediatric emergency care cart, *J Emerg Nurs* (14)2:91–94, 1988.
*Although it is recommended that all equipment possible be actually in or on the cart, these items are very bulky and could be stored within the emergency department if space on the cart was not available. However, there should be a notation on the cart itself exactly where the items are to be found, and these items should be accounted for each shift when the cart is checked.

---

emergency physicians; some of the most frequently required courses include the following:
- The American Heart Association/American Academy of Pediatrics' Pediatric Advanced Life Support (PALS) course is a 2-day assessment-based course that focuses on assessment of respiratory distress and shock in pediatric patients and on pediatric resuscitation.[6] The course is taught by instructors who have completed a training course in PALS, and it has been given to thousands of health care providers nationally. It emphasizes acquisition of skills and knowledge in a nonthreatening, supportive environment.
- The Advanced Pediatric Life Support (APLS) course for physicians was developed by the AAP and the ACEP. This 3-day course covers resuscitation and the medical treatment of the critically ill and injured child.[46] The course is expensive and is less widely available than the PALS course, but it provides a solid knowledge base for emergency medical care of the pediatric patient, including the treatment of the most common life-threatening pediatric illnesses and injuries. Nurses may attend the APLS course, but do not participate or receive a certificate of completion.

Pediatric emergency medicine is now a recognized subspecialty; fellowship training programs in pediatric emergency medicine may include an EMS rotation.

Nurses. Several continuing education courses are available in pediatric emergency nursing. The ENA provides two programs for nurses; other national organizations offer education in resuscitation and trauma care using a team approach.
- The Emergency Nursing Pediatric Course (ENPC) is a 2-day course given in seminar format with skills stations. Content covers assessment, resuscitation, and nursing management of acutely ill and injured pediatric patients. Both skills and knowledge are emphasized in this course. A core of trained and certified instructors is necessary to provide the course. 19.2 hours of continuing education (CE) credit is given for successful completion of the ENPC.[22]
- The *Pediatric Emergency Nursing Manual* is a self-learning text for emergency nurses, covering assessment and intervention for pediatric illness and injury. The manual is designed to be used individually or in a group format with a facilitator. The manual is published by Springer Publishing Co., is distributed by ENA and the publisher, and offers 10.8 hours of CE from ENA for successful completion of a multiple-choice test.[26]
- The PALS course is useful for nurses because it emphasizes a team approach to pediatric resuscitation. The format is designed to provide a realistic simulation of emergency situations, with health care providers assuming roles appropriate to their professional capacities. Although the PALS course was not originally intended for prehospital providers, the latest edition includes prehospital care scenarios.

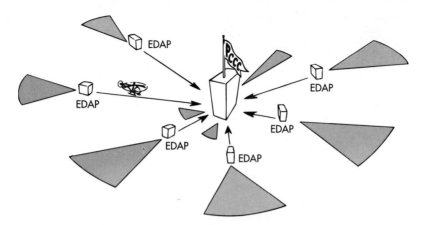

FIG. 1-1. Urban EMSC system. In urban areas, pediatric patients are triaged according to seriousness of illness or injury to either an EDAP or a PCCC. Critically ill and injured patients may bypass other hospitals to be transported directly to a PCCC from the field. (Redrawn from Haller JA: *Emergency medical services for children,* Report of the 97th Ross Conference on Pediatric Research, Columbus, Ohio, 1989, Ross Laboratories.)

Other nursing courses have been developed and are provided on a smaller scale. Several were developed with funding from MCHB. The Children's National Medical Center in Washington, D.C., developed a 25-hour course combining lectures, skills stations, and case simulations. This course, the Pediatric Emergency Nursing Education Program (PENEP), was designed for nurses working in community emergency departments. Other courses include the Emergency Nursing Advanced Pediatric Management (EN-APM) course developed by the Florida EMSC Project,[48] a preceptorship program for emergency nurses developed by the Alaska EMSC project, and the pediatric emergency nursing course developed by the North Carolina EMSC Project.[27]

INTENSIVE CARE/SPECIALIZED CARE

Characteristics and requirements of levels of pediatric care may vary with the population base and the facilities available. In some areas, specifically rural and semi-rural areas where transport times can be an hour or longer, an additional level of care may be required to stabilize patients before transport to definitive care (Figs. 1-1 and 1-2). An intermediate level of care may also be required for children in communities lacking intensive care units. In all cases, the emergency care system must include access to referral centers for the small number of the critically ill and injured pediatric patients who need the highest level of care.

REHABILITATION

There are many repercussions of hospitalization, both physical and psychologic, for the child and for the family. In addition to the obvious stresses of illness, injury, and hospitalization, patient transfer brings with it the added stress of displacement. Traveling to regional centers may pose problems for families, and the absence of familiar support systems may weaken customary coping mechanisms. Regional centers caring for seriously ill and injured children should address the long-term effects of the disease process from the moment of entry into the system and should address the needs of the child and family.

In addition to care in the hospital, provisions should be made in an emergency care system for children with special needs after their return to the community. Wisconsin EMSC and New Mexico EMSC have developed programs that link the hospital to the community by providing information about children with special needs to prehospital providers.

▮ REGIONAL DEVELOPMENT

Ideally, both urban and rural communities should have access to a regional or tertiary care center. Regionalization of certain types of care occurred during the 1960s with support from EMS block grant funding: trauma, burns, spinal cord injury, poisoning,

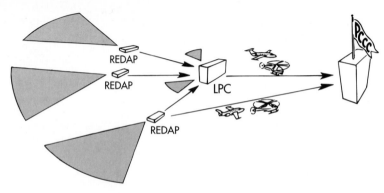

FIG. 1-2.   Rural EMSC transport system. In rural areas, a critically ill or injured patient may be transported by air directly from the rural emergency department approved for pediatrics (RE-DAP) to a PCCC. In very remote or inaccessible areas, the REDAP may provide initial stabilization of pediatric patients and transport the patient by ambulance to the local pediatric center (LPC) or fixed wing aircraft or helicopter transport to a PCCC. (Redrawn from Haller JA, ed: *Emergency medical services for children,* Report of the 97th Ross Conference on Pediatric Research, Columbus, Ohio, 1989, Ross Laboratories.)

high-risk infants and mothers, and behavioral emergencies. There was little recognition of the special needs of children until research showed a higher-than-normal mortality and morbidity in areas where there were no tertiary centers.[44] Pediatric intensive care was not included at that time. Since then, several states have regionalized certain aspects of pediatric care, including pediatric trauma and intensive care. In many areas of the United States, however, pediatric emergency and tertiary care is still not regionalized. When regionalization of care is mentioned, there is often an assumption that a competitive process will occur—this is not necessarily true.

There are several methods of regionalizing care: *categorization* usually involves voluntary assessment and compliance with standards, *verification* or *confirmation* implies a process of review and meeting of standards, *accreditation* requires the stamp of approval of a certifying body, and *designation* is a process in which there is a formal evaluation and a limited number of facilities are selected.[13] To develop a regionalized system of care for pediatric patients, several elements of the system must be addressed, including inter/intrastate agreements, hospital care, transport and transfer issues, follow-up information, and reimbursement. The American College of Surgeons guidelines state that 1000 patients per year is the number of admissions for a level I trauma center. The catchment areas for regional pediatric centers should be planned to provide care for a similar minimum

number of pediatric patients.[34] In some areas, the catchment area may include a large geographic region, and in other, more densely populated areas, the geographic region may be much smaller. A regional center should draw from a large population base to include sufficient numbers of patients for hospital personnel to maintain skills and for facilities to justify costs.

HOSPITAL AGREEMENTS

With EMSC development, hospitals providing a higher level of care to pediatric patients can be identified. Research has shown that when critically ill or injured children are kept in midlevel facilities, morbidity and mortality is significantly higher.[39] Hospitals in a given region should have some guidelines for transfer, and the modes of transfer and time frames for transfer to higher levels of care should be clearly defined. A "hotline" provided by the tertiary facility receiving the patient may be helpful in providing information and transfer instructions. In all instances there must be clear accountability at each stage of the transfer.[13]

INTERFACILITY TRANSPORT EQUIPMENT AND TRAINING

Interfacility transport providers should all be well trained and able to handle any type of pediatric emergency. Some emergency departments, usually regional centers or pediatric facilities, have pediatric interfacility transport teams, with highly skilled professionals providing an advanced level of care. When a child requires transport from a facility in a remote area, the transport team may be less well trained. These providers, whether transporting by ground or air, should have received pediatric education and training and should have the proper equipment available to care for pediatric patients. Transport teams with specialized education and training in pediatric emergency care may need to be used selectively for pediatric transfers.

INTER/INTRASTATE AGREEMENTS

In some regions, the nearest pediatric tertiary care facility is out of state. There may also be geographic barriers, such as mountains or a lack of infrastructure, that cause difficulty when transporting a child from one region to another. For these reasons written interfacility transport agreements should be available. This is particularly true when reimbursement issues for interstate transport may cause unnecessary delay in the transport or transfer of children.

TRANSFER CHECKLISTS

Continuity of care requires the provision of essential information when a child is transferred from one health care provider to another. The development of a transfer checklist will ensure that the center receiving the patient has sufficient information to care for the child. Included in the checklist are such items as the medical record, patient demographic data, and diagnostic data (e.g., x-rays, laboratory results). Model programs have been developed linking regional facilities by fax machine, providing immediate access to critical information.[53]

FOLLOW-UP INFORMATION

When a pediatric patient is transferred to a tertiary facility, the sending facility and the primary care provider should be given follow-up information regarding the patient's condition and treatment. This serves to close the loop and provide feedback about possible areas for improvement in initial care. It also assists community health care providers such as primary care providers to prepare for care of the child after the return home. When a child has special needs, the local prehospital providers and receiving facility should be informed in advance of the special problems in caring for the child.

REIMBURSEMENT

Although reimbursement for critical illness and injury can be complex for adults, it may be less difficult for children because of the availability of private and public agencies dealing specifically with pediatric care. Interfacility and interstate transport does complicate reimbursement, however. Advance planning is necessary to help expedite the transfer of pediatric patients and reimbursement for their care.[45] When the closest tertiary center for pediatric care is across state lines, standard reimbursement agreements should be developed in advance of need and should be outlined in a comprehensive plan.

PUBLIC EDUCATION AND ACCESS TO EMS

INJURY PREVENTION

The most effective way to lower mortality and morbidity in the pediatric age group is injury prevention. Programs to increase the use of seat belts, child car seats, safety helmets, and safety catches in homes have all been shown to be effective in lowering injury rates.[21] Ongoing programs can be developed and promoted through hospitals, by EMS providers, or by community agencies. Use of flyers, brochures, and informational packets developed by national and regional agencies and institutions can keep the cost of these programs to a minimum. Many injury prevention programs for children have been developed through federal funding and are in the public domain. Emergency departments (EDs) may also be useful in promoting injury prevention. Parents may be very receptive to injury prevention instruction and educational materials when a child with a preventable injury is being discharged from the ED. In Santa Cruz, California, injury prevention materials were developed for use in parent education when a child is brought in with a preventable injury.[16] Schools, churches, and local civic groups may also be interested in providing hospital tours and distributing injury prevention materials for children to take home.

9-1-1 ACCESS

Identification of ill and injured children requires an educated public with knowledge of how and when to access the emergency care system. Instructions for parents and caretakers may be provided through community groups, public service announcements, and by primary care providers.

CARDIOPULMONARY RESUSCITATION (CPR) AND FIRST AID

Community education in CPR and first aid procedures may be helpful in early identification of and assistance to children before the arrival of prehospital providers. Educational programs for the general public should include information on what constitutes an emergency, some basic first aid procedures, and the fastest way to obtain emergency care. Early initiation of CPR for a submersion injury, for instance, may be lifesaving. Educational programs for school-age children and adults are provided through the American Red Cross, the American Heart Association, and other organizations. Schools should be encouraged to include first aid training in their health programs—this can often be an effective outreach program given by a community hospital. Hospitals are also often able to provide CPR and baby safety courses for new parents. The Red Cross, the American Heart Association, and other agencies should be included in a community's efforts to improve emergency medical services for children.

RESEARCH/PUBLICATION

Information about pediatric emergency care and injury prevention may be disseminated to other professionals through journals and conferences and to the public through popular magazines and public service announcements. Schools, hospitals, and local community agencies may form coalitions to assess the needs of the region and to plan and implement improvements in emergency care for children.

▌QUALITY IMPROVEMENT

Continuous quality improvement (CQI) programs are a vehicle to review prehospital, emergency department, hospital, and rehabilitative care. Since the CQI concept is relatively new to the health care arena, EMS systems have not yet demonstrated that care can be improved by this mechanism. Without this type of monitoring, however, there is little hope for determining what may be effective.

PREHOSPITAL CARE

Every EMS system should gather essential data elements as a means of reviewing care and assessing the epidemiology of pediatric illness and injury. These data elements should be consistent throughout the EMS system, from prehospital care through discharge. The Rochester EMSC Targeted Issue grant provides a model for data collection system-wide.[35] The EMSC projects, the Joint Commission on the Accreditation of Healthcare Organizations, and the American College of Surgeons have all developed data elements for collection by EMS systems. A comparison of these three is included in Appendix A. Mechanisms for peer review should be included when possible (or review by members of other health care disciplines), with close follow-up of problem cases. Good data collection and analysis can assist in ensuring adherence to protocols and offers the greatest potential for system improvement.

EMERGENCY CARE

Emergency departments should review the care of pediatric patients on a timely basis. All deaths and patients requiring CPR are reviewed by most facilities accepting pediatric patients. In addition, mechanisms should be in place to review patient transfers and instances in which child abuse is suspected. It should be remembered that bad outcomes may not be related to defective care but are a means of deciding what cases should be reviewed for errors in management. In Los Angeles, pediatric liaison nurses (PdLNs) have developed a list of generic screens to review care. Some suggestions for generic screens are outlined in Box 1-7. Consistent and ongoing review of pediatric care is the best method of ensuring continued improvement. Nurses should be active participants in this process, assisting in review of nursing care and working collaboratively to develop standards for pediatric emergency care.

▌A SUCCESSFUL EMSC SYSTEM (EDAP)

Research conducted in the 1980s raised questions about the adequacy of pediatric care in emergency settings. In Los Angeles, this research resulted in a

---

Box 1-7   Generic Screens for Pediatric Emergency Care

Focus on high-risk, high-volume, problem-prone aspects of care.

Some "occurrences" for screening:

1. Cardiopulmonary resuscitation was performed on patient.
2. Patient was dead on arrival.
3. Patient died in the emergency department or within 48 hours of admission.
4. Caretaker(s) refused treatment for child, left without completion of treatment, or refused hospitalization.
5. Suspicion or allegation of child abuse, sexual abuse, or rape.
6. Patient had symptoms of pain in neck, headache, or seizure with fever; no lumbar puncture performed.
7. Patient had abdominal pain; no CBC or urinalysis done.
8. Emergency physician's interpretation of x-rays differed from radiologist's.
9. Patient returned to emergency department within 48 hours for same complaint.
10. Patient was sent home before results of x-rays or lab tests were obtained.
11. Lab tests were in critical range, and patient was discharged.
12. Major invasive procedures: chest tubes, subclavian catheters, intubation, lumbar punctures performed.
13. Patient had laceration or puncture wound; no documentation of immunization.
14. Patient was given blood or blood products.
15. Patient's visit lasted more than _____ hours.
16. Referral or transfer to another facility for emergency care.

---

collaborative effort between the Los Angeles County Department of Health, EMS Division, and the Los Angeles Pediatric Society to develop standards for pediatric training and equipment in emergency departments. The standards were met on a voluntary basis by 88 of 104 receiving hospitals in Los Angeles County. These hospitals became the first emergency departments approved for pediatrics (EDAPs). Hospitals providing a higher level of care, including a

pediatric intensive care unit, met standards for pediatric critical care centers (PCCCs). Prehospital providers were instructed to take all pediatric patients to EDAPs or PCCCs. Patients were selectively triaged to an EDAP or PCCC on the basis of specific criteria (see Table 1-2). Key features of the EDAP standards were requirements for education and training of physicians and nurses and availability of pediatric equipment. Another important feature was that each facility was required to have a PdLN who would be available as a resource to emergency department staff and review pediatric emergency care on an ongoing basis. Meeting the standards for EDAPs or PCCCs was strictly voluntary on the part of the hospitals, and any hospital meeting those standards was included in the system. After confirmation of the hospitals, a 2-day course in pediatric emergency care was given, with each facility in the EDAP system sending two nurses. This voluntary system has been successful for 10 years; the standards were updated in 1996, and this model has been used for implementing EMSC in many states.

THE IDEAL PEDIATRIC EMERGENCY DEPARTMENT

When children need emergency care, the entire family is affected. Both parents and children have needs, including the need for information, physical comfort, and emotional support. Parents or caretakers who are confused, uncomfortable, anxious, and upset will have a negative effect on their child. It may not be possible to meet ideal standards in a busy emergency department, but a few simple measures may go a long way toward improving the family's experience during this painful time. Emergency departments can be designed to increase the comfort of pediatric patients, lessen their frightening isolation, and provide a humane and compassionate environment for the family.

Additionally, the attitude of health care providers in the emergency setting is of paramount importance in developing rapport with children and their families and ensuring the best experience possible. There are several ways to provide a family-centered environment.

PHYSICAL COMFORT OF FAMILIES

In all of the studies regarding the needs of families of hospitalized patients, the need for physical comfort is ranked near the top of the list. Traditionally, emergency department waiting areas have rows of seats or benches, often lined up against the walls. This arrangement discourages conversation and closeness among family members. When waiting areas have chairs grouped in L-shaped clusters, more seating can be provided and a more private, intimate atmosphere is created. Drinking fountains and bathrooms should be readily accessible to the waiting area as minimum necessities. Handicapped-accessible telephones should be provided. When possible, a machine or snack bar to provide coffee, tea, cocoa, juices, and light snacks for caretakers should be available nearby. Many emergency departments offer television or videos in the waiting area—some provide health care information and injury prevention programs. Reading materials can be donated by local bookstores or newspaper stands from left-over stock.

Play Areas

Play areas for children who wait with their parents should be simple and accessible. A low platform with a table at which children can kneel and a partition with an opening that can be used for peeking through or as a puppet theater may be sufficient to encourage safe play and cannot be easily destroyed by active children. Child-size chairs and tables in the waiting area indicate to children that they are expected and welcome. Soft, disposable toys should be provided for the play area when possible—local toy stores may be willing to donate items for this purpose. Children's books can also be donated by local libraries or commercial establishments.

Safety

Safety of both children and adults should be considered in ED waiting areas and treatment rooms. Needle containers should not be at levels accessible to children, hot water should be no warmer than 120° F, and electrical outlets should be covered when possible.

Treatment Rooms

The emergency department treatment areas should provide privacy but allow for constant monitoring of children. Individual treatment rooms permit privacy and may be especially helpful when a procedure is being performed, but most families resist being left in rooms alone with doors closed. Treatment areas should have seating for parents to hold their children,

as well as enough chairs to enable health professionals to sit down with the family. Some ethnic groups expect to have several family members assist in decision making—when this is a common expectation, larger treatment rooms should be used. When children are treated in adult emergency departments, privacy should be ensured for both the adults and the children. Small children may be frightened by the sights and sounds of an adult emergency department; having a separate room available for pediatric patients is ideal. If the emergency department is set up as a large room with individual cubicles, the use of sturdy curtains is important and they should be on tracks that provide complete privacy. Many children, especially adolescents, are embarrassed to be seen unclothed and often are unwilling to express their embarrassment. When single treatment rooms are used, glass doors are useful in permitting children and their families to view the medical staff, and vice versa, while controlling spread of infection and keeping noise to a minimum; curtains can be used around the bed to ensure privacy when necessary. When automatic doors are used, sideways sliding doors rather than doors that swing inward or outward prevent the risk of injury to children.

Privacy

When a child is brought to the emergency department with a life-threatening condition, the child's caretakers are often overwhelmed with emotion and need privacy to attempt to gain control. A private room close to the treatment area can serve this purpose. Tissues, a telephone, and a bathroom should be made available. Many emergency departments do not have a room dedicated for this purpose, but a nearby office or physician sleeping quarters can be used. Social workers and/or chaplains or other religious support personnel can be available to support families with critical illnesses or injuries.

Child-Life Programs

Some hospitals have child-life specialists on staff. These professionals have received advanced training in preparing children for procedures, and in some hospitals they are available to assist during procedures, using behavioral interventions such as visualization, distraction, and relaxation to lessen the trauma. In some studies these techniques have been found to be more effective than medication in reducing pain perception and behavioral distress for children undergoing painful procedures.[29] Although it may not be possible to finance a full-time child-life position, it may be possible for a child-life specialist to assist in training emergency department staff in the use of behavioral techniques.

CARING FOR CHILDREN IN ADULT EMERGENCY DEPARTMENTS

When children are cared for in combined adult-pediatric emergency departments, some of the following suggestions may facilitate and humanize nursing care.

ENVIRONMENT

- The triage desk should be low enough to enable personnel to assess pediatric patients easily. There should be enough room for the parent to hold the child in his or her lap or for the child to stand next to the parent.
- A specific room or rooms can be designated for pediatric patients and decorated with decals and/or colorful designs. If the room is used for both adults and children, bright colors without a pediatric theme may be sufficient. At least one chair should be available so that the caretaker can sit with the child.
- A play area can be designated for children; it should be in plain view of ED staff so they can intervene if necessary.
- Scales for weighing children should be readily accessible in or near the triage area. Both a scale for small children and a stand-on scale for larger children are necessary.
- Small soft toys can be made available to comfort children. Rewards such as stickers or toys can be offered after procedures. Community groups are sometimes willing to supply these toys.

SUPPLIES AND EQUIPMENT

Pediatric resuscitation equipment should be placed in one location, such as a special crash cart. Systems such as the Broselow tape, which indicates correct medication dosages and pediatric equipment based on the length of the patient, are especially helpful.[32] The hospital pharmacy may be able to supply a list of medication dosages by weight on short notice. Once the patient has been weighed, a computer printout may be available. Dosages by weight may be obtained in advance and placed in a book for use during codes. Charts and tables with lists of medications by weight can be made readily available on or in the crash cart or on the wall in the resuscitation room.

TRAINING

A guideline recommended for adult emergency departments that treat children is that at least one nurse per shift should have received special training in pediatric emergency care (such as PALS or ENPC). This nurse serves as a resource for other nursing staff[25] and attends pediatric continuing education courses yearly.

POLICIES AND PROCEDURES

In addition to the usual emergency department policies and procedures, some advance planning should be made to ensure a family-centered approach when caring for children. Some of the psychosocial issues that should be addressed are discussed in the following sections.

Presence of family members in treatment rooms. Policies regarding who is allowed in treatment rooms should be agreed to collaboratively among nurses, physicians, and other health care providers. Studies have shown that parents prefer to stay with the child and do not present a problem when rules are clear and adequate preparation is given.[54] A study of parents during attempted resuscitation of their child showed that a great majority of parents felt it was a valuable experience.[12] Despite the fact that the resuscitation was unsuccessful, parents felt it was useful in helping them in their grieving process. Health care professionals may be uncomfortable with parents observing in treatment rooms, however, so clear guidelines should be available.

Child neglect and maltreatment. Policies and protocols should be clearly outlined for handling child abuse, child sexual abuse, and child neglect. When and how to obtain consultation and reporting issues should be covered.

Death of a child. Helping the family whose child has died in the emergency department is a team effort requiring a systematic approach. The family should be given both a list of referrals to community agencies for support and the name of a person to call in the emergency department when there are questions regarding the child's death (see Chapter 9).

FUNDING FOR EMSC

Ongoing support for EMSC programs should be available in all states and can be built into EMSC as it is integrated into EMS.

FEDERAL SUPPORT

Since 1985, federal funding has been made available through grants from MCHB for integration of EMSC into EMS systems. In the first 2 years, awards were given to states for demonstration grants to develop different methods of integrating pediatric emergency care into EMS systems. Later grants were provided for adaptation and implementation of these models. To date, 44 states, U.S. Territories, and the District of Columbia have received EMSC funding. Currently, applications for several types of EMSC grants are offered through MCHB in collaboration with NHTSA; these include planning grants, implementation grants, targeted issue grants, enhancement grants, and grants for national centers for EMSC. Some of the highlights of projects undertaken by grantees include the following:

- Implementation of EMSC in rural and urban areas (California EMSC)
- Development of injury prevention projects for Native Americans (New Mexico EMSC) and playground safety (Maine EMSC)
- Interventions for pain management for children in the emergency department (Missouri EMSC)
- Evaluation of pediatric prehospital airway management—the largest prospective study of pediatric prehospital care (California Airway Management Project)
- Provision of information about children with special needs (Wisconsin and New Mexico EMSC)
- Education for prehospital providers in rural areas using mobile interactive videodisk training (Idaho EMSC)
- A training program for emergency personnel in suicide prevention for adolescent suicide attempters (Columbia University)
- Injury prevention for emergency departments (California EMSC)

- Development of a regional, population-based pediatric emergency data surveillance system that includes both ED and hospital outcome data (Rochester EMSC Targeted Issue Grant)
- Cultural sensitivity training for emergency personnel (Washington EMSC, District of Columbia EMSC)
- Resource catalogues for all aspects of pediatric emergency care (National EMSC Resource Alliance)

Many of the products developed by these projects are available through the National EMSC Resource Alliance in Torrance, California; others are available directly through EMSC grant contacts (see Appendix B).

The federal EMSC program continues to receive widespread support. To ensure continued implementation of EMSC, MCHB developed a 5-year plan in 1995 addressing specific goals and objectives, many of which include nursing care.[52] This document includes areas where there are opportunities for nurses to play important roles in improving the care of children.[24]

LEGISLATION

One of the most effective ways of ensuring funding for continuing EMSC services is to provide legislative support for EMSC development and integration. In New Jersey, legislation established the Emergency Medical and Injury Prevention Systems for Children (EMIPSC) Program within the Office of Emergency Medical Services. The function of the EMIPSC is to oversee EMSC activities, including education of prehospital providers, development of standards and guidelines, solicitation of funding, and EMSC development throughout the state.[2] Other states such as Colorado, Hawaii, Louisiana, Oklahoma, Texas, and Utah have developed legislation to support ongoing EMSC functions. Sample templates for EMSC legislation have been developed based on the New Jersey model.[36] To assist in developing legislation at the state level, the AAP's Committee on Pediatric Emergency Medicine (COPEM) has drafted sample legislation to be used as a model for institutionalizing EMSC.

THE INSTITUTE OF MEDICINE (IOM) REPORT

In 1991, the U.S. Department of Health and Human Services, Maternal and Child Health Branch, in collaboration with the Department of Transportation, National Highway Traffic Safety Administration, funded a 2-year study of EMSC by the National Institutes of Health, Institute of Medicine. This study conducted by a multidisciplinary committee reviewed the literature, EMS research, and past and present EMSC projects. The result was a 396-page report with specific recommendations for EMSC (see Appendix B). The resulting report will have an enduring effect on pediatric emergency care. Recommendations included establishing a substantial federal role in EMSC, including the funding of grants, research, and national centers for dissemination of information about EMSC. Currently, there are three resource centers: the National EMSC Resource Alliance in Torrance, California; the National Resource Center in Washington, D.C.; and the National EMSC Data and Resource Center in Salt Lake City, Utah.

Nurses' Roles in EMSC

Nurses play an important role nationally in EMS systems, through direct care, education, and administration.

Prehospital care.   In some areas nurses are direct providers of prehospital care and in others they are an essential link to prehospital personnel via telephone or radio communication, providing medical direction and assisting with triage decisions. In the emergency department, nurses often review prehospital care to obtain information from prehospital personnel about the patient's mechanism of injury and the conditions surrounding the incident.

Education.   Nurses with special education and training in pediatric emergency care are a great asset to emergency departments. They serve as resources to prehospital providers, to ancillary staff, to physicians, and to other emergency department nurses. Promotion of continuing education in pediatric emergency care, assistance with PALS and other pediatric course instruction, and providing information to other staff members regarding educational opportunities are all important nursing functions.

Injury prevention.   The traditional role of nurses in injury prevention activities is especially important in the emergency department. Important injury prevention activities for nurses include monitoring the incidence of trauma to assist in appropriate targeting of injury prevention programs, working with commu-

nity programs in violence prevention, and providing injury prevention information to patients and their families.[16]

Quality improvement.   Pediatric liaison nurses serve as continuous quality improvement reviewers in many emergency departments nationally. When EMSC has not been integrated into the EMS system, nurses can still be responsible for reviewing care given to pediatric patients, determining which charts need additional review, and setting up generic screens and monitoring mechanisms within emergency departments.

Coalition building.   Local and national nursing organizations can work together to improve pediatric emergency care. The Pediatric Committee of the ENA has been instrumental in developing educational materials in pediatric emergency care, and state ENA chapters have formed pediatric committees that meet on a regular basis. Nurses should become involved in these activities by participating in local and national committees involved in pediatric emergency care. Networking and building coalitions with other organizations to influence legislation and educate public officials have been very effective in promoting and supporting pediatric emergency care issues.

Research.   There are tremendous opportunities for research in pediatric emergency care. Emergency department nurses are in an ideal position to study the relationship between prehospital and emergency department care, triage decisions, transport issues, and the effectiveness of emergency interventions on the outcomes of pediatric patients. As the price of health care increases, emergency nurses can demonstrate the cost effectiveness of nursing interventions such as patient discharge teaching and injury prevention.

Patient advocacy.   Nurses have always played a critical role in serving as advocates for children and their families in emergency settings. With awareness of the psychosocial issues in health care, they help to keep families together and work with other health care professionals to develop policies and procedures to ensure humane, family-centered care in the emergency department.

▋ Summary

As EMS systems become more sophisticated with the availability of advanced technology, improved communication, and better-trained personnel, more patients are receiving a higher level of care in the field and in emergency departments. Although the majority of patients seen in emergency settings are adults, EMS systems must give equal attention to the needs of pediatric patients. The special needs of children should be addressed throughout EMS systems, from the moment of identification through rehabilitation and return to the community. Nurses have consistently performed an essential role in providing care and advocacy for children in prehospital settings, in hospitals, and in home care. They will certainly continue to find creative and innovative ways to ensure that children's needs are met in all varieties of emergency settings.

REFERENCES

1. American Academy of Pediatrics: *Guidelines for air and ground transport,* Elk Grove, 1993, AAP.
2. Barden RC, et al: Emergency medical care and injury/illness prevention systems for children, *Harvard J Legisl* 30(1):461–497, 1992.
3. Baxt WG, Jones G, Fortiage D: The trauma triage rule: a new resource-based approach to the prehospital identification of major trauma victims, *Ann Emerg Med* 19(12):1401–1406, 1990.
4. Benedict K, Hiatt D, Ward P: *Santa Cruz County EMSC: ALS protocols and policies manual,* Santa Cruz, Calif, 1991, Health Services Agency, County of Santa Cruz.
5. Boyd CR, Tolson MA, Copes WS: Evaluating trauma care: the TRISS method, *J Trauma* 27(4): 370–378, 1987.
6. Chameides L, Hazinski MF: *Textbook of pediatric advanced life support,* Dallas, 1994, *American Heart Association.*
7. Champion HR: Field triage of trauma patients, *Ann Emerg Med* 11(3):160–161, 1982.
8. Champion HR et al: A revision of the trauma score, *J Trauma* 29(5):623–629, 1989.
9. Champion HR et al: Assessment of injury severity: the triage index, *Crit Care Med* 8(4):201–208, 1980.
10. Committee on Ambulance Equipment and Supplies, National EMSC Resource Alliance: Guidelines for pediatric equipment and supplies for basic and advanced life support ambulances, *Pediatric Emergency Care* 12(6):452–453, 1996.
11. Dieckmann RA et al: *Paramedic pediatric education guidelines,* Dallas, 1993, American College of Emergency Physicians.
12. Doyle CJ, et al: Family participation during resuscitation: an option, *Ann Emerg Med* 16(6):673–675, 1987.
13. Durch JS, Lohr KN, eds: *Emergency medical services for children,* Washington, DC, 1993, National Academy Press.
14. Eichelberger MR et al: A comparison of the trauma score, the revised trauma score, and the pediatric trauma score, *Ann Emerg Med* 18(10):1053–1058, 1989.
15. Eichelberger MR et al: Trauma score versus revised trauma score in TRISS to predict outcome in children with blunt trauma, *Ann Emerg Med* 18(9):939–942, 1989.
16. Ellerby P, Ward P: Development of a pediatric injury prevention program for emergency departments, *J Emerg Nurs* 15(3):224–228, 1988.
17. Emerman CL, Shade B, Kubincanek J: Comparative performance of the Baxt trauma triage rule, *Am J Emerg Med* 10(4):294–297, 1992.
18. Gabram SG et al: Airway intubation in injured patients at the scene of an accident, *Conn Med* 53(11):633–637, 1989.
19. Gausche M et al: Pediatric deaths and emergency medical services (EMS) in urban and rural areas, *Pediatr Emerg Care* 5(3):158–162, 1989.
20. Gormican SP: CRAMS scale: field triage of trauma victims, *Ann Emerg Med* 11(3):132–135, 1982.
21. Guyer B, ed: *Injury prevention: meeting the challenge,* New York, 1989, Oxford University Press; American Journal of Preventive Medicine.
22. Haley K, Baker P: *Emergency nursing pediatric course,* Park Ridge, Ill, 1992, Emergency Nurses Association.
23. Haller JA: *Emergency medical services for children,* Report of the 97th Ross Conference on Pediatric Research, Columbus, Ohio, 1989, Ross Laboratories.
24. Henderson D: Implementation of the recommendations of the Institute of Medicine report, emergency medical services for children: registered nurses, *Pediatr* 96(1):194–198, 1995.
25. Henderson DP: The Los Angeles pediatric emergency care system, *Emerg Nurs* 14(2):96–100, 1988.
26. Henderson DP, Brownstein D: *Pediatric emergency nursing manual,* New York, 1994, Springer Publishing Co.
27. Henderson DP, Seidel JS: *EMSC product catalogue,* Torrance, Calif, 1993, National EMSC Resource Alliance.
28. James HE, Anas NG, Perkin RM: *Brain insults in infants and children,* Orlando, Fla, 1985, Grune & Stratton.
29. Jay SM et al: Behavioral management of children's distress during painful medical procedures, *Behav Res Ther* 23(5):513–520, 1985.
30. Kane G et al: Empirical development and evaluation of prehospital trauma triage instruments, *Trauma* 25(6):482–489, 1985.

31. Kitchen L, Haubner LM: Guidelines for the triage of pediatric trauma patients, *J Emerg Nurs* 15(5):414–415, 1989.

32. Lubitz DS et al: A rapid method for estimating weight and resuscitation drug dosages from length in the pediatric age group, *Ann Emerg Med* 17(6):576–581, 1988.

33. Luten R, Foltin G: *Pediatric resources for prehospital care*, ed 3, Arlington, Va, 1993, National Center for Education in Maternal and Child Health.

34. Matlak ME: *Current problems in the management of pediatric trauma*. Paper presented at the Emergency Medical Servies for Children: Report of the 97th Ross Conference on Pediatric Research, Columbus, Ohio, 1989.

35. National Center for Education in Maternal and Child Health and the National EMSC Resource Alliance: *Emergency medical services for children: abstracts of active projects FY 1994*, Arlington, Va, 1994, National Center for Education in Maternal and Child Health.

36. National EMSC Resource Alliance: *EMSC legislation*, Torrance, Calif, 1996, National EMSC Resource Alliance.

37. Reference deleted in proofs.

38. Ornato J, et al: Ineffectiveness of the trauma score and CRAMS scale for accurately triaging patients to trauma centers, *Ann Emerg Med* 14(11):1061–1064, 1985.

39. Pollack MM et al: Improved outcomes from tertiary center pediatric intensive care: a statewide comparison of tertiary and nontertiary care facilities, *Crit Care Med* 19(2):150–159, 1991.

40. Ramenofsky ML et al: Maximum survival in pediatric trauma: the ideal system, *J Trauma* 24(9):818–823, 1984.

41. Rice T, Engelbaugh S: *Prehospital basic level assessment and treatment guidelines*, 1990, Madison, WI, Wisconsin Department of Health and Social Services, Section of Emergency Medicine.

42. Seidel JS: EMS-C in urban and rural areas: the California experience. In Haller JA Jr, ed: *Emergency medical services for children*, Report of the 97th Ross Conference on Pediatric Research, Columbus, Ohio, 1989, Ross Laboratories.

43. Seidel JS, Henderson DP, eds: *Emergency medical services for children: a report to the nation*, Washington, DC, 1991, National Center for Education in Maternal and Child Health.

44. Seidel JS et al: Emergency medical services and the pediatric patient: are the needs being met? *Pediatr* 73(6):769–772, 1984.

45. Seidel JS et al: Pediatric prehospital care in urban and rural areas, *Pediatr* 88(4):681–690, 1991.

46. Silverman BK, ed: *Advanced pediatric life support*, ed 2, Elk Grove Village, Ill, 1993, AAP.

47. Smith J Jr, Bartholomew MJ: Trauma index revisited: a better triage tool, *Crit Care Med* 18(2):174–180, 1990.

48. Taylor M, Soud T: Florida pediatric emergency nursing education project, *J Emerg Nurs* 17:3, 152–155, 1991.

49. Teasdale G, Jennett B: Assessment of coma and impaired consciousness: a practical scale, *Lancet* 2(872):81–84, 1974.

50. Tepas JJ et al: The pediatric trauma score as a predictor of injury severity: an objective assessment, *J Trauma* 28(4):425–429, 1988.

51. Tsai A, Kallsen G: Epidemiology of pediatric prehospital care, *Ann Emerg Med* 16(3):284–292, 1987.

52. US Department of Health and Human Services, Health Resources and Services Administration, Maternal and Child Health Bureau: *5-year plan for EMSC*, Washington, DC, 1995, EMSC National Resource Center.

53. Yamamoto LG, Wiebe RA: Improving medical communication with facsimile (fax) transmission, *Am J Emerg Med* 7(2):203–208, 1989.

54. Zeltzer LK, Jay SM, Fisher DM: The management of pain associated with pediatric procedures, *Pediatr Clin North Am* 36(4):941–964, 1989.

CHAPTER 2

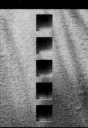

Legal and Ethical Considerations

Melissa Stimler

■ LEGAL CONSIDERATIONS

INTRODUCTION

The practice of emergency medicine carries with it exposure to many legal risks and ethical issues that are further complicated when a child is the patient. The purpose of this chapter is to identify these issues and provide the emergency nurse with basic knowledge necessary to function as a caregiver and advocate for the child in the emergency medical system.

LEGISLATIVE AND REIMBURSEMENT ISSUES

The Consolidated Omnibus Budget Reconciliation Act (COBRA).   A series of decisions made by Congress in the past few years has required that Medicare-participating hospitals operating emergency departments (EDs) be held liable for refusing to treat anyone with a medical emergency. The most notable legislation is the 1985 Consolidated Omnibus Budget Reconciliation Act (COBRA), often referred to as the "antidumping law".[11] This law prevents the transfer to another institution of unstable patients, women in active labor, or anyone having an emergency medical condition for economic reasons. The purpose of this legislation is to restrain hospitals or physicians from "dumping" patients who lack the funds to pay for care.

COBRA requires any Medicare-participating hospital with an emergency department to provide an appropriate screening examination, which is defined as "within the capability of the emergency room," to anyone requesting care. The law does not state who is responsible for performing the screening exam, and therefore in some facilities the triage nurse or a physician extender performs the exam. The purpose of the medical screening examination is to determine whether the patient suffers from an "emergency medical condition" or is in "active labor." When either of these conditions exists, the hospital must initiate appropriate medical care. If the institution is not capable of providing ongoing care, the patient may be transferred to a facility that is capable of providing care.[7,21]

"Transfer" is defined as the movement of an individual outside a hospital's facilities at the direction of any person employed by or affiliated with the hospital. COBRA legislation does make allowances for the transfer of patients before stabilization if a facility is unable to provide necessary treatment. However, a physician must certify, in writing, that the medical benefits of transferring the patient outweigh the risks to the individual from effecting the transfer.

For a medically appropriate transfer to occur, the *receiving* hospital must (1) have available space; (2) have qualified personnel for the treatment of the patient; and (3) agree to accept the patient. The *sending* hospital is responsible for ensuring all requirements are met before transferring the patient. These include (1) requesting acceptance of the patient from the receiving hospital; (2) providing the receiving hospital with complete medical records of the examination and treatment given; (3) using qualified personnel and transportation equipment for the transfer; and (4) providing appropriate life-support equipment during transfer. In many institutions a form is used to document compliance with COBRA/OBRA regulations (Fig. 2-1).

Penalties for knowingly violating COBRA laws are severe. The facility or physician may be fined up to $50,000 for each violation. Hospitals may also be terminated or suspended from receiving Medicaid

PATIENT TRANSFER FORM

I.   Transfer Request Prior to Stabilization of Emergency Medical Condition

I acknowledge that my medical condition has been evaluated and *explained to me* by the Emergency Department physician or other qualified medical person and/or my attending physician who has recommended and offered to me further medical examination and treatment. The potential benefits of such further medical examination and treatment as well as the potential risks associated with transfer to another facility have been explained to me and I fully understand them. In spite of this understanding, I refuse to consent to the further medical examination and treatment which has been offered to me, and request transfer to: _____

(Name of Facility)

I understand that my medical record for this visit will be copied and sent to the receiving facility.

I release the hospital, the physician(s) and any other persons caring for me from all responsibility of liability for any injury or ill effects that may result from my transfer and agree to accept all responsibility for the consequences of my refusal.

_____   _____
Signature of patient or legally responsible individual signing on patient's behalf   Witness

_____   _____
Relationship to patient   Date and time

II.   Transfer Refusal

I acknowledge that my medical condition has been evaluated and *explained to me* by the Emergency Department physician or other qualified medical person and/or my attending physician, who has recommended that I be transferred to the service of Dr. _____ at _____. The potential benefits of such transfer, the potential risks associated with transfer, and the probable risks of not being transferred have been explained to me and I fully understand them. Even though Dr. _____ believes it is in my best interests to be transferred. I refuse to be transferred and request instead to continue receiving treatment at: _____

I release the hospital, the physician(s) and any other persons caring for me from all responsibility of liability for any injury or ill effects that may result from my transfer and agree to accept all responsibility for the consequences of my refusal.

_____   _____
Signature of patient or legally responsible individual signing on patient's behalf   Witness

_____   _____
Relationship to patient   Date and time

III.   Transfer Consent

I acknowledge that my medical condition has been evaluated and *explained to me* by the Emergency Department physician or other qualified medical person and/or my attending physician, who has recommended that I be transferred to the service of Dr. _____ at _____. The potential benefits of such transfer, the potential risks associated with such transfer, and the probable risks of not being transferred have been explained to me and I fully understand them. With this knowledge and understanding, I agree and consent to be transferred.

I understand that my medical record for this visit will be copied and sent to the receiving facility.

_____   _____
Signature of patient or legally responsible individual signing on patient's behalf   Witness

_____   _____
Relationship to patient   Date and time

If the patient cannot sign or any of the above signatures cannot be obtained, explain why: _____

_____

Patient Label

19-794NC 4/94

FIG. 2-1.   Patient transfer form.

Continued.

PATIENT TRANSFER FORM
PHYSICIAN ASSESSMENT AND CERTIFICATION FOR TRANSFER

Patient Condition

1. _____ The patient has been stabilized such that within reasonable medical probability, no material deterioration of the patient's condition or the condition of the unborn child(ren) is likely to result from transfer.

2. _____ The patient's condition has not stabilized.

3. _____ The patient is pregnant and having contractions.

Transfer Requirements

1. _____ The receiving facility, _____has available space and
   Name of facility
   qualified personnel for treatment as acknowledged by:

   _____
   Name/Title/Phone No.   Time

2. _____ The receiving facility has agreed to accept transfer and to provide appropriate medical treatment acknowledged by:

   _____
   Physician Name/Phone No.   Time

3. _____ Appropriate medical records of the examination and treatment of the patient are provided at the time of transfer.

   _____   _____
   Signature as completed   Print Signature

4. _____ The patient will be transferred by qualified personnel and transportation equipment as required, including the use of necessary and medically appropriate life support measures.

   _____
   Transport Agency

5. _____ A nurse has called report to _____ at the receiving facility.

   _____   _____
   Nurse's Signature   Print Signature

Provider Certification

I have examined the patient and explained the following risks and benefits of being transferred/refusing transfer to the patient: _____

_____

_____

Based on these reasonable risks and benefits to the patient and/or the unborn child(ren), and based upon the information available at the time of the patient's examination, I certify that the medical benefits reasonably to be expected from the provision of appropriate medical treatment at another medical facility outweigh the increased risks, if any, to the individual's, and in the case of a patient in labor, to the unborn child's medical condition from effecting the transfer.

This transfer is medically appropriate and necessary.

_____   _____
Signature of physician or other qualified medical person   Date   Time

_____
Title

Patient Label

19-794NC 4-94

Fig. 2-1, cont'd. Patient transfer form.

funding. Individuals suffering personal harm as a direct result of a COBRA violation may also file suit against the transferring hospital and responsible physician.[20,24]

Omnibus Budget Reconciliation Act (OBRA). In July 1990 Congress enhanced COBRA legislation, enacting even more stringent laws relating to the transfer of patients. The Omnibus Budget Reconciliation Act (OBRA) demands hospitals provide medical screening examinations, including all ancillary services normally available to emergency departments, before inquiry about payment status.[11] For example, a child arriving in an emergency department with a head injury is entitled to have x-rays, laboratory tests, or any other test offered by the facility that will adequately eliminate the possibility of an emergency, regardless of ability to pay for the procedures or studies.

OBRA requires transfer records be kept for 5 years. The records must (1) document the name of any on-call physician who refused or failed to provide treatment; (2) describe the condition of the patient, including signs and symptoms, preliminary diagnosis, treatment provided, and the results of any tests; and (3) include a copy of the informed written consent or physician certification that transfer was necessary. COBRA/OBRA legislates the posting of signs and information, in all languages common to the patient population, informing individuals of their right to treatment.

As a result of OBRA, receiving hospitals with specialty care units (e.g., burn units, neonatal intensive care centers, trauma centers) cannot refuse the appropriate transfer of patients needing special services unless they do not have the capacity to treat the individual ("appropriate" is not defined). Hospitals and physicians failing to comply with the revised antidumping law are subject to loss of Medicare funds and penalties of up to $50,000 for each violation.[19]

Health Maintenance Organizations (HMOs) and Hospital Insurance Plans (HIPs). The goal of health maintenance organizations (HMOs) and hospital insurance plans (HIPs) is to reduce costs of health care by assigning patients to a primary care provider. Some HMOs or HIPs will not authorize payment for treatment in an emergency department unless the patient's primary care provider is notified and approves the visit before any emergency department interventions.[21] It is, however, a violation of the COBRA law if the hospital fails to provide a screening examination, even if the HMO's authorizing physician

or nurse ("gatekeeper") recommends sending the patient home or refers the patient to a private clinic or physician's office.[7] Even delaying the screening examination long enough for the gatekeeper to call back may be a violation of federal law.

Hospitals have elected to deal with the issue of nonauthorization by an insurance company in different manners. Some explain that although the provider has not authorized payment, the patient is still entitled to a medical screening examination. If they choose to leave, patients are asked to sign a statement that they have not been denied treatment by the emergency department. Other hospitals do not make the call to insurance gatekeepers. To comply with federal law, the hospital accepts the financial burden to seek payment retrospectively when treating the HMO patient.[7] Unfortunately, many contracts between HMOs and HIPs are negotiated without consideration of responsibilities placed on the facility to comply with federal and state law imposed by COBRA and OBRA. Emergency department nurses and physicians should examine emergency department admission procedures to be certain of compliance with federal and state mandates and keep the hospital administration informed of changes in legislation that might affect future HMO or HIP contracts.

CONSENT FOR TREATMENT

Introduction. The concepts of consent and informed consent are key points in the care of any patient. These issues present particular problems when an emergency situation involves a child. Although the issues are discussed broadly in many texts, laws governing consent vary in detail from state to state. Hospital policies are written in accordance with these laws; however, each facility determines how its employees are to comply with the law. The application of consent laws changes with differing clinical situations. Emergency nurses must be well informed about the consent laws within their states and the policies of the institutions in which they practice.

Definition/Categories of consent. Consent is the legal right (based on constitutionally protected rights of privacy and personal autonomy) that allows competent adults to have control over their own bodies by making choices about medical treatment.[23,44] In most states, individuals 18 years of age or older are considered adults. A few states still use 19 or 21 years of age as the age of majority. (The Nurse Practice Act or State Nurses Association can be consulted for laws governing each state.) Generally, children below the age of majority must have a legal guardian or parent exercise the right of consent.

There are three types of consent: express, implied, and surrogate. Express consent is consent that is given verbally, by signature, or by conduct (e.g., one who brings a child in for treatment and gives no objection to the treatment offered).[23] Implied consent arises by reasonable inference from the conduct of the patient or when a patient submits voluntarily to a procedure with knowledge of what is to occur.[41] Implied consent in the case of a minor is demonstrated when a legal guardian is not available to give permission to treat a child whose life, health, or physical function may be endangered without care. In this situation caregivers assume that the legal guardian would, if present, act in the best interest of the child by consenting to treatment. Surrogate consent is permission given by a parent, court, or guardian (Table 2-1).[23]

Informed consent involves both legal and ethical issues. Parents or caregivers have the right to make decisions about their child after receiving all of the information surrounding the child's illness. Nurses and physicians presenting an issue to parents should not withhold information to "protect" the parent or child or attempt to sway a decision in one direction or another.

When an informed consent is obtained, parents or surrogates must be given (1) a thorough explanation about the child's condition; (2) an explanation about the risks and benefits of the recommended treatment; (3) information about alternative courses of action; and (4) an explanation about the child's expected outcome if treatment is withheld (Box 2-1).[23,44]

Children's right to give assent. Legally, an emergency nurse must gain permission for treatment for any minor from the adult guardian of that child. Ethically, the nurse must also attempt to gain "assent"—agreement or acceptance—from any child who is old enough to understand (usually 7 years or older). Gaining assent means that the child has (1) a developmentally appropriate understanding of the health problem; (2) been informed of what is going to occur during the treatment; and (3) demonstrated willingness to receive the treatment. Although it is not a legal requirement to gain assent, it is ethically sound to encourage participation from children in decisions affecting their own health care.[6]

Notification of parents/caregivers. Caring for children in emergent situations poses additional problems concerning consent. The caretaker of a child may not actually be a parent or legal guardian. Aunts, uncles, siblings, grandparents, or others often provide physical care of the child but are not legal guardians unless designated by the parents in writing or by court order, as required in some states. In these cases an attempt to gain legal consent must be made. If, however, delay of an intervention may cause lasting

TABLE 2-1	Consent	
TYPE	**DEFINITION**	**EXAMPLES**
Express	Given verbally, by signature, or by conduct.	A parent brings a 2-year-old boy to the emergency department because he has a laceration on his foot. The parent signs a form giving the physician the authorization to give care as needed.
Implied	A parent submits voluntarily to a procedure or treatment with knowledge of what is to occur.	A parent takes a child to the pediatrician's office to have blood drawn for a monospot. Although no signature is required to authorize phlebotomy, the parent knows what will occur and does not verbally object.
Surrogate	Consent given by a parent, a court, or guardian for a child.	A parent signs permission for a child to have a spinal tap. A Jehovah's Witness child needs a blood transfusion. A court appoints a guardian to act in the best interest of the child by giving consent for the transfusion.

harm or impairment, care may begin under the auspices of implied consent. In such instances, two physicians should document in the medical record that delay in treatment will place the child in jeopardy. At the same time, continued efforts should be made to contact the legal guardian, and all efforts should be documented in the medical record.[23] In some instances, it may be necessary to involve the police in notifying legal guardians. Court rulings have consistently supported physicians who have treated minors for the nonnegligent emergency care of a child without parental consent.[25]

Because parents may not be physically present at the time emergent care is required, consent may be obtained by telephone. The telephone conversation should be witnessed and all pertinent data should be documented, including the times, persons spoken to, and identity of the witnesses.

Emancipated and mature minors. In every state there are minors who are legally allowed to act as adults and are able to give consent for their own treatment. Criteria for this emancipation differs among states and may include court order, marriage, and active-duty status in the armed forces.

Pregnancy emancipates a minor, although in some states minors do not retain the status after the birth of the child. The minor parent does, however, have the authority to consent to treatment for the child and for any condition related to the pregnancy. In some states, pregnant minors must have parental permission to treat a condition unrelated to the pregnancy. For example, the minor may need parental permission for treatment of a sore throat but does not require permission for treatment of vaginal bleeding.

"Mature minor statutes" have been enacted in many states, allowing a minor the authority to consent to medical care in specific situations. These instances include treatment for drug abuse or sexually transmitted diseases. Minors who live apart from their parents

---

Box 2-1   Informed Consent

- Complete explanation of child's condition
- Description of risks and benefits of treatment
- Review of alternative courses of action
- Child's expected outcome if treatment is withheld

---

may, in some states, be considered mature minors empowered to consent to health care.[41]

In summary, consent laws vary from state to state; therefore it is important for emergency nurses to be well informed about statutes setting parameters for the treatment of illness or injury within their states. Hospital policies defining role expectations and procedures to follow when gaining consent should be readily available in all emergency departments.

REPORTABLE INCIDENTS

All 50 states mandate that health care providers report suspected child abuse or neglect, including sexual abuse, to an appropriate child protective agency. There are wide variations in the definitions of child abuse, sexual abuse, and neglect from state to state;[43] however, the following may help nurses in clinical settings.

Child abuse may be defined as "the willful infliction of bodily harm onto a child under the age of 18 by a parent, a person acting as a parent, a family member, or a legal guardian."[43] Although the definition of abuse varies from state to state, most exclude injury to a child by a *noncaregiver* (someone other than a parent acting as a parent). Teachers, day care workers, and hospital workers are included in some definitions.

Sexual abuse may be defined as "the involvement of children and adolescents in sexual activities they cannot comprehend because of their developmental level; to which they are unable to give informed consent; or that violate the social taboos of family or society."[12] Examples of sexual abuse are activities that cause physical injuries; genital touching; genital exposure of an adult to a child; or photographs of unclothed children engaging in sexual activity.[12]

Neglect may be defined more broadly as actions taken or not taken that place a child under the age of 18 in actual or potential risk of harm. Neglect may result in harm through negligent treatment such as failure to provide adequate food, shelter, clothing, medical care and treatment, and emotional support. The individual responsible may be a parent, a person acting as a parent, a family member, or a legal guardian.[43]

Requirements for reporting of child abuse are different from state to state. Some require telephone reports to be followed by a written report. Failure to report may carry criminal penalties, civil liabilities, and loss of licensure for health care providers. Additionally, health care providers failing to report an incident may be held liable if the same child (or another child in the family) suffers further injury. It can be argued that the incident could have been avoided had the original case been reported.

As long as a reportable incident is made in good faith, persons with a duty to report are given immunity from liability for a mistaken report or if abuse or neglect is not substantiated.[23] Policies written for emergency departments must conform to state and federal laws. For a complete discussion of child abuse see Chapter 25.

MEDICAL NEGLIGENCE/MALPRACTICE

Introduction. *Medical negligence* or *malpractice* with regard to emergency medicine is defined as the failure of a nurse or physician to provide the accepted standard of care that a reasonable nurse or physician of ordinary learning, judgment, or skill would do, or the doing of something that a reasonable and prudent nurse or physician would not do in the same or similar circumstances.[8,9] The great volume and high acuity of patients who enter emergency departments put this area at high risk for medical malpractice suits.

The care of children increases the risks of litigation for emergency nurses for many reasons, including (1) direct communication with young children is very difficult; (2) parents are usually frightened and upset and may be very young themselves; (3) parent's judgment may be impaired as a result of drug or alcohol use; (4) parents may be poor historians of the child's illness or injury; (5) the atmosphere of the emergency department is noisy and chaotic; (6) there is little time to establish trust and rapport between staff and families; (7) long delays exist due to the high volume of patients; and (8) language barriers often exist.[13,23] These issues tend to "set the emergency team up" for legal recourse if there is any perception on the part of the parents of wrong doing (Box 2-2).

Nursing malpractice lawsuits fall into four major categories: (1) treatment; (2) failure to notify a physician of changes in signs, symptoms, and patient status; (3) medication; and (4) monitoring, observing, and supervising (Table 2-2).[33] To succeed in a medical malpractice suit, a plaintiff must prove four elements: (1) the provider had a duty to meet a certain standard of care; (2) the provider failed to meet that accepted standard of care; (3) there was harm to the child; and (4) there was a link between the breach of duty and the harm sustained by the child.[23,39]

Regardless of the quality of care, some children will die or be left with serious deficiencies after an emergent illness or injury. Parents are, of course, devastated. Filing a lawsuit against the staff of an emergency

> **Box 2-2 Factors That Increase the Risk of Litigation in Pediatric Emergency Care**
>
> - Communicating with young children is difficult
> - Parents may be very frightened
> - Parents are sometimes very young themselves
> - Parents' judgment may be impaired
> - Parents may be poor historians
> - The ED environment is noisy and chaotic, leaving little time to develop rapport with the family
> - The child's care may be delayed while other, more acutely ill patients are seen
> - Language barriers may exist

department or the treating facility may be the result of this devastation.

Prevention of litigation. The possibility of litigation may be reduced if nurses display excellent communication skills, stay current in their specialty, are cognizant of legislation affecting emergency care, and employ proper standards of practice when caring for children.

Orientation of new personnel is an important step to reduce the risk of malpractice litigation. An effective orientation program must address expectations for documentation, the care of children and the most common presenting complaints, and the correct use of equipment and drugs. Records should be kept for each employee documenting components of the orientation program, and managers should evaluate the performance of each employee as guided by hospital policy.

All nurses should keep up to date with hospital policies and procedures, as well as legislation that pertains to the practice of emergency nursing. In addition, nurses should stay current in the practice of emergency nursing by attending conferences or reviewing literature. Courses such as the American Heart Association's Pediatric Advanced Life Support (PALS) program or the Emergency Nurses Association's Emergency Nursing Pediatric Course (ENPC),[16] may help prepare nurses to care for the special needs of the pediatric patient, thus reducing the risk of malpractice.

Communication plays a significant role in reducing the risk of liability. Taking the time to speak with the

TABLE 2-2	Four Major Categories of Nursing Malpractice Suits	
TYPE	**EXAMPLES**	
Treatment	An apnea monitor alarms. The nurse ignores the alarm. The infant suffers brain damage as a result of anoxia.	
Communication	A 2-year-old with asthma in an emergency department becomes less responsive to the guardian. The nurse notes this in the nursing notes but fails to report the decline in status to a physician. The patient progresses to respiratory arrest, is intubated, and later dies.	
Medication	In flushing an IV line, a nurse mistakenly uses potassium chloride instead of normal saline through the central line. The child arrests and dies.	
Monitoring, observing, and supervising	A nurse instructs a nursing student to care for a child with a compound fractured forearm. The student fails to monitor radial pulses, which are absent. The child loses the use of the right hand as a result.	

child and family and carefully explaining delays or procedures will show care and concern. In addition, the nurse should always take the concerns of a sick child's parents seriously. Parents know their child best and will often give the most accurate assessment of the severity of a child's symptoms when asked the right questions. Communication is enhanced when a multidisciplinary approach is used (e.g., involving other professionals such as a social worker, chaplain, or patient advocate) to bridge gaps that are often forgotten in a busy emergency department.

Statute of limitations. The statute of limitations on malpractice suits is by definition the "length of time after medical care has been rendered that a lawsuit can be instituted";[9] however, the length of time in which a lawsuit can be filed varies from state to state. Emergency personnel treating children are susceptible to malpractice claims for longer periods of time than those treating adults. Although parents have the authority to pursue legal action for their children, children also have the right to file claims on their own behalf for a period after the age of majority. A child suffering a birth injury may (in some states) sue for malpractice at 18 years of age. Thorough documentation of the care of children becomes even more critical when viewed in the light that claims may not be filed for many years after care is rendered.

TELEPHONE ADVICE

Parents often telephone an emergency department (as they would a pediatrician's office) to gain advice about treating an illness or injury. In the majority of cases, there is rarely an ongoing relationship between the

> **Box 2-3 Recommendations Regarding Telephone Advice**
>
> - Parents of children recently discharged from the emergency department may request additional explanation about discharge instructions, medications, or referrals.
> - It is acceptable to provide recommendations for first aid or instructions about accessing emergency care.
> - Only qualified medical professionals informed about the legal ramifications of providing telephone advice should provide this service.
> - Policies, protocols, documentation, and quality assurance programs must be in existence to monitor the quality of advice given by telephone.
>
> From American College of Emergency Physicians (ACEP), Professional Liability Committee, Position Statement: Providing telephone advice from the emergency department, *Ann Emerg Med* 19:600, 1990.

staff of the emergency department and the caller. Because it is difficult to adequately assess a patient from a description of symptoms over the phone, the safest response to a request for telephone advice is an offer to evaluate the child in the emergency department. In 1990 the American College of Emergency Physicians established guidelines regarding telephone advice.[1] These are reviewed in Box 2-3.

Telephone orders from private physicians. Physicians who see children in an office may not be able to provide treatment needed in the outpatient setting or during normal office hours. The physician may telephone orders to the emergency department and send the child for treatment stating that an assessment by the emergency department physician is unnecessary. The emergency physician, the private physician, and the emergency facility may experience significant liability in these situations should the child suffer an adverse outcome.[22] This is because the physician-patient relationship is established between the emergency department physician and the patient, even if the patient is not examined by the emergency physician.[22] For this reason, the American College of Emergency Physicians recommends that patients be seen and evaluated by an emergency physician before instituting telephone orders,[1] although this approach is not uniformly practiced.

With specific regard to telephone orders, it is always best for orders to be written by a physician; however, in reality, transcribing telephone orders is often a part of the emergency nurse's responsibility. To prevent miscommunication or misunderstanding the nurse should read the order back to the physician to be certain there are no errors in transmission. Nurses also need to be aware that drug enforcement administration regulations prohibit the dispensation of controlled substances from emergency department stocks when ordered by telephone.

REFUSAL OF CARE

Introduction. Occasionally, a parent may refuse consent when a child's medical condition is actually or potentially serious. Refusal to allow care may result from fear or religious, cultural, or personal beliefs. If the child's condition will not deteriorate immediately, hospital counsel should be contacted at once to petition the court for permission to treat.

Religious beliefs. Few times are as disturbing to the emergency team than when parents refuse medical care for a child based on religious beliefs. These instances raise both ethical and legal issues. The Constitution grants the freedom to practice religion of choice, and it is assumed that parents will act in the best interest of their child. At times, however, the parent's religious beliefs are in contrast to what society would consider in the best interest of the child. When a child has a life-threatening illness or injury the courts may override parental wishes with regard to religious beliefs.

The issue of treatment for any child revolves around the seriousness of the child's illness or injury. When the parents refuse treatment in *nonemergency* situations, the hospital's legal counsel and ethics committee should be consulted. In this situation, emergency physicians may be held liable for negligence if they disregard a parent's wishes.[17,45,47] The decision to involve the court system in these cases should be made jointly by the hospital attorney and the treating physician.

When *emergent* intervention is necessary to save a child's life or prevent disability, a court order is necessary to override a parent's refusal for care; however, emergency treatment should begin even in the absence of parental permission. As therapy is instituted, the hospital attorney can pursue a legal ruling. Court orders can be obtained in a relatively short time. Court cases have affirmed the legal acceptability of allowing treatment for minors with emergent medical needs in circumstances when a child's life is jeopardized or when there is risk of disability.[28]

Jehovah's Witness. The most frequent context in which religious issues arise in the emergency department is the refusal of a blood transfusion for a child by parents who are Jehovah's Witnesses. The believers of this fundamentalist Christian faith firmly feel transfusion of whole blood, packed red blood cells, white blood cells, plasma, or platelets will prevent the child from receiving eternal life after death.[26] Life extended by transfusion is regarded as meaningless and lacking in spiritual purpose because the hope for everlasting life is lost.[28,38] Jehovah's Witnesses do, however, seek medical care for illnesses and injuries not requiring transfusion of blood (Box 2-4).

In a 1944 precedent-setting case, parents who were Jehovah's Witnesses refused to consent to lifesaving medical treatment for their child. A court ruled "neither the right of religion nor the rights of parenthood are beyond limitation . . . parents may be free to make martyrs of themselves but they are not free to make martyrs of their children before they have reached the age when they can make that choice for themselves."[37] This concept has been upheld in a number of court cases reinforcing the stand that parents do not have the right to withhold standard medical care and subject children to ill health.[27,34,47]

Summary. Emergency medical teams following accepted standards of care may be relatively certain that claims of negligence made by parents who have refused consent will be deemed unreasonable by the legal system.[28] Additionally, medicolegal risks can be

---

Box 2-4   Acceptable and Unacceptable Transfusion Methods for Jehovah's Witnesses

1. Transfusions of whole blood, packed red blood cells, white blood cells, platelets, and plasma (fresh or frozen) are forbidden.
2. The use of albumin, immune globulin, and hemophilia preparation is a decision left up to the individual.
3. Nonblood plasma expanders such as saline solution, Ringer's lactate, and hetastarch are acceptable.
4. Banking of the person's own blood or salvage from suction is forbidden, because Witnesses believe that blood that has left the body should be discarded.
5. There is no restriction in handling blood, and Witnesses may give blood for a sample.

From Thurkauf GC: Understanding the beliefs of Jehovah's Witnesses, *Focus Crit Care* 16(3):199–204, 1989.

---

minimized by establishing policies and guidelines to follow when such decisions must be made—before they occur. These should include accurate and meticulous documentation of the event. Every emergency nurse and physician should know how to access the legal system so that judicial assistance can be obtained quickly when the life of a child is at risk.[28]

RISK MANAGEMENT

In recent years, greater consumer awareness, court decisions that allow contingency fees instead of fee for service for attorneys, and a large number of inexperienced attorneys willing to take cases refused by more experienced attorneys have contributed to increased litigation against hospitals, nurses, and physicians.[13] For these reasons, emergency departments must have an active risk-management program to protect children from harm and reduce the risk of liability to providers of emergency care. A review of incident reports, patient complaints, and identified poor outcomes is essential to identifying high-risk situations (e.g., high numbers of febrile children with meningitis who are misdiagnosed).

Incident reports. An incident (occurrence) report is a form used to document events that are not consistent with hospital policy, deviate from routine or standard practice, or involve environmental accidents or circumstances that could result in poor outcome. The report should be completed as soon as possible after an occurrence to relate an accurate and thorough account.

Emergency department staff completing incident reports should record only the facts and never draw conclusions about fault or harm. Because incident reports contain extremely sensitive information, they should be kept strictly confidential. An incident report must never be mentioned in a patient's chart or record and should never be duplicated. An established hospital procedure describing the appropriate channels through which reports are to be filed should be familiar to all staff. Incident report forms may be kept from discovery in litigation if they are worded to comply with state statutes and kept confidential.[10,13,49]

Incident reports serve several purposes. They notify hospital officials of potential or actual situations of liability. They are a useful method to gather data for recognizing trends that may result in policy or procedural changes, employee educational programs, or system changes. The reports are also an excellent method of evaluating new system changes that may impact patient care (e.g., Has a reduction in staffing had an impact on the number of patients who leave without being seen or decreased turnaround time?).

Patient complaints. Even the best emergency departments receive complaints as a result of lengthy waits, perception that staff members are uncaring, the high cost of emergency care, or other highly charged emotional situations. At times, negative outcomes occur even if emergency care is exemplary. A proactive system of handling complaints from angry parents is one method of monitoring the quality of emergency services provided.

All complaints should be investigated promptly by telephone, letter, or in a face-to-face meeting. It is best if one or two employees are assigned this task. The complaints should be recorded in a log book or monthly report so trends may be identified and tracked to resolution through a quality-management program.

When speaking to a parent or caretaker about a complaint, one should actively listen, showing concern and sympathy. It is best not to accuse parents of being wrong in their complaint nor to admit guilt on the part of the emergency provider. The goal is for parents to feel confident their issue has been heard and will be investigated.

Documentation. Thorough documentation of all events, including legal and ethical issues, must be made a part of the medical record. The legal standard is that if something is not charted, it was not done or did not exist.[23] Quality care cannot be proven if it is undocumented.

Every page of an emergency department treatment record should clearly identify the patient. Documentation should describe the mode of transportation and the name and relationship of the person accompanying the child. All prehospital care must be addressed in the record.

Soon after the child's arrival in the emergency department, the nurse should document a thorough history of the presenting complaint. It is important to note any past medical history that may affect the child's treatment or outcome. A complete physical examination, including weight, vital signs, physical findings, or clinical observations, made by the nurse or physician should be accurately recorded. Abnormal findings, for example, an elevated temperature, pain, change in mental status, or delayed capillary refill, should be reassessed at intervals and clearly acknowledged in writing by the emergency team.

Orders, interventions, or procedures performed in the emergency department should be documented. The record should clearly identify when an order was begun and completed, and it should include the name of the staff member completing the order. When interventions such as medications or procedures are required, the child's physical or emotional response should be recorded. The standard of care for any given situation must be reflected in the medical record.

Before admitting, transferring, or discharging a child, the emergency nurse should reassess the child's current physical and emotional status, as well as findings reflected in the nursing documentation. When a child is to be admitted or transferred, the record should reflect the name of the person receiving the report to document transference of the responsibility for care.

The discharge process deserves special attention in an emergency department record. First, documentation of a child's final disposition and condition on discharge should be reflected. Second, copies of the after-care instructions signed by parents attesting to an understanding of instructions and a willingness to follow them are recommended for inclusion in the medical record. Discharge instructions should be given in the patient's native language.

▌ETHICAL CONSIDERATIONS

Ethics is a branch of philosophy defined as a "principle of right or good conduct or a system of moral principles or values."[3] Ethical decision making is difficult for the caregiver; however, this responsibility is further complicated when children are involved—they are vulnerable, often unable to participate in the decision-making process, and are legally considered minors. It is further complicated because the emergency medical team has little time to establish rapport and trust with parents or children needing care.

The following recent societal changes have influenced ethical decision making:

1. Public policy once supported care for all who sought it. Currently, the ability to pay affects the quality and quantity of health care offered.[46]

2. Advances in medical technology offer opportunities for manipulating patient destiny by controlling vital functions or altering body parts. There is rarely a single treatment modality for an illness or injury. Families must consider each option with its different side effects, degrees of intrusiveness, and implications for resulting way of life.[5]

3. More than 10% of the gross national product is spent on health care, resulting in major criticisms of the system.[46] In an attempt to control rising costs, the federal government has introduced a system of managed care that has affected the entire approach to health care.

4. There has been a redefinition of the roles of health care providers. Families no longer consider nurses and physicians to be the "unchallenged decision makers" for their child and expect professionals to share knowledge with them as a basis of informed consent.[5,46]

ETHICAL DECISION MAKING

By nature of practice, nurses, more than any other discipline, are in constant contact with pediatric patients and parents. As a result, the emergency nurse often assumes the role of advocate for sick and injured children. Nurses may be asked to provide information that will guide families in making decisions based on their individual belief and cultural systems. In providing this information, the emergency nurse must weigh the principles of beneficence and nonmaleficence, respect, and justice.[42]

BENEFICENCE AND NONMALEFICENCE

The issues of beneficence (doing good) and nonmaleficence (avoiding harm) are considerations when determining treatment alternatives. It may not be possible to do good without also causing harm. For example, the nurse may cause pain to a child by injecting drugs or fluids and passing a nasogastric tube; however, these procedures may be essential to the child's survival.[5] The nurse acts as advocate when providing information about treatment alternatives. As long as legal issues are followed, parents and children must be given the opportunity to define "good" and "harm" within the framework of their own beliefs and culture.

It is considered in the "best interest" of a child to favor life over death; however, when the chance of survival is minimal, some feel treatments that are burdensome (those causing pain, suffering, physical and emotional isolation, or immobilization) should not be performed.[30] When the child's parents and health care team decide that the burdens of treatment outweigh the benefits of life, priority of care becomes the alleviation of pain. The American Nurses Association Position Statement on Promotion of Comfort and Relief of Pain in Dying Patients[4] supports pain relief at the end of life, reminding nurses to advocate pain relief in dying patients even if life is secondarily shortened (Box 2-5).

RESPECT FOR PERSONS

Another important principle in decision making involves respect for the child. Respect implies certain rights, including prevention from harm, the right to be told the truth, the right to informed consent, and the right to receive or refuse treatment.[5] Children are not autonomous or self-determining; therefore decisions should be made by someone representing their best interests. Parents are usually this surrogate decision maker because of the strong bonds of affection and love for the child. When there is no parent, or when the parent is unwilling or unable to act as a surrogate, the health care team is obliged to find an alternative to protect the child's interests.[42]

JUSTICE

Children must be treated fairly, or justly, as individuals. Some feel decisions about treatment should not be made on the basis of race, age, sex, ability to pay, diagnosis, or socioeconomic status. Others argue that just decision making considers society as a whole, not only the person in question. For example, should a severely mentally retarded child who is a ward of the state receive astronomically expensive treatment for a terminal illness, or should the limited funds be spent to care for a mildly retarded child who may grow to be a productive citizen? Health care professionals should work to create fair systems for the distribution of limited resources.[42] Emergency nurses may find themselves in the position of helping others decide how to divide resources in a fair, equitable manner.

SPECIFIC ETHICAL DECISIONS

The terminally ill child. When a terminally ill child arrives in the emergency department it is traumatic not only for the parent and child but also for the health care team. Occasionally these children are well known to the staff, but too frequently this may be the first contact the parent/child has with the ED staff. In these cases prehospital care providers, physicians, and nurses have little information about a child's past medical history or a family's belief and value system.

Although in most cases the ED team reflexively acts to save a child's life, in the case of a terminally ill child the team may wrongly assume the parents of a child with a clear-cut problem (e.g., severe motor or mental retardation, inoperable heart lesions, or a terminal malignancy) do not want the child resuscitated, and the team may choose not to act. Ideally, the decision not to resuscitate, or to provide only a certain level of care to a terminally ill child, is made by parents who have been fully informed by the child's physician—before an emergency room visit. For this reason, physicians who care for terminally ill children in the community should be encouraged to draft letters describing each child's circumstances and the parents' wishes.

When letters are drafted, two copies should be made—one for the parents and one for the medical record. Parents should keep the letter in their possession at all times and bring it to the emergency department if their child is seen; the emergency team rarely has access to the medical record quickly enough to aid in decision making.

Parents who bring a letter should be asked if they still agree with their earlier decisions. Parents who had previously decided a child should not be resuscitated during a terminal event may change their decision when confronted with the actual situation. In this case, the emergency team is obligated to

Box 2-5   American Nurses Association Position Statement on Promotion of Comfort and Relief of Pain in Dying Patients

Summary: The American Nurses Association (ANA) believes that the promotion of comfort and aggressive efforts to relieve pain and other symptoms in dying patients are obligations of the nurse. Nurses should not hesitate to use full and effective doses of pain medication for the proper management of pain in the dying patient. The increasing titration of medication to achieve adequate symptom control, even at the expense of life, thus hastening death secondarily, is ethically justified.

Background: Nursing has been defined as the diagnosis and treatment of human responses to actual or potential health problems.[1] When the patient is in the terminal stage of life, when cure or prolongation of life in individuals with serious health problems is no longer possible, the focus of nursing is on the individual's response to dying and palliative care. Diagnosis and treatment then focuses on the promotion of comfort which becomes the primary goal of nursing care.

One of the major concerns of dying patients and their families is the fear of intractable pain during the dying process. It is widely acknowledged that pain is commonly undertreated and that many patients experience inadequate pain management.[2] Indeed, overwhelming pain can cause sleeplessness, loss of morale, fatigue, irritability, restlessness, withdrawal, and other serious problems for the dying patient.[3,4,5] Nurses play an extremely important role in the assessment of symptoms and the control of pain in dying patients because they often have the most frequent and continuous patient contact. In planning nursing care of dying patients, "the patient has a right to have pain recognized as a problem, and pain relief perceived by the health care team as a need."[6,7]

The assessment and management of pain should be based on a thorough understanding of the individual patient's personality, culture and ethnicity, coping style and emotional, physical and spiritual needs, and on an understanding of the pathophysiology of the disease state.[8] The main goal of nursing intervention for dying patients should be maximizing comfort through adequate management of pain and discomfort as this is consistent with the expressed desires of the patient. Toward that end, the patient should have whatever medication, in whatever dosage, and by whatever route is needed to control the level of pain as perceived by the patient.[9]

Careful titration of pain medication is essential to promote comfort in dying patients. The proper dose is "the dose that is sufficient to reduce pain and suffering."[10] Tolerance to pain medications often develops in patients after repeated and prolonged use. Thus, both adults and children may require very high doses of medication to maintain adequate pain control.[11] These doses may exceed the usual recommended dosages of the particular drug for patients of similar age and weight.[12,13,14] Additionally, regular dosing (or administration) of pain medication has been shown to be more effective than PRN use.[15] Caregivers frequently fear hastening patients' death, causing addiction or professional/legal sanctioning which can interfere with the appropriate relief of pain in dying patients.[16,17]

While it is well known that pain medications often have sedative or respiratory depressant side effects, this should not be an overriding consideration in their use for dying patients as long as such use is consistent with the patient's wishes. It should be recognized that pain may continue even when a patient is unresponsive and at the end hours of life when respirations decline. Pain relief should continue unless there is a reason to believe that the physiologic cause of pain is no longer present.[18] The increasing titration of medication to achieve adequate symptom control, even at the expense of maintaining life or hastening death secondarily, is ethically justified. Nurses should not hesitate to use full and effective doses of pain medication for the proper management of pain in the dying patient.

Nurses can seek to remove barriers that impede the goals of appropriate pain and symptom management. The availability of pain management experts, supportive care teams and other resources can be helpful in devising and maintaining a plan of care to meet the patient's comfort needs. Additionally, mechanisms should be available (e.g., ethics committees) when there are conflicts around the appropriate relief of pain and other symptomatology.

References

1. American Nurses Association. (1995). *Nursing: a Social Policy Statements*. Washington, D.C.: Author.
2. U.S. Department of Health and Human Services. (1994). *Management of Cancer Pain*. Clinical Practice Guidelines, #9. Rockville, MD.
3. Spross, J.A., (1985). Cancer pain and suffering: clinical lessons from life, literature, and legend, *Oncology Nursing Forum, 12,* 23-31.
4. Amenta M. & Bohnet, N.L. (Eds.) (1986). *Palliative care nursing*. New York, Little, Brown, and Company.
5. Melzack, R. (1990). The tragedy of needless pain. *Scientific American, 262,* 27-33.
6. Spross, J.A., McGuire, D.B. & Schmitt, R.N. (1990). Oncology Nursing Society position paper on cancer pain, part one. *Oncology Nursing Forum, 17*(4), 595-606.
7. Spross, J.A., McGuire, D.B., & Schmitt, R.M. (1990b). Oncology Nursing Society Position paper on cancer pain, part two, *Oncology Nursing Forum, 17,* 751-760.
8. Dalton, J.A. & Fenerstein, M. (1988). Biobehavioral factors in cancer pain. *Pain, 33,* 137-147.
9. Wanzer, S.H., et. al. (1989). The physician's responsibility toward hopelessly ill patients: a second look. *The New England Journal of Medicine, 320,* 884-889.
10. Ibid.
11. Kachoyenos, M.K. & Zollo, M.B. (1995). Ethics in pain management of infants and children. *Maternal Child Nursing, 20,* 142-147.
12. Eland, J.M. (1989). Pharmacologic management of pain. In B. Martin (Ed.) *Pediatric Hospice Care: What Helps*. Children's Hospital of Los Angeles.
13. Foley, K. (1989). Controversies in cancer pain: medical perspectives. *Cancer, 63* (supplement), 2257-2265.
14. Inturrisi, C.E. (1989). Management of cancer pain: pharmacology and principles of management. *Cancer, 11,* 2308-2320.
15. American Pain Society. (1992). *Principles of analgesic use in the treatment of acute pain and cancer pain,* 3rd ed. Skokie, IL: Author.
16. Solomon, M.Z., et. al. (1993). Decisions near the end-of-life: professional views on life sustaining treatments. *American Journal of Public Health, 83,* 14-23.
17. Buchan, M.L. & Tolle, S.W. (1995). Pain relief for dying persons: dealing with physicians fears and concerns. *The Journal of Clinical Ethics, 6*(1), 53-61.
18. Coyle, N., Cherny, N. & Portenoy, R. (1995). Pharmacologic management of cancer pain. In McGuire, D.B., Yarbro, C.H., & Ferrell, B.R. (eds). *Cancer Pain Management.* Jones & Bartlett, Boston, MA.

Effective Date:	September 5, 1991, rev. 1995
Status:	Position Statement
Originated by:	Task Force on the Nurse's Role in End-of-Life Decisions
	Center for Ethics and Human Rights
Adopted by:	ANA Board of Directors

Related Past Action: 1. *Code for Nurses with Interpretive Statements,* 1985

American Nurses Association
600 Maryland Avenue, S.W.
Suite 100
Washington, DC 20024
(202) 651-7000

From American Nurses Association (ANA): *Position statement on promotion of comfort and relief of pain in dying patients,* Washington, DC, 1996, ANA.

honor the wishes of the parent. Regardless of the decision, the emergency nurse and physician should document the events leading to the decision. Documentation should include conversations with the parents, the child (when possible), and the child's personal physician. Copies of all written documents accompanying the child should be mentioned in the progress notes.

At times, a child with a terminal condition may be brought to the emergency department with a treatable illness. For example, a child with terminal cancer may be brought in by ambulance with dehydration and vomiting. At first glance, the emergency team may assume the child is dying from the cancer. A careful history and examination may reveal a treatable gastrointestinal disorder. The decision not to resuscitate during such times could unnecessarily shorten the life span and rob the child and parents of many happy experiences. Do not resuscitate orders are not applicable in terminal children with treatable illnesses.[40]

The emergency team should not let personal definitions of "quality of life" influence the mode of treatment offered to a terminally ill child. It is important to be well informed about hospital policy, legal issues, and the wishes of children and their caretakers when making ethical decisions about those with terminal illnesses.

THE CHILD'S RIGHT TO DIE

Before the 1950s and the advent of miracle drugs, immunizations, and technologic advances, 50% of all deaths occurred in homes among familiar surroundings. The dying were attended by loved ones, friends, and family doctors. An estimated 80% of all deaths now occur in hospitals under impersonal conditions.[36] Death often is a decision to separate the body from machines and tubes rather than a failure of organs to function. Death is the final act of living. Children have the right to death with dignity.

Advanced directives. The Patient Self-Determination Act (advanced directives or living wills) allows adults the right to determine treatment by stating their wishes in written form. Children are not legally allowed to have an advanced directive; however, this right may be extended to emancipated or mature minors.[5] In the rare instance when a minor does have an advanced directive, emergency department nurses and physicians are obligated to honor this request.

When to stop resuscitation/care. In some states, prehospital personnel are obligated to begin resuscitation of any living patient when dispatched to the scene of an accident or to a home. When to terminate an ongoing resuscitation is a complicated decision for the emergency team, even if the medical standard for ceasing resuscitative efforts is brain death or cardiovascular unresponsiveness. Some states (Minnesota, Alaska, Colorado) have provided models for prehospital providers outlining times when resuscitation need not be considered. These models give prehospital personnel permission to simply transport a dying patient who does not desire resuscitative efforts.

Once cardiopulmonary resuscitation (CPR) has been initiated in the field, however, only a physician can make the decision to terminate efforts, because termination is equivalent to determining death.[2] As long as the provider is physically able, or until care is transferred to another qualified person, nonphysicians must continue CPR.

Guidelines for cessation of CPR have been proposed by different sources utilizing specified periods of apnea, pulselessness, and resuscitation efforts to determine predictability of cardiac recovery.[15] Studies, however, have demonstrated physicians interpret clinical data differently when deciding to terminate CPR.[15,35]

BRAIN DEATH

The issue of brain death has been a topic in legal, medical, religious, and ethical discussions for years. The legal definition of death (the total cessation of cardiac and respiratory function) has been expanded to include brain death. *Brain death* is defined as the irreversible cessation of cerebral and brain stem functioning.[18] The determination of brain death is important primarily because of the ability to retrieve and transplant organs.

ORGAN DONATION

Religious, social, cultural, and metaphysical beliefs affect opinions on the morality of organ transplants or the transfer of body tissues from one person to another.[5] Some compare a body to a machine and view transplantation as replacing defective parts.[5] Others, such as Jehovah's Witnesses, consider the transfer of any tissue as a moral impunity.[31]

Regardless of beliefs, the Uniform Anatomical Gift Act of 1968, adopted by every state, requires all hospitals to establish protocols for the identification of potential organ donors.[40] Provisions of the legislation require hospital personnel to ask the next of kin to donate the organs or tissues of patients who have expired or been pronounced brain dead. Failure to comply with this legislation can result in loss of Medicare or Medicaid reimbursements to the facility.

The emergency nurse may be reluctant to add to the grief of parents whose child is dying by inquiring about organ donation. However, studies have indicated that families who were asked about organ donation responded that it eased their grief. Some were even upset if no one gave them the opportunity to choose organ donation.[40]

Occasionally the emergency nurse is required to care for the child for whom the sole purpose of care is to keep the organs alive for future transplantation. At this time, alleviation of pain and suffering of the child and supporting the grieving family become the priorities of care.

Nursing care.   Children are expected to outlive their parents and grandparents; therefore the sudden death of a child is a highly charged emotional event for not only the parents but also the emergency department staff. Factors that may contribute to the staff's inability to cope with death or a brain death determination and communication with the family include reluctance to accept brain death as meaning death with no hope of recovery, personal beliefs that are in conflict with the decision to shift care from the needs of the dying child to those of an unknown organ recipient, and the perception that approaching the grieving parents will add to their grief.

There are, however, approaches that can help both the parents and the ED staff cope with the brain death determination of a child. These include giving the parents—and staff—time to deal with the impending death, explaining the meaning of brain death, and allowing the parents to say "goodbye" to the child. To assist in communicating with the family, the transplant coordinator should be notified as soon as the brain death determination is made.

Parents and the health care team may be helped by hearing the positive aspects of organ donation. Explanations concerning the logistics of the actual procedure and the meaning of brain death may allay some fears that the child will suffer pain or indignity during the retrieval. Some parents have said that organ donation has helped them find meaning and comfort after their child's death. For a complete discussion of the care of the dying child, see Chapter 9.

ALTERNATIVE HEALTH CARE PRACTICES

Nurses are likely to encounter families in the emergency setting who follow alternative health care practices. Alternative therapies may be referred to as "holistic," "alternative," "nontoxic," "folk," or "traditional"; allopathic therapies are called "western," "conventional," or "traditional"[48] (Table 2-3).

Alternative practices focus on the interrelationship between the mind, body, and spirit, with the belief that the body can heal itself.[48] Examples of alternative practices include acupuncture, chiropractic, reflexology, therapeutic touch, herbalism, feldenkrais (gentle massage to relax muscle tension and allow the body to move more freely), homeopathy, vegetarianism, and vitamin therapy. Alternative health practices can overlap allopathic therapies (e.g., vitamin C is given to promote healing); be in disagreement with allopathic therapies (e.g., using diet rather than antibiotics to cure an ear infection); or not affect allopathic therapy.[48]

Unfortunately, there is often criticism between groups that practice alternative methods of healing and those who practice allopathic medicine. The beliefs promoted by alternative practitioners are not completely foreign to nursing. In her *Notes on Nursing*, Florence Nightingale wrote that the job of nursing "is to put the patient in the best condition for nature to act upon . . ."[32] Thus the nurse may feel comfortable in the role of advocate, both for the beliefs of the parents and child and for the practice of allopathic medicine.

Parents may choose alternative methods of therapy for several reasons: (1) there is an opportunity for parents to take an active role in the healing of their child; (2) there is a perceived lack of harmful side effects, because alternative methods are viewed as "natural"; and (3) these methods of therapy may offer cures for conditions that allopathic medicine does not treat (e.g., the common cold).[48]

Parents who are using alternative therapies and who perceive disapproval on the part of nurses and physicians may hide the practice or abandon allopathic medicine altogether for their children. Nurses can help parents and physicians coordinate the care of a child using the positive attributes of both disciplines. At times, education of the parents is necessary to help prevent harm from alternative methods, as may happen if large doses of vitamins or iron are given to a child.

It is ethically sound to allow families the right to practice their beliefs as long as the beliefs do

TABLE 2-3	Alternative Health Care Practices	
ALTERNATIVE HEALTH CARE PRACTICE	**THEORY**	**NURSING INTERVENTIONS**
Acupuncture	Based on Oriental system of energy "meridians" throughout the body. Treatment uses small needles inserted into the skin to stimulate flow of "chi" (energy).	There are physician and nonphysician acupuncturists. All are licensed. Acupuncturists vary in their approach. Some have a "first aid" approach, whereas others follow patients in health and illness. Discuss with the family what they are looking for in a practioner.
Bodywork Chiropractic	Health problems are the result of vertebrae being subtly out of alignment. Treatment focuses on realigning vertebrae through spinal manipulation.	Advise parents to check the background of their practitioner. All chiropractors must be state licensed.
Feldenkrais	Bodies become locked into patterns of movement that preserve muscle tension. Sessions of gentle massage allow the body to move freely.	Feldenkrais practitioners are certified by their national organization after lengthy training courses.
Reflexology	Points throughout the body are affected by massaging specific points on the hands and feet.	As long as the child's condition does not preclude use of touch, reflexology can be relaxing to both the child and the parent, who may feel relieved at being able to help.
Therapeutic touch	Healing modality initiated by Delores Krieger, PhD, RN, and Dora Kunz whereby practitioner utilizes system of centering and assessment to transfer energy to the recipient. It is effective in reduction of pain and anxiety and promotion of healing.	It is important that the practitioner has had adequate training in the use of T.T. and has had experience working with children.
Herbalism	Herbs in various form (capsules, teas, poultices, etc.) can be effective treatments for a variety of ailments. Herbs are generally thought of as "safe" and without the dangerous side effects that can be seen with allopathic treatments, although side effects and toxic doses are possible.	Ask about intake of herbs during the diet history. Find out if herbs are bought from a reputable store, or are hand picked. If hand picked, pollution of source is possible, as is the possibility that the wrong herb may be chosen. Note that herbs bought in a health food store as capsules and extracts need to be verified as "standardized," (which means they are free of pesticides and have a guaranteed dosage). Pediatric dosages should be specified on each container. Dosage cannot be guaranteed by using teas and poultices. Recommend that family receives guidance from a health care practitioner who uses herbs for treating children.

From Zagorsky ES: Caring for families who follow alternative health care practices, *Pediatr Nurs* 19(1):71-75, 1993.

Continued.

TABLE 2-3	Alternative Health Care Practices—cont'd	
ALTERNATIVE HEALTH CARE PRACTICE	**THEORY**	**NURSING INTERVENTIONS**
Homeopathy	"Like cures like." Scientific method wherein a practitioner prescribes extremely dilute amounts of an extract of animal, vegetable, or mineral to heal the patient's underlying condition. The extremely dilute amounts (the more dilute the remedy, the more potent it is) and natural substances trigger the immune system to respond.	Homeopathy has been used in Europe for over 100 years, and there is a growing body of health care practitioners who incorporate homeopathy into their practice. Remember that the more dilute the dose, the more potent it is. Make sure that the family is receiving guidance in using homeopathy, as some doses/remedies may exacerbate problem. Proper role of self-medicating at home is for mild/moderate conditions. Chronic, emergent, or severe health problems require the care of an experienced homeopath.
Mind/Body/ Spirit balance	Imagining the body as healing itself, or totally healed, stimulates the immune system to achieve the desired result. Also, the mind is where all illness starts, and it is there that illness can be changed to wellness. People who stay sick are unwilling or unable to look honestly at why they became sick in the first place.	Encourage imagery for patient relaxation (i.e., have patient imagine being in a relaxing environment). Discourage blaming of oneself if illness recurs, or is not relieved.
Vegetarianism/ Veganism	For religious, social, ethical, spiritual, or political reasons, it is better not to eat meat. Lacto-ovo-vegetarians eat milk and egg products. Vegans eat only plant-based food.	Dietician consult on admission if hospital does not offer food options that meet the patient's needs. If patient is not on a restricted diet, encourage family to bring food from home. Vitamin B_{12} is only available from animal sources. Deficiency is noted after several years of veganism in adults. Supplementation is necessary.
Vitamin therapy	The modern diet does not provide adequate nutrition, and therefore must be supplemented, and/or vitamins in large doses are therapeutic in the same ways that allopathic medications are.	Include supplement intake on admission diet history. Note potentially toxic doses, especially of fat-soluble vitamins (that is A, D, E, and K). Ask parents to bring in empty vitamin bottles, or bottle labels, to help ensure accurate reporting. Coordinate and provide input with dietician about potentially dangerous practices. Do not suddenly withdraw patient from any vitamin (even stopping large doses of Vitamin C can cause rebound deficiency.*

From Zagorsky ES: Caring for families who follow alternative health care practices, *Pediatr Nurs* 19(1):71-75, 1993.
*Scheider W: *Nutrition, basic concepts, and applications,* New York, 1983, McGraw Hill.

not promote harm to the child. Alternative methods of healing used in conjunction with allopathic medicine may prove the best course of treatment for a child.

SUMMARY

The future is sure to bring new and more complex ethical dilemmas to the forefront of emergency nursing practice. The costs of emergency care to both the individual and society are staggering. The American Nurses Association Code for Nurses can guide emergency nurses in ethical conduct and patient advocacy. When caring for a child in the emergency department, nurses cannot rely on emotional responses to ethical questions. Participation in hospital ethics committees, attending seminars, and reading current literature on ethics can prepare nurses for the difficult day-to-day situations that arise.

REFERENCES

1. American College of Emergency Physicians (ACEP), Professional Liability Committee, Position Statement: Providing telephone advice from the emergency department, *Ann Emerg Med* 19:600, 1990.
2. American Heart Association: *Pediatric advanced life support,* Dallas, 1994, American Heart Association.
3. *The American heritage dictionary,* second college edition, Boston, 1991, Houghton Mifflin Co.
4. American Nurses Association (ANA): *Position statement on promotion of comfort and relief of pain in dying patients,* Washington, DC, 1991, American Nurses Association.
5. Bandman EL, Bandman B: *Nursing ethics through the life span,* Norwalk, Conn, 1990, Appleton & Lange.
6. Bernardo L: Ethical and legal considerations in emergency care of children. In Haley K, ed: *Emergency nursing pediatric course, provider manual,* Chicago, 1993, Kap Graphics.
7. Bitterman R: A critical analysis of the federal COBRA hospital "antidumping law": ramifications for hospitals, physicians, and the effects on access to healthcare, *University of Detroit Mercy Law Review* 70(1):126–155, 1992.
8. *Black's law dictionary,* ed 5, St Paul, 1979, West Publishing Company.
9. Bowerman C: Malpractice and civil case law. In Henry G, ed: *Emergency medicine risk management: a comprehensive review,* Philadelphia, 1991, JB Lippincott.
10. Cales RH: Medical direction and quality assurance. In Grossman M, Dieckmann RA, eds: *Pediatric emergency medicine: a clinician's reference,* Philadelphia, 1991, JB Lippincott.
11. Consolidated Omnibus Budget Reconciliation Act (COBRA), Ammended Dec 19, 1989, Publ No 101-239, 6211, HR 3299, 140–44, 1985 (effective July 1990).
12. Coulter KP: Sexual abuse. In Grossman M, Dieckmann RA, eds: *Pediatric emergency medicine: a clinician's reference,* Philadelphia, 1991, JB Lippincott.
13. DeHass-Harper P: Risk management. In Frank IC, ed: *Managing emergency nursing services,* Rockville, Md, 1989, Aspen.
14. Eliastam M: When to stop cardiopulmonary resuscitation, *Top Emerg Med* 1:109, 1979.
15. Eliastam M et al: Cardiac arrest in the emergency medical services systems, guidelines for resuscitation, *J Am Coll Emerg Phys* 6:525–529, 1977.
16. Emergency Nurses Association: *Emergency nursing pediatric course (ENPC),* ed 1, Chicago, 1993, ENA.
17. Fontanarosa PB: Informed consent in emergency medicine: principles, practice and pitfalls, *Top Emerg Med* 14:2, 1992.
18. Fost N: Death and dying. In Fuhrman BP, Zimmerman JJ, eds: *Pediatric critical care,* St Louis, 1992, Mosby.
19. Frew S: *Patient transfers, how to comply with the law,* Dallas, 1991, American College of Emergency Physicians.
20. Gardner PC: Patient dumping: recovering under federal law, *Trial* May, 42–47, 1991.
21. Goldman P: Discharge to private physician's office. In Henry G, ed: *Emergency medicine risk management: a comprehensive review,* Dallas, 1991, American College of Emergency Physicians.
22. Goldman P: Telephone orders from private physicians. In Henry G, ed: *Emergency medicine risk management: a comprehensive review,* Dallas, 1991, American College of Emergency Physicians.
23. Gough AR: Medicolegal issues. In Grossman M, Dieckmann RA, eds: *Pediatric emergency medicine: a clinician's reference,* Philadelphia, 1991, JB Lippincott.
24. Hamilton JD, Lydon DR: Significant legal developments affecting the practice of emergency medicine in the last year, *Emerg Legal Brief* 4(4):25–31, 1993.
25. Holder AR: *Legal issues in pediatrics and adolescent medicine,* ed 2, New Haven, 1985, Yale University Press.
26. *Jehovah's Witnesses and the question of blood,* New York, 1977, Watchtower Bible and Tract Society of Pennsylvania.
27. Jonsen AR: Blood transfusion and the Jehovah's Witnesses, *Crit Care Clin* 2:91–100, 1986.
28. Kolodzik PW: Religious beliefs and emergency medical care. In Henry G, ed: *Emergency medi-*

cine risk management: a comprehensive review, Dallas, 1991, American College of Emergency Physicians.

29. Reference deleted in proofs.

30. Macklin R: Who speaks for the child? The problems of proxy consent. In Gain W, Macklin R, eds: *Return to the best interests of the child,* New York, 1982, Plenum Press.

31. McCormick R: Organ transplants: ethical principles. In Reich W, ed: *Encyclopedia of bioethics,* New York, 1978, The Free Press.

32. Nightingale R: *Notes on nursing,* London, 1859, Harrison and Sons.

33. Northrup CE: Nursing actions in litigation, *Qual Rev Bull* 13(10):343–347, 1987.

34. Nusbaum P: Compulsory medical treatment and a patient's free exercise of religion, *Medico-Legal Bull* 24:1–10, 1975.

35. O'Marcaigh AS et al: Cessation of unsuccessful pediatric resuscitation: how long is too long? *Mayo Clin Proc* 68:332–336, 1993.

36. President's Commission for the Study of Ethical Problems in Medicine and Biomedical and Behavioral Research: *Making health care decisions: a report on the ethical and legal implications of informed consent in the patient-practitioner relationship,* Washington, DC, 1982, US Government Printing Office.

37. *Prince v Massachusetts,* 321 US 158, 166–167, 1944.

38. Quintero C: Blood administration in pediatric Jehovah's Witnesses, *Pediatr Nurs* 19(1):46–48, 1993.

39. Rice MM: Legal issues in emergency medicine. In Rosen P, Barkin RM, eds: *Emergency medicine: concepts and clinical practice,* St Louis, 1992, Mosby.

40. Rosen P, Honigman B: Life and death. In Rosen P, Barkin RM, eds: *Emergency medicine: concepts and clinical practice,* St Louis, 1992, Mosby.

41. Roseoff AJ: Consents. In *Hospital law manual: attorney's volume II,* Gaithersberg, Md, 1983, Aspen.

42. Rushton CH et al: End of life care for infants with AIDS: ethical and legal issues, *Pediatr Nurs* 19(1): 79–83, 1993.

43. Sheridan D: Family violence. In Kitt S, Kaiser J, eds: *Emergency nursing: a physiologic and clinical perspective,* Philadelphia, 1990, WB Saunders.

44. Siegel DM: Patient consent. In Henry G, ed: *Emergency medicine risk management: a comprehensive review,* Philadelphia, 1991, JB Lippincott.

45. Thurkauf GC: Understanding the beliefs of Jehovah's Witnesses, *Focus Crit Care* 16(3):199–204, 1989.

46. Walleck CA: Ethical concerns in trauma care. In Cardona V et al, eds: *Trauma nursing: from resuscitation through rehabilitation,* Philadelphia, 1988, WB Saunders.

47. Winer R: Emergency consent, *J Kansas Med Soc* 10:458–462, 1981.

48. Zagorsky ES: Caring for families who follow alternative health care practices, *Pediatr Nurs* 19(1):71–75, 1993.

49. Zeller CL: Occurrence (incident) reports. In Henry G, ed: *Emergency medicine risk management: a comprehensive review,* Philadelphia, 1991, JB Lippincott.

CHAPTER 3

Unique Characteristics of Children

Janice S. Rogers

INTRODUCTION

Emergency department visits are stressful experiences for sick or injured children and their families. Normal childhood fears can be magnified by the unfamiliar sights, sounds, smells, and personnel in the emergency department (ED). The suddenness of the illness or injury, the seriousness of the child's condition, and the need for diagnostic and therapeutic interventions also produce varying degrees of stress. Much can be done to promote effective coping and diminish the physiologic and psychologic effects of stress on both the child and family. To facilitate positive outcomes, health care providers need to understand the unique characteristics of children.

Children are not small adults. Physiologic, cognitive, and psychosocial differences affect a child's perceptions, reactions to illness or injury, communication patterns, and coping abilities. To determine a child's health status and individual needs, knowledge of normal growth and development, careful observation of behavioral and physiologic cues, and listening to the primary caregiver are important.

Developmental variations are not the only factors influencing a child's reaction to an ED visit. Past experiences, the nature of the current illness/injury, cultural background, personality style, and available support systems can alter the child's perceptions and response to illness and hospitalization. For example, a stoic child with appendicitis may exhibit less behavioral evidence of pain than an expressive child with a mild gastroenteritis. To accurately assess the child's pain level, the typical developmental response and individual factors, such as culture and personality, must be considered.

Although the primary focus of emergency care is the physiologic stabilization of acutely ill or injured children, psychologic well-being is also important. Emergency staff can easily incorporate psychosocial interventions into their plan of care to minimize the emotional impact of an ED visit. For example, keeping parents with the child during procedures, as well as including them in the care of their child, alleviates stress and facilitates the assessment.

The ED experience can be growth producing for children.[39] Potentially positive outcomes include learning new coping mechanisms; increasing knowledge of body functioning, illness/injury, and prevention strategies; fostering parent-child relationships; and becoming better health care consumers. One 7-year-old child stated that she was glad that she had stitches, because now she knew that if she had to have stitches again, they "weren't so bad." This child increased her self-esteem by recognizing that she could cope with a stressful situation.

PEDIATRIC GROWTH AND DEVELOPMENT

Knowledge of growth and development facilitates interpretation of the pediatric physical assessment, understanding of children's perceptions and reactions, and effective communication. Developmental milestones provide standards of reference that assist the health care provider in differentiating between normal and abnormal signs, symptoms, and behaviors.

Although development proceeds in an orderly, linear sequence, individual variation occurs. Heredity is a major determinant of physical, intellectual, and emotional development. Other factors, such as injury, illness, nutrition, socioeconomic level, social stimulation, and parenting behaviors, can also have a significant effect on children's development. Delays may occur in physical, cognitive, and/or psychosocial aspects of development. Knowing the child's baseline helps the ED nurse determine the impact of the present illness or injury on the child's health status.

Developmental theories provide explanations of behavior and offer useful guidelines for pediatric care. Many child-development theories have been described but only Erikson's, Piaget's, and Freud's theories will be reviewed in this chapter. Specific applications of each theory are included in each age-related section.

Erik Erikson's psychosocial developmental theory defines personality traits that emerge at eight critical stages of human life, five of which occur in childhood.[7,21] Positive resolution of each stage or "crisis" allows successful management of later problems with that particular conflict, such as trust or autonomy. Failure to resolve a stage results in the development of the negative trait of the stage (e.g., mistrust or shame and doubt). Erikson's theory incorporates the effects of psychologic, social, and biologic influences on development and has been used extensively as the basis for pediatric assessments and interventions.

Piaget's theory of cognitive development describes intellectual development, that is, how children think and learn.[24,25] According to Piaget, cognitive development proceeds as a fixed sequence of orderly changes in the child's ability to process information. Development of logical thought occurs in four major phases as increasingly complex methods of structuring thought and new ways of problem solving emerge. Piaget's theory provides a framework for understanding children's perceptions, communicating with them, and preparing them for procedures.

Freud's psychosexual developmental theory describes the interrelationships between the child's ego (sense of self), the id (primitive urges), and the superego (conscience), emphasizing the power of the unconscious in motivating behavior.[9,10] Psychologic development occurs in stages that are linked with sexual urges, such as the oral, anal, and phallic drives. Difficulties in any stage may result in fixation of the personality at that level. Freud's theory emphasizes the importance of childhood experience and the role of the environment in developing adult personality.

▌ Developmental Stages

Infant Development (0-1 Year)

Although newborn infants are vulnerable and dependent, they possess simple protective reflexes, rudimen-

tary communication abilities, and the capacity to learn. From birth, infants engage in social interactions, establish eye contact, discriminate among various sounds and smells, and convey their feelings in a rudimentary way (Table 3-1).[34]

Exceptionally rapid growth and development occurs during infancy. In 1 year, most infants learn to walk, say a few meaningful words, feed themselves, convey particular needs and desires, and exert some control over their environment. Physical care alone is not sufficient for optimal growth and development. A secure and loving relationship with a primary caregiver is also essential, as evidenced by research on attachment, maternal deprivation, and failure to thrive.[1,2,3,6a,13,29]

Psychosocial development. According to Erikson, the first developmental crisis to be resolved is trust vs. mistrust. A positive relationship with a primary caregiver promotes the development of a sense of well-being and basic trust in an infant. When physical needs are consistently met, infants learn to trust both themselves and their environment. With a well-developed sense of trust, infants can better tolerate unfamiliar or unknown situations.

Behavioral indicators of positive parental attachment include close physical contact, good eye contact, and responsiveness to the infant's needs. The astute emergency nurse can identify ineffective parent-child interactions and make appropriate referrals. Identification of dysfunctional relationships is particularly important in suspected abuse or neglect situations.

Besides obvious physical characteristics, infants display differences in sleep/wake patterns, sociability, temperament, and self-consoling behaviors. Some infants are good-natured; others are difficult to console. Some infants are interactive socially; others are placid. These variations can have potent positive or negative effects on parent/child relationships and the infant's growth and development.

Intellectual/language development. During Piaget's sensorimotor period, infants learn by using their senses and observing the effect of their actions on objects or persons. Active exploration by touching, kicking, chewing, and biting reveals the characteristics of objects. Repetition commits the information to memory. Through this learning process, infants begin to differentiate themselves from others and their environments. This marks the beginning of the child's process of separation from parents, which culminates in adolescence.

TABLE 3-1	Infant Development (1 Month to 1 Year)	
PHYSICAL AND MOTOR DEVELOPMENT	**PSYCHOSOCIAL DEVELOPMENT**	**INTELLECTUAL/LANGUAGE DEVELOPMENT**
The first year *Period of most rapid growth* *Infant weight gain 1 oz/day* *Weight doubles by 6 months;* *triples by 1 year*	*Oral stage (Freud)* *Trust vs. mistrust (Erikson)* *Common fears (after 6 months)* *Separation* *Strangers*	*Sensorimotor period (Piaget)*
1-2 months Lifts head momentarily from prone position Moro reflex brisk Responds to sounds	Totally dependent on adults to meet needs Social smile Maximal sucking needs Derives satisfaction and pleasure from tactile stimulation, rocking, cuddling Quiets when picked up	Recognizes familiar face Makes cooing sounds Follows moving objects/persons with eyes Uses crying, body language, tone of voice to convey wants/needs
3-4 months Rolls over Carries object to mouth Grasps objects with both hands In prone position, supports upper body with arms Begins to drool Moro reflex diminishing	Laughs Still has great sucking needs Demands attention by fussing; enjoys attention Interest in mother heightens Ceases crying when mother enters room	Actively interested in environment Recognizes familiar faces and objects: no object permanence Shows awareness of strange situations Babbling, cooing
5-6 months Sits with support Picks up small objects easily Grasps, holds, manipulates objects Reaches persistently	Beginning sense of self Beginning ability to postpone gratification Other family members become important Enjoys play with people and objects	Able to discriminate strangers from family Beginning object permanence: will briefly search for lost object Great interest in babbling
7-8 months Transfers objects from one hand to another Sits without support Creeps/crawls Gums or mouths solid food Rudimentary self-feeding Teething	Strong attachment to mother; shows signs of distress when mother leaves or in presence of strangers Orally aggressive in biting and mouthing	Repeats activities that are enjoyed Drops and picks up objects in exploration Searches for "lost" objects Lively curiosity about world

Data from Mott, 1990; Pontious, 1982 Waechter and Blake, 1985.

Continued.

TABLE 3-1	Infant Development (1 Month to 1 Year) — cont'd	
PHYSICAL AND MOTOR DEVELOPMENT	**PSYCHOSOCIAL DEVELOPMENT**	**INTELLECTUAL/LANGUAGE DEVELOPMENT**
9-10 months Pulls to standing Drinks from cup Pincer grasp	Separation anxiety—reacts violently to actual or threatened loss of parent Beginning fears of going to bed and being alone; nighttime rituals important Powerful urge toward independence in locomotion, feeding Experiences joy when achieving a goal or mastering a fear	Explores objects by sucking, chewing, biting Imitates others' actions/speech Looks at pictures in book Responds to simple verbal requests Plays peek-a-boo, patty-cake Responds to own name Inhibits behavior in response to "no-no" First words
11-12 months "Cruises" around furniture Walks with or without assistance Uses spoon in feeding Babinski disappears	Reacts to restrictions with frustration, but has ability to master new situations *with help* Able to show emotions of fear, anger, affection, jealousy, anxiety	Heightened curiosity and drive to explore environment Works to get toy that is out of reach Communicates by pointing to objects desired Experiments to achieve goals Jabbers; few simple words

Thought and reasoning processes emerge as infants develop the concept of object permanence. By approximately 7 to 8 months of age, infants learn that objects or persons continue to exist even when they cannot be seen, and they actively seek out objects that have disappeared. Games such as peek-a-boo are not only great fun for infants of this age but also help reinforce the concept of object permanence.

The infant's primary mode of communication is nonverbal. Sounds, babbling, and words are primarily imitation. Wants or needs are conveyed by crying, body language, and tone of voice. Mothers become very adept at interpreting their own infant's communication. For example, a mother can usually identify whether her infant's cry indicates pain, boredom, hunger, or illness.

Common fears. Intellectual development and attachment to the primary caregivers give rise to the major fears of infancy. As infants become more aware of themselves as individuals, differentiate between familiar and unfamiliar persons, and recognize the permanence of objects, separation and stranger anxiety peak. Older infants will cry inconsolably when their primary caregiver leaves the room as they grieve for the loss of their main source of security.[3] The infant's poorly developed concept of time contributes to the protest, because the infant does not understand when or if the parent will return. Strangers are identified as "not-self" and are threatening to the child.[32] When approached by unfamiliar persons, many infants cling to their parents, protest vehemently, and resist contact with the stranger.

Approach to infants (Table 3-2). Developing a trusting relationship is difficult in the emergency department, largely because of its short-term and intensive nature. However, it is vital to foster a trusting relationship with both the infant and parent or caregiver. Parental anxiety can have a negative effect on the infant's emotional and physical well-being. Therefore, measures to meet the parents' needs and allay their anxiety promote positive outcomes for the infant. For example, a croupy infant's stridor can often be

TABLE 3-2	**Approach to Infants**	
GOALS	**APPROACH**	
Develop a trusting relationship.	Approach the infant slowly and calmly. Use a quiet, soothing voice. Provide for parents' needs and allay anxieties; decreasing parental fear will make the infant feel more secure. *Never* perform a painful procedure on a sleeping child; give some warning.	
Decrease separation and stranger anxiety.	Keep the primary caregiver with the infant as much as possible. Provide comfort measures (e.g., warmth, pacifiers). Avoid inserting IVs in locations which will impede the infant's ability to suck favorite thumb/fingers. Allow the infant to hold security object.	
Facilitate assessment of the infant and safe, efficient procedures.	Examine older infant on caregiver's lap. Distract the infant to gain cooperation with physical assessment. Observe the infant first. Do most distressing components last (i.e., intrusive procedures such as taking a rectal temperature). Let older infant handle simple equipment such as the stethoscope.	

significantly diminished by the comforting measures provided by a parent who has been supported and reassured by the nurse.

No one can replace the importance of the primary caregiver in providing a sense of security and well-being for infants, especially in times of stress. Therefore it is best for infants to have parents/caregivers with them throughout the ED visit, especially during procedures, even if the infant appears more distressed when the parents are present. Security objects can provide comfort for infants when the parents are not at the bedside.

The separation and stranger anxiety experienced by older infants frequently interferes with the health care provider's ability to assess the infant. Decreasing, or at least circumventing, infants' fears improves the quality of the physical exam, facilitates cooperation, and diminishes psychologic stress.

TODDLER DEVELOPMENT (1–2 YEARS)

Toddlers are both exciting and challenging. Their growing mobility and independence expand the environment they can explore—and the trouble they can unwittingly get into (Table 3-3). Many negative attributes have been associated with toddlers. However, these are merely immature expressions of their growing autonomy. Hospitalized toddlers are the age group at greatest risk for permanent emotional sequelae.[27] Although the impact of a short emergency department visit has not been studied, toddlers are probably most vulnerable to the risk of emotional sequelae from an ED visit because of their developmental characteristics and immaturity in dealing with stress.

Psychosocial development. The developmental crisis of toddlers is autonomy vs. shame and doubt. Toddlers want the autonomy of making their own decisions and of controlling their own bodies. If this developmental crisis is not positively resolved, the child experiences a personal sense of shame and doubts his or her ability to succeed.[7]

The negativism seen in toddlers is exemplified by the frequent use of the word *no,* even when they mean *yes.* Although it is a normal expression of budding autonomy, negativism is often interpreted by parents as willful defiance and can be extremely frustrating. Much patience and effort is needed to allow the child some independence, while gaining compliance with the limits necessary for safety and acceptable behavior. Toddlers continuously test these limits, resulting in injuries or temper tantrums when they have exceeded their typically low frustration threshold.

With increased mobility and muscle maturity, toddlers discover increasing control over many body functions. Toilet training is a major task that begins during these years. Erikson's stage of autonomy corresponds with Freud's anal/retentive stage, wherein the toddler is challenged by the developing abilities to

TABLE 3-3	Toddler Development (1 to 2 Years)	
PHYSICAL AND MOTOR DEVELOPMENT	**PSYCHOSOCIAL DEVELOPMENT**	**INTELLECTUAL/LANGUAGE DEVELOPMENT**
Growth Rate significantly slows down, accompanied by a decrease in appetite	**Anal stage (Freud)** **Autonomy vs. shame and doubt (Erikson)** **Common fears** Separation Loss of control Altered rituals Pain Physical restraint	**Sensorimotor period (Piaget)** Cognition and language not yet sophisticated enough for toddler to learn through thought processes and verbal communication
General appearance Potbellied Exaggerated lumbar curve Wide-based gait Increased mobility is a hallmark of physical development in the toddler		
18 months Walks without support and with balance Runs, climbs Walks upstairs; creeps down Better fine motor control; scribbles spontaneously	Imitates parents' behavior Beginning to test limits Increasing autonomy; still highly dependent on parents, especially in times of stress Begins to exert some control over body functions and activities Indicates wet pants; most not ready for potty-training Play is a learning mechanism; plays "pretend games"; "into everything"	Uses some words to indicate wants; mainly gestures Follows simple directions Egocentrism in thought and behavior Short attention span Beginning sense of time Magical thinking
2 years Protruding abdomen decreasing 16-20 teeth Steady gait Walks up and down stairs Jumps in place	Temper tantrums Negativism Resistant to bedtime; dawdles Transitional objects decrease anxiety Rituals and routines provide consistency and security Extremely resistant to restrictions on freedom May be ready for potty-training Extreme reaction to separation Very possessive with toys	2-3 word sentences Increasing vocabulary Beginning to learn time sequences Searches for new ways to solve problems Increasing attention span Symbolic thought Magical thinking Relates cause and effect No concept of danger

Data from Pontious, 1982; Waechter and Blake, 1985; Wieczorek and Natapoff, 1981.

"hold on" and to "let go." Getting urine specimens from toddlers can be a challenge for even the most experienced pediatric nurse if the potty-trained toddler refuses to urinate in a cup and protests the use of a urine-collection bag.

Toddlers need to experience the joy and stimulation of exploring their environment while still maintaining the support of their "anchor" or primary caregiver. Stress intensifies the toddler's usual dependency on caregivers for physical care and emotional security. Toddlers will often cling to their parents and vigorously protest examination and procedures.

Play is an integral part of children's lives. It provides a nonthreatening means of learning and an outlet for feelings. The toddler's cooperation during an examination can be enhanced through the use of play. Playing peek-a-boo with younger toddlers or giving them a small toy to play with during a physical exam engages their interest, distracts them from other activities, and helps build a rapport with the health care provider.

Intellectual/language development. Toddlers complete Piaget's sensorimotor period and advance to the preoperational stage at approximately 2 years of age. Cognition and language are rapidly developing, but their intellectual development is still not sophisticated. Learning primarily occurs through the physical senses, such as vision and touch. Verbal descriptions are meaningless. While memory is beginning to develop, toddlers do not yet have the capacity to generalize their knowledge to different situations. Repetitive teaching, for example, about hospital equipment or house rules, is necessary, because they cannot easily remember or generalize from past experiences. Because of this, toddlers can be told "no" over and over yet still continue to do the forbidden activity.

Magical thinking, egocentricity, and some understanding of causality and time begin to develop in older toddlers. However, misconceptions are common. If the cause of an event is not readily apparent, the toddler will usually invent an illogical reason. For example, many toddlers feel that illnesses or injuries are caused by their bad thoughts or actions. They are not yet able to understand true cause and effect.

Toddlers like consistency. They have difficulty adjusting to disruptions in their schedules. Regression and sleep disturbances may occur after an emergency department visit, especially those involving intrusive procedures or a prolonged stay. It is helpful to inform parents of possible behavioral sequelae and assure them that these are temporary reactions.

The toddler's ability to communicate is continuously improving. Vocabulary expands rapidly, and simple sentences are formed. Wants or needs are now more easily understood by health care providers, but often parents are needed to "interpret" their child's communications.

Common fears. Separation from primary caregivers continues to be a major concern for toddlers. Parental contact is crucial for a toddler's well-being, especially in times of stress. Absence of parents in the ED, even for short periods of time, may be interpreted by the toddler as punishment or complete desertion.

Loss of control from altered rituals, physical restraints, and pain threatens a toddler's sense of security. Intrusive procedures are particularly frightening to toddlers, because the child has a poorly defined concept of body boundaries and does not comprehend normal body functions. Fearful toddlers typically react with physical resistance, aggression, negativism, and regression.

Approach to toddlers (Table 3-4). Toddlers' immature psychosocial and cognitive abilities enhance their vulnerability to the stresses of an ED visit. Overcoming toddlers' fears and anxieties often seems like an insurmountable task. However, there are many approaches and interventions that can diminish the ED impact on the toddler and promote more positive outcomes.

As the toddler's attention span increases with age, simple directions, such as "open your mouth wide like a lion," can be followed. Capitalizing on the child's magical thinking can make health care fun for the child. Cooperation and rapport is improved when the examiner "feels" a peanut butter sandwich during an abdominal exam or "hears" birds singing in the child's chest.

PRESCHOOL DEVELOPMENT (3–5 YEARS)

Psychosocial development. Preschoolers are more secure in their sense of self. With greater autonomy and independence, the preschooler reaches out into the environment and initiates individual activities rather than just imitating others (Table 3-5). This stage is Erikson's initiative vs. guilt. Preschoolers are increasingly able to separate from their parents for short periods of time. However, in stressful situations they react similarly to toddlers, with an intense need for their parents.

Preschoolers want to please. They are much more

TABLE 3-4	Approach to Toddlers	
GOALS	**APPROACH**	
Develop a trusting relationship.	Use a playful approach.	
	Use behavioral cues to guide the approach; if possible, let child get used to you before doing the physical exam.	
	Talk with parent before touching the child; this decreases parental anxiety and gives the toddler time to adjust to your presence.	
	Be honest with the toddler and caregiver.	
Minimize fear and anxiety.	Keep the primary caregiver and security object, if available, with the toddler as much as possible.	
	Examine the toddler on the parent's lap or in the parent's arms.	
	Make the ED environment less threatening with bright posters, toys, or videotapes.	
	Let the child handle equipment; use equipment, such as stethoscope, first on dolls or stuffed animals.	
	Set limits; children have not yet mastered control of their impulses and need protection from harm.	
	Use restraints judiciously.	
Allow the toddler to maintain autonomy.	Offer limited choices, only when a choice truly exists.	
	Acknowledge positive behavior with rewards, praise, or stickers.	
Facilitate assessment and safely perform procedures.	Observe the child first. Save the most distressing procedures for last.	
	Restrain the child firmly and talk to the child during procedures.	
	Prepare the toddler immediately before the procedure; perform the procedure as quickly as possible, then provide comfort.	
	Provide explanations in simple, concrete terms.	

cooperative than toddlers during physical exams and procedures. When they don't live up to their own or others' expectations, however, they feel embarrassed and guilty.

Many questions about male/female differences and sex roles arise during the preschool years. Freud describes this age as the phallic stage, during which the child begins developing sex-role identification. Preschoolers' awareness of the various societal roles are exhibited in their play.

Play is also a mechanism for children to learn to share and get along with others. As the superego or conscience develops, preschoolers exhibit their growing knowledge of right and wrong and expect rigid adherence to "the rules." Dolls or other children will often be admonished for doing something naughty.

Intellectual/language development. During Piaget's preoperational period, children learn by trial and error. Logical or abstract thought is not yet possible. Because of these cognitive limitations, preschoolers cannot be adequately prepared for proce-

dures or other events merely by verbal descriptions. Explanations should be concrete and described in terms of their senses, such as what they will feel, smell, see, or hear.

The egocentric preschooler lives in a world of magic, unable to discriminate between fantasy and reality. Imaginary friends, dramatic play, and fascination with monsters and super-heroes are prevalent. These fantasies can be harmful when they result in exaggerated, bizarre, and frightening explanations for injuries, illnesses, or treatments. Young children may view illness in themselves or others as retribution for "bad" behavior or thoughts. They may invent a story or refuse to give the details of a situation in which an injury occurred during a forbidden activity. Misconceptions must be identified and clarified.

Most 4- to 5-year-old children speak clearly in compound sentences and use an extensive vocabulary. Because preschoolers feel that nothing happens by chance and want to know the purpose and cause of everything, they incessantly ask "why" questions. The inquisitive preschooler is best answered with simple

TABLE 3-5	Preschool Development (3 to 5 Years)	
PHYSICAL AND MOTOR DEVELOPMENT	**PSYCHOSOCIAL DEVELOPMENT**	**INTELLECTUAL/LANGUAGE DEVELOPMENT**
Growth Weight gain approximately 2 kg/yr Height gain approximately 6-8 cm/yr **General appearance** "Baby fat" and protuberant abdomen disappears	**Phallic stage (Freud)** **Initiative vs. Guilt (Erikson)** Greater autonomy and independence Still intense need for parents when under stress Initiates activities rather than just imitating Age of discovery, curiosity, developing social behavior Sense of self as individual **Fears (common at this age)** Bodily injury, mutilation, castration Loss of control Death Dark Ghosts and monsters The unknown	**Preoperational (Piaget)** Trial-and-error learning Egocentric—believes own perspective is the only viewpoint Understand explanations only in terms of real events or what their senses tell them No logical or abstract thought; coincidence confused with causation Magical thinking Difficulty distinguishing between reality and fantasy Imaginary friends; fascination with super-heroes, monsters
3 years Walks down stairs, alternating feet Balances, hops on one foot Fine motor control increasing; enjoys painting, coloring Eruption of deciduous teeth complete Picky eaters; over time, usually eats a well-balanced diet	Dramatic play; imaginative Begins to share Beginning awareness of social roles, including sex roles Wants to conform to parents' expectations Decrease in ritualistic behavior Bladder control fairly reliable; occasional accidents	Increased attention span Can give first and last name "Why" questions Centers attention on one aspect of a situation Can carry out complex commands Many misconceptions and fears about illness/injuries
4 years Increased coordination and articulation of small muscle movements, as in writing Balances well on toes More coordinated body movements Enjoys stunts	Dresses, undresses self, ties shoes Masters own toileting Prefers to play with 2-3 other children Enjoys playing simple board games, ball Strict ideas of "right and wrong"	Most infantile speech patterns gone Often interprets expressions and slang literally Boasts, exaggerates, threatens Can carry out complex commands Knows age, one or more colors; counts to 4 Converses with imaginary friends

Data from Waechter and Blake, 1985; Wieczorek and Natapoff, 1981.

Continued.

TABLE 3-5	Preschool Development (3 to 5 Years)—cont'd	
PHYSICAL AND MOTOR DEVELOPMENT	**PSYCHOSOCIAL DEVELOPMENT**	**INTELLECTUAL/LANGUAGE DEVELOPMENT**
5 years Throws and catches ball well Jumps rope Walks backward heel to toe Skips, hops Prints name	Nighttime bladder control complete Castration complex; any injury, surgery, or procedure in area of genitalia is particularly traumatizing Initiates contact with strangers Likes to tell stories Peer relations becoming more important Assumes rigid sex roles	Thinks that thoughts and feelings will happen Asks meaning of words 90% of speech is intelligible

explanations that define objects in terms of their functions. For example, the question "why do I have skin?" could be appropriately answered with "to keep the dirt out of your body."

Cooperation with physical exams and procedures is facilitated by the preschooler's increased attention span and ability to carry out complex commands. However, sometimes misperceptions of the health care provider's explanations increase a preschooler's fear and resistance. Table 3-6 gives some examples of children's literal or concrete perceptions of common hospital terminology. Clear and nonthreatening terms are suggested.

Common fears. With their limited cognitive abilities and abundant fears, such as the dark, ghosts, and the unknown, preschoolers have difficulty with many common events such as bedtime and health care experiences. Fear of mutilation, along with incomplete understanding of how body parts work, leads to many misconceptions concerning illness and injuries. For example, many preschoolers fear if they are cut, their "insides" will leak out. Loss of control and fear of death are normal fears that take on more real connotations during an emergency experience.

Around age 5, the castration complex appears.[10] Boys fear castration as punishment for misdeeds or bad thoughts. Procedures or health problems involving the genital area, such as urinary catheterization or testicular torsion, are frequently very traumatic for preschool boys. Vigorous resistance is common. Care-

ful explanations of exactly what will and will *not* happen diminish a preschooler's fear and improve cooperation.

Approach to preschool children (Table 3-7). Actively including preschoolers in their health care and carefully explaining all procedures contribute to feelings of control and self-esteem. Choices, however small, should be given whenever possible. Only choices that truly exist should be given. For example, a child may decide whether to drink the medicine from a cup or use a syringe to squirt it into the mouth, but refusing the medicine is not an option.

SCHOOL-AGE DEVELOPMENT (6–10 YEARS)

Psychosocial development. School-age children engage in physical activities, team sports, hobbies, reading, projects, and a variety of other pastimes. This is Erikson's stage of industry vs. inferiority, the age of accomplishment, increasing competence, and mastery of new skills (Table 3-8). Through successful accomplishments, children develop self-esteem and self-control.

The peer group is increasingly important to school-age children. Any actual or perceived separation from friends is threatening. Children worry that chronic illness or disfiguring injuries may set them apart from their friends. Although they still need parental support, especially in times of stress, they may be unwilling to ask for this support. Sometimes, caught in this

TABLE 3-6	Considerations in Choosing Language

Words that have different meanings can be confusing. If it is likely that the child will hear the standard medical expressions used, these words should be explained or defined. Ideally the child should be asked if he or she knows what nurses and doctors mean when they say these words. Compare, for example, the phrases in the left column with the suggested alternatives in the right.

POTENTIALLY AMBIGUOUS	CLEARER
Shot: When people get shot, they're really badly hurt. Are they trying to hurt me?	Medicine through a (small, tiny) needle.
CAT Scan: Will there be cats? Or something that scratches?	Describe in simple terms, and explain what the letters of the common name stand for.
ICU: I see you?	Explain, as above.
Move you to the floor: Why are they going to put me on the ground?	Unit; ward. Explain why the child is being transferred, and where.
Take a picture (X-rays, CT, and MRI machines are far larger than a familiar camera, move differently, and don't yield a familiar end product.)	A picture of the inside of you. Describe appearance, sounds, and movement of the equipment.

Words can be experienced as "hard" or "soft" according to how much they increase the perceived threat of a situation. For example, consider the following word choices:

HARD	SOFT
This part will hurt.	You may feel sore, achy, tight, snug, full. (Words such as scratch, poke, or sting might be familiar for some children and frightening to others.)
The medicine will taste (or smell) bad.	The medicine may taste different than anything you have tasted before. After you take it, will you tell me how it was for you?
As big as . . . (e.g., size of an incision).	Smaller than . . ..
As long as . . . (e.g., for duration of a procedure).	For less time that it takes you to . . ..

Note: Words or phrases that are helpful to one child may be threatening for another. Health care providers must listen carefully and be sensitive to the child's use and response to language.

POTENTIALLY UNFAMILIAR	CONCRETE EXPLANATION
Take your vitals (or your vital signs)	Measure your temperature; see how warm your body is; see how fast and strongly your heart is working.
Intravenous, IV	Medicine that works best when it goes right Into a Vein (IntraVenous). It's the quickest way to help you get better. First ask child if he or she knows what a vein is, and why some medicine is OK to take by mouth and others work best into a vein.
Anesthesia	The doctor will give you medicine. It will help you go into a very deep sleep. You will not feel anything at all. The doctors know just the right amount of medicine to give you so you will stay asleep through your *whole* operation. When the operation is over the doctor stops giving you that medicine and helps you wake up.

Modified from Gaynard L et al: *Psychosocial care of children in hospitals: a clinical practice manual from the ACCH child life research project,* Bethesda, MD, 1990, Association for the Care of Children's Health.

TABLE 3-7	Approach to Preschool Children	

GOALS	APPROACH
Develop a trusting relationship.	Introduce self by name. Direct questions to both the parent(s) and the child. Be honest.
Minimize fears and anxieties.	Identify child's understanding of events and clarify misconceptions. Prepare child for *all* procedures in simple concrete terms, emphasizing the sensory experience. Make things fun for the child; capitalize on magical beliefs (e.g., "see" elephant tracks in ears, "feel" a hot dog in their tummies).
Teach child about health care practices.	Reinforce simple explanations about body structures and function and safety and preventive strategies. Teach child what to do to cooperate with treatments.
Promote communication on the child's level.	Use simple, clear, and concrete terminology (see Table 3-6). Avoid using analogies (e.g., like a bee sting), since they may have a different meaning for the child.
Augment child's feelings of control and body integrity.	Give realistic choices. Use adhesive bandages and dressings freely; reassure child when removing bandages or stitches that the "insides" will not leak out.

dilemma, they become angry and irritable with the very people from whom they need support.

Intellectual/language development. At about 7 years of age, children enter Piaget's stage of concrete operations. This is a decisive turning point in cognitive development, the beginning of logical thought. School-age children still operate in the present, but deductive reasoning (if . . . then) is now part of their repertoire. Since abstract thinking is not yet developed, school-age children cannot reason through hypothetical situations. However, they are able to comprehend the relationship of parts to the whole and have a more sophisticated understanding of time and causality. This increases their flexibility and diminishes their need for rigid routines.

Before age 9, children are not cognitively able to understand the anatomic structures and physiologic functioning of their bodies, and misconceptions are common. Clarifying the child's understanding of an illness or injury is therefore important. Health teaching not only expands a child's knowledge but also enhances their cooperation, compliance, and coping mechanisms. School-age children are very receptive to learning.

School-age children interpret words and sayings at face value. Medical phrases, idioms, and abbreviations often represent very different meanings. Also, since

they want to act and be treated as adults, school-age children may not want to admit that they do not understand something they think they are expected to know.

Common fears. School-age children are particularly vulnerable to situations in which they feel a loss of control. "Saving face" is critical to their self-esteem. They want to live up to the perceived expectations of significant others and as a result will deny pain or illness to protect their image and not appear babyish. For example, denial of pain may be an attempt to avoid a painful shot.

Physical disability is more worrisome than pain to the school-age child. They fear limitations of their usual activities and alterations in their peer group status. An improved concept of time allows the school-ager to think in terms of what will happen tomorrow, as well as today. An awareness of possible long-term consequences of illnesses or injuries increases concerns about bodily injury or illness.

The school-age child's response to stress may range from depression, withdrawal, or passive acceptance to hostility or frustration. Magical rituals may still be used to cope with stressful or painful situations.

Approach to school-age children (Table 3-9). Since the school-age child's level of understanding is

TABLE 3-8	School-Age Development (6 to 10 Years)	
PHYSICAL AND MOTOR DEVELOPMENT	**PSYCHOSOCIAL DEVELOPMENT**	**INTELLECTUAL/LANGUAGE DEVELOPMENT**
Growth Relatively latent period	**Latency (Freud)** **Industry vs. inferiority (Erikson)** **Common fears** Separation from friends Loss of control Bodily injury; disability Death	**Preoperational to concrete operations (Piaget)**
6-7 years Larger, stronger muscles Can't sit for prolonged time Unable to precisely control small muscles Knows right from left	Increased interaction with peers Able to handle basic impulses, separation from parents; adapts to new situations Rigidly adheres to rules	Preoperational thinking until age 7 Interested in learning about body functions
7-8 years Somewhat clumsy Improving balance Tries new physical activities cautiously Eye-hand coordination not fully developed Very energetic	Peer groups firmly established; same sex Sets own elaborate rules and moral codes	**Concrete Operations** Beginning of logical thought; deductive reasoning Understands cause and effect Improved time concept; aware of possible long-term consequences Interprets phrases and idioms at face value Can appreciate others' thoughts and feelings, but tends to hide own
8-10 years Organized sports Coordination and fine motor control improves	Wants to act and be treated as grownups Decreased fantasy and aimlessness	Able to understand anatomy and body functions Able to consider internal factors, such as feelings

Data from Pontious, 1982; Waechter and Blake, 1985; Wieczorek and Natapoff, 1981.

increasingly developed, preparation for procedures should be more extensive. Educating older children about their illness, tests, and treatments not only expands their knowledge but also allays their fears and helps them cope. Friendly conversation about school, friends, hobbies, or pets puts school-age children at ease and distracts them from painful or frightening procedures. Explaining what to expect during the ED stay, as well as what is not expected to happen, is also helpful. For example, telling a child that you don't expect any shots to be necessary, but that you'll be sure to let him or her know what needs to be done before it happens, can decrease the child's fears and improve cooperation. At all times, it is important to be honest.

School-age children do not want to act like "babies," but they often regress in stressful situations and need additional family and nursing support. Reassuring children that crying or other such behavior is normal and acceptable under the

Table 3-9	Approach to School-Age Children	
Goals	**Approach**	
Develop open and trusting communication.	Be honest. Be nonjudgmental. Provide privacy.	
Support child's self-esteem.	Acknowledge positive behavior. Let the child know it's OK to cry.	
Decrease fear and anxiety.	Explain all procedures. Give the child time before the procedure to "get ready." Tell child when normal activities can be resumed.	
Teach child to be a good health care consumer.	Encourage child to ask questions. Ask child to describe symptoms. Encourage child to participate in own care.	

circumstances supports their self-esteem. Teaching children coping strategies helps them maintain control over the situation and allays their anxiety.

Adolescent Development (11-18 Years)

Despite adultlike appearance, adolescents have not yet reached maturity. With the onset of puberty, adolescents enter into a time of phenomenal developmental changes (Table 3-10). There is a prominent differentiation between younger and older adolescents in their concerns and behaviors, as well as their physical maturity.

Psychosocial development. Erikson describes the developmental crisis of adolescence as identity vs. role confusion. Adolescents must separate from parents, adapt to a rapidly changing body, develop a sense of identity, and learn to function autonomously. With this developmental upheaval, it is not surprising that adolescents exhibit labile behavior. They respond to the phenomenal developmental changes with mood swings, depression, periodic regression, and mild antisocial behavior. Family dissension frequently occurs. Often adolescents rebel against family traditions or values to assert independence and self-identity. Peer group influence initially flourishes as the parents' impact on an adolescent's actions and decisions wanes. As *older* adolescents become more secure in their identity, self-esteem, independence, and sexual relationships, then peer group influence, behavioral lability, and family disruption diminishes. The adolescent's

priorities then shift to career development and role definition.

Body image is particularly important, especially to younger adolescents. Anything that differentiates the adolescent from the peer group is regarded as a major tragedy. Visible injuries (such as facial lacerations) create more stress than nonvisible but perhaps more serious injuries. Adolescents worry about how illness/injury will affect their appearance, function, mobility, and status in their peer group. Their perception of illness and its significance may be distorted because of a heightened concern for appearance and self-preoccupation.

Coping with increasing sexual urges, pubertal changes, and budding sexual identity is developmentally stressful. The prevalence of teenage pregnancy, STDs, AIDS, and date rape illustrates the conflicts that adolescents face in today's world.

Intellectual/language development. During adolescence thought processes are maturing and becoming more complex. Many but not all teens reach Piaget's formal operations stage. Abstract thinking is the hallmark of this stage. The adolescent becomes capable of projecting to the future and understanding the potential consequences of actions and illnesses or injuries. Although understanding of illnesses, treatments, and outcomes is more sophisticated, misconceptions still exist and feelings are hidden to save face. Denial of pain can hinder adequate pain control, as well as prevent making an accurate diagnosis. To intervene appropriately, nurses should observe the adolescent for behavioral cues and encourage sharing of feelings and concerns.

TABLE 3-10	Adolescent Development (11 to 18 Years)	
PHYSICAL AND MOTOR DEVELOPMENT	**PSYCHOSOCIAL DEVELOPMENT**	**INTELLECTUAL/LANGUAGE DEVELOPMENT**
Growth Females—growth spurt begins at approximately age 9½ Males—growth spurt begins at approximately age 10½	**Genital stage (Freud)** **Identity vs. role confusion (Erikson)** Transition from childhood to adulthood Quest for independence often leads to family dissension Need to establish identity and mature sexual orientation Risk-taking behavior	**Concrete to formal operations (Piaget)** Memory fully developed Concept of time well understood Adolescent can project to the future and imagine potential consequences of actions and illness Some adolescents do not achieve formal operations
Puberty Secondary sex characteristics begin to develop between the ages of 8 and 13 for females; 10-14 for males	**Common fears** Changes in appearance; disfigurement Dependency; loss of control Separation from peer group Pain	
11-14 years *Male* Beginning growth of pubic hair Enlargement of testicles Wet dreams *Female* Continued breast development Growth of axillary and pubic hair Menstruation may begin	**Body image** Self-conscious; acutely aware of body appearance and imperfections Anything that differentiates self from peers is a major tragedy Visible injuries more stressful than nonvisible Increased somatic complaints Sexual urges, fantasies; often result in guilt and shame May sublimate sex drive through aggressive sports, hobbies, and group activities	Beginning to think abstractly; thinks about concepts outside own experiences Self-centered May view illness in terms of changes in appearance and functions
	Family relationships Negativism as manifestation of rejection of family's values and seeking own identity Test parental controls	
	Peers Important for psychologic support and social development Early adolescents: same-sex relationships Middle adolescents: heterosexual interests Mood swings, periodic regression, antisocial behavior, depression	

Data from Waechter and Blake, 1985; Wieczorek and Natapoff, 1981.

Continued.

TABLE 3-10	Adolescent Development (11 to 18 Years)—cont'd		
PHYSICAL AND MOTOR DEVELOPMENT		**PSYCHOSOCIAL DEVELOPMENT**	**INTELLECTUAL/LANGUAGE DEVELOPMENT**
15-18 years Continued development of secondary sex characteristics		**Body image** Less of a concern than in younger adolescents	Thinks abstractly Deductive thinking and formal logic used in problem solving Idealistic Future goals become more clear
Males Increased size of penis, testes, scrotum Growth of body hair Voice change		**Family relationships** Increasing independence and identity formation Critical of family's morals and traditions	
Females Enlarged breasts Broadened pelvic bones Growth of body hair Menstruation		**Peer relationships** Group social activity and/or individual dating Heterosexual relationships predominate Sexual relationships may move from physical emphasis to one of emotional commitment Increasingly secure in self-esteem, independence, and heterosexual relationships	

Adolescents frequently engage in risk-taking behaviors, believing that nothing bad will happen. Educating adolescents about the dangers of reckless behavior, such as drinking and driving, is not always effective, largely because of these feelings of invincibility. When these behaviors result in injuries, the adolescent usually recognizes responsibility and experiences guilt and grief. If these feelings are unresolved, extreme depression may result.

Common fears. Adolescents are vulnerable to feelings of loss of control and loss of independence. Pain or the fear of pain is very distressing to them. Younger adolescents worry how illness or injury will affect their body image or their status in their peer group. Older adolescents are threatened by the potential effect on career and life-style goals or plans.

Approach to adolescents (Table 3-11). Many health care providers feel that adolescents can be treated as adults. Although the physical appearance and physiology of adolescents are more like adults than children, adolescents do have special needs. Although they expect to be treated as adults, adolescents have most of the fears and concerns of younger children. Independence and body image are very tenuous and sensitive issues. Interactions with adolescents should occur in a manner that supports their self-esteem. A respectful and nonjudgmental attitude creates an atmosphere in which the adolescent can share concerns. Actively involving an adolescent in care and encouraging personal responsibility for health is extremely important.

COPING STRATEGIES

Children's coping mechanisms are highly individualistic and may be positive or negative. Particular coping strategies tend to be used by different age groups. For example, aggression, fantasy, and motor activity are more common with preschool children, whereas intellectualization and displacement are more common with adolescents. Withdrawal and denial are coping mechanisms used by both age groups. Regression is a common coping mechanism in young children. It may, however, be observed in stressed adolescents. Regression is evidenced by the reappearance of self-comforting measures, such as thumb-sucking, which

TABLE 3-11	Approach to Adolescents

GOALS	APPROACH
Develop open and trusting communication.	Communicate with both adolescent and parent; ask to interview adolescent alone. Be honest. Be nonjudgmental. Provide privacy; this is critical for the adolescent. Tell adolescent that information will be kept confidential unless something is revealed that is life threatening (e.g., suicidal intent).
Foster independence and self-esteem.	Acknowledge positive behavior. Let adolescents know it's OK to express feelings (e.g., crying). Encourage adolescents' participation in their health care.
Promote positive body image.	Tell adolescents all normal physical findings or behavior, as well as what is abnormal. Give adolescents realistic information concerning their diagnosis and its implications.
Decrease fear and anxiety.	Explain all procedures. Allow time before procedure starts to "get ready." Allow choices whenever possible.
Encourage good health care consumer behaviors.	Encourage adolescent to ask questions. Ask adolescent history questions; have parent fill in the information the adolescent doesn't know. Encourage responsibility for own care (e.g., taking medicines).

helps a young child deal with stress, or the loss of recently acquired skills, such as the use of the toilet in toddlers. Regression is usually a temporary reaction, and with time and support the child will regain lost skills or behavior.

PARENT INVOLVEMENT

Children are inherently part of a family, whether it be traditional or nontraditional. Parents or primary caregivers provide for the child's emotional well-being and play a vital role in helping the child cope with illness or injury. In the parents' absence, however, the child's tenuous control over the situation may deteriorate.

Despite anxiety during an ED visit, parents must understand and manage their child's illness, support their sick child, and continue to provide for their own and other family members' needs. This can be very difficult when the parent is faced with a childhood injury or illness. Anxiety not only affects the parent's ability to cope and provide for family needs but can also can be conveyed directly to the child. This "emotional contagion" intensifies the child's fear and

anxiety[38] and can negatively affect the child's physical and emotional well-being. Interventions designed to diminish parental or caregiver anxiety enable the parent to provide effective care and support for the child. The resulting reduction in the child's anxiety facilitates their recovery and emotional well-being.

To effectively support parents, the sources of parental stress must be identified. Situational factors, such as the suddenness of admission, seriousness of the child's condition, intensity of the interventions, and degree of uncertainty of outcomes affect a parent's perception of the event. Other factors, such as personality, coping abilities, culture, and concurrent life events, also significantly contribute to the parent's reaction. An exhausted mother caring for a colicky baby may bring her child to the emergency department. To the ED staff, the mother's anxiety may seem inappropriate; however, upon questioning, the nurses find that the woman's husband recently lost his job. Recognizing and respecting the parent's perception of a situation and the varying levels of tolerance of a perceived crisis situation are important components of pediatric ED care.

Parental anxiety cannot be totally eliminated, but nurses can recognize typical stress responses and intervene accordingly. Parents often blame themselves for their child's problem, feel helpless, and displace angry feelings onto the staff. Psychologic defenses are weakened or absent. Stressed people often behave in typical, but seemingly inappropriate, ways. Sedgwick (1975) identified seven responses to stress that interfere with a parent's ability to cope with a stressful situation. (Table 3-12) lists these responses and suggested nursing interventions that can help parents cope with stress.

NURSING INTERVENTIONS TO DECREASE PARENTAL STRESS

Suggested nursing interventions to decrease parental stress include providing ongoing information regarding the child's condition, procedures to be performed, test results, and the expected course of events in understandable terminology. When necessary an interpreter (e.g., non–English speaking parent or deaf parent) should be used. Unrealistic expectations about the child's condition should not be supported, but parents do need to maintain some hope of positive outcomes if any exists. Parents may benefit from assistance in identifying and mobilizing their own resources for such things as child care arrangements for siblings, transportation, or emotional support. Physical comfort measures can be provided or arranged, such as food, medicines, or a breast pump.

Disruption of the parent-child relationship may be more anxiety-provoking than the hospital environment or illness/injury itself. In the PICU setting parents have identified "being with their child" as their most important need.[19,23] Parents should be given the option of staying with their child for procedures. Because children often show more protest when the parent is present, some health care professionals feel it is better to ask parents to leave the room

TABLE 3-12	Parental Responses to Stress and Nursing Interventions	
RESPONSES	**NURSING INTERVENTIONS**
Decreased ability to absorb incoming information, especially threatening information.	Offer constant repetition and consistent reinforcement of information. Provide written instructions.
	Give only the information that is currently necessary; for example, long-term consequences can usually be discussed at a later time.
Decreased ability to think clearly and problem solve.	Assist the family in resolving problems such as child care for other children.
	Involve Social Services when appropriate.
Reduced ability to master tasks.	Give parents clear, concrete directions or have another family member accomplish the task if possible (e.g., admitting office or parking car).
Decreased sense of personal effectiveness (sense of helplessness, loss, incompetence).	Suggest ways in which the parents can help their child (e.g., hold child, give fluids). Rocking is very soothing to both the infant and parent.
Reduced ability to make effective, constructive decisions.	Give the parents time, whenever possible, to assimilate information and make decisions (e.g., informed consent).
Heightened or decreased sensitivity to self (e.g., somatic symptoms or inattention to personal needs such as eating).	Encourage and help parents to meet their own personal health needs.
	Provide comfort measures such as coffee and chairs.
Decreased sensitivity to the environment (may miss cues in their child, spouse, or staff).	Use straightforward communication.

Data from Montagu, 1971; Norris and Grove, 1986; Sedgwick, 1975; Wright and Dyck, 1984.

during procedures. However, the child's anxiety may be so intense when the parent leaves that the child is unable to express his or her feelings. On the other hand, in the parents' presence the child may feel secure enough to express feelings of distress. This outlet can be very healthy.

In some instances, parents may need to be encouraged to participate in their child's care. They may be frightened of hurting the child or interfering with medical and nursing care. Nurses can identify specific tasks the parents can perform to help their child, such as initiating comfort measures, offering fluids, or reading the child a story. However, not all parents are able or ready to participate in their child's care. Some parents may be unable to stay during various procedures. Their wishes should be respected. Other situations may occur in which the parent's presence may be detrimental to the child's welfare, such as an inebriated or violent parent. Each situation is individually assessed and the best interests of the child considered. Older children and adolescents may not want their parents to stay during all aspects of care. Children in this age group can be given a choice.

Other staff behaviors that support parental coping include sensitive and quick response to the child's needs and showing genuine concern and understanding. Merely acknowledging the difficulty of the situation is beneficial. Sometimes acknowledging the parent's feelings in a nonjudgmental way can be difficult, especially when parental behaviors put the child at risk (e.g., abusive situations). In fact, a nurse's feelings about the family or child can influence the nurse's level of involvement.[17] To avoid the detrimental effects of judgmental feelings, nurses can examine their own attitudes and recognize that there is usually more to the situation than "meets the eye." With this approach the nurse can control his or her reactions, be respectful of families, and provide quality care to the child.

CULTURE

Cultural beliefs affect an individual's perception of health problems and treatments, as well as reactions to illness, injury, and hospitalization. By identifying and respecting individual health beliefs and developing mutually agreeable plans of care, nurses can incorporate non-traditional remedies into the plan of care—as long as they are not harmful to the child.[28,30]

Awareness of various cultural beliefs facilitates assessment, increases compliance, and improves relationships between health care providers and families.[28] An uninformed American health care provider may mistakenly identify the effects of alternative treatments, such as coin rubbing, cupping, and pinching, as child abuse. Referring such a patient to Child Protective Services, instead of providing education, may alienate the family. Alternatively, a culturally aware health care provider will recognize these differences in health care beliefs and promote a positive relationship with the family. When conflict occurs, an explanation of the disease process and traditional therapeutic interventions, while maintaining respect for the parents' cultural beliefs, may facilitate compliance.

PREVENTION/SAFETY EDUCATION

Emergency nurses not only play an integral role in the care of children with illnesses and injuries but they can also foster prevention. Individual parent/child teaching can be performed verbally or through written handouts. Bulletin board displays will inform the "captive audience" in the waiting room. The emergency nurse's expertise can be taken to schools, community groups, or shopping malls to educate the public about such issues as bike safety, the use of car seats, the importance of immunizations, childproofing strategies, and poison control (Table 3-13). A variety of excellent sources for prevention are available, including preprinted educational material, posters, and videotapes.

ANATOMIC AND PHYSIOLOGIC DIFFERENCES IN CHILDREN

Growth of the child from birth to adulthood results in profound changes in anatomy and physiology. These differences affect the prevalence and severity of various illnesses or injuries, as well as the child's physiologic reactions and clinical presentation. For example, a 6 month old with respiratory syncytial virus (RSV) usually has signs and symptoms of bronchiolitis, whereas the 6-year-old child with RSV exhibits signs of a cold. The following discussion is a brief review of the anatomic and physiologic differences in children (Table 3-14). Comprehensive information is described in each systems overview chapter.

PHYSICAL GROWTH

The first year of life heralds tremendous changes in an infant's size. The average infant's birth weight doubles

TABLE 3-13	Common Injuries by Development Level	
DEVELOPMENTAL CHARACTERISTICS	COMMON INJURIES	PREVENTIVE MEASURES
Infant		
Increasing mobility	Falls	Do not leave infant alone on tables, beds, etc.
Puts everything in mouth	Aspiration or ingestion	Keep crib rails up
Reaches for interesting	of foreign bodies	Use gates by stairs
objects	Burns	Remove all small items or toys with removable
	Drowning	parts from infant's environment
		Do not feed infant small solid items such as peanuts and hot dogs
		Keep hot or other harmful substances out of reach
		Cover electrical outlets
		Never leave infant alone in tub or near a body of water
		Use car seats
		Post Poison Control and EMS phone numbers
		Encourage CPR classes
Toddler		
Highly mobile	Falls	Provide adequate supervision
Unaware of danger	Burns	Use stair gates
Climbs furniture or stairs	Drowning	Keep child in enclosed play area if an adult is
with ease	MVC	not present
Curious; avidly investigates	Pedestrian	Turn handles of pots and pans on stove out of
environment	Passenger	reach
Imitates adults	Ingestion or aspiration	Use car seats
Puts almost everything in	of harmful substances	Keep harmful substances (medicines, cleaning
mouth	or items	supplies) out of reach
	Suffocation	Cover electrical outlets
		Use age-appropriate and safe toys
		Never leave toddler alone in tub or near water
		Role model safe behaviors
Preschooler		
Able to open doors	Falls	Teach child safety rules concerning traffic,
Runs and climbs with ease	Drowning	playground, and home
Investigates drawers,	Burns	Teach swimming and water safety
cupboards, closets	MVC	Keep harmful items out of reach; lock up
Rides tricycle	Pedestrian	firearms
Uses playground	Passenger	Teach safety with matches, fire
equipment	Playground injuries	Provide safe play equipment and toys
		Use car seats for children <4 yrs or <40 lbs; seat belts for larger children
		Caution against talking to strangers
		Teach sexual abuse prevention

Modified from Wong, 1997.

TABLE 3-13	Common Injuries by Development Level—cont'd	
DEVELOPMENTAL CHARACTERISTICS	**COMMON INJURIES**	**PREVENTIVE MEASURES**
School-age Adventurous Increased motor skills and strength Needs physical activity Needs peer approval	Falls Sports injuries MVC Pedestrian Bicycle Passenger Alcohol and drug abuse	Teach safety rules for traffic, bicycles, skateboarding, pools, etc. Provide safety equipment for sports activities (e.g., bike helmets) Keep firearms locked up except under adult supervision Teach fire safety
Adolescent Strong need for peer approval Risk-taking behaviors Increased independence	MVC Driver Passenger Pedestrian Alcohol and drug abuse Suicide Drowning	Teach motor vehicle safety Educate about hazards of drug and alcohol abuse Teach safe use of sports equipment and encourage use of protective padding or helmets Recognize the signs of depression

by 5 to 6 months of age and triples by 1 year of age. This rapid growth rate slows to an annual weight gain of approximately 2½ kg during the preschool and school-age years.[5] With approaching adolescence, significant growth spurts occur.

Because of the wide variances between children in each age group, accurately estimating body weight in the child is extremely difficult. In the ED (as in pediatrics in general), all children are weighed before the initiation of fluids or medications. If the weight cannot be obtained (e.g., if the child is on a backboard), standardized growth charts or parental history may be used to estimate the weight. In emergent situations, an accurate method of estimating body weight (e.g., Broselow tape) should be used (see Chapter 8, Fig. 8-4).

Body proportions differ between infants, young children, and adults. For example, the midpoint of the infant's height is the umbilicus, compared to the symphysis pubis in the adult. This difference results in a higher center of gravity in the infant. Perhaps the best illustration of the difference in proportions is the large size of the infant's head in relation to the body. Because of the increased surface area of the head, infants can lose a significant amount of heat through their scalp. Also, the relatively large head, coupled with a higher center of gravity, predisposes the child to a higher center of gravity, predisposes the child to head injuries as a result of falls or other traumatic events.

METABOLISM AND FLUID AND ELECTROLYTE BALANCE

Fluid distribution, metabolism, and body surface area vary widely between infants, young children, and adults. In the infant, 75% of body weight is water, compared to 60% to 70% in the adult. Additionally, extracellular fluid represents a larger proportion of fluid in the infant than in the older child or adult. Daily turnover of water in the infant is more than half the extracellular fluid volume, compared to one fifth in the adult[15] (Table 3-15).

Other differences include a large body surface area (BSA) to weight ratio, which promotes heat and insensible water losses, and immature kidneys (in young infants), which are unable to adequately concentrate urine and thus reabsorb needed fluids.

The metabolic rate in infants and young children is higher than the metabolic rate in the older child and adult. In fact, the metabolic rate in the infant is two to three times that of the adult. These differences contribute to the increased fluid, caloric, and oxygen requirements in children.

Increased fluid requirements and a propensity for

TABLE 3-14	Pediatric Anatomic and Physiologic Differences	
PEDIATRIC DIFFERENCES	**CLINICAL SIGNIFICANCE**
Neurologic	
Babinski reflex present until the child starts walking	Babinski reflex is abnormal after 2 years of age.
Immature infant reflexes	Absence, exaggeration, or prolonged presence can indicate a neurologic problem.
Infant posture is primarily flexion	Poor motor tone and absence of flexed posture is abnormal
Head	
Proportionally larger head in relation to body	Increased surface area for heat loss; greater propensity for head injuries
Cranial sutures not fused until approximately 16-18 months of age; anterior fontanel closes between 9-18 months	Gradual increases in intracranial pressure can be accommodated
Brain continues to grow: 25% of its mature adult weight at birth; 75% by age 2½ years; 90% by 6 years of age	Difficult to predict extent of recovery after a neurologic insult in young children
Cranial nerves, spinal cord reflexes, and protective reflexes are intact at birth	Protected from various environmental factors (e.g., can sneeze, cough, blink, gag)
Immature autonomic nervous system	Limited ability to control body temperature and other autonomic functions
Eyes, ears, nose, throat	
Newborns can see clearly up to 12 inches away	Should follow a light and fix gaze from birth
Infants have immature eye muscles	Disconjugate gaze, crossed eyes common in infancy—usually resolves by 6 months of age
Eustachian tubes shorter, straighter, more horizontal	Increased vulnerability to otitis
Children's tonsils and adenoids are usually larger than adolescents' or adults'	Potential for increased airway resistance/obstruction; adenoid tissue can obstruct eustachian tubes
Gastrointestinal	
Immature abdominal muscles	Provide little protection for internal abdominal organs
Liver and spleen are proportionally larger than in adults	Increased susceptibility to injury
Infants younger than 6 months of age have immature lower esophageal sphincter	Gastroesophageal reflux and "spitting up" are common
Immature liver enzyme synthesis and degradation in infants	Decreased ability to metabolize toxic substances; affects drug metabolism
Genitourinary	
Kidneys are highly vascular and poorly protected	Increased vulnerability to renal trauma
Immature kidneys have altered ability to excrete various substances, such as toxic substances	Increased susceptibility to acid-base imbalances and drug toxicity

Data from Dobbing and Sands, 1973; Haley and Baker, 1993; Hauser and Holbrook, 1988; Hazinski, 1992; Wilson, 1986.

TABLE 3-14	Pediatric Anatomic and Physiologic Differences—cont'd	

PEDIATRIC DIFFERENCES	CLINICAL SIGNIFICANCE
Musculoskeletal	
Incompletely calcified bones are more pliable and porous	Bones able to absorb large amounts of energy from traumatic forces; damage can easily occur to underlying structures without the presence of fractures; greenstick and buckle fractures are common
Thicker periosteum	Contributes to rapid healing
Active growth plates	Severe injury can arrest bone growth
Hematologic and Immune System	
Neonates	
Relatively high hematocrit; decreases over first 2-3 months to a physiologic low	Variations in lab values; hematocrit should start to rise after 3 months of age
Red blood cells more fragile with shorter life span than adult red blood cells	
Infants	
Immature immune system	Increased susceptibility to disease
IgG actively produced; adult levels not reached until approximately 4 years of age	Infants rely on maternal immunoglobulins transferred during pregnancy for first several months after birth
Insufficient viral immunity and immature T-cell function	Children will not produce antibodies to specific diseases, such as varicella, until they've been exposed; increased frequency of respiratory and other viral infections

Data from Dobbing and Sands, 1973; Haley and Baker, 1993; Hauser and Holbrook, 1988; Hazinski, 1992; Wilson, 1986.

TABLE 3-15	Differences in Pediatric Fluids and Electrolytes*	

DIFFERENCES	CLINICAL SIGNIFICANCE
Greater total body weight is water: 75% water in full-term infants; 60% to 70% water in adults	Greater potential for dehydration
Infants' body water is mostly extracellular	Increased vulnerability to fluid loss
Higher metabolic rate	Increased fluid requirements
Increased body surface area/weight	Increased heat and water loss
Kidney immaturity in infants	Inability to concentrate urine; cannot efficiently adjust to fluid changes

Data from Haley and Baker, 1993; Hazinski, 1992.

fluid loss predispose the child to rapid fluid deficits during periods of decreased fluid intake and/or increased fluid losses. If the child cannot maintain adequate fluid intake to meet normal daily requirements and replace additional fluid losses, dehydration rapidly follows. Physical problems such as fever or burns, as well as therapeutic interventions such as radiant warmers, can exacerbate fluid loss in children.

Metabolic demands coupled with immature organ development affect the child's ability to metabolize and excrete drugs and toxins. For example, the metabolism of a drug such as acetaminophen in the immature liver of an infant may take longer than in an older child or adult. These factors should be taken into account each time a drug is administered to a child. Although drug dosages are most commonly calculated based on the child's weight, the most effective method is to use the child's body surface area, which correlates more closely with the child's metabolic rate.

Beyond the neonatal period, normal serum electrolyte levels and arterial blood gas values are the same for children and adults. However, certain imbalances, such as hypoglycemia, hypocalcemia, and hyponatremia, and hypernatremia, do tend to be more common and/or potentially more harmful in children. During the first year of life, metabolic acidosis more commonly occurs, because the low renal threshold for bicarbonate limits renal compensation.

PULMONARY SYSTEM

Newborns are normally endowed with adequate pulmonary structures to support oxygenation and ventilation. The child's small airway size and immature immune system, however, increases susceptibility to airway obstruction and respiratory disorders (Table 3-16). As the pulmonary system develops, vulnerability to respiratory illness diminishes. By 8 years of age, the child's respiratory anatomy and physiology approximates that of an adult.

Airway. The upper and lower airways of the infant and small child are significantly smaller than those of the adult. Tracheal diameter is approximately the size of the infant's little finger. Small amounts of mucus, soft tissue edema, or the presence of a foreign body can affect airway patency. Additionally, infants

TABLE 3-16	Pediatric Respiratory Differences	
DIFFERENCE	**CLINICAL SIGNIFICANCE**
Airway	
Small airway diameter (tracheal diameter approximates that of the infant's little finger)	Easily obstructed by small amounts of mucus, foreign bodies, edema
Greater amount of soft tissue surrounding airway	Prone to obstruction from airway edema
Soft laryngeal cartilage	Airway tends to collapse with hyperextension or hyperflexion
Obligate nose breathers (first several months of life)	Obstruction of nasal passages leads to respiratory distress
Proportionally large tongue	Easily obstructs airway
Incompletely developed pathways of collateral ventilation (intraalveolar pores of Kohn and bronchoalveolar canals of Lambert)	Limited ability to compensate for airway obstruction; increased risk of atelectasis and compromised gas exchange
Close proximity of tongue, hyoid bone, and epiglottis	Easy to aspirate
Cricoid is narrowest part of airway	Creates a natural seal for endotracheal tubes without a cuff
Pulmonary	
Fewer and smaller alveoli	Decreased gas exchange surface
Less supportive pulmonary elastic and collagen tissue	Increased susceptibility to atelectasis or air leaks
Cartilaginous sternum and ribs	Increased chest wall compliance; retractions commonly associated with respiratory distress
Poorly developed intercostal and accessory muscles	Relies primarily on diaphragmatic breathing
Thin chest wall	Poorer protection for heart and lungs; easily transmitted breath sounds may be misleading

Data from Haley and Baker, 1993; Hazinski, 1992; Soud, 1992.

are obligate nose breathers for the first several months of life. Nasal congestion can therefore produce signs of respiratory distress in young infants.

Breathing. Infants and young children have fewer and smaller alveoli than adults. This diminishes pulmonary reserve. The ribs are cartilaginous and soft and provide less support for the lungs than in older children and adults. The diaphragm is the primary muscle of respiration in the child, because poorly developed intercostal muscles contribute little to chest wall movement during inspiration. During periods of respiratory distress, the combination of diaphragmatic breathing and pliable ribs causes the chest wall to move inward, or retract, with inspiration. Because the child has less pulmonary compensatory reserves and higher oxygen requirements than the adult, untreated respiratory distress can rapidly progress to respiratory failure.

CARDIOVASCULAR SYSTEM

The normal child's cardiovascular system is relatively healthy; however, anatomic and physiologic differences alter the child's response to stress (Table 3-17). To meet metabolic demands, the child's cardiac output (CO) is normally higher than an adult's. The child's stroke volume (SV), however, is limited by a relatively small heart size, less contractile mass, and decreased myocardial compliance. Children therefore rely primarily on increasing their heart rate (HR) to compensate for increasing metabolic demands caused by illness or injury ($CO = HR \times SV$). When the limits of HR compensation are exceeded, CO falls precipitously and signs of shock will develop. Sustained bradycardia is an ominous sign of circulatory failure. Conversely, an excessive HR (>200-220 infant; >160-180 child) can also decrease CO by compromising ventricular filling.[16]

Children can maintain normal blood pressure for prolonged periods of time despite relatively large losses of extracellular fluid volume. For example, up to 25% of circulating blood volume can be lost before hypotension occurs.[4] The blood pressure is maintained by an increase in peripheral vascular resistance, but this is often at the expense of peripheral perfusion. Signs of early shock, therefore, include changes in peripheral perfusion such as decreased capillary refill and diminished peripheral pulses, while the blood pressure remains normal. Once compensatory mechanisms fail and the blood pressure drops, children rapidly progress to circulatory and subsequent cardiorespiratory failure.

NEUROLOGIC SYSTEM

During infancy the soft, pliable bones of the cranium are connected by fibrous tissue called sutures. Soft

TABLE 3-17	Pediatric Circulatory Differences	
DIFFERENCES	**CLINICAL SIGNIFICANCES**
Myocardium—less contractile mass and less compliant	Limited stroke volume Cardiac output is heart-rate dependent; sustained bradycardia is ominous
Strong compensatory mechanisms; able to maintain cardiac output for long periods of time	Can remain normotensive until 25% of blood volume lost Rapid deterioration after compensatory mechanisms exhausted
Less total circulatory blood volume than adult Neonates: 85-90 ml/kg Infants: 75-80 ml/kg Children: 70-75 ml/kg Adolescent/adult: 65-70 ml/kg	Small blood losses can compromise circulation
Incompletely developed sympathetic nervous system in neonates	Very sensitive to parasympathetic stimulation (suctioning, defecating); produces transient bradycardia

Data from Haley and Baker, 1993; Hazinski, 1992; Soud, 1992.

unossifed membranous spaces (fontanels) are located anteriorly and posteriorly, where several cranial bones meet. Although the posterior fontanel may be closed at birth or shortly thereafter, the anterior fontanel remains open for 9 to 18 months. Open sutures and fontanels allow for normal brain growth. However, gradual abnormal increases in intracranial pressure are also accommodated. This often protects infants from the deleterious effects of increased intracranial pressure (ICP) but may also delay recognition of the problem.

The major structures of the infant's neurologic system are present at birth, but they are incompletely developed. Immature corticospinal pathways are reflected by the presence of primitive reflexes (such as the Moro and Babinski reflexes). Incomplete development of the autonomic nervous system is evidenced by temperature instability and marked sensitivity to parasympathetic stimulation in infants (e.g., propensity toward bradycardia with defecation or deep suctioning). Myelinization of some motor nerves is also incomplete, accounting for the uncoordinated movements and frequent small tremors normally seen in young infants. Cognitive function is largely undeveloped.

THERMOREGULATION

Infants and small children have difficulty maintaining their body temperature due to increased heat loss from their relatively large body surface area per weight and their limited ability to produce heat. The proportionally large head size accounts for much of the exposed surface area and heat loss. Infants under 6 months of age cannot shiver. They rely on non-shivering thermogenesis to produce heat. This process increases oxygen consumption and may lead to hypoxia, especially in stressed infants. Other serious complications of hypothermia in infants and small children may include lactic acidosis, hypoglycemia, pulmonary vasoconstriction, and right-to-left intracardiac shunting.

▮ SUMMARY

Numerous developmental and individual differences in children contribute to the uniqueness of pediatric patients. Biophysical, psychosocial, and cognitive differences have been described in this chapter. Knowledge of these developmental variations provides a foundation for emergency nursing care of the child.

REFERENCES

1. Ainsworth M: Attachment: retrospect and prospect. In Parkes C, Stevenson-Hinde, eds: *The place of attachment in human behavior,* New York, 1982, Basic Books.
2. Ainsworth M: The effects of maternal deprivation: a review of findings and controversy in the context of research strategy. In *Deprivation of maternal care: a reassessment of its effects,* Public Health Papers No 14, Geneva, 1962, World Health Organization.
3. Bowlby J: Attachment and loss: retrospect and prospect, *Am J Orthopsychiatr* 52 (4):664–678, 1982.
4. Chameides L, Hazinski MF: *Textbook of pediatric life support,* Dallas, 1994. American Heart Association.
5. Chow MP et al: *Handbook of pediatric primary care,* New York, 1979, John Wiley and Sons.
6. Dobbing J, Sands J: Quantitative growth and development of human brain, *Arch Dis Child* 48:757, 1973.
6a. Durand B: Failure to thrive in a child with Down's syndrome, *Nurs Res* 24(4):272–286, 1975.
7. Erikson E: *Childhood and society,* ed 2, New York, 1963, WW Norton.
8. Flavell JH: *Cognitive development,* Englewood Cliffs, NJ, 1977, Prentice-Hall.
9. Freud S: *The ego and the id,* New York, 1960, WW Norton.
10. Freud S: *A general introduction to psychoanalysis,* New York, 1963, Pocket Books.
11. Gaynard L et al: *Psychosocial care of children in hospitals: a clinical practice manual from the ACCH child life research project,* Bethesda, Md, 1990, Association for the Care of Children's Health.
12. Haley K, Baker P, eds: *Emergency nursing pediatric course instructor manual,* 1993, Chicago Emergency Nurses Association.
13. Harlow H, Harlow M: The affectional systems. In Schrier A, Harlow H, Stollnitz , eds: *Behavior of nonhuman primates,* vol 2, New York, 1965, Academic Press.
14. Hauser GJ, Holbrook PR: Immune dysfunction in the critically ill infant and child, *Crit Care Clin* 4:711, 1988.
15. Hazinski MF: Children are different. In Hazinski MF: *Nursing care of the critically ill child,* ed 2, St Louis, 1992, Mosby.
16. Hazinski MF, Barkin RM: Shock. In Barkin RM, ed: *Pediatric emergency medicine, concepts and clinical practice,* St Louis, 1992, Mosby.
17. Hickey M, Lewandowski LA: Critical care nursing role with families: a descriptive study, *Heart Lung* 17:670, 1988.

18. Kaspar JW: The perceived needs of parents of children in the pediatric intensive care unit: a descriptive study, master's thesis, Los Angeles, 1986, UCLA.
19. Reference deleted in proofs.
20. Montagu A: *Touching,* New York, 1971, Harper and Row.
21. Mott S: Developmental theories: how the child grows. In Mott SR, James SR, Sperhac AM: *Nursing care of children and families,* Redwood City, Calif, 1990, Addison-Wesley.
22. Norris LO, Grove SK: Investigation of selected psychosocial needs of family members of critically ill adult patients, *Heart Lung* 15:194–199, 1986.
23. Philichi LM: Supporting the parents when the child requires intensive care, *Focus Crit Care* 15:34, 1988.
24. Piaget J: *The language and thought of the child,* ed 3, New York, 1967, Humanities Press.
25. Piaget J: *The origins of intelligence in children,* New York, 1952, International Universities Press.
26. Pontious SL: Practical Piaget: helping children understand, *Am J Nurs* 82 (1):114–117, 1982.
27. Robertson J: *Young children in hospitals,* New York, 1969, Basic Books.
28. Rosenberg JA: Health care for Cambodian children: integrating treatment plans, *Pediatr Nurs* 12 (2) : 118–125, 1986.
29. Rutter M: Maternal deprivation, 1972-8: new findings, new concepts, new approaches, *Child Dev* 50:283–305, 1979.
30. Satz KJ: Integrating Navajo tradition into maternal-child nursing, *Image* 14(3):89–91, 1982.
31. Sedgwick R: Psychological responses to stress, *J Psychiatr Nurs* 13:20, 1975.
32. Skerrett K, Hardin SB, Puskar KR: Infant anxiety, *MCN J* 12(1):51–9, 1983.
33. Soud T: Airway, breathing, circulation, and disability: what is different about kids? *JEN* 18(2):107–116, 1992.
34. Tronick ED, Als H, Brazelton TB: The infant's capacity to regulate face-to-face interaction, *J Comm* 27:74, 1977.
35. Waechter EH, Blake FG: *Nursing care of children,* ed 9, Philadelphia, 1985, JB Lippincott.
36. Wieczorek R, Natapoff J: *A conceptual approach to the nursing of children: health care from birth to adolescence,* Philadelphia, 1981, JB Lippincott.
37. Wilson CB: Immunologic basis for increased susceptibility of the neonate to infection, *J Pediatr* 108:1, 1986.
38. Wolfer JA, Visintainer MA: Pediatric surgical patients' and parents' stress responses and adjustment as a function of psychologic preparation and stress-point nursing care, *Nurs Res* 24(4):244–55, 1975.
39. Wong DL: *Whaley and Wong's Essentials of pediatric nursing,* ed 5, St Louis, 1997, Mosby.
40. Wright K, Dyck S: Expressed concern of adult cancer patients' family members, *Cancer Nurs* 7:371–374, 1984.

CHAPTER 4

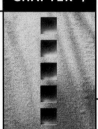

Pediatric History and Physical Examination

Valerie L. Benjamin

INTRODUCTION

Pediatric emergency care has evolved dramatically over the past decade as emergency care providers have recognized that children are individuals with unique health care needs. Some institutions that provide emergency care to both adults and children are even creating separate treatment areas for children and their families. Many have begun to employ professionals with pediatric expertise.

In addition to these changes, economic trends have impacted the emergency department (ED) population and the degree of pathology seen. Children are presenting with conditions of varying acuity ranging from simple primary care problems such as ear infections and colds to complex illnesses such as sickle cell disease and diabetes. Nurses caring for children must therefore be familiar not only with common childhood illness but also with complex life-threatening conditions.

The goal of the pediatric assessment is no different from that of the adult. It is to identify actual or potential emergencies in children and adolescents and to intervene accordingly. This chapter describes the pediatric history and physical and will help the emergency nurse learn to identify physical problems commonly seen in children and adolescents.

OBSTACLES TO PATIENT CARE

There are obstacles to providing optimum patient care in most settings, but this is particularly true in the emergency department, where patient census and acuity is unpredictable. Staffing estimates, which are usually based on patient census, may seem high one hour and dangerously low the next. Personnel who are available to fill gaps in staffing may have little experi-

ence in caring for pediatric patients. This lack of knowledge, coupled with an increasing census and decreasing communication as the activity level increases, can lead to errors in care.

Ways to offset these obstacles include the development of systems to provide pediatric care such as primary or team nursing; establishing back-up coverage (e.g., on-call nurses); providing pediatric orientation programs for all nurses, but particularly those who "float" or are part time in the emergency department; and offering ongoing pediatric educational programs for all emergency department staff (Table 4-1).

PEDIATRIC HISTORY

Protocols for performing a nursing history and physical vary from institution to institution. Some emergency department nurses perform comprehensive assessments, and others perform brief assessments. In all settings the examination is usually based on the chief complaint and unusual physical findings. Unlike the primary care setting, the goal of this focused assessment is to identify the most seriously ill or injured children and intervene before the condition becomes life threatening.

The interview is the beginning of an entire process of communication between the child, parent, and emergency care team, and it usually begins in the triage setting. These interactions set the tone for the entire ED visit. During the interview a wealth of information can be obtained—beyond that verbalized by the parent or child. How the child and parent conduct themselves will reveal their personal resources such as their state of mind and coping skills. With experience, the nurse will develop a "sixth sense" or a certain perceptiveness about children and their unique situations.

TABLE 4-1	Approach to Pediatric Assessment—Common Problems	
SAMPLE PROBLEMS	**SOLUTION**	
Anxious child/parent	Take care of child's most urgent needs (ABCs, etc.)	
	Allow child to remain with and be held by parent when possible	
	Allow child to play with toy, read a book	
	Take time to listen to parent's concerns and questions	
	Communicate frequently with parent; avoid medical jargon; contact translator if necessary	
	Contact social service worker, chaplain	
	Encourage parent to take a break	
Physical environment problems	Provide quiet, comfortable environment (e.g., rocking chair for parents with infants and toddlers, close door, pull curtain)	
	Knock or announce yourself before entering room/curtained area	

APPROACH TO THE PEDIATRIC HISTORY

An emergency department visit is usually stressful for the child and parent. Fear and uncertainty surrounding the child's condition, coupled with a loss of control of the situation, add to that stress. Positive, caring interactions with the child and parent help to alleviate stress and facilitate the history-taking process.

The timing and length of the interview will depend on the circumstances. If the child is medically or surgically unstable during the primary survey, a detailed history may be delayed until the child has been stabilized.

The interview should optimally begin with an introduction and the exchange of a few social pleasantries that include the child. This interaction personalizes the encounter and facilitates the flow of information. While obtaining the history the nurse can simultaneously perform a general survey of the child and observe family dynamics.

The importance of the history cannot be overstated. Obtaining an exact description of signs and symptoms, chronology, surrounding circumstances, and actions taken to alleviate the problem paves the way for an accurate diagnosis and appropriate management (Box 4-1).

INTERVIEWING THE PARENT

Active listening is a fundamental part of the history-taking process. Initially the nurse should note the order in which the parent/caregiver presents the chief complaint(s), because signs and symptoms are often revealed according to the parent's level of concern.

Box 4-1 Interviewing Hints

Interviewing parent
- Perform introductions; introduce self, giving name and title
- Exchange a few pleasantries to personalize the encounter
- Identify chief complaint and symptoms of most concern to the parent/caregiver
- Observe the manner in which the parent relays the information (e.g., eye contact, tone of voice, facial expressions)

Interviewing child
- Talk to the parent first, while observing the child for nonverbal cues
- Use a tone of voice based on child's responses to interviewer (i.e., gregarious or quiet)
- Engage the child in dialogue regarding things important to him or her (e.g., favorite animated characters)
- Use familiar terms and ask simple questions

Interviewing teens
- Interview the teen initially
- Allow the parent to supplement the history
- Ask the parent to leave when discussing sensitive information (e.g., sexual history)

Frequently parents will dwell on the aspect of the chief complaint that worries them most. For example, if the nurse inquires about the child's runny nose, the parent may briefly discuss the runny nose before restating concerns about the child's loud nighttime cough. The parent may continue to do this well after the nurse has taken a thorough history of the cough. After completion of the history, information collected is reviewed with the parent and child to clarify any misinformation and to let the child and parent know that their concerns have been heard.

The nurse should note the ease with which the parent/caregiver presents the information, as well as the tone of voice. The tone of voice and the urgency with which the history is presented can reveal much about the parent's state of mind.

Sometimes parents present the chief complaint as a diagnosis when they have already formed an opinion (e.g., "My child's got an ear infection!"). When this happens the nurse might ask the parent to describe the signs and symptoms that led to that conclusion.

Occasionally the person bringing a child into the emergency department is not the primary caregiver. A number of different approaches can be used to obtain historical information in these situations. Initially, the nurse may attempt to collect the information by phoning the parent. If the child was previously treated at the hospital, the medical record will also be helpful. Occasionally the nurse (or ED physician) may need to call the primary care physician and/or specialist to obtain a more thorough history. This is particularly important if the child is being followed for a chronic medical condition. If the child arrives by rescue from a day care or school, the school nurse, teacher, or other students may be questioned.

INTERVIEWING CHILDREN

Historical information relating to infants and toddlers is generally obtained from the parent or caregiver. However, preschoolers and early school-age children can be very good historians with appropriate questioning. Although they generally cannot give a detailed history or chronology, they can often describe how they feel, particularly when given multiple choices to help describe their symptoms.

Most preschoolers and early school-age children are initially apprehensive about being interviewed. As the child gets used to the interviewer this fear tends to lessen. By allowing a child to remain with the parents and observing the child for nonverbal cues the nurse can often determine how a child will respond to being interviewed.

The nurse's tone of voice should mirror the child's reactions. The gregarious and outgoing child may respond well to a happy, flamboyant tone, whereas the shy or withdrawn child may respond better to a quiet, gentle tone. Children generally respond when they see that the nurse can relate to things that matter to them. For example, if the child is wearing a T-shirt with a cartoon character on it, the nurse can compliment the shirt and let the character be a starting point for engaging in conversation. Once the ice is broken the nurse can ease into taking the history. When phrasing questions, simple, familiar terms should be used, such as, "Your mommy tells me that your tummy hurts. Does it hurt right now?"

INTERVIEWING ADOLESCENTS

Adolescents are developmentally advanced enough to provide a detailed history. The parent can offer supplemental information as needed. Because the adolescent may be reluctant to discuss sensitive information, such as sexual history, in the presence of the parent or other family member, the nurse may politely ask the parent to step out of the room while performing the history and physical. Most parents understand this sensitivity and will not object.

Questions must be phrased in a nonjudgmental fashion. Passing judgment or using embarrassing language will damage the lines of communication and undermine the opportunity to obtain an accurate and complete history. Occasionally, embarrassment, temperament, or anxiety can emerge in the form of hostility or closed behavior. When this occurs, the adolescent must be reassured that the emergency staff's role is to find the source of the illness or injury.

PEDIATRIC PHYSICAL EXAMINATION

The traditional physical examination proceeds from head to toe and uses the techniques of inspection, auscultation, palpation, and percussion. However, the approach to the pediatric physical examination varies depending on the age and developmental level of the child. Most young children are frightened by the ED environment; they are further frightened and less likely to cooperate when invasive procedures, such as taking a rectal temperature or looking in the ears, are performed early during the examination. Therefore, procedures considered invasive are reserved for last. If the child has an area of pain or discomfort, it is

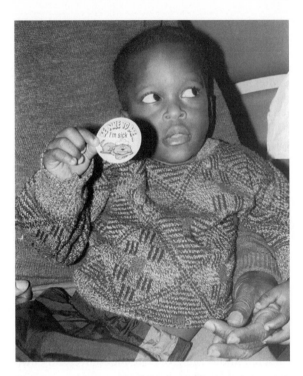

FIG. 4-1. Reward the child for tolerating the examination.

Box 4-2   Quick Tips for Gaining the Young Child's Cooperation During the Physical Examination

- Explain examination to child and caregiver.
- Examine as much as possible from a distance.
    Primary survey
    Neurologic status
    Respiratory effort
- Involve caregivers.
    Allow child to sit in parent's lap whenever possible
    Allow parent to perform gentle palpation or range-of-motion during examination of extremities
- Make examination fun for the child.
    Use imagery with favorite characters (e.g., "Let's see if I can feel Mickey Mouse in your tummy.")
    Allow child to inspect and touch equipment
    Blow out the "birthday candle" (penlight) during respiratory assessment
    Distract child with whistling or clicking noises made with tongue
- Progress from least distressing to most distressing.
    Inspection of scalp first; inspection of genitalia last

also assessed at the end of the exam. After the examination the child should be rewarded for tolerating the procedures (Fig. 4-1).

PARENTAL INVOLVEMENT

Young children identify strongly with their parents and for this reason should not be separated from the parent. Additionally, by involving the parent several goals are accomplished. It eases the child's anxieties about being in a strange place and being touched by strangers, it allows the parent to learn more about the child's illness or injury, and it helps the parent feel a part of the child's care.

Parents may be encouraged to hold young children during the examination, because the child feels more secure when in the parent's arms. Much of the examination can be conducted while the child is being held. When the child resists certain portions of the exam (e.g., auscultation), the parent may hold the stethoscope against the child's chest. To restrain the child's head for the otoscopic examination, the child can straddle the parent as if hugging. To assess a painful extremity, the parent may gently touch the region in question.

Occasionally a child resists the entire examination and is scolded by the parent. When this happens the parent should be reminded that the child's reactions are normal. Some children have a higher level of stranger anxiety than others. Regardless of the degree of cooperation the child is given a reward such as a sticker for tolerating the entire experience.

TECHNIQUES FOR GAINING THE CHILD'S COOPERATION

Infants.   The key to obtaining an accurate assessment of an infant is to keep the infant calm during the examination (Box 4-2). Allowing the parent to hold or feed the infant when appropriate provides the infant with warmth and comfort. When an infant whimpers or cries the parents can offer effective calming tech-

Box 4-3 Age-Appropriate Responses to Hospital Situations

0–3 months
Infants have little ability to discriminate or move in an organized fashion. Discomfort, pain, and sudden loud noises cause crying.

4–6 months
Infants begin to develop perceptual ability, distinguishing the strange from the familiar.

7–12 months
Perceptions are more discriminating. Responses are better organized and more predictable. By end of the first year, a baby can predict unpleasant situations based on recent unpleasant experiences. For instance, older infants may cry when placed on the examination table or when hands are restrained for the ear examination. Sight of strangers and strange objects may arouse fear. Older infants tend to be fearful of rapidly approaching objects or people.

Beyond first year
Child can increasingly foresee unpleasant situations based on prior experience, taking precautionary measures such as hiding face with hands, running away, and kicking.[2]

niques. Sounds such as popping, clicking, kissing, or whistling will distract most infants long enough for the nurse to auscultate the chest and abdomen (Box 4-3).

Toddlers. Toddlers are fearful of strangers and look to their parents for comfort and support. When possible allow the child to remain in the parent's lap during the examination. Play is often an effective diversion for children in this age group and can be used to distract the child from the examination (Fig. 4-2). Many children will cooperate with the examination if allowed to touch and play with the equipment and when the examination is made fun (e.g., ask the child to blow out the light on a penlight or blow bubbles). If a child remains upset, the examination should be carried out as quickly as possible. Because the otoscopic, oral, and genitourinary examiniations are generally the most distressing parts of the exam, they are performed last.

Preschoolers. Preschoolers are also fearful of the environment, but with some encouragement they are usually more cooperative than toddlers. They are curious and like to handle equipment such as the stethoscope and will often actively participate in the exam by doing things such as holding the stethoscope to their chest. Games such as "What's in your belly?", "Let's see how far you can stick out your tongue," and "Can you jump up and down?" make the examination fun for the child and more pleasant for the examiner. When possible, give the child choices. For example, "Do you want me to look in this ear or that ear first?" Avoid questions that require a *yes* or *no* answer, such as, "Can I look in your ears?" As with toddlers, the most invasive portion of the exam is reserved for last.

School-age children. Many of the techniques used to examine younger children are effective in the school-age child. They remain very dependent on their parents, and therefore parents should stay while the child is being examined. Before the examination the child is given a brief explanation of what will occur. Children in this age group are inquisitive, and questions should be answered honestly.

Adolescents. The physical exam is easier to perform in adolescents, because they are usually cooperative. Privacy is very important, and they often prefer that their parents not be present during questioning or during the examination. The examination is explained before initiation and all questions are answered honestly (Table 4-2).

GROWTH PARAMETERS

Growth parameters are an important component of the pediatric assessment. Initially the child is weighed. In some rare circumstances the child's height and head circumference may be required. Though most professionals who exclusively work with children become skilled in quickly determining the achievement of normal growth parameters by simple observation, using standardized growth charts helps confirm findings (see Appendix D).

Growth parameters vary from child to child and are most effectively evaluated when trended over time. Growth charts are used to determine not only where the child falls in relation to other children but also whether the child is maintaining a consistent growth pattern such as maintaining a growth rate at the 5th percentile. Gross abnormalities in trending (e.g., the

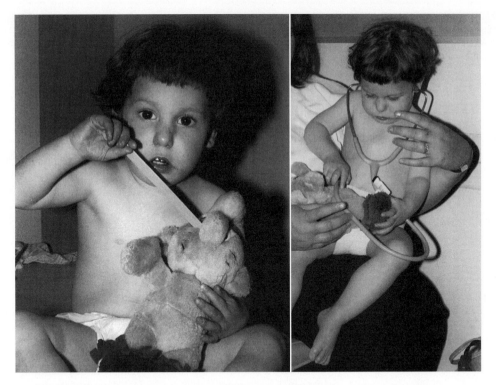

FIG. 4-2. Encouraging play before the examination helps prepare the child.

child who tracks along at the 75th percentile and suddenly drops below the 5th percentile) may indicate serious illness or certain childhood conditions such as cardiac or endocrine disorders.

GENERAL SURVEY

The general survey evaluates the child's activity level, interaction with the environment, and outward appearance and affect. The appearance and affect of the parent(s) must also be considered (Box 4-4).

Initially the child is examined from a distance, because the personal space of a young child tends to be much wider than that of an older child. Immediately violating that child's personal space may bring on agitation, complicating the clinical picture. The child's level of activity provides the first clues to the degree of illness. A child who is awake, alert, running around the examination area, playing, or babbling is not in distress. A child who is lying on the examination table or in the parent's lap or who is drowsy or unarousable despite stimulation may be seriously ill.

Young infants are somewhat harder to examine. Their primary activities are limited to sleeping and eating. Gentle stimulation of the infant may be used to elicit normal developmental responses. These include maintaining eye contact with the parent or examiner, tracking objects or faces, grabbing objects, smiling, or cooing. Other assessment parameters include muscle tone, consolability, and arousability. The infant who is not acutely ill should be willing to engage in the environment and should be easily consoled when crying. The crying infant is signaling to the parent that a physiologic need is unmet. The infant may be hungry, sleepy, in pain, or may not feel well. Parents become very astute at interpreting the infant's cry and can relate the infant's need to the emergency nurse.

Toddlers and older children can offer verbal clues to their physical or emotional discomfort; however, observation of their behavior provides important clues to the seriousness of the illness. The toddler or preschooler who does not feel well or is frightened usually clings to the parent for comfort. When seriously ill these children usually cannot be distracted

TABLE 4-2	Age-Specific Approaches to Physical Examination During Childhood	
Position	**Sequence**	**Preparation**
Infant		
Before sits alone: supine or prone, preferably in parent's lap; before 4 to 6 months: can place on examining table	If quiet, auscultate heart, lungs, abdomen	Completely undress if room temperature permits
After sits alone: use sitting in parent's lap whenever possible	Record heart and respiratory rates	Leave diaper on
If on table, place with parent in full view	Palpate and percuss same areas	Gain cooperation with distraction, bright objects, rattles, talking
	Proceed in usual head-toe direction	Smile at infant; use soft, gentle voice
	Perform traumatic procedures last (eyes, ears, mouth [while crying])	Pacify with bottle of sugar water or feeding, or pacifier
	Elicit reflexes as body part examined	Enlist parent's aid for restraining to examine ears, mouth
	Elicit Moro reflex last	Avoid abrupt, jerky movements
Toddler		
Sitting or standing on/by parent	Inspect body area through play: "count fingers," "tickle toes"	Have parent remove outer clothing
Prone or supine in parent's lap	Use minimal physical contact initially	Remove underwear as body part examined
	Introduce equipment slowly	Allow to inspect equipment; demonstrate use of equipment
	Auscultate, percuss, palpate whenever quiet	If uncooperative, perform procedures quickly
	Perform traumatic procedures last (same as for infant)	Use restraint when appropriate; request parent's assistance
		Talk about examination if cooperative; use short phrases
		Praise for cooperative behavior
Preschool child		
Prefer standing or sitting	If cooperative, proceed in head-to-toe direction	Request self-undressing
Usually cooperative prone/ supine	If uncooperative, proceed as with toddler	Allow to wear underpants
Prefer parent's closeness		Offer equipment for inspection; briefly demonstrate use
		Make up "story" about procedure: "I'm seeing how strong your muscles are" (blood pressure)
		Give choices when possible
		Expect cooperation; use positive statements: "Open your mouth"

From Wong DL: *Whaley & Wong's essentials of pediatric nursing,* ed 5, St Louis, 1997, Mosby.

TABLE 4-2	Age-Specific Approaches to Physical Examination During Childhood—cont'd		
POSITION	**SEQUENCE**	**PREPARATION**	

School-age child

Prefer sitting	Proceed in head-to-toe direction	Request self-undressing
Cooperative in most positions	Examine genitalia last in older child	Allow to wear underpants
Younger child prefers parent's presence	Respect need for privacy	Give gown to wear
Older child may prefer privacy		Explain purpose of equipment and significance of procedure, such as otoscope to see eardrum, which is necessary for hearing
		Teach about body functioning and care

Adolescent

Same as for school-age child	Same as older school-age child	Allow to undress in private
Offer option of parent's presence		Give gown
		Expose only area to be examined
		Respect need for privacy
		Explain findings during examination: "Your muscles are firm and strong"
		Matter-of-factly comment about sexual development: "Your breasts are developing as they should be"
		Emphasize normalcy of development
		Examine genitalia as any other body part; may leave to end

into engaging actively in the environment. Facial expressions, eye contact, demeanor, and body language provide important clues to the child's degree of illness.

Another component of the general survey is the child's appearance. Observation of the child's clothes, hair, and cleanliness can reflect the home situation and the degree of care provided within that home. The emergency nurse should remember, however, that parents often rush their children to the emergency department when accidents have occurred and the child may be dirty from playing. In the adolescent, dress and grooming often reveal life-style and habits.

Observing the parents' or guardians' interactions with the child, as well as their degree of cleanliness and dress, provides additional clues to the home situation. For example, is the parent wearing tattered, dirty clothes; does the parent smell of tobacco or alcohol; is the parent nurturing, punitive, or disinterested when relating to the child?

HEAD

Anatomy and physiology. The neonate's head accounts for one third of body weight and one fourth of body length, with an average head circumference of 32.5 to 37.5 cm. In the newborn the sutures can be

Box 4-4   The General Survey

General appearance of the child
- Rapid evaluation of airway, breathing, and circulation
- Age-appropriate behavior (neurologic assessment)
- Hygiene
- Affect and mood
- Quality of speech or cry
- Facial expression
- Posture and motor activity
- Odors (breath, skin)

General appearance of the parent/caregiver
- Hygiene
- Interactions with the child
- Affect and mood
- Evidence of smoking, drinking, or drugs

palpated as ridges and the fontanels (anterior and posterior) as indentations. The sutures are palpable up to the age of 4 months. The anterior fontanel, which is found at the junction of the frontal and parietal bones, is approximately 2.5 × 2.5 cm at birth and closes between 9 and 19 months of age. The posterior fontanel is found at the junction of the occipital and two parietal bones, with an average size of 1 × 1 cm at birth. It closes by 4 months of age. Brain growth is at its highest rate from birth until age 2 years, at which time the sutures have fused and the fontanels closed (Fig. 4-3).

Evaluation. The head and face are inspected for size and shape, evidence of trauma, presence of masses, hair character and distribution, dysmorphic features, or other pathologies. When observing the child the features of the parents and siblings should be considered. Head circumference is obtained if the child has dysmorphic features or if the head appears small or large for age. Measurements are plotted on the growth chart to identify deviations from normal.

Normal features of the head and face vary by age. The newborn skull may show evidence of birth trauma, which can include cranial molding or an elongated head. Occasionally a benign soft mass over the occipitoparietal region is found in the early newborn period. One such mass, a caput succedaneum, is swelling of the soft tissue of the scalp. Another mass, a cephalohematoma, is a collection of blood beneath the skull's periosteum; it is therefore bound by the suture line.[3] Both masses usually resolve within a few days after birth; however, a cephalohematoma can take months. Other signs of birth trauma to the head include round indentations or masses at the zygomatic or parietal regions. These may be from the pressure of forceps.

As the child develops, abnormalities in size or shape of the skull can indicate CNS pathology or genetic disorders. The child with spina bifida and hydrocephalus may have an unusually large head; conversely the child with cerebral palsy and inadequate brain development may have an unusually small head. Dysmorphic features such as a triangular face, low-set ears, or widely spaced eyes may indicate genetic disorders. Prominent bony ridges over one or more suture lines with an abnormal head shape may indicate premature closure of a suture, which is called craniosynostosis. Craniosynostosis can lead to impared neurologic development and complications such as increased intracranial pressure, particularly when more than one suture is involved.[1]

The suture lines and fontanels of the infant and young child are palpated while the child is upright and calm. Assessing the fontanel while the child is screaming or recumbent yields false information. The anterior fontanel should be flat and soft, although a fontanel that is mildly full and soft or mildly depressed is also acceptable. A fontanel that is unquestionably full and tense or depressed is abnormal. A tense, bulging fontanel is caused by increased intracranial pressure, whereas a sunken fontanel is caused by dehydration. The remainder of the skull is palpated for masses, step-offs, crepitus, and areas of tenderness.

Percussion of the skull is rarely indicated; however, percussion over the frontal and maxillary sinuses is indicated when a child complains of pain over the sinuses, frequent headaches and cold symptoms, and facial trauma. The area over the mastoid region is percussed for tenderness associated with mastoiditis (Box 4-5).

EYES

Anatomy and physiology. Visual acuity varies depending on the age of the child. At birth the immature eyes are limited in their ability to accommodate and focus on an object for any length of time. During this period visual acuity is reported to be between 20/100 and 20/400, depending on

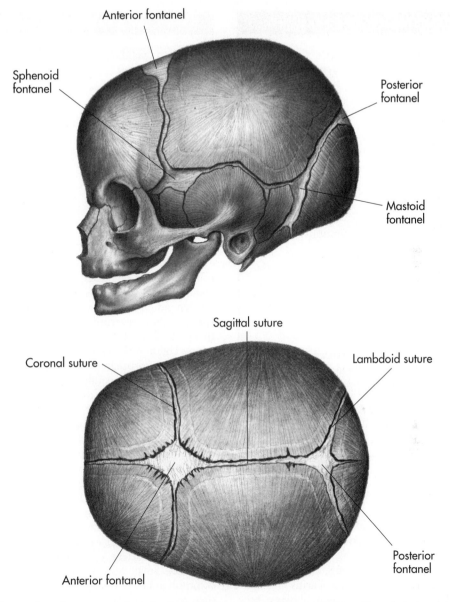

Anterior fontanel

Sphenoid
fontanel

Posterior
fontanel

Mastoid
fontanel

Sagittal suture

Coronal suture

Lambdoid suture

Posterior
fontanel

Anterior fontanel

FIG. 4-3. Fontanels and sutures on the infant's skull. (From Seidel HM et al: *Mosby's guide to physical examination,* ed 3, St Louis, 1995, Mosby.)

the technique used; therefore newborns only distinguish objects within 8 to 10 inches.[5] Fixation on close objects and faces begins at birth. Tracking objects begins at age 5 to 6 weeks. Hand-eye coordination begins around age 3 months.

With development, visual acuity improves. The visual acuity of a 3 year old is $\pm 20/40$; the acuity of a 4 to 5 year old is $\pm 20/30$; and the acuity of a 6-year-old child or older is $\pm 20/20$.

Evaluation. Initially the eyes are inspected for positioning. During the emergency department physical exam, however, gross abnormalities are usually observed first (such as redness, swelling, or crusted

Box 4-5   Examination of the Head and Neck

Head
Symmetry, hair, skull, facial structures, fontanelles, sutures

Eyes
Position and alignment
Pupillary size and reaction to light
Color of sclera and conjunctiva
Drainage: color, consistency, amount
Visually tracts object

Ears
Position and symmetry
Drainage: color, consistency, amount
Ability to hear

Nose
Nasal drainage: color, consistency, amount, from one or both nares
Nasal flaring

Mouth
Color of lips and mucous membranes
Moistness of mucous membranes and lips
Mouth breathing vs. nose breathing

Neck
Lymph nodes, masses: pain, color, mobility
Tracheal alignment

Box 4-6   Abnormalities of the Eyes

Sunken eyelids
• Dehydration
• Malnutrition

Eyelid edema
• Congestive heart failure
• Periorbital cellulitis
• Conjunctivitis
• Allergies
• Angioedema
• Renal disease
• Trauma
• Prolonged crying

discharge). Additionally, eyelid edema; masses; or excessive, infrequent, or asymmetric blinking may be seen.

The child with redness, swelling, and a discharge along the lid margin may have blepharitis and conjunctivitis. The child with excessive blinking may simply have a nervous habit or may have an irritant in the eye. Infrequent blinking and/or ptosis may indicate muscle weakness or nerve paralysis.

The eyes can be used as a barometer of hydration in infants and young children with moderate to severe changes readily noted. Sunken eyes generally mean dehydration or poor nutrition. Eyelid edema can indicate one of several illnesses, including congestive heart failure, periorbital cellulitis, allergies, angioedema, renal disease, and trauma. It can also indicate prolonged crying or inadequate rest, or it can simply be a variation of normal. It is often helpful to ask the parent if the child's eyes appear different (Box 4-6).

Depending on the child's symptoms and chief complaint the structures beneath the eyelid may need to be checked. This can be difficult in infants and young children who actively resist efforts to separate the eyelids. Fortunately, most structures beneath the eyelid can be successfully observed when the child's eyes are open and while distracting the child with a toy or other attractive object.

In older children the conjunctivae can be inspected by manipulating the eyelids and having the child look in the opposite direction. Smoothness, moisture, color, blood vessel dilation, and evidence of trauma or a foreign body are all observed. The sclera should be white; however, a light blue color is normal in the newborn because the sclera is very thin. Some abnormal findings include cobblestoning, which is seen in conjunctivitis caused by the herpesvirus, and yellow-tinged sclera, which is seen in newborns with jaundice. Small subconjunctival hemorrhages are common in newborns as a result of the birth process; they resolve spontaneously. Subconjunctival hemorrhages in older infants and children are seen in trauma, bleeding disorders, harsh coughing, and abuse. Abuse should be considered in any child with subconjunctival hemorrhages.

The cornea is inspected for clouding, enlargement, ulceration, irritation, and injury. The pupils are inspected for size and reactivity, which is more evident in a dimly lighted room. The pupils of the newborn contract and dilate more slowly than in older infants, children, and adults. The iris and anterior chamber are observed for color or evidence of trauma.

TABLE 4-3	Testing Visual Acuity in the Child	
AGE	**ASSESSMENT**	
Young infant	Hold penlight 10 inches from face. Look for blinking. Infants >1 month old should track light.	
Older infant	Tracks brightly colored objects. Good hand-eye coordination.	
Toddler	Names objects on age-appropriate eye chart. Accurate hand-eye coordination.	
School-age child	Age-appropriate eye chart, Snellen chart. Test both eyes, affected eye, then normal eye.	

Visual acuity should be tested on all children with a chief complaint of headache, head trauma, eye injury, eye discharge, chemical or thermal burns to the eye, or other neurologic problems. In infants, visual acuity is tested with a bright light held approximately 10 inches away from the eyes. Blinking, pupillary constriction, and tracking are observed. Hand-eye coordination can be tested in older infants by observing whether they reach for a toy or colored object placed in front of them.

Assessing the visual acuity in toddlers and preschoolers is mostly a matter of observation, because the child's cooperation is required to perform the examination. This is particularly true of the toddler. Several charts can be used to test the young child's visual acuity; some of these are included in Chapter 19.

Testing each eye separately can be difficult in young children, because the child may resist attempts to cover one eye. If available, use disposable cardboard eyeglass occluders or "special sunglasses" to gain the child's cooperation. Assist the child or parent in holding the hand-held visual acuity charts the proper distance from the child's eyes. Allow the child to name the objects, letters, or numbers on the chart line by line.

School-age children and adolescents can use the Snellen chart traditionally used to assess visual acuity in adults. The chart must be placed in an area where the lighting is adequate and the flow of traffic is minimal. If the problem involves only one eye, test the visual acuity of the affected eye first by covering the good eye (Table 4-3).

EAR

Anatomy and physiology. The basic shape of the ear and hearing do not change across the life span. However, as the child grows the cartilage of the ear becomes less flexible and the ear canal elongates and changes position relative to the tympanic membrane.

Evaluation. The external structures of the ear are inspected for position, alignment, and shape. Abnormal findings include swelling, discharge, evidence of trauma, displacement of the pinna, and visibly enlarged cervical or occipital lymph nodes. Other findings can include skin tags in the preauricular area (which are generally benign) or sinuses, which can become infected.

Because the positioning of the ear canal changes as the child develops, the pinna must be manipulated accordingly to best view the tympanic membrane. In infants the tympanic membrane is best seen by gently pulling the pinna downward and outward. In older children the tympanic membrane is best seen by gently pulling the pinna outward and upward.

The otoscopic examination requires that the child hold the head still. The nurse may need to assist the diagnostician in safely restraining the infant or young child during this examination (Fig. 4-4).

A brief test of the child's hearing acuity is also important. The newborn usually blinks, startles, or cries in response to sudden loud noises. Older infants may briefly cease activity as if listening in response to sounds. Infants with good head control and older children usually turn in response to loud sounds or familiar voices, grossly demonstrating intact hearing. Language development is also associated with intact hearing. Poor language development is an indication for referral for further testing of speech and hearing.

Structures of the ear should be palpated for tenderness and the helix and lobe *gently* tugged. The mastoid region should be percussed for tenderness associated with mastoiditis or trauma.

NOSE

Anatomy and physiology. The functions of the nose depend on patency and include smell, filtration, humidification, and warming of inspired air. New-

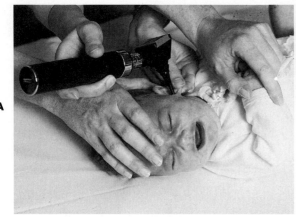

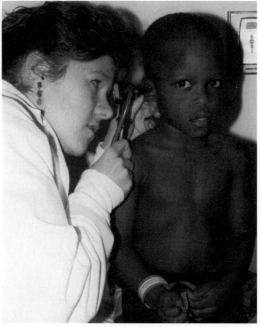

FIG. 4-4. Positioning for examination of the ear. **A,** Infant. **B,** Child. (**A** from Wong DL: *Whaley & Wong's essentials of pediatric nursing,* ed 5, St Louis, 1997, Mosby.)

borns and young infants are obligate nose breathers and become agitated when they cannot breathe through their noses.

Evaluation. The shape and size of the nose is inspected, as are visible internal structures. Observe for swelling, ecchymosis, discharge, lacerations, and foreign bodies. Depending on the chief complaint each nare may be checked for patency by having the child obstruct one nare, close the mouth, and breathe in and out of the open nare.

Nasal congestion is a frequent complaint voiced by parents in the emergency department. The etiology of nasal congestion and discharge is usually infectious. Viral nasopharyngitis (the common cold) is a frequent etiology in children of all ages. In the newborn, infection with *Chlamydia trachomatis* must be ruled out when both eye and nasal discharge are present. Bacterial causes are more common in older children with sinusitis. Nasal discharge after head trauma may be a sign of cerebrospinal fluid leakage and a basilar skull fracture. Unilateral nasal discharge is seen in the child with a nasal foreign body. Allergic rhinitis is seen in older infants and children, along with sneezing and watery eyes.

MOUTH/THROAT

Anatomy and physiology. Major structures of the mouth are present at birth, with the exception of the teeth (Fig. 4-5). As the infant develops, teeth begin to erupt. Although teething is a part of physical development, the timing of dentition is quite variable. The tongue is larger in relation to the oral cavity in the young child when compared to the adult, and the tonsils of the school-age child are generally larger than in the adult.

Evaluation. The mouth examination yields information about cranial nerve function, dentition, and the presence of infection. The lips, buccal mucosa, dentition, tongue, hard and soft palate, uvula, tonsillar pillars, tonsils, and posterior pharynx are inspected. Signs of infection include swelling, masses, redness, and exudate (Fig. 4-6).

Infants and toddlers commonly resist attempts to open the mouth, whereas preschoolers enjoy cooperating during the mouth examination—if their fears are verbally allayed. Most children respond when the examination is made fun. Using such phrases as "Show me how pretty your teeth are" or "Let's see

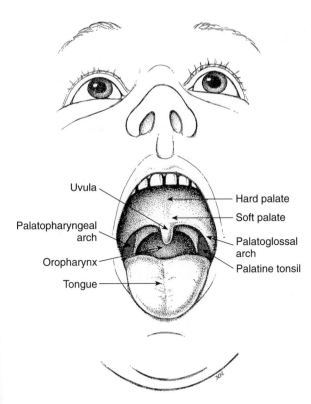

FIG. 4-5. Interior structures of the mouth. (From Wong DL: *Whaley & Wong's essentials of pediatric nursing,* ed 5, St Louis, 1997, Mosby.)

Labels on figure:
- Uvula
- Palatopharyngeal arch
- Oropharynx
- Tongue
- Hard palate
- Soft palate
- Palatoglossal arch
- Palatine tonsil

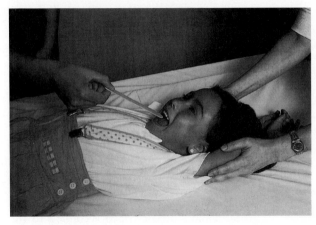

FIG. 4-6. Positioning the child for examining the structures of the mouth. (From Wong DL: *Whaley & Wong's essentials of pediatric nursing,* ed 5, St Louis, 1997, Mosby.)

if Mickey Mouse is hiding at the back of your throat" will often gain the child's cooperation.

If a tongue depressor is needed to view the posterior pharynx, prepare the child. Frightened children may cooperate if the tongue depressor is called a "popsicle stick" of the child's favorite flavor. Avoid gagging the child if possible. If it is necessary to gag the child to view posterior structures, do so quickly and gently. Save this unpleasant maneuver for last. Prepare to quickly rotate the child to the side to avoid aspiration in case of vomiting. Allow the child to be comforted by the parent soon after the examination is complete.

NECK

Anatomy and physiology. The neck of young infants is very short, making anatomic landmarks sometimes difficult to identify. Infants younger than 3 to 4 months of age have limited head control, but as they develop head control improves. By 6 months of age the infant can hold the head erect and steady.

Evaluation. The neck is inspected for size, shape, asymmetry, range of motion, and posture, as well as tenderness, masses, jugular venous distention, and tracheal deviation. Abnormalities in the shape of the neck include webbing, the presence of masses, and edema. Asymmetry may indicate torticollis or nerve palsy. Cervical adenopathy, in the absence of other physical findings, is often a variation of normal in preschoolers and school-age children.

The neck is palpated for lymph nodes or masses. Size, mobility, tenderness, and firmness of the nodes or mass should be noted. Lastly, the neck may be auscultated for bruits.

CHEST

Anatomy and physiology. The shape of the chest of young infants is fairly round. In the newborn the chest circumference is about 1 inch less than the head circumference. With age, the transverse diameter increases to nearly one and a half times the anteroposterior diameter. By the toddler years, head circumference almost equals the chest circumference. After this period, the chest circumference exceeds the head circumference and abdominal girth.

Changes in breast appearance occur primarily in the newborn period and at the onset of puberty. These changes are regulated by hormonal influence.

Evaluation of the chest. Examination of the thorax yields information about the ribs, lungs, heart, and breast development. The chest is inspected for size, shape, symmetry, and respiratory effort. Abnormal shape and size of the chest may indicate underlying pathology of the lung(s), heart, or bony structures. Widening of the anteroposterior diameter, or barrel chest, is seen in children with chronic lung diseases, such as severe asthma, cystic fibrosis, or restrictive lung disease secondary to severe scoliosis. Protrusion of the sternum is known as *pigeon chest* (pectus carinatum), and sternal depression is called *funnel chest* (pectus excavatum).

When masses, injured areas, or deformities of the chest are identified they should be palpated for size, tenderness, and mobility.

Physical findings are described according to the landmarks of the chest. Imaginary lines of the anterior chest include the anterior axillary, midclavicular, and midsternal lines. Imaginary lines of the side include the anterior axillary, the midaxillary, and the posterior axillary lines. Imaginary lines of the back include the posterior axillary, scapular, and vertebral lines.

Physical findings can also be described according to their proximity to the ribs and sternum. Ten ribs can be palpated anteriorly, and all twelve may be palpated on a very thin child posteriorly. The nipple line can be estimated at the fourth intercostal space on a child in whom breast development has not occurred. Posteriorly the tip of the scapula lies near the eighth rib.

Evaluation of respiratory effort. The evaluation of respiratory effort includes observing the child's level of consciousness, as well as looking for obvious signs of an increase or decrease in the work of breathing. The child with wheezing and retractions who is smiling and running around the examination area is generally in minimal respiratory distress. The child who is posturing, mouth breathing, and has an anxious appearance is in more serious distress.

Chest movements should be symmetric and coordinated with breathing. Asymmetry in movements, such as "seesaw" respirations, represents severe respiratory distress and requires prompt medical attention. Retractions also represent respiratory distress in the infant and young child. The severity of retractions directly represents the degree of respiratory effort. They may be seen intercostally, sternally, suprasternally, subcostally, or in the clavicular region. Intercostal, subcostal, and supraclavicular retractions are typically seen in lower airway obstruction. Sternal and suprasternal retractions are

often seen in upper airway obstruction such as with croup or narrowing of the airway. Diminished respiratory effort or respiratory distress in the child with an altered level of consciousness is a sign of respiratory failure.

The anterior chest, posterior chest, and axillary region are auscultated for heart and lung sounds. Breath sounds should be of equal intensity on each side of the chest. They diminish naturally toward the base of the thorax. Because the chest wall and musculature of infants and young children are fairly thin, breath sounds in this age group will be louder. The breath sounds in older children and adolescents are more faint.

In infants and young children with nasal congestion it may be difficult to distinguish between sounds produced by nasal secretions in the upper airway and sounds produced in the chest. To facilitate the distinction, remove nasal secretions with a bulb syringe. Saline nose drops can be used to loosen secretions. Compare sounds auscultated at the cheek and neck with sounds auscultated in the chest. The harsh sounds of secretions will be louder at the cheek and neck if produced in the upper airway.

The inspiratory and expiratory phases of respiration are fairly equal. A prolonged expiratory phase is seen in conditions with air trapping and the inability to exhale efficiently. Such conditions include asthma and bronchiolitis.

Evaluation of the heart. When auscultating the heart, the first heart sound is identified and evaluated. Next the second heart sound is evaluated. Heart sounds should be singular and distinct. The amplitude, rate, and rhythm should be noted. With the exception of soft, functional murmurs and physiologic splitting, additional sounds are generally abnormal. If a child does have a murmur, it is accentuated when the child is febrile. Most heart murmurs heard in the child occur after the first heart sound. If a murmur is present, its location is described in relation to the first and second heart sounds. For example, systolic murmurs occur after the first (systolic) heart sound. Diastolic murmurs occur after the second (diastolic) heart sound.

To complete the evaluation of the cardiovascular status, note the quality of central and peripheral pulses, capillary refill time, and blood pressure. Orthostatic blood pressure readings are indicated for children experiencing syncope or dizziness. Blood pressure readings of all extremities are indicated if congenital heart disease is suspected.

ABDOMEN

Anatomy and physiology. Abdominal organs are more easily examined in the child because the abdominal wall is relatively thin, the abdominal muscles are less well developed than in the adult, and there is less subcutaneous tissue. The protuberant abdomen and relatively exposed organs, however, are more likely to sustain serious injuries from relatively mild trauma.

Evaluation. The size and shape of the abdomen is inspected with the child reclining. Abnormal findings include evidence of trauma such as bruising, rashes, asymmetry, distention, or peristaltic activity. Because the abdomen is protuberant in young infants, normal anatomic findings must be distinguished from abdominal distention. Peristaltic waves are seen in small infants with intestinal obstruction.

Auscultation of the abdomen is performed before palpation. All four quadrants are auscultated for the presence and quality of bowel sounds. Bowel sounds are normally heard every 10 to 13 seconds. Hyperactive, hypoactive, or absent bowel sounds are noted.

The abdomen is palpated for tenderness, size of the organs (particularly the liver and spleen), and masses. This is best accomplished with the knees flexed to promote relaxation of the abdominal wall (Fig. 4-7). The abdomen of an infant or toddler is soft and protuberant. Organ position and musculature varies according to the child's age; however, underlying structures are usually easily palpated because the abdominal muscles have not fully strengthened. Many infants have umbilical hernias of various sizes. Ordinarily they are not problematic, and they resolve spontaneously with increasing strength of the abdominal muscles.

Abdominal pain or tenderness is describe by location, quality, radiation, and intensity. Children with debilitating abdominal pain require rapid evaluation. Rebound tenderness is a sign of peritoneal irritation and is elicited with gentle but deep pressure to the abdomen, which is rapidly released. On release the child experiences sharp abdominal pain.

The location and size of the liver and spleen are palpated. The liver border is usually palpable 2 to 3 cm below the right costal margin in the child, and the spleen, which is more difficult to palpate, is felt at the left costal margin. Tenderness of either organ is abnormal. A palpable spleen in a child with sickle cell anemia may be caused by splenic sequestration, which

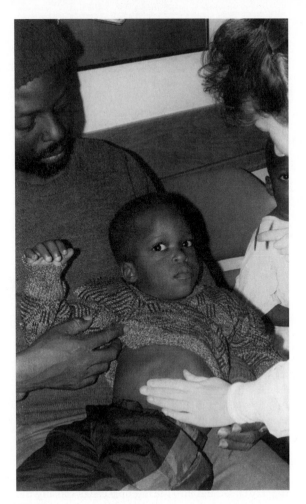

FIG. 4-7. An abdominal exam on a young child.

is considered a medical emergency. When symptoms suggest an underlying pathology, the nurse may attempt to palpate for associated masses. For example, an "olive" felt in the upper right quadrant of an infant with vomiting and weight loss may be indicative of pyloric stenosis; a "sausage-shaped" mass may be indicative of intussusception.

GENITOURINARY SYSTEM

Anatomy and physiology. The components of the male and female genitalia are present at birth and grow incrementally at varying rates until puberty. At puberty the sexual organs begin to enlarge, and pubic hair appears. Initially pubic hair is soft and straight, but with development it becomes coarse and curly. Menstruation (menarche) usually occurs in female adolescents between 8 and 16 years of age.

The urinary system develops early in gestation. The kidneys, though developed at birth, continue to mature during the first year of life. Until then the kidneys are unable to concentrate urine effectively. Bladder capacity increases proportionately as the child develops.

Evaluation. Before the genitourinary examination the procedure is explained to the child. Children are extremely modest, and their privacy should be ensured by keeping them covered with a gown and the genitalia covered with a sheet or gown until the area is to be examined. The exam room curtains should be pulled and/or the door closed.

The genitals are inspected for abnormalities such as rashes, lesions, swelling, masses, evidence of trauma, discharge, color, or odor. Common complaints related to the genitourinary system include diaper rash, vaginal discharge, swelling and/or pain in the inguinal region, and testicular pain. Variations in genital development and findings depend on the age of the child. Premature female infants tend to have prominent labia majora and clitorises. Newborn females may have a small amount of bloody discharge that resembles a menstrual period due to the presence of maternal hormones. The hymenal opening of preschool, school-age, and adolescent females may vary in size.

Males have penile erections throughout the life span. Male infants may have testes that "float" out of the scrotal sac and into the inguinal canal, causing the scrotum to look flat or empty. In older males the testes are fairly apparent in the scrotum.

The suprapubic region is palpated for tenderness. If the child has been a victim of multiple trauma the pelvis is checked for stability. Abnormal masses are palpated for pain, tenderness, and mobility.

RECTUM

Anatomy and physiology. The rectal examination yields information about neurologic function, as well as the presence of intestinal pathology such as parasitic infestation and gastrointestinal bleeding. The rectum is normally tightly closed and slightly hyperpigmented.

Evaluation. A rectal examination is recommended on all children with a chief complaint of abdominal pain. Like the genitourinary examination, this exam is performed with respect for the child's privacy. The exterior of the rectum is inspected for rashes, protrusions, lesions, and evidence of trauma. The buttocks may be stretched apart to check for fissures. Stool may be tested for blood when the chief complaint is abdominal pain, diarrhea, or rectal or abdominal trauma.

Internal rectal palpation is usually done by a physician or advanced practice nurse. Infants and young children are best examined in the prone position and can be allowed to straddle the parent's waist. Older children and adolescents can lie on either side with the uppermost leg flexed at the waist. Stool obtained from this examination is tested for blood.

EXTREMITIES

Anatomy and physiology. The bones of the infant and young child are porous and flexible, and bone growth occurs at epiphyseal-metaphyseal junctions called *growth plates*. These developmental differences predispose the child to a unique array of injuries, including growth plate injuries, cortical fractures, greenstick fractures, and bent or bowed bones with no evidence of a fracture.

Evaluation. When inspecting an injured extremity the nurse should first observe whether the child uses the limb and if so to what degree. Findings are compared to the opposite side. Swelling, redness, or deformity is abnormal. Common chief complaints related to the extremities include pain, swelling and deformity associated with trauma, and abnormal use of an extremity. Variations of normal are usually seen in the lower extremities such as mild bowlegs or knock knees.

The most painful area of the extremity is palpated at the end of the examination, with areas proximal and distal to the injury palpated first. Tenderness, crepitus, swelling, heat, and induration are abnormal findings. Pulses distal to the area in question are palpated. Color, sensation, and degree of movement of the extremity are evaluated. If a joint is involved, range of motion of the entire extremity is tested.

SKIN

Anatomy and physiology. The texture of the child's skin changes with age; as hair follicles proliferate, skin thickens and toughens due to friction. Birthmarks, including café-au-lait spots, hemangiomas, Mongolian spots, and nevi, are common in children. These may or may not be associated with underlying systemic pathology.

TABLE 4-4	Pediatric Immunizations—Sample Schedule*	
AGE	**DISEASE**	**VACCINE**
0 to 1 month	Hepatitis	(HB)
2 months	Diphtheria, tetanus, acellular pertussis	(DTaP #1)
	Polio	(OPV or IPV #1)
	H. influenza B	(HiB #1)
	Hepatitis	(HB #2)
4 months	Diphtheria, tetanus, acellular pertussis	(DTaP #2)
	Polio	(OPV or IPV #2)
	H. influenza B	(HiB #2)
6 months	Diphtheria, tetanus, acellular pertussis	(DTaP #3)
	†H. influenza B	(HiB #3)
	‡Polio	(OPV #3)
6 to 18 months	Hepatitis	(HB #3)
12 months	Varicella	(Var)
12 or 15 months	Measles, mumps, rubella	(MMR #1)
	H. influenza B	(HiB #4)
15 or 18 months	Diphtheria, tetanus, acellular pertussis	(DTaP #4)
	‡Polio	(OPV or IPV #3)
4 to 6 years	Diphtheria, tetanus, acellular pertussis	(DTaP #5)
	Polio	(OPV or IPV #4)
	Measles, mumps, rubella	(MMR #2)
14 years	Diphtheria, tetanus (adult vaccine)	

OPV = live oral polio vaccine.
IPV = inactivated polio vaccine.
*Several variations of this schedule are acceptable based on CDC and American Academy of Pediatrics recommendations.
†Hib: the 3rd dose at 6 months of age may be omitted depending on the type of conjugate vaccine administered.
‡Polio: the 3rd dose of polio may be given at 6 months (OPV) or 15-18 months (OPV or IPV).

Evaluation. Inspect skin color and texture, and observe for evidence of trauma or the presence of lesions and rashes. Describe skin lesions and rashes by distribution and character. Normal skin should be warm, smooth, and without excessive moisture. Common chief complaints related to the skin include rashes, diaper rash, impetigo, and rashes associated with childhood illness (e.g., chicken pox).

Exanthems are common in the pediatric population. An accurate history of onset, evolution, changes in distribution, pain, and pruritus is helpful in identifying the etiology of a rash. Children with rashes of an infectious nature must be identified and separated from other patients within the emergency department. A Wood's lamp may be used to identify fungal skin rashes. While most skin rashes do not constitute an emergency, petechial and purpuric rashes are associated with life-threatening illnesses and require emergent interventions.

The skin is palpated for temperature, moisture, and turgor. Skin lesions are palpated for warmth, tenderness, and texture. Light pressure to the lesion will determine if the lesion blanches. The reddish purple rash that is not raised and does not blanch with pressure is petechial or purpuric.

WELL CHILD CARE RECOMMENDATIONS

The American Academy of Pediatrics has made recommendations on the frequency, timing, length, and priorities of well child visits to a primary care provider. These recommendations are based on the immunization schedule and other health screening requirements (Table 4-4). During these visits a comprehensive examination of the physical, developmental, and psychosocial status of the child or adolescent is performed. At the same time the parent is given anticipatory guidance on expected developmental achievements, as well as the management of common childhood illnesses. In addition to acute health problems, the primary care provider is prepared to address issues such as temper tantrums, accident prevention, nutrition, and adolescent sexuality.

▍SUMMARY

The differences in the physical examination between children and adults are based on the child's age and stage of physical development. There are many chief complaints and physical findings that are seen exclusively in childhood, as well as complaints and findings seen exclusively in adulthood.

The purpose of the nursing assessment of the child in the emergency department is twofold. The first purpose is for the nurse to perform an initial brief history and physical examination and report abnormal or potentially life-threatening findings to a diagnostician promptly. The second purpose is for the nurse to be able to evaluate, document, and report the child's progress during the emergency department visit, particularly during and after interventions.

REFERENCES

1. Behrman RE: *Nelson textbook of pediatrics,* ed 4, Philadelphia, 1992, WB Saunders.
2. Bowlby J: *A secure base: parent-child attachment and healthy human development,* New York, 1988, Basic Books.
3. Seidel HM et al: *Mosby's guide to physical examination,* ed 3, St Louis, 1995, Mosby.
4. Tanner JM: *Growth and adolescence,* ed 2, Oxford, England, 1962, Blackwell Scientific Publications.
5. Wong DL: *Whaley & Wong's essentials of pediatric nursing,* ed 5, St Louis, 1997, Mosby.

CHAPTER 5

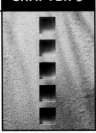

Pediatric Triage

Treesa Soud, Connie Andry

▌INTRODUCTION

The goal of pediatric triage is the same as that of adult triage, which is to identify seriously ill or injured patients and patients *at risk* so they can receive priority care. In pediatric patients, however, this determination can be somewhat difficult. Developmental and physiologic variations between a range of ages make communication, assessment, and the identification of serious illness or injury quite different when compared to adult triage. The purpose of this chapter is to review some of these developmental variations, outline triage assessment techniques that are useful in children, and describe the "red flags" associated with pediatric triage.

▌TRIAGE SETTING

Triage is performed in a variety of settings within hospital emergency departments (EDs), ranging from small semiprivate areas within the waiting room to private areas physically separate from the waiting area. A few EDs place the child directly in an examination room, eliminating the need for a formal triage area. In these settings, however, the priority of care must still be determined when other patients are waiting to be seen.

Regardless of the location of the triage area, children require privacy as much as adults. Even if triage is performed in a designated area within the waiting room, privacy can be maintained with a screening device. Young children and adolescents are modest and struggling with their new-found body image; exposing them in the chaotic ED environment does little to allay their fears or to gain their cooperation.

Children are less frightened of the unusual surroundings if the triage area is decorated in a childlike motif with wall hangings and/or colorful wallpaper. Nurses may choose not to wear white or monotone scrubs but instead wear colorful tops and pants that depict a friendly environment. The child who is at ease in the environment is usually more cooperative and can be assessed more rapidly.

WAITING AREA

Ideally the waiting area should be visible from the triage desk. Although this is not always possible, staff should be aware that children can become progressively ill while waiting to be seen. With continuous monitoring of the waiting area, these children can be identified.

Emergency departments treating significant numbers of adults and children should provide a separate waiting area for children. The busy ED can be a frightening place for a small child as patients and families rush in frightened, crying, or demanding care. Waiting rooms dedicated to children provide an environment more appropriate to the child. If a separate area is not possible, and the current waiting area is large enough, a section may be segregated for use by children.

▌APPROACH TO TRIAGE

STAFFING

Triage is performed by a variety of personnel, including nurses, physicians, and paramedics. Although nurses triage patients in most institutions, some busy emergency departments use pairs of personnel (e.g., while the nurse interviews a parent an EMT or nursing assistant obtains vital signs).[22] Other hospitals use a tiered approach to triage, particularly those treating large numbers of adults and children, who may have lengthy waits. Using this system a triage nurse briefly examines or "eyeballs" all patients and assigns a triage priority. Later the child is reassessed by a nurse to evaluate the level of care assigned and to determine if the priority of care should be upgraded. Regardless of the system used, the final triage decision should be made by an experienced emergency nurse with some knowledge of pediatrics, using pediatric triage criteria.

For the child's and parent's well-being, and from a public relations point of view, every child presenting to an emergency department should be evaluated by a caring, concerned health care provider. This individual should be able to initiate minor interventions such as splinting and applying ice to a suspected fracture and must be allowed to exercise judgment when performing tasks in the triage arena.

TRIAGE NURSE

The role of the triage nurse is to rapidly prioritize care for patients by determining the urgency of the illness or injury. This ability is dependent upon the nurse's experience, skill, and clinical judgment and the ability to set priorities in a sometimes chaotic environment.[23] In addition, the triage nurse is usually the child's and family's first contact in the emergency department, and it is this interaction that often sets the tone for the remainder of the ED visit.[19]

The triage nurse's responsibility does not end with the triage decision. Once the child has been evaluated and assigned a triage category, the nurse must continue to evaluate the child while waiting to be seen. Signs and symptoms of serious illness or injury can change rapidly, increasing the risk of rapid decompensation. Without frequent assessments, serious conditions can easily be missed.

To effectively triage infants and children, pediatric knowledge and experience is required. Nurses with little pediatric experience must first learn the differences between adult and pediatric anatomy and physiology, the developmental milestones of childhood, and the most common emergency department presentations. Additionally, pediatric assessment skills should be practiced over and over with a skilled pediatric preceptor. Pediatric triage classes are extremely useful in facilitating this process and enhance the learning process. In the long run, however, there is no substitute for practice and experience, which is why many emergency departments require 6 months to 1 year's worth of experience before a nurse is allowed to triage children (Box 5-1).

TRIAGE ASSESSMENT

The location of the triage area, the skills of the personnel manning the area, the number of staff available, and the average activity level seen within the ED all play a role in the degree of assessment performed during triage. The approach may be as simple as performing an eyeball assessment while focusing on the chief complaint to as complex as performing and documenting a complete nursing

---

Box 5-1 Sample Content for Pediatric Triage Training Program

Philosophy of pediatric triage
- Creating a child-friendly environment
- Approaching the child
- Approaching the parents/caregivers

Emergency department policies and procedures
- Triage admission procedures
- Standing orders/protocols

Legal considerations
- COBRA legislation/state laws
- Documentation
- Suspected child abuse or neglect

Dealing with violent or disruptive behavior
- Use of the panic button
- Defusing anger

Infection control

Review of child development
- Characteristics of psychosocial development
- Characteristics of physical development
- Tips for gaining the child's cooperation

The pediatric assessment
- The "across the room" assessment
- The triage history
- The triage physical
- Triage vital signs
- Pediatric red flags

The triage classification system
- Categories of classification
- Description of categories

Workshop—triage case studies

history and physical, including vital signs (or any variations of the above).

Institutions with a relatively small patient census or with adequate triage staffing may elect to perform a complete nursing history and physical at triage, alleviating the need for an additional nursing assessment once the child is placed in an examination room. With this approach a clerk or nursing assistant places the nonemergent child in an examination room. Other institutions with a high patient volume and limited triage staff may use the abbreviated triage approach. This system allows the nurse to rapidly assess or "eyeball" the child to rule out the presence of a life-threatening illness or injury before making the triage decision. With this approach the complete nursing assessment is performed by an emergency nurse once the child is placed in an examination room.

In EDs where a complete assessment is performed during triage, specialized equipment such as pulse oximetry; an automated blood pressure machine; Doppler device; rectal, oral, and tympanic thermometers; pediatric blood pressure cuffs; and/or a blood glucose monitor should be available. If the triage area is occasionally used by the physician or advanced nurse practitioner to examine a child, equipment such as an otoscope and ophthalmoscope should also be available (Box 5-2).

TRIAGE INTERVENTIONS

Triage interventions include splinting an injured extremity, applying ice to a fracture or sprain, controlling bleeding, or fully immobilizing a child after head or neck trauma. To improve patient flow many EDs

---

Box 5-2 Pediatric Triage Supplies and Equipment

Equipment
Clock
Desk
3 Chairs
Telephone
Examining table (optional)
Sink
Intercom to ER and to waiting area
Privacy screen (optional)
Wastebasket
Cart or cabinets for supplies
Laundry hamper
Blood pressure device (automated, or wall-mounted or hand-held sphygmomanometer)
Blood pressure cuffs (infant to adult sizes)
Doppler device
Infant and child scales
Thermometers (tympanic, rectal, and oral)
Pulse oximeter (optional)
Ophthalmoscope and otoscope (optional)

Supplies*
Pediatric cervical collars
Ice bags
Pediatric splints
Pediatric slings
Gauze pads (4 × 4 and 2 × 2)
Kling

Adhesive bandages
Examination gloves
Emesis basins
Wash basins
Normal saline for irrigation
Sterile water for irrigation
Betadine solution
Hydrogen peroxide
Alcohol preps
Contamination box
Sheets
Gowns (infant, child, adult)
Towels
Washcloths
Blankets
Diapers (small, medium, large)
Swabs for throat cultures (optional)
Urine collection cups
Urine collection bags (small and large)
Acetaminophen suspension, tablets, and suppositories
Ibuprofen suspension and tablets
Medicine droppers or syringes for oral administration
Medicine cups
Ammonia capsules
Universal Precautions supplies

*Also consider "latex-free" supplies (e.g., gloves, dressings)

have instituted standing orders or protocols that allow the triage nurse (or the nurse examining the child once in the ED) to obtain x-rays of injured extremities, bag a child for urine, administer antipyretics, and/or obtain a throat culture while the child is waiting to be seen. These procedures assure the parents that something is being done, even while they are waiting. They also speed up the assessment process once a health care provider is available to examine the child (Table 5-1).

TRIAGING OUT OF THE ED

Many parents seek emergency medical care when the child has a minor illness or injury because of a lack of access to or knowledge of primary care. The result is a costly, ineffective system of emergency care. Reimbursements for emergency department care do not match the costs, patient waiting times increase, costly tests may be performed on children on whom the health care provider has little background knowledge, and there is no guarantee of follow-up or ongoing care.

One unique, yet effective approach to triage has been instituted in a few settings that allow nonurgent children with primary care complaints to be triaged to outside agencies.[11,13,24] With this system seriously ill children receive prompt care within the emergency department, whereas children with primary care problems are referred to a primary care physician or clinic.

When referring children to outside agencies the triage nurse must be able to perform a comprehensive patient assessment (including vital signs) and adequately identify children with nonurgent complaints. Referrals include making phone calls to the child's primary care physician or enrolling

children in community clinics. Discharge teaching emphasizes follow-up with an appropriate primary care provider.[35] Strict triage criteria must be established, and adequate staffing is required because nursing interventions can exceed 20 to 30 minutes.[13,35]

Emergency departments using this system have observed a decrease in costs—even when patients are not charged for the triaging examination, and patient satisfaction has increased—even when parents do not seek follow-up care.[8,13,24] The concern that the nurse may triage seriously ill children away from the emergency department has not been realized. In fact one study compared the physician's diagnosis with the triage nurse's diagnosis and found they were in agreement, or the physician felt the child was less seriously ill than the nurse, in 93.4% of the patients.[24]

Variations in the interpretation of the COBRA law from state to state have made this approach attractive in some areas and less attractive in others. Although COBRA clearly states that all patients must receive a medical screening examination, the qualifications of personnel performing the examination are not defined. In Florida the state Access to Care law is quite strict and does not equate triage with a medical screening examination. To institute this type of program an institution must develop formal rules and regulations regarding the medical screening examination, must specify the qualifications of the person performing the examination, and must develop referral protocols with primary care providers and community clinics. From a legal standpoint, the institution must be able to prove that the medical screening examination performed at triage met the same standard of care as would be afforded any other patient within the institution, regardless of ability to pay.

TABLE 5-1	Extremity Trauma Sample Protocol	
INITIAL INTERVENTIONS	**EXCEPTIONS**
1. Immobilize and elevate the injured extremity.	Angulated deformities should be treated urgently.
2. Apply ice to the injured extremity.	
3. Assess neurovascular function in the extremity, including color, movement, sensation, capillary refill, and pulses. Compare the injured and noninjured extremities.	Signs of neurovascular compromise require the child be seen emergently.
4. Place sterile dressings on open wounds.	
5. Order x-rays according to protocol.	All open fractures are treated emergently.

▌TRIAGE CRITERIA

Triage criteria are developed within each emergency department to assist emergency department staff in determining the priority of care when multiple patients are waiting to be seen. Many similarities exist between triage tools (e.g., the apneic child is treated emergently in all institutions); however, a nurse's ability to interpret the triage criteria is related to that nurse's degree of pediatric knowledge and experience. If the nurse has limited experience, strict interpretation of the triage criteria is required, as the intuitive ability, judgment, and assessment skills necessary to identify the acutely ill or injured child may not yet be developed. In institutions where nurses possess strong pediatric skills, the approach to triage may be less "criteria" or "vital signs" oriented, allowing the nurse latitude in making decisions based on observations and physical findings.

In the majority of emergency departments triage priorities are divided into three categories, which are defined as emergent, urgent, and nonurgent for both adults and children. Using this system the child falling within the emergent category has a life- or limb-threatening illness or injury, the child in the urgent category requires care within the next 2 hours, and the child in the nonurgent category may safely wait longer than 2 hours (Table 5-2). Some emergency departments have adopted systems that include four or five categories of care. The following is an example of a five-category system:

Category 1—resuscitation

Category 2—life-threatening illness or injury

Category 3—may be seriously ill, requires medical care within the next 2 hours

Category 4—requires care, but not necessarily the specialized care of an emergency department

Category 5—requires teaching and/or education

APPROACHES TO DEVELOPING A PEDIATRIC TRIAGE SYSTEM

Multiple approaches are used when developing triage categories and the criteria defining those categories. Triage criteria most often address physiologic parameters, such as vital signs and an assessment of the ABCs, and historical data to identify children at risk, such as premature infants or children with sickle cell disease or cystic fibrosis. Some may describe subtle findings that are consistent with serious illness, such as the child who does not respond appropriately to the environment for age. Others may list specific chief complaints that would serve as red flags, such as the neonate with a fever. Most institutions use a combination of all of these approaches.

Occasionally triage systems use specific tools for categorizing the priority of care, for example, the use of a form for scoring findings, which then automatically assigns the level of care. Others use algorithms to guide the nurse through the triage process (Fig. 5-1). Although the use of these tools can be time consuming, the ultimate goal is to assist the nurse in forming a triage decision and to justify or validate that decision.[26,36] These tools are especially useful in illustrating to the inexperienced nurse some of the nuances of triage decision making in general and pediatric triage in particular. (See Table 5-3 for a sample approach to triage and Box 5-3 for important points.)

TABLE 5-2	Triage Categories	
CATEGORY	**DESCRIPTION**	
Emergent	Children requiring major resuscitation or immediate intervention to avoid loss of life or permanent disability	
Urgent	Children requiring prompt, but not immediate care. Children with conditions in which a delay of up to 2 hours will not compromise life or limb. Children in this category must be closely monitored while awaiting care.	
Nonurgent	Minor illness or injury; these children may safely wait over 2 hours without an increase in morbidity or mortality.	

From Haley K, Baker P: *Emergency nursing pediatric course,* ed 1, Chicago, Ill, 1993, Emergency Nurses Association.

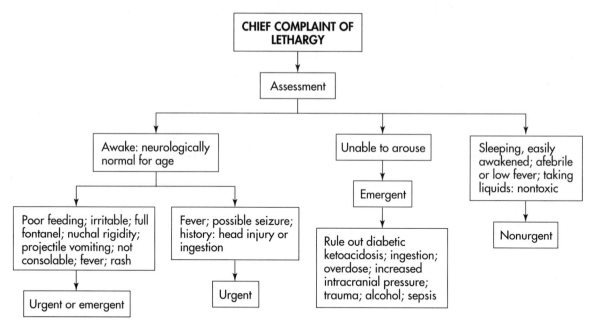

FIG. 5-1. Algorithm for chief complaint of lethargy. (Modified from Campbell LS in Thomas DO: Pediatric triage and assessment. In Sheehy SB, ed: *Emergency nursing: principles and practice,* ed 3, St Louis, 1992, Mosby.)

TABLE 5-3	Sample Approach to Triage Using Physiologic Criteria
CRITERIA	**DESCRIPTION**
Level I/emergent	
Airway/breathing	Bradypnea; apnea; gasping respirations; resting respiratory rate >60 (any age child); grunting respirations; ↓ inspiratory/expiratory breath sounds; inspiratory stridor; significantly increased work of breathing; positioning for air entry (tripod or "sniffing" position)
Circulation	
Peripheral pulses	Thready; weak; absent
Capillary refill	>2 seconds, with other significant findings
Skin color	Dusky; mottled; cyanotic; petechiae or purpura
Pulse rate	Absent; bradycardia for age; resting pulse >180 (any age child)
Blood pressure	Hypotension for age
Disability	
Muscle tone	Weak (floppy); absent
Fontanel	Sunken; bulging
Level of consciousness	Unusual irritability; extreme lethargy; unconscious; decreased response to pain; inability to recognize parents; weak or high-pitched cry
Temperature	Hypothermia (≤95° F or 35° C) or hyperthermia (≥107° F or 42° C)

Box 5-3 Important Points to Remember Regarding Pediatric Triage

- The purposes of triage are prioritization, efficiency, treatment, and public relations.
- The single most important means of prioritizing pediatric patients is accurately assessing "general appearance."
- Rigid adherence to the principle of "first-come, first-seen unless very sick" is incompatible with an efficient emergency room.
- Standing orders should enable the emergency room nurse to initiate certain therapies, such as acetaminophen for fever or splinting of suspected fractures.
- The triage nurse must anticipate and address patient concerns such as waiting time, pain, and disability. However, information offered by the triage nurse must be accurate. Reassurance that the physician will examine the child "within a few minutes" aggravates the situation if it does not occur.
- The triage nurse has a responsibility to prepare the child in such a way that maximal cooperation with the physician's examination can be obtained.
- Triage requires much thought and judgment. Rigid rules that require, for example, a full set of vital signs on all patients are no substitute for and are often an impediment to thoughtful judgment.

Author unknown.

Box 5-4 Components of the Pediatric Triage Assessment

"Across the room" assessment
- Does the child "look well," "look sick," or appear to "feel bad"?

The triage history
- Are there any underlying illnesses or psychosocial issues that may alter the initial triage impression? Are there cultural issues that require special attention during the assessment?

The triage physical
- Are the ABCDEs within normal limits?

The triage decision
- Based on history and physical findings, triage criteria, and previous knowledge and experience.

▌TRIAGE EXAMINATION

Pediatric triage consists of a series of assessment parameters that are used to determine the seriousness of a child's illness or injury. Although these are discussed separately in this chapter, in reality they are evaluated simultaneously. For example, while obtaining a history the nurse is observing the child's respiratory status and neurologic status. The triage examination can be separated into four categories: (1) the "across the room" assessment; (2) the triage history; (3) the triage physical, which includes the ABCDEs of assessment; and (4) the triage decision (Box 5-4).

"ACROSS THE ROOM" ASSESSMENT

The "across the room" assessment, or "eyeball" examination is a rapid evaluation of the child's status to identify the presence of a serious illness or injury that requires emergent care. It is a subjective impression of the child's status in which the nurse determines if the child "looks well," "feels bad," or "looks sick." Observational findings that support this subjective impression include the patency of the child's airway and the child's breathing pattern, color, and neurologic status (Table 5-4).

This *impression* is usually formed while the parent is relaying the chief complaint to the triage nurse. During this time, much information is derived by simply *looking* at a child. For example, the smiling, playful, bright-eyed infant has a patent airway, has adequate respirations, and is neurologically intact. This child "looks well." However, the pale, listless child who does not recognize the parent and is unaware of the surroundings "looks sick." This child is neurologically compromised and requires emergent interventions. Further triage evaluation will simply delay care.

Many children appear to "feel bad." It is these children that the ED nurse with limited pediatric experience has the most difficulty assessing. The

TABLE 5-4	The "Across the Room" Assessment
ASSESSMENT	**EXPLANATION**
Initial subjective impression	Does the child "look well," "feel bad," or "look sick"?
Airway	Is the airway clear, compromised, or obstructed?
Breathing	Is breathing normal, or is there an increase or decrease in the work of breathing?
Circulation	Is skin color pink, pale, mottled, or cyanotic?
Disability (neurologic status)	Is the child alert and active, quiet and withdrawn, crying continuously, unconcerned with the surroundings, or unresponsive?

TABLE 5-5	The CIAMPEDS History
FORMAT	**QUESTIONS**
(C) Chief complaint	*Why was the child brought to the emergency department?* What is the primary problem/concern and duration of complaint?
(I) Immunizations	*Are they up to date?* When were they last given? Table 4-4 lists the ACIP immunization schedule.
Isolation	*Has the child recently been exposed to any communicable diseases?*
(A) Allergies	*Does the child have any known allergies?* Is the child allergic to any medications? What was the child's reaction to the medication?
(M) Medications	*Is the child taking any prescription drugs or over-the-counter drugs* (e.g., acetaminophen)? When was the last dose administered and how much was given? Is the child on immunosuppressive medications?
(P) Past medical history	*Does the child have a history of any significant illness, injury, or hospitalization?* Does the child have a known chronic illness?
Parent's impression of child's condition	*What is different about the child's condition that concerns the caregiver?*
(E) Events surrounding the illness or injury	*How long has the child been ill? Was the onset rapid or slow?* Has anyone else in the family been ill? If the emergency visit is for an injury, when did the injury occur, was it witnessed, and what happened?
(D) Diet	*How much has the child been eating and drinking?* When was the last time the child ate or drank?
Diapers	*When was the child's last void?* How much was it? When was the child's last bowel movement? What did it look like and how large was the stool?
(S) Symptoms associated with the illness or injury	*What other symptoms are present?* When did the symptoms begin? Has the condition gotten better or worse?

From Haley K, Baker P: *Emergency nursing pediatric course,* ed 1, Chicago, Ill, 1993, Emergency Nurses Association.

febrile toddler may be quiet and appear flushed yet may be observant of the surroundings. Determining the seriousness of the illness in this child will require astute pediatric assessment skills, which include knowledge of normal development and illnesses common within this age group. However, even the best pediatric nurse, without additional historical information or the ability to perform a complete examination, cannot determine whether this child simply has an ear infection or is exhibiting early signs of bacteremia.

These children require a more comprehensive evaluation, and their triage assignment may be upgraded (see the following sections).

HISTORY

After the "across the room" assessment, and assuming the child is not emergently ill, further evaluation is indicated. The triage history and physical may be abbreviated or comprehensive depending on hospital protocols. For the purposes of discussion, a comprehensive triage history and physical is included in this chapter (see also Chapter 4).

The triage history consists of open-ended questions regarding the nature of the visit, duration of the illness or injury, and associated signs and symptoms (Table 5-5). Additional important questions include immunization status, allergies, exposure to infectious diseases, variations in normal activity and behavior, and pertinent past medical history. Medications taken routinely or since the illness or injury should also be determined, with specific reference made to over-the-counter medications such as antipyretics. Parents often think only of prescription drugs when asked about medications. If the infant is a neonate, questions regarding the pregnancy and delivery, birth weight, and length of stay in the hospital are appropriate. In adolescent females who have begun menstruating, the date of the last menstrual period is important.

Historical findings will reveal some children who should be seen immediately, regardless of the initial clinical impression. These children may be at risk of rapid decompensation because of the nature of the illness or injury, or they may have an underlying medical condition that could rapidly progress. A child may also be at increased risk of contracting a serious illness from other children while waiting to be seen. Examples of children who should be seen emergently based on historical findings include the reported ingestion of a toxic material or substance, a history of unconsciousness and/or recent seizures, potential anaphylaxis, a history of high impact trauma, or evidence of child abuse or sexual assault with the risk of flight from the ED.[34] Chronic conditions that may place the child at higher risk of rapid decompensation include a history of congenital heart defect, sickle cell disease, cystic fibrosis, or bronchopulmonary dysplasia (BPD). The immunosuppressed child on chemotherapy is also at risk of serious illness and requires priority care. Even if this child arrives in the ED with an occluded central line port, the history (e.g., parental report of the presence of neutropenia or fever) will

---

Box 5-5   Red Flags: Children Who May Require Emergent Management and/or Isolation Based on Historical Findings

- History of communicable illness (e.g., chicken pox or measles)
- History of an underlying medical condition (e.g., congenital heart defect, muscular dystrophy, sickle cell disease)
- Possible immunosuppression (e.g., child on chemotherapy)
- Neonate with fever
- History of child maltreatment with risk of flight from ED
- History of ingestion of toxic substance
- History of unconsciousness and/or seizures
- History consistent with potential to develop anaphylaxis

---

guide the emergency nurse's decision. This child may be provided either a private waiting room, to decrease the risk of contracting an illness from other children waiting to be seen, or may be placed directly in an examination room for immediate evaluation.

While obtaining the history the triage nurse may identify a child who must be isolated from other children because of the presence of a suspected contagious illness (e.g., chicken pox or measles). These children may be placed in a private waiting area or in an examination room with a door. Long delays in triage to obtain a lengthy history or perform a complete physical simply increase the risk of other children contracting the illness. For this reason many EDs without private waiting rooms place these children in either the emergent category or a "send back" category simply to provide isolation, even though the child may not require priority care (Box 5-5).

PHYSICAL ASSESSMENT

Young children are frightened by strangers and unusual surroundings; therefore efforts should be made to allay or ease the child's fears. The triage evaluation can be quite fun when a child is cooperative and helpful and almost impossible to perform when the child is crying and protesting. Not only are vital signs skewed in the crying child, but other children waiting to be seen also become frightened. By allowing the parent to hold the child, and by *observing* the child while obtaining the history from the caregiver, the child has a few minutes to become familiar with the triage nurse, and the nurse may have a few minutes to observe the child in a calm state. The "hands-on" part of the examination, including vital signs, is the most frightening portion of the assessment and is therefore performed at the end of the evaluation. Often, during the first few minutes of discussion with the parent the child begins to feel at ease with the examiner and will cooperate with the hands-on portion of the examination.

Helpful tips for performing the pediatric physical examination are described at length in Chapter 4. In the triage arena, however, the nurse has little time to gain the child's trust and cooperation. Some techniques that are useful in triage include placing stickers or small stuffed animals on the stethoscope, referring to the stethoscope as a telephone, and playing guessing games (e.g., "Let me guess what you ate for breakfast?"—while listening to the child's chest) (Table 5-6).

Airway. During the triage evaluation the child's airway is assessed for patency. Because the upper and lower airways of the child are significantly smaller than those of the adult, small amounts of mucus in the airway or edema of the soft tissue surrounding the airway can significantly affect the infant or small child's ability to ventilate.

Signs and symptoms of an upper airway obstruction include the presence of an audible inspiratory stridor, drooling, and dysphagia (drooling is normal in infants after the age of 2 to 3 months). In addition to these findings, older children may maintain an erect position to facilitate air entry. They will usually sit in the "tripod" position, using both hands to stay erect, or they will sit in the sniffing position with the chin thrust slightly forward. Infants and children in significant respiratory distress from an upper airway obstruction will exhibit tachypnea, tachycardia, severe retractions, nasal flaring, inspiratory stridor, and the use of the accessory muscles of respiration. Children with these symptoms are triaged emergently (Table 5-7).

Neonates and young infants are obligate nose breathers; therefore nasal congestion can produce signs of respiratory distress and complaints of "difficulty breathing" or a "rattling chest." To make a triage determination the nares should be suctioned and the infant reassessed for the continued presence of respiratory symptoms. If signs of significant respiratory distress persist, the infant is triaged emergently.

Breathing. Ventilatory status is initially assessed during the across the room assessment with observations of the child's skin color and neurologic status.

TABLE 5-6	Tips for the Pediatric Triage Assessment	
AGE	TIPS
Infants	Allow parent/caregiver to hold child during the assessment
	Uncover only as necessary—avoid chilling
	Look, listen, then FEEL
	Obtain vital signs, particularly the rectal temperature, LAST
Toddlers	As above
	Talk to parents/caregivers first, while observing child
	Allow child to touch equipment
	Play games
Preschoolers	As above
	Stay at eye level (sit or squat), avoid sustained eye contact
	Use distraction techniques (e.g., ask the child to tell a story about a favorite cartoon character or experience)
School-age children	As above, but may stand or sit by parent
	Engage the child in interactions (e.g., questions, games, brief explanations)
Adolescents	Provide brief, honest explanations as desired
	Respect privacy

However, when the chief complaint is "difficulty breathing" or the nurse has reason to believe the child's breathing may be compromised—or the nurse is not sure (e.g., history of cold symptoms or fever)—a more thorough assessment is performed.

Triage assessment of the child's ventilatory status includes auscultating breath sounds and observing chest wall movement by lifting the child's shirt. *Simply looking at the infant or child's chest through the shirt reveals little information.* When observing the child's chest, the work of breathing is assessed by noting the child's breathing pattern, rate of respirations, and respiratory effort. When auscultating the chest, inspiratory and expiratory air exchange is assessed, as well as the presence of adventitious breath sounds (e.g., wheezing, crackles). The absence of adventitious sounds or the absence of air exchange in the child with signs of respiratory distress (e.g., the asthmatic who is not wheezing) is not normal and may indicate impending respiratory failure.

Signs and symptoms of respiratory distress in the child include retractions, grunting, tachypnea, tachycardia, pallor or mottled skin, and/or the use of the accessory muscles of respiration. Retractions are considered a hallmark sign of respiratory distress in the child and are observed when an upper or lower airway obstruction causes negative intrathoracic pressure to "cave in" or retract the child's compliant chest wall during inspiration. The location (supraclavicular, intercostal, substernal) and severity (mild, moderate, severe) of retractions, coupled with an assessment of the child's neurologic status, color, and air exchange, can assist in making the triage decision. Mild intercostal retractions in an alert, talkative 2 year old are not as concerning as supraclavicular, intercostal, and substernal retractions in another child who is pale and listless.

TABLE 5-7	The ABCDEs of Pediatric Triage	
ABCDEs	**ASSESSMENT PARAMETERS**	**RED FLAGS**
Airway	Patency	Audible airway sounds such as stridor, wheezing
	Posture	Positioning for best air entry (tripod position or "sniffing" position)
Breathing	Respiratory pattern	Grunting respirations
	Respiratory rate	Abnormal resting respiratory rate for age in the afebrile child
	Respiratory effort	Retractions, nasal flaring, anxious facial expression
	Breath sounds	Adventitious sounds; decreased air movement
Circulation	Skin color and turgor	Pale, mottled, or cyanotic skin, presence of skin tenting
	Peripheral pulses	Weak or absent peripheral pulses
	Capillary refill	Capillary refill time >2 seconds
	Heart rate	Bradycardia: tachycardia for age
Disability (neurologic status; discomfort/pain)	Arousability	Slow to arouse or unusual irritability
	Consolability	Unable to console yet quiet when left alone
	Response to environment	Unaware or unconcerned with surroundings, unresponsive
	Fontanel (infants)	Bulging, tense fontanel when upright and not crying, sunken in the presence of other signs of dehydration
	Pupils	Unreactive
	Muscle tone	Weak; floppy; absent
Exposure/ environment	Skin temperature	Cool/clammy/cold skin
	Skin color	Pallor, mottling, cyanosis
	Skin abnormalities	Injuries, wounds, bruises, petechiae, purpura, rashes

Modified from Soud T, Taylor ML: Assessment and triage. In Henderson DP, Brownstein D, eds: *Pediatric emergency nursing manual,* New York, 1994, Springer Publishing Co.

Grunting is a sign of severe respiratory distress in the young child and is evidenced by an audible expiratory grunt coupled with inward movement of the lower chest wall. Grunting can also be produced by nonrespiratory illnesses such as cardiac conditions (e.g., congestive heart failure and myocarditis), fevers in excess of 38.5° C (101.3° F) that may be associated with bacteremia or sepsis, and a variety of other serious conditions such as pyelonephritis, intussusception, or peritonitis.[21,30] Respiratory causes of grunting produce severe respiratory distress and usually indicate an interstitial or alveolar disease (e.g., pneumonia or pulmonary edema).[10] Children with grunting respirations are triaged emergently.

Late and ominous findings that indicate respiratory failure or impending respiratory arrest include decreased respiratory effort and rate and/or cyanosis. A decrease in the rate and depth of retractions in the child with previous signs of significant respiratory distress may indicate the child is fatigued and can no longer maintain an increase in the work of breathing. Cyanosis is not relied on to determine the presence of hypoxia, because almost 50% of the relatively anemic child's blood must be deoxygenated for the blue color to be evident. In the hypoxic adult only 30% of the blood must be deoxygenated. Children with signs of central cyanosis or with signs of decreasing respiratory rate or effort are triaged emergently (Box 5-6).

Circulation. Infants and young children have larger surface area to volume ratios than adults, higher metabolic rates, and greater insensible fluid losses. Additionally, the young child has less circulating blood volume, is relatively anemic, and has a smaller stroke volume than in the adult. All of these differences influence the triage assessment of the pediatric patient.

For example, because insensible fluid losses are greater in the child, fever and diaphoresis coupled with ongoing fluid losses such as vomiting and diarrhea can rapidly lead to dehydration.[31] Therefore the triage assessment in a child with a history of fever, vomiting, diarrhea, and/or decreased fluid intake should include observation for signs of dehydration (Table 5-8).

Young children are better able to physiologically compensate for both fluid and blood losses than the adult by peripheral vasoconstriction and tachycardia, which maintain cardiac output and blood pressure. Tachycardia is the infant and young child's principal method of increasing cardiac output when perfusion is

---

Box 5-6   Red Flags: Respiratory Signs and Symptoms in the Infant and Child

- Retractions
- Use of accessory muscles of respiration
- Nasal flaring
- Tachypnea
- Head bobbing with respirations
- Drooling
- Grunting
- Positioning for air entry (tripod position or sniffing position)
- Inspiratory stridor
- Audible wheeze
- Apnea, gasping respirations, or decreasing respiratory effort
- Bradypnea
- Cyanosis
- Altered mental status

TABLE 5-8   Signs and Symptoms Associated with Degrees of Dehydration

ASSESSMENT PARAMETERS	MODERATE (URGENT)	SEVERE/SHOCK (EMERGENT)
Weight loss	6% to 10%	11% to 15%
Skin turgor	Normal	Tenting
Mucous membranes	Sticky/dry lips	Dry
Fontanel (infants)	Normal to depressed	Sunken
Eyes	Normal to sunken	Sunken, without tearing
Blood pressure	Normal	Normal to decreased
Urine output	Normal to decreased	Significantly decreased to absent
Neurologic status	Normal to mildly lethargic, with age-appropriate behavior	Decreased LOC/no response to pain

compromised, and unlike in the adult the child can maintain a tachycardic heart rate for a prolonged period of time. When the heart rate exceeds 180 to 200 beats per minute, however, ventricular filling time is compromised and cardiac output—and therefore peripheral perfusion—will decrease. Conversely, a bradycardic heart rate in an infant or young child—because of the child's limited stoke volume—produces an immediate and life-threatening drop in cardiac output.

Emergent management is required for any child exhibiting signs of decreased cardiac output such as pallor, mottled skin, cool extremities (associated with other signs of shock), diminished or absent peripheral pulses, delayed capillary refill (>2 seconds), or an altered mental status (lethargy or decreased response to pain). Late signs of circulatory compromise include hypotension, bradycardia, and hypothermia (Box 5-7).

Disability (neurologic status). Assessment of neurologic status is one of the most important yet overlooked components of the triage assessment. Perhaps this is because nurses with limited experience cannot relate findings to normal developmental milestones of childhood and are instead focused on overt, measurable findings such as vital signs. With childhood development, however, cognitive, language, and motor skills change; knowledge of age-appropriate behavior can provide important clues to a child's neurologic status (Table 5-9).

When a parent arrives at the triage desk the emergency nurse first observes the child's activity level, age-appropriate response to the environment, and level of consciousness. This observation often sets the tone for the rest of the examination. If a previously normal child is limply lying the parent's arms and

---

TABLE 5-9	Quick Review of Normal Developmental Parameters
AGE	**ACTIVITY**
Birth to 1 month	Visually tracks objects
	Startle reflex (Moro)
	Turns head side to side
	Responds to sounds
1-2 months	Lifts chin
	Coos
	Smiles socially
	Reaches for objects
4-5 months	Babbles/laughs/squeals
	Rolls over
	Visually follows objects 180°
	Moro reflex gone
	Grasps toys
	Pulls to sitting with little head lag
6-8 months	Reaches for objects
	Turns to voice
	No head lag
	Hand-to-mouth activity
	Transfers objects
	Sits with support
	Sits alone
9-11 months	Plays pat-a-cake
	Says "Mama" or "Dada"
	Crawls or scoots
	Tries to find hidden objects
	Pulls to stand/cruises/walks
12-17 months	Drinks from a cup
	Pincer response
	Tosses or rolls a ball
	Speaks two to three words
18-23 months	Walks well
	Three or more words
	Feeds self
2 years	Runs
	Observes pictures
	Climbs stairs
3 years	Knows first name
	Counts three objects
	Stands momentarily on one foot
6 years	Knows colors
	Counts to ten
	Balances on one foot

Modified from Soud T, Taylor ML: Assessment and triage of the pediatric patient. In Henderson DP, Brownstein D, eds: *Pediatric emergency nursing manual*, New York, 1994, Springer Publishing Co.

Box 5-7   Red Flags: Circulatory Compromise in the Infant and Child

- Pallor, mottled skin, cyanosis
- Decreased, thready, or absent peripheral pulses
- Delayed capillary refill (>2 seconds)
- Cool extremities
- Decreased or absent urinary output
- Altered mental status
- Hypotension
- Bradycardia

does not appear to be aware of or concerned with the ED environment, the child is emergently ill and further triage assessment is not required. On the other hand, if a child runs up to the triage desk and asks, "What's your name?", the child is probably not seriously ill.

The neurologic examination can be complicated in some children by an underlying medical disorder that affects neurologic development (e.g., cerebral palsy, mental retardation). Unless the child is well known to the emergency department staff, the best assessment of the child's current neurologic status, compared to baseline, is made by the parents or caregivers. Questions regarding normal activity levels can provide important clues to the seriousness of the illness or injury in these children.

In normal children, objective tools to measure neurologic status, such as the Glasgow Coma Score (GCS), Pediatric Glasgow Coma Score (PGCS) (see Tables 7-4 and 7-5), and AVPU score, are also useful at triage. Although the GCS and PGCS scores (spontaneous eye opening, verbal response, motor response) were originally developed to assess the victim of head trauma, they are useful in other children as well, because they provide the nurse with specific, measurable assessment parameters. They do not always work effectively, however, because frightened young children may refuse to cooperate with the examination. At triage the most rapid and easily performed tool is the AVPU score, which includes Alert, responds to Verbal stimulation, responds to Painful stimulation, or is Unresponsive.

Infants are more difficult to evaluate neurologically than older children. However, an examination of the infant's daily routine, including feeding pattern, elimination pattern, and activity level, provides clues to the infant's status. For this reason the history provided by the caregiver or parent is often considered more important than a lack of overt physical or neurologic findings on examination. Positive historical findings include less-than-normal intake over the past 24 hours, a history of decreased activity, a history of fewer than four wet diapers in the past 24 hours, and a history of increased drowsiness.[10] Observational findings that indicate the need for emergent care include changes in the quality of the child's cry (weak, moaning, or high-pitched cry), an abnormal reaction to the parents (crying continually with no response to comforting; barely responding), decreased response to social overtures (dull or expressionless face), and changes in state variation or arousability (difficult to arouse, barely responds, or will not arouse).[18]

An additional assessment parameter in the infant is the anterior fontanel, which closes between 9 and 18 months of age. A bulging fontanel in the quiet, upright infant may indicate increased intracranial pressure, whereas a sunken fontanel may indicate dehydration (Box 5-8).

Disability (discomfort/pain). Another important component of the triage evaluation is the assessment of pain or discomfort, which should be added to the ABCDEs of assessment.[33] Pain may be a symptom of a significant underlying illness or injury such as the severe lower abdominal pain associated with appendicitis or volvulus, or pain may be related to an obvious pathologic process such as the pain associated with a deformity caused by a fracture.

When pain is a symptom of an illness or injury, the triage nurse should determine the onset of the pain, the location of the pain, and the character of the pain. A determination of the child's demeanor (e.g., stoic or crying) and observation and palpation at the site of the pain are also required. Crying is often assumed to be caused by fear and anxiety during the initial assessment and may be overlooked as a symptom of pain.

Children, unlike adults, often attempt to hide the degree of pain associated with an illness or injury to avoid a perceived unpleasant sequela such as a shot. Clues to the presence and degree of pain include a stoic

---

Box 5-8   Red Flags: Neurologic Compromise in the Infant or Child

- Difficult to arouse
- Unaware or unconcerned with the environment
- Decreased or absent response to pain
- Does not recognize the parents/caregivers
- Inconsolable crying when held and quiet and listless when left alone*
- Bulging anterior fontanel (infant)
- High-pitched, moaning, or whimpering cry
- Abnormal pupillary response
- Unequal pupils (unless normally unequal—anisocoria)
- Decreased or absent muscle tone
- Nuchal (back of the neck) rigidity

*This finding is called *paradoxic irritability* and can reflect involvement of the CNS. It is most commonly observed in infants with meningitis.

child who sits quietly and refuses to move, the child who vigorously denies pain yet physical evaluation reveals an obvious source of pain, and children who are unable or unwilling to walk (the otherwise ambulatory child who arrives at triage in a wheelchair).

Many emergent conditions that would cause pain are obvious (e.g., a traumatic amputation or serious burn). These conditions are treated emergently because they are life threatening, not because of the severity of the pain. Other conditions may be life threatening but are more subtle. The child who cries despite attempts at comforting and is quiet and listless when left alone may be exhibiting signs of a CNS disease such as meningitis. The infant who cries uncontrollably and draws up the lower legs but then stops abruptly may be exhibiting signs of volvulus or intussusception.

Whether or not a child in pain is treated emergently, urgently, or nonurgently depends on presenting signs and symptoms, historical findings, suspicion of a serious underlying condition, and the policies of the emergency department regarding the treatment of pain in children. Because pain severity can sometimes be difficult to evaluate in the child, and because pain management practices in children have been found to be inadequate,[6,33] the presence of an overt condition that would cause pain (e.g., an obvious fracture) may place the child in a higher category of care than the child without pain. (For a complete discussion of pain management in the child, see Chapter 29.)

Exposure/environment. Depending on the chief complaint and the triage nurse's initial impression of the child, an examination of the abdomen, chest, back, and/or extremities may be required to observe the child's breathing pattern, a wound, or to palpate an injured area such as a fracture. Of course exposing the child depends on the child's age, the degree of exposure required, the ability to provide privacy, and the suspected underlying condition. Examples of children who may require exposure to further evaluate signs of illness or injury include children with possible fractures, victims of suspected child abuse, children with a history of respiratory distress, children with a history of significant fever and no other focal signs of infection (e.g., runny nose or ear pain), and children with rashes.

The presence of a rash may indicate a communicable illness that requires isolation, such as chicken pox, or it may indicate the presence of a significant underlying infection. If the child presents with a significant fever and/or a history of fever and an altered level of consciousness, the trunk should be examined for the presence of petechiae. Petechiae are small purplish, hemorrhagic spots that do not blanch and may indicate meningococcemia or a *Haemophilus influenzae* infection, both of which can be life threatening (and are therefore emergent) and both of which require isolation.

When an injured extremity is evaluated for a suspected fracture, not only is the injured area palpated, but the distal portion of the extremity is also palpated. Signs of neurovascular compromise such as a decreased or absent pulse, decreased or absent sensation, delayed capillary refill, extreme pallor, or coolness of the extremity indicate the need for emergent care. Open fractures are always treated emergently.

VITAL SIGNS/MONITORING

Heart rate and respiratory rate (Table 5-10). Triage leveling rarely relies solely on abnormal vital signs in the child—unless they are grossly abnormal—because vital signs are less valuable indicators of the severity of an illness or injury than in adults. Many factors such as fear, anxiety, pain, or crying can produce significant tachycardia and tachypnea in the otherwise normal, healthy child. Fever also produces a rise in the child's heart rate and respiratory rate. In fact, the respiratory rate rises approximately 10% for every one-half degree centigrade above normal.[14] If the infant or young child is frightened or crying, the respiratory rate can easily approach 60 breaths per minute.

Although vital signs are rarely relied on to make the triage decision, there are a few notable exceptions.

TABLE 5-10	Normal Pediatric Vital Signs		
AGE	HR (BEATS/ MIN)	RR (BREATHS/ MIN)	BP (SYSTOLIC, MM HG)
Newborn	100-160	30-60	50-70
1-6 wk	100-160	30-60	70-95
6 mo	90-120	25-40	80-100
1 yr	90-120	20-30	80-100
3 yr	80-110	20-30	80-110
6 yr	70-100	18-25	80-110
10 yr	60-90	15-20	90-120

From Siedel JS, Henderson DP: *Prehospital care of pediatric emergencies,* Los Angeles, 1987, Pediatric Society, American Academy of Pediatrics, and Calfornia EMS-C Project.

HR, Heart rate; *RR,* respiratory rate; *BP,* blood pressure.

Bradycardia produces a significant drop in cardiac output in the infant and small child and requires emergent management. Conversely, extreme tachycardia that compromises ventricular filling time (e.g., supraventricular tachycardia [SVT]) will also cause a significant drop in cardiac output. In both of these cases the heart rate, however, will only confirm what the nurse should have already identified on clinical assessment (i.e., signs of decreased peripheral perfusion evidenced by weak, thready, or absent peripheral pulses; delayed capillary refill [>2 seconds]; extreme pallor, mottling, or cyanosis; and an altered mental status).

Blood pressure. Blood pressure is another important monitoring parameter depending on the age of the child and the chief complaint. The usefulness of blood pressure measurements at triage is debatable, because hypotension is a late sign of shock in the young child and if a child is hypotensive clinical signs are usually evident. Additionally, accurate blood pressure measurements can be difficult to obtain in the young, active child; can be time consuming; and require the use of a properly sized cuff—which should cover two thirds of the upper arm. Serial blood pressure measurements are extremely valuable, however, in evaluating the course of illness in a seriously ill or injured child. Therefore obtaining a baseline blood pressure at triage is often a routine protocol in children at risk. Examples of children considered at risk include those with a history of significant trauma, particularly of the abdomen or head, and children with a history of fluid loss coupled with neurologic findings not consistent with the child's developmental level (e.g., the child unconcerned or unaware of surroundings). Because hypotension is a late sign of compromise in the child, it is always treated emergently.

Temperature. Temperature measurements may be taken rectally, orally, axillary, or via tympanic thermometer. The rectal and oral routes are the most accurate methods of evaluating the core body temperature, and the axillary route is the least reliable method beyond the neonatal period.[2,4,27] (See Chapter 26, Box 26-5.) There is continuing debate over the accuracy of the tympanic thermometer in determining core body temperature.[3,25,27,28] In general, the tympanic thermometer can be used to screen for temperature in the older child in whom the degree of fever is not a factor in determining the seriousness of the illness (e.g., the child with a laceration). When an accurate temperature

is required to make the triage decision, such as the neonate with possible fever, a rectal temperature is the most reliable method.[28] If obtaining a rectal temperature at triage is not feasible, a reliable history of fever from the parent (e.g., the parent documented the presence of a fever by taking the child's temperature) may be used to make the triage decision in infants younger than 2 months of age.

Whether or not the presence of a fever is associated with a serious illness depends on the child's clinical presentation, history, and age. Because of limited immunity, febrile neonates are more susceptible to serious illnesses than older infants and children. Therefore febrile infants (temperature >38° C or 100.4° F) younger than 1 month of age are always treated emergently. Although febrile infants between 1 and 3 months of age may also be seriously ill, most present with benign illnesses. However, because of the increased risk of serious illness, these infants are always seen either emergently or urgently. The age definition (e.g., <2 months = emergent) is dependent upon the assessment skills of the staff and physician preference. In emergency departments where personnel infrequently treat children, febrile infants younger than 2 to 3 months of age should be classified as emergent or "send backs." (For a discussion of specific risks and suggested criteria, see Chapter 26.)

Beyond early infancy the height of the fever is often considered a determinant of triage leveling. Although some studies have indicated that fevers in excess of 40° C (104° F) are more commonly associated with serious bacterial infections in children younger than 2 years of age,[16,17] one recent study found there is no relationship between the degree of fever and the seriousness of the illness.[1] Whether or not the height of the fever is considered in the triage determination depends on the child's presenting signs and symptoms, the history, the pediatric assessment skills of the triage personnel, the ability to provide antipyretics at the triage desk, and the ability to frequently evaluate the child while waiting to be seen. Many EDs have established arbitrary triage criteria of a fever of 39.4° C (103° F) as an urgent category simply because of the anticipated need for antipyretic therapy.

Hypothermia, defined as a core temperature of ≤95° F (35° C), is perhaps a more specific indication of serious illness in the infant or child than fever. It may develop from prolonged exposure to the environment, it may signal a serious underlying infection such as sepsis, or it may signal an insult to the hypothalamic temperature regulating mechanism in the brain. Hypothermia produces metabolic acidosis, decreased respiratory effort, decreased perfusion, and ultimately cardiorespiratory arrest.[34] For these reasons the hypothermic child is triaged emergently. True hyperthermia caused by heat illnesses such as heat exhaustion and heat stroke is also treated emergently. As temperatures approach and exceed 107.2° F (42° C), CNS disturbances result and cellular damage occurs.

Pulse oximetry. Many institutions now have pulse oximetry available in the triage area. Pulse oximetry is a rapid, noninvasive and therefore painless method of determining oxygen saturation within the blood (Sao_2). It is most commonly used to determine the severity of a respiratory illness that produces respiratory symptoms such as asthma.[15]

Normal pulse oximetry readings should reflect an arterial oxygen saturation of 95% to 100%, at sea level. When pulse oximetry readings indicate a decrease in oxygen saturation, the partial pressure of oxygen in the blood drops dramatically. For example, a drop in oxygen saturation to 85% may reflect a drop in the partial pressure of oxygen in the blood to 55%. (See Chapter 6, Fig. 6-1.) In general, the child with signs of significant respiratory distress and an Sao_2 of less than 93% is triage emergently.

Pulse oximetry does have some drawbacks. It does not measure carbon dioxide content in the blood, nor does it measure acid-base balance, both of which may be required to definitively identify the presence of respiratory failure.[5] In addition, patient conditions and environmental factors may affect pulse oximetry readings. Patient movement, decreased perfusion states (e.g., hypovolemia or hypothermia), stray ambient lighting, elevated bilirubin levels, and the presence of nail polish on the nailbeds can all affect the accuracy of the data.[5] Despite these limitations, pulse oximetry is a valuable screening tool at triage when correlated with a child's history and physical findings.

▍ SUMMARY

Pediatric triage requires knowledge of developmental parameters of the child and astute assessment skills. Nurses who triage children should seek educational programs to learn the differences between children and adults and the "red flags" associated with the pediatric patient. As the nurse "practices" with pediatric patients, assessment skills will improve. Subjective impressions and intuition will become second nature, and the nurse will recognize the "sick" child.

REFERENCES

1. Alpert G, Hibbert E, Fleisher GR: Case control study of hyperpyrexia in children, *Pediatr Infect Dis J* 9(3):160–161, 1990.
2. Anagnostakis D et al: Rectal-axillary temperature difference in febrile and afebrile infants and children, *Clin Pediatr* 32(5):268–272, 1993.
3. Bernardo LM et al: A comparison of aural and rectal temperature measurements in children with moderate and severe injuries, *JEN* 22(5):403–408, 1996.
4. Brown RD et al: A probability nomogram to predict rectal temperature in children, *Clin Pediatr* 31(9): 523–531, 1992.
5. Durren M: Getting the most from pulse oximetry, *J Emerg Nurs* 18(4):340–342, 1992.
6. Friedland L, Kulick R: Emergency department analgesic use in pediatric trauma victims with fractures, *Ann Emerg Med*, 23:203–207, 1994.
7. Haley K, Baker P: *Emergency nursing pediatric course*, ed 1, Chicago, Ill, 1993, Emergency Nurses Association.
8. Hansagi H: Referral of non-urgent cases from an emergency department; patient compliance, satisfaction and attitudes, *Scand J Soc Med* 18:249–255, 1990.
9. Harrahill M: Pulse oximetry: pearls and pitfalls, *J Emerg Nurs* 17(6):437–439, 1991.
10. Hewson PH et al: Markers of serious illness in infants under 6 months old presenting to a children's hospital, *Arch Dis Child* 65:750–756, 1990.
11. Kelly KA: Referring patients from triage out of the emergency department to primary care settings: one successful emergency department experience, *J Emerg Nurs* 20(6):458–463, 1994.
12. Koziol-McLain J, Oman K, Edwards G: Ear temperatures: making research-based clinical decisions, *J Emerg Nurs* 22(1):77–79, 1996.
13. Kuensting LL: Triaging out children with minor illnesses from an emergency department by a triage nurse: where do they go? *J Emerg Nurs* 21(2):102–108, 1995.
14. Levin R, Nahlen BL, Kent D: Diagnosis of the child with fever in the emergency department, *J Emerg Nurs* 14(6):359–364, 1988.
15. Mayefsky JH, El-Shinaway Y: The usefulness of pulse oximetry in evaluating acutely ill asthmatics, *Pediatr Emerg Care* 8(5):262–264, 1992.
16. McCarthy PL, Dolan TF: Hyperpyrexia in children—eight year emergency room experience, *Am J Dis Child* 130:849, 1976.
17. McCarthy PL, Jekel JF, Dolan TF: Temperature greater than or equal to 40° C in children less than 24 months of age: a prospective study, *Pediatr* 59:663–668, 1977.
18. McCarthy PL et al: Observation scales to identify

serious illness in febrile children, *Pediatr* 70(5):802, 1982.

19. McMillan JR et al: Satisfaction with hospital emergency department as a function of patient triage, *Health Care Manage Rev* 3:21, 1986.

20. Ogle KA: Problems in the management of respiratory distress. In Luten RL, ed: *Problems in pediatric emergency medicine,* New York, 1988, Churchill Livingstone.

21. Poole SR, Chetham M, Anderson M: Grunting respirations in infants and children, *Pediatr Emerg Care* 11(3):158–161, 1995.

22. Purnell LD: A survey of emergency department triage in 185 hospitals: physical facilities, fast track systems, patient classification systems, waiting times, and qualification, training, and skills of triage personnel, *J Emerg Nurs* 17(6):402–407, 1991.

23. Rice M, Abel C: Triage. In Sheehy, SB, ed: *Emergency nursing: principles and practice,* ed 3, St Louis, 1992, Mosby.

24. Rivara FP et al: Pediatric nurse triage, *AJDC* 140:205, 1986.

25. Romano MJ et al: Infrared tympanic thermometry in the pediatric intensive care unit, *Crit Care Med* 21(8):1181–1185, 1993.

26. Rowe JA: Nurse educator: triage assessment tool, *J Emerg Nurs* 18(6):540–544, 1992.

27. Schuman AJ: The accuracy of infrared auditory canal thermometry in infants and children, *Clin Pediatr* 32(6):347–354, 1993.

28. Selfridge J, Shea SS: The accuracy of the tympanic membrane thermometer in detecting fever in infants aged 3 months and younger in the emergency department setting, *J Emerg Nurs* 19(2):127–130, 1993.

29. Siedel JS, Henderson DP: *Prehospital care of pediatric emergencies,* Los Angeles, 1987, Pediatric Society, American Academy of Pediatrics, and California EMS-C Project.

30. Singer JI: Grunting respirations: chest or abdominal pathology, *Pediatr Emerg Care* 8(6):354–358, 1992.

31. Soud T: Airway, breathing, circulation, and disability: what is different about kids? *J Emerg Nurs* 18(2):107–116, 1992.

32. Soud T, Taylor ML: Assessment and triage of the pediatric patient. In Henderson DP, Brownstein D, eds: *Pediatric emergency nursing manual,* New York, 1994, Springer Publishing Co.

33. Tanabe P: Recognizing pain as a component of the primary assessment: adding D for discomfort to the ABCs, *J Emerg Nurs* 21(4):299–304, 1995.

34. Thomas DO: The ABC's of pediatric triage, *J Emerg Nurs* 14(3):154–159, 1988.

35. Vixby M: Personal communication, Cardinal Glennon Children's Hospital, St Louis, Nov 1995.

36. Wiebe R, Rosen LM: Triage in the emergency department, *Emerg Med Clin North Am* 9:491–505, 1991.

CHAPTER 6

Respiratory Failure and Shock

Treesa Soud

INTRODUCTION

The two most common conditions leading to cardiopulmonary arrest in the child are respiratory failure and shock. Unlike the adult who suffers an acute cardiopulmonary arrest from a disorder of the cardiovascular system (e.g., myocardial infarction), conditions leading to respiratory failure or shock in the child are most commonly preceded by a prodromal stage in which all of the child's physiologic reserves are exhausted. By the time a cardiopulmonary arrest occurs and physiologic reserves are depleted, the child's chance for survival is diminished. Therefore the key to survival is early recognition and intervention of conditions that lead to respiratory failure or shock. The purpose of this chapter is to describe the pathophysiology, clinical presentation, and treatment of the child once respiratory failure or shock is identified. Respiratory distress, including severe respiratory distress, and dehydration are reviewed in subsequent chapters.

RESPIRATORY FAILURE

DEFINITION

Respiratory failure is a clinical condition characterized by impaired gas exchange within the lungs causing metabolic demands of the body to go unmet. It is represented by inadequate oxygenation of the tissues and/or inadequate elimination of carbon dioxide.

ETIOLOGY

Respiratory failure can be caused by any illness, injury, or congenital defect that affects ventilation. Etiologies are classified as conditions that affect the lungs, such as pneumonia; the airways, such as croup or asthma; the

nervous system, such as head trauma or the ingestion of a respiratory depressant; the respiratory muscles, such as muscular dystrophies; or the thorax, such as a ruptured diaphragm (Table 6-1).

In children the most common causes of respiratory failure are conditions that directly affect either the upper or lower respiratory tract. These include pneumonia, bronchiolitis, asthma, foreign bodies, and croup.

PATHOPHYSIOLOGY

The respiratory system is comprised of lung tissue, the respiratory muscles, ribs, the airways, and the central nervous system. The high incidence of respiratory failure in the pediatric population is attributed to many different factors directly related to the child's unique respiratory anatomy and physiology. For example, the child's small, compliant airways are prone to obstruction or collapse from mucus or edema. When obstructed these small airways produce a significant increase in airway resistance which increase the work of breathing and oxygen consumption. The chest wall, including the respiratory muscles and rib cage, is less well developed than in the adult and collapses inward on inspiration (retractions). In addition, the immature musculature is prone to rapid fatigue. And lastly, oxygen consumption is higher in the child than in the adult, predisposing the child to rapid decompensation when oxygen supply is decreased. (For a more complete review of respiratory physiology, see Chapter 10.)

Respiratory control of ventilation. The respiratory center, located in the brainstem, controls ventilatory function and is highly sensitive to carbon dioxide (CO_2) levels and hydrogen ion (H^+) concentration. Excesses of either—as occurs during respira-

TABLE 6-1	Causes of Respiratory Failure in Children
SYSTEMS	**EXAMPLES**
Central nervous system depression	
Immaturity	Apnea of prematurity
Infection	Sepsis
	Meningitis
Intoxication	Phenobarbital
	Narcotics
Anoxia or increased intracranial pressure	Head trauma
	Near drowning
Musculoskeletal disorders	
Neuromuscular	Reye syndrome
	Muscular dystrophies
	Guillian-Barré
	Poliomyelitis
Skeletal	Scoliosis
	Severe pectus excavatum
	Congenital thoracic dystrophy
Thoracic disorders	Flail chest
	Ruptured diaphragm
	Diaphragmatic hernia
Respiratory tract disorders	
Upper airway obstruction	Croup
	Epiglottitis
	Foreign body
Lower airway obstruction	Asthma
	Bronchiolitis
	Foreign body

From Soud T: Respiratory failure and shock. In Haley K, Baker P, eds: *Emergency nursing pediatric course,* Chicago, Ill, 1993, Emergency Nurses Association.

tory failure—produce a direct effect on the respiratory center, increasing the rate of ventilation. As the rate of ventilation increases, carbon dioxide levels drop as CO_2 is blown off. If the child has an acute obstructive disorder that would increase the rate of ventilation, such as asthma, this normal compensatory response should produce a lower than normal CO_2. However, as the obstruction worsens CO_2 levels will begin to rise to normal or above normal levels and signs of respiratory failure will be observed.

Oxygen does not significantly affect the respiratory center but instead acts on chemical receptors called *chemoreceptors* located in the carotid and aortic bodies. Chemoreceptors are sensitive to oxygen levels, carbon dioxide levels, and hydrogen ion concentrations; however, they are most strongly stimulated when arterial Pao_2 falls into the 30 to 60 mm Hg range.[13]

Gas exchange. Gas exchange occurs both within the lung tissue and at the cellular level. In the lungs any one of three mechanisms can diminish gas exchange, including inadequate alveolar ventilation, mismatching of alveolar ventilation and pulmonary perfusion, and abnormal diffusion of gases at the alveolar capillary interface. Alveolar ventilation is dependent upon all of the components of the respiratory system. Failure of any of these systems, such as decreased CNS input, respiratory muscle fatigue, or increased airway resistance, can lead to respiratory failure in the child.

Ventilation and perfusion are expressed as a ratio of ventilation (V) to pulmonary blood flow (Q), which reflects the degree of gas exchange that takes place in the pulmonary beds. Conditions that may affect the V:Q ratio and produce respiratory failure in the child include those in which pulmonary capillary blood flow is decreased, such as low cardiac output states (shock), or conditions in which alveolar ventilation is compromised, such as airway obstruction.

Diffusion is the ability of oxygen and carbon dioxide to move across the alveolar-capillary membrane and is affected by the surface area of the alveolar capillary membrane and the pressure difference between alveoli and pulmonary capillaries. Conditions that affect the amount of gas diffusing through the capillary membrane include interstitial edema, pneumonia, and bronchiolitis.

Oxygen transport. Oxygen moves through the bloodstream in either the dissolved state (Pao_2 = partial pressure of oxygen) or bound to hemoglobin (Sao_2 = oxygen saturation). Nearly all oxygen in the serum, approximately 97%, is bound to hemoglobin. The amount of bound oxygen is directly affected by the hemoglobin concentration in the serum and the affinity of oxygen for hemoglobin. The relationship of oxygen-bound hemoglobin to dissolved oxygen is expressed by the oxygen-hemoglobin saturation curve (Fig. 6-1). On the flat portion of the curve (at the top of the illustration) a reduction in dissolved oxygen (Pao_2) has little effect on oxygen saturation (Sao_2)—in fact, hemoglobin is nearly 100% saturated between the

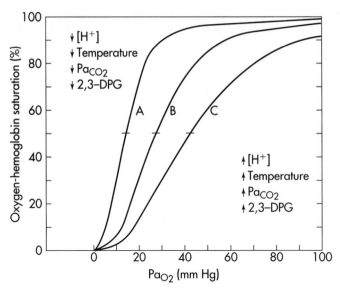

FIG. 6-1. Oxygen-hemoglobin saturation curve. *A,* Shift of curve to left, resulting in reduced O_2 dissociation from hemoglobin; the effect is increased O_2 saturation for any given Pao_2 value. *B,* Oxygen-hemoglobin saturation curve. Note the flat portion of the curve, where a reduction in Pao_2 has little effect on O_2 saturation, and the steep portion, where a reduction in Pao_2 significantly diminishes O_2 saturation. *C,* Shift of curve to right (with factors responsible for the phenomenon), resulting in increased O_2 dissociation from hemoglobin; the effect is a reduced O_2 saturation for any given Pao_2 value. (From Blumer JL: *A practical guide to pediatric intensive care,* ed 3, St Louis, 1991, Mosby.)

TABLE 6-2	Normal Mean Arterial Blood Gas Values for Children			
	NEWBORN (AGE 24 HRS)	**INFANT (1-24 MOS)**	**CHILD (7-19 YRS)**	**ADULT**
pH	7.37	7.40	7.39	7.40
Pao_2 (mm Hg)	70	90	96	100
$Paco_2$ (mm Hg)	33	34	37	40
BE (mEq/liter)	−6.0	−3.0	−2.0	0.0
HCO_3 (mEq/liter)	20	20	22	24

From Helfaer MA, Nichols DG, Rogers MC: Developmental physiology of the respiratory system. In Rogers MC, ed: *Textbook of pediatric intensive care,* vol 1, ed 2, Baltimore, 1992, Williams & Wilkins.

Pao_2 ranges of 70 to 100 mm Hg. Once Pao_2 drops below 70 mm Hg (illustrated by the steep portion of the curve), there is a dramatic drop in Sao_2.

Conditions such as acidosis or alkalosis, increases or decreases in body temperature, and changes in carbon dioxide levels will affect the oxyhemoglobin saturation curve, shifting it to the left or right. Conditions that shift the curve to the left increase the affinity of oxygen for hemoglobin, and conditions that shift the curve to the right decrease the affinity of oxygen for hemoglobin. Therefore, in the child with an increasing $Paco_2$ and/or acidosis, the curve shifts to the right, decreasing the oxygen affinity for hemoglobin (and therefore Sao_2). However, the off-loading of oxygen to the tissues is increased. Conversely, hypothermia causes the curve to shift to the left, increasing the oxygen

affinity for hemoglobin and decreasing the off-loading of oxygen to the tissues.

Acid-base balance. The respiratory system and the renal system work in unison to maintain acid-base balance. In general the acid-base balance remains constant from childhood to adulthood with very minor average differences within the normal ranges (Table 6-2). Although a comprehensive discussion of acid-base balance is covered in Chapter 14, a brief review of acid-base disorders as they relate to respiratory failure follows.

Under normal conditions, tissue metabolism produces carbon dioxide, which is carried by the bloodstream to the lungs, where it is eliminated. Conditions that impair alveolar ventilation by obstructing

| Box 6-1 | The Bicarbonate/Carbonic Acid Buffer System[8] |

$$CO_2 + H_2O \longleftrightarrow H_2CO_3 \longleftrightarrow H^+ + HCO_3^-$$

Carbon dioxide   Water   Carbonic acid   Hydrogen ion   Bicarbonate

the airways, such as asthma or croup, or by hypoventilation caused by ingestion of a CNS depressant decrease the ability of the alveoli to expel carbon dioxide. As carbon dioxide levels rise, carbonic acid is produced, which subsequently dissociates into bicarbonate (HCO_3^-) and hydrogen ions (H^+) (Box 6-1). With increased hydrogen ion production the renal system attempts to regulate the pH by excreting hydrogen ions and reabsorbing bicarbonate ions. The degree of regulation (or compensation) is reflected in the serum pH, $Paco_2$, bicarbonate, and the amount of base excess or deficit. When compensatory mechanisms fail, uncompensated respiratory failure is observed. The most common acid-base abnormality of the child in the emergency department is acute, uncompensated respiratory acidosis defined by an increase in $Paco_2$ and a decreasing pH.

The determination of respiratory failure can be difficult in children with chronic respiratory conditions, particularly when blood gas findings are nonspecific and the child's normal clinical state is unknown. For example, the child with a chronic lung disease such as bronchopulmonary dysplasia (BPD) may have a normal pH in the presence of a "normally" high $Paco_2$ and low Sao_2—chronic, partially compensated respiratory acidosis. In these children the history, serial blood gases, and continuous monitoring of clinical status (e.g., level of consciousness, respiratory rate, respiratory effort, color, capillary refill, and parental report of normal activity levels for the child) are required to make the diagnosis of respiratory failure.

CLINICAL PRESENTATION

The presentation of respiratory failure can vary significantly depending on etiology. Children with respiratory disease such as asthma may exhibit obvious signs of respiratory distress that can lead to failure, whereas the child who has ingested a drug causing respiratory depression will show no overt signs of respiratory distress such as retractions or grunting.

In all cases the initial diagnosis of respiratory failure should be based on historical data and clinical findings—not blood gas analysis. Historical findings should include the cause of the illness or injury (e.g., trauma, ingestion, foreign body aspiration), symptoms associated with the illness (e.g., rapid or slow breathing, retractions, lethargy), length of the illness, significant past medical history (e.g., musculoskeletal disorder, respiratory disease), previous hospitalizations, and medications (e.g., bronchodilators, steroids).

Although it is sometimes difficult to distinguish between severe respiratory distress and respiratory failure, clear cut physical findings associated with respiratory failure include decreased or absent breath sounds, decreasing respiratory rate and effect, a decreasing level of consciousness, decreased response to pain, poor muscle tone, and/or a weak to absent cough reflex. Cyanosis is a late and ominous sign of respiratory failure in the child; therefore its presence or absence is not relied on to make the diagnosis.

EMERGENCY DEPARTMENT INTERVENTIONS

Diagnostic testing performed on the child with suspected respiratory failure includes blood gases and a chest x-ray. Additional testing is performed based on additional clinical findings and the suspected underlying etiology. Blood gas analysis is important in determining the degree of acidosis; when submitted to the lab it must be accompanied by a notation of the child's temperature (remember that hypothermia or hyperthermia may shift the oxygen-hemoglobin saturation curve) and the amount of supplemental oxygen being administered to the child.

Because respiratory failure is a clinical diagnosis, definitive treatment for obvious signs of respiratory failure, including positive pressure ventilation, is not delayed while awaiting blood gas results. In addition, blood gas analysis may be unreliable in the vigorously crying child or may be misinterpreted if the child has a normal $Paco_2$ in the presence of severe respiratory distress (e.g., asthmatic).

NURSING CARE AND EVALUATION OF THE CHILD IN RESPIRATORY FAILURE

Children arriving in the emergency department with clear signs and symptoms of respiratory failure are treated emergently. The child with decreasing respiratory effort and an altered level of consciousness is immediately placed in the jaw thrust or head-tilt, chin-lift position, and bag-valve-mask (BVM) ventilation with 100% oxygen is begun. The child in severe respiratory distress may initially be placed in a position of comfort and receive supplemental oxygen via a nonrebreather face mask while the underlying cause is addressed (e.g., albuterol for the asthmatic). If the response to therapy is not immediate, however (e.g., improved oxygenation, decreased work of breathing), assisted ventilation is required. While ventilatory status is being stabilized the child is placed on the pulse oximeter and cardiac monitor, and venous access is achieved.

Nursing interventions to decrease oxygen consumption and carbon dioxide production include instituting temperature control measures (e.g., over-bed warmers for hypothermia or prompt administration of antipyretics for fever), the recognition and treatment of pain, and promoting a calm and reassuring atmosphere for the child. If the child has not been intubated but continues to exhibit signs of severe respiratory distress, continuous monitoring for signs of deteriorating status, including bradycardia, decreasing respiratory effort, and alterations in consciousness (such as extreme agitation or frank lethargy), is indicated.

RAPID SEQUENCE INDUCTION (RSI)

Rapid sequence induction may be used to induce anesthesia and neuromuscular blockade in fully or partially conscious children before proceeding with intubation. It is indicated in children requiring emergent intubation in the emergency department, such as those with respiratory failure, status epilepticus with inadequate airway control, or conditions producing increased intracranial pressure (ICP) (such as head trauma). Because the nature of the illness/injury requires emergent management, these children have rarely fasted prior to arrival, and they have an intact gag reflex. RSI facilitates intubation by placing the child in a fully relaxed state, using a combination of sedatives, muscle relaxants (to induce paralysis), and atropine (to block vagal stimulation). Although numerous drugs have been used in various combinations to produce RSI, the most common are listed in Table 6-3. Other

drugs occasionally used include morphine, fentanyl, lorazepam, atracurium, and pancuronium.

Nursing care and evaluation. Before RSI the emergency nurse places the child on a cardio-respiratory monitor and pulse oximeter and assembles all intubation equipment, including a correctly sized laryngoscope and blade, endotracheal tube (uncuffed if the child is younger than 8 years of age), suction equipment (suction catheters and tonsil suction), a bag-valve-mask device connected to 100% oxygen, stylet, and oral and nasal airways. Because few children requiring RSI have fasted prior to intubation, nasogastric tube insertion may be required to guard against regurgitation and the possibility of aspiration.

The steps required for RSI include preparing the equipment, preoxygenating the child with 100% oxygen for 2 to 5 minutes (by nonrebreather if the child is breathing spontaneously or BVM if the child is apneic or hypoventilating), administering pharmacologic agents for sedation and premedication, and administering pharmacologic agents for muscle relaxation.[20] Throughout the procedure the emergency nurse monitors the child's heart rate (a declining heart rate most often indicates hypoxia), oxygen saturation (via pulse oximeter), and clinical status (skin color, perfusion, capillary refill). If signs of hypoxia develop during the intubation, the physician is notified and positive pressure ventilation with a BVM device and 100% oxygen is initiated. Once the child is intubated, confirmation of tube placement and continuous monitoring of the child's status are required (refer to Chapter 8).

┃ SHOCK

DEFINITION

Shock is a clinical syndrome characterized by acute dysfunction of the cardiovascular system. Shock is caused by either a deficiency in blood volume or an expanded capacity of the vascular system. The result is inadequate delivery of oxygen and nutrients to the cells and inadequate removal of metabolic substrates.

ETIOLOGY

Shock is categorized based on etiology. Categories of shock include hypovolemic shock (characterized by overall circulating volume loss), cardiogenic shock (caused by myocardial damage or dysfunction), obstructive shock (caused by vascular compression or

TABLE 6-3	Common Drugs Used for RSI		
	DOSE	**INDICATIONS**	**PRECAUTIONS**
Premedication			
Atropine	0.02 mg/kg IV Min dose 0.1 mg Max dose 0.5 mg	Used for all children less than 1 year of age to prevent vagally mediated bradycardia Should be considered for use in all children <6-7 years of age Used for all children receiving succinylcholine	May mask hypoxic-induced bradycardia
Lidocaine	1.5 mg/kg IV (also may be given via oral mucosa, aerosol, or IM injection)	Used to blunt the increased ICP response to intubation and suppress the cough reflex Primarily used when increased ICP is suspected	
Sedatives			
Thiopental (Pentothal)	3-5 mg/kg IV	Depresses the CNS, producing sedation and hypnosis—does not provide analgesia Drug of choice for children with head injury because it reduces cerebral blood flow and cerebral oxygen consumption	May cause hypotension Should be avoided in children in hypovolemic shock—dose may be lowered if child is not hypotensive (1-2 mg/kg)
Ketamine	1-2 mg/kg IV Most commonly administered IM 4-7 mg/kg	Produces analgesia, amnesia, and dissociation from the environment with protection of respiratory drive and airway reflexes Drug of choice for children with asthma and respiratory failure; or shock	When administered IV, must be administered slowly—over 1 minute—to prevent respiratory depression Is contraindicated in infants <3 months of age (increased incidence of laryngospasm) and children >11 years of age (increased incidence of hallucinations) Increases ICP Increases salivation

TABLE 6-3	Common Drugs Used for RSI—cont'd		
	DOSE	**INDICATIONS**	**PRECAUTIONS**
Sedatives			
Diazepam	0.25-0.4 mg/kg Max dose 10 mg	Produces sedation but has no analgesic properties	Can produce cardiorespiratory depression
Midazolam	0.1-0.2 mg/kg Max dose 5 mg	Produces sedation with no analgesic properties Is faster acting, but of shorter duration than diazepam	Can produce cardiorespiratory depression
Muscle relaxants			
Succinylcholine (Anectine)	1-1.5 mg/kg IV (>10 kg) 1.5-2 mg/kg IV (<10 kg)	Rapid acting depolarizing agent with a short duration of action (4-10 minutes) Produces muscle fasciculations in muscular children and adolescents—a defasciculating dose of a nondepolarizing agent should be given before succinylcholine administration	Contraindicated in children with burns and upper motor neuron diseases (increased risk of hyperkalemia) Contraindicated in children with head injury and suspected increased ICP (increases intraocular pressure, intragastric pressure, and ICP)
Vercuronium (Norcuron)	0.1-0.3 mg/kg IV Defasciculating dose 0.01 mg/kg	Rapid onset nondepolarizing agent with longer duration than succinylcholine (90-120 minutes)	May produce tachycardia

Data from Silverman, 1993; Yamamoto, Yim, and Britten, 1990.

obstruction), and distributive shock (characterized by massive vasodilation) (Table 6-4). Although these categories describe distinct etiologies, shock is a dynamic state that may encompass several categories. For example, the child with septic shock will also lose circulating volume (hypovolemic shock) as cellular damage contributes to "third-spacing" of fluids. As the shock state progresses to multisystem organ failure, cardiogenic shock results from damage to the myocardium.

PATHOPHYSIOLOGY

Autonomic nervous system. Autonomic nervous system control of cardiovascular function is regulated by the hypothalamus. Signals from the hypothalamus stimulate cardiovascular control centers located in the medulla oblongata and the pons. These centers receive impulses from the heart by means of a reflex loop, primarily baroreceptors, and send signals to target organs throughout the sympathetic and parasympathetic systems.

TABLE 6-4	Categories of Shock	
ETIOLOGY	PATHOLOGY	CAUSES
Hypovolemic shock	Overall decrease in circulating blood volume. Results in decreased ventricular filling (preload) and decreased cardiac output (CO).	Hemorrhage Severe dehydration Burns Diabetes Third-spacing of body fluids
Cardiogenic shock	Inability of the myocardium to produce adequate CO. Caused by damage or dysfunction of the myocardium.	Dysrhythmias Electrolyte disturbances Myocarditis Congenital heart defect Ischemia
Obstructive shock	Inadequate perfusion despite normal intravascular volume and myocardial function. Caused by vascular compression or obstruction	Pericardial tamponade Tension pneumothorax Pulmonary or systemic hypertension Coarctation or interrupted aorta

Distributive shock
  Septic shock
  Neurogenic shock
  Anaphylactic shock
	Massive vasodilation of the vascular bed, although blood volume remains normal, results in a general maldistribution of blood flow.	Sepsis
		Loss of sympathetic tone
		Antigen-antibody reaction

Baroreceptors are stretch receptors located in the walls of the aorta and carotid arteries. With baroreceptor stimulation, impulses are transmitted to the brain stem, resulting in increased or decreased vasomotor stimulation of the autonomic nervous system. An increase in baroreceptor stimulation produces a cardioinhibitory effect, producing vasodilation, hypotension, bradycardia, and decreased cardiac output. A decrease in baroreceptor stimulation, as occurs during hypotension, reduces vagal tone and stimulates a sympathetic response, including an increase in heart rate and both arterial and venous constriction.

The sympathetic and parasympathetic systems play major roles in the regulation of heart rate, contractility, and blood flow. Stimulation of the sympathetic system causes norepinephrine and epinephrine to be released and act on alpha, beta, and dopaminergic receptors. This results in an increase in S-A nodal discharge, excitability of all portions of the heart, and the force of contractions. Additionally, an increase in the tone of vascular smooth muscle surrounding arteries and arterioles affects the rate of blood flow through the tissues and organs (Fig. 6-2).

In early compensated shock, this compensatory vasomotor response shunts blood from the skeletal, splanchnic, and cutaneous vascular beds to the heart and brain. Therefore, cardiac output and blood pressure remain normal, although tachycardia will be observed. In children the relatively healthy cardiovascular system is capable of maintaining adequate cardiac output through tachycardia for prolonged periods. Children, however, have limited circulating volume and increased oxygen demands compared to adults and are prone to rapid unexpected cardiovascular decompensation.

Intrinsic autoregulation. Autoregulation of cardiovascular function occurs in response to changes in blood volume flowing to the heart. As central venous return fills the heart, cardiac muscle fibers stretch. The degree to which these fibers stretch (ventricular preload) affects the force of the contraction (contractility) and the amount of blood being pumped each minute (cardiac output). The intrinsic ability of the healthy heart to adapt to blood flow changes in venous return is called the *Frank-Starling law.*

The neonatal myocardium is less compliant and contains less contractile mass than the adult myocardium, limiting both stroke volume and contractility. Since cardiac output equals heart rate times stroke volume, tachycardia becomes the infant/child's pri-

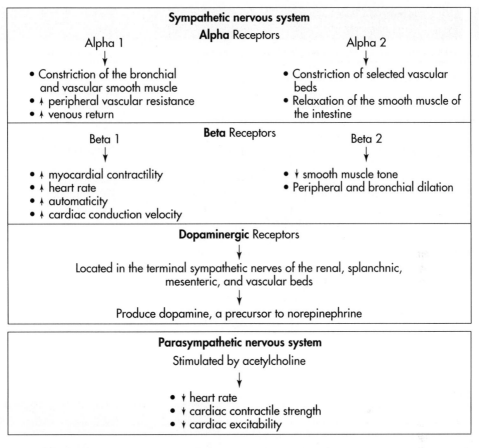

FIG. 6-2. Stimulation of the sympathetic and parasympathetic nervous systems.

mary means of increasing cardiac output during the shock state.

$$Cardiac\ output\ (CO) = Heart\ rate\ (HR) \times Stroke\ volume\ (SV)$$

As volume depletion continues and the heart rate approaches 180 to 200 beats per minute, ventricular filling time is compromised and cardiac output will begin to fall.

Renal regulation. The kidneys secrete renin when there is a decrease in arterial pressure and subsequent decrease in renal blood flow. As renin is secreted the angiotensin-aldosterone system is activated. Angiotensin produces marked constriction of the peripheral arterioles, moderate constriction of the veins, and constriction of the renal arterioles causing the kidneys to retain water. It also stimulates the release of aldosterone, which causes the kidneys to retain sodium. As serum osmolality increases with sodium retention, the hypothalamus and posterior pituitary gland release the antidiuretic hormone (ADH) also known as *vasopressin*. Vasopressin exerts a direct vasoconstrictive effect on the peripheral arterioles and promotes water reabsorption in the kidneys.

The initial result of activation of the renin-angiotensin-aldosterone system during the shock state is the maintenance of peripheral vascular resistance and blood pressure. However, with prolonged shock, intense vasoconstriction can cause ischemic renal damage and peripheral hypoperfusion.

Cellular metabolism. Cellular metabolism is dependent upon oxygen delivery. The components of oxygen delivery include the hemoglobin concentration, percentage of hemoglobin oxygen saturation, dissolved plasma oxygen, and cardiac output. When

TABLE 6-5	Signs and Symptoms of Shock		
COMPENSATED SHOCK	**UNCOMPENSATED SHOCK**	**LATE-STAGE SHOCK**
Normal blood pressure	Hypotension	Hypotension
Tachycardia	Tachycardia	Tachycardia/bradycardia
Tachypnea	Tachypnea	Tachypnea/bradypnea
Normal to delayed capillary refill*	Delayed capillary refill	Capillary refill >5 sec
Normal to weak peripheral pulses*	Weak or absent peripheral pulses	Absent peripheral pulses
Strong central pulses	Strong to weak central pulses	Weak to absent central pulses
Skin: pink, pale, or mottled*	Skin: pallor, mottling/cyanosis; petechiae and/or purpura*	Mottling, peripheral and central cyanosis
	Areas of regional coolness	Cold, clammy skin; hypothermia
Agitation or lethargy	Lethargy/decreased response to pain	Coma
Normal urine output (1-2 ml/kg/hr)	Oliguria	Oliguria/anuria

*In early septic shock capillary refill will be brisk, peripheral pulses may be bounding, and skin may be warm, flushed, ruberous, or mottled. Petechiae and purpura may be observed early in septic shock depending on etiology.

tissue oxygen demands go unmet, cellular hypoxia produces cellular damage, stimulating anaerobic glycolysis. This results in the production of lactic and pyruvic acid. Cellular damage contributes to the development of capillary leak and the release of vasoactive mediators. Impaired perfusion compromises the removal of these waste products, further contributing to the acidotic state and cellular damage. As the pH falls, the oxyhemoglobin curve is shifted to the right; therefore hemoglobin has less affinity for oxygen and more readily delivers oxygen to the tissues, provided oxygen saturation is maintained. This phenomenon, known as the *Bohr effect*, initially ameliorates the adverse effects of acidemia by aiding in the unloading of oxygen to the tissues.

CLINICAL PRESENTATION

Assessment of the child in shock requires an evaluation of the child's vital signs, peripheral perfusion (e.g., peripheral pulses, skin color and temperature, capillary refill), neurologic status, and urine output (Table 6-5). Specific presentations vary depending on the etiology and stage of shock and are reviewed later in this chapter.

TABLE 6-6	Systolic Blood Pressure Calculation in Children	
AGE	**SYSTOLIC BLOOD PRESSURE**
Normal newborn	60-90 mm Hg
After 1 year of age:	
Normal values	$90 + (2 \times \text{age in years}) =$ Systolic B/P
Lower limit of normal	$70 + (2 \times \text{age in years}) =$ Systolic B/P
Example: 2 year old	$90 + (2 \times 2 \text{ yrs}) =$ 94 mm Hg

Although blood pressure is commonly used to determine the degree of shock in the adult, findings can be deceiving in the child. First, the ability of the cardiovascular compensatory response to volume loss in the child allows the maintenance of an adequate blood pressure, even in the face of impending cardiovascular collapse. Second, normal blood pressures vary in children depending on age; therefore normal pediatric values must be known (Table 6-6).

HYPOVOLEMIC SHOCK

ETIOLOGY

Hypovolemia is the most common cause of shock in children. It represents a decrease in intravascular fluid volume and consequently a decrease in venous return. As ventricular filling is compromised, cardiac output falls below normal. The most common cause of hypovolemia—and subsequent death—in children throughout the world is vomiting and diarrhea. Hemorrhagic shock from trauma-related injuries is the most common cause of hypovolemia in children in the United States. Hypovolemic shock can result from either direct or indirect fluid losses and can occur acutely or over time. Examples of direct losses include hemorrhage, prolonged vomiting or diarrhea (often combined with decreased fluid intake), or diuresis as seen in diabetic ketoacidosis. Indirect losses may occur when fluids are sequestered or "third-spaced" as is observed in septic shock. Children with severe burns are susceptible to hypovolemic shock from both evaporative fluid losses and from massive fluid sequestration.

Box 6-2   Hypovolemia: Comparison of Acute and Gradual Fluid Losses

Example: 10-kg child   Circulating blood volume in young children is approximately 80 ml/kg. In a 10-kg child circulating volume would be 800 ml.

Acute blood losses (e.g., hemorrhage)
10% Blood loss = 80 ml blood loss
20% Blood loss = 160 ml blood loss
30% Blood loss = 240 ml blood loss

Gradual fluid losses (e.g., vomiting or diarrhea)
5% Weight loss (50 ml/kg) = 500 ml fluid loss
10% Weight loss (100 ml/kg) = 1000 ml fluid loss
15% Weight loss (150 ml/kg) = 1500 ml fluid loss

PATHOPHYSIOLOGY

Infants and children are particularly susceptible to hypovolemia for several reasons. Among these is the fact that children have larger body surface to volume ratios than adults. This means that a higher metabolic rate is required to maintain body temperature, which results in a daily turnover rate of fluids that represents more than half of the child's extracellular fluid volume—compared to one fifth in the adult. Additionally, the child has less circulating volume than the adult; therefore small blood losses can represent large percentages of total circulating volume.

In acute hemorrhagic shock, a rapid drop in cardiac output stimulates an immediate sympathetic nervous system response, producing increased peripheral vascular resistance and tachycardia. Initially cardiac output and blood pressure are maintained. In adults blood volume deficits approaching 15% to 20% will be evidenced by acute peripheral circulatory compromise and a fall in systolic blood pressure. Young children, however, are able to maintain vascular tone and peripheral vascular resistance until blood loss approaches 25% of circulating volume.[20]

Volume loss in infants and young children who have not suffered an acute loss of vascular volume most commonly results from vomiting and/or diarrhea.

Although losses may be classified as "gradual," when compared to hemorrhage they can occur rapidly in young children because of the increased metabolic rate and daily fluid requirements. These gradual losses are referred to as *dehydration,* which reflects a total fluid and electrolyte output that exceeds fluid intake. The degree of dehydration in children is based on the percentage of body weight lost. Mild dehydration is classified as less than 5% weight loss, moderate dehydration is classified as 5% to 10% weight loss, and severe dehydration is classified as greater than 10% weight loss. In the child, a 10% weight loss represents a fluid loss of 100 ml/kg of body weight. If the child weighs 10 kg, total body fluid losses would approach 1000 ml—when the child's total circulating blood volume is estimated to be only 800 ml (Box 6-2).

The reason children can lose total body fluid amounts that exceed circulating blood volume is that while fluid loss is occurring—either acutely or gradually—fluid is being shifted from the interstitial space into the vascular space to maintain vascular volume. If these losses continue, both intracellular and interstitial fluids will be depleted. Young children, however, are able to compensate for these losses longer and with fewer clinical signs than adults.

This is because water comprises a greater proportion of body weight than in the adult and a higher percentage of body water is located in the interstitial space.

CLINICAL PRESENTATION

Clinical manifestations of hypovolemic shock vary depending on the etiology and the degree of volume loss. In acute hypovolemic shock, the compensatory response produces an immediate increase in heart rate and the maintenance of peripheral perfusion. With gradually evolving dehydration certain clinical characteristics, including weight loss, and changes in heart rate, capillary refill, skin turgor, and urine output, are used to define the degree of fluid loss (see Table 14-3). As volume loss continues and peripheral vasoconstriction shunts blood from the skin to cerebellar and coronary beds, pallor, delayed capillary refill, weak peripheral pulses, and cool extremities will be observed. Initially, neurologic status will be maintained, evidenced by normal cognition that progresses to lethargy. As volume depletion continues and compensatory mechanisms are unable to maintain cardiac output, both neurologic status and cardiovascular status will be compromised. When approximately 25% of circulating volume is lost, hypotension will result.

EMERGENCY DEPARTMENT INTERVENTIONS

Emergent management of the child in hypovolemic shock requires immediate fluid resuscitation to expand intravascular volume. Initially a 20 ml/kg bolus of normal saline or lactated Ringer's solution is administered. Additional bolus therapy of 20 ml/kg is based on the child's clinical response. When hypovolemia has occurred gradually, the total volume of replacement fluids will often exceed the child's circulating volume. When hemorrhage is the cause of hypovolemic shock, the child may ultimately require blood replacement therapy.

CARDIOGENIC SHOCK

ETIOLOGY

Cardiogenic shock represents a failure of the myocardium to maintain cardiac output either by a direct insult to the myocardium or myocardial dysfunction. The most common conditions that lead to cardiogenic shock in children are congenital heart disease, postoperative open heart surgery, and the advanced stages of septic shock. Other etiologies include heart rate abnormalities such as supraventricular tachycardia (SVT) and bradyarrhythmias, immunologic disorders such as acute rheumatic fever, inflammatory processes such as myocarditis, traumatic injuries such as myocardial contusion, and cardiomyopathies that follow hypoxic-ischemic injuries such as near drowning. Cardiogenic shock is observed in late-stage shock of any origin.

PATHOPHYSIOLOGY

When cardiac output drops a number of physiologic compensatory responses are stimulated to conserve circulating volume and maintain blood flow to the vital organs. These physiologic responses may have short-term beneficial effects in the child, but over the long term they may produce undesirable effects. For example, the initial physiologic response to a decrease in cardiac output is baroreceptor simulation of the sympathetic nervous system, producing tachycardia and an increase in systemic vascular resistance. Although children can maintain tachycardia and increases in systemic vascular resistance for longer periods than adults, they cannot do so with a failing heart. As systemic vascular resistance rises, blood pressure may remain normal but the workload of the heart increases (afterload—or resistance against which the failing ventricle must contract). This increase in workload also causes an increase in myocardial oxygen consumption. At the same time ventricular distention limits filling of the coronary arteries, producing myocardial ischemia. As afterload rises, left ventricular end-diastolic volume and pressure continue to rise. This increase in pressure is passively transmitted to the pulmonary bed and contributes to the development of pulmonary edema and congestive heart failure. Additionally, decreases in renal perfusion stimulate the renin-angiotensin-aldosterone system, resulting in sodium and water retention (even though fluid volume may be normal), further contributing to the development of congestive heart failure.

CLINICAL PRESENTATION

Signs of cardiogenic shock are observed much earlier in the shock state, because compensatory responses may be short lived. Additionally, signs will be observed with varying degrees of severity as cardiac output falls. Decreased tissue perfusion is initially evidenced by skin pallor that progresses to mottling and eventually cyanosis. Skin may be cool and clammy and peripheral pulses weak and thready. Neurologically the child may appear "tired" or be frankly lethargic. Hypotension and oliguria will be observed. As the shock state progresses, signs of congestive heart failure (CHF) will be manifested, including tachypnea, hepatomegaly, and pulmonary crackles. Peripheral edema may be evidenced by periorbital or sacral edema in the infant but is rarely an early finding in the emergency department (ED). Jugular venous distention as a sign of CHF may be difficult to detect because of the infant's relatively short neck and overlying fat. (For a complete discussion of CHF, see Chapter 11.)

EMERGENCY DEPARTMENT INTERVENTIONS

The treatment and degree of diagnostic testing performed on the child with cardiogenic shock depends on the underlying etiology and symptomatology. For example, when the cause of shock is known to be SVT, diagnostic testing—other than placing the child on an ECG monitor—is generally unnecessary. SVT is treated with electrical cardioversion or adenosine. Suspected myocarditis requires a complete workup, including a CBC with differential, blood cultures, ESR, ECG, chest x-ray, and echocardiogram. Treatment in these children depends on the seriousness of the clinical presentation. (NOTE: Cardiovascular disorders and their management are reviewed in Chapter 11.)

When the etiology of shock is unknown, initial ED management includes fluid resuscitation with a 20 ml/kg bolus of isotonic solution. Many times cardiogenic shock is identified only after the child has failed to respond to emergent fluid therapy or only after the history reveals a previously diagnosed congenital heart defect or recurrent arrhythmias.

Once cardiogenic shock is suspected, pharmacologic management is required to counteract the compensatory response and improve cardiac function. Afterload reducing agents such as nitroprusside and nitroglycerin may be required to lower systemic vascular resistance associated with the administration of α-adrenergic agents. Angiotensin-converting enzyme inhibitors may be used to block the renin-angiotensin system, and diuretics may be given to reverse abnormal fluid retention.

▌ SEPTIC SHOCK

ETIOLOGY

Septic shock is the most common form of distributive shock observed in children.[1] It is defined as

an acute systemic response to an infectious organism, or to toxins produced by the organism. The result is massive vasodilation, increased capillary permeability, and maldistribution of blood flow. Gram-negative organisms account for the majority of cases of septic shock in children; however, gram-positive organisms such as Group B β-hemolytic streptococci and *Staphylococcus aureus* are not uncommon. Other causes include fungi, rickettsia, and viruses. Children at risk for the development of septic shock include (1) neonates, because of immune system immaturity; (2) children with conditions that affect the immune system and/or cellular integrity, such as sickle cell disease or HIV, or who are on steroids or chemotherapeutic agents; (3) children who have sustained a disruption in the integrity of the skin, caused by burns, trauma, or cellulitis; and (4) hospitalized children exposed to invasive diagnostic procedures and hemodynamic monitoring (Table 6-7).

PATHOPHYSIOLOGY

Organisms that produce sepsis or septic shock gain access to the bloodstream through a variety of mechanisms, in some cases without any identified predisposing condition. Exactly what triggers the cascade of

TABLE 6-7	Common Pathogens Causing Septic Shock in Children
AGE	PATHOGENS
Neonates	Group B β-hemolytic streptococci
	Enteric bacteria (e.g., *E. coli*)
	Listeria monocytogenes
	Staphylococcus aureus
Infants	*Haemophilus influenzae*
	Streptococcus pneumoniae
	Staphylococcus aureus
Childen	*Streptococcus pneumoniae*
	Neisseria meningitidis
	Staphylococcus aureus
	Enteric bacteria
Immunocompromised	Enteric bacteria
	Staphylococcus aureus
	Pseudomonas
	Candida albicans

From Wetzel RC: Shock. In Rogers MC, ed: *Textbook of pediatric intensive care,* vol 1, Baltimore, 1987, Williams & Wilkins.

events that leads to septic shock is not well understood; however, once the organism enters the bloodstream and is destroyed by the body's defense mechanisms, toxic substances contained within their cell walls (gram positive—peptidoglycans; gram negative—endotoxic lipopolysaccharides) are released. These substances activate proinflammatory cytokines (e.g., tumor necrosis factor, interleukin-1), which are believed to be the stimulus for the development of the systemic inflammatory response characteristic of septic shock.[4,10,23] With these events numerous biochemical and physiologic responses are activated, including stimulation of the complement system, which can further exacerbate the inflammatory response and tissue injury; activation of the coagulation system, which can lead to the development of disseminated intravascular coagulation (DIC); production of β-endorphins, which can contribute to vasodilation and hypotension; and the activation of polymorphonuclear leukocytes, which

can mediate vascular injury and potentiate the development of capillary leak syndrome.(Fig. 6-3). In addition, oxygen delivery and consumption are disrupted. Decreased oxygen delivery is the result of decreased perfusion; however, during septic shock tissues are unable to effectively utilize oxygen delivered to them, even when they receive adequate oxygenation.[11,17,25]

Because of the complexity of these responses and the variability in clinical findings, Bone (1991) suggested uniform terminology for adult patients. In 1993 Saez-Llorens and McCracken further defined these events as they relate to children. They defined *sepsis* as an acute systemic response to an organism exhibited by fever or hypothermia, tachycardia, tachypnea, and white blood cell count abnormalities; *sepsis syndrome* results when sepsis presents with the above symptoms, plus signs of altered organ perfusion such as changes in mental status, oliguria, hypoxemia, and increased plasma

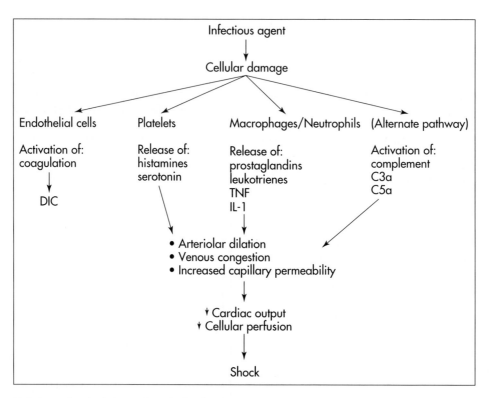

FIG. 6-3. Cellular pathophysiology of septic shock. (Redrawn from Cotran RS, Kumar V, Robbins SL: *Robbins pathologic basis of disease,* ed 4, Philadelphia, 1989, WB Saunders.)

lactate; *early septic shock* is chacaracterized by hypotension and delayed perfusion that responds promptly to fluid therapy and pharmacologic management. In children, early-stage septic shock is characterized by the maintenance of or an increase in cardiac output—referred to as a *hyperdynamic state.* These children will initially present with a widened pulse pressure and warm, flushed skin. Hypotension occurs late in the course of illness in children; therefore as the shock state progresses signs of decreasing tissue perfusion will be evidenced by pallor, weak pulses, mottled skin, and delayed capillary refill. *Refractory septic shock* is shock that lasts for more than 1 hour despite vigorous therapeutic interventions. *Multiple organ dysfunction syndrome (MODS)* describes impaired organ function in combination with signs of biochemical derangement such as DIC, adult respiratory distress syndrome (ARDS), renal failure, hepatic failure, or acute CNS dysfunction.

CLINICAL PRESENTATION

In early sepsis normal physiologic responses produce a compensated, "hyperdynamic" state characterized by an increase in cardiac output and cardiac index. Clinical signs of early hyperdynamic shock include tachycardia, tachypnea, brisk capillary refill, bounding peripheral pulses (wide-pulse pressure), and warm flushed skin. Initially, urine output and blood pressure may be normal; however, if this stage goes unrecognized urine output and blood pressure will decline. Other findings may include petechiae or purpura, which result as cellular damage stimulates the coagulation cascade. Petechiae are often seen in conjunction with bacterial invasion by a gram-negative organism such as *Haemophilus influenzae* or *Neisseria meningitidis.*

Uncompensated shock occurs when sympathetic stimulation can no longer maintain an adequate cardiac output, evidenced by a drop in blood pressure. Signs of uncompensated shock include hypotension, tachycardia, weak or absent peripheral pulses, delayed capillary refill, mottled skin with areas of regional skin coolness, decreased response to pain, ARDS, oliguria, and depressed myocardial contractility (cardiogenic shock).

EMERGENCY DEPARTMENT INTERVENTIONS

Diagnostic testing generally includes arterial blood gases; a complete blood count and differential; serum electrolytes; serum glucose; renal, hepatic, and cardiac function studies; and serum lactate. Additional testing includes a chest x-ray to identify cardiomegaly and/or pulmonary congestion. An ECG may be ordered to assist in the evaluation of cardiac involvement, and an echocardiogram may be ordered to identify cardiac malformations and evaluate systolic function.

Children in septic shock have tremendous fluid needs as systemic vasodilation and capillary leak exacerbate the shock state. Emergent management requires the administration of a 20 ml/kg bolus of normal saline or lactated Ringer's solution. Further bolus therapy is based on the child's clinical response; however, aggressive fluid volume therapy within the first hour of resuscitation has been associated with a high survival rate.[6]

The goal of drug therapy is to maximize cardiac output and cardiac index, increase peripheral vascular resistance, and improve oxygenation of the tissues. Drugs used to treat shock are reviewed later in this chapter.

Antibiotic therapy is initiated in all these children. When feasible, cultures are obtained from the blood, urine, spinal fluid, and/or other potentially infected sites before therapy. If the child is unstable definitive therapy may take precedence over the obtaining of cultures. When the offending organism is unknown therapy is based on the most likely organism for history, age, and risk factors. Gram-positive organisms are treated with penicillins and cephalosporins, and gram-negative organisms are treated with penicillins, aminoglycosides, and/or cephalosporins.

ADDITIONAL APPROACHES TO THERAPY

Numerous experimental therapies are under investigation for the treatment of septic shock. Among these are drugs that inhibit the release of vascular mediators that produce the vasodilating effects of septic shock; opiate antagonists such as Narcan, which counteracts the effects of endogenous opiates that further contribute to hypotension; and monoclonal antibodies that react to the endotoxin or bind to vascular mediators such as tumor necrosis factor or interleukin-1. Thus far these therapies have little efficacy in the emergency department.

The use of steroids in septic shock is not recommended, because several studies have demonstrated a higher mortality rate in steroid-treated adults.[3,22]

NURSING CARE AND EVALUATION OF THE CHILD IN SHOCK

AIRWAY AND BREATHING

Children in shock require the administration of high-dose supplemental oxygen to improve oxygen saturation and tissue oxygenation. Septic children, because of the tissues' inability to effectively utilize oxygen, will require supranormal levels of oxygen.[5,25] Airway maintenance and the delivery of assisted ventilations depends on the child's initial presentation and the suspected underlying etiology. The child who is unable to maintain a patent airway because of an altered level of consciousness will require airway positioning, and the child with signs of respiratory failure will require assisted ventilation with a bag-valve-mask device. Infants and children in septic shock are intubated to provide the highest dose of oxygen, to decrease oxygen consumption, and to provide positive end-expiratory pressure (PEEP) should pulmonary edema develop (Box 6-3).

CIRCULATION

Vascular access is obtained via two large-bore peripheral venous catheters. When this route cannot be obtained rapidly the intraosseous route may be required (see Chapter 8). The goal of fluid therapy in the hypovolemic child is to maintain peripheral perfusion

---

Box 6-3	Initial Approach to the Child in Shock

- Establish airway
- Administer 100% oxygen
- Provide ventilatory support, as indicated
- Establish vascular access; obtain lab work and ABGs
- Administer fluid bolus (20 ml/kg isotonic crystalloid)
- Reassess perfusion
- Administer pharmacologic support, as indicated
- Monitor response to pharmacologic agents
- Administer specific therapy (e.g., antibiotics, blood replacement)
- Maintain normothermia

---

and thus oxygen delivery to the tissues. Initially an isotonic crystalloid solution (lactated Ringer's solution or normal saline) is administered at 20 ml/kg of body weight. After the first bolus, the child's blood pressure, capillary refill, peripheral pulses, skin color, mental status, and heart rate are reassessed. Additional 20 ml/kg boluses are administered based on the child's clinical response. Improvement in clinical status after one or two boluses of fluid indicates a positive response to therapy.

Central lines. Central lines are occasionally initiated in the emergency department to monitor central venous pressure (CVP), to administer large fluid volumes, and to administer certain drugs directly into the central circulation. This procedure can be time consuming and is therefore attempted only after venous access has been rapidly achieved by another route. Central lines in children are placed in the internal or external jugulars or the femoral vein. In young children the subclavian route is not accessed emergently, because this route is associated with a high incidence of complications, particularly pneumothorax.[7]

The goal of central line management is to monitor preload augmentation and to protect against volume overload. This is particularly important with capillary leak syndrome. CVP monitoring is augmented with continuous evaluations of clinical status, blood pressure readings, and urine output, because CVP readings do not reflect left ventricular function or perfusion status. Ideally, CVP readings should be maintained at about 10 mm Hg. However, if CVP readings approach or exceed 10 mm Hg with fluid administration and no apparent improvement in peripheral perfusion, myocardial dysfunction should be suspected.

Crystalloids and colloids. Both crystalloids and colloids are used to improve vascular volume during the shock state. Crystalloid fluid administration produces an immediate clinical improvement. Crystalloid fluids, however, rapidly diffuse into the interstitial space and can therefore contribute to the development of pulmonary and peripheral edema with capillary leak syndrome. Colloids have a higher oncotic pressure and remain in the vascular space longer. They also tend to exert an intravascular oncotic force that stimulates the movement of interstitial fluid into the vascular space. The main disadvantages of colloids are that they are expensive and patients may develop sensitivity reactions to them (Table 6-8).

Blood administration. The primary indication for blood administration is shock secondary to hemorrhage. The criteria for blood administration in children varies; however, a conservative approach is the rule. Blood volume in children is significantly less than in adults; therefore small blood losses can represent relatively large percentages of total circulating volume. Blood volume is generally calculated as 100 ml/kg in neonates, 80 ml/kg in children 1 month to 2 years, and 70 ml/kg in children greater than 2 years of age.[16]

When the child requires blood administration, type and cross matched or type and screened blood is ordered. If the child requires an immediate transfusion, group O negative packed red blood cells (PRBC) may be given at 10 ml/kg. The following formulas may be used to calculate additional transfusion requirements: transfusion of 1 ml of PRBC per kilogram of body weight increases the hematocrit by 1%, 3 ml/kg of PRBC raises the hemoglobin level by 1 g/dl.[16]

Pneumatic antishock garments. Pneumatic antishock garments (PASGs) are occasionally used in children, although their use is controversial. With inflation the PASG improves peripheral vascular resistance, affecting afterload. Current guidelines suggest that PASGs may be useful in children with major pelvic fractures; however, their use in children with mild or moderate hypotension may actually worsen the outcome.[7,8] When PASG devices are used in children inflation of the abdominal compartment is not recommended, because the device may impair diaphragmatic function.

PHARMACOLOGIC MANAGEMENT

The goal of pharmacologic therapy is to optimize ventricular preload using fluid administration; increase or improve cardiac contractility using inotropic support; and then manipulate compliance and distribution of blood volume to the vital organs using individual or combinations of drugs such as inotropic, chronotropic, and/or vasodilator therapy. Because shock is complex and dynamic, no single formula can be used to determine pharmacologic needs. In addition, electrolyte and acid-base disturbances and tissue ischemia all contribute to variable responses to therapy (Table 6-9).

TABLE 6-8	Colloid Solutions Available for Volume Resuscitation
SOLUTION	**DESCRIPTION**
Human plasma	Uncoagulated, unconcentrated plasma Contains all plasma proteins, including albumin Contains clotting factors
Plasma protein fraction (e.g., Plasmanate)	5% Solution of human plasma proteins in normal saline Contains albumin α and β-globulins Sodium 130-160 mEq/L Potassium 1-2 mEq/L
Albumin	5% Albumin 50 g/L Sodium 130-160 mEq/L 25% Albumin 250 g/L Sodium 130-160 mEq/L
Dextran	Low molecular weight: 10% solution of glucose polysaccharides with average molecular weight of 40,000 High molecular weight: 6% solution of glucose polysaccharides with molecular weight of 70,000
Hetastarch	6% Solution containing synthetic polymar of hydroxethyl starch

From Perkin RM, Levin DL: General major system failure. In Levin DL, Morriss FC: *Essentials of pediatric intensive care,* St Louis, 1990, Quality Medical Publishing.

TABLE 6-9	Pharmacologic Agents Commonly Used in Pediatric Shock		
DRUG	**DOSAGE**	**RECEPTORS**	**USUAL EFFECT**
Dopamine	0.5-3 µg/kg/min	Dopaminergic	Dilation in renal, mesenteric, cerebral vasculature
	5-10 µg/kg/min	β-adrenergic	Mostly inotropic (increased cardiac output)
	10-20 µg/kg/min	α-adrenergic	Increased heart rate, vascular resistance, blood pressure
Dobutamine	1-20 µg/kg/min	β-adrenergic	Mostly inotropic; some vasodilation
Epinephrine	0.02-0.1 µg/kg/min	Mostly β	Mostly inotropic
	0.1-1 µg/kg/min	α and β	Increased heart rate, vascular resistance, blood pressure
Norepinephrine	0.05-0.3 µg/kg/min	Mostly α	Increased vascular resistance
Amrinone	0.75-5 mg/kg (loading dose—slowly) 5-10 µg/kg/min	β-adrenergic	Mostly inotropic; some vasodilation
Isoproterenol	0.05-1.5 µg/kg/min	β-adrenergic	Rapid increase in heart rate; some vasodilation

Modified from Corneli, H: Evaluation, treatment, and transport of pediatric patients with shock, *Pediatr Clin North Am* 40:(2): 310, 1993.

Sympathomimetics. Low-dose *dopamine* improves renal perfusion, urine output, and mesenteric perfusion. As the dose is increased, beta-1 effects predominate, including increased myocardial contractility and increased heart rate. At very high doses (greater than 20 µg/kg/min), alpha effects dominate, improving blood pressure at the expense of perfusion. Dopamine is inactivated by alkaline solutions and should not be administered in the same tubing as sodium bicarbonate.

Dobutamine acts primarily on beta receptors and increases myocardial contractility and heart rate. It is, however, less likely than epinephrine or isoproterenol to produce ventricular dysrhythmias. Because dobutamine also produces mild peripheral vasodilation, it is not recommended for the hypotensive child. Dobutamine is incompatible with alkaline solutions.

Epinephrine is an endogenous catecholamine that can produce both alpha and beta effects. At low doses the effects are mostly inotropic; however, as the dose

increases both alpha and beta effects are exhibited. Because of the alpha response (vasoconstriction) associated with high-dose epinephrine it is often administered with low-dose dopamine to maintain splanchnic and renal blood flow. Epinephrine increases myocardial oxygen consumption at any dose.

Isoproterenol acts primarily on beta receptors, increasing myocardial contractility and heart rate and producing peripheral and bronchial vasodilation. Isoproterenol significantly increases myocardial workload and oxygen consumption, and its use in infants has been associated with myocardial ischemia.[12,14] In addition, peripheral vasodilation is nonselective; therefore blood flow to nonessential vascular beds (e.g., cutaneous flow) may be increased. Because of its beta-2 effects, isoproterenol should not be used in the hypotensive child.

Norepinephrine has both alpha and beta effects but is predominantly alpha. Because of its potent vasoconstrictor effects, blood pressure is elevated at the expense of pulmonary, peripheral, renal, and splanchnic blood flow. During conditions when peripheral vascular resistance is low (e.g., septic shock) norepinephrine enhances peripheral vasomotor tone. When used in these situations, continuous hemodynamic monitoring is required to assess the positive and negative effects of therapy.

Amrinone is a noncatecholamine inotropic agent that increases ventricular contractility and produces a direct relaxant effect on smooth muscles. Peripheral vasodilation makes it useful in children with congestive heart failure or cardiogenic shock, but it is not recommended for children who are hypovolemic.

ACID-BASE IMBALANCES

Metabolic acidosis is treated first with oxygen administration and volume expansion to improve tissue oxygenation and to reverse anaerobic metabolism. Sodium bicarbonate administration in the face of impaired tissue perfusion may actually worsen acidemia by increasing circulating carbon dioxide levels. Other buffers that may be used include tris-hydroxymethyl-aminomethane (THAM), dichloroacetate, and carbicarb.

When acidosis is severe, pH correction may be required before tissue perfusion can be restored. Sodium bicarbonate 1 to 2 mEq/kg or one of the other buffers may be administered. In infants the 4.2% solution of sodium bicarbonate, rather than the 8.4% solution, is used because of the hyperosmolar effects of the solution and the associated risk of intraventricular hemorrhage.

Outcomes of untreated metabolic acidosis include depressed myocardial contractility, decreased response to catecholamines, inhibition of glycolysis, and increased pulmonary vascular resistance.

ELECTROLYTE DISTURBANCES

Ionized calcium levels fall during conditions associated with inadequate tissue perfusion, although total circulating calcium levels may remain normal. Since ionized calcium is essential to myocardial contractility, decreasing levels will impair myocardial function. The treatment for documented hypocalcemia is calcium chloride 20 to 25 mg/kg (0.2 ml to 0.25 ml/kg). Calcium is administered no faster than 100 mg/min (and the child is placed on a heart rate monitor), because rapid administration can produce bradycardia and dysrhythmias.

Potassium levels rise during shock as cellular damage releases potassium into the intravascular space. Additionally, metabolic acidosis contributes to hyperkalemia as circulating hydrogen ions are exchanged for intracellular potassium. Although circulating levels of potassium may be normal or slightly elevated, overall potassium stores are often low. Alterations in potassium levels will adversely affect cardiac contractility and conduction.

Glucose is rapidly depleted during periods of stress in the infant and small child. This, coupled with the child's limited glycogen stores, predisposes the child to hypoglycemia. Blood glucose is therefore evaluated at the onset of resuscitative management of the child in shock and monitored throughout the child's stay in the emergency department.

Box 6-4   Nursing Care of the Child in Shock

Monitor respiratory status
- Airway patency
- Breath sounds
- Effort
- Rate

Monitor hemodynamic status and perfusion
- Heart rate—rhythm
- Skin color
- Skin temperature (central and peripheral)
- Pulses (central and peripheral)
- Capillary refill
- Central venous pressure
- Blood pressure

Monitor neurologic status
- Level of consciousness
- Motor response
- Pupillary responses

Monitor urine output
- Infant 2–4 ml/kg/hr
- Child 1–2 ml/kg/hr
- Adolescent 0.5–1 ml/kg/hr

Evaluate responses to fluid and drug therapy
Monitor core temperature and institute measures to maintain normothermia
Observe for coagulation abnormalities (petechiae or purpura)
Monitor for and address issues related to pain, fear, and anxiety
Monitor serum glucose
Monitor for acid-base and electrolyte abnormalities
Observe for signs of multisystem organ failure

ONGOING CARE AND EVALUATION (BOX 6-4)

Ongoing care of the child in shock requires continuous monitoring of the child's airway and breathing, circulatory status, and neurologic status. The intubated child is continuously monitored for the development of pulmonary edema. If pulmonary edema is present, frequent suctioning and higher PEEP is required. If the child is not intubated, continuous observations for a decreasing level of consciousness (and therefore an unprotected airway) or an increase or decrease in the work of breathing are required. Vital signs are taken at least hourly—more often if the child is unstable. All intake and output are recorded. A urinary catheter is required to monitor urine output, and all IV fluids and drips are placed on IV pumps. Signs of multisystem failure or coagulation anomalies such as oliguria or anuria, decreased or absent response to pain, decreasing perfusion (cardiac output) despite fluid therapy and inotropic support, and petechiae or purpura are reported immediately to the ED physician.

Throughout management, efforts are made to decrease oxygen consumption and increase oxygen delivery to the tissues. Nursing measures to decrease oxygen demand include warming all fluids administered, providing supplemental warming measures such as overbed warmers, addressing pain and fear by comforting the child and administering pain medications as ordered, titrating inotropic drug administration appropriately, and immediately notifying the physician of changes in the child's vital signs or perfusion.

▮ SUMMARY

Caring for the child in shock or respiratory failure is a challenge. The emergency nurse must first be able to recognize conditions that can lead to respiratory failure or shock and must also respond emergently to prevent cardiopulmonary arrest. When either condition leads to cardiopulmonary arrest, the child has little chance for survival.

REFERENCES

1. Blumer JL: *A practical guide to pediatric intensive care*, ed. 3, St Louis, 1991, Mosby.
2. Bone RC: Let's agree on terminology: definitions of sepsis, *Crit Care Med* 19:973, 1991.
3. Bone RC et al: A controlled clinical triage of high dose methylprednisolone in the treatment of severe sepsis and septic shock, *N Engl J Med* 317:653–658, 1987.
4. Cannon JG et al: Circulating interleukin-1 and tumor necrosis factor in septic shock and experimental endotoxin fever, *J Infect Dis* 161:79–84, 1990.
5. Carcillo JA: Management of pediatric septic shock. In Holbrook PR, ed: *Textbook of pediatric critical care*, Philadelphia, 1993, WB Saunders.
6. Carcillo JA, Davis AI, Zariski A: Role of early fluid resuscitation in pediatric septic shock, *JAMA* 226: 1242, 1991.
7. Chameides L, Hazinski MF: *Textbook of pediatric advanced life support*, Dallas, 1994, American Heart Association.
8. Cooper A et al: Efficacy of MAST use in children who present in hypotensive shock, *J Trauma* 33:151, 1992 (abstract).
9. Corneli H: Evaluation, treatment, and transport of pediatric patients with shock, *Pediatr Clin North Am* 40(2):310, 1993.
10. Dinarello CA: The proinflammatory cytokines interleukin-1 and tumor necrosis factor and treatment of the septic shock syndrome, *J Infect Dis* 163:1177–1184, 1991.
11. Epstein CD, Henning RJ: Oxygen transport variables in the identification and treatment of hypoxia, *Heart Lung* 22(4):328–344, 1993.
12. Finley JP et al: Transient myocardial ischemia of the newborn infant demonstrated by thallium myocardial imaging, *J Pediatr* 94:263, 1979.
13. Guyton AC: *Textbook of medical physiology*, ed 8, Philadelphia, 1991, WB Saunders.
14. Kurland G, Williams J, Lewiston NJ: Fatal myocardial toxicity during continuous infusion intravenous isoproterenol therapy of asthma, *J Allergy Clin Immunol* 63:407, 1979.
15. Reference deleted in proofs.
16. Patel RI: Blood use and coagulation. In Eichelberger MR, ed: *Pediatric trauma: prevention, acute care, rehabilitation*, St Louis, 1993, Mosby.
17. Perkin RM, Levin DL: General major system failure. In Levin DL, Morriss FC: *Essentials of pediatric intensive care*, St Louis, 1990, Quality Medical Publishing.
18. Reference deleted in proofs.
19. Saez-Llorens X, McCracken GH: Sepsis syndrome and septic shock in pediatrics: current concepts of terminology, pathophysiology, and management, *J Pediatr* 123(4):497–508, 1993.
20. Silverman BK: *Advanced pediatric life support*, Elk Grove Village, Ill, 1993, American Academy of Pediatrics, Dallas, 1989, American College of Emergency Physicians.
21. Soud T: Respiratory failure and shock. In Haley K, Baker P, eds: *Emergency nursing pediatric course*, Chicago, Ill, 1993, Emergency Nurses Association.

22. Veterans Administration Systemic Sepsis Cooperative Study Group: Effect of high-dose glucocorticoid therapy on mortality in patients with clinical signs of systemic sepsis, *N Engl J Med* 317:659, 1987.

22a. Wetzel RC: Shock. In Rogers MC, ed: *Textbook of pediatric intensive care,* vol. 1, Baltimore, 1987, Williams & Wilkins.

23. Whitfield JM, Dobyns E, Webb S: Neonatal sepsis. In Holbrook PR, ed: *Textbook of pediatric critical care,* Philadelphia, 1993, WB Saunders.

24. Yamamoto LG, Yim GK, Britten AG: Rapid sequence anaesthesia induction for emergency intubation, *Pediatr Emerg Care* 6(3):200–213, 1990.

25. Yu M et al: Effect of maximizing oxygen delivery on morbidity and mortality rates in critically ill patients: a prospective, randomized, controlled study, *Crit Care Med* 21(6):830, 1993.

CHAPTER 7

Life-Threatening Neurologic Emergencies

Marianne Chiafery

■ INTRODUCTION

Neurologic emergencies can be frightening for both the nurse and family. The nervous system coordinates all body functions and determines personal individuality. Injury or disease affecting this system can cause devastating sequelae. Rapid, accurate assessment and treatment are required for any child presenting with neurologic dysfunction.

The purpose of this chapter is to describe common pediatric neurologic emergencies, emergency room treatment, and the role of nursing in patient care. Topics to be addressed are status epilepticus, coma, and increased intracranial pressure.

■ STATUS EPILEPTICUS

ETIOLOGY

Seizures are abnormal, uncontrolled electrical discharges from the neurons of the cerebral cortex resulting in disturbances of motor movement, sensation, and/or level of consciousness. Status epilepticus (SE), a serious complication of seizures, results from prolonged neuronal discharge in the brain. Generalized tonic-clonic seizures that persist for longer than 20 minutes are termed *status epilepticus*. Other seizures, including nonconvulsive, that occur repetitively for at least 30 minutes in the child who does not regain consciousness are also considered status epilepticus.

Status epilepticus is often associated with an underlying problem (Box 7-1). A common etiology of SE is the sudden withdrawal of anticonvulsant drugs in patients with known seizure disorders.[17] Serum anticonvulsant levels fall below the therapeutic range for a variety of reasons, including lack of compliance, insufficient dosage due to a growth spurt, or interactions with other medications. However, other neurologic, metabolic, or infectious disorders must also be ruled out. Possible neurologic problems include infections, intracranial tumors, and trauma. Metabolic disorders that may present with seizures include hypoxia, electrolyte disturbances, and toxic ingestions. Febrile seizures, common in children under 5 years of age, may result in SE. In many instances, however, no cause can be identified for SE.

Any uncontrolled seizure activity can result in status epilepticus. Generalized tonic-clonic SE, involving multiple areas of the brain, is life threatening. Death may occur from complications, overmedication, or the underlying disease. SE with partial seizures, involving a localized area of the brain, is less serious. However, untreated partial seizures may progress to generalized SE. The various types of seizures are described in Chapter 12.

PATHOPHYSIOLOGY

With prolonged generalized motor seizure activity, the child develops systemic abnormalities that contribute to poor outcomes. Hypoxia and lactic acidosis result from poor ventilation and oxygenation. Decreased oxygenation of the brain and cardiac compromise due to acidosis can result in permanent neurologic sequelae or death. Increased motor movement and stress increase glucose utilization. The young child who has poor glycogen stores can quickly develop hypoglycemia. Hyperthermia is common due to continuous motor movement.

CLINICAL PRESENTATION

The child in status epilepticus presents in a state of continuous seizures or frequently recurring seizures

Box 7-1   Common Causes of Status Epilepticus in Children

Idiopathic
Anticonvulsant medication withdrawal
Febrile seizures
Infectious
   Meningitis
   Encephalitis
Toxic-Metabolic
   Hypoxia
   Hypoglycemia
   Electrolyte imbalances
   Toxic ingestion
Chronic encephalopathy
CNS degenerative disease
Tumors
Congenital abnormalities
Trauma

Box 7-2   History of the Seizing Child
Seizure description • Duration • Presence of aura • Eye movements • Cyanosis • Incontinence • Loss of consciousness during seizure • Focal vs. generalized movements **Acute precipitating factors** • Fever • Trauma • Ingestion • Exposure to toxins • Medical illness, such as diarrhea **Past medical history** • Previous seizures • Neurologic disorder • Other chronic disorders such as hypertension, renal disease, diabetes mellitus • Medications, including anticonvulsants • Head trauma **Family history of seizures**

without regaining consciousness. Generalized tonic-clonic seizures involve a period of tonic contractions of all muscles (tonic phase), followed by rhythmic contracting and relaxing muscle movement (clonic phase). The airway may be occluded by the tongue, vomitus, mucus, or blood. Breathing may be shallow, ineffective, or totally absent. As the jaw muscles contract, the soft tissue of the mouth may be injured. Bladder and bowel sphincter control are often lost.

History. A complete history is required to determine the cause of the seizure, but stabilization of the child is never delayed while obtaining a history. Pertinent information includes the details of the current seizure, past medical history, and signs and symptoms of possible acute precipitating factors (Box 7-2).

EMERGENCY DEPARTMENT INTERVENTIONS/NURSING CARE AND EVALUATION

Status epilepticus is a medical emergency; therefore initial interventions require stabilization of the ABCs and control of the seizure activity. Additional interventions include preventing or reversing systemic

abnormalities associated with SE, determining the etiology of the seizures, treating the underlying problem(s), and preventing seizure recurrence (Box 7-3).

ABCs. The airway is of primary concern; however, in the seizing child maintaining a patent airway is a challenge because the jaw is often clenched. Force should not be used to insert any solid object(s), including an oral airway, into the mouth. Nasal airways are easy to insert and may be all that is required until the seizure is controlled. Intubation is indicated if the seizure activity is prolonged, if the child cannot be adequately ventilated with a bag-valve-mask, or before general anesthesia is initiated. Additional airway interventions include keeping the airway clear of secretions by suctioning and preventing aspiration by turning the child on the side (unless there is evidence of head or neck trauma).

Box 7-3 Nursing Care of the Child in Status Epilepticus

Airway
Maintain C-spine if suspicion of trauma
Suction secretions
Insert nasal airway
Position child on side if possible
Prepare for possible intubation

Breathing
Give oxygen by nonrebreather mask
Bag-valve-mask if hypoventilating
Place child on pulse oximeter

Circulation
Establish vascular access
Administer fluids as ordered
Place child on a cardiac monitor

Disability (neurologic)
Establish seizure precautions
Administer medications to control seizures as
   ordered

Expose
Remove child's clothing

Fahrenheit
Keep child warm but prevent hyperthermia

Get vital signs
Obtain vital signs, including rectal or core
   temperature

History
Talk to family, EMS, witnesses

Head-to-toe
Complete physical assessment
Look for signs of abuse

Diagnostic tests
Bedside blood glucose
Obtain lab specimens
Accompany child to radiology
Prepare for possible septic workup

Treat systemic abnormalities
Correct acidosis with ventilation
Administer $NaHCO_3$ for persistent acidosis
Administer dextrose 25% for hypoglycemia
Administer antibiotics if infection is suspected

Family care
Keep family informed
Provide emotional support

Oxygenation is maximized by administering 100% oxygen via a nonrebreather mask. Bag-valve-mask (BVM) ventilation with 100% oxygen is indicated when the child's ventilatory efforts are ineffective. Intubation should be anticipated, and supplies must be readily available. Pulse oximetry is helpful in monitoring the child's oxygenation. Arterial blood gases (ABGs) may be obtained to assess the severity of metabolic acidosis and the effectiveness of oxygenation and ventilation. When BVM ventilation is initiated, a nasogastric tube should be inserted to remove gastric contents and air from the stomach. This prevents emesis and facilitates ventilation, especially in small children.

Rapid sequence induction (RSI) anesthesia is the safest method of intubating a child in status epilepticus (see Chapter 6). A sequence of drugs, including a short-acting barbiturate, atropine, and a paralyzing agent, are administered for sedation, paralysis, and prevention of procedural complications. Sometimes lidocaine is given to decrease the transient rise in intracranial pressure (ICP) that occurs with intubation. Although paralyzing agents may appear to stop seizure activity, they merely block all skeletal muscle movement, eliminating the clinical manifestations of seizure activity. The nurse caring for a child who is chemically paralyzed must remain with the child at all times. Endotracheal tube patency and placement must be assessed frequently.

After stabilization of the airway and breathing, cardiovascular status is assessed. Vascular access is required to treat the seizure and any underlying disorders. Intravenous (IV) access may not be easily achieved on a seizing child; therefore the intraosseous (IO) route is sometimes indicated. The IO route provides a rapid and highly effective alternative for the infusion of fluids and antiepileptic drugs. If signs of shock are present, a fluid bolus of 20 cc/kg normal saline (NS) or lactated Ringer's solution (LR) may be infused to improve perfusion. If the child's perfusion is normal, intravenous fluids is restricted until cerebral edema and head trauma are ruled out. All fluid intake and output requires strict monitoring.

Seizure precautions. The seizing child should be protected from injury by careful monitoring of the child's immediate environment. Potentially harmful objects such as equipment and needles should be kept off the bed. The child is not forcibly restrained; however, side rails can be padded and placed in the up position. Airway management equipment must be readily available at the bedside.

Seizure control. Anticonvulsant medications are administered to stop the seizures as quickly as possible and to prevent their recurrence (Table 7-1). Emergency anticonvulsant drugs are administered via the port closest to the insertion site of the IV/IO catheter and flushed with 2 to 3 cc NS to ensure rapid delivery into the systemic circulation. If vascular access is not readily established, diazepam or lorazepam may be administered per rectum, although the absorption is slower and more variable than the intravascular route. A lubricated 1-cc syringe can be directly inserted into the rectum to deliver the medication, or a feeding tube may be used. If a feeding tube is used, the medication must be flushed out of the tubing. The intravascular route is preferred whenever possible.

Benzodiazepines (lorazepam and diazepam) are first-line medications for the treatment of SE. Lorazepam (Ativan) and diazepam (Valium) readily cross the blood-brain barrier for a rapid onset of action. Unfortunately, they have a short duration of action, and the risk of seizure recurrence is high.

Lorazepam is preferred for the acute management of status epilepticus, because it has a longer duration of action than diazepam, with similarly rapid onset.[10,21] Diazepam enters the brain rapidly, but serum concentration falls to 50% within 15 minutes after administration.[3] If either lorazepam or diazepam is ineffective, it may be repeated.

Administration of the benzodiazepines can cause respiratory depression or arrest. It is necessary, therefore, to closely monitor respiratory status and have emergency airway equipment readily available. Positioning of the child's head and/or insertion of a nasal airway helps maintain airway patency and may prevent respiratory arrest.

Long-acting anticonvulsants are often given in conjunction with benzodiazepines. An IV loading dose of phenytoin (Dilantin) 15–20 mg/kg (up to 1000 mg) is initially administered to quickly achieve serum levels.[17] *Phenytoin* must be administered in normal saline because it precipitates in glucose solutions. It is given slowly (max rate of 50 mg/min) to prevent hypotension and cardiac dysrhythmias. Cardiac and blood pressure monitoring and frequent vital signs are required during the administration of a phenytoin bolus. *Phenobarbital* is a long-acting barbiturate that does not cause cessation of seizures until 10 to 20 minutes after the drug is infused. Therefore it is not a first-line medication in the control of seizures, but it does help prevent recurrence of seizures.

If seizure activity persists for more than 1 hour, the child requires more aggressive treatment in an intensive care environment. Treatment may require general anesthesia induced by inhalation agents or barbiturates, such as pentobarbital, thiopental, or phenobarbital. During these interventions, the child must be chemically paralyzed, mechanically ventilated, and closely monitored.

Treat/Prevent systemic abnormalities. Systemic abnormalities often result from prolonged seizure activity. Therefore interventions are initiated to not only treat actual problems but also prevent abnormalities secondary to the seizure activity. Examples of systemic abnormalities include hypoxia, acidosis, hypoglycemia, and hyperthermia. Hypoxia and acidosis can be prevented or corrected with adequate ventilation and oxygenation as described in the section on ABCs.

Frequent bedside blood glucose determinations are required, because hypoglycemia may either cause or be precipitated by seizures. Hypoglycemic children are given 1 to 2 ml dextrose 25% slow IV push. A maintenance dextrose solution may then be continuously infused to prevent further hypoglycemia.

Hyperthermia is another problem created by prolonged seizures. The child's rectal or core temperature is continuously monitored and active methods of cooling are initiated as indicated.

Evaluate and treat underlying cause. While seizure control interventions are being undertaken, a search for the underlying cause of the seizure activity is conducted. This includes obtaining a thorough history (see Box 7-2) and performing a complete physical exam. The exam must include observation for signs of child abuse such as retinal hemorrhage, an indication of "shaken baby syndrome." Another finding that may indicate intracranial pathology is a bulging fontanel on an infant. Diagnostic tests such as lumbar puncture or nuclear imaging studies may be performed depending on the history and clinical findings (Box 7-4). If infection is the suspected cause of the seizure activity, antibiotics are begun, even if the septic workup is not complete.

Family care. Seizures are frightening events to witness, and parents may be very upset on their child's arrival in the emergency department (ED). Whenever possible, parents should be allowed to remain with their child; however, if ED protocol or physician

TABLE 7-1	Medications for Status Epilepticus				
DRUG	DOSAGE*	ROUTE	ONSET OF ACTION†	DURATION†	COMMENTS
Lorazepam	0.05-0.1 mg/kg/ dose over 2 min (up to max of 4 mg/dose) May repeat q 10-15 min Adult: 4 mg/dose; max dose 8 mg/ over 12 hrs	IV IO PR	2-3 min Slowly absorbed from rectal route	24-48 hr	Has longer half-life than diazepam May cause respiratory depression Rectal route less effective than for diazepam
Diazepam	0.2-0.5 mg/kg; rate not to exceed 2 mg/min 0.5 mg/kg per return (PR) Adult: 5-10 mg/ dose May repeat q15-30min up to a max dose: <5 yrs: 5 mg >5 yrs: 10 mg Adult: 30 mg	IV IO PR	IV or IO 1-3 min PR 6-10 min	5-15 min	May cause respiratory depression, hypotension Precipitates easily; inject as close to IV insertion site as possible Use with caution in patients with glaucoma, shock, and depression
Phenytoin	15-20 mg/kg (loading dose) Rate not to exceed 0.5 mg/kg/ min or 50 mg/ min (adult) Max 1000 mg/ 24 hr	IV IO	10-30 min after infusion complete	12-24 hr	May cause bradycardia, hypotension, or cardiac dysrhythmias; toxicity related to rapid infusion rates Dilute in NS only Contraindicated in heart block or sinus bradycardia
Phenobarbital	15-18 mg/kg (loading dose) infants/ children/adults Rate not to exceed 1 mg/kg/min May give additional 5 mg/kg q15-30min up to 30 mg/kg	IV IO	IV 10-20 min IM 2-4 hr	1-3 days	May cause respiratory depression or hypotension Profound effect on mental status Dilute in NS only Contraindicated in hepatic or renal disease or porphyria (disorder of blood pigment metabolism)

*Dosages (may vary according to local protocols) from Barone M: *The Harriet Lane handbook,* ed 14, St Louis, 1996, Mosby.
†From Tunik MG, Young, GM: Status epilepticus in children: the acute management, *Pediatr Clin North Am* 39(5):1007-1030, 1992.

Box 7-4   Diagnostic Tests for Status Epilepticus

Frequent bedside glucose determinations
Serum glucose
Serum electrolytes
Calcium
ABG
WBC with differential

Obtain the following based on child's history and physical exam:
   LP (for signs/symptoms of meningitis; may need to be postponed until child is stabilized and increased ICP ruled out)
   Blood cultures (if febrile)
   Anticonvulsant drug levels (if currently taking anticonvulsants)
   Toxicology screen (if any question of accidental or intentional ingestion)
   Nuclear imaging studies (if concerned about trauma or masses)

Box 7-5   Altered Levels of Consciousness

Lethargy: Drowsy, but follows simple commands
Stupor: Difficult to arouse and responds inconsistently to verbal commands
Semicoma: Does not follow commands, but demonstrates purposeful movement to noxious stimuli
Coma: No purposeful movements; cannot be aroused by verbal or noxious stimuli

TABLE 7-2	Etiologies for Coma
CATEGORY	**ETIOLOGIES**
Congenital	Hydrocephalus
	Arteriovenous malformation
	Arnold-Chiari malformation
Metabolic	Diabetic ketoacidosis
	Hypoglycemia
	Severe dehydration
	Vitamin deficiency
	Toxic ingestions
	Intrinsic metabolic disorders
	Myxedema
	Uremia
	Hypoxic-ischemic insult
Infectious	Sepsis
	Encephalopathy
	Reye's syndrome
	Meningitis
Vascular	Intracranial hemorrhage
Intracranial	Tumor
	Trauma
	Infarction
	Abscess

preference requires they leave the room, they must be continuously informed of their child's progress. Concerns about etiology, long-term prognosis, and immediate care needs are common. Parents may express feelings of guilt about missing signs of the child's illness or delays in seeking attention. Honesty is essential and reassurances, if appropriate, are helpful.

Documentation. The seizure history, initial physical assessment, interventions, and ongoing assessments should be accurately documented. When child abuse is suspected, documentation must also reflect objective, nonjudgmental findings, including conflicting or changing stories or an injury that does not correlate with the history. A description of caregiver affect, parenting behaviors, and the physical condition of the child should also be included. Photographs of obvious injuries provide accurate and objective evidence when child abuse is suspected.

▌COMA

ETIOLOGY

A coma is a state of unconsciousness from which the patient cannot be aroused by verbal or noxious stimuli. The comatose patient has no purposeful movements.

There are other less profound altered states of consciousness, which can be difficult to categorize, including lethargy, stupor, and semicoma (Box 7-5). These terms are subjective and open to interpretation.

The bewildering array of potential etiologies for coma present a challenging puzzle to health care providers (Table 7-2). Coma can be caused by traumatic or nontraumatic causes such as metabolic, hormonal, or electrolyte abnormalities; anoxic damage; or exogenous toxins.

PATHOPHYSIOLOGY

The reticular activating system, located within the brain stem, acts in tandem with the cerebral cortex to maintain consciousness and easy arousability. Coma results from extensive damage to both cerebral hemispheres or the reticular activating system.[20] Whatever the etiology, however, a common final pathway results in the comatose state and is indicative of dangerous pathology.

Brain stem compression from either traumatic or nontraumatic coma etiologies can lead to herniation, a life-threatening displacement or compression of brain tissue. Cerebral herniation can occur laterally from one side of the brain to the other across the falx cerebri, through the foramen magnum into the posterior fossa (transtentorial or central) or from the supratentorial to the infratentorial compartment (uncal) (Fig. 7-1). Ultimately brain stem compression will lead to respiratory arrest, bradycardia, and death (Table 7-3).

CLINICAL PRESENTATION

The comatose child's clinical presentation provides diagnostic clues to the severity of cerebral dysfunction, as well as the affected area of the brain. Signs and symptoms vary based on the underlying pathology and the child's age (Box 7-6).

Level of consciousness. Children may present to the ED with varying levels of conscious-

ness. The Glasgow Coma Scale is an objective, standardized tool that helps measure and interpret the adult and older child's level of consciousness (Table 7-4). Modifications of the Glasgow Scale have been made for preverbal children (Tables 7-4 and 7-5), but they are not as widely accepted. A Glasgow coma score (GCS) of less than 7 generally indicates a comatose state; the lowest score of 3 is associated with deep coma.[22] Periodic evaluation of the child's GCS is required to determine changes in the child's status.

Motor movement. Motor response to command or painful stimuli is measured by the Glasgow Coma Scale. Purposeful movements to ward off painful stimuli are positive signs, whereas flaccidity is an ominous sign of diffuse brain dysfunction. Spontaneous movement, muscle strength, tone, and symmetry must also be assessed serially; these may range from normal to absent. Spontaneous movements may be completely absent or there may be tremors, muscle spasms, purposeless plucking, or repetitive movements. Combative behavior is sometimes present.

Decorticate and decerebrate posturing are abnormal motor responses (Fig. 7-2). Decorticate posturing indicates damage to the basal ganglia, thalamus, or cerebral hemisphere with brain stem function intact. Decorticate posturing involves flexion of the arms and wrists on the chest, adduction of the upper extremities, and extension and adduction of the lower extremities. Damage to the brain stem at the level of the midbrain or pons is evidenced by decerebrate rigidity including rigid extension, abduction, and hyperpronation of the upper and lower extremities.

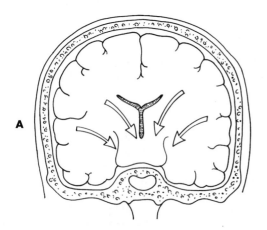 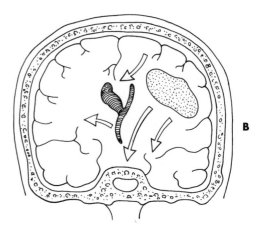

FIG. 7-1. **A,** Central downward herniation. **B,** Uncal herniation.

Eyes. The eye exam reveals extensive information about both the etiology and severity of the comatose child's illness. Best eye opening in response to stimuli helps identify the child's level of consciousness in the GCS. Fundoscopic exam may reveal retinal hemorrhages consistent with trauma, or papilledema, a sign of increased ICP. Spontaneous or induced eye movements should be noted.

Pupillary responses in comatose patients vary. The size and the reactivity to light provide helpful diagnostic clues to the etiology of coma. Table 7-6 reviews some of the common pupillary responses and associated disorders.

Reflexes. A neurologically intact child has normal reflex responses. Abnormal deep tendon reflexes (DTRs) indicate spinal cord injury and are not helpful in determining the level of a brain injury, because the reflex arc only involves the spinal cord. Decreased or absent DTRs may indicate an electrolyte or metabolic abnormality. Reflexes that are useful in assessing brain stem function are the oculocephalic, oculovestibular, corneal, and other protective reflexes.

The oculocephalic, or "doll's eyes," reflex is evaluated by watching the child's open eyes as the head is quickly turned from midline position to one side, then the other. Normally the patient's eyes move symmetrically in the opposite direction from which the head is turned. If the eyes turn with the head in the direction of the turn, an abnormality of the brain stem or the third cranial nerve is indicated. This test is contraindicated in any patient with a possible cervical spine injury.

The oculovestibular response, or "cold calorics," is elicited by the instillation of 20 cc of ice water into the external auditory canal, causing vestibular stimula-

TABLE 7-3	Clinical Manifestations of Brain Herniation Syndromes	
TYPE	**DESCRIPTION**	**CLINICAL MANIFESTATIONS**
Central	Downward displacement of brain tissue through the tentorium onto the diencephalon and brain stem	Early (diencephalon involvement): Depressed LOC Cheyne-Stokes respirations Small reactive pupils Abnormal flexion posturing Intact oculocephalic and oculovestibular reflexes Late (brain stem involvement): Apnea or slow, irregular respirations Fixed, dilated pupils Decerebrate posturing to flaccidity No oculocephalic or oculovestibular reflexes Death
Uncal	Unilateral displacement of temporal lobe (uncus) laterally and downward across tentorial edge and onto brain stem	Early: Ipsilateral dilated, unreactive pupil from compression of 3rd nerve Depressed LOC Impaired oculocephalic or oculovestibular reflexes Contralateral hemiparesis to hemiplegia Plantar extensor responses (Babinski) Late: If process not reversed, progressive diencephalon and brain stem compression occurs with clinical signs as noted above

Box 7-6   Signs and Symptoms Indicating Cerebral Dysfunction or Increasing ICP

Infants
Tense, bulging fontanel; lack of normal pulsations
Separated cranial sutures
Macewen (cracked-pot) sign
Irritability
High-pitched cry
Increased occipital-frontal circumference
Distended scalp veins
Changes in feeding
Cries when held or rocked
"Setting sun" sign

Children
Headache
Nausea
Vomiting—often without nausea
Diplopia, blurred vision
Seizures

Personality and behavior signs
Irritability (toddlers), restlessness
Indifference, drowsiness, or lack of interest
Decline in school performance
Diminished physical activity and motor performance
Increased complaints of fatigue; tiredness; increased time devoted to sleep
Significant weight loss possible from anorexia and vomiting
Memory loss if pressure is markedly increased
Inability to follow simple commands
Progression to lethargy and drowsiness

Late signs
Lowered level of consciousness
Decreased motor response to command
Decreased sensory response to painful stimuli
Alterations in pupil size and reactivity
Sometimes decerebrate or decorticate posturing
Cheyne-Stokes respirations
Papilledema

From Wong DL: *Whaley and Wong's essentials of pediatric nursing,* ed 5, St Louis, 1997, Mosby.

tion. The eyes of a child with an intact brain stem symmetrically deviate toward the irrigated ear. Nystagmus is often observed. This test is painful and for obvious reasons is not performed on a child who is awake.[22]

The corneal reflex is tested by gently stroking the peripheral area of the cornea with a wisp of cotton. If the brain stem is intact, the child will blink. The absence of cough and gag reflexes signifies the child's inability to maintain and protect the airway. The gag reflex can be tested by inserting a suction catheter into the oropharynx. Airway management is essential in the absence of the gag reflex.

Vital signs.   Vital sign changes are sensitive, but often nonspecific, indicators of various disorders that cause coma. For example, fever or hypothermia may be associated with infections such as meningitis or sepsis. Tachycardia is an early, sensitive indicator of shock, but it may also be caused by fever, stress, or increased activity. Respiratory patterns correlate with the level of brain involvement and in combination with pupillary findings, posturing, and reflexes can indicate the severity of the coma (Fig. 7-3). Hypotension is an ominous sign of late-stage shock. Cushing's triad of bradycardia (tachycardia in infants), widened pulse pressure, and alteration in the respiratory pattern occurs late in the course of increased ICP.

EMERGENCY DEPARTMENT INTERVENTIONS/NURSING CARE AND EVALUATION

When a comatose child arrives in the ED, the health care team works collaboratively to stabilize the ABCs, and search for an etiology (Box 7-7). Because many interventions and the history are performed simultaneously, the basics of stabilization should not be overlooked.

Airway.   As with any critically ill patient, assessment of the airway and ventilation is the first priority of care. The comatose child is particularly prone to airway problems, since an altered level of consciousness can allow the tongue to fall back and occlude the airway. Manual positioning of the head and the use of oral or nasal airways temporarily assist in maintaining the airway. Early, definitive control of the airway through intubation is required if ventilatory status is compromised, the gag and swallow reflexes are absent,

TABLE 7-4	Glasgow Coma Scale	
CATEGORY	PATIENT RESPONSE	SCORE
Best eye opening	Spontaneous	4
	To speech	3
	To pain	2
	No response	1
Best motor response	Obeys commands	6
	Localizes pain/purposeful movements	5
	Withdraws (pain)	4
	Abnormal flexion (decorticate)	3
	Abnormal extension (decerebrate)	2
	No response	1
Best verbal response	Oriented	5
	Confused conversation	4
	Inappropriate words	3
	Incomprehensible sounds	2
	No response	1

TABLE 7-5	Pediatric Glasgow Coma Scale		
0-1 YEAR	>1-5 YEARS	>5 YEARS	
Best eye opening			
4 Spontaneous	Spontaneous		
3 To voice/shout	To verbal command		
2 To pain	To pain		
1 No response	No response		
Best motor response			
6 Normal spontaneous movements	Obeys commands		
5 Localizes pain	Localizes pain/purposeful movements		
4 Flexion withdrawal	Flexion withdrawal (pain)		
3 Abnormal flexion (decorticate)	Abnormal flexion (decorticate)		
2 Abnormal extension (decerebrate)	Abnormal extension (decerebrate)		
1 No response	No response		
Best verbal response			
5 Cries appropriately, smiles, coos	Appropriate words/sounds	Oriented and converses	
4 Cries	Inappropriate words/sounds	Disoriented and converses	
3 Inappropriate crying/screaming	Cries/screams	Inappropriate words	
2 Grunts, moans	Grunts, moans	Incomprehensible sounds	
1 No response	No response	No response	

Modified from Barkin R: *Pediatric emergency medicine,* ed 2, St Louis, 1996, Mosby.

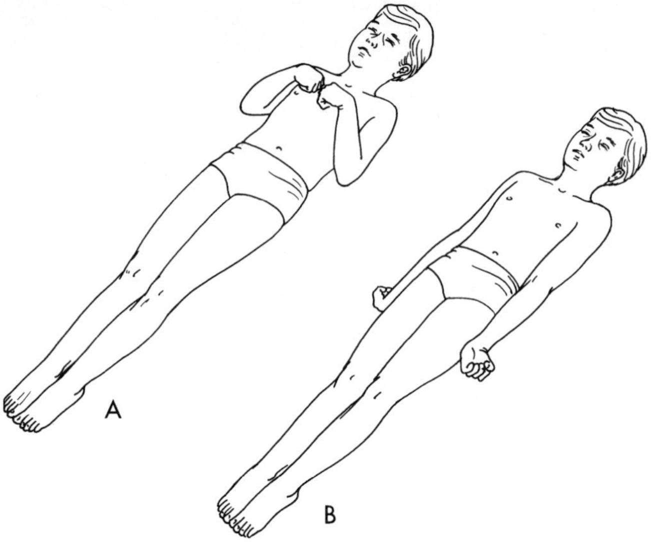

Fig. 7-2. Decorticate (**A**) and decerebrate (**B**) motor responses.

TABLE 7-6	Pupillary Abnormalities in Coma
PUPILLARY FINDINGS	**ASSOCIATED ABNORMALITY**
Dilated, reactive to light	Drug use or toxic ingestion
Regular, no light reaction	Midbrain lesion
Pinpoint or small, reactive to light	Damage to pons area of brain stem Metabolic disorders Opiate or barbiturate ingestion
Dilated or pinpoint, sluggish reaction to light	Increased ICP
Dilated and unreactive to light	Herniation, brain stem damage, especially when pupils "fixed" Third cranial nerve damage—may be unilateral Hypothermia, anoxia, poisoning with atropine-like substances

Data from Fuchs et al., 1992; Matthew, 1971; Wong, 1997.

or prolonged airway maintenance is necessary. C-spine precautions must be maintained if there is any suspicion of trauma. Because the comatose child may be unable to manage secretions, suction equipment must be readily available. In addition, positioning the child on either side will facilitate drainage of secretions. Gastric decompression by means of an orogastric or nasogastric tube will prevent aspiration due to vomiting or reflux.

Breathing. An assessment of respiratory rate, effort, and pattern is required in the comatose child. Oxygen administration via nonrebreather mask is always indicated during the acute stage of coma. Bag-valve-mask ventilation with 100% oxygen is indicated if the child is apneic or hypoventilating. Pulse oximetry is used to monitor oxygenation.

Circulation. Heart rate, cardiac rhythm, blood pressure, and perfusion is continuously monitored. Vascular access will be required to administer fluids and medications. If the comatose child is hypotensive or has poor perfusion, immediate fluid resuscitation (10 to 20 cc/kg NS or LR) is initiated, along with vasopressor support as needed. If the child is normotensive and perfusing well, circulatory status is maintained by judicious administration of fluids. Children with suspected intracranial hypertension require close neurologic monitoring during fluid administration, because liberal crystalloid infusion

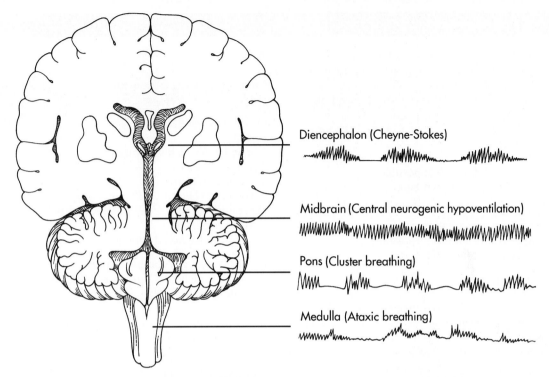

Diencephalon (Cheyne-Stokes)

Midbrain (Central neurogenic hypoventilation)

Pons (Cluster breathing)

Medulla (Ataxic breathing)

FIG. 7-3. Respiratory patterns correlated with brain function level. As the influences of higher areas of the brain are removed through ischemia or compression, characteristic breathing patterns are found.

can create a shift of free water into the brain tissue, worsening intracranial hypertension.

Disability (neurologic). Once the ABCs are stabilized, a quick neurologic exam is performed, including pupillary responses and level of consciousness. As time permits, a more detailed neurologic assessment is required and is often performed during the head-to-toe exam.

The Glasgow Coma Scale is an objective assessment of the patient's best verbal response, motor response, and eye opening. Because children are more likely to respond to a familiar voice, it is best to ask the parents' help in eliciting responses. If the child is partially paralyzed or injured, the unaffected extremities are tested to determine the best response. The GCS ranges from a total score of 15, indicating a fully alert, conscious patient to a minimum of 3, which is total unresponsiveness. A change of 2 points or more indicates a true improvement or deterioration of patient status. The modified Glasgow Coma Scale is used to evaluate young children and infants with limited verbal capabilities.

Vital signs. A complete set of baseline vital signs, including a rectal temperature, is required. Vital signs that are abnormal for the child's age should be correlated with clinical findings. Transient changes are usually not as concerning as prolonged abnormalities. For example, transient bradycardia may occur in response to suctioning, whereas prolonged bradycardia suggests ominous pathology, such as intracranial lesions, hypoxia, or a dysfunctional cardiac conduction system.

Head-to-toe assessment. Valuable clues to the etiology of coma can be identified while conducting a head-to-toe assessment. Further treatment and prioritization of care is often dictated by the results of this exam. For the nurse to perform an adequate exam, the child must be fully exposed; however, the child must be kept warm.

Box 7-7   Nursing Care of the Comatose Child

Airway
Position the airway; sniff position for infant or jaw thrust for child
Maintain C-spine precautions if suspicion of trauma
Suction secretions; simultaneously check for gag reflex
Insert an oral or nasal airway
Position child on side if possible
Prepare for possible intubation

Breathing
Give oxygen by nonrebreather mask
Bag-valve-mask if hypoventilating
Place child on pulse oximeter

Circulation
Establish vascular access
Administer fluids (bolus, maintenance, or restricted) as needed
Put child on a cardiac monitor
Vasopressor support if indicated

Disability (neurologic)
Assess pupils and GCS

Expose
Remove child's clothing

Fahrenheit
Keep child warm or control fever

Get vital signs
Include rectal or core temperature

History
Talk to family, EMS, witnesses

Head-to-toe
Complete physical assessment
Look for signs of abuse

Diagnostic tests
Bedside blood glucose
Obtain baseline lab specimens
Blood, urine cultures
Toxicology screen
Accompany child to CT/x-ray
Defer lumbar puncture until increased ICP ruled out
EEG for undiagnosed patients

Identify etiology/complications
Assess for evidence of herniation, increased ICP, meningitis, poisoning, intracranial lesions

Interventions
Insert an orogastric/nasogastric tube to prevent aspiration and facilitate ventilation
Insert indwelling bladder catheter
Immediately treat possible herniation
Treat increased ICP if present (see Box 7-8)
Administer trials of glucose and naloxone
Treat for poisoning if indicated
Correct fluid and electrolyte abnormalities
Administer broad-spectrum antibiotics if meningitis or sepsis suspected

Family care
Keep family informed
Provide emotional support

Transfer to ICU
Continuously monitor the child
Reassess before transfer

A variety of findings that indicate high-risk situations or a particular etiology may be elicited during the head-to-toe exam. Examples include bruises in various stages of healing or injuries that are not consistent with the history, fulminating meningitis if the child presents with a purpuric rash and altered level of consciousness, or fruity breath odor consistent with diabetic ketoacidosis. All findings must be evaluated in light of the entire clinical picture.

History. Parents should be questioned about prodromes, access to toxic substances, signs and symptoms of infection, chronic illnesses, congenital anomalies, and recent trauma. Ambulance personnel and other witnesses often have pertinent information that can assist in the diagnosis and treatment of the child. A description of the environment may also provide clues about toxic substances or unsafe conditions. Meticulous documentation of the history is

---

Box 7-8   Measures to Control Increased Intracranial Pressure

Hyperventilation (keep Paco$_2$ between 25 and 30 mm Hg)
Fluid restriction (two-thirds maintenance)
Diuretics: mannitol (0.5–1 gm/kg) and/or furosemide (1 mg/kg/dose)
Steroids, controversial (1–2 mg/kg)
Intracranial pressure monitoring
Barbiturate coma

---

important, especially since the etiology may not be readily apparent.

Diagnostic tests.   A variety of diagnostic tests are indicated depending on the child's history and presentation. Bedside blood glucose measurement is performed as soon as possible and baseline laboratory specimens are obtained. These may include a complete blood cell count (CBC) and differential, serum electrolytes, BUN, coagulation studies, liver function tests, arterial blood gas, and toxicology screen. Blood and urine cultures are required for any child with suspected infection, preferably before antibiotics are given.

If intracranial pathology is suspected, a CT scan is indicated to determine the diagnosis and subsequent interventions, such as surgery or medical management. All children with an altered LOC are accompanied to CT or x-ray. STAT EEGs may be helpful for patients without clear-cut diagnoses. A lumbar puncture may be deferred until increased ICP is ruled out, because a sudden decompression within the spinal cord can cause herniation and acute deterioration.

Procedures.   Definitive therapies for the comatose child are dependent upon the specific etiology of the coma. Until the diagnosis is obtained, therapies are initiated on a symptomatic basis.

An indwelling bladder catheter is inserted to accurately assess urine output. If not yet done, a nasogastric tube is inserted. Possible herniation or increased ICP is treated immediately (Box 7-8). Intravenous administration of glucose may be necessary to correct hypoglycemia. Frequently, trials of glucose and naloxone may be administered, whether or not documented hypoglycemia or drug abuse

is present. Temperature extremes and fluid and electrolyte imbalances are corrected. Broad-spectrum antibiotics are administered as soon as cultures are obtained or immediately if the child is emergently ill. Ingestions or other problems are treated symptomatically.

Psychosocial care.   Although the comatose child seems oblivious of the environment, it is unknown what the child is truly experiencing. Anecdotal reports of children who remember statements, songs, and procedures that they experienced while in a coma abound. Thus it behooves all personnel and family members to act as if the child can hear and feel everything. Simple explanations of procedures, gentle conversation, provision of pleasant diversions (such as stories or music), and pain medications before procedures should be routine elements of nursing care.

Family needs must also be addressed. The uncertainty of diagnosis and outcome makes this an extremely difficult situation for family members. They may be frightened to hear that the medical establishment does not immediately *know* what is wrong. The lay public often expects instant answers and finds it difficult to accept that medicine does not always have the answers. Much support is necessary during this uncertain time, including honest answers and frequent updates of the child's condition.

Prognosis.   Reversal of coma and a return to baseline neurologic function are primarily dependent upon the etiology of the comatose state, timing of definitive management, and prevention of complications. The prognosis of a comatose child is generally better than that of a comatose adult, especially in cases of trauma.[8] It is very difficult, however, to predict the outcome for individual children.

INCREASED INTRACRANIAL PRESSURE

ETIOLOGY

A variety of causes can produce increased ICP, including trauma, infection, structural abnormalities, and anoxia. In chronically ill children, a common etiology of increased ICP is ventriculoperitoneal (VP) shunt malfunction (see Chapter 12). Box 7-9 provides a partial list of potential etiologies for increased ICP.

Box 7-9 Etiologies for Increased Intracranial Pressure

Trauma
Head trauma
  Closed
  Penetrating
Multiple trauma

Bleeds
Intracerebral hemorrhage
Subdural hemorrhage
Subarachnoid bleed
Epidural bleed

Infection
Meningitis
Intracranial abscess

Encephalopathy
Diabetic ketoacidosis
Reye's syndrome
Hepatic failure

Hydrocephalus
Arnold-Chiari malformation
Ventriculoperitoneal shunt malfunction

Miscellaneous
Hypertension
Occlusion of cerebral venous outflow
Hyperemia
Hypoxic-ischemic event
Tumors
Status epilepticus

Pathophysiology

The contents of the intracranial vault are enclosed in the rigid, nondistensible skull. Pressure is exerted by three major components of the intracranial vault: brain tissue, circulating blood volume, and cerebrospinal fluid (CSF). Normally ICP is less than 15 mm Hg. Small, transient increases in ICP can occur with normal activities of daily living, such as sneezing. However, the healthy body is able to adjust for these normal fluctuations.

Expansion of any component of the intracranial vault can increase the pressure within the skull. Compensatory mechanisms, to a certain extent, adjust the volume of other components to maintain ICP at a steady state (Monro-Kellie principle). Autoregulatory measures that maintain normal ICP include increased CSF reabsorption by the arachnoid villi, decreased CSF formation, and vasoconstriction of the blood vessels. These compensatory mechanisms are generally effective for mild injury or illness but are quickly overwhelmed by moderate to severe disturbances.

As pressure in the intracranial vault climbs, the brain tissue expands through any possible outlet. Herniation is the syndrome of brain tissue being displaced from the intracranial vault through the tentorium, foramen magnum, or falx cerebri (see Fig. 7-1). As brain tissue is displaced, compression and destruction of vital centers for life function occur, and the patient suffers neurologic death.

Children seem to tolerate increased ICP more readily than adults, although the reasons for this are unclear. Infants have the advantage of an easily distensible skull, due to open sutures and fontanels, allowing the intracranial contents room to expand. Another possible factor may be the lower blood pressure in children, which diminishes the incidence of cerebral edema.[9] Children respond to head injury differently than adults. Whereas adults develop localized edema, children tend to have diffuse brain swelling. In children, cerebral hyperemia, an increase in cerebral blood volume, is commonly seen in the first hours after a head injury and may contribute to the development of cerebral edema.[15]

Two processes cause brain tissue swelling: cytotoxic edema and vasogenic edema. Cytotoxic edema results from a failure of the sodium-potassium pump at the cellular level. The osmotic gradient is disturbed, allowing water to flow into the cell. The resulting increase in cell size causes swelling of brain tissue. Vasogenic edema results from disruption of the blood-brain barrier, with increased fluid leak between the brain cells. Decreased density is seen on the CT scan, because water is less dense than brain tissue or blood.

Clinical Presentation

Increased ICP may occur rapidly or slowly, depending on the etiology. Early signs and symptoms are often very subtle and may be confused with other illnesses.

Because early signs of increased ICP are subtle, the caregivers' assessment of their infant or child is extremely important. Alterations in normal behavior and activities of daily living may be the earliest signs of increasing ICP. Signs of increasing ICP in the infant differ from those in the child and include irritability, a high-pitched cry, a tense or bulging fontanel, and/or separated cranial sutures. The child may be lethargic, confused, agitated, or disoriented; older children may complain of a headache (see Box 7-6). Early morning headaches with vomiting may be an indication of intracranial tumor, which is compressing the medulla. Blurred vision or diplopia may occur from direct pressure on the optic nerve. Regardless of cause, if the ICP continues to increase without intervention, the child's condition will deteriorate.

Late signs of increased ICP are more dramatic and indicate the need for immediate intervention. Marked changes in the child's level of consciousness will be observed. Seizures may also occur and are frequently the presenting complaint. The development of a dilated, nonreactive pupil, resulting from direct compression of the third nerve, is an ominous sign, indicating imminent or actual tentorial herniation. Bilateral pupil dilation unresponsive to light indicates brain stem herniation (see Table 7-3).

Changes in vital signs are a late indication of increased ICP. Cushing's triad, consisting of bradycardia, widened pulse pressure, and respiratory irregularities, may be seen in older children. Young children and infants often become tachycardic rather than bradycardic with increased ICP.

EMERGENCY DEPARTMENT INTERVENTIONS/NURSING CARE AND EVALUATION

When the child with an altered level of consciousness and suspected increased ICP presents to the ED, stabilization of the ABCs is the first priority of care. In addition, measures to decrease ICP must be initiated rapidly and underlying pathology identified and treated.

Early control of the airway with endotracheal intubation is required if the child is obtunded or comatose, respiratory function is inadequate, or the airway cannot be protected. Maximizing oxygenation to ensure adequate oxygen delivery to the brain tissue is essential. Oxygen saturation should be maintained at normal or slightly supernormal levels.

Hyperventilation. Prolonged hypercarbia in the first hours after a brain insult has been shown to increase morbidity and mortality rates.[5] Hyperventilation by controlled mechanical ventilation is a standard protocol for decreasing CO_2 and therefore ICP (see Box 7-8). Decreasing the $Paco_2$ with hyperventilation causes cerebral vasoconstriction, with a subsequent decrease in intracranial blood vol-

ume. Some physicians prefer mild hyperventilation ($Paco_2$ = 30 to 34 mm Hg) as the initial intervention, anticipating that further vasoconstriction may be necessary when the ICP peaks at 24 to 72 hours after the injury. As ICP rises, the patient's $Paco_2$ is lowered into the 25 to 30 mm Hg range. Other physicians prefer to immediately hyperventilate the patient to the lower $Paco_2$ range. Hyperventilation, although rapidly effective, is thought to have only transient effects.[8]

Fluid management/diuretics. If hypovolemia is present (e.g., from traumatic, hemorrhagic shock), aggressive fluid resuscitation is required to support perfusion. If perfusion is normal, fluid restriction and diuretic therapy are indicated to decrease the fluid volume in the brain. When diuretic therapy is initiated, a Foley catheter is inserted into the bladder to monitor urine output.

Mannitol is a hyperosmolar agent that is administered IV push at a dose of 0.5 to 1 gm/kg.[18] The goal of mannitol use is to achieve a serum osmolality of 300 to 320 mOsm/L.[11] This facilitates diffusion of free water from brain tissue into the serum, thus causing cells to shrink and the ICP to decrease. Complications of mannitol administration include dehydration and circulatory collapse. Mannitol can also increase the size of an intracranial bleed. Furosemide (Lasix) is a loop diuretic that has been shown to potentiate the action of mannitol.[16] The usual dose of furosemide is 1 mg/kg/dose. A combination of colloids and furosemide can effectively reduce ICP without producing hypovolemia.[11]

Steroids. The effectiveness of steroids such as dexamethasone (Decadron) and methylprednisolone is controversial. Steroids are thought to decrease or prevent cerebral inflammation and edema, although studies have not clearly established any benefits in patients with generalized cerebral edema.[8] Steroids are most effective in managing increased ICP in patients with intracranial tumors.[2] Increased risk of infection, syndrome of inappropriate antidiuretic hormone (SIADH), and hyperglycemia may occur with the use of steroids.

Barbiturates. Barbiturates are thought to reduce ICP and prevent ischemic brain damage by decreasing metabolic needs and oxygen consumption by the brain. Barbiturates are most often used in patients with increased ICP that is not responsive to the other therapies. Potential side effects include hypotension, which can compromise cerebral perfusion, and blunting of the neurologic exam. Etomidate, a hypnotic barbiturate, has been shown to lower ICP by decreasing oxygen demand, without myocardial depression.[4,7]

Intracranial pressure monitoring. An intracranial pressure device may be inserted to monitor changes in intracranial pressure and cerebral perfusion pressure (CPP) in response to fluid therapy and ventilatory management (Fig. 7-4). Although ICP is an important value to assess, cerebral perfusion pressure is more important because children with a normal ICP may have decreased systemic arterial blood flow, which can produce cerebral ischemia (CPP = mean arterial pressure [(MAP)] − ICP). Generally, cerebral ischemia occurs if the CPP falls below 50 mm Hg.

The three most commonly used intracranial pressure monitors include the ventricular drain, subarachnoid screw, and fiberoptic catheter. With a unilateral injury, the monitoring device is placed on the same side as the lesion, since the ICP is often higher under the injured area.[13] To ensure accurate ICP readings, the transducer is positioned level with the top of the auricle of the ear, approximating the level of the lateral ventricle.

In addition to directly measuring the ICP, the ventricular drain, which is inserted into the lateral ventricle, allows for sampling and drainage of CSF when ICP rises to greater than 15 to 20 mm Hg. Unless otherwise ordered by the physician, the drip chamber, as well as the transducer, must be placed at the level of the lateral ventricle (the ear). If the drip chamber is placed too low, excessive CSF will drain and the ventricles will collapse; if it is placed too high, CSF will not drain and the ICP will rise. The nurse should document the color of the drainage and the number of times the patient requires draining of CSF. Since the ventricles make approximately 200 ml of CSF each day, the actual volume of fluid drained is not as important as monitoring the frequency of draining. A major disadvantage of the ventricular catheter is the risk of infection, because it passes through brain tissue.

The subarachnoid or subdural screw and fiberoptic catheter have a lower risk of infection than the ventricular catheter. They are useful for measuring ICP if the ventricles cannot be tapped due to compression by edema. Unfortunately the screw cannot be easily placed in infants because of their thin skulls.

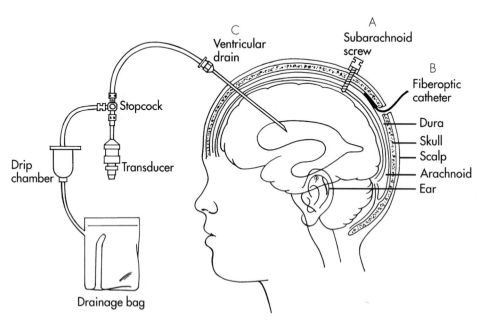

FIG. 7-4. Anatomic positions of *A,* subarachnoid screw; *B,* fiberoptic catheter; and *C,* ventricular drain. Note position of transducer and drip chamber.

The fiberoptic catheter consists of a tiny glass filament, which if bent or crushed will render the catheter useless.

The nurse must never rely totally on the ICP monitor for evaluation of neurologic status. As always, the patient's clinical exam is more important than the number on the monitor. A monitor placed in the supratentorial region may not accurately reflect pressures in the infratentorial region. Thus herniation can occur even with ICP values in the normal range.

Uncontrolled increased intracranial pressure. Uncontrolled intracranial hypertension that is refractory to the usual treatment protocols requires more aggressive management. In these cases, barbiturate coma may be induced to decrease metabolic demand of the brain. This procedure is only undertaken with a well-controlled airway and central venous pressure monitoring.[8] Surgical management of intractable intracranial hypertension includes shunt placement, insertion of a ventricular catheter, burr holes, or removal of a piece of the skull to allow for expansion of the contents of the intracranial vault. Emergency surgery may also be necessary for depressed skull fractures or rapidly expanding lesions.

Patient care measures. The patient with increased ICP requires delicate handling by health care providers to prevent sharp rises in ICP. These measures include providing a calm therapeutic environment (e.g., discussions at the patient's bedside should be limited to positive interactions, and noxious stimuli should be limited).

To facilitate venous return the child's head is maintained in a neutral, midline position and the head of the bed elevated 30 degrees.[6] If a cervical collar is in place, it should not be applied so tightly that it compromises venous return.

Because suctioning increases ICP, it is performed only when absolutely necessary, with no more than two passes of the suction catheter each time.[19]

Temperature extremes are treated aggressively. The shivering and muscle contraction of hypothermia and the increased metabolic demands of fever will elevate ICP. If the child is febrile, the source of the fever is sought and antibiotics administered if bacterial infection is suspected. Central hyperthermia, a common finding in children with damage to the hypothalamic area of the brain, is generally unresponsive to antipyretic drugs such as acetaminophen or ibuprofen.

In these children, cooling blankets are more effective in reducing body temperature.

ADDITIONAL INTERVENTIONS

Several drugs have been suggested for use in reducing ICP. Tham (tromethamine) is an alkalizing agent that lowers CSF lactate levels and decreases ICP.[18] The efficacy of glycerol 30%–sodium ascorbate 20% (GLIAS) as an osmotic diuretic to decrease ICP has also been the subject of study. GLIAS has been shown to effectively decrease ICP and increase intracerebral compliance without significant side effects.[14]

COMPLICATIONS

Because the brain is responsible for all body functions and homeostatic regulation, injury to the nervous system can wreak havoc with other body systems. Complications that may present in the ED include SIADH, diabetes insipidus (DI), neurogenic adult respiratory distress syndrome (ARDS), respiratory depression or failure, cardiac dysrhythmias, or coagulopathies.

SIADH results from pituitary damage causing inappropriate antidiuretic hormone (ADH) release, which decreases urine output, increasing fluid retention. The result is low serum osmolality (<280 mOsm/L) and low serum sodium. The dangers of SIADH are water intoxication which increase cerebral edema, and dilution of serum electrolytes. The only therapy for SIADH is fluid restriction.

Diabetes insipidus also results from pituitary damage. It is characterized by the inability to concentrate urine. These children will present with massive diuresis, dilute urine (specific gravity <1.003), and urine osmolality 50% or less of the serum value. The greatest danger is hypovolemia. Treatment includes fluid replacement and administration of a synthetic antidiuretic hormone such as vasopressin.

Another complication is neurogenic ARDS, which is thought to result from massive catecholamine release that leads to pulmonary vasoconstriction and pulmonary capillary leak. As capillary integrity is lost, fluid leaks into the alveoli, causing hypoxia, which is often unresponsive to oxygen administration.

Because these complications are not unusual in the child with increased ICP, frequent nursing assessments for changes in neurologic status and for signs of complications are required. Abnormal findings are reported to the physician immediately.

▌SUMMARY

Life-threatening neurologic disorders are complex and often involve multiple body systems. Early signs and symptoms may be subtle or difficult to interpret. Early and aggressive intervention is imperative to prevent death or permanent neurologic damage. Knowledge of pediatric responses to neurologic disorders, astute assessment skills, and the ability to intervene rapidly are important nursing skills.

REFERENCES

1. Barone M: *The Harriet Lane Handbook,* ed 14, St Louis, 1996, Mosby.
2. Barron TF: Increased intracranial pressure. In Hoekelman, RA, ed, *Primary pediatric care,* ed 3, St Louis, 1997, Mosby.
3. Booker H, Celesia G: Serum concentrations of diazepam in subjects with epilepsy, *Arch Neurol* 29:191, 1973.
4. Chesnut R, Marshall L: Management of head injury: Treatment of abnormal ICP, *Neurosurg Clin North Am* 2(2):267–84, 1991.
5. Elias-Jones A et al: Management and outcome of severe head injuries in the Trent region 1985–1990, *J Arch Dis in Childhood,* 67(12):1430-1435, 1992.
6. Feldman Z et al: Effect of head elevation on ICP, cerebral perfusion pressure and cerebral blood flow in head-injured patients, *J Neurosurg* 76:207-211, 1992.
7. Frizzell R et al: The effects of etomidate on cerebral metabolism and blood flow in a canine model for hypoperfusion, *J Neurosurg* 74(2):263-269, 1991.
8. Fuchs SM et al: Neurologic disorders. In Barkin RM, ed: *Pediatric emergency medicine: concepts in clinical practice,* St Louis, 1992 Mosby, pp 889-936.
9. Go KG et al: The development of oedema in the immature brain, *Psychiat Neurol Neurochir* 76:427-437, 1973.
10. Govoni M, Wilson B: *Drugs and nursing implications* Norwalk, Ct, 1992, Appleton Lange.
11. Hayek D, Veremakis C: Intracranial pathophysiology brain injury. *Problems in critical care: resuscitation following acute brain injury.* 5:156-186, 1991.
12. Kraus J, Fife D, Conroy C: Pediatric brain injuries: the nature, clinical course, and early outcomes in a defined United States population, *Pediatrics* 79:501, 1987.
12a. Matthew H: Acute poisoning: some myths and misconceptions, *Br Med J* 1:519-522, 1971.
13. Mindermann T et al: Significant lateralization of supratentorial ICP after blunt head trauma. *J Acta Neurchir* 116(1):60-61, 1992.
14. Oppido P et al: Brain oedema and intracranial hypertension treatment by GLIAS, *J Acta Neurchir* 55:40-42, 1992.
15. Pilmer SL, Duhaime A, Raphaely RC: Intracranial pressure control. In Eichelberger, MR, (ed): *Pediatric trauma: prevention, acute care, rehabilitation,* St Louis, 1993, Mosby, pp 200-216.
16. Pollay M et al: Effect of mannitol and furosemide on blood-brain osmotic gradient and intracranial pressure, *Neurosurg* 59:945, 1983.
17. Roddy SM, McBride MC: Status epilepticus. In Hoekelman, RA (ed): *Primary pediatric care,* ed 3, St Louis, 1997, Mosby, pp 1774-1775.
18. Rosner MJ et al: Prospective, randomized trial of THAM therapy in severe brain injury: Preliminary results. In Hoff JT, Betz AL, eds, *Intracranial pressure VII,* Berlin, SpingerVerlag, p 611.
19. Rudy E et al: Endotracheal suctioning in adults with head injury, *Heart Lung* 20(6):667-674, 1991.
20. Steinhart CM, Pearson-Shaver AL: Coma in the pediatric patient. In Fuhrman, BP & Zimmerman, JJ eds: *Pediatric critical care,* St Louis, 1992, Mosby, pp 589-594.
21. Tunik MG, Young GM: Status epilepticus in children: The acute management, *Pediatr Clin North Am* 39(5):1007–1030, 1992.
22. Wong DL: *Whaley and Wong's essentials of pediatric nursing,* ed 5, St Louis, 1997, Mosby.

CHAPTER 8

Pediatric and Neonatal Resuscitation

Mary Fran Hazinski, Saniyyah Mahmoudi

INTRODUCTION

This chapter provides an overview of pediatric and neonatal resuscitation, including the principles, techniques, equipment, and skills needed during resuscitation. The content is written with the assumption that spontaneous ventilation is absent and cardiac compressions are required. For additional information regarding shock and respiratory failure and cardiovascular emergencies, see Chapters 6 and 11.

EPIDEMIOLOGY OF PEDIATRIC AND NEONATAL CARDIOPULMONARY ARREST

The epidemiology of pediatric and neonatal cardiopulmonary arrest is quite different from the epidemiology of arrest in the adult. Adult cardiopulmonary arrest is often cardiac in origin and typically results from a sudden cardiac dysrhythmia associated with myocardial infarction.[11] By comparison, primary cardiac arrest is relatively uncommon in children. In fact, malignant ventricular dysrhythmias are observed in less than 15% of children under the age of 15 when a prehospital cardiopulmonary arrest has occurred.[12,22,23,31]

Hypoxia-induced respiratory arrest is the most common form of pediatric arrest, and bradycardia is the most common terminal cardiac rhythm observed in infants and children.[8] In the newborn, hypoxia caused by respiratory depression or arrest is the most common etiology of bradycardia. If hypoxic bradycardia is not treated, asystolic cardiac arrest develops as a secondary event.

ETIOLOGY OF ARREST IN THE FIELD AND PRIORITIES OF CARE

In an adult the appropriate treatment of sudden ventricular tachycardia/fibrillation cardiac arrest is early defibrillation and support of cardiovascular function.[11,32] Therefore, when an adult is found to be unresponsive by a layperson the American Heart Association recommends "phone first," because definitive treatment requires prompt defibrillation.[9] In the child this approach is inappropriate, because malignant ventricular dysrhythmias are relatively uncommon[4] and because the most common prearrest conditions are respiratory compromise and hypoxic bradycardia.[33] Definitive treatment in the child is therefore the prompt initiation of ventilatory assistance. For this reason the American Heart Association recommends lay rescuers provide basic life support for approximately 1 minute in the child *before* the emergency medical services (EMS) system is activated.[9]

OUTCOME OF RESUSCITATION

In the adult victim of a sudden prehospital cardiac arrest, survival approaches 30%. Most adult survivors are neurologically intact as long as basic life support was initiated after a *witnessed* arrest, defibrillation occurred within 4 minutes of the arrest, and advanced life support was initiated within 8 minutes of the arrest.[11] By comparison, the outcome of pediatric prehospital cardiac arrest is dismal. Survival averages 7% to 11% in most studies, and the majority of survivors are neurologically devastated.[4,16,24] If prehospital *respiratory* arrest is detected *before* cardiac arrest develops, survival may be as high as 50% to 75%, and most survivors are neurologically intact.[33]

An exception to the previous statistics is the pediatric victim of near-drowning. In these children survival approaches 35% and most survivors are neurologically intact when the following conditions are met: the child is submerged for less than 5 minutes; the child receives prompt basic life support at the scene; and the child then receives prompt advanced life support, including intubation.[18,20,25] Poor prognostic signs in pediatric submersion victims include absence of perfusing cardiac rhythm on arrival in the emergency department (ED) despite prehospital basic life support (BLS), a Glasgow Coma Score of less than 4 with unresponsive pupils during the initial 12 to 24 hours in ICU, a submersion duration of greater than 5 minutes in non–icy waters, and a CPR duration of greater than 25 minutes.[18,20,25]

RECOGNITION OF PREARREST CONDITIONS

Pediatric or neonatal cardiorespiratory arrest typically results from progressive deterioration of the child in respiratory failure or shock. In the delivery room, hypoxic respiratory failure is presumed to be present if bradycardia or asystole is observed. In older infants and children many other conditions are potential etiologies of arrest.

Respiratory failure may result from airway, pulmonary, or neuromuscular disease or injury that impairs oxygen exchange or elimination of carbon dioxide. Pulmonary etiologies can produce inadequate gas flow, an increase in the work of breathing, and/or impaired gas diffusion with hypoxemia or respiratory acidosis. Neurologic disease or injury can impair the respiratory drive or compromise the child's ability to protect the upper airway (Fig. 8-1).

Signs of *potential* respiratory failure in children include a respiratory rate that is too fast or too slow for age and/or an increase in the work of breathing. *Actual* respiratory failure is documented by arterial blood gas analysis and clinical examination. It is characterized by hypoxemia despite oxygen administration, increased work of breathing—or inappropriate slowing of respirations, evidence of an increasing intrapulmonary shunt, and/or respiratory acidosis (hypercarbia associated with acidosis). However, any interpretation of arterial blood gases requires knowledge of the child's baseline condition (e.g., the presence of an underlying pulmonary disorder) and a determination of the child's response to therapy.

Causes of shock beyond the newborn period include inadequate intravascular volume relative to the vascular space (hypovolemic shock), myocardial dysfunction (associated with congenital or inflammatory heart disease, electrolyte imbalance, or toxins), or maldistribution of blood flow (septic or anaphylactic shock). Hypovolemic shock, resulting from dehydration or trauma, is the most common form of shock in

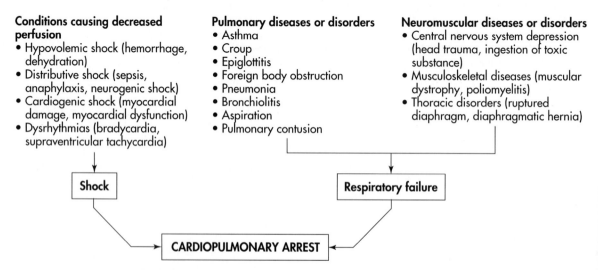

Conditions causing decreased perfusion
- Hypovolemic shock (hemorrhage, dehydration)
- Distributive shock (sepsis, anaphylaxis, neurogenic shock)
- Cardiogenic shock (myocardial damage, myocardial dysfunction)
- Dysrhythmias (bradycardia, supraventricular tachycardia)

Pulmonary diseases or disorders
- Asthma
- Croup
- Epiglottitis
- Foreign body obstruction
- Pneumonia
- Bronchiolitis
- Aspiration
- Pulmonary contusion

Neuromuscular diseases or disorders
- Central nervous system depression (head trauma, ingestion of toxic substance)
- Musculoskeletal diseases (muscular dystrophy, poliomyelitis)
- Thoracic disorders (ruptured diaphragm, diaphragmatic hernia)

Shock

Respiratory failure

CARDIOPULMONARY ARREST

FIG. 8-1. Etiologies of cardiopulmonary arrest in the child.

children. Clinical signs of shock include evidence of inadequate cardiac output and oxygen delivery, evidenced by decreased peripheral perfusion and altered organ function (e.g., oliguria), an altered level of consciousness, and lactic acidosis. Shock may be present despite a normal, low, or high blood pressure—in fact, in children, normotension may persist until cardiopulmonary arrest occurs. Once hypotension is present, *decompensated shock* has developed (see Chapter 6).

▌ BASIC LIFE SUPPORT

The sequence of basic life support is identical in infants and children. Because hypoxia is the most common cause of respiratory arrest, the priorities of care emphasize opening the airway and establishing oxygenation and ventilation. The procedures for BLS (e.g., the hand/finger position for chest compressions) are based on the child's age—infants are less than 1 year of age, and children are between 1 and 8 years of age. Although BLS is defined as resuscitation without the use of adjuncts, performance of ventilation and compression in the ED with the use of a bag and mask will be presented in this section. Resuscitation in the delivery room is summarized later in the chapter.

The following information is based on the recommendations of the American Heart Association.[8,9]

DETERMINE RESPONSIVENESS

The child with impending or actual arrest will be unresponsive to even painful stimuli. When a child is found to be unresponsive in the prehospital setting, the lone rescuer shouts for help. If a second rescuer is present, that rescuer ensures that the EMS system is activated. When the prehospital rescuer is alone, and trauma has not occurred, the rescuer may carry the child to a telephone while initiating resuscitation, in order to activate the EMS system. If head or neck trauma is suspected, the child is not moved unless the cervical spine is completely immobilized.

If the child has arrested or an arrest is imminent in the ED, the nurse calls for assistance and begins resuscitation.

AIRWAY

The most common cause of an airway obstruction in the infant or child is the tongue, particularly if the child has an altered level of consciousness. Other causes of an airway obstruction include foreign bodies, secretions, or inflammatory tissue. When an infant or child

is found unresponsive in the prehospital or ED setting, the airway is opened using the head tilt–chin lift or jaw-thrust maneuver (Fig. 8-2). If trauma is suspected, the jaw-thrust maneuver is performed and the cervical spine completely immobilized. The jaw thrust requires lifting the angles of the mandible bilaterally to move the jaw outward. Suction equipment should be immediately available to clear the airway of secretions.

BREATHING

Assessment. After the airway is opened, the rescuer looks, listens, and feels for evidence of spontaneous ventilation by observing the chest for rise and fall, listening for exhaled air, and feeling for exhaled air flow from the mouth. If spontaneous breathing is present in the prehospital setting, the patent airway is maintained and the child is transported to the hospital. If spontaneous respirations are observed after opening the airway in the hospital setting, consideration is given to intubation or insertion of an oral or nasal airway to maintain patency.

Rescue breathing. If no spontaneous breathing is detected, ventilation is provided. In the prehospital setting, the lay rescuer provides two breaths via mouth-to-nose-and-mouth (in the infant) or mouth-to-mouth (in the child) rescue breathing. A barrier device such as a mask with one-way valve is used when available. The professional rescuer should be equipped with a mask with a one-way valve or other infection control barrier or with a resuscitation bag and mask and 100% oxygen.

The correct force and volume for each rescue breath is that which causes visible chest expansion. If the chest does not rise, the child is not effectively ventilated. Although the airways of young children provide high resistance to flow, the tidal volume required is relatively small. Therefore the volume required is the minimal amount to cause the chest to rise. These breaths are delivered over 1 to 1½ seconds. If breaths are provided rapidly, using significant force and high pressure, gastric inflation will also occur and may result in elevation of the diaphragm, which compromises ventilation and stimulates regurgitation. These consequences may be avoided by delivering the breaths slowly, using low pressure.[8,9]

CIRCULATION

Assessment. For the lay rescuer in the prehospital setting or the professional responder without benefit of a cardiac monitor, assessment of pulses in the

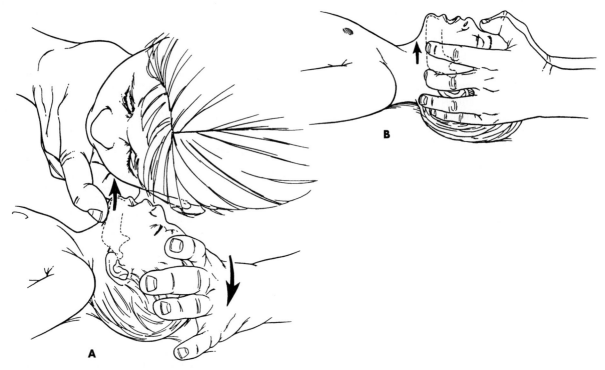

FIG. 8-2. **A,** Airway opening in the child using the head tilt–chin lift maneuver. One hand is used to tilt the head, extending the neck. The index finger of the rescuer's other hand lifts the mandible outward by lifting on the chin. Head tilt should not be performed if a cervical spine injury is suspected. **B,** Airway opening in the child using the jaw-thrust maneuver, with simultaneous cervical spine stabilization. (From Chameides L, Hazinski MF, eds: *Textbook of pediatric advanced life support,* Dallas, 1994, American Heart Association.)

unresponsive, nonbreathing infant or child has been deemphasized for three reasons. First, lay rescuers cannot reliably locate pulses or determine the pulse rate.[6,21] Second, the unconscious, nonbreathing infant or child is likely to be bradycardic or pulseless, so compressions are likely to be indicated. Third, the incidence of complications resulting from chest compressions appears to be very low in infants and children; rib fractures have not been documented after resuscitation of infants or children.[13,27]

To assess pulses the rescuer palpates the brachial pulse in the infant and the carotid pulse in the child. Professional rescuers may also palpate the femoral pulse. If a pulse is not palpated within a few seconds, it is likely the child has pulseless arrest or bradycardia. The lay rescuer is instructed to begin chest compressions if the pulse is absent. The professional rescuer begins chest compression if the pulse rate is less than 60 beats per minute with evidence of poor systemic perfusion. If pulses are present but no spontaneous respirations are observed, rescue breathing or ventilation with a bag and mask continues at a rate of approximately 20 per minute.

Chest compressions. Serial, rhythmic chest compressions are provided during CPR in an attempt to circulate oxygen-containing blood to vital organs. In children, the mechanism of blood flow has not been determined. Blood flow may occur as a result of direct compression of the heart, or it may result from changes in intrathoracic pressure occurring during chest compression and relaxation.[8]

The infant's chest is compressed approximately one finger-breadth below the nipple line, and the child's chest is compressed over the lower half of the sternum (Fig. 8-3). The xiphoid process should be avoided. The proper depth or force of chest compression has not been experimentally determined in infants and children; however, the compression force should be sufficient to depress the sternum approximately one

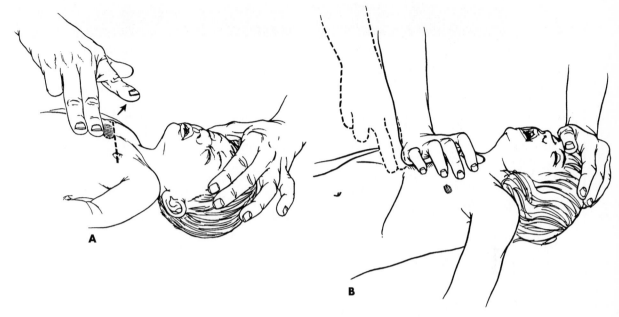

FIG. 8-3.   **A,** Locating proper finger position for chest compression in the infant. Note that the rescuer's other hand is used to maintain head position to facilitate ventilation. **B,** Locating hand position for chest compression in the child. Note that the rescuer's other hand is used to maintain head position to facilitate ventilation. (From Chameides L, Hazinski MF, eds: *Textbook of pediatric advanced life support,* Dallas, 1994, American Heart Association.)

third to one half the depth of the chest. This force approximates ½ to 1 inch in the infant and 1 to 1½ inches in the child, although these measurements are not precise.[8]

The infant compression rate is at least 100 per minute, and the child compression rate is approximately 100 per minute. With pauses for ventilation, the actual number of compressions delivered is lower. Compressions and ventilations are provided in a 5:1 ratio. When rescue breathing is provided to the unintubated infant or child, a slight pause after every fifth compression enables delivery of a rescue breath; once the child is intubated, no pause is necessary for delivery of the breath.

ACTIVATION OF THE EMS SYSTEM

During prehospital resuscitation of the infant or child, the EMS system is activated after approximately 1 minute of rescue support. This rescue support may consist of airway opening only; airway opening and rescue breathing; or airway opening, rescue breathing, and compressions (Table 8-1).

RELIEF OF FOREIGN BODY AIRWAY OBSTRUCTION

Foreign body airway obstruction (FBAO) should be suspected in any child who demonstrates the sudden onset of coughing, gagging, stridor (high-pitched, noisy sound), or wheezing. If signs of a *complete* airway obstruction are present, attempts to relieve the obstruction are necessary until the object is expelled or the victim loses consciousness. Signs of complete airway obstruction include ineffective cough (and loss of sound), increased work of breathing associated with stridor, cyanosis, and/or loss of consciousness.

Relief of FBAO in the conscious infant.   In the conscious infant with an airway obstruction the infant is held prone, with the head down, straddled over the rescuer's forearm, and five back blows are provided between the shoulder blades. The infant is then supported and turned supine, and five *chest thrusts* are provided in a manner identical to chest compressions but at a slower rate. The pharynx is then inspected, and if an object is visualized it is removed. If the object is not visualized, a blind finger sweep is contraindicated

TABLE 8-1	Summary of BLS Maneuvers in Infants and Children	
MANEUVER	**INFANT (<1 YEAR)**	**CHILD (1 TO 8 YEARS)**
Airway	Head tilt–chin lift (if trauma is present, use jaw thrust)	Head tilt–chin lift (if trauma is present, use jaw thrust)
Breathing		
Initial	Two breaths at 1 to 1½ seconds/breath	Two breaths at 1 to 1½ seconds/breath
Subsequent	20 breaths/min (approximate)	20 breaths/min (approximate)
Circulation		
Pulse check	Brachial/femoral	Carotid
Compression area	Lower half of sternum	Lower half of sternum
Compression width	2 or 3 fingers	Heel of 1 hand
Depth	Approximately one third to one half the depth of the chest	Approximately one third to one half the depth of the chest
Rate	At least 100/min	100/min
Compression-ventilation ratio	5:1 (pause for ventilation)	5:1 (pause for ventilation)
Foreign-body airway obstruction	Back blows/chest thrusts	Heimlich maneuver

From Chameides L, Hazinski MF, eds: *Textbook of pediatric advanced life support,* Dallas, 1994, American Heart Association.

because the object may be pushed further into the airway. Back blows and chest thrusts continue until the object is expelled or the victim loses consciousness.

Relief of FBAO in the unconscious infant. Once the infant loses consciousness, the rescuer opens the airway using a tongue-jaw lift, looks for the object, and removes it if one is present. Ventilation is then attempted. If ventilation is unsuccessful, the head is repositioned and a second attempt at ventilation is made. If the airway obstruction persists (chest expansion is not produced by rescue ventilation), the back blows and chest thrusts are alternated with visualizing the oropharynx and attempts at ventilation until ventilation is successful.

If an infant is found to be unconscious and the presence or absence of a FBAO has not been determined, the sequence of BLS is initiated. When ventilation is unsuccessful after the airway is opened, the head is repositioned and ventilation is reattempted. If ventilation is still unsuccessful (ventilation fails to produce chest expansion), five back blows and five chest thrusts are provided. The mouth is then opened using a tongue-jaw lift and any object seen is removed. Ventilation is attempted and the sequence is repeated until ventilation is successful.

Relief of FBAO in the conscious child. In the conscious child with an airway obstruction *abdominal thrusts* are provided until the object is expelled or

the victim loses consciousness. Abdominal thrusts (Heimlich maneuver) are performed with the rescuer standing behind the child and encircling the child's chest with the rescuer's arms. One hand is formed into a fist with the thumb side next to the child's body and the other hand is placed over the fist. The fist is placed on the child's abdomen slightly above the navel and below the level of the xiphoid process. Rapid, distinct upward thrusts are used with the intent of relieving the obstruction.[8]

Relief of FBAO in the unconscious child. Once a child loses consciousness, the rescuer kneels next to the child and places the child supine. The mouth is then opened using a tongue-jaw lift. The object is removed if seen. Rescue breathing is attempted; if it is unsuccessful (fails to produce chest expansion), the head is repositioned and ventilation is reattempted. If ventilation is still unsuccessful, abdominal thrusts are performed. These thrusts are created utilizing the heel of one hand in the midline of the abdomen, between the umbilicus and the xiphoid process. The rescuer's second hand is placed on top of the first, and five upward thrusts are delivered. The mouth is then opened, and the object removed if visualized. Ventilation is then reattempted. If ventilation is unsuccessful the series is repeated until ventilation is successful.

If the child is found unconscious and the presence or absence of an FBAO has not been determined, the victim is placed in a supine position and the sequence of BLS is initiated. When ventilation is unsuccessful after the airway is opened, the head is repositioned and ventilation is reattempted. If ventilation is still unsuccessful (ventilation fails to produce chest expansion), five abdominal thrusts are delivered as described above. The mouth is then opened using a tongue-jaw lift, and the object is removed if seen. Ventilation is attempted and if unsuccessful, the head is repositioned and ventilation is reattempted. If the airway remains obstructed, the sequence of abdominal thrusts, opening of the mouth, removing the object (when visible), and attempt and reattempt of ventilation is repeated until ventilation is successful.

| SECTION I | **Pediatric Resuscitation: Advanced Life Support** |

When a child requires resuscitation, 100% oxygen is administered and venous access obtained as quickly as possible. Some therapies must be performed immediately and should not be delayed if venous access is difficult to achieve. For example, decompensated shock caused by supraventricular tachycardia (SVT) requires immediate synchronized cardioversion if venous access has not been established.

TEAM MEMBER RESPONSIBILITIES

In the prehospital setting, resuscitation activities must be prioritized because the number of rescuers is limited. Although activities are also prioritized in the ED setting, in reality the resuscitation team performs numerous tasks simultaneously. Preassigned roles and responsibilities provide each member with a set of tasks to accomplish with which they can become proficient. These preassigned roles allow the resuscitation to progress efficiently and without confusion.

The following division of responsibilities may be helpful in assigning resuscitation team responsibilities; however, many variations exist depending on the number of personnel available and their skill levels.

Nurse #1: Airway and breathing
  If the responsibility is taken by a respiratory therapist or physician, the nurse may assist with intubation and suction the airway and endotracheal tube as indicated
Nurse #2: Circulation
  Provide cardiac compressions and obtain relief as needed
Nurse #3: Monitoring, medications, venous access OR
  Nurse # 2 may perform these tasks if compressions are performed by other personnel
  Place child on the ECG monitor and pulse oximeter; obtain vascular access
  Obtain medications and supplies from the code cart

Nurse #4: Recorder
  Record activities of code
Physician #1: Direct code activities
  May intubate the child or assign this responsibility
Physician #2: Complement the activities of physician #1
  Intubate child or establish intravenous/intraosseous access (IO)

SEQUENCE OF RESUSCITATION ACTIVITIES

The sequence of resuscitation activities is determined by the presentation of the patient, including the precipitating factors (usually respiratory failure or shock) and the cardiac rhythm. Because hypovolemic shock is one of the most common causes of shock and cardiorespiratory deterioration, this chapter addresses shock as a presenting form of arrest. Other forms of arrest are categorized by the presenting rhythm. In general, airway and ventilation (with 100% oxygen) must be established, intubation accomplished, intravenous/intraosseous access achieved, and cardiorespiratory monitoring established early in the resuscitation sequence. Epinephrine is the first-line drug during pediatric resuscitation, because it is indicated for both bradycardia and pulseless arrest. Therefore epinephrine and other commonly utilized resuscitation drugs will be presented. Finally, management of the most common pediatric cardiac rhythms is presented.

RESUSCITATION EQUIPMENT

A length-based tape can facilitate selection of appropriate equipment sizes and drug dosages during resuscitation (Fig. 8-4). The tape is stretched from the top of the child's head to the child's heel. The length at the child's heel corresponds to a blue or white box,

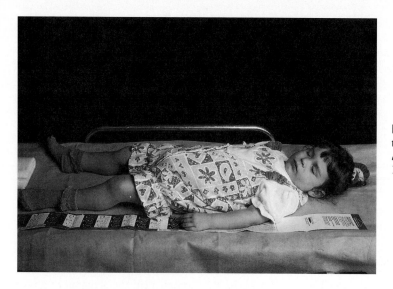

FIG. 8-4. The Broselow resuscitation tape. (From Aehlert B: *PALS: pediatric advanced life support study guide,* St, Louis, 1994, Mosby.)

which contains that child's resuscitation drug dosages. On the opposite side of the tape a color-coded box indicates resuscitation equipment sizes for the child. Resuscitation equipment can then be organized in color-coded baskets or bags. Equipment sizes based on a color-coded resuscitation tape are listed in Table 8-2.

AIRWAY AND VENTILATION

Airway patency is maintained by the jaw-thrust maneuver or the head tilt–chin lift procedure. When bag-mask ventilation is initiated, both the bag and the mask must be of appropriate size (Fig. 8-5). The fingers of the hand holding the mask to the child's face should also lift the angle of the jaw to maintain airway patency during hand ventilation. It may be necessary to move the head (unless cervical spine injury is suspected) through a range of positions to determine the position of optimal airway patency and ease of ventilation.

Self-inflating resuscitation bags. Resuscitation bags are of two major types, the self-inflating and the non–self-inflating. The self-inflating bags may provide ventilation with room air without any supplementary gas source, making them perfect for initiating resuscitation in the prehospital setting or away from an oxygen source. A reservoir must be attached to the bag to deliver oxygen concentrations of greater than 80%. The self-inflating bag recoils between compressions and does not enable evaluation of lung compliance.

Most of these bags contain a fish-mouth valve, preventing gas flow to the patient unless the bag is compressed; as a result, these bags should be used only for hand ventilation and should not be used to provide supplemental oxygen through a mask during spontaneous respirations (Fig. 8-6).

Many self-inflating bags are equipped with a pressure pop-off valve to prevent ventilation with high pressure. During bag-mask ventilation, however, it is often necessary to occlude the pressure pop-off valve of the bag to enable delivery of adequate tidal volume.

The administered tidal volume is approximately 10 to 15 ml/kg. In general, the smallest bag that should be used for resuscitation of full-term neonates or infants is a 450-ml bag. A 1000-ml bag should be used for children older than approximately 8 years of age. To obtain the highest possible concentration of oxygen within the bag a minimal gas flow of 10 to 15 L/min is required.

Non–self-inflating ("anesthesia") resuscitation bags. Non–self-inflating bags inflate only if a gas source is provided, but they can deliver 100% oxygen without the addition of a reservoir. They do require skill to operate.

Oxygen flows into the bag and out an expiratory gas outlet; resistance may be altered in this expiratory outlet to create positive end-expiratory pressure during hand ventilation (Fig. 8-7). These bags are very compliant and enable evaluation of the child's lung compliance during hand ventilation. Because oxygen is continuously flowing into the bag, this bag may be

TABLE 8-2 Pediatric Emergency Department Supplies*

Color on Broselow Pediatric Resuscitation Tape	INFANT (3-7 KG) RED	SMALL CHILD (8-11 KG) PURPLE	CHILD (12-14 KG) YELLOW	CHILD (14-17 KG) WHITE	CHILD (18-23 KG) BLUE	SMALL ADULT (24-30 KG) ORANGE	ADULT (32-34 KG +) GREEN
Bag valve device	Infant	Child	Child	Child	Child	Child/adult	Adult
O₂ mask	Newborn	Pediatric	Pediatric	Pediatric	Pediatric	Adult	Adult
Oral airway	Infant/small child	Small child	Child	Child	Child/small adult	Child/small adult	Medium adult
Laryngoscope blade	0-1 straight	1 straight	2 straight or curved	2 straight or curved	2 straight or curved	2-3 straight or curved	3 straight or curved
ET tubes	Premie 2.5 mm Term 3.0 mm Infant 3.5 mm uncuffed	4.0 mm uncuffed	4.5 mm uncuffed	5.0 mm uncuffed	5.5 mm uncuffed	6.0 mm cuffed	6.5 mm cuffed
ET tube length (cm at lip)	10-10.5 cm	11-12 cm	12.5-13.5 cm	14-15 cm	15.5-16.5 cm	17-18 cm	18.5-19.5 cm
Stylet	6 Fr.	6 Fr.	6 Fr.	6 Fr.	14 Fr.	14 Fr.	14 Fr.
Suction	8 Fr.	8 Fr.	8-10 Fr.	10 Fr.	10 Fr.	10 Fr.	12 Fr.
BP cuff	Newborn-infant	Infant-child	Child	Child	Child	Child-adult	Adult
IV: Catheter	22-24 G	20-24 G	18-22 G	18-22 G	18-20 G	18-20 G	16-20 G
Butterfly	23-25 G	23-25 G	21-23 G	21-23 G	21-23 G	21-22 G	18-21 G
NG tube	5-8 Fr.	8-10 Fr.	10 Fr.	10-12 Fr.	12-14 Fr.	14-18 Fr.	18 Fr.
Urinary catheter	5-8 Fr.	8-10 Fr.	10 Fr.	10-12 Fr.	10-12 Fr.	12 Fr.	12 Fr.
Chest tube	10-12 Fr.	16-20 Fr.	20-24 Fr.	20-24 Fr.	24-32 Fr.	28-32 Fr.	32-40 Fr.

*Adapted from the Broselow Pediatric Resuscitation Tape. Reproduced with permission from Vital Signs, Totoda NJ, 07512.

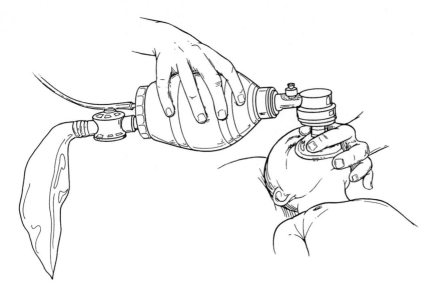

FIG. 8-5. One-handed face mask application technique. Note that the fingers avoid pressure on the soft tissues of the neck, which could cause laryngeal/tracheal compression. (From Chameides L, Hazinski MF, eds: *Textbook of pediatric advanced life support*, Dallas, 1994, American Heart Association.)

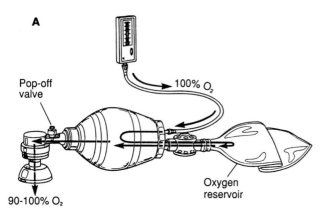

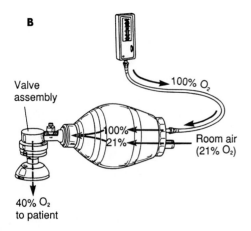

FIG. 8-6. Self-inflating resuscitation bags with (**A**) and without (**B**) an oxygen reservoir. Oxygen is entering both bags in this illustration. (From Chameides L, Hazinski MF, eds: *Textbook of pediatric advanced life support*, Dallas, 1994, American Heart Association.)

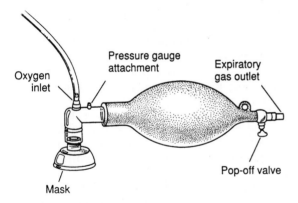

FIG. 8-7. Anesthesia ventilation bag. (From Chameides L, Hazinski MF, eds: *Textbook of pediatric advanced life support,* Dallas, 1994, American Heart Association.)

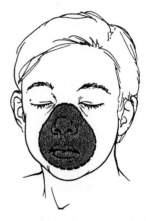

FIG. 8-8. Proper area of the resuscitation face mask application. Note that no pressure is applied to the eyes. (From Chameides L, Hazinski MF, eds: *Textbook of pediatric advanced life support,* Dallas, 1994, American Heart Association.)

used to provide supplemental oxygen to a mask during spontaneous ventilation. Fresh gas flow of at least 2 L/min is required for infants weighing less than 10 kg, at least 4 L/min is required for patients weighing 10 to 50 kg, and at least 6 L/min is required for children weighing more than 50 kg.

Resuscitation masks. The appropriate mask size is that which will cover the nose and mouth without covering the eyes or the chin (Fig. 8-8). Most masks contain an inflatable rim to facilitate creation of a tight seal between the child's face and the mask.

INTUBATION

Intubation should be performed as quickly as possible by medical personnel skilled in pediatric intubation. Indications for intubation include inadequate central nervous system control of ventilation, loss of protective airway reflexes, functional or anatomic airway obstruction, excessive work of breathing, respiratory arrest, need for mechanical ventilation or high peak inspiratory pressure, or the potential for any of these conditions if patient transport is needed.

Equipment. Before intubation, all necessary equipment should be gathered at the bedside. Equipment includes a source of 100% oxygen, a bag and mask device, suction equipment, an ECG monitor, a pulse oximeter, a laryngoscope blade and handle, a stylet, and an assortment of endotracheal tubes. The bag and mask is used before and between intubation attempts. After successful intubation, the bag is used

to provide hand ventilation while tube location is assessed.

Suction equipment includes a large suction catheter or rigid tonsil suction device to suction the pharynx and a suction catheter of appropriate size to pass through the endotracheal tube should it become occluded.

Continuous ECG monitoring with a bedside monitor is required, and an audible alarm should be set to indicate mild bradycardia. If possible, audible QRS tones should be heard, so bradycardia is immediately apparent during intubation. Pulse oximetry is an additional useful monitor during intubation.

A laryngoscope blade and handle are required, and the bulb on the blade should be checked for function and brightness. A stylet is often used to facilitate passage of the endotracheal tube through the vocal cords. If nasotracheal intubation is performed, a McGill forceps will be used to advance the endotracheal tube from the posterior nasopharynx to the vocal cords.

Endotracheal tube (ETT) selection. In general, oral intubation is performed using an uncuffed tube for children younger than 8 years of age. Cuffed tubes are unnecessary, because anatomic narrowing of the pharynx at the level of the cricoid cartilage will form a natural seal around an endotracheal tube. A cuffed tube may be used in older children, but the cuff is generally deflated during resuscitation.

Endotracheal tube size (internal diameter [ID]) is typically selected for patients on the basis of age. Term neonates are generally intubated with a 3 or 3.5 mm tube, and infants 6 months to 1 year of age are intubated with a 4 mm tube. Beyond 1 year of age tube size can be estimated by the following formula:

$$\text{ET tube size (mm ID)} = \frac{\text{Age (in years)}}{4} + 4$$

However, proper tube size more reliably corresponds to a child's length than age. As a result, use of a resuscitation tape such as the Broselow Resuscitation Tape facilitates tube selection (see Fig. 8-4 and Table 8-2).

The depth of tube insertion in centimeters can be estimated by multiplying the internal diameter of the tube by 3. For example, if a 4.5-mm ID tube is inserted, the depth of insertion will be approximately 13.5 cm. Of course, proper tube insertion depth should be evaluated by clinical exam and chest radiograph.

Suction catheters. The size of the suction catheter that passes easily through the endotracheal tube can be estimated by doubling the ID (mm) of the endotracheal tube. In general, even the next French size suction catheter passes easily through the endotracheal tube.

Pharmacologic preparation. Sedatives, hypnotics, or neuromuscular blockers may be administered before the intubation attempt. Neuromuscular blockers alone should never be administered to the awake patient—sedatives should also be provided. The choice of agents is determined by the child's condition (awake vs. unconscious, quiet vs. struggling), physiologic condition (e.g., head injury with suspected increased intracranial pressure), and physician preference (see Chapter 6). Atropine may be administered to prevent the development of bradycardia during intubation (particularly if succinylcholine is administered). However, its use may prevent the development of bradycardia, which signals hypoxia during the intubation attempt. If atropine is administered, close observation and continuous monitoring of oxygen saturation using pulse oximetry are required.

Monitoring during intubation. Before each intubation attempt, the child is ventilated with 100% oxygen. If the child is not in full arrest, this is done until the heart rate and color are satisfactory. During the intubation attempt, the child's heart rate and color are monitored continuously. The intubation attempt is interrupted if bradycardia, hypoxemia, or other deterioration is observed—and the child is ventilated using a bag-mask device until heart rate and clinical status improve.

Pressure over the cricoid cartilage (the Sellick maneuver) may facilitate entrance of the endotracheal tube into the trachea. In addition, such pressure may prevent passive regurgitation during intubation.

Evaluation of endotracheal tube placement. Once the tube is inserted, chest expansion and breath sounds are evaluated during hand ventilation. The chest should visibly rise and breath sounds should be readily heard over all lung fields, including the lateral and posterior chest wall and under the axillae. Prominent breath sounds should not be heard over the stomach. If an end-tidal CO_2 monitor is available, the CO_2 should be detectable and appropriate for clinical condition.

When the child is stable, endotracheal tube position is evaluated by chest radiograph. The tip of the tube should be at the level of the third rib and approximately 1 to 2 cm above the carina. Endotracheal tube position is always evaluated in light of the child's head position—the tip of the tube will move in the same direction as the child's chin if the neck is flexed or extended.

CIRCULATION

Intravenous (IV)/Intraosseous access (IO). During a resuscitation, intravenous access is established using the largest catheter placed in the largest vein possible. A protocol should be used during resuscitation requiring the establishment of an intraosseous catheter in children younger than 6 years of age if intravenous access is not achieved within 90 seconds or three attempts, whichever comes first. Intraosseous access utilizes the noncollapsible venous plexus in the tibia of the young child for the delivery of intravenous medications, fluids, or blood products.

In the past, central venous access or upper extremity access was thought to be preferable for the administration of resuscitation drugs. However, more recent evidence suggests that peripheral venous or intraosseous administration of drugs during pediatric resuscitation results in drug levels comparable to central venous administration. This is provided the drugs are followed by a flush of at least 5 ml to move them into the central circulation.[2,14] Any vascular route used for drug delivery must be secure, because extravasation of resuscitation drugs may produce chemical burns and can compromise intravenous drug delivery. Therefore the infusion site should be closely monitored for evidence of extravasation and an alternative site chosen if it is detected.

Intraosseous access can be readily established using an intraosseous needle placed in the anterior surface of the tibia. After the site is cleansed with an antiseptic solution, the needle is inserted approximately 1 to 3 cm below and medial to the tibial tuberosity. The needle is inserted perpendicular to the long axis of the bone or slightly caudad (toward the toes), using a firm twisting or drilling motion (Fig. 8-9). During insertion of the needle the leg should be held firmly, but the provider's hand *should not rest behind the tibia*.

When a sudden decrease in resistance is sensed during advancement of the needle, the needle has penetrated the periosteum and bony cortex of the tibia and entered the marrow. The needle will remain upright without support. Fluid usually flows freely through the needle, without evidence of any subcutaneous infiltration. If infiltration is observed, the needle is withdrawn. When intraosseous access is still required, the contralateral tibia is used.

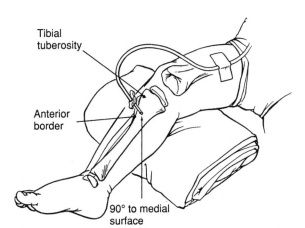

FIG. 8-9. Intraosseous cannulation technique. (From Chameides L, Hazinski MF, eds: *Textbook of pediatric advanced life support*, Dallas, 1994, American Heart Association.)

MANAGEMENT OF HYPOVOLEMIA

Cardiopulmonary arrest can be caused by hypovolemia and should be the suspected cause of an arrest in the pediatric victim of trauma or the dehydrated child. In these children volume administration must be rapidly administered. Intravenous or intraosseous isotonic crystalloids (normal saline or lactated Ringer's solution) are administered at a volume of 20 ml/kg. If significant blood loss has occurred, blood products are administered (10 ml/kg of packed red blood cells or 20 ml/kg of whole blood). In general, crystalloids and colloids/blood are administered in a 3:1 ratio for trauma victims. During emergent conditions, unmatched blood (O negative) is administered until matched blood is available.

When a child presents with the history of a prehospital cardiac arrest of unknown etiology and fails to respond to initial resuscitation, fluid administration may be considered. Occult child abuse, internal bleeding, or septic shock may be responsible for hypovolemia, which is difficult to detect when the initial presentation is cardiopulmonary arrest.

Rapid volume administration is facilitated by placement of a stopcock in the intravenous tubing. A large syringe (e.g., 30 or 60 ml) is used to pull fluid from an intravenous bag and administer it as a rapid IV push to the child.

MANAGEMENT OF DYSRHYTHMIAS

Symptomatic bradycardia. Symptomatic bradycardia is a heart rate that is too slow to maintain adequate cardiac output and is therefore associated with signs of inadequate systemic perfusion. Because hypoxemia is the most common cause of symptomatic bradycardia, treatment initially consists of the administration of 100% oxygen and establishment of an adequate airway and effective ventilation. Vascular access is also established as quickly as possible. If the heart rate is less than 60 beats per minute and is associated with poor systemic perfusion (diminished peripheral pulses, altered level of consciousness, respiratory distress, and possible hypotension), chest compressions should be performed.

If symptomatic bradycardia persists despite effective ventilation of the child with 100% oxygen, administration of epinephrine is indicated (0.01 mg/kg IV/IO or 0.1 mg/kg ET tube) and should be repeated every 3 to 5 minutes as long as bradycardia persists. Atropine sulfate may also be administered

(0.02 mg/kg with a minimum dose of 0.1 mg and a maximum single dose of 0.5 mg for children and 1.0 mg for adolescents). The atropine dose may be repeated once.

If heart block is not present, esophageal pacing may be attempted to correct the symptoms. Transthoracic pacing may be effective even in the presence of heart block, but data in pediatric patients is limited. Isoproterenol administration (continuous infusion, 0.01 to 0.1 μg/kg/min) may be considered for the treatment of symptomatic bradycardia associated with heart block, because the isoproterenol will accelerate ventricular pacers.

Symptomatic supraventricular tachycardia. Symptomatic SVT is associated with signs of shock. Treatment requires the administration of 100% oxygen. If intravenous access is already established, adenosine 0.1 mg/kg is administered as a rapid IV bolus into the injection port *nearest* the child. The maximum single dose of adenosine is 12 mg. The onset of action of adenosine is almost immediate.

If intravenous access is not available, synchronized cardioversion with 0.5 J/kg is performed immediately. Ideally, intubation and ventilation with 100% oxygen are performed before cardioversion, but cardioversion should *never be delayed* when shock is present.

Verapamil is occasionally used for the treatment of SVT, but its use in infants has been associated with the development of hypotension, bradycardia, and asystole. For this reason it should not be used in the ED for the treatment of infants with SVT, in children with myocardial failure or depression, in children receiving beta-adrenergic blocking agents, or in children who may have SVT associated with a bypass tract.

Ventricular tachycardia and ventricular fibrillation. Ventricular tachycardia is uncommon in pediatric patients. If it is associated with pulses, synchronized cardioversion at a dose of 0.5 J/kg is performed. If the dysrhythmia persists the dose may be doubled for a second attempt.

Pulseless ventricular tachycardia and ventricular fibrillation are managed identically. Hyperventilation is accomplished with 100% oxygen, and cardiac compressions are performed while the defibrillator is prepared. Intravenous/intraosseous access should be achieved and intubation accomplished, but these procedures should not delay defibrillation.

Defibrillation is performed up to three times in rapid succession at doses of 2 J/kg, 4 J/kg, and 4 J/kg. If the dysrhythmia persists, compressions are continued and the first dose of epinephrine is provided (0.01 mg/kg by IV/IO route or 0.1 mg/kg by ET route). Defibrillation is repeated (4 J/kg) 30 to 60 seconds after the epinephrine dose. If the dysrhythmia persists, "high-dose" epinephrine is administered (0.1 mg/kg by IV, IO, or ET route), followed by defibrillation at 4 J/kg within 30 to 60 seconds. If the dysrhythmia persists, "high-dose" epinephrine is administered every 3 to 5 minutes, and additional drugs may be given, including lidocaine (1 mg/kg) or bretylium (5 mg/kg first dose, then 10 mg/kg). Each medication should be followed within 30 to 60 seconds by a defibrillation attempt at 4 J/kg.[8]

Asystole. Asystolic arrest is associated with a dismal prognosis; therefore, resuscitation interventions must begin immediately. Hyperventilation is provided with bag and mask, and 100% oxygen and cardiac compressions are provided. Intravenous or intraosseous access is achieved. Epinephrine is administered by IV/IO route at an initial dose of 0.01 mg/kg or, if IV/IO access has not been achieved, by ET route at a dose of 0.1 mg/kg. Epinephrine is administered every 3 to 5 minutes, and after the first IV/IO dose all doses are "high dose" (0.1 mg/kg).

Electromechanical dissociation (narrow QRS pulseless electrical activity). Electromechanical dissociation (EMD) is a form of pulseless electrical activity characterized by narrow QRS complexes. The management of this form of pulseless arrest is identical to the management of asystole. Simultaneous with the management of asystole, reversible causes of the EMD should be sought and treated if found. These potential reversible causes include severe hypoxemia, severe acidosis, severe hypovolemia, tension pneumothorax, cardiac tamponade, and profound hypothermia.

DEFIBRILLATION AND CARDIOVERSION

The technique of paddle placement and discharge of the defibrillator unit is the same for defibrillation or synchronized cardioversion; however, the indications for each are different. Before use, the unit must be programmed for synchronized cardioversion to deliver a current that is in synchrony with the child's ventricular depolarization.

Defibrillation is the untimed delivery of electrical current to the myocardium to produce depolarization of a critical mass of myocardium in an attempt to restore organized electrical activity, which should result in organized contraction. The dose used is 2 J/kg, which may be increased, if unsuccessful, to 4 J/kg.

Synchronized cardioversion is delivery of a current timed to coincide with the patient's intrinsic myocardial electrical activity. Synchronized cardioversion is designed to gain control of a tachydysrhythmia. The dose used for synchronized cardioversion is lower than that used for defibrillation, beginning at 0.5 J/kg. Subsequent doses may be increased to 1 J/kg. The synchronizer circuit must be activated in the unit to ensure synchronized cardioversion.

Procedure and paddle placement. For defibrillation, the paddles used can be the monitoring type or plain paddles. For synchronized cardioversion, the paddles must be of the monitoring type, or the unit must be joined by cable to the bedside monitor to enable synchronization of the delivered energy with the patient's intrinsic myocardial electrical activity.

Paddles used are the largest that will allow good chest contact over the entire surface of the paddle and good separation between paddles. "Infant" paddles are recommended for use in infants up to 1 year of age or 10 kg, and "adult" paddles are recommended for use in children beyond 1 year of age or larger than 10 kg.

A low-impedance interface medium, such as self-adhesive defibrillation pads or electrode cream or paste- or saline-soaked gauze pads, should be placed between the defibrillator paddles and the chest wall. Sonographic gel or alcohol pads should not be used. "Bridging" (contact between the interface medium under one paddle and the medium under the second paddle) must be prevented, or the current will bypass the patient and pass from paddle to paddle.

Paddles are most commonly placed on the anterior chest. One paddle is placed on the upper right chest just below the clavicle, and the other is placed on the left chest, to the left of the left nipple in the anterior axillary line. If dextrocardia is present, the left-right position is reversed. Anterior-posterior paddle placement may also be used for small infants if the paddles are too large to enable placement on the anterior chest without overlapping or touching.

Safety. Before discharging the paddles, the operator looks around the bed to ensure that everyone is clear. The American Heart Association suggests the operator state the following before the paddles are discharged: "One—I am clear; two—you are clear; three—everyone is clear." During defibrillation, the paddles deliver the energy as soon as the discharge buttons are pushed. During synchronized cardioversion, delay in energy delivery may occur until the energy can be synchronized with the patient's intrinsic electrical activity.

PEDIATRIC RESUSCITATION DRUGS

Endotracheal drug delivery. When intravenous and intraosseous access cannot be achieved, lipid-soluble resuscitation drugs (LEAN: lidocaine, epinephrine, atropine, and naloxone) may be administered by endotracheal route. However, pediatric data regarding this route of delivery during resuscitation is minimal, and the optimal dose and method of delivery of endotracheal drugs have yet to be established. Most recent studies in small animals suggest that optimal endotracheal drug distribution is enhanced if the drug is diluted to a minimal volume of 3 to 5 ml before instillation.[17] This volume may have to be divided into two doses, with positive pressure breaths provided after each portion.

An alternative method of delivery involves injection of the medication through a suction catheter or small feeding catheter inserted through the endotracheal tube. Any medication instilled should be followed by irrigation with 5 ml of normal saline and by several positive pressure breaths. Since the intravenous/intraosseous route is preferable to the endotracheal route, medications should be administered by intravenous/intraosseous route as soon as access can be achieved.

Epinephrine. Epinephrine is the most useful drug during pediatric resuscitation because its alpha- and beta-adrenergic effects are useful in treating bradycardia and pulseless arrest. The alpha-adrenergic actions increase systemic vascular resistance and elevate systolic and diastolic blood pressure. These effects elevate both blood pressure and coronary artery perfusion pressure and enhance the delivery of oxygen to the heart. The beta-adrenergic effects increase cardiac automaticity, heart rate, and myocardial contractility.[8]

Two concentrations of epinephrine may be utilized during pediatric resuscitation. "Standard" concentration is the 1:10,000 dilution and is utilized to deliver a "standard-dose" epinephrine. "High" concentration of epinephrine is 1:1000 dilution and is utilized to deliver "high-dose" epinephrine. Regardless of the dilution of epinephrine desired, the volume of drug administered is always 0.1 ml/kg.

TABLE 8-3	Epinephrine Doses for Resuscitation of Infant and Child			
INDICATION	ROUTE	DOSE	CONCENTRATION	VOLUME
Bradycardia	IV/IO	0.01 mg/kg	1:10,000	0.1 ml/kg
Bradycardia	ET	0.1 mg/kg	1:1000	0.1 ml/kg
Pulseless arrest	IV/IO (first)	0.01 mg/kg	1:10,000	0.1 ml/kg
Pulseless arrest	IV/IO (second and subsequent)	0.1 mg/kg	1:1000	0.1 ml/kg
Pulseless arrest	ET	0.1 mg/kg	1:1000	0.1 ml/kg

"Standard-dose" epinephrine is 0.01 mg/kg and is utilized for the IV/IO treatment of bradycardia and for the first IV/IO dose of epinephrine during the resuscitation of pulseless arrest. "High-dose" epinephrine is 0.1 mg/kg and is utilized for all endotracheal doses of epinephrine and for second and subsequent IV/IO doses of epinephrine for treatment of pulseless arrest (Table 8-3).

Atropine. Atropine may be administered for the treatment of vagally induced symptomatic bradycardia (Table 8-4). There is no evidence that atropine is useful in the treatment of pulseless arrest. A dose of 0.02 mg/kg is administered, with a minimal dose of 0.1 mg required to prevent a paradoxical bradycardia. The maximum single atropine dose is 0.5 mg for the child and 1 mg for the adolescent. The atropine dose may be repeated once for a maximum total dose of 1 mg for the child and 2 mg for the adolescent.

Naloxone. Naloxone is a narcotic antagonist that may be administered to reverse the undesirable side effects of narcotic poisoning, including respiratory depression. It acts rapidly and has a shorter half-life than the narcotics it reverses, so it is often necessary to repeat the dose as frequently as every 2 minutes (a continuous infusion may be provided). The recommended dose is 0.1 mg/kg for infants and children up to 5 years of age or 20 kg body weight and 2 mg for children over 5 years of age or more than 20 kg body weight. A continuous IV infusion of 0.04 to 0.16 mg/kg may also be administered and titrated to patient response. This drug is administered with caution to the newborn of an addicted mother, because it may precipitate narcotic withdrawal and seizures.

Sodium bicarbonate. Sodium bicarbonate administration during resuscitation may actually worsen central nervous system acidosis. It is therefore not considered a first-line resuscitation drug. Its use may be considered for the treatment of documented metabolic acidosis (pH < 7.25 in the presence of normocarbia or hypocarbia). Administration may also be considered during prolonged resuscitation, because acidosis is likely to be present. The dose is approximately 1 mEq/kg. Before the administration of sodium bicarbonate, effective ventilation and oxygenation must be established.

Calcium. Calcium is essential for excitation of nerves and muscles and for muscle contraction. However, during cardiopulmonary arrest and resuscitation there is evidence that calcium accumulates in the cytoplasm and calcium entry into the cell occurs during cell death. For this reason, calcium is no longer administered as a first-line resuscitation drug—it is not recommended as a routine part of resuscitation for the patient with asystole or electromechanical dissociation. Its use is indicated to treat documented total or ionized hypocalcemia, hyperkalemia, hypermagnesemia, and calcium channel blocker overdose. It may be administered if ionized hypocalcemia is strongly suspected, as in children with sepsis or septic shock, or in children who have received blood preserved with citrate-phosphate-dextran. Calcium chloride is the supplemental calcium salt most frequently used during resuscitation. The dose is 0.2 to 0.25 ml/kg of 10% calcium chloride solution, which provides approximately 20 to 25 mg/kg of calcium chloride.

Glucose. Glucose is another resuscitation drug that is no longer a first-line drug but may be administered under certain conditions. Glucose is the major substrate utilized by the newborn myocardium, and it provides a significant myocardial energy source for older children. Infants have high glucose needs and low glycogen stores, so the serum glucose concentra-

TABLE 8-4	Drugs Used in Pediatric Advanced Life Support	
DRUGS	**DOSAGE (PEDIATRIC)**	**REMARKS**
Adenosine	0.1-0.2 mg/kg Maximum single dose: 12 mg	Rapid IV bolus
Atropine sulfate*	0.02 mg/kg	Minimum dose: 0.1 mg Maximum single dose: 0.5 mg in child, 1 mg in adolescent
Bretylium	5 mg/kg; may be increased to 10 mg/kg	Rapid IV
Calcium chloride 10%	20 mg/kg	Give slowly
Dopamine hydrochloride	2-20 µg/kg per min	α-Adrenergic action dominates at ≥15-20 µg/kg per min
Dobutamine hydrochloride	2-20 µg/kg per min	Titrate to desired effect
Epinephrine for bradycardia*	IV/IO: 0.01 mg/kg (1:10,000; 0.1 ml/kg) ET: 0.1 mg/kg (1:1000; 0.1 ml/kg)	Be aware of total dose of preservative administered (if preservatives are present in epinephrine preparation) when high doses are used
Epinephrine for asystolic or pulseless arrest*	**First dose:** IV/IO: 0.01 mg/kg (1:10,000; 0.1 ml/kg) ET: 0.1 mg/kg (1:1000; 0.1 ml/kg) IV/IO doses as high as 0.2 mg/kg of 1:1000 may be effective **Subsequent doses:** IV/IO/ET: 0.1 mg/kg (1:1000; 0.1 ml/kg) Repeat every 3-5 min IV/IO doses as high as 0.2 mg/kg of 1:1000 may be effective	Be aware of total dose of preservative administered (if preservatives are present in epinephrine preparation) when high doses are used
Epinephrine infusion	Initial at 0.1 µg/kg per min Higher infusion dose used if asystole present	Titrate to desired effect (0.1-1 µg/kg per min)
Lidocaine*	1 mg/kg	
Lidocaine infusion	20-50 µg/kg per min	
Naloxone*	If ≤5 years old or <20 kg: 0.1 mg/kg If >5 years old or >20 kg: 2 mg	Titrate to desired effect
Sodium bicarbonate	1 mEq/kg per dose or 0.3 × kg × base deficit	Infuse slowly and only if ventilation is adequate

From Chameides L, Hazinski MF, eds: *Textbook of pediatric advanced life support,* Dallas, 1994, American Heart Association.
*For ET administration dilute medication with normal saline to a volume of 3 to 5 ml and follow with several positive-pressure ventilations.

tion may fall rapidly if the neonate or infant is stressed. However, in the past, hypoglycemia was treated empirically, with large bolus doses of glucose. Data from adult animal models and pediatric trauma victims suggest that hyperglycemia may be as harmful to the ischemic brain as hypoglycemia is to the myocardium. For this reason, glucose is administered to treat documented hypoglycemia or to encourage intracellular potassium movement for the patient with severe hyperkalemia.

The dose of glucose is 0.5 to 1 g/kg or 2 to 4 ml/kg of the 25% solution administered slowly via IV or IO line. If the 50% solution is used, it must be diluted 1:1 with sterile water. In neonates the 50% solution must be diluted 1:4 (see the following section). A continuous glucose infusion is probably preferable to intermittent boluses of large amounts of hypertonic glucose, because the infusion will produce less fluctuation in serum glucose concentration and serum osmolality.

SECTION II	**Neonatal Resuscitation**

INTRODUCTION

The purpose of this section is to outline the interventions required when caring for the neonate immediately after delivery and to describe the components of the neonatal resuscitation. Chapter 28 includes a complete discussion of care of the neonate within the first month of life and includes common conditions of the neonate.

Few newborn infants require resuscitation. In fact the majority require only the maintenance of temperature, mild stimulation, and suctioning of the airway.[8] A small number require ventilatory assistance, and an even smaller percentage require advanced life support measures such as intubation and the administration of resuscitative medications. Even so, most health care professionals agree that the ideal environment for delivering a neonate is in a controlled setting such as the delivery room. In the delivery room, personnel are skilled in pediatric resuscitation and have supplies and equipment readily available if the neonate becomes distressed. Unfortunately, however, precipitous deliveries occasionally occur in the emergency room or in the prehospital setting. Thus emergency personnel must be trained to assist the neonate in the transition from intrauterine to extrauterine life. The relationship of interventions and priorities is depicted in the inverted pyramid, which illustrates the relative frequency with which specific interventions are required. Regardless of the degree of stimulation or resuscitation required, all interventions proceed sequentially as outlined by this pyramid (Fig. 8-10).

PHYSIOLOGY

At birth significant physiologic changes take place that affect the neonate's transition to extrauterine life. The lungs, which are filled with fluid and are nonfunctional in utero, expand and fill with air with the first breaths, forcing the fluid from the interstitium. As the partial pressure of oxygen increases, the arteries surrounding the alveoli dilate, decreasing pulmonary vascular resistance. With increased pulmonary blood flow, volume and pressure in the left heart increases and right-to-left circulatory shunting (fetal circulation) decreases (see Chapter 11).

Serious complications can occur during any of the stages of transition and may lead to the need for resuscitation. Neonates with apnea or a weak initial respiratory effort may not adequately clear the lungs of fluid or elevate their Pao_2 enough to expand the pulmonary arteries, impairing oxygenation. Because pulmonary perfusion does not increase and blood flow to the left heart does not increase, fetal circulation or right-to-left shunting may persist.

ADVANCE PREPARATIONS

Neonatal resuscitations are best conducted in well-equipped and well-staffed delivery rooms by experienced personnel. If time does not permit or it is not feasible or safe to delay the birth until the mother is transported to a delivery room, a well-rehearsed plan for the safe delivery of the infant is required. In the emergency department this plan should include the identification of and delegation of responsibilities of

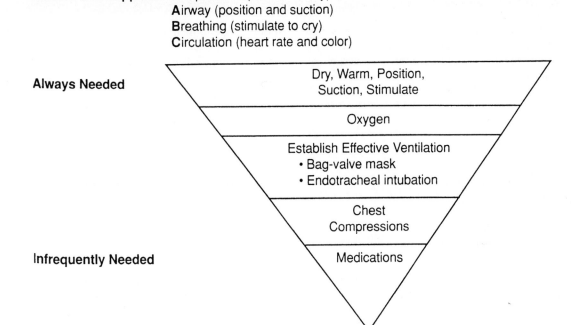

Assess and Support: Temperature (warm and dry)
Airway (position and suction)
Breathing (stimulate to cry)
Circulation (heart rate and color)

Always Needed

Dry, Warm, Position, Suction, Stimulate

Oxygen

Establish Effective Ventilation
• Bag-valve mask
• Endotracheal intubation

Chest Compressions

Medications

Infrequently Needed

FIG. 8-10. Inverted pyramid reflecting relative frequencies of neonatal resuscitation effort for the newborn who does not have meconium-stained amniotic fluid. Note that a majority of newborns respond to simple measures. (From Chameides L, Hazinski MF, eds: *Textbook of pediatric advanced life support,* Dallas, 1994, American Heart Association.)

resuscitation team members, the preparation of resuscitation supplies and equipment, and the arranging of neonatal transport. In the field, delegation of responsibilities, preparation of supplies and equipment, and identification of an appropriate referral facility are required.

NEONATAL RESUSCITATION TEAM

In the emergency department neonatal resuscitation is most effective when performed by a designated, knowledgeable, and coordinated team. Therefore personnel responsible for participating in neonatal resuscitations should obtain and maintain a certification in pediatric and/or neonatal resuscitation and practice neonatal resuscitation skills on a regular basis using mock scenarios.

Ideally at least one person skilled in neonatal resuscitation should be available at every delivery. This person must be able to perform a complete resuscitation if required and direct the actions of other team members. Immediately after the delivery this individual's only responsibility is to provide care to the infant.

When the delivery of a depressed newborn is anticipated in the field or in the hospital, two caregivers skilled in neonatal resuscitation can work as a team during the resuscitation. In the hospital, additional personnel are often available to assist in obtaining equipment, administering medications, and documenting interventions as required. When only two team members are available, one of the team members dries, suctions, and stimulates the infant and provides bag-mask ventilation and chest compressions as indicated. The other team member may assist with compressions or take on the additional steps of performing endotracheal intubation, obtaining vascular access, and administering medications.

RESUSCITATION EQUIPMENT

Neonatal resuscitation equipment must be immediately available and in working order in any ED or

Box 8-1   Neonatal Resuscitation Supplies and Equipment

Radiant warmer and/or warm blankets
Stethoscope, blood pressure monitor and cuffs
Cardiopulmonary monitor, pulse oximeter, temperature monitor
Masks with shields, gloves, gowns
OB kit (blankets, sterile blade or scissors, cord clamp)

Suction equipment
Bulb syringe
Mechanical suction apparatus
Suction catheters (5 or 6 Fr, 8 Fr, 10 Fr)
Meconium aspirator

Ventilation equipment
Neonatal resuscitation bags (240, 450, and 750 ml) with a pressure-release valve or pressure gauge and capability of delivering 90% to 100% oxygen
Face masks, oral airways (newborn and premature sizes)
Oxygen with flow meter and tubing
Laryngoscopes with straight (Miller) blades (No. 00, 0, and 1)
Endotracheal tubes, uncuffed (2.5, 3.0, 3.5, 4.0 ID)
Stylet, scissors

Adhesive tape ½ inch
Blood gas syringes
Feeding tubes (5, 8 Fr)

Medications
Epinephrine 1:10,000
Naloxone hydrochloride (0.4 mg/ml or 1 mg/ml)
Volume expanders (5% albumin, normal saline, Ringer's lactate)
Sodium bicarbonate 4.2%
Dextrose 10%, 250 ml

Vascular access supplies
Syringes (1, 3, 5, 10, 20, 50 ml), needles (25, 21, 18 gauge)
Umbilical catheterization tray, umbilical catheters (3.5, 5 Fr), umbilical tape
Three-way stopcocks, T-connectors, adhesive tape, IV pumps and tubing
Alcohol sponges, sterile gloves (different sizes), blood sample tubes, bedside glucose monitor
Normal saline 10 ml vials, heparin flushes (10 unit/ml)
Vascular access catheters (24 Fr) and intraosseous needles

---

prehospital unit that may potentially deliver a newborn. Ideally, a radiant warmer should be kept in the emergency department and personnel must be oriented to its use. Specific neonatal resuscitation equipment and supplies that should be immediately available include a bulb syringe, suction with manometer, oxygen with flow meter and tubing, neonatal resuscitation bags with face masks, an OB kit, and a resuscitation tray. Once stocked these supplies must be checked regularly and replenished as needed (Box 8-1).

Prehospital Transport

Neonatal transport teams. The delivery of preterm and high-risk infants should take place at perinatal centers. In rural areas this is not always feasible. In these situations local hospitals and prehospital caregivers should have established transport protocols with the nearest perinatal center and a neonatal transport/resuscitation team, when available.

The requirements for a neonatal resuscitation/transport team vary from state to state; however, these teams usually consist of at least two personnel. Both may be registered nurses or one may be a registered nurse and the other may be a physician, registered respiratory therapist, or paramedic. Each team member has a clearly identified role and works jointly with the referring institution and other team members to provide care and plan the safest and most expedient mode of transport.

Transport. Neonates may be transported to a definitive care facility via ground transport or air. Factors to be considered when choosing a mode of transport include the condition of the neonate, the distance to be traveled, traffic, weather conditions, availability of the crew, and cost effectiveness. The transport unit must be equipped with neonatal resuscitation supplies and should be able to carry additional neonatal transport equipment such as a transport incubator with portable power supply, portable ventilator, portable oxygen tanks, and a source of compressed air.

Before transport, the referring institution communicates to the receiving institution the condition of the neonate, the estimated time of arrival, and any special needs of the neonate on arrival. When the neonate arrives at the receiving hospital a verbal and written report is given, which includes maternal ante/intrapartum history, neonatal resuscitative steps required, the infant's condition during transport, and any other pertinent information (see Chapter 1).

▌NEONATAL RESUSCITATION

In general, neonatal resuscitation follows the ABC format presented earlier in this chapter. However, some of the interventions and their sequencing differ during a neonatal resuscitation. For example, in the normal newborn, drying, warming, positioning, suctioning, and stimulating the infant are performed before initiating specific airway interventions (see Fig. 8-10). In other situations, interventions may be altered depending on the neonate's condition at the time of delivery. If a neonate presents with thick meconium staining, suctioning of the mouth and nose is performed before stimulation. The goals of neonatal resuscitation are to prevent hypothermia and stimulate effective respirations.

The information contained in this chapter is based on recommendations of the American Heart Association and the American Academy of Pediatrics.[5,7,8]

OBSTETRIC HISTORY

Before any delivery a comprehensive obstetric history is obtained to identify risk factors that may point to the need for a resuscitation (Box 8-2). In the field and in the emergency department, because of time constraints and the need for emergent care, this is not always feasible. Often only a brief history can be obtained. Several key questions include (1) the possibility of multiple births; (2) the presence of meconium in the amniotic fluid; (3) the presence of premature labor; and (4) a history of drug abuse or the recent administration of narcotics. Other information that should be obtained as time permits includes (1) a history of prenatal care; (2) the presence of maternal infections; (3) medication history; and (4) prolonged rupture of the membranes.[8]

Box 8-2 Factors Associated with an Increased Risk for Neonatal Resuscitation

Antepartum maternal or fetal factors
Age: >35 or <16
No prenatal care
Toxemia
Diabetes mellitus
Hypertension
Pulmonary disease
Cardiac disease
Bleeding, anemia
Substance abuse
Drug therapy (e.g., magnesium, lithium carbonate)
Multifetal gestation
Oligohydramnios
Diminished fetal activity
Fetal malformation identified by ultrasound
Acute febrile illness

Intrapartum maternal or fetal factors
Prematurity (<37 weeks) or postmaturity (>42 weeks)
Abnormal fetal heart rate pattern
Intrauterine growth retardation
Immature lecithin-sphingomyelin (L/S) ratio
Meconium-stained amniotic fluid
Blood group isoimmunization
Breech or other abnormal presentation
Abnormal pattern or length of labor (prolonged or precipitate)
Prolonged rupture of membranes
Prolapsed cord
Maternal sedation
Operative delivery
Multiple births

STIMULATION AND TEMPERATURE CONTROL

When delivery of an infant is imminent all resuscitation equipment and personnel must be immediately available to assist both the mother and the newborn. With the emergence of the infant's head, the mouth and then nose is suctioned using a bulb syringe. Once the neonate is delivered, the umbilical cord is clamped and cut. The newborn is received on a warm towel or blanket and placed under a radiant warmer or in an isolette. The head and body are dried thoroughly to remove amniotic fluid and to prevent evaporative heat loss. Wet towels or blankets are removed from contact with the infant and the infant is wrapped in a dry towel or blanket. A stockinette or cap is placed on the infant's head. If a radiant warmer or isolette is not available, the newborn is placed undressed against the mother's body and both are covered with a blanket.[8,15]

One of the most important interventions after the delivery of any neonate is the maintenance of body heat. Neonates are particularly sensitive to cold and can rapidly lose body heat when exposed to the environment. In addition, they are limited in their ability to compensate for heat loss by generating body heat. With the development of cold stress, oxygen consumption increases, accentuating signs of hypoxia and respiratory distress, the metabolic rate increases, and acidosis develops.[15]

Airway

The airway is maintained by placing the newborn supine under the radiant warmer or on the side with the head in a neutral position. If the infant is supine the neck is slightly extended; however, hyperextension is avoided because the cartilaginous trachea may collapse and obstruct the airway. A blanket or towel folded to a 1-inch thickness can be placed under the infant's shoulders to maintain the correct head position.[8]

A manual bulb syringe is used to suction the mouth first and then the nose. The mouth is suctioned initially to prevent aspiration should the infant gasp during nasal suctioning. A mechanical suctioning device may also be used to suction the infant using an 8 Fr or 10 Fr suction catheter; however, these devices must be used with caution and negative pressures should not exceed 80 to 100 mm Hg. Deep suctioning of the oropharynx should be avoided, because it may stimulate a vagal response producing reflex bradycardia and/or apnea.[8] With either method, suctioning time should not exceed 5 seconds per attempt and the infant's heart rate must be monitored.

In the majority of newborns the acts of drying, warming, and suctioning provide gentle stimulation that initiates or helps to maintain respirations. If warming, drying, and suctioning the neonate are not immediately effective in producing spontaneous respirations, additional tactile stimulation is indicated. This may include rubbing the infant's back quickly and firmly once or twice and flicking the heels or slapping the soles of the feet. If after 5 to 10 seconds the infant fails to respond to these interventions, additional actions are indicated. (Note that suctioning precedes tactile stimulation such as drying and warming when a neonate is meconium stained—see p. 175.)

Apgar score. The infant who is effectively transitioning from intrauterine to extrauterine life will by this point in the delivery be breathing spontaneously and effectively. To objectively evaluate this transition an Apgar score is obtained at 1 minute and 5 minutes after birth. The Apgar score assesses five objective parameters, including the heart rate, respirations, muscle tone, reflex irritability, and color.[3] The maximum possible Apgar score that can be obtained is 10; however, newborn infants rarely receive this score at 1 minute. Any score of greater than 7 reflects an infant who is effectively transitioning to extrauterine life. Infants who are not effectively transitioning to extrauterine life are usually evident before obtaining the 1-minute Apgar score. For this reason the score is not useful in determining the need for resuscitation, which should be initiated immediately once it becomes evident the infant requires assistance[8] (Table 8-5).

Table 8-5	Apgar Score		
Sign	**0**	**1**	**2**
Heart rate per minute	Absent	Slow (less than 100)	Greater than 100
Respirations	Absent	Slow, irregular	Good, crying
Muscle tone	Limp	Some flexion	Active motion
Reflex irritability (catheter in nares)	No response	Grimace	Cough or sneeze
Color	Blue or pale	Pink body with blue extremities	Completely pink

From Apgar V: A proposal for a new method of evaluation of the newborn, *Anesth Analg* 32:260-267, 1953.

BREATHING

The infant's color, respiratory effort, and heart rate are reassessed after each of the interventions previously described. In the majority of infants these interventions are all that are necessary. When an infant is apneic or gasping, has a heart rate of less than 100, or has persistent central cyanosis despite the administration of 100% oxygen, positive pressure ventilation is provided immediately.[8] The infant is oxygenated for 15 to 30 seconds at a rate of 40 to 60 breaths per minute and reevaluated.

Because the tidal volume in the neonate is significantly less than in the older infant or child (6 to 8 ml/kg compared to 10 to 15 ml/kg), the pressure and volume of the initial ventilations must be closely monitored by observing chest wall movement. The best indicators of adequate ventilation are expansion of the chest wall and improvement in the infant's color and heart rate.

To effectively deliver positive pressure ventilation the bag and mask must be appropriately sized to the infant. The mask should form a tight seal around the nose and mouth without covering the eyes. Masks with inflatable or cushioned rims are ideal. Two types of positive pressure ventilation bags are available for use. One is a flow-inflating bag (anesthesia bag), and the other is a self-inflating bag. A pressure gauge attached to the bag is useful to monitor the pressure of breaths delivered. Normally pressures should not exceed 30 to 40 cm of H_2O; however, the initial breaths may require slightly higher pressures to overcome decreased pulmonary compliance.[8] Bags with a pressure-release valve may not provide adequate pressure in these infants and should therefore have a mechanism by which the pressure-release or "pop-off" valve can be bypassed.

When using a self-inflating bag the 240-ml volume bag is used only for premature infants, and the 450- to 750-ml bags used for full-term infants. Flow-inflating bags require the use of compressed air or oxygen to inflate the bag. Because they require specialized equipment, as well as skill and practice, they are rarely used in the emergency department or in the field.

Gastric decompression. An orogastric tube is inserted whenever an infant requires positive pressure ventilation with a bag-valve-mask device for longer than 2 minutes. With bag-mask ventilation, air is forced into the oropharynx where it is free to enter both the trachea and the esophagus. As air is forced into the stomach, abdominal distention compresses the diaphragm and prevents full expansion of the lungs. Additionally, gastric distention places the neonate at risk for regurgitation of gastric contents and aspiration.

Intubation. Endotracheal intubation is indicated (1) when prolonged positive pressure ventilation is required; (2) when bag-mask ventilation is ineffective—inadequate chest rise or continuing low heart rate; (3) when tracheal suction is required to clear the trachea (e.g., meconium staining); (4) when a diaphragmatic hernia is suspected; or (5) when a preterm infant (<1000 grams) is delivered.[5,8]

Before intubation all necessary supplies must be assembled. The infant is placed supine with the neck slightly extended but not hyperextended. To maintain the correct position a towel roll may be placed under the infant's shoulders. Because the endotracheal tube is small and flexible and because the trachea is slightly anterior in position, a stylet may be required to facilitate insertion of the endotracheal tube. During the intubation suction must be immediately available to clear the pharyngeal area of secretions.

The neonate's heart rate, which correlates with oxygenation, is monitored throughout the intubation attempt, which should not exceed 20 seconds. If the 20-second period elapses or the infant becomes bradycardic, the intubation attempt is halted and the infant ventilated with 100% oxygen using a bag-mask device until the heart rate is within normal limits. After successful intubation the ET tube is held firmly in place at the level of the lips while the laryngoscope blade and the stylet (if used) is removed and the ET tube is attached to a resuscitation bag. The infant is then ventilated and the tube position assessed.

Tube placement is assessed by observing the chest for bilateral, equal chest rise and auscultating the chest for bilateral, equal breath sounds. The abdomen is auscultated to determine if air is entering the stomach. Clinical parameters that should be observed include an improvement in the infant's color and heart rate. After confirming tube placement the centimeter mark on the ET tube is noted at the level of the upper lip, and the tube is secured with adhesive tape. X-ray confirmation of ET tube placement is performed as soon as feasible.

Complications of the intubation procedure include (1) hypoxia caused by prolonged intubation or incorrect placement of the ET tube; (2) bradycardia/apnea due to hypoxia, or vagal response; (3) pneumothorax caused by overventilation of one lung; (4) contusions or lacerations to the mouth area or pharynx; (5) perforation of the trachea or esophagus because of inappropriate placement of the stylet; and (6) infection caused by the introduction of organisms via equipment or hands [5] (Box 8-3, Table 8-6, and Fig. 8-11).

Box 8-3   Intubation Supplies

- Laryngoscope with blade: No. 1 (term infants) or No. 0, 00 (premature infants).
- ET tubes: Size (2.5, 3.0, 3.5, and 4.0 ID, uncuffed).
- Stylet: Use of a stylet is optional. If used, insert stylet in ET tube, making sure the tip does not protrude from the end of the ET tube. Secure the stylet so that it cannot advance further into the tube during intubation.
- Suction: This includes an oropharyngeal device with a 10 Fr or larger suction catheter.
- Adhesive tape: Tape should be cut and ready to use for securing ET tube after intubation.
- Resuscitation bag and mask: Resuscitation bag should be connected to oxygen and ready to deliver 100% oxygen.

CIRCULATION

Heart rate is an important indicator of both ventilatory and circulatory status. The heart rate is evaluated by auscultating apical heart sounds and by palpating the pulse at the base of the umbilical cord or by palpating the brachial or femoral arteries. If the heart rate is greater than 100 beats per minute, spontaneous respirations are present, and the infant is pink in color or has acrocyanosis, no further interventions are required. Acrocyanosis or peripheral cyanosis is common in newborn infants immediately after birth and represents decreased blood flow to the extremities.[15] It is usually of no clinical significance.

The presence of central cyanosis, cyanosis involving the entire body, necessitates the administration of 100% oxygen. If the heart rate is less than 100 beats per minute, even in the presence of spontaneous respiratory effort, positive pressure ventilation with 100% oxygen is begun immediately. Chest compressions are indicated when the heart rate is less than 60 or is between 60 and 80 and is not rising despite effective ventilation with 100% oxygen.[8] The ventilation-to-compression ratio for neonates is 1:3, delivering at least 100 compressions and 30 ventilations per minute.

Chest compressions. To perform chest compressions on a neonate, pressure is applied to the lower third of the sternum, just below an imaginary line between the two nipples, using the thumb or two-finger technique (Fig. 8-12). With the thumb technique, the two thumbs are used to depress the

TABLE 8-6	Neonatal Intubation Supplies by Weight			
NEONATE WEIGHT	FACE MASK SIZE	ET TUBE SIZE (INSIDE DIAMETER IN MM)	SUCTION CATHETER SIZE	LARYNGOSCOPE AND STRAIGHT (MILLER) BLADE SIZE
<1 kg	Premature	2.5	5 Fr.	00,0
1 kg	Premature	2.5	5 Fr.	0
2 kg	Premature	3.0	5 Fr.	0
3 kg	Newborn/infant	3.5	8 Fr.	0,1
4 kg	Infant	3.5-4.0	8 Fr.	1

$$\text{Approximate ET tube size in mm} = \frac{\text{Post conceptual age in weeks}}{10}$$

Bag-valve-mask device (240, 450, and 750 ml)

Modified from Chameides L, Hazinski MF, eds: *Textbook of pediatric advanced life support*, Dallas, 1994, American Heart Association.

sternum, with the hands encircling the torso and the fingers supporting the back. With the two-finger technique, the tips of the middle finger and either the index or ring finger of one hand are used to compress the sternum. The other hand is used to support the infant's back, unless the infant is on a very firm surface. Using either technique, the chest is compressed ½ to ¾ inches.

After 30 seconds of chest compressions, the heart rate is reevaluated for a maximum of 6 seconds. The 6-second heart rate is then multiplied by 10 to determine the rate per minute. Chest compressions are discontinued if the heart rate is 80 beats per minute or greater; however, ventilations are continued until the heart rate is above 100 beats per minute and the infant is breathing spontaneously. Chest compressions and ventilations are continued if the heart rate remains less than 80 beats per minute (Fig. 8-13).[5,8]

Umbilical catheterization. During neonatal resuscitation vascular access is required to administer fluids and medications. Vascular access can be achieved using the peripheral route, IO route, or umbilical vein. Both the peripheral route and intraosseous route are reviewed earlier in this chapter. In the neonate the preferred route for obtaining vascular access during resuscitative management is the umbilical vein, because it is readily available and is easily identified and cannulated.[8] Either the umbilical artery (UA) or vein (UV) can be cannulated, and both can be used to administer fluids and medications and to obtain blood samples. Umbilical venous lines can also be used to monitor central venous pressure, whereas arterial lines are used to monitor the blood pressure and blood gases.

When insertion of an arterial or venous umbilical catheter is planned the supplies necessary to perform

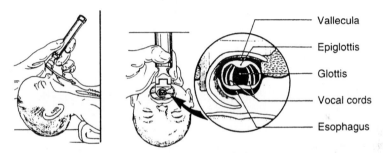

FIG. 8-11. Correct position of laryngoscope. (From Bloom R, Cropley C, AHA/AAP Neonatal Resuscitation Program Steering Committee: *Textbook of neonatal resuscitation*, Dallas, 1994, American Heart Association.)

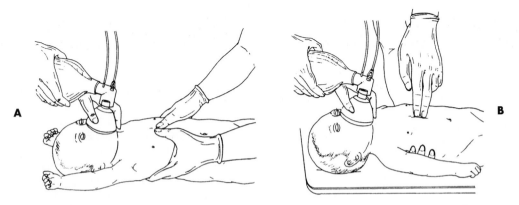

FIG. 8-12. Bag-valve-mask ventilation and chest compression in the newborn. **A,** Thumb method: Use the fingers to support the infant's back, and use both thumbs to compress the sternum. **B,** Two-finger method: Use the tips of two fingers of one hand to compress the sternum, and use the other hand or a firm surface to support the infant's back. (From Bloom R, Cropley C, AHA/AAP Neonatal Resuscitation Program Steering Committee: *Textbook of neonatal resuscitation*, Dallas, 1994, American Heart Association.)

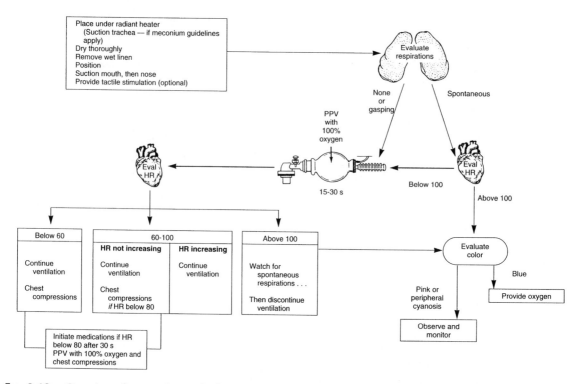

FIG. 8-13. Overview of neonatal resuscitation. (From Bloom R, Cropley C, AHA/AAP Neonatal Resuscitation Program Steering Committee: *Textbook of neonatal resuscitation,* Dallas, 1994, American Heart Association.)

Box 8-4   Umbilical Catheterization Equipment and Supplies

Appropriate umbilical catheters (No. 5 Fr catheter for infants weighing more than 1250 g, No. 3.5 Fr for infants less than 1250 g) or needle-over-the-catheter
Three-way stopcock
Umbilical tape placed around base of cord to be restricted if bleeding occurs
Heparin solution (1 unit per ml) to flush catheter before insertion
Intravenous fluids and tubing
Sterile scalpel, drapes, and gauze
Tape, sutures

---

the procedure must be gathered (Box 8-4). Because this is a sterile procedure, sterile technique including a gown (when possible) and gloves is used. The umbilical catheter is prepared by attaching a three-way

stopcock and syringe to the distal end and flushing the tubing with sterile saline. When an umbilical catheter is not available a catheter-over-the-needle can be used—after removing the needle. If an umbilical arterial line is to be inserted a heparinized solution may be used.

To perform the procedure umbilical tape is placed around the base of the cord and the cord is cut with a sterile scalpel 1 to 2 cm above the base. The umbilical vein and the two arteries are identified. The umbilical arteries are small, thick-walled, and constricted, whereas the umbilical vein is larger, thin-walled, and may continue to bleed after being cut. If a UA is to be cannulated, iris forceps are used to dilate the desired vessel before catheter insertion.

Umbilical artery catheters are inserted to the "high line," which is at the level of the eight to tenth thoracic vertebrae, or at the "low line," which is at the level of the third to fourth lumbar vertebrae[10] (Fig. 8-14). Umbilical venous lines are inserted only a few centimeters (1 to 4 cm) into the UV or inferior vena cava, until blood flow is obtained. The UV line should not lie in the portal vein, because liver injury can result.[8,28]

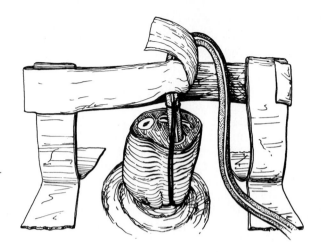

FIG. 8-14. Umbilical vessel catheterization. The cord is cut 2 cm from the base after placement of a cord tie. If umbilical artery catheterization is performed, an iris forceps or bent 22-gauge needle is used to hold open the vessel lumen. Umbilical artery catheters are inserted to the "high line" or "low line" (see text). An umbilical venous catheter is inserted only 1 to 4 cm—until blood flow is obtained. The line is then secured with tape and suture. (From Ruddy RM. In Fleisher GR, Ludwig S, eds: *Textbook of pediatric emergency medicine,* ed 2, Baltimore, Md, 1988, Williams & Wilkins.)

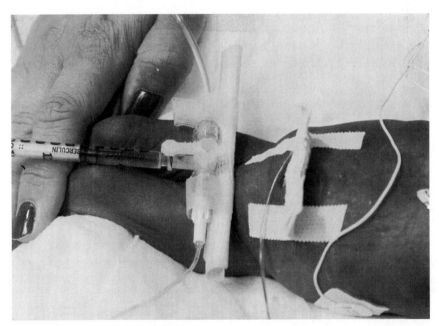

FIG. 8-15. An umbilical artery line secured using the "H" technique. Note the three-way stopcock connected to the distal end of the umbilical artery line.

Once the line is in the desired position, blood is aspirated to confirm placement and the line is flushed with normal saline or heparinized saline solution. The line is then secured using a "goalpost" or "H" technique (Fig. 8-15). An abdominal x-ray is performed to confirm catheter placement. After the procedure the nurse should monitor the infant's feet, legs, and buttocks for signs of vascular compromise.

FLUIDS AND MEDICATIONS (TABLE 8-7)

Required medications can be administered via the ET tube or the peripheral, IO, or UV routes. Ideally, medications are administered centrally rather than endotracheally, because the neonatal lungs are filled with fluid at birth, which may delay the absorption and action of the drugs.[5a] However, in the absence of a peripheral line, medications are administered via the endotracheal route. Medications that can be administered via the ET tube include lidocaine, epinephrine, atropine, and naloxone, which are referred to using the mnemonic LEAN.

Epinephrine. Epinephrine is the drug of choice in the neonate for asystole or when the heart rate is below 80 beats per minute despite adequate oxygenation, ventilation, and chest compressions. Epinephrine increases the strength and rate of cardiac contractions and causes peripheral vasoconstriction, which may play a role in increasing blood flow through the coronary arteries, as well as the brain.[5]

The dose of epinephrine during neonatal resuscitation is 0.01 to 0.03 mg/kg or 0.1 to 0.3 ml/kg of the 1:10,000 solution given rapidly IV or IO; it may also be diluted with 1 to 2 ml of normal saline and given via the ET tube. The dose can be repeated every 3 to 5 minutes as necessary. The efficacy of high doses of epinephrine in neonates has not been established, and it is felt that prolonged hypertension may result from its use. However, epinephrine 0.1 mg/kg *may be considered* in the infant without venous access who has failed to respond to positive pressure ventilation with 100% oxygen and a standard endotracheal dose of epinephrine.[8]

Naloxone hydrochloride. Naloxone hydrochloride is a narcotic antagonist used to reverse respiratory depression induced by narcotics administered to the mother within 4 hours before delivery.

Prompt and adequate ventilatory support must always be provided before the administration of naloxone. If the mother used narcotics chronically during the pregnancy, naloxone can induce a withdrawal reaction and seizures in the neonate. Naloxone is available in two preparations: 0.4 mg/ml or 1 mg/ml. The dose is 0.1 mg/kg rapid IV or IO push or via the ET tube, repeated as necessary every 2 to 3 minutes. The effects of the narcotics may outlast the duration of action of naloxone which is only 1 to 4 hours; therefore repeated doses of naloxone may be required.[5] Naloxone may also be administered subcutaneously or intramuscularly; however, a delayed onset of action should be expected.

Sodium bicarbonate. Sodium bicarbonate is used to correct metabolic acidosis. Its administration is discouraged during brief resuscitations, but it may be used during prolonged arrests and in infants not responding to other therapies.[8] Sodium bicarbonate is administered only after effective ventilation and oxygenation have been achieved. In neonates the 4.2% (0.5 mEq/ml) solution is used. The dose is 2 mEq/kg given IV or IO push *slowly* over at least 2 minutes, or at a rate of 1 mEq/kg per minute.

Glucose. Glucose is used to correct hypoglycemia in the neonate, especially in the postresuscitation phase of care. Hypoglycemia occurs rapidly in newborns recovering from asphyxia and in infants with diminished glycogen stores, such as pre-

TABLE 8-7	Neonatal Resuscitation Medications						
NEONATE WEIGHT	EPINEPHRINE (1:10,000) IV, ET, IO* 0.01-0.03 MG/KG	VOLUME EXPANDERS IV, IO* 10 ML/KG	NARCAN IV, IM, ET, SQ, IO 1 MG/ML	0.4 MG/ML	SODIUM BICARBONATE IV, IO (4.2%) 2 MEQ/KG		
1 kg	0.1-0.3 ml	10 ml	0.1 ml	0.25 ml	1 kg	4 ml
2 kg	0.2-0.6 ml	20 ml	0.2 ml	0.5 ml	2 kg	8 ml
3 kg	0.3-0.9 ml	30 ml	0.3 ml	0.75 ml	3 kg	12 ml
4 kg	0.4-1.2 ml	40 ml	0.4 ml	1 ml	4 kg	16 ml
	Administer rapidly	Give over 5-10 minutes	Administer rapidly		Administer slowly over at least 2 minutes	

Modified from Bloom R, Cropley C, AHA/AAP Neonatal Resuscitation Program Steering Committee: *Textbook of neonatal resuscitation*, Dallas, 1994, American Heart Association.
ET drugs should be diluted with a volume of 1-2 ml of saline before administration.
*IO route should be used only when other routes cannot be established.

mature and intrauterine-growth–retarded infants.[19] (Box 8-5). Hypoglycemia depresses myocardial function in the neonate and produces symptoms of shock, including tachycardia, decreased peripheral perfusion, and hypotension.

Although glucose administration is important in the hypoglycemic neonate, its use can lead to serious side effects such as hyperglycemia or intraventricular hemorrhage. Hyperglycemia can result from rapid infusions of glucose and may increase lactate production and contribute to cerebral injury.[30] Additionally, the administration of hyperosmolar solutions such as glucose is associated with intraventricular hemorrhage. Glucose is therefore administered only to the neonate with documented hypoglycemia (a blood glucose level < 30 mg/dl), with a blood glucose level between 30 and 40 mg/dl and symptoms consistent with hypoglycemia, or when a depressed infant is at risk for hypoglycemia—but only after the ABCs of care have been addressed.[8]

The concentration of glucose administered to neonates should not exceed 12.5%.[8] A $D_{10}W$ IV solution is ideal, but when it is not available the 50% solution can be diluted 1:4 with sterile water, which will produce a 10% solution. The dose is 0.5 to 1.0 g/kg of body weight or 5 to 10 ml/kg of the 10% solution. Glucose is administered *slowly*, over 20 minutes. Preterm infants (<25 to 27 weeks gestation or <1000 grams) are particularly susceptible to the development of hyperglycemia with glucose administration, be-

cause their glucose utilization rate is low. In these infants the D_5W solution is used and a continuous drip of 70 to 80 ml/kg/day is begun.[29]

Volume expanders. Volume expanders are indicated when there is evidence of hypovolemia or a suspicion of acute blood loss with signs of hypovolemia. Normal saline, Ringer's lactate, 5% albumin (or other plasma substitute), or whole blood (O-negative blood cross matched with the mother's blood) may be given to counteract the effects of hypovolemia by increasing vascular volume and improving tissue perfusion. The dose is 10 ml/kg of volume expander, administered over 5 to 10 minutes.[8]

SPECIAL RESUSCITATIVE SITUATIONS

MECONIUM ASPIRATION

Meconium aspiration syndrome is a major cause of neonatal morbidity and mortality. It is estimated that approximately 11% of all pregnancies are complicated by the passage of meconium and that 2% of infants have some degree of aspiration syndrome, which ranges from minor initial tachypnea to severe meconium-aspiration pneumonia with pulmonary hypertension.[29] Meconium present in the amniotic fluid can be thin and watery with a greenish hue or thick and particulate with the appearance of "pea soup." The presence of meconium in the amniotic fluid indicates that the infant has been distressed at some period of time during the labor or delivery.

During the delivery, if thin and watery meconium staining is observed, the infant's nasopharynx (mouth first, and then nose) is suctioned at the perineum as soon as the head is delivered and before the chest is delivered. The mouth, nose, and pharynx are suctioned using a large-bore suction catheter (12 or 14 Fr) before the first breath. Once the oropharynx is cleared, and if the infant exhibits no signs of respiratory distress, no further special management is needed.[8] These infants should, however, be closely observed for the development of respiratory distress and increased oxygen demands.

When thick meconium is present the newborn's mouth, nose, and posterior pharynx are suctioned with a large-bore suction catheter at the perineum, before the shoulders and thorax are delivered. Once the body is delivered, the newborn is placed supine in a prewarmed environment. Before drying or stimulat-

---

Box 8-5 Neonatal Risk Factors for Hypoglycemia

- Small for gestational age
- Large for gestational age
- Weight < 6 pounds (2.7 kg)
- Weight > 8 pounds (3.6 kg)
- Premature (<37 weeks gestation)
- Infant of a diabetic mother (chronic or gestational)
- Sepsis
- Dehydration
- Shock
- Hypothermia
- Respiratory distress

From Haley K, Baker P: *Emergency nursing pediatric course,* Chicago, 1993, Emergency Nurses Association.

ing the infant to breathe, the hypopharynx is visualized with a laryngoscope and any residual meconium is suctioned. The trachea is then intubated and the lower airway is suctioned. Suction may be applied directly to the ET tube using a special adapter or by using a meconium aspirator device. As suction is applied directly to the ET tube, the tube is slowly withdrawn. In the presence of large amounts of thick meconium, the trachea may be repeatedly intubated and suctioned until clear secretions are obtained. Occasionally a nasogastric tube is inserted to clear the stomach of meconium.

Once the trachea is clear of meconium, stimulation and drying of the infant are initiated. If the infant fails to breath spontaneously, positive pressure ventilation using 100% oxygen may be used. If the infant does not respond and continues to show signs of deterioration, the ABCs of resuscitative care are followed as described earlier in this chapter.

Preterm Deliveries

Resuscitation of the preterm infant who is less than 1000 grams or less than 25 to 27 weeks gestation requires a high level of skill. Preterm infants are fragile and require gentle handling. They are at high risk for the development of respiratory depression and cold stress. To minimize heat loss they are immediately dried well and placed under a radiant warmer. Their temperatures are constantly monitored.

Many preterm infants require immediate intubation. Some centers routinely intubate all preterm infants to enhance the clearance of lung water and the release of surfactant.[29] Once the infant is intubated and ventilated, caution must be taken not to overinflate the lungs and create a tension pneumothorax. Ventilated gases delivered should be humidified and warmed.

Vascular access and fluid management in preterm infants also require special consideration. Umbilical artery or venous catheterization may be required for the administration of fluids and medications, as well as blood gas monitoring (see p. 171). The administration of hyperosmolar solutions or large boluses of volume expanders should be avoided.[8] Rapid changes in blood pressure and fluctuations in serum osmolality place the preterm infant at risk for developing an intracranial hemorrhage. Nursing management includes continuous monitoring of the infant's temperature, heart rate, and respiratory status, as well as maintaining a strict record of intake and output.

Tension Pneumothorax

The development of a pneumothorax or tension pneumothorax is a potential complication whenever resuscitation and positive pressure ventilation is performed. A pneumothorax develops when alveolar air ruptures into the pleural space resulting in partial or complete collapse of the affected lung. A tension pneumothorax results as progressive pressure on the affected side puts pressure on the opposite lung and a mediastinal shift toward the unaffected side results. A spontaneous tension pneumothorax develops in 1% to 2% of all term newborns and in 10% of infants with retained fetal lung fluid.[29] Infants with a history of meconium aspiration, difficult delivery, and fetal distress and infants requiring intubation, resuscitation, or positive pressure ventilation are at increased risk for developing a tension pneumothorax.

A tension pneumothorax should be suspected when asymmetric chest expansion is noticed; unequal breath sounds and distant heart sounds are auscultated; the infant develops signs of respiratory distress; the infant develops signs of compromised systemic perfusion, bradycardia, hypoxia, or hypocapnia; or when an infant who has been improving during resuscitative efforts suddenly decompensates.

Transillumination with a strong light source such as a fiberoptic transilluminator may be used, if available, to detect the pneumothorax. A chest x-ray is another diagnostic method that may be used; however, it is time consuming and may interfere with the resuscitative process. Diagnostic studies should not delay definitive therapy in the unstable neonate with a suspected pneumothorax.

When a pneumothorax is suspected in the critically ill infant with respiratory distress and hemodynamic compromise, a diagnostic/therapeutic thoracentesis is performed immediately. A 22-gauge scalp vein needle attached to a three-way stopcock and a large syringe is inserted along the anterior axillary line over the top of the third or fourth rib on the affected side. When suction is applied with the syringe a rapid flow of air will result, evacuating the pneumothorax if present and providing temporary relief. A chest tube connected to suction is then inserted on the affected side for continuous relief.

▮ Summary

Neonatal resuscitation requires the skills of specially trained personnel, as well as the availability of specific neonatal resuscitation supplies and equipment. Therefore emergency department staff should prepare for unexpected deliveries. This can be done by participating in neonatal educational programs, obtaining needed supplies and equipment, developing a consultation program for obtaining assistance, and developing a referral network with a transport system and a neonatal ICU.

REFERENCES

1. Aehlert B: *PALS: pediatric advanced life support study guide,* St Louis, 1994, Mosby.
2. Andropoulos AB, Soifer SJ, Schreiber MD: Plasma epinephrine concentration, after intraosseous and central venous infusion, *J Pediatr* 116:312–315, 1990.
3. Apgar V: A proposal for a new method of evaluation of the newborn, *Anesth Anagl* 32:260–267, 1953.
4. Appleton GO et al: CPR and the single rescuer: at what age should you "call first" rather than "call fast"? *Ann Emerg Med* 25:492–494, 1995.
5. Bloom R, Cropley C, AHA/AAP Neonatal Resuscitation Program Steering Committee: *Textbook of neonatal resuscitation,* Dallas, 1994, American Heart Association.
5a. Burchfield D, Berkowitz I, Berg R, Goldberg R: Medications in neonatal resusitation. *Ann Emerg Med* 22:(2)435-437, 1993.
6. Cavallaro DL, Melker RJ: Comparison of two techniques for detecting cardiac activity in infants, *Crit Care Med* 11:189–190, 1983.
7. Chameides L, AHA/AAP Neonatal Resuscitation Program Steering Committee: *Textbook of neonatal resuscitation,* Dallas, 1990, American Heart Association.
8. Chameides L, Hazinski MF, eds: *Textbook of pediatric advanced life support,* Dallas, 1994, American Heart Association.
9. Chandra NC, Hazinski MF, eds: *Textbook of basic life support for healthcare providers,* Dallas, 1994, American Heart Association.
10. Cloherty J, Stark A: *Manual of neonatal care,* Boston, 1991, Little, Brown.
11. Cummins RO, ed: *Textbook of advanced cardiac life support,* Dallas, 1994, American Heart Association.
12. Eisenberg M, Bergner L, Hallstrom A: Epidemiology of cardiac arrest and resuscitation in children, *Ann Emerg Med* 12:672–674, 1983.
13. Feldman KW, Brewer DK: Child abuse, cardiopulmonary resuscitation and rib fractures, *Pediatr* 73:339–342, 1984.
14. Fleisher G, Caputo G, Baskin M: Comparison of external jugular and peripheral venous administration of sodium bicarbonate in puppies, *Crit Care Med* 17:251–254, 1989.
15. Haley K, Baker P: *Emergency nursing pediatric course,* Chicago, 1993, Emergency Nurses Association.
16. Hazinski MF et al: Outcome of cardiovascular collapse in pediatric blunt trauma, *Ann Emerg Med* 23:1229–1235, 1994.
17. Jasani MS et al: Endotracheal epinephrine administration technique effects in pediatric porcine hypoxic-hypercarbic arrest, *Crit Care Med* 22:1174–1180, 1994.
18. Kallas HJ, O'Rourke PP: Drowning and submersion injuries in children, *Curr Opin Pediatr* 5:295–302, 1993.
19. Kenner C, Brueggemeyer A, Gunderson L: *Comprehensive neonatal nursing: a physiologic perspective,* Philadelphia, 1993, WB Saunders.
20. Kyriacou DN et al: Effect of immediate resuscitation on children with submersion injury, *Pediatr* 94:137–142, 1994.
21. Lee CJ, Bullock LJ: Determining the pulse for infant CPR: time for a change? *Mil Med* 156:190–199, 1991.
22. Losek JD et al: Prehospital countershock treatment of pediatric asystole, *Am J Emerg Med* 7:571–575, 1989.
23. Mogayzel C et al: Etiologies and outcomes of the pulseless, nonbreathing pediatric patient presenting with ventricular fibrillation, *Ann Emerg Med* 21:484–491, 1995.
24. O'Rourke PP: Outcome of children who are apneic and pulseless in the emergency room, *Crit Care Med* 14:466–468, 1986.
25. Quan L et al: Outcome and predictors of outcome in pediatric submersion victims receiving prehospital care in King County, Washington, *Pediatr* 86:586–593, 1990.
26. Ruddy RM. In Fleisher GR, Ludwig S, eds: *Textbook of pediatric emergency medicine,* ed 2, Baltimore, Md, 1988, Williams & Wilkins.
27. Spevak MR et al: Does cardiopulmonary resuscitation cause rib fractures in infants? Postmortem radiologic-pathologic study, *Radiology* 177P:162, 1990, (abstract).
28. Strauss RH: Pediatric vascular access. In Fuhrman BP, Zimmerman JJ, eds: *Pediatric critical care,* St Louis, 1992, Mosby.
29. Taeusch H, Ballard R, Avery ME: *Diseases of the newborn,* ed 6, Philadelphia, 1991, WB Saunders.
30. Vannucci RC: Experimental biology of cerebral hypoxia-ischemia: relation to perinatal brain damage, *Pediatr Res* 27:317, 1990.
31. Walsh CK, Krongrad E: Terminal cardiac electrical activity in pediatric patients, *Am J Cardiol* 51:557–561, 1983.
32. Weaver WD et al: Use of automatic external defibrillator in the management of out-of-hospital cardiac arrest, *N Engl J Med* 319:661–666, 1988.
33. Zaritsky A et al: CPR in children, *Ann Emerg Med* 16:1107–1111, 1987.

CHAPTER 9

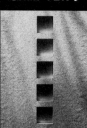

Crisis Intervention and Death

Donna Thomas

INTRODUCTION

A visit to a busy emergency department (ED) can be stressful to both parent and child. The sights, smells, sounds, and occasional long wait can be unnerving. When the wait is long, the parent's concern for the child intensifies. During this time ED staff are usually busy and may not have the time to develop a relationship with or to keep the family informed about why they are waiting and how long it might be. Usually the nurse is unaware of the family's perceptions, fears, and past experiences.

Although an ED visit is usually stressful for the parent and child, it may not always result in a crisis situation. The terms *stress* and *crisis* are not synonymous. A crisis situation is usually precipitated by serious illness, injury, or the death of a child. Because of the unexpected nature of the illness or injury, parents have little time to prepare for the event.

Serious illness, injury, or death of a child is often rated as a major cause of stress for emergency department nurses as well. The fast pace of the ED allows little time for nurses to interact with and support families and even less time for their own recovery. Another patient is always waiting.

The purpose of this chapter is to define events that may precipitate a crisis and discuss common reactions to crisis in the family of the pediatric patient in the ED. The ED nurse's role in assessment and intervention will be presented, along with interventions to prevent stress from developing into crises. Helping staff cope with the stress of dealing with families in crisis will be reviewed in the section on critical incident stress management. Finally, selected pediatric emergencies that may result in a crisis will be reviewed.

CRISIS

DEFINITIONS

Crisis refers to an acute emotional upset arising from situational, developmental, or social sources resulting in a temporary inability to cope by one's usual problem-solving devices.[15a] Examples of crisis situations are sudden illness or injury and death.

Stress is defined as tension, strain, or pressure, such as the stress of waiting to be seen for extended periods of time, or being overwhelmed by conflicting demands and stimuli.[15a] Although the terms refer to different conditions, increasing stress with no relief can lead to a crisis.

Crisis management refers to the entire process of working through the crisis to its endpoint—crisis resolution. Crisis intervention is a short-term helping process that focuses on the resolution of the immediate problem through the use of personal, social, and environmental resources. The positive or negative resolution of a crisis often depends on crisis intervention. Whether or not a stressful event precipitates a crisis depends on the family's interpretation of the events, coping ability and previous experiences, and social and personal resources.[17]

By definition, an ED visit is usually precipitated by an event (trauma incident or illness) that is unanticipated and over which the family has no direct control. The parents' previous experience, involvement in other stressful events, and significance of this event will determine how they react and cope with the current situation (Box 9-1).

Even the serious illness or death of a child with preexisting illness or injury can precipitate a crisis.

Box 9-1 Event Characteristics that Influence Stress Level

- Whether onset of the event is gradual or sudden
- Whether the event is anticipated
- Whether individual feels he or she has some control over the event
- Whether the event is similar to other events experienced in the past or is new and unique
- Whether event is in isolation or combination with other stressful events
- Meaning and significance attached to event

Compiled from Solursh DS: The family of the trauma victim, *Nurs Clin North Am* 25:155, 1990.

TABLE 9-1 Behavioral and Physiologic Signs and Symptoms of the Family in Crisis

BEHAVIORAL	PHYSIOLOGIC
Withdrawal, isolation	Tachycardia
Demanding behavior, restlessness, pacing	Sweaty palms
	Dry mouth
Speaking loudly, quickly, profanely	Hyperventilation
	Chest pain
Poor eye contact	Nausea
Loud crying, shouting, banging on walls or tables	Headache
	Fainting
Violent behavior, threats against family members or members of the health care team	Lethargy
Self-destructive behavior	
Blaming others	
Stated feelings of helplessness and increased frustration, decreased ability to make decisions	

Compiled from ENA, 1991; ENA, 1993.

Despite some preparation for the death, the family may react in a highly emotional manner. Although the family may have decided beforehand that resuscitative measures not be performed, they may change their mind at the last minute, or they may be alarmed if resuscitative measures are initiated.

SIGNS AND SYMPTOMS OF THE FAMILY IN CRISIS

While assessing the child and interviewing the family, the ED nurse should observe family interactions. Signs and symptoms of crisis include both behavioral and physiologic signs and symptoms, which may vary depending on the situation (Table 9-1).

Anger is commonly observed in the family in crisis. It may be expressed by the caregiver, toward other family members, or toward other persons involved with the child or with the incident. Anger at the nursing staff and/or medical staff for being incompetent or uncaring may also be exhibited by family members, and they may accuse or lash out. Emergency department staff should not take these comments personally but should instead explore them with the family for clarification. Because anger is a coping mechanism, it should be allowed as long as it does not result in violent behavior.

By recognizing the stages of emotional distress, the ED nurse can intervene on a corresponding level, averting unnecessary hostility while providing the most therapeutic response to the family's emotional needs.[2]

APPROACH TO CRISIS: CRITICALLY ILL OR INJURED CHILD

Emergency department interactions are brief and intense. How the nurse interacts with the family during these encounters can positively influence the parent's ability to deal with the situation. Because sudden, unanticipated events are more likely to result in a crisis, the ED nurse should evaluate the situation based on knowledge of the event and recognize factors that might cause these events to escalate into a crisis.

COMMUNICATION

When a child is seriously ill or injured, anxiety can be reduced if ongoing information is regularly conveyed to the family regarding the child's condition and treatment. Communication should begin as soon as the child is admitted to the ED and can be initiated by a nurse, social worker, physician, or chaplain.

If the family is not at the hospital when the child arrives, informing them is the first step.[15] When telephoned, the parents should be told that the child is critically ill and that everything is being done that can be done. They should be told to come to the ED immediately. Suggest the family find someone to drive them and ask if they would like anyone else notified, such as their pediatrician. The family should be given directions to the ED and the name of a person to ask for on arrival. This establishes a communication link. If the child has died, informing the family over the telephone should be avoided.

CRISIS INTERVENTION: INITIAL INTERVIEW

On the parents' arrival in the ED a brief history should be obtained to assist in the diagnosis and treatment of the child. Providing this history can be a therapeutic experience for the family. While conveying the history, parents often feel they are participating in the child's treatment, giving them more control over the situation.[11] Stress is lessened when the family is given some control over the situation and allowed to make choices where possible. In addition, while interviewing the family the ED staff will become familiar with the family's perceptions of the situation, previous coping abilities, and past experience—further guiding interactions (Box 9-2).

CRISIS INTERVENTION: FAMILY

When the parents/caregivers of a critically ill or injured child arrive in the ED they should immediately be escorted to a private area where they will not be interrupted by others. Many EDs have consultation rooms, but if none are available an office or empty exam room can be used. As soon as possible, the ED physician should be introduced as the person in charge of the child's care. Additionally, one nurse or social worker should serve as a liaison to provide the family with continuous information about the child's condition. The number of ED personnel providing information to the family should be limited to avoid inconsistencies or discrepancies. Talking with a family whose child is about to die is difficult for health care professionals, and it is often easier for the ED staff to focus on the clinical aspects of care. However, family members need and appreciate the contact of someone who is involved in the care of their child (Box 9-3). Often the nurse need only sit with the family and listen. Although families may not seem comforted at the time, they will later remember everything that was said and often find comfort from the support given.

When communicating with the family, allow them to talk, and listen to their perceptions of the illness or injury. Expressions of guilt are common, even if there was no way the illness or injury could have been prevented. If the parents are responsible for an injury,

---

Box 9-2 Components of the Nursing History of the Family in Crisis

- Family's perception of the event or situation
- Availability of support systems
- Previous illness or injury of the child
- Concurrent maturational crisis within the family
- Family's current level of functioning, past experiences, and usual coping mechanisms
- Drug and/or alcohol use by the family, especially if associated with the child's injury
- Family's religious preference
- Level of education

Modified from Emergency Nurses Association: *Emergency nursing pediatric course, provider manual,* Chicago, 1993, Award Printing Company.

Box 9-3 Support of the Family of a Critically Ill or Injured Child

- Introduce self; use family name and the child's name
- Give accurate, honest information
- Provide privacy
- Meet the family's physical needs (bathroom, water, tissues, telephone)
- Do not eliminate all hope while resuscitation is still underway
- Ask about the need for clergy or religious rites
- Give brief, frequent updates on the child's condition
- Consider allowing the family to observe the resuscitation

From Henderson DP: Death of a child. In Barkin R, ed: *Pediatric emergency medicine: concepts & clinical practice,* ed. 2, St Louis, 1997, Mosby.

ED staff should try to remain nonjudgmental and instead help the family deal with guilt feelings and accept the facts of the injury.

CRISIS INTERVENTION: CHILD

Children require the comfort of family members regardless of the degree of illness or injury—or whether they are conscious or unconscious. Yet in the midst of clinical care the child's emotional needs are often overlooked.[15] Recognizing these needs, nursing staff should allow parents to remain with their child whenever possible.

When the child is conscious, anxiety and fear should be expected. To establish rapport one staff member should be assigned to care for the child during medical interventions and to provide emotional support (e.g., talking quietly to the child, touching or holding the child's hand, and providing age-appropriate information to the child).

CRISIS INTERVENTION: RESUSCITATION

Family presence during a resuscitation is controversial; however, experience has shown that family presence can be beneficial. Although not all parents may be able to cope with observing resuscitation activities, others are thankful when given the opportunity to say "goodbye" to their child. Others are assured from the activity level that "everything that could have been done was done." Examples include the following:[31]

1. A father who kissed his daughter just after she was intubated and prepared for surgery. Although her condition was stable at the time, during surgery her injuries were found to be fatal and she died. The father later thanked the ED staff for allowing him to remain with his daughter while she was still alive.
2. A father allowed to remain in the room with his teenage son during a resuscitation responded later by saying, "Being in the room gave me a chance to say goodbye while I thought he might still hear me."

A survey performed at one hospital ED that allows family presence during resuscitations indicated 76% of the families interviewed felt that adjustment to the death of their loved one was made easier by their presence in the room.[14] In addition, 64% of the families felt that their presence was beneficial to the dying person.[14] Another study surveyed parents who had remained with their child during invasive procedures, including intubations, and found that 91% found it to be beneficial.[24]

When the decision is made by ED staff to allow family presence during resuscitations, guidelines must be established and agreed upon by all staff members. Policies should include (1) giving the family a choice to be in the room; (2) informing the family of the activities or interventions they might see; (3) assigning a member of the team (nurse, social worker, clergy) to be with the family member at all times; (4) determining which family member(s) should be included; and (5) dealing with emotionally charged situations or potential violence.[14]

CRISIS INTERVENTION: VIOLENT BEHAVIOR

Risk of violence in the Emergency Department. The nature of the ED is conducive to violence for many reasons. Some of these include the following:[22]

1. Accessibility—The ED is open 24 hours a day to anyone requiring medical care
2. Physical environment—EDs are often noisy, crowded, and conducive to unrest
3. Characteristics of patients and families—EDs are open to all socioeconomic and cultural groups, each of which may exhibit varying responses to stress and crisis. Even normally calm people may become fearful when they or a family member is in pain or is seriously ill or injured
4. Characteristics of ED staff—ED nurses often cope with long hours, understaffing, repeated harassment, and frustration

Although preventing a crisis from escalating into violent behavior is preferable, it is not always possible. However, staffing behavior that provokes potentially hostile, angry family members can increase the likelihood and frequency of violence. Instead, ED staff should recognize risk factors that might lead to violence and intervene to prevent a crisis from escalating into violent behavior (Box 9-4).

Interventions for potentially violent behavior. Remaining calm, confident, and nonjudgmental when confronted with a family who is angry or abusive may help to defuse the situation. In addition, dealing with the family one on one is preferable; however, a path of easy escape should be maintained and the nurse should remain within shouting distance of help.[2]

Sometimes simply having a staff member listen will calm a family member; therefore the ED nurse should

Box 9-4   Risk Factors that may Lead to Violent Behavior

- Repeat visits to the ED
- Alcohol or drug use by family members
- Male gender
- Age less than 30
- History of violent behavior
- Physical signs: pacing, clenched fists, tense posture
- Verbal signs: anger, demands, threats

From Kinkle S: Violence in the ED: how to stop it before it starts, *Am J Nurs* 93:22, 1993.

initially listen rather than talk. When speaking, not only what is said but also how it is said can make a difference in a family member's response.[2] A calm, quiet voice should be used regardless of the language or loudness of the family's responses.

Setting realistic limits is another important element for controlling a family member's behavior. For example, "I really want to listen to you, but your shouting is upsetting to your child and other children."

Once a family member becomes physically abusive, the potential for harm to the ED staff is high, and the person must be controlled quickly. Team intervention using security and a prearranged plan for dealing with violent behavior is the only safe recourse.[2] Unless trained, the ED nurse should never attempt to restrain a violent patient or family member.

All EDs should develop protocols for both the prevention of violent behavior and for intervening when necessary. A team approach involving hospital security, ED staff, and the local police is required to protect staff, other patients, and family members.

DEATH OF A CHILD IN THE EMERGENCY DEPARTMENT

INTRODUCTION

When a child dies unexpectedly in the ED the family experiences an acute grief reaction, because sudden death eliminates the opportunity for anticipatory grief that usually prepares survivors for death following a long illness.[9,41] Thus survivors are at higher risk for prolonged or complicated grief.

DEFINITIONS

Grief can be defined as the reaction of the bereaved to a loss.[6] The expression of grief varies from person to person but is almost always influenced by a person's cultural background (Box 9-5).[40] Forms of grief include anticipatory grief and unresolved or pathologic grief. Anticipatory grief is a normal reaction in preparation for a loss and allows for absorbing the reality of the loss over time.[32] Unresolved or pathologic grief refers to an abnormally prolonged duration or intensity of reactions, which may result in personal disability.[41] Certain situations may predispose survivors to the development of pathologic grief, including sudden or unexpected death, death of an infant or child, death involving homicide or suicide, or death caused by the survivor.[41]

Denial, anger, and guilt are common reactions to grief.[41] Calmness, another response, may be difficult for the ED staff to understand and may be misinterpreted as uncaring. For example, an uncle of a child who died said he "wasn't very close to the child anyway." Viewed as uncaring by the staff, he was later discovered sobbing uncontrollably outside the emergency department.

Although varied expressions of grief should be recognized and accepted by the ED staff, grief reactions that result in violence directed toward another family member or the ED staff require immediate intervention by hospital security or according to existing hospital policy.

Mourning is the process of coping with grief, together with the expected behaviors or interpersonal rituals of individual societies.[6] The mourning process may begin in the ED, or if the child has been chronically ill it may have begun when the illness was first diagnosed. The four tasks of mourning after a death include the following.[43]

1. Accepting the reality of the loss. This involves coming full face with the reality that the child is dead.
2. Experiencing the pain of grief. During this stage it is necessary to acknowledge and work through this pain or it will manifest itself through some symptom or other form of aberrant behavior.
3. Adjusting to an environment without the child.

Box 9-5 Cultural Influences Affecting the Grieving Process

Native Americans
- Consider children of great value
- Grief tends to be family and even community oriented
- Religion and healing are inseparable
- Parents may find native healers more acceptable than medical approach
- Burial practices may vary; some forbid leaving the deceased alone and insist that a family member remain in attendance until the burial
- Expressions of grief may range from quiet and stoic to dramatic and hysterical
- Parents may feel that talking about the death or mentioning the child's name detracts from the child's spirituality and may bring bad luck
- Parents may deny autopsy, because they value the integrity of the body
- Parents may be suspicious of health professionals

Mexican Americans
- Loss of children represents loss of hope and expectations for future
- Help must be directed toward entire family, which may include friends and extended family
- Family structure is patriarchal
- Concepts of death are rooted in Roman Catholicism
- May consider death and hardship "God's will"

Southeast Asians
- Family is basis of society, large families are valued
- Father is head of the family, and eldest male often has key role in family; health professionals must acknowledge key role of eldest and direct interventions to the family as a whole
- Death of an infant is deeply mourned
- Religious beliefs influence all aspects of life
- Expressions of grief vary

Modified from Valk Lawson L: Culturally sensitive support for grieving parents, *MCN* 15:76, 1990.

---

4. Withdrawing emotional energy and reinvesting it in another relationship.

NURSING INTERVENTIONS: FAMILY

A family member's ability to successfully resolve grief is greatly affected by what occurs during the time immediately surrounding the death of a child.[9] Therefore interactions cannot be rushed. How the family is told and what is said can affect their psychological well-being[41] (Table 9-2).

Adjusting to the environment without the child and reinvesting emotional energy is a long process that will vary from family to family. These tasks begin when the family leaves the ED. Other family members such as grandparents and baby-sitters, who may have been present when a child died, may also need special attention and follow-up with counselors.

Immediately after the death, family members should be informed in a private area, away from the noise of ED activity. A social worker, chaplain, or nurse should remain with the family and may offer to call other family members or close friends when appropriate. The family should be offered the opportunity to see the child and hold and/or caress the child as long as necessary to assist in the grieving process (Box 9-6).

If the child is from an unfamiliar culture, the ED nurse may ask the family what would be helpful; watch family members, especially parents, for cues as to what is acceptable (body space, speaking of the dead); help the family identify resources within their culture in the community; and find an interpreter to translate if the parents do not speak English.[40]

Parents often fear what will happen to the body of their child and may be reluctant to leave. They should be reassured their child will be in good hands.

Before a family leaves the department the following interventions may be helpful and appropriate:

1. Funeral arrangements. ED staff (nurse, social worker or chaplain) can assist the family with funeral arrangements and answer questions about details such as how the body will get to the funeral home if an autopsy is being done.
2. Follow-up. Parents may be given the name of a local support group or a social worker for follow-up. Sometimes subsequent calls are made by a social worker or nurse at intervals such as 2 weeks, 6 months, and 1 year. The family may be provided with the phone number of an ED staff member whom they can contact if they have questions or if they wish to talk.

TABLE 9-2	Informing the Family about a Child's Death: Some Do's and Dont's	
DO		**DON'T**
Tell the family immediately.		Don't say, "I know how you feel."
Sit down with family—physically join them unless the situation is hostile.		Don't imply guilt (of parents, medical care, or others).
Be kind, but direct. Speak directly to the person closest to the child (mother or father).		Don't use euphemisms (e.g., "Your child has passed away" or is "gone").
Give a brief explanation of what was done in the ED and the suspected cause of the death, if known.		Don't offer meaningless comfort such as "It was God's will" or "He is in a better place."
Provide physical comfort (by touching the family, if you are comfortable doing this).		Don't tell them they can always have another child. This may not be true, and another child will not replace the one who has died.
Ask the parent(s) what their perception of the death is—reassure them that they are not at fault (unless this is not true).		Don't tell the family how they should or should not feel. Grief is individual.
Allow family to express pain.		
Stay long enough to answer questions.		Don't offer sedatives, because this may delay some of the grief process for later.
Say you are sorry.		

Compiled from Frader and Sargent, 1992; Hamilton, 1988, McQuay, 1995.

3. Written material. Parents may not process or remember much of the information that has been discussed or given to them. Handouts concerning the grieving process, support groups, and who should be contacted may be useful after the initial shock wears off.

When possible, ED staff should arrange transportation home for family members and accompany them to the car. Watching a family whose child has died leave the ED, and knowing that they must go home and face all of the child's belongings can be very emotional. After the family leaves the ED, all interventions and follow-up recommendations should be documented. A useful tool is a prepared death packet consisting of all necessary forms. This packet helps to prevent errors of omission and facilitates the completion of paperwork.

Siblings. Children's understanding of the concept of death varies depending on their age. Therefore the approach to a child should be matched to that child's developmental level. This recommendation may not be helpful to parents who may lack the energy or creativity for this effort in the midst of intense grief. General guidelines include offering the child the chance to see the sibling, encouraging parents to include the child in the sibling's funeral and burial,

discouraging parents from trying to "protect" the child from sadness or grief, and answering questions honestly[11] (Box 9-7).

NURSING INTERVENTIONS: STAFF

The death of a child often triggers intense emotional reactions among the ED staff. This is especially true if the death was caused by a careless accident, self-destructive behavior, or criminal violence.[41]

Perhaps nothing is more painful or stressful to the staff than telling a family their child has died. Medical and/or nursing education usually does not include this information. Further complicating the interaction is the required discussion of emotional issues such as organ donation and the autopsy.[36]

Although the physician in charge of the child's care should inform the family of the child's death, the nurse is often present. In some situations the nurse must inform the family; there are important considerations when informing a family of a child's death. The family should be told as soon as possible after the child is pronounced dead. If possible, all family members should be told as a group. If all family members cannot be told together, the staff should communicate directly with each family

---

Box 9-6   Helping a Family After the Death of a Child

1. Give the family a choice of viewing the body
   - Prepare the family for how the child will look and feel. Explain any tubes that are left in place.
   - Provide privacy.
   - Remain with the family if they request you to do so.
   - Allow them ample time to be with the child.
   - Give family permission to leave.
   - Have one nurse remain with the child when the family leaves.
2. Provide mementos
   - Provide hand and/or footprints and a lock of hair.
   - Provide a picture if requested.
   - If the family viewed and held the body, give them the blanket that the child was wrapped in.
3. Provide help with cessation of breast-feeding
   - Allow mother to use a breast pump (usually available in a hospital nursery).
   - Refer to family physician or obstetrician for further instructions.
   - Refer to La Leche League or lactation specialist, if available.
4. Provide help with siblings
   - Talk with siblings to find out their perception of the death—be honest with them. Reassure them that they were not to blame. Using euphemisms such as "your brother has gone to sleep" will only make the child fearful of going to sleep—he or she might die too.
   - Encourage parents to include siblings in funeral arrangements and burial and to answer questions honestly.
   - Give literature or refer to support group.
5. Provide information about autopsy
   - Answer questions—parents may agree to an autopsy to find out why their child died.
   - Let parents know who will contact them about results.
   - Obtain consent, if necessary.

Box 9-7   Approach to the Sibling After the Death of a Child

- Offer the child the chance to see the sibling in the ED. The child should never be forced to see or touch the body. Because children often imagine death to be worse than reality, seeing the body helps their understanding.
- Encourage parents to involve siblings in the funeral and burial. To say goodbye, let go, and get on with reinvesting in life, the child needs a clear understanding of what has happened.
- Discourage parents from attempting to protect siblings from sadness. Children are perceptive and will know something is wrong by the way the parents are acting. Children excluded from the grief may believe that they somehow are at fault for the death.
- Explain normal responses to the loss of a loved one to the child. They should be told that it is OK for them to be sad and cry.
- Answer questions honestly. Children often have the need to talk and ask questions, and they also need to be reassured.

Modified from Frader and Sargent, 1993; Papadatou and Papadatos, 1991.

---

member to prevent misinformation. Family members cannot be expected to accurately absorb, recall, and then transmit information to other family members (Figs. 9-1 and 9-2).

Showing emotion is appropriate and can indicate to the parents that the ED staff care. Excessive emotion, however, will prevent the nurse from helping the family. The best intervention is to be with the family, listen, and acknowledge their pain. This can be difficult, as the family's anguish is often painful to observe. The desire to help can cause the nurse to talk needlessly when all that is necessary is to say, "I am sorry."

Organ donation.   Despite the fact that requesting organ donation is the law in most states, it is done infrequently, perhaps because it has been identified as a significant source of stress for the ED staff.[36] However, health care professionals are responsible for

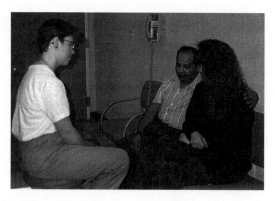

FIG. 9-1. The family should be told as soon as possible after the child's death in a private area, away from the noise and confusion of a busy emergency department.

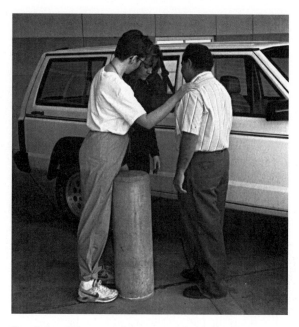

FIG. 9-2. When possible a member of the emergency department staff should arrange transportation home for the family and accompany them to their car.

offering the family or next of kin the opportunity to consider organ donation.[30]

Most hospitals have protocols for requesting organ donation that describe who is responsible for communicating with the family. With so much media attention, families are often aware that organ donation is an option and may find comfort in helping someone else—and even feel cheated if not given the chance. In general, almost every patient who dies can be considered a tissue or organ donor (excluding patients with systemic infectious disease).[30] Therefore, every child who dies in the ED can be considered a potential tissue donor.

Autopsy. Although an autopsy is required in all cases of sudden and unattended death, health care professionals are reluctant to discuss autopsy with grieving family members. In fact, discussing autopsy information has been identified as a significant source of stress for the ED staff.[36]

When possible, the ED physician or nurse who has established rapport with the family should request the autopsy. Ideally, and if present, the family physician may request the autopsy. When an autopsy is required by law, the family should be given an explanation as to why it is necessary. Whether the autopsy was requested by the physician or required by law, some families find comfort in the explanation that the autopsy may provide information that could be useful to other family members (e.g., by identifying genetic abnormalities) or may provide information helpful to other parents and children.[11]

Common concerns regarding the autopsy include the questions of how the autopsy will affect the appearance of the child and who will inform the family of the results. In many emergency departments the physician is responsible for notifying the family of autopsy results; however, in some institutions conveying autopsy results is the responsibility of the medical examiner. When a private physician is involved, he or she may convey the information to the family. Regarding the appearance of the child, in most cases a viewing is still possible.

CRITICAL INCIDENT STRESS MANAGEMENT (CISM)

INTRODUCTION/DEFINITIONS

Dealing with pediatric death, critical illness, and other crisis situations takes its toll on ED nurses. Because a busy ED allows very little time for recovery of staff after these events, feelings related to the incident may be repressed. A *critical incident* is any event that has sufficient emotional power to overcome the usual coping abilities of emergency personnel.[27]

Critical incident stress management (CISM) pro-

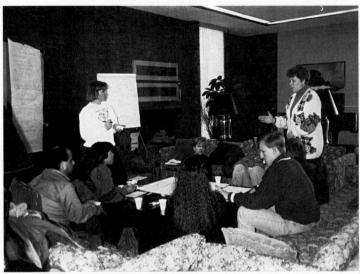

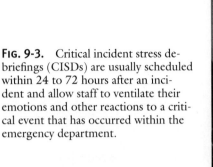

FIG. 9-3. Critical incident stress debriefings (CISDs) are usually scheduled within 24 to 72 hours after an incident and allow staff to ventilate their emotions and other reactions to a critical event that has occurred within the emergency department.

vides "care for the health care professional" after an emotional and/or stressful event and consists of defusings and debriefings.[9] Defusings are gatherings following a stressful situation that are primarily informational.[9] They are usually much shorter, less formal, and less structured than debriefings. For example, ED staff involved in a death may take a few minutes to briefly discuss the case, evaluate their performance, and comfort each other.

Critical incident stress debriefing (CISD) is an organized approach to the management of stress responses.[25] Debriefing teams consist of dedicated, trained mental health professionals who combine expert knowledge with specially trained EMS peer support personnel.[26] Debriefings are usually scheduled within 24 to 72 hours after an incident and are designed to allow ventilation of emotions and other reactions to a critical event.[9] The goal is to provide immediate crisis intervention to ED staff, prevent or lessen the impact of a critical incident, and allow staff to return to normal functioning (Fig. 9-3 and Box 9-8).

EMERGENCY STAFF RESPONSE TO STRESS

The impact of critical events can lead to such reactions as denial, emotional numbing, hostility, anger, anxiety, fear, helplessness, frustration, sleep problems, and

---

Box 9-8   Additional Suggestions for Helping ED Staff Cope with Death or Critical Incidents

- Written protocols or checklists describing the treatment of children and families
- Education on the grieving process and dealing with death
- Evaluation of one's feelings concerning death
- Evaluations of staff performances after each death, not only in resuscitative efforts but also in dealing with the family
- Recovery time after death in the ED, even if only for a few minutes
- Acceptance of peer's responses to death and recognition that everyone reacts differently
- A sympathy card signed by all ED staff involved
- ED staff need to take care of themselves by getting plenty of rest, exercise, and proper nutrition
- Remember that most children get better and go home
- Realize that being responsible for a child's life is *not* the same as being responsible for a child's death

flashbacks.[34] It is impossible for staff to remain emotionally unaffected, but they must be able to contain their emotions so they can deliver the expertise needed for the critical patient.[10]

The following case study illustrates an ED staff's response to a situation that resulted in the need for a CISD.

A woman and her two children were found wandering around an airport. The children were dressed inappropriately for the weather and the woman was mumbling incoherently. The children were brought to the ED to be evaluated for protective custody placement.

While the mother was being interviewed by the police, she excused herself to use the restroom. When she didn't return in a reasonable amount of time, a nurse knocked on the bathroom door. There was no answer, and the door was locked. A key to this lobby restroom was not available and security personnel were called to open the door. When the door was opened, the mother was found on the floor in a pool of blood. She had lacerated her wrists and her neck with scissors and was bleeding profusely. She was resuscitated and admitted to an adult facility.

Staff involved reported not being able to sleep. "I kept seeing that white face turn towards me, and those eyes looking at me. I couldn't imagine someone losing so much blood and still being alive." Another nurse commented, "I tried to pull her out of there [the bathroom] and kept slipping on the blood. My shoes were covered. I felt I would never be clean again." Other feelings reported were anger and ambivalence. Some nurses wished the staff would have let her die. One said, "I wish that the scissors were sharper!" The head nurse, who was not present, described feelings of anger at this woman for putting the ED staff through such emotional trauma.

A debriefing was held within the same week, and staff reported it was very helpful.

▌SELECTED EMERGENCIES

SUDDEN INFANT DEATH SYNDROME

Etiology. Sudden infant death syndrome (SIDS) is the sudden death of an infant younger than 1 year of age, for which postmortem exam, investigation of the death scene, and a review of the case history fail to establish a cause.[44] The peak incidence is 2 months of age, with SIDS rarely occurring in infants younger than 1 month of age. Of all infant deaths between the ages of 1 week and 1 year, a third are attributable to SIDS.[39] In the United States, the rate of SIDS is two deaths per 1000 births, or approximately 7000 infants each year.[39] Most deaths occur in the winter months.

Although no single cause of SIDS has been identified, SIDS tends to be more common in babies whose mothers are younger than 20 years of age, have had at least one other child, have received poor prenatal care, and smoke during pregnancy and after birth.[3] Narcotic or methadone use is also a risk factor. Risk factors for the infant include prematurity and low birth weight, and SIDS is more predominant in males.

Pathophysiology. Many theories have been and continue to be researched regarding the cause of SIDS. Although there is no consensus regarding the etiology of SIDS, there is agreement that there is no single cause of SIDS. Instead, the diagnosis includes infants who may have died from several different causes. Commonalities include that the death was unexpected and that the cause could not be determined by clinical history, autopsy, or a death scene investigation.[3]

Current theories regarding the causes of SIDS include abnormalities in respiratory control, small airway occlusion, cardiovascular abnormalities, defects of metabolism, infection, delayed neural development, and abnormal sleep and arousal states.[3,6]

Because of numerous studies from abroad that indicate an increased risk of SIDS in infants sleeping in the prone position, the American Academy of Pediatrics (AAP) added sleeping in the prone position to the risk factors for SIDS.[1] The AAP now recommends that all normal infants be placed on their sides or their backs instead of on their stomachs. The side position is best if the infant has been recently fed. Since this recommendation the mortality attributed to SIDS has decreased significantly in Northern Europe and Australia where the prone position has been recommended for several years.[42]

Clinical presentation. The victim of SIDS is usually found apneic and pulseless with a pink, frothy drainage from the mouth and nose. If prehospital providers respond to the scene, CPR may be initiated before transport to the ED. Some states have developed criteria that allow for death to be pronounced in the home. In these cases the medical examiner may be called to the scene.

On arrival in the ED, parents typically relate a history of a healthy baby who was put down for a nap or for the night. The infant may have had a slight cold and may have recently been seen by a physician for a minor illness. No warning signs and symptoms will have been evident.

Emergency Department and nursing care. Resuscitative measures in the ED usually prove unsuccessful. A heart rate may be obtained for a short time, long enough for the child to be admitted to the intensive care unit, but the outcome is usually the same. Despite what seems to be a futile resuscitation, parents often say they were glad to have the additional time in the intensive care unit to prepare for the death and contact family members.

After the death, nursing interventions are focused on the family. Families react to the sudden, unexpected death of their infant in many different ways. Some become accusatory, others withdraw, and others experience intense guilt. Siblings also grieve, often feeling guilty for jealously wishing their brother or sister would go away. The general nursing approach to caring for the family after the death of a child is reviewed earlier in this chapter. Specific interventions for the family of the victim of SIDS are described in Table 9-3.

HOMICIDE AND VIOLENCE

Epidemiology of violence against children. Almost daily the news media describes incidents of violence against children, many of which are directly related to the home environment. Others occur within the community and include societal violence—particularly when drug use or gang issues are involved.[12] With this trend the epidemiology of pediatric ED visits has changed, as have pediatric morbidity and mortality statistics.[9] For example, a growing number of children are joining gangs. Once a child or adolescent is associated with a gang, violence is often inevitable. The resulting injuries are commonly caused by penetrating trauma, which in years past was rarely seen in the pediatric population.[9]

Children living in neighborhoods experiencing gang violence display distress reactions, somatic symptoms, difficulty in routine functioning, and acting out, similar to children living in war zones.[33] Some children shut down emotionally and become desensitized to violence.

Epidemiology of homicide. Homicide is the leading cause of death related to injury in the first year

of life.[21] Approximately one fourth of all reported childhood homicide deaths occur in children less than 5 years of age, with the most common injuries being beatings, arson, burns, and neglect.[4] Estimates of child abuse homicides vary, depending on the source of the data, but national estimates cite approximately 5000 fatalities annually as a result of all forms of child abuse.[21] Most childhood victims of homicide are injured by their parents.

Handgun injuries in the pediatric patient have increased since 1986. The number of pediatric gunshot wounds reported by urban trauma centers has increased by 300%.[5] The death rate from pediatric firearm injuries is 12%—three times the death rate for severe trauma in general.[5]

Clinical presentation of survivors. For the survivors of the murdered child, the grief is often overwhelming. This grief takes on a special quality when the parents know or may have known the murderer—many murders are committed by family members, friends, or acquaintances. Regardless of the identity of the murderer, the drive for revenge is often a central issue for the parents.[19]

Parents have special problems as a result of the murder of their child, including the following:[20]

1. Fear that it will happen again. Parents may become overly protective of other children and family members.
2. Fear that a family member will seek revenge for the death.
3. Anger directed at the event, the murderer, and the criminal justice system.
4. Guilt at not having protected the child.
5. Marital difficulty due to lack of communication and support. Many marriages may end in divorce.

Emergency Department and nursing care. After the death of a child nursing interventions generally consist of communicating with the family. However, if the child was a victim of homicide, evidence collection is crucial. In these situations, the nurse must not only communicate with the family but also be familiar with procedures for preserving/collecting evidence for the medical examiner. These procedures should be included in ED policy manuals.

Parents whose child has been a victim of homicide require the same support as other parents whose children die in the ED (Box 9-9). If the situation is suspicious for child maltreatment, talking with

TABLE 9-3	Interventions for the Family of the Child Dying of SIDS
INTERVENTIONS	**COMMENTS**
Explain the diagnosis of SIDS to the parents and that the diagnosis is only probable.	The final diagnosis will not be confirmed until an autopsy is done.
Give the family the option to say goodbye before stopping the resuscitation, if possible.	Parents may be comforted to know that everything was done that could have been and may appreciate the time to say goodbye.
Provide mementos.	Because children who die of SIDS are so young, often parents do not have any pictures or memories. They will treasure hand and/or footprints and a lock of hair mounted on heavy paper.
Allow parents to hold the child.	Prepare family for what they will see (some bloody drainage from the nose and mouth and any marks from the resuscitative efforts). Wrap the child in a warm blanket or quilt, and allow the family to take the quilt home with them.
Provide assistance for the nursing mother.	Refer to La Leche League, other lactation specialists, or pediatrician for assistance in stopping lactation.
Provide SIDS literature.	Although the family may not read literature immediately, it may offer some comfort later.
Answer any questions about the death.	Often parents have misconceptions that the child froze to death, cried too long, was hurt by a sibling, or died from some medication they were taking.
Allay feelings of guilt as much as possible. Tell parents there was nothing they could have done to prevent SIDS.	Feelings of guilt are universal in most deaths but are especially prominent in SIDS parents because the child was previously healthy and a cause cannot be pinpointed.
Refer the family to a local SIDS support group or give them information on how to contact one.	Most states have support groups, but if information is not available, the family can be referred to the National SIDS Alliance or the National SIDS Clearing House.*
Answer questions concerning the autopsy.	An autopsy is required to confirm the diagnosis.
Give the family the phone number of the medical examiner.	The medical examiner may call the family with the results, but the family may have questions that occur before they are called.

Modified from Jezierski, 1989; Thomas, 1991; Thomas, 1992.
*National SIDS Alliance, 10500 Little Patuxent Parkway, Suite 420, Columbia, MD 21044, (800)221-SIDS; National SIDS Clearing House, 8201 Greensboro Drive, Suite 600, McLean, VA 22101, (703)821-8955.

the family can be difficult because staff members may experience feelings of anger, sadness, and guilt. In addition, the potential for violence should be anticipated and precautions (such as having a security guard present) taken to protect the staff.

The following guidelines are recommended when communicating with families suspected of child abuse:[7]

1. Remain nonjudgmental when obtaining information. The parents may not be responsible for the abuse.

> **Box 9-9** Nursing Interventions for Survivors of the Child Who is Murdered
>
> • Implement policies and procedures to protect the family from the media, who will try to gain access to the child's family.
> • Refer the family for immediate counseling, because they will require help in dealing with their grief, anger, and desire for revenge against the murderer.
> • Provide the family with phone numbers for support groups such as Compassionate Friends. Some areas have support groups called Parents of Murdered Children.
> • Provide information about the autopsy and how the family may obtain results.
>
> Compiled from ENA, 1993; Klass, 1988; Knapp, 1983.

2. Give the family the respect and compassion extended to the parents of the child with accidental trauma or illness. Reactions from parents may be the same, more subdued, or more exaggerated. Fear of being accused may be prominent.
3. Inform parents of the need to report circumstances to legal authorities and what they should expect from authorities.

If the death or injury is thought to be related to gang violence, the following precautions should be taken to protect the patient, family, and ED staff.[33]

1. Notify security to provide surveillance for other gang members.
2. Disrobe the child entirely to check for weapons.
3. Observe for signs of imminent violence by family members or visitors.
4. Limit access to the patient and family.
5. Develop reporting policies for the media to avoid publicizing information that could endanger the family or the victim.

The grief of parents whose child has been murdered is often prolonged by the criminal justice system. Because the justice system is designed to protect the rights of the accused, it has become a maze of legal rules and procedures. Parents need help in understanding the system, and then they need help in demanding their place within the justice system.[19] The ED nurse may remind parents to discuss these issues

with the investigating officer while in the emergency department or obtain the name of a contact person who can keep them informed and answer questions as they arise.

SUMMARY

A visit to the emergency department can be a stressful event for both the child and family. This stress can escalate into a crisis when serious illness, injury, or death occurs. How ED staff interact and intervene with the family can influence the family's reaction to the crisis. These interactions include communicating with the family in a sensitive, honest manner while assessing the family's current coping mechanisms and past experiences with crisis situations. When a child dies, ED staff should be prepared to expect varying expressions of grief from the family and intervene in a therapeutic manner. Helping the family deal with grief may prevent the later development of pathologic grief.

The death of a child in the ED is a tragic event that often leaves staff feeling angry, hopeless, or depressed. Nursing education rarely includes instruction on how to deal with the family in a crisis situation or what to say to a family whose child has died. Critical incident stress debriefing is a healthy way to work through feelings concerning a death. Even if a formal debriefing is not possible, ED staff can take a few moments between patients to discuss their feelings and support each other. It is helpful for ED staff to remember to take care of themselves by getting plenty of rest, exercise, and proper nutrition. Also, keeping the following points in mind will help put crisis events into perspective:

1. Most children get better and go home.
2. Being responsible for a child's life is *not* the same as being responsible for a child's death.

REFERENCES

1. American Academy of Pediatrics: *To lessen SIDS risk, AAP recommends infants sleep on side or back,* Elk Grove Village, Ill, 1992, AAP (news release).
2. Bjorn P: An approach to the potentially violent patient, *JEN* 17:336, 1991.
3. Carroll J, Loughlin G: Sudden infant death syndrome, *Pediatr Rev* 14:83, 1993.
4. Christoffel KK: Child abuse fatalities. In Ludwig S, Kornberg A, eds: *Child Abuse. A medical reference,* ed 2, New York, 1992, Churchill Livingstone.
5. Committee on Injury and Poison Prevention: Firearm injuries affecting the pediatric population, *Pediatr* 89:788, 1992.

6. Cork CA, Fuller H, Barnickol CA, eds: *Sudden infant death syndrome. Who can help and how,* New York, 1991, Springer Publishing.

7. Dieckman R: Death of a child in the emergency department. In Grossman M, Dieckman R, eds: *Pediatric emergency medicine: a clinician's reference,* Philadelphia, 1991, JB Lippincott.

8. Emergency Nurses Association: Psychosocial aspects of trauma care. In *Trauma nursing core course provider manual,* ed 4, Chicago, 1995, Award Printing Company.

9. Emergency Nurses Association: *Emergency nursing pediatric course provider manual,* Chicago, 1993, Award Printing Company.

10. Feinstein D, Raatowski C, Reagan L: Hartford hospital trauma support program, *Critical Care Nursing Clinics of North America* 7(3):535–540, 1995.

11. Frader J, Sargent J: Sudden death or catastrophic illness: family considerations. In Fleisher GR, Ludwig S, eds: *Textbook of pediatric emergency medicine,* Baltimore, 1993, Williams & Wilkins.

12. Gyulay J: Grief responses, *Issues Compr Pediatr Nurs* 12:1, 1989.

13. Hamilton G: Sudden death in the ED: telling the living, *Ann Emerg Med* 17:382, 1988.

14. Hanson C, Strawser D: Family presence during cardiopulmonary resuscitation: Foote hospital emergency department's nine-year perspective, *JEN* 18:104, 1992.

15. Henderson DP: Death of a child. In Barkin R, ed: *Pediatric emergency medicine: concepts and clinical practice,* ed. 2, St Louis, 1997, Mosby.

15a. Hoff LA: *People in crisis. Understanding and helping,* ed 3, Redwood City, Calif, 1989, Addison-Wesley.

16. Jezierski M: Infant death: guidelines for support of parents in the emergency department, *JEN* 15:475, 1989.

17. Johnson L, Mattson S: Communication: the key to crisis prevention in pediatric death, *Crit Care Nurs* 12(8):23–27, 1992.

18. Kinkle S: Violence in the ED: how to stop it before it starts, *Am J Nurs* 93:22, 1993.

19. Klass D: *Parental grief. Solace and resolution,* New York, 1988, Springer Publishing.

20. Knapp RJ: *Beyond endurance: when a child dies,* New York, 1983, Schocken.

21. Levitt C, Smith W, Alexander R: Abusive head trauma. In Reece RM: *Child abuse: medical diagnosis and management,* Philadelphia, 1994, Lea and Febiger.

22. Mahoney BSL: The extent, nature and response to victimization of emergency nurses in Pennsylvania, *JEN* 17:282, 1991.

23. McQuay J et al: "Death telling" Research project, *Critical Care Nursing Clinics of North America* 7(3):549–555, 1995.

24. Mellick L, ed: Jersey ED surveys parents who witness resuscitations, find positive results, *ED Management* 8:11, 1996.

25. Mitchell JT: Development and functions of a critical incident stress debriefing team, *JEMS* 43, Dec 1988.

26. Mitchell JT: The history and future of critical incident stress debriefings, *JEMS* 47, Nov 1988.

27. Mitchell JT: When disaster strikes. The critical incident stress debriefing process, *JEMS* 36, Jan 1983.

28. Mitchell J, Bray G: *Emergency services stress,* Englewood Cliffs, NJ, 1990, Prentice-Hall.

29. Papadatou D, Papadatos C, eds: *Children and death,* New York, 1991, Hemisphere Publishing.

30. Pederson ME: Tissue and organ donation. In Sheehy SB, ed: *Emergency nursing. Principles and practice,* ed 3, St Louis, 1992, Mosby.

31. Post H: Letting the family in during a code, *Nurs 89,* 43, March 1989.

32. Rando T: *Grief, dying, and death,* Champaign, Ill, 1984, Research Press Company.

33. Rollins J: Nurses as gangbusters: a response to gang violence in America, *Pediatr Nurs* 19:559, 1993.

34. Rubin JG: Critical incident stress debriefing: helping the helpers, *JEN* 16:255, 1990.

35. Solursh DS: The family of the trauma victim, *Nurs Clin North Am* 25:155, 1990.

36. Swisher L et al: Death notification in the emergency department: a survey of residents and attending physicians, *Ann Emerg Med* 22:102, 1993.

37. Thomas DO: Every parent's worst nightmare, *RN* 34, Sept 1992.

38. Thomas DO: *Quick reference to pediatric emergency nursing,* Gaithersburg, 1991, Aspen Publishers.

39. Valdes-Dapena MA: The phenomenon of sudden infant death syndrome and its challenges. In Cork CA et al., eds: *Sudden infant death syndrome. Who can help and how,* New York, 1991, Springer Publishing.

40. Valk Lawson L: Culturally sensitive support for grieving parents, *MCN* 15:76, 1990.

41. Walters D, Tupin J: Family grief in the emergency department, *Emerg Med Clin North Am* 9:189, 1991.

42. Willinger M: SIDS prevention, *Pediatric Annals* 24(7):358–364, 1995.

43. Worden WJ: *Grief counseling and grief therapy: a handbook for the mental health practitioner,* New York, 1982, Springer Publishing.

44. Zylke J: Sudden infant death syndrome: resurgent research offers hope, *JAMA* 262:1565, 1989.

CHAPTER 10

Respiratory System

Janice S. Rogers

INTRODUCTION

Respiratory disorders account for approximately one half of all illnesses in children less than 5 years of age and one third of illnesses in children between 5 and 12 years.[90] Anatomic differences in the pediatric respiratory tract and immaturity of the pulmonary and immune systems are primarily responsible for the child's increased susceptibility to respiratory infection and airway obstruction.

Respiratory etiologies vary with age. Pneumonia, bronchiolitis, asthma, croup, foreign body aspiration, congenital heart disease, sepsis, and congenital airway anomalies are the most common causes of respiratory distress in children less than 2 years of age. Older children are more likely to present with asthma, pneumonia, ingestions, near-drownings, trauma, or cystic fibrosis.

ANATOMY AND PHYSIOLOGY

Pulmonary function depends on the adequacy of the respiratory muscles and chest wall, the mechanical properties of airways and alveoli, the systemic and pulmonary perfusion, and central nervous system control. The respiratory system grows and matures until approximately 8 years of age, when pulmonary anatomy and physiology approximates that of an adult (Fig. 10-1).

AIRWAYS

Full-term infants have a full complement of conducting airways. However, these airways are much smaller than those of adults. Because airway resistance is inversely related to the radius of the airway, small airways normally have a high resistance to air flow. Any

reduction of airway radius will therefore significantly increase the resistance to air flow.

Other important characteristics of the pediatric airway include a proportionally large tongue, increased soft tissue surrounding the airway, and soft laryngeal cartilage (Table 10-1). Young infants are obligate nose breathers and can exhibit signs of respiratory distress with copious nasal secretions. Incompletely developed small airway muscles and supporting airway cartilage in infants and young children may contribute to the development of lower airway obstruction from bronchospasm during illnesses such as bronchiolitis.

ALVEOLI

The exchange of oxygen and carbon dioxide occurs within the alveoli. Newborns have fewer and smaller alveoli than older children and adults (24 to 50 million at birth compared to 300 to 400 million in the average adult).[67] The availability of alveolar surface for gas exchange is therefore less than in the adult. Although most alveolar development is complete by 2 years of age,[82] the size of the alveoli continues to grow.[54] Despite proportionally less gas exchange surface, infants can normally provide for their daily oxygen needs. However, because of their limited reserve, any condition that produces an increase in the metabolic rate (e.g., respiratory distress or fever) may cause oxygen demand to exceed supply.

CHEST WALL

The pediatric chest wall is comprised of soft, cartilaginous ribs and incompletely developed intercostal muscles. The diaphragm is the primary muscle of

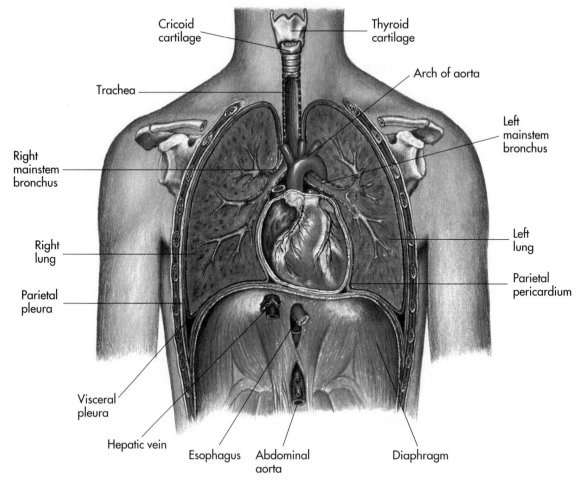

FIG. 10-1. Chest cavity and related anatomic structures. (Modified from Seidel et al: *Mosby's guide to physical examination,* ed 3, St Louis, 1995, Mosby.)

respiration in the child and adult; however, increased compliance and the horizontal (rather than oblique) orientation of the child's ribs and diaphragm limit elevation of the chest wall during inspiration. Pressure on the diaphragm from above or below (e.g., pneumothorax or abdominal distention) can impede respiratory excursion and increase the work of breathing.

CENTRAL NERVOUS SYSTEM CONTROL OF BREATHING (SEE CHAPTER 6)

LUNG TISSUE

Lung tissue compliance is determined by surfactant and elasticity, which keep the alveoli open at the end of expiration. Young children have less supportive pulmonary elastic and collagen tissue than adults, resulting in a relatively low lung compliance and a high chest wall compliance. The result is decreased ability to maintain alveolar patency during periods of respiratory distress and an increased incidence of atelectasis, air leaks, and pulmonary edema in young children.

PULMONARY FUNCTION

Pulmonary function depends on adequate ventilation and perfusion of the lungs. Ventilation is the product of the respiratory rate and the tidal volume (TV). Infants normally have less TV and lower residual capacities, which provide minimal reserves of oxygen.

TABLE 10-1	Anatomic Differences in the Pediatric Airway and Their Clinical Implications
ANATOMIC CHARACTERISTIC	**CLINICAL IMPLICATION**
Small airway diameter	Greater resistance to air flow Easily obstructed by small amounts of mucus, edema, or foreign bodies
Young infants are obligate nose breathers	Nasal secretions or malformations can easily obstruct air flow and contribute to respiratory distress
Tongue proportionally larger	Increased susceptibility to mechanical airway obstruction, especially if level of consciousness is altered
Soft laryngeal cartilage	Hyperextension or hyperflexion of the neck can compress and obstruct the airway; use the "sniff" position or "jaw thrust" to open the airway
Shorter trachea (4-5 cm in newborn; 7 cm in 18 month old)	Maintaining endotracheal tube (ETT) placement more difficult; slight movement can dislodge tube Easy to intubate right mainstem bronchus
Larynx more anterior and cephalad	Esophageal intubations common Easy to aspirate
Cricoid is narrowest part of larynx until age 8 years	Cricoid provides a natural seal for *uncuffed* ETTs

Data from Haley and Baker, 1993; Hazinski, 1992; Semonin-Holleran, 1993; Soud, 1992.

Therefore infants cannot tolerate even brief interruptions in oxygen supplies.

PROTECTIVE MECHANISMS

Lung tissue is protected from invasion by foreign substances, including pathogens, by a variety of mechanisms. The mucociliary escalator mechanism is the primary protector of the pulmonary system in the healthy child and clears all parts of the lung down to the alveolar ducts. Beyond the terminal bronchiole, the phagocytic system ingests and kills bacteria and the lymphatic system transports particles from the lungs. The epiglottal reflex and cough reflex prevent aspiration and expel aspirated material, respectively.

NURSING HISTORY AND ASSESSMENT

HISTORY

When the child presents to the emergency department (ED) in respiratory distress or with a respiratory illness, historical information assists with the triage

decision and guides initial interventions. Depending on the child's age and clinical presentation, information regarding the birth history (e.g., full term or premature), past medical history, onset and length of the current illness, and associated signs and symptoms (e.g., cough, fever) may be obtained. Information regarding prematurity may lead the nurse to suspect such illnesses as bronchopulmonary dysplasia (BPD). The past medical history may reveal frequent hospitalizations for respiratory-related illnesses such as asthma or a chronic disorder such as cystic fibrosis. The onset and length of the current illness, as well as the signs and symptoms associated with the illness, provide clues to the seriousness of the illness. For example, the child with epiglottitis, may present with an acute onset of fever, upper airway obstruction, and dysphagia, whereas the young child with a lower respiratory infection may present with mild respiratory distress and nonspecific symptoms such as vomiting, fever, or abdominal pain.

PHYSICAL EXAMINATION

Initial emergency nursing assessment. The initial respiratory examination requires a general assess-

Box 10-1   Signs and Symptoms of Respiratory Distress and Failure

Respiratory distress
Labored respirations
Dyspnea
Retractions—mild to moderate
Use of accessory muscles
Tachypnea, tachycardia
Nasal flaring
Mouth breathing
Positioning for air entry (tripod or sniffing position)

Impending respiratory failure
Restlessness, irritability
Diminished level of consciousness (e.g., lethargy)
Central cyanosis
Inadequate or maximal respiratory effort
Decreasing respiratory rate without clinical improvement
Poor air entry, weak cry
Grunting respirations, head bobbing
Stridor or severe retractions at rest
Poor muscle tone
Tachycardia progressing to bradycardia

ment of the child's appearance, position of comfort, mental status, respiratory rate, and respiratory effort. If during this assessment the infant or child exhibits signs or symptoms of significant respiratory distress or impending respiratory failure, emergent management is required.

Signs of significant respiratory distress include labored respirations, retractions, nasal flaring, grunting respirations, and significant tachypnea and tachycardia. Impending respiratory failure is exhibited by signs of severe respiratory distress and end-organ dysfunction including diminishing respiratory effort, diminished breath sounds, decreasing level of consciousness or pain response, decreased muscle tone, pallor, or cyanosis. Bradycardia due to hypoxemia is an ominous sign of impending cardiorespiratory arrest (Box 10-1).

Observation

Color.   Color reflects perfusion and oxygenation. Cyanosis, a bluish discoloration of the skin and mu-

cous membranes, is produced by desaturated capillary blood and is best observed in areas with thin epidermis, minimal pigment, and abundant capillaries[2] such as the tongue and mucous membranes (central cyanosis). Peripheral cyanosis (of the distal extremities) is a less reliable indicator of hypoxemia, because it may result from a cold environment or decreased perfusion rather than from hemoglobin desaturation.

The absolute amount of reduced hemoglobin in the blood determines the degree of cyanosis. Color change from hypoxia is not evident until 5 g/dl of desaturated hemoglobin is present.[37] Because pediatric hemoglobin levels are lower than adult, a greater percentage of children's total hemoglobin must be desaturated before cyanosis occurs. Anemic children may not develop cyanosis despite profound hypoxemia. Thus cyanosis is an unreliable and late sign of hypoxia in children.

Chest and abdomen.   The chest and abdomen of the child are observed for shape and symmetry and for signs of an increase in the work of breathing. Retractions are one of the hallmark findings in the child with respiratory distress. Retractions occur during inspiration as negative intrathoracic pressure increases to facilitate air movement into the lungs. The result is collapse or retraction of the child's soft chest wall. Common areas where retractions are observed include the intercostal, subcostal, substernal, suprasternal, and supraclavicular spaces. Retractions compromise the child's ability to generate adequate tidal volume or maintain functional residual capacity, further increasing the work of breathing (Fig. 10-2).

Grunting is another finding specific to children and is evidenced by an audible expiratory sound or grunt, coupled with abrupt inward movement of the upper abdomen. Expiratory grunting is a sign of moderate to severe respiratory distress. Physiologically, grunting is thought to force expired air against a partially closed glottis, thereby increasing intrapulmonary pressure, which keeps the alveoli open at the end of expiration.

Auscultation.   The quality, symmetry, timing, and clarity of breath sounds are evaluated by auscultation. When listening to breath sounds, both inspiratory and expiratory sounds are first evaluated to determine the degree of air exchange. Breath sounds in infants and young children are usually harsh and loud, because sounds are easily transmitted throughout the small chest cavity and thin chest wall. Interpretation of findings, particularly adventitious (abnormal) breath sounds, can be difficult for this reason. For

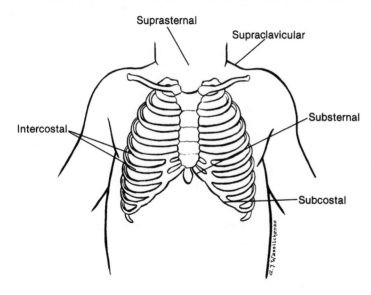

Suprasternal

Supraclavicular

Intercostal

Substernal

Subcostal

FIG. 10-2. Location of retractions. (From Wong DL: *Whaley & Wong's nursing care of infants and children,* ed 5, St Louis, 1995, Mosby.)

TABLE 10-2	Adventitious Breath Sounds		
ADVENTITIOUS SOUND	**INSPIRATORY**	**EXPIRATORY**	**DESCRIPTION**
Sibilant wheezes	+	+++	Musical, high-pitched continuous sounds resulting from turbulent air flow through narrowed small airways
Sonorous wheezes (rhonchi)	+	+++	Musical, low-pitched continuous sounds with snoring quality resulting from turbulent air flow through narrowed large airways (upper airway obstruction or obstruction in the tracheobronchial passages)
Crackles (rales)	+++	+	Fine or coarse nonmusical, discontinuous "popping" sounds created by air movement through secretions in small airways or by the opening of previously closed airways
Stridor	+++ Suggests supraglottic obstruction	+ Suggests obstruction below the larynx	Harsh sound produced by turbulence of air flow around a partial airway obstruction in the large airways

Compiled from Bates, 1991; Letourneau, Schuh, and Gausche, 1992.
+ = Heard least commonly.
+++ = Heard most commonly.

example, upper airway sounds caused by congestion are often transmitted throughout the chest and do not represent significant respiratory pathology. In contrast, the absence of breath sounds (in a particular area of consolidation or obstruction) may be difficult to appreciate because the absence of air exchange may not be recognized. When auscultating breath sounds, concentrating on the pitch rather than the intensity (or loudness) of breath sounds will assist in the evaluation.

Adventitious sounds usually indicate respiratory disease or obstruction and are described as inspiratory, expiratory, or both. The quality and location of the sounds assists both the diagnosis and the evaluation of the severity of the obstruction. Upper airway obstructions caused by a foreign body or edematous narrowing of the large airways (e.g., croup) are usually exhibited by an inspiratory stridor, although a low-pitched expiratory wheeze is sometimes heard. Lower airway obstructions (e.g., asthma, bronchiolitis) are more commonly exhibited by expiratory sounds such as high-pitched wheezing. Fine or coarse discontinuous sounds referred to as *crackles* or *rales* are also heard with lower respiratory pathology (e.g., pneumonia). They are most often auscultated during inspiration as collapsed alveoli open (Table 10-2).

Vital signs. The respiratory rate, heart rate, blood pressure, and temperature are taken in the child with signs of respiratory distress. The respiratory rate is auscultated for 1 full minute. Tachypnea is a sensitive sign of respiratory distress when coupled with physical findings and a positive history. However, factors other than respiratory pathology, such as fever, pain, anxiety, or central nervous system disorders, can adversely affect the respiratory rate (Table 10-3).

TABLE 10-3	Normal Respiratory Rates in Children*	
AGE	**RATE (BREATHS PER MIN)**	
Infants	30-60	
Toddlers	24-40	
Preschoolers	22-34	
School-age children	18-30	
Adolescents	12-16	

From Hazinski MF: Children are different. In Hazinski MF: *Nursing care of the critically ill child*, St Louis, 1992, Mosby.
* The child's respiratory rate is expected to increase in the presence of fever or stress.

Pulse oximetry is often used during the initial evaluation of a child's respiratory status. As a valuable noninvasive monitor, it transcutaneously measures the oxygen saturation of hemoglobin. Limitations to its usefulness include patient movement, abnormal hemoglobin levels, and low perfusion states (Box 10-2). Pulse oximetry does not provide information on ventilatory status or acid-base balance. The best locations for pulse oximetry measurement include the fingertips, toes, and earlobes. Readings are reliable only when the heart rate measured by the oximeter correlates with the child's pulse rate.

NURSING CARE OF THE CHILD IN RESPIRATORY DISTRESS (SEE BOX 10-3)

UPPER RESPIRATORY INFECTION (URI): THE COMMON COLD

Etiology. The common cold or upper respiratory infection (URI) is an acute viral infection of the upper respiratory tract. URIs are most commonly caused by a rhinovirus but may also be caused by parainfluenza, coronavirus, or adenovirus. Infants and young children are prone to frequent colds because of the numerous types of rhinoviruses, the child's increased susceptibility to infection, limited previous exposure to infectious organisms, and close contact with other children in schools and day care settings.

Box 10-2	Clinical Situations that may Limit Effectiveness of Pulse Oximetry

Patient motion
Abnormal hemoglobin
  • Carboxyhemoglobin
  • Methemoglobin
Low perfusion states
  • Hypovolemia
  • Hypothermia
  • Excess pressure at or proximal to sampling site
Excess ambient light
Nail polish

Modified from Durren M: Getting the most from pulse oximetry, *JEN* 18(4):340–342, 1992.

Pathophysiology. Viral invasion of the mucous membranes of the upper respiratory tract triggers an inflammatory response. This results in vasodilation of the nasal passages, edema, and mucus formation. Complications of the common cold include otitis media and lower respiratory tract infections such as pneumonia. Older children may develop sinusitis.

Clinical presentation. Cold symptoms include nasal congestion, rhinorrhea, coughing, and sneezing. Nasal discharge commonly changes consistency over the course of the illness from watery to thick. Fever, if present, is usually low grade. Respiratory distress is rarely associated with a simple URI. Additional symptoms in younger children may include irritability, restlessness, sleep disturbance, diarrhea, or vomiting (especially after feedings). Emesis usually contains large amounts of mucus. Older children may complain of dryness or irritation of the nose and throat, muscular aches, headache, and cough.

Emergency Department interventions. The diagnosis of a URI is based on clinical findings, after more serious illnesses have been ruled out. Diagnostic testing such as a chest x-ray, CBC, and differential may be ordered depending on the age of the child and associated symptoms.

Treatment is symptomatic and includes rest, humidification of air, ample fluids, and antipyretics as needed. The efficacy of over-the-counter decongestants, antihistamines, antitussives, and expectorants is debatable, especially in young children. Use of topical nasal decongestants is limited to a few days only, because prolonged use can result in rebound congestion.[84] Cough suppression is not recommended if increased mucus production is present, unless the cough is interfering with sleep. Antitussives may be helpful for children with dry, nonproductive coughs that disturb sleep. Codeine is the most effective cough suppressant, but it is associated with reduced mucokinesis, dizziness, sedation, nausea, vomiting, and constipation. Dextromethorphan, a nonnarcotic derivative of codeine, is often effective as an antitussive.

Nursing care and evaluation. Nursing care is primarily supportive and focuses mainly on discharge teaching. Because young infants are obligate nose breathers, copious nasal secretions can produce mild to moderate respiratory distress. These infants should be suctioned frequently with a bulb syringe to facilitate breathing, feeding, and sleep. Saline nose drops may be used to loosen thick secretions.

Attention to the child's hydration status is required, and clear liquids should be administered frequently. A cool mist vaporizer or shallow pan of water near the heat register will increase environmental humidity and soothe inflamed mucous membranes.

Box 10-3 Nursing Care of the Infant or Child in Respiratory Distress

Airway

Assess airway patency

Maintain infant's head in the neutral position

Suction nose and oral pharynx with a bulb syringe or gentle mechanical suction

Insert an oral or nasal airway as needed to maintain airway patency

Breathing

Assess respiratory rate and effort, breath sounds, color

Check pulse oximetry

Allow child to maintain position of comfort; elevate infant's head with blankets or pillows

Administer humidified oxygen to maintain oxygen saturation greater than 95%

Circulation

Assess heart rate and rhythm, perfusion, color, blood pressure

Place on cardiac monitor for moderate to severe distress

Disability

Assess neurologic status, including age-appropriate response to environment and parents, and response to pain

Maintain normothermia to minimize oxygen and fluid requirements

Prepare airway management equipment/supplies—have readily accessible

Reduce parent and child's anxiety: explain procedures, keep caregiver with child

---

ACUTE UPPER AIRWAY INFECTIONS

Although there are many causes of upper airway infections in children, none is more concerning to the health care professional than those which cause an acute obstruction to air flow. This section of the chapter specifically focuses on croup syndromes, which are upper airway infections that can produce obstruction.

VIRAL CROUP (LARYNGOTRACHEOBRONCHITIS)

Etiology. Viral croup (laryngotracheobronchitis) is the most common cause of upper airway obstruction in children.[22,23] It is characterized by subglottic and tracheal swelling. Parainfluenza viruses account for the majority of cases; however, respiratory syncytial virus (RSV), influenza, and adenovirus can also cause croup.

Children between 3 months and 5 years of age are susceptible to viral croup, with a peak incidence between 1 and 2 years of age. Viral infections such as laryngotracheobronchitis predominantly occur in the fall and winter. Transmission results from direct contact with respiratory secretions through droplets or fomites. The incubation period is 2 to 6 days.

Pathophysiology. The viral infection produces inflammation and swelling of the mucosa that lines the subglottic region of the larynx. Turbulent air flow through the obstructed airway creates the stridor typical of moderate to severe croup. Vocal cord swelling and pharyngeal irritation produce a characteristic barking cough and hoarseness. A significant obstruction can produce negative intrapleural pressure sufficient to alter the hydrostatic and oncotic balance in the pulmonary vasculature. When this occurs pulmonary edema may result.[23]

The small airways may also become inflamed with croup. This inflammation can result in increased secretions, atelectasis, and mucus plugging. The resultant ventilation-perfusion inequality can lead to hypoxia and carbon dioxide (CO_2) retention.

Clinical presentation. Croup symptoms are usually preceded by several days of progressive upper respiratory symptoms. On the second or third day of illness, a hoarse cry and barking or "seal-like" cough develops with varying degrees of respiratory distress. Fever, if present, is usually low grade. Inspiratory stridor, which may be present only with crying, is not affected by posture. Stridor at rest, expiratory stridor, severe retractions, hypoxemia with lethargy or agitation, tachycardia, and tachypnea develop with severe obstruction. Croup symptoms are typically worse at night (Table 10-4).

Emergency Department interventions. Croup is diagnosed based on clinical findings. Diagnostic testing such as a CBC, cultures, chest x-ray, AP and lateral neck x-ray may be ordered depending on the child's presentation. The chest x-ray is usually negative, and the classic subglottic "steeple" sign seen on the AP film is visible in only 40% to 50% of children. [22] The lateral neck x-ray is more valuable and may show variable subglottic narrowing and distention of the hypopharynx.

The treatment of croup depends on the severity of the child's presentation. In all cases attempts are made to keep the child calm and prevent crying, which will worsen the obstruction. Allowing the parent to remain with and hold the child and offering diversionary activities such as toys are helpful interventions. Since anxiety is contagious, measures to reduce parental stress are also helpful.

Mild croup (no stridor at rest) usually responds to cool, humidified air, which soothes inflamed membranes, moistens secretions, and offers symptomatic relief. Moderate to severe croup requires the administration of cool humidified air with supplemental oxygen, if the child's oxygen saturation is less than 95%. Children with moderate to severe croup or children who fail to respond to humidified air receive nebulized racemic epinephrine, which produces mucosal vasoconstriction, reducing subglottic swelling. The recommended dose of a 2.25% solution of racemic epinephrine is 0.05 ml/kg/dose (0.5 ml maximum) diluted to 3 ml with normal saline. The effects of racemic epinephrine occur within 10 to 30 minutes of administration and last for approximately 2 hours.[76] Because the symptoms can return to the original severity when the drug wears off, continuous monitoring either in the ED or an inpatient unit is required for at least 3 to 4 hours after drug administration. The child with severe respiratory distress despite pharmacologic interventions requires endotracheal intubation. The recommended endotracheal tube is one size less than expected for age/weight/length because of airway edema. Less than 1% of children hospitalized for viral croup require intubation.[23]

Parenterally administered steroids can decrease the severity of croup symptoms within 12 to 24 hours after treatment.[41] Steroids decrease inflammation and edema by reducing capillary permeability and stabilizing lysosomal membranes.[21] Because these effects are not evident for at least 3 hours, steroids are not substituted for racemic epinephrine.

Helium-oxygen mixtures have been successfully used as an alternative approach to croup management.

TABLE 10-4	Comparison of the Clinical Presentation of Croup, Epiglottitis, and Bacterial Tracheitis		
CLINICAL MANIFESTATIONS	CROUP (LARYNGOTRACHEOBRONCHITIS)	EPIGLOTTITIS	BACTERIAL TRACHEITIS
Cough	Loud barking cough	Absent	May have paroxysms of productive coughing
Stridor	Harsh, inspiratory	Soft, inspiratory	Progressively worse stridor unaffected by position
Sore throat	+/−	Intensely sore Pain on swallowing Drooling	+/− Swallowing not affected No drooling
Fever	Low grade (<38.5° C)	High (>38.5° C)	High
Toxicity	Nontoxic appearance	Toxic appearance	Toxic appearance
Voice	Hoarse voice, cry	Muffled voice	Hoarse voice; noisy breathing
Respiratory distress	Variable	Variable	Severe
Other	Symptoms worse at night	Tripod position Restless, anxious, agitated	Thick purulent tracheal secretions Tend to lie flat Older children may have burning substernal pain

Because helium is less dense than air, it is thought to flow better through the narrow airway. Helium-oxygen therapy may cause ventilation-perfusion inequalities that results in hypoxia.[12] This therapy should only be used by experienced practitioners.

Most children with croup are discharged from the emergency department. Discharge instructions include conveying signs of respiratory distress to the parents, as well as providing follow-up care information. Supportive measures include humidification, hydration, and antipyretics. Parents can be informed that future episodes of croup may initially be treated by placing the child in a bathroom where steam has been created after running a hot shower or taking the child outside in the cool night air. If these actions do not alleviate respiratory distress, the parent should seek medical care.

EPIGLOTTITIS

Etiology. Epiglottitis (supraglottitis) is a fulminating, life-threatening bacterial infection of the epiglottis and other supraglottic structures. It is most commonly seen in children between 2 and 5 years of age with a peak incidence of 3 to 4 years of age. Because most pediatric cases are caused by *Haemophilus influenzae* type B, the incidence of epiglottitis has significantly declined since the *H. influenzae* type B conjugate vaccine (Hib) became available.[31] Rare causes of epiglottitis include Group A beta-hemolytic streptococcus (GAβHS) (tends to affect older children), pneumococcus, and staphylococcus.

Pathophysiology. Direct invasion by the bacterial organism causes inflammation of the supraglottic structures, including the epiglottis, aryepiglottic folds, and arytenoids. The vocal cords and subglottic structures are usually not affected. Inflamed, swollen supraglottic structures can significantly reduce air flow and rapidly lead to a complete airway obstruction. Pneumonitis, pulmonary edema, and circulatory collapse are rare.

Clinical presentation. Children with epiglottitis typically have a history of abrupt onset of high fever and an intensely sore throat. Characteristic signs and symptoms of epiglottitis include difficulty swallowing, drooling, slight tachypnea, a toxic appearance, and soft inspiratory stridor. Epiglottitis differs from croup in that there is an absence of spontaneous cough, in the presence of drooling and agitation. Atypical presentations can occur, especially in infants and older children. Some children with epiglottitis have a barky cough and prodromal upper respiratory symptoms, while drooling and dysphagia are absent.[11,23]

Respiratory distress is exhibited by suprasternal, supraclavicular, and substernal retractions and inspiratory stridor. Older children typically assume a tripod position (child sits upright, leaning forward and supporting upper body with hands, the chin thrust out) to maintain an airway. Decreased muscle tone, an altered level of consciousness, and cyanosis are signs of impending respiratory arrest.

Emergency Department interventions. The diagnosis of epiglottitis is based on classic physical findings. Diagnostic testing is delayed until the airway has been secured, because agitation from venipunctures or other disturbing procedures can precipitate a complete airway obstruction. Direct laryngoscopy with visualization of a distinctive large, cherry-red, edematous epiglottis is diagnostic; however, the anxiety caused by the throat examination can also precipitate a complete airway obstruction.

A lateral neck x-ray is recommended, but only if the diagnosis is uncertain. Because of the danger of complete obstruction, portable radiography is preferred. The classic x-ray finding is a "thumbprint like" swollen epiglottis, but this sign is present in only 50% of children with endoscopically proven epiglottitis.[22]

Children with suspected epiglottitis require emergent management. Airway equipment, including endotracheal intubation supplies, must be at the child's bedside should a complete obstruction occur. Blow-by oxygen may be administered if it does not produce unnecessary agitation. Parents are allowed to remain with the child and should be kept informed of all treatment plans. The fearful parent can convey anxiety to an already frightened child. These children require continuous monitoring. If a complete airway obstruction occurs, the child can often be successfully ventilated with a bag-valve-mask (BVM) device. Only when BVM ventilation is unsuccessful will a cricothyroidotomy be performed.

Personnel skilled in airway management must accompany the child during all transfers, and intubation equipment must be immediately available. The child who is sent to another institution should be intubated before transfer to avoid the development of an airway obstruction en route.

Definitive treatment requires endotracheal intubation. This is best performed in a controlled setting (such as the operating room) by the provider who is most skilled at pediatric intubation. After intubation, the child is kept sedated and paralyzed to protect the airway.

Intravenous antibiotics are administered as soon as the airway has been secured. A second or third generation cephalosporin, such as ceftriaxone, cefotaxime, or cefuroxime, is most commonly given for 5 to 7 days. The majority of children completely recover from epiglottitis if the airway has been protected. Recurrences are rare.

BACTERIAL TRACHEITIS

Etiology. Bacterial tracheitis is an infection of the laryngeal and tracheal mucosa. It primarily occurs in children age 1 month to 6 years. The most common cause of bacterial tracheitis is *Staphylococcus aureus*. Less common etiologies include Group A beta-hemolytic streptococci, *H. influenzae* type B, Streptococci, or *Moraxella catarrhalis*. Although it is a rare disease, bacterial tracheitis (also known as pseudomembranous croup or membranous laryngotracheitis) is associated with serious consequences, including airway obstruction and respiratory arrest.

Pathophysiology. Inflammation of the laryngeal and tracheal mucosa produces airway edema and airway obstruction. Formation of adherent pseudomembranes over the inflamed mucosa is common. The epiglottis may also be inflamed.

Clinical presentation. Bacterial tracheitis presents with a several-day history of a croup-like upper respiratory illness that progresses to severe respiratory distress, high fever, and copious thick purulent tracheal secretions. Early symptoms include a barking cough and inspiratory stridor that is unresponsive to croup therapy. The child rapidly becomes toxic with progressive respiratory decompensation. Worsening stridor clinically mimics epiglottitis and is unaffected by position. Unlike epiglottitis, however, there is an absence of drooling and the child tends to lie flat. A hoarse voice, noisy breathing, tachypnea, retractions, and coarse rhonchi are commonly present.

Emergency Department interventions. The diagnosis of bacterial tracheitis is clinically confirmed during intubation or bronchoscopy by the presence of copious thick secretions and pseudomembranes in the airway. The pathogen can be identified by tracheal cultures and gram stain. Blood cultures are rarely positive.

The classic x-ray finding is clouding of the tracheal air column or an irregular tracheal margin created by the pseudomembranes. Subglottic narrowing may be visible, but the supraglottic structures are normal unless epiglottitis is also present. Approximately 50% of children with bacterial tracheitis have lung infiltrates, especially if the illness has lasted more than 24 hours.[22]

Effective treatment of bacterial tracheitis requires early recognition and aggressive interventions similar to that of epiglottitis (see previous section). Broad-spectrum antibiotics that cover *S. aureus, S. pneumoniae*, and *H. influenzae* are initially administered. These may include nafcillin (or clindamycin in penicillin-allergic children) and chloramphenicol, or a third-generation cephalosporin alone may be given.[22,32] Treatment is typically more prolonged, and the child may remain in the ICU for up to 1 week. Intubation and frequent suctioning are almost universally necessary. On rare occasions a tracheostomy may be indicated if the endotracheal tube is repeatedly obstructed by thick secretions or if prolonged intubation is required. Recovery is usually uncomplicated, although lower respiratory involvement (focal atelectasis, pneumonitis, and edema), sepsis, and cardiac arrest from airway obstruction can occur. Late sequelae may include the development of granulation tissue and tracheal stricture.

NURSING CARE AND EVALUATION OF THE CHILD WITH AN ACUTE UPPER AIRWAY OBSTRUCTION

The child with a suspected upper airway infection that has the potential to cause an obstruction is treated emergently. Because the airway in these children can rapidly and unexpectedly obstruct, protocols for management are required to guide emergent nursing interventions. Once the child is placed in an examination room attempts are made to keep the child (and parents) calm and to decrease anxiety. Invasive interventions such as venipuncture are avoided, because agitation and crying can precipitate an obstruction. The parents are allowed to remain with the child and the child is allowed to maintain a position of comfort. Supplemental oxygen may be administered if it does not cause undue anxiety. Often the parents can administer oxygen via blow-by. Pulse oximetry and cardiac monitoring are required, but attempts to place probes on the child may cause agitation and crying.

These children are continuously monitored, and a bag-valve-mask device and intubation equipment should be immediately accessible. Frequent vital signs and observation for signs and symptoms of increasing airway obstruction and respiratory failure (e.g., increasing stridor at rest, severe retractions, and a decreased level of consciousness) are essential. The child with an altered level of consciousness requires airway positioning using the jaw-thrust or sniffing position, and the child with signs of respiratory failure despite supplemental oxygen administration will require BVM ventilation (see Chapter 8).

A nurse or physician must accompany the child for any diagnostic testing (e.g., x-rays) or during patient transfers (e.g., to the OR). Ventilatory equipment, including oxygen, a bag-valve-mask device, laryngoscope blade and handle, stylet, and appropriately sized endotracheal tubes, must also accompany the child.

An airway obstruction is frightening to both the parents and the child. Although difficult to offer during emergent management, a calm, quiet environment can help to allay anxiety and prevent crying. Staff in the child's room should be limited to those essential to providing care.

▌ ACUTE LOWER AIRWAY INFECTIONS

PNEUMONIA

Etiology.   Pneumonia is a lower respiratory tract infection that can be caused by bacteria, viruses, fungi, parasites, or atypical organisms (e.g., *Mycoplasma pneumoniae, Chlamydia trachomatis, Mycobacterium tuberculosis*). Although any of these organisms can produce pneumonia in any child, certain etiologies are more prevalent in specific age groups.

The most common causes of neonatal pneumonia are *C. trachomatis* and Group B streptococci (GBS). In neonates Group B streptococci is associated with a greater than 50% mortality rate.[44,66] The most common etiologies in the 1- to 3-month-old child include *S. pneumoniae, H. influenzae,* and *C. trachomatis.*

Viral etiologies such as RSV, parainfluenza, influenza, and adenovirus are the most prevalent cause of pneumonia in children between the ages of 3 months and 5 years. The most common bacterial pathogen in children 3 months to 2 years of age is *S. pneumoniae*. Before the initiation of the Hib vaccine, *H. influenzae* was the most common bacterial etiology in this age group.

In school-age children and young adults the atypical organism *M. pneumoniae* becomes the most common etiology, with a peak incidence in the 10 to 12-year-old age group. Of the bacterial pathogens, *S. pneumoniae* is the most prevalent in this older age group.

Because of its high communicability and brief incubation period, viral pneumonia often occurs in epidemic proportions in the winter and spring months. Atypical pneumonia is more prevalent in areas of crowded conditions, such as schools and day cares. The annual incidence of childhood pneumonia ranges from 40 per 1000 in children less than 5 years old to 7 per 1000 in 12 to 15 year olds.[9]

Pathophysiology. Infants and young children are particularly susceptible to pneumonia because of their pulmonary and immunologic immaturity. Pneumonia occurs when pulmonary defense mechanisms are altered, allowing pathogens to invade the lung tissue. The result is inflammation of the interstitium or alveoli.

Viral infections are the most common cause of altered pulmonary defense mechanisms, and these infections often precede bacterial pneumonias. The virus enters the upper respiratory tract, proliferates, and spreads to the lower respiratory tract. The infected epithelium loses its ciliary appendages and sloughs into the airways, where mucus and cellular debris accumulates. Airway obstruction, altered capillary membranes, and decreased surfactant production by infected alveolar lining cells lead to atelectasis and pulmonary edema.

Bacteria usually invade the lung via the nasopharynx. Occasionally bacteria that enters the bloodstream from inflamed nasal mucosa or infected ears or sinuses may spread to the lungs hematogenously. Bacterial invasion of the lungs triggers an inflammatory response that results in hyperemia of the lower respiratory mucosa, exudation, edema, and infiltration of the alveoli with white blood cells. Tissue destruction and abscess formation occurs with some organisms, such as *S. aureus* and *Klebsiella pneumoniae*.

Clinical presentation. Clinical manifestations vary with age, etiology, and host factors. Older children tend to have cough, fever, pleuritic chest pain, and dyspnea or tachypnea. The child may also complain of abdominal pain. Young children and infants usually exhibit nonspecific symptoms such as fever, tachypnea, irritability, poor feeding, decreased physical activity, vomiting, diarrhea, and apnea spells. Because these children tend to swallow the mucus as it is coughed from the lungs, emesis frequently contains large amounts of mucus.

Children with pneumonia usually exhibit signs and symptoms of respiratory distress. The degree of distress varies with the severity of the illness. Tachypnea at rest, tachycardia, nasal flaring, and retractions are consistent with respiratory compromise. Grunting respirations may be heard if air trapping or atelectasis is present. Signs of dehydration may result from increased insensible water loss associated with fever and tachypnea, decreased intake, and vomiting.

Auscultatory findings vary. Rales or moist crackles are a highly specific sign of pneumonia but are not always present. Wheezing may be heard, especially with nonbacterial pneumonias. Decreased breath sounds and dullness to percussion may be evident over areas of consolidation or pleural effusion.

Differentiation of the etiology of pneumonia is assisted by particular clinical findings. Bacterial pneumonia is characterized by an abrupt onset of cough, high fever, chills, crackles, decreased breath sounds, and often pleuritic pain. Viral pneumonia is typically preceded by 1 to 2 days of upper respiratory symptoms, followed by an insidious onset of low-grade fever, cough, and variable pulmonary findings (Table 10-5).

Host factors affect the severity of pneumonia. Children with underlying diseases such as congenital heart disease, chronic pulmonary disorders, or immune deficiencies tend to have more severe and even fatal pneumonias. Opportunistic pathogens are common in these children.

Emergency Department and nursing interventions

Diagnosis. The diagnosis of pneumonia is usually based on clinical findings. Diagnostic testing may confirm the presence of pneumonia and assist in identifying the etiology. The number of diagnostic tests performed depends on the suspected underlying etiology, the age of the child, and the severity of the symptoms.

The most useful initial test is the chest x-ray. Radiographic patterns of pulmonary infiltrates on chest x-ray may suggest the cause of pneumonia but are not necessarily diagnostic. Lobar consolidation

TABLE 10-5	Differentiation of Types of Pneumonia			
	BACTERIAL	**VIRAL**	**ATYPICAL**	
Pathogens	*S. pneumoniae* *H. influenzae* *S. aureus*	RSV Parainfluenza Influenza Adenovirus Rhinovirus	*M. pneumoniae*	*C. trachomatis*
Typical age group	>3 Months	3 Months to 5 years	School-age Adolescent	<6 Months
Clinical presentation				
Fever	High, chills	Usually low grade	Low grade	None
Cough	Productive	Slight; usually nonproductive early in disease	Dry progressing to mucoid or mucopurulent; paroxysmal, often at night	Staccato-like cough; posttussive cyanosis with increasing tachypnea
Toxicity	High	Usually low	Low	
Breath sounds	Crackles, decreased breath sounds	Few crackles or wheezes	Wheezes	Wheezes
Associated symptoms	Pleuritic pain	Malaise, myalgia	Malaise, myalgia, headache, sore throat	Conjunctivitis
Treatment	Antibiotics	Supportive	Erythromycin	Erythromycin or sulfonamide

and pleural effusions are more common with bacterial etiologies, and diffuse perihilar or peribronchial infiltrates, air trapping, or atelectasis are more common with viral etiologies. The WBC may assist in the differentiation of bacterial from nonbacterial pneumonias. Greater than 15,000 cells/mm³ with increased band cells suggests bacterial pneumonia. A low WBC (fewer than 5000 cells/mm³) may indicate an overwhelming infection.

Bacterial culture results of the sputum and blood may help identify the etiology of pneumonia. In the child, however, obtaining a satisfactory sample of nasopharyngeal secretions and sputum can be difficult. Contamination with mouth flora can make culture results difficult to interpret. Blood cultures are useful, because bacteremia is seen in a significant number of cases.[66] Counterimmune electrophoresis (CIE) or latex agglutination may

also be performed on the blood or sputum to identify specific bacterial antigens.

Rapid antigen detection techniques for identifying common respiratory viral pathogens (e.g., RSV, influenza) and *C. trachomatis* may be ordered, although false-positive and false-negative results can occur. Because these organisms are rarely carried in normal upper respiratory secretions, their presence in nasal aspirates is highly suggestive of the disease etiology. Positive cold agglutinins suggest but do not confirm the presence of *M. pneumoniae*.

Treatment. Most children with pneumonia are not seriously ill and can be treated on an outpatient basis. Seriously ill children who are toxic appearing or who exhibit significant signs of respiratory distress require airway management, supplemental oxygen administration, and hospital admission. Inhaled bronchodilators may be necessary if pneumonia is accompanied by bronchospasm.

The treatment for viral pneumonia is primarily supportive, although some antiviral medications are available for seriously ill or compromised children. Antibiotics do not alter the course of the illness.

Children with bacterial pneumonia or pneumonia caused by one of the atypical organisms are treated with antibiotics. The choice of antibiotics depends on the presence of allergies and known bacterial sensitivity patterns. Although treatment regimens can vary, the most common approaches follow. Suggested antibiotics in the neonatal population are ampicillin and gentamicin. In the 1- to 3-month-old child ampicillin or cefotaxime is preferred. In children 3 months to 5 years of age either amoxicillin, a cephalosporin, or a β-lactamase–resistant drug such as amoxicillin-clavulanate (Augmentin) is prescribed. School-age children and adolescents are usually given erythromycin. Any child with a suspected staphylococcal infection is treated with nafcillin. Bacterial pneumonia has also been successfully treated with one to two doses of IM/IV ceftriaxone and subsequent oral antibiotics.[24]

If the child is to be discharged, parents can be told to treat fever with antipyretics and to administer plenty of fluids. Signs and symptoms of significant respiratory distress are discussed and parents are notified to contact their primary care provider or return to the emergency department should these symptoms appear. Parents often worry about the effect of cough on the child's ability to rest. However, expectorants, antihistamines, and cough suppressants are of little value in the management of pneumonia. Antitussives with codeine or dextromethorphan are sometimes prescribed for use before bed or nap time to facilitate sleep. To prevent future episodes, obtaining the annual influenza vaccine is encouraged. Pneumococcal vaccine is recommended for high-risk children. Cigarette smoking in the household must be avoided, because exposure doubles the risk of pneumonia and bronchitis in infants.[18]

BRONCHIOLITIS

Etiology. Bronchiolitis is an acute lower respiratory infection that affects the small airways. RSV is responsible for most cases of bronchiolitis. Other etiologies include adenoviruses, influenza, and parainfluenza viruses.

Bronchiolitis is seen in children less than 2 years of age, with the highest incidence occurring in infants less than 1 year of age. Premature infants; infants with compromised cardiac, pulmonary, or immune func-

tion; and immunocompromised children are at the highest risk for severe disease. Factors associated with an increased incidence of bronchiolitis include crowded living conditions, low socioeconomic status, and passive exposure to cigarette smoke.[87] Bronchiolitis is most prevalent in the winter and early spring.

Pathophysiology. Viral invasion of the lower respiratory tract produces a relatively superficial and reversible necrosis of the bronchiolar epithelium with associated peribronchiolar inflammation. Proliferation of nonciliated epithelial cells results in ineffective clearance of inflammatory mucus and exudate. The inflammatory secretions and submucosal edema obstruct small airways. Airway obstruction interferes primarily with expiration, leading to patchy areas of air trapping and atelectasis. Air trapping results in hyperinflation, which increases the functional residual capacity, decreases lung compliance, and increases the work of breathing. Atelectasis produces ventilation-perfusion mismatching, abnormal gas exchange, and hypoxemia. In addition, a peribronchial interstitial pneumonitis develops from the inflammatory involvement of the interalveolar walls.

Respiratory syncytial virus (RSV). RSV is a highly contagious respiratory pathogen that is transmitted by direct contact with infected respiratory secretions or contaminated objects. The virus enters the body via contact of the hands with the nose, eye, or other mucous membranes. Aerosol spread occurs but is less common. The child with RSV is probably contagious during the 24 to 48 hours before the onset of symptoms and for several days thereafter.[87] Conclusive evidence is not available on the incubation period of RSV, but it is thought to be about 5 days.

RSV affects all age groups; however, adults and older children generally develop only an upper respiratory illness. Lower respiratory involvement, in the form of bronchiolitis, occurs primarily in infants less than 1 year of age. Virtually all children develop an RSV infection in the first 2 to 3 years of life, and because immunity to the virus is short lived, repeated infections are possible.[35] Subsequent infections tend to be less severe than the initial episode.

Clinical presentation. The clinical manifestations of bronchiolitis range from mild URI symptoms to severe lower respiratory tract symptoms. Typically, a several-day history of rhinorrhea, dry cough, and sometimes a low-grade fever precedes the development of lower respiratory symptoms. Fever usually disappears with the onset of lower respiratory symptoms. Expiratory wheezing develops and cough becomes more frequent and severe. The infant may improve after a mild illness or progress to signs of respiratory distress and even failure. Life-threatening symptoms that result from hypoxemia include air hunger, cyanosis, and lethargy. An apnea spell may be the first sign of bronchiolitis in infants less than 3 months of age. Apnea occurs in approximately 20% of hospitalized infants with RSV.[35] Bronchiolitis is particularly severe in infants with BPD.

Emergency Department and nursing interventions

Diagnosis. The diagnosis of bronchiolitis is based on clinical findings. Wheezing infants with a several-day history of URI symptoms, particularly during peak season, are assumed to have bronchiolitis rather than asthma. Forty to fifty percent of infants with bronchiolitis have recurrent wheezing episodes until 2 to 3 years of age.[87] Not all of these children will develop classic asthma.

Diagnostic testing for the infant with mild respiratory symptoms associated with bronchiolitis is not always necessary. Infants with more serious symptoms may receive a chest x-ray, an antigen detection test, and a CBC. The CBC is not particularly useful, however, because the WBC is usually only mildly elevated or normal—unless a rare coexisting bacterial infection is present.

Classic chest x-ray findings in the child with bronchiolitis include a "shaggy" heart border. Hyperinflation with flattening of the diaphragm and patchy areas of atelectasis are also seen. Diffuse interstitial infiltrates similar to viral pneumonia are commonly seen, but hyperinflation is a differentiating factor.

Reliable, rapid antigen detection tests have been developed to identify RSV. Enzyme-linked immunosorbent assay (ELISA) and direct fluorescent antibody (DFA) are greater than 90% sensitive and 95% specific for RSV.[61] Samples of respiratory secretions may be obtained by nasopharyngeal swabs or nasal washings. To obtain a nasal wash, 2 to 4 ml of sterile saline solution is inserted into one nostril and is then aspirated and placed in transport medium. To obtain a nasopharyngeal specimen, the swab is inserted through the nares into the nasopharynx. A cough is usually elicited when the swab reaches the nasopharynx. Secretions are then transferred from the swab to viral transport media.

Treatment. Most infants with bronchiolitis are mildly ill and merely require supportive care. Infants with signs of moderate to severe respiratory distress may require oxygen therapy and admission. The decision to hospitalize the infant is based on severity of illness, reliability of parents, duration of present illness, and likelihood of adequate follow-up. The best predictors of the need for hospitalization are an oxygen saturation less than 95% and a toxic appearance.[72] Other factors supporting the decision to admit include gestational age less than 34 weeks, current age less than 3 months, respiratory rate greater than 70, x-ray with atelectasis, associated dehydration,[72,87] and/or the presence of underlying health problems—especially BPD.[42]

Aerosolized bronchodilators may be used to treat infants with bronchiolitis, but the response to therapy varies. A trial dose of an aerosolized beta-adrenergic agent (e.g., albuterol) may be given; if improvement is noted, subsequent doses may be administered. During administration the infant is monitored for tolerance of the drug, including observations of the work of breathing, respiratory rate, and heart rate. Discharge instructions may include the administration of albuterol via nebulizer, oral syrup, or inhaler for up to 5 to 7 days.

The hospitalized infant with severe disease (e.g., requires assisted ventilation) or high-risk factors (e.g., BPD or congenital heart defect [CHD]) may be treated with aerosolized ribavirin. Ribavirin, a synthetic nucleoside that inhibits viral replication, decreases the severity of RSV bronchiolitis and improves oxygenation.[34,77]

Infection control is required to prevent the spread of RSV. Strict hand washing is the most effective method of prevention. In the ED these infants should be placed in a private room—or at least separated from other patients. Gowns and masks are of little value, although gowns may decrease fomite spread during close contact with an infected infant.[35] If the child is discharged the parents are informed that transmission occurs with direct contact of contaminated secretions from the hands, contaminated surfaces, or person-to-person. Viral shedding usually lasts from 3 to 8 days; however, in young infants it may last for up to 4 weeks.[19] Immunocompromised children may shed the virus for prolonged periods. Additional discharge teaching includes instructions on follow-up care, attention to the infant's hydration status, fever-control measures, and when to seek immediate care (e.g., signs and symptoms of worsening respiratory distress).

Additional approaches to care. RSV vaccines are currently under investigation but are not expected to be available in the near future.[27] An intravenous immunoglobulin preparation with high titers of RSV-neutralizing antibody is also being investigated to prevent RSV infection in high-risk infants.[87] Breast milk contains antibody to RSV and may provide temporary protection for the infant.[5]

PERTUSSIS (WHOOPING COUGH)

Etiology. Pertussis is a highly contagious respiratory infection caused by *Bordetella pertussis* (a gram-negative rod). The incidence of pertussis has increased dramatically over the past decade as many parents have refused to immunize their children against pertussis because of concern over possible neurologic damage. Although this vaccine is thought to be safe,[33,45,74,86] an acellular vaccine that has equal effectiveness and fewer minor adverse reactions has recently been approved for use in infants and children.

Forty percent of the reported cases of pertussis occur in infants less than 1 year old, and almost 70% of cases are seen in children less than 4 years of age.[28,63] The greatest risk of morbidity and mortality is among young infants. Adults and older children can contract pertussis even if they were immunized as children, because immunity wanes over time. However, adolescents and adults with the disease generally have a mild illness with nonspecific symptoms. A single attack of pertussis confers lifetime immunity.

Pathophysiology. *B. pertussis* attaches to the ciliated respiratory epithelium, where it rapidly proliferates. Toxins trigger an inflammatory response with lymphocytic and granulocytic infiltration, edema of the mucosal lining of the respiratory tract, and increased mucus production. Diminished ciliary function causes mucus and cellular debris to accumulate, producing bronchiolar congestion, obstruction, and necrosis. Mucus plugging can lead to atelectasis and pneumothoraces. Bronchopneumonia is the most common complication and the most frequent cause of death in infants with pertussis.

Toxins also affect the functioning of certain target cells in the body, including lymphocytes, myocardial cells, and pancreatic islet cells. Pathologic effects include lymphocytosis, increased susceptibility to histamine and serotonin, and increased insulin activity resulting in decreased blood glucose levels. Seizures or encephalopathy may develop from toxin-mediated effects, CNS hypoxia, or alkalosis caused by persistent vomiting.

Forceful, prolonged coughing may rupture alveoli and cause subcutaneous emphysema. Epistaxis, subconjunctival hemorrhages, hernias, rectal prolapse, or rupture of the diaphragm may also occur secondary to coughing and vomiting.

Transmission. Pertussis is transmitted by direct contact with infected respiratory secretions, droplet spread from an infected person, or indirect contact with freshly contaminated articles. The period of communicability is greatest during the catarrhal stage (before the onset of paroxysmal cough) but may extend throughout the paroxysmal stage. The incubation period is 6 to 20 days, with 7 to 10 days being most common.

Clinical presentation. Pertussis symptoms range from mild upper respiratory complaints in the adult to severe respiratory distress in infants. There are typically three stages of pertussis spanning a 6 to 8-week period (Table 10-6). Children seen during the first stage, or *catarrhal stage,* are typically diagnosed with an upper respiratory infection. These children later return during the *paroxysmal stage* with spells of short, rapid coughs followed by a sudden inspiration

TABLE 10-6	Clinical Stages of Pertussis	
STAGE	**DURATION**	**CLINICAL FEATURES**
Catarrhal	1-2 Weeks	Rhinorrhea, lacrimation, mild cough, fever (usually low grade)
Paroxysmal	2-4 Weeks	Paroxysmal cough, neurologic and respiratory complications
Convalescent	1-4 Weeks	Gradual improvement in symptoms; paroxysmal cough may persist for up to 6 months

From Felter RA: Infectious disorders. In Barkin RM, ed: *Pediatric emergency medicine: concepts and clinical practice,* St Louis, 1992, Mosby.

associated with a "whooping" sound. The "whooping" sound is not always present, especially in infants less than 6 months of age. During this stage, fever is usually absent. Apnea spells frequently accompany pertussis in young infants. Thick nasal secretions may obstruct air passages, further impeding breathing. The *convalescent stage* is characterized by gradual improvement in symptoms, but the cough may persist for up to 6 months.

Coughing is a characteristic finding with pertussis and is usually worse at night. During violent or prolonged coughing spells, the child's cheeks may become red or cyanotic, the eyes bulge, and the tongue protrudes. Coughing often continues until a thick mucus plug is dislodged. Vomiting brought on by coughing is common. After a coughing spell the infant may be listless and apathetic.

Emergency Department and nursing interventions

Diagnosis. When pertussis is suspected, nasopharyngeal secretions are either directly plated onto appropriate media at the bedside or placed in transport media and immediately sent to the laboratory.[43] Growth of *B. pertussis* on the culture media confirms the clinical diagnosis, but the organism is difficult to grow and results may not be available for 3 to 7 days. Fluorescent antibody (FAB) testing yields rapid results, but specificity and sensitivity are unpredictable. The polymerase chain reaction (PCR) is a new rapid diagnostic test that can accurately identify *B. pertussis*.[15]

The white blood cell count is frequently greater than $15,000/mm^3$ with an associated lymphocytosis. Eosinophilia, although uncommon, suggests the possibility of pertussis. Serum electrolytes are indicated if the child appears dehydrated. ABGs are reserved for severe disease only.

There are no characteristic chest x-ray findings in pertussis. However, atelectasis or pneumonia with associated peribronchial thickening, infiltrates, and a "shaggy" heart border may be present.

Treatment. Infants in the paroxysmal stage of the disease may present with moderate to severe signs of respiratory distress. Humidified oxygen may be administered as necessary to maintain an oxygen saturation above 95%. Mist should be avoided, because it can trigger paroxysmal coughing. Suctioning of thick airway secretions may be required to maintain airway patency, but deep suctioning can precipitate coughing spells.

Nursing care of the child with pertussis is primarily supportive (Box 10-4). Oxygen saturation, respiratory status, and hydration status are monitored continuously. Signs of respiratory failure are immediately reported to the emergency physician. Venous access is achieved and a bedside blood glucose is obtained, because hypoglycemia is common. Respiratory isolation is initiated and maintained until antibiotic therapy has been given for 5 days.

Erythromycin or erythromycin estolate is the drug of choice for eradicating pertussis from the respiratory tract and decreasing the spread of the disease. It does not hasten clinical improvement unless it is started before the paroxysmal stage begins. A 14-day course is suggested for treatment, as well as prophylaxis for close contacts—regardless of immunization status.[19] Albuterol and corticosteroids may decrease the severity and frequency of coughing spells. Cough suppressants are avoided. Hospital admission is recommended for children who are less than 6 months of age, are dehydrated, or have complications.

If the child is to be discharged, instructions should include information about the disease and its communicability, medications, hydration, nutrition, and follow-up care. Vomiting is common and may clear some of the secretions and facilitate subsequent feedings. Gentle nasal suctioning before feedings will also clear secretions. Reducing environmental triggers such as dust, smoke, sudden changes in temperature, activity, and excitement may decrease coughing. Because pertussis has a prolonged course, a public health nurse referral may be helpful for ongoing care and support.

TUBERCULOSIS

Etiology. Tuberculosis (TB) is a communicable disease caused by *Mycobacterium tuberculosis,* a small, nonmotile, slow-growing organism. High risk factors for TB include poverty and overcrowded living conditions. Chronic medical conditions such as AIDS, diabetes mellitus, and immunosuppressive therapy also increase the risk of TB.

In the United States the incidence of TB has been increasing in both adults and children since 1985.[75] Between 1988 and 1993, there was a 40% increase in TB in U.S. children.[80] The vast majority of pediatric cases occur in children from racial and ethnic minorities.[79]

Pathophysiology. Once the tuberculosis organisms enter the respiratory tract they begin to

Box 10-4 Nursing Considerations for the Infant with Pertussis

Observe for and treat respiratory distress or failure

Administer supplemental oxygen to maintain a saturation > 95%

Avoid mist, as it may trigger paroxysmal coughing

Suction thick airway secretions—avoid deep suctioning

Initiate respiratory isolation

Evaluate hydration status and administer fluids as necessary

Monitor bedside glucose

Obtain diagnostic testing as ordered

Initiate erythromycin or erythromycin estolate therapy as ordered

Address prophylaxis needs of the parents and close contacts

Notify the local health department as required

multiply in the alveoli and establish a primary focus of infection or tubercle (asymptomatic TB infection). Tubercles may lie dormant, resolve and disappear, calcify and form a Ghon complex, or become necrotic. The Ghon complex consists of the initial alveolar infection site, the infected lymph nodes, and the associated lymphangitis. Although most primary infections resolve, viable TB organisms may be harbored in the focal lesions and reactivated months to years later.[60]

Bacilli may spread from the primary focus to the regional lymph nodes and then to other parts of the body. Approximately 25% of children less than 15 years of age will develop extrapulmonary disease.[19] Miliary tuberculosis, a generalized disease resulting from hematogenous spread from the lungs to multiple organs, and tuberculous meningitis are the most serious extrapulmonary complications.

With disease progression, the primary focus enlarges and liquid pus may empty into one or more bronchi, leaving a residual cavity. Pus may spread to other areas of the lung or may be coughed up, thus exposing others to infection. Enlarged peribronchial lymph nodes may obstruct bronchi, especially in children less than 2 years of age. With airway obstruction hyperaeration and atelectasis can result. Pleural effusion may be present in children older than 2 years of age.

Transmission. Tuberculosis is spread via airborne droplets expelled from persons with active TB of the lungs or larynx. Sometimes TB is spread by direct contact with infected discharges such as saliva, sputum, or urine or by heavily contaminated fomites. Because children rarely develop active laryngeal or pulmonary TB with cavitation, it is unusual for them to transmit the disease. Most children contract TB from infected adults. The incubation period from TB exposure to a positive TB skin test is usually 2 to 10 weeks.

Clinical presentation. The clinical manifestations of TB depend on the quantity and virulence of the tuberculous bacilli, the age, immunocompetence, susceptibility of the host, and the degree of extrapulmonary involvement. Unlike adults, children exhibit few signs and symptoms of tuberculosis. In most cases signs and symptoms are nonspecific and may include low-grade fever, mild cough, malaise, weight loss, or wheezing. The child with miliary TB may have a persistent high fever, hepatosplenomegaly, and rales or crackles. TB meningitis may progress from nonspecific signs such as irritability to specific signs of meningeal irritation and increased intracranial pressure.

Emergency Department and nursing interventions

Diagnosis. Asymptomatic children with TB are usually identified during routine tuberculin skin testing or the screening of adult contacts. Although few children develop active disease, TB should be considered in high-risk children with persistent fevers and cough. Diagnostic testing may include a Mantoux skin test, a chest x-ray, and cultures of the blood, sputum, and urine. In young children the best sputum specimen is an early morning gastric aspirate, because young children often swallow their secretions. Other tests may include a CBC, erythrocyte sedimentation rate, urinalysis, and serum liver enzymes.

Chest x-rays in children with asymptomatic primary tuberculous infections are usually negative. The primary complex may be visible on chest x-ray within the first several months after infection, especially in small children and infants. Healed, calcified lesions do not appear on x-ray for at least 6 months.

Treatment. Most children with tuberculosis do not require emergent management. In fact, because the signs and symptoms of TB in children are nonspecific the presence of this disease may not be recognized

Box 10-5   AFB Isolation

1. Masks are indicated only when patient is coughing and does not reliably cover mouth.
2. Gowns are indicated only if needed to prevent gross contamination of clothing.
3. Gloves are not indicated.
4. Hands must be washed after touching the patient or potentially contaminated articles and before taking care of another patient.
5. Articles should be discarded, cleaned, or sent for decontamination and reprocessing.

Diseases requiring AFB isolation
• This isolation category is for patients with current pulmonary TB who have a positive sputum smear or a chest x-ray appearance that strongly suggests current (active) TB. Laryngeal TB is also included in this category. In general, infants and young children with pulmonary TB do not require isolation precautions because they rarely cough and their bronchial secretions contain few AFB.

From Committee on Infectious Disease: *1994 Red Book: Report of the Committee on Infectious Disease,* ed 23, Elk Grove, Ill, 1994, American Academy of Pediatrics.

until the history, physical, and diagnostic testing have been performed. Although most children with the disease are not contagious, they may be accompanied by the "source" of their infection. Once tuberculosis is suspected the child is placed on AFB (acid-fast bacilli) isolation (Box 10-5). Accompanying adults must also adhere to isolation precautions, and their status regarding the disease should be determined when the history is obtained. Laws in all states require that cases of tuberculosis be reported to local health departments.

Pharmacologic management. Although most TB is treatable, an increase in multidrug-resistant organisms has complicated treatment regimens. In addition to drug resistance, other factors used to determine treatment regimens include the presence of active or inactive TB and the presence of extrapulmonary disease. In children without active disease, isoniazid (INH) 10 mg/kg is administered once daily. Children who have been exposed to contacts with INH-resistant *M. tuberculosis* or children who are at high risk from the consequences of the infection are

additionally given rifampin 10 mg/kg daily.[40] In addition to the above drugs, children with tuberculous meningitis, miliary TB, suspected multiple-drug–resistant (MDR) TB, and HIV are also given a 6-month regimen of pyrazinamide.[40] If initial drug resistance is suspected in these children, ethambutol or streptomycin is also administered.[19] Side effects to antituberculous medications include hepatotoxicity and peripheral neuritis, but these findings are rare in American children.[78]

The bacillus Calmette-Guérin vaccine (BCG) is a safe method of prevention of the disease, but its efficacy is variable. Although BCG may not prevent the infection, it may prevent the progression of the disease or the development of miliary TB and tuberculous meningitis in children. In the United States BCG may be used for uninfected children who have close contact with an adult with active pulmonary TB and who are unlikely to be compliant with INH therapy, uninfected children with frequent exposure to MDR TB, or children with asymptomatic HIV infection and likely exposure to TB.[40] Children must have a negative Mantoux tuberculin skin test and a negative chest x-ray within 2 weeks before administration of the vaccine.

Discharge teaching. A major problem limiting successful treatment of TB is poor compliance with the treatment regimen. Parents are instructed to strictly follow treatment protocols and comply with follow-up care requirements. Community health nurses are often consulted to monitor compliance and response to therapy. Parents are also instructed to observe for the development of side effects of antituberculous drugs, including jaundice, rash, visual disturbances, gastrointestinal symptoms, or unexpected deterioration. Isolation is not usually required if the child is compliant with the medication protocol. However, good general health habits such as covering the nose and mouth when sneezing and thorough hand washing are encouraged.

NONINFECTIOUS RESPIRATORY DISORDERS

REACTIVE AIRWAY DISEASE (ASTHMA)

Etiology.   Asthma is a chronic inflammatory lung disease characterized by recurrent episodes of lower airway obstruction that are reversible either spontaneously or with treatment.[52,73] It is a multifactorial disease with both genetic and environmental influences, although the relative contributions of each are unclear. A variety of risk factors correlate with the development of asthma, including family history, allergen exposure and allergies, low socioeconomic status, low birth weight, young maternal age, and race.[8,48] There is a higher incidence in blacks than whites.

Asthma is the most common chronic disease in children, and it affects approximately 5% to 10% of all children.[6] Asthma morbidity and mortality have been increasing over the past decade, despite advancements in treatment.[26,52] Suggested reasons for the increased incidence of asthma include changes in the definition of asthma, air pollution, poor access or underutilization of health care, and underuse of steroids. Mortality risk factors include severe disease, poor self-care, severe depression, and other psychologic problems. Approximately half of all children with asthma outgrow the disease by 14 years of age.[26]

Pathophysiology. Asthma is characterized by three interrelated features: airway obstruction, airway inflammation, and airway hyperresponsiveness. Airway obstruction is usually reversible either spontaneously or with treatment. However, a variable degree of airway obstruction and inflammation may be chronically present. Asthmatic airways are hyperresponsive to a variety of stimuli or triggers, including allergens, environmental irritants, cold air, viral infection, and exercise. Viral infections are the most common triggers in young children, whereas allergies and exercise are more common triggers in older children and adolescents. The degree of airway hyperreactivity usually correlates with the severity of asthma and the need for medications.[16,52,64]

An asthma exacerbation is simply a worsening of the underlying pathophysiology. Exposure to "triggers" most likely stimulates the release of inflammatory mediators such as histamine and prostaglandins. These mediators cause airway smooth muscle contraction and infiltration of the airway by inflammatory cells, which results in epithelial damage. Bronchoconstriction, mucus plugging, and edema obstructs the airways. Decreased expiratory air flow results in air trapping and hyperinflation as the work of breathing increases to ventilate the obstructed and hyperaerated alveoli. Increased oxygen consumption and the mismatching of ventilation and perfusion leads to the development of hypoxia. Pulmonary vascular resistance increases during severe exacerbations secondary to hypoxia and pulmonary hyperinflation. Decreasing ventilatory effort and airway obstruction lead to hypercapnia.

Clinical presentation. Clinical presentation varies depending on the severity of the disease. Children with a history of previous intubation or ICU admission, frequent hospitalizations or ED visits within the past year, or current use of systemic corticosteroids are at highest risk for serious life-threatening asthma exacerbations. However, a child may arrive in the ED with severe respiratory distress and no previous history of asthma.

The severity of symptoms ranges from mild wheezing and respiratory distress to respiratory failure (Table 10-7). Typical symptoms of asthma include expiratory wheezing; dyspnea; a dry, tight, nonproductive cough; prolonged-expiration; tachypnea; retractions; and accessory muscle use. Older verbal children may complain of shortness of breath or chest tightness. They may speak in short, panting phrases.

Wheezing may be audible without a stethoscope or auscultation may reveal end-expiratory wheezes. Inspiratory wheezing is associated with more severe exacerbations. If inspiratory and expiratory sounds are decreased, wheezing may be diminished or absent. A "silent lung," in which air movement and, wheezing cannot be heard despite increased respiratory effort, is a sign of impending respiratory failure.

Emergency Department interventions

Diagnosis. Recommended diagnostic tests for the wheezing child vary with respect to age, past medical history, severity of disease, and associated signs and symptoms. Pulse oximetry is measured on all wheezing children. ABGs may be obtained in the child with obvious hypoventilation, cyanosis, or severe respiratory distress that has not responded to initial treatment. Chest x-rays are not routinely ordered but may be obtained to rule out other causes of wheezing such as foreign body aspiration or pneumonia, or to rule out serious complications such as pneumomediastinum. Classic chest x-ray findings in the asthmatic child include hyperaeration, increased bronchial markings, and atelectasis. Other tests such as a CBC or blood culture may be ordered to identify a coexisting illness.

Spirometry or peak expiratory flow meters may be used to objectively measure the severity of an asthma exacerbation and the response to treatment. Because the reliability of spirometry and peak expiratory flow rate (PEFR) depends on the child's effort and cooperation during the testing, it is best performed in children older than 5 years of age. Pretend games such

TABLE 10-7	Estimation of Severity of Acute Exacerbations of Asthma in Children		
SIGN/SYMPTOM	MILD	MODERATE	SEVERE
PEFR*	70-90% predicted or personal best	50-70% predicted or personal best	<50% predicted or personal best
Respiratory rate, resting or sleeping	Normal to 30% increase above the mean	30-50% increase above the mean	Increase over 50% above the mean
Alertness	Normal	Normal	May be decreased
Dyspnea†	Absent or mild; speaks in complete sentences	Moderate; speaks in phrases or partial sentences; infant's cry softer and shorter, infant has difficulty suckling and feeding	Severe; speaks only in single words or short phrases; infant's cry softer and shorter, infants stops suckling and feeding
Work of breathing	No retractions to mild retractions	Moderate intercostal retraction with tracheosternal retractions; use of sternocleidomastoid muscles; chest hyperinflation	Severe intercostal retractions, tracheosternal retractions with nasal flaring during inspiration; chest hyperinflation
Color	Good	Pale	Possibly cyanotic
Auscultation	End expiratory wheeze only	Wheeze during entire expiration and inspiration	Breath sounds becoming inaudible
Oxygen saturation	>95%	90-95%	<90%
P_{CO_2}	<35	<40	>40

Modified from National Asthma Education Program, Expert Panel Report: *Executive summary: guidelines for the diagnosis and management of asthma,* Bethesda, Md, 1991, National Heart, Lung, and Blood Institute, National Institutes of Health, Pub No 91-3042A.
NOTE: Within each category, the presence of several parameters, but not necessarily all, indicates, the general classification of the exacerbation.
*For children 5 years of age or older.
†Parents' or physicians' impression of degree of child's breathlessness.

as blowing out birthday candles may facilitate the younger child's cooperation. Spirometry measures the volume of air exhaled during a maximal expiratory effort. Results reflect the functional ability of the lungs. During asthma exacerbations, the initial PEFR may not be helpful unless baseline results have been previously established. However, the PEFR may help evaluate the response to treatment.

Treatment. Treatment goals for acute asthma exacerbations include rapid reversal of air-flow obstruction, correction of hypoxemia, and reduction of the rate of recurrent severe asthma symptoms.[52]

Repetitive administration of inhaled beta₂-agonists (usually albuterol) is the most effective treatment for the rapid reversal of air-flow obstruction.[52] Albuterol dilates the airways and improves air flow by relaxing smooth muscle. Inhaled aerosolized beta₂-agonists are delivered directly to the airways and usually provide better bronchodilation, faster onset, and fewer side effects at lower doses than the oral or parenteral route. The onset of action for inhaled beta₂-agonists is less than 5 minutes (Table 10-8).

Systemic corticosteroids alleviate airway inflammation with subsequent reduction in mucus secretion, edema, and possibly airway reactivity.[4] They are given

TABLE 10-8	Medications Used in the Treatment of Asthma Exacerbations in Children		
MEDICATION	**DOSE**	**ACTION/INDICATION**	**SIDE EFFECTS**
Beta$_2$-Agonists		Bronchodilator	
Inhaled		Used for the immediate reversal of bronchospasm in acute exacerbations	
Albuterol Nebulizer 0.5% (5 mg/ml)	0.15 mg/kg/dose up to 5 mg q20min for 1-2 hours, then q1-2h prn (minimum: 1.25 mg/dose) Continuous nebs: 0.5 mg/kg/h (maximum: 15 mg/h)		Cardiovascular stimulation, tachycardia, skeletal muscle tremor, elevated blood pressure, nervousness, anxiety
Metered-dose inhaler (MDI) (90 μg/puff)	Two puffs every 5 minutes for total of 12 puffs, then 4 puffs q1h if improved		
Systemic		Inhaled beta$_2$-agonist preferred	
Epinephrine 1 : 1000 (1 mg/ml)	SQ: 0.01 mg/kg up to 0.3 mg q20min × 3		Epinephrine has beta 1 effects on cardiovascular system: significant tachycardia and cardiac toxicity
Terbutaline (1 mg/1 ml)	SQ: 0.01 mg/kg up to 0.3 mg q2-6h prn IV: 10 μg/kg over 10 min (loading dose), followed by 0.4 μg/kg/min; increase prn by 0.2 μg/kg/min (expect to use 3-6 μg/kg/min)	May be used in the hospitalized child with severe asthma	
Steroids		Antiinflammatory Used to treat moderate to severe acute exacerbations Prolonged daily use of corticosteroids should only be used for severe asthma that cannot be controlled with high-dose inhaled steroids	Reversible abnormalities in glucose metabolism, increased appetite, fluid retention, weight gain, rounding of face, mood alterations, hypertension, peptic ulcer, aseptic necrosis of femur; adrenal suppression; immunosuppression

TABLE 10-8	Medications Used in the Treatment of Asthma Exacerbations in Children—cont'd		
MEDICATION	**DOSE**	**ACTION/INDICATION**	**SIDE EFFECTS**
Steroids—cont'd			No need to taper short-burst therapy (3-5 days)
Oral Prednisone Prednisolone	1-2 mg/kg/day in single or divided doses for outpatients; 1-2 mg/kg q6h for inpatients	Onset of action: 3 hours; peak effectiveness 6-12 hours	
Parenteral Methylprednisolone	ED: 1-2 mg/kg/dose q6h		
Anticholinergics Ipratropium bromide (Atrovent)		Bronchodilator; slower onset of action with peak at approximately 60 min	
MDI	5-10 puffs with spacer q4-6h	May be used in conjunction with beta-agonists, if poor response to optimal beta-agonist therapy	
Nebulizer (0.025% solution)	0.025-0.05 mg/kg (max 5 mg) q6h	Give with caution in children with severe asthma who have poor response to beta-agonist and aminophylline	
Methylxanthines IV: aminophylline	Loading dose: 6mg/kg (if patient not currently taking theophylline)	Bronchodilator Third-line drug used in hospitalized patients with moderate to severe asthma	Early signs of toxicity: nausea, headache, tachycardia, irritability Late signs of toxicity: seizures, encephalopathy, cardiac dysrhythmias, GI bleeding
	Continuous infusion: 0.5-1.2 mg/kg/hr depending on age	Infrequently used due to narrow therapeutic window and high iatrogenic complications	
	Dosage to achieve serum level of 15 μg/ml; check blood levels 1 hour after loading dose		

Compiled from Murphy and Kelly, 1991; National Asthma Education Program, 1991; Zahr, Connolly, and Page, 1989.

early in the course of asthma exacerbations that do not respond to the initial nebulized beta$_2$-agonist treatment. The onset of action of systemic corticosteroids is approximately 3 hours, with peak effectiveness between 6 and 12 hours after administration. Parenteral steroids are given if the child cannot tolerate oral medications.

Anticholinergics may be given when the child has a poor response to albuterol and steroid therapy. Anticholinergics may also be mixed with albuterol in the nebulizer and administered every 20 minutes.[69] Anticholinergics produce bronchodilation by decreasing vagal tone to the airways. Ipratropium is preferred over atropine, especially when used in combination with beta$_2$-agonists, because of its more rapid onset and minimal side effects.[49,53]

Theophylline, which has mild to moderate bronchodilator effects, is not recommended for the care of children with asthma exacerbations in the emergency department. It has a high potential for serious toxicity when used with frequently administered beta$_2$-agonists and lacks additional bronchodilation effect.[25,52] Theophylline may be helpful in children who are admitted for severe asthma.[52,53]

Aggressive medication therapy is initiated in children with severe status asthmaticus to avoid respiratory failure and the need for mechanical ventilation. Medications may include continuous administration of nebulized beta$_2$-agonists, continuous intravenous infusions of beta$_2$-agonists (e.g., terbutaline) and aminophylline, infusions of magnesium sulfate, or the administration of ketamine. Intravenous magnesium sulfate may be used to treat moderate to severe asthma in children who do not respond well to beta$_2$-agonist therapy.[47,50] Magnesium sulfate causes smooth muscle relaxation and bronchodilation and is administered at 40 mg/kg over 20 minutes. During administration continuous ECG monitoring, frequent vital signs including blood pressure, and observation for seizure activity is required. Ketamine, single dose (1 to 2 mg/kg) or continuous infusion (1 to 2.5 mg/kg/hr), has also been advocated for use in children with refractory status asthmaticus.[68,81] Ketamine is thought to relax bronchial smooth muscle and increase catecholamine levels. When used in the presence of other beta-agonists, the rise in catecholamine levels can increase the risk of dysrhythmias.[39]

Prevention. The goals of long-term therapy include control of chronic symptoms, elimination or reduction of asthma triggers, and the prevention of exacerbations. Medications used to treat the underlying pathology and control chronic symptoms may include antiinflammatory agents such as inhaled steroids and cromolyn, and long-acting bronchodilators such as oral theophylline or inhaled salmeterol.

Nursing care and evaluation. Initial management of the child depends on presenting signs and symptoms. The child with mild to moderate signs of respiratory distress, low risk factors, and no other concurrent illnesses can be treated urgently. The child with signs of severe respiratory distress is treated emergently. Supplemental oxygen is administered via a nonrebreather mask, and the administration of continuous nebulized albuterol therapy and steroids is anticipated. Airway management and intravenous access supplies should be readily accessible.

Young children are not able to hold the mouthpiece or mouth breathe when receiving nebulized medications. Therefore a face mask (or blow-by if the face mask is not tolerated) is the best method of administering nebulized medications to children less than 5 years of age. Making a game of the treatment often improves cooperation with young children.

Ongoing care requires frequent evaluation of the child's cardiac, respiratory, and neurologic status, particularly after each bronchodilator treatment. Occasionally bronchodilator therapy worsens the ventilation-perfusion mismatching from pulmonary vascular dilation, causing an increase in hypoxia. In the stable child, pulse oximetry is checked at least hourly. If the child is unable to maintain an adequate oxygen saturation between treatments, continuous pulse oximetry is required and supplemental oxygen is administered to maintain the oxygen saturation greater than 95%.

Supportive nursing interventions include hydration and emotional support. Adequate fluids are necessary to replace increased fluid losses from hyperventilation and diaphoresis and to thin mucus secretions. Clear fluids at room temperature can be encouraged, but cold liquids may trigger bronchospasm. Measures that decrease stress and anxiety include offering information and reassurance to the child and family, providing for comfort needs, and allowing parents to remain with their child.

Discharge teaching with written instructions promotes compliance with outpatient therapy (Box 10-6). Children and parents who understand the disease process, individual triggers, early signs and symptoms of exacerbations, and use of medications are more likely to intervene early and appropriately when symptoms develop. It is helpful to refer to the child's

---

Box 10-6   Discharge Teaching for Asthma in Children*

Review the pathophysiology of asthma.

Discuss factors that "trigger" the child's exacerbations, such as viral infections, cigarette smoke, wood stoves, pets, dust, seasonal pollens, and cold air.

Discuss environmental controls to reduce exposure to common irritants and allergens.

Identify initial signs and symptoms of asthma exacerbation to promote early recognition and interventions.

Teach proper use of peak flow meter and interpretation of results.

Give clear written instructions of prescribed medications. Discuss indications, routes of delivery, and possible side effects.

Teach proper use of metered-dose inhalers and spacers as indicated.

Specify and encourage appropriate follow-up care.

Provide educational resources (see inside cover).

*Discharge teaching includes both parent and child; age-appropriate terminology and materials should be used.

---

presenting signs and symptoms to clarify signs of respiratory distress for the parents. If extensive education or reinforcement is necessary, the family is referred to their primary caregiver or asthma specialist.

FOREIGN BODY ASPIRATION

Etiology.   The aspiration of a foreign body can occur in adults and children of any age, but the incidence of foreign body aspiration (FBA) increases in children less than 4 years of age. Several developmental characteristics contribute to this finding, including infants' and toddlers' tendency to put everything into their mouths and the inability to adequately chew food until the molars have erupted. Commonly aspirated objects include nuts, hot dogs, vegetables and fruits (carrots, raisins, grapes), candy, popcorn, and small toys—or pieces of toys. Children with debilitating diseases such as cerebral palsy have a greater risk of aspirating food and oral secretions.

Pathophysiology.   Foreign bodies that lodge in the upper airways can completely or partially obstruct the airway and cause a life-threatening emergency, but many foreign bodies pass through the larynx and trachea to the peripheral airways. The right mainstem bronchi is more commonly affected because of the larger size and straighter deviation from the trachea.

The location, configuration, type of object ingested, and length of time since the ingestion affect physiologic responses. Smooth, conforming, and occlusive spheres are associated with the highest number of fatal outcomes.[65] Large objects or chunks of food or items with sharp, irregular edges tend to get caught in the larynx. Retained foreign bodies will produce an inflammatory response and lead to a persistent or recurrent infection distal to the object. Air trapping may result from an object that allows air to be inspired but not expired. Atelectasis may develop from a complete obstruction. Objects that swell, such as popcorn or beans, can lead to progressive airway obstruction. Caustic ingestions (e.g., disc battery leakage) or sharp objects can lead to airway perforation. Some small, foreign bodies can lodge in the bronchus and stimulate an irritant reflex that produces bronchoconstriction in both lungs. Lipoid pneumonia can result from the ingestion of oily substances such as peanuts and chips.

Clinical presentation.   The child who has aspirated a foreign body may present with a complete or significantly obstructed airway evidenced by apnea or decreased air entry in all lung fields, inability to speak or cry, severe stridor, cyanosis, an altered level of consciousness, and signs of severe respiratory distress. Most children presenting to the ED with an FBA have a partial airway obstruction. Initial signs and symptoms vary with the size, location, and nature of the foreign body. Physical findings may include inspiratory and expiratory stridor, wheezing, retractions, coughing, drooling, diminished breath sounds distal to the obstruction, or hoarseness. Respirations may be asymmetrical with an expiratory lag on the obstructed side. Signs and symptoms may change if the foreign body changes position.

The child with a foreign body that is not expelled may become asymptomatic. The person who observed the FBA may assume that the foreign body has been coughed out of the respiratory tract and swallowed. Greater than 25% of foreign bodies are not detected for more than a week.[38] The asymptomatic period may last for hours, days, or months, after which complications such as atelectasis, pneumonia, or pulmonary

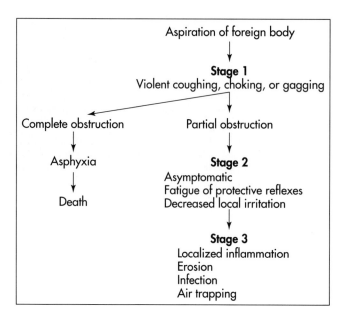

FIG. 10-3.   Stages of foreign body aspiration.

abscess develop. Secondary signs and symptoms are usually related to an infection distal to the retained foreign body and may include recurrent or persistent cough, hemoptysis, fever, rales, wheezing, croup, and focal decrease in breath sounds (Fig. 10-3).

Emergency Department interventions

Diagnosis.   FBA is considered in the differential diagnosis of any previously well child presenting with either an acute onset of choking, coughing, or wheezing or a nonspecific chronic respiratory complaint. Although a positive history is supportive of the diagnosis, a negative history is common.

Most aspirated foreign bodies are not radiopaque; therefore initial chest x-rays are often normal. Nonspecific signs may be visible on the chest x-ray 24 hours after the event. These signs, which include localized air trapping, atelectasis, hyperlucency, mediastinal shifts, or infiltrates, may also be present with asthma, pneumonia, or mucus plugging. Lateral decubitus x-rays may show more specific localized hyperinflation distal to a foreign body. Fluoroscopy may be used to detect and localize foreign bodies in the bronchi.

Treatment.   The treatment for an FBA depends on the degree of airway obstruction. Complete and partial airway obstructions are treated using the basic life support techniques described in Chapter 8. The child with a complete obstruction will require imme-

diate removal of the foreign body by direct laryngoscopy or bronchoscopy. A cricothyroidotomy may be required to oxygenate the child until the object is removed.

The child with a partial airway obstruction also requires the prompt removal of the foreign body. Bronchoscopy to remove the object is ideally performed under general anesthesia in a controlled setting, such as the operating room. Most children who have aspirated a foreign body are treated and released.

Antibiotics are indicated to treat secondary infections, such as pneumonia. If generalized wheezing is present due to reflex bronchoconstriction triggered by an FBA, asthma may be mistakenly diagnosed and treated. In this situation, bronchodilators and steroids will decrease wheezing and improve air flow in the unaffected side only.

Nursing care and evaluation.   Nursing care varies depending on the presentation of the child. If the child has a completely obstructed airway and cannot cough, speak, or cry, obstructed airway maneuvers are performed. Otherwise, coughing is the most effective way of clearing the airway of a foreign object. Blind finger sweeps are not recommended, because the object may be pushed further into the airway (for a complete discussion, see Chapter 8).

If the airway is partially obstructed, the child is placed on a heart rate monitor and pulse oximeter and is closely observed for deteriorating respiratory status, while awaiting bronchoscopic removal of the foreign body. The child is kept quiet and calm to prevent further descent of the foreign body to more inaccessible airways. Oxygen is administered as needed.

Discharge teaching focuses on prevention. Because most pediatric aspirations occur at home, preventive measures primarily focus on home safety. Parents of preschoolers are instructed to keep small objects away from children's reach, cut food into small pieces, avoid hazardous foods or objects such as nuts or hot dogs, and teach their child to chew thoroughly and to avoid putting objects in their mouths. Children should not talk, run, or play with food or objects in their mouths.

NEAR-DROWNING

Etiology. Drowning is defined as death from asphyxia due to submersion in a liquid. Near-drowning refers to survival, at least temporarily, after asphyxia caused by submersion. The most common factors contributing to drowning incidents in the pediatric population are a lack of supervision of younger children and infants and risk-taking behavior and alcohol use in the adolescent population. For these reasons the highest incidence of drowning occurs in children younger than 5 years of age and in adolescents older than 15 years of age. Cervical spine injuries resulting from diving into unknown depths are often associated with near-drowning incidents in adolescent boys. Child maltreatment may also be associated with submersion injuries. Most drownings or near-drownings occur in swimming pools; however, submersion injuries can happen in any body of water, including bathtubs, toilets, pails of water, ponds, and lakes. In infants less than 1 year of age bathtub drownings are most common.

Drowning is the third most common cause of death in children between the ages of 1 and 14 in the United States.[55] It is more common in males, in low-income groups (except middle-class children with pools and boats), and in black children over the age of 3 years.[29,72] The incidence of near-drowning is uncertain, because many events are not reported.

Pathophysiology. With submersion, the child's initial response is breath-holding. Within minutes, the increasing P_{CO_2} level overrides voluntary control of respirations and an involuntary gasp may allow water to enter the larynx. At this point water may be aspirated (wet drowning), or laryngospasm may prevent water from entering the trachea (dry drowning) (Fig. 10-4).

Wet vs. dry drownings. Wet drownings are the more common type of drowning incident. They are associated with the aspiration of water and debris, such as emesis, mud, algae, sewage, and bacteria, which enter the lower airways and damage the alveoli. The result is pulmonary edema, atelectasis, pneumonitis, and intrapulmonary shunting. These conditions exacerbate the asphyxia and hypoxia.

Approximately 10% of near-drowning incidents are dry drownings, where no water enters the trachea. These "dry drownings" are thought to result from severe laryngeal spasm caused by a parasympathetic response to water in the larynx.[62,72] Hypoxia occurs primarily by asphyxiation.

Salt vs. fresh water drownings. Ultimately, the aspiration of both salt water and fresh water results in surfactant deficiencies, hypoxia, and decreased lung compliance. Aspirated hypertonic salt water fosters fluid movement from the plasma to the alveoli, where it dilutes surfactant and washes it out of the alveoli. Fresh water denatures surfactant. The deficiency of functional surfactant results in alveolar collapse and intrapulmonary shunting. Frothy fluid that is produced by alveolar injury is present in the airways and diminishes ventilation in both types of drowning.

Salt water and fresh water submersion injuries are not associated with life-threatening electrolyte imbalances. The amount of fluid aspirated is rarely large enough to affect electrolyte levels. However, large amounts of swallowed fresh water, if not removed promptly, may cause a dilutional hyponatremia.

Hypothermia. Several children have survived prolonged submersion in icy cold water (<20° C). Rapid cooling of the brain is thought to decrease the cerebral metabolic rate, thus protecting the brain from anoxic injury. Children cool faster than adults because of their large surface area to weight ratio. Vasodilation caused by vigorous muscle use during the initial struggle (or alcohol consumption) also enhances heat loss. Rapid cooling is thought to contribute more to prolonged survival after submersion in icy water than the controversial diving reflex theory.[58,72] The diving reflex, which may be triggered in humans by the stimulation of face receptors with icy cold water, preserves function and prolongs survival by causing bradycardia and severe peripheral vasoconstriction with preferential shunting of blood to the heart and brain.

Complications. Children may survive the initial hypoxic event, ischemic tissue damage, or other com-

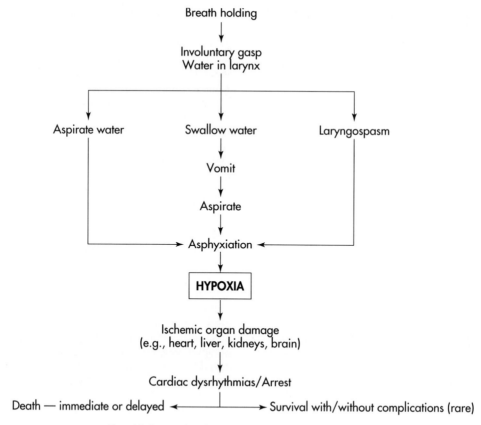

Breath holding

↓

Involuntary gasp
Water in larynx

Aspirate water   Swallow water   Laryngospasm

Vomit

↓

Aspirate

↓

→ Asphyxiation ←

↓

HYPOXIA

↓

Ischemic organ damage
(e.g., heart, liver, kidneys, brain)

↓

Cardiac dysrhythmias/Arrest

Death — immediate or delayed ←———————→ Survival with/without complications (rare)

FIG. 10-4. Pathophysiology of submersion incidents.

plications but later die from permanent sequelae. The brain is most vulnerable to lack of oxygen. Cerebral neurons sustain irreversible damage after 4 to 6 minutes of submersion, whereas the heart and lungs can survive up to 30 minutes.[89] Cerebral edema, herniation, and brain death resulting from anoxia and ischemia are the most common causes of later mortality after near-drowning events.[29] Other complications include dysrhythmias, acute tubular necrosis, liver failure, necrotic bowel, disseminated intravascular coagulation, pneumothorax, pneumomediastinum, and pneumonia.

Clinical presentation. The presentation of near-drowning victims in the ED ranges from cardio-pulmonary arrest to completely asymptomatic depending on the length of submersion, the physiologic response of the child, the degree of immersion hypothermia, and the efficacy of initial resuscitation attempts (Box 10-7). Pulse and respiration may be present due to the initiation of CPR in the prehospital setting or spontaneous recovery after the child was removed from the water. An altered level of consciousness and loss of reflexes may result from cerebral hypoxia, especially if the child was submerged for more than 4 minutes. Pupil size and reactivity varies from normal to fixed and dilated. Hypothermia is almost universal. Severely hypothermic near-drowning victims may appear pulseless due to bradycardia and peripheral vasoconstriction. Ventricular fibrillation may occur because of the irritability of the hypothermic heart. Associated injuries due to abuse, diving or falling (spinal cord or head injuries), or animal bites or stings may be present.

Emergency Department interventions

Diagnosis. Diagnostic testing depends on the child's clinical presentation and the history of the event. However, a baseline chest x-ray and ECG are

---

Box 10-7 Clinical Manifestations of Near-Drowning

Directly related to the degree of consciousness following rescue and resuscitation

Category A: Awake (minimum injury)
  Fully conscious
  May have mild hypothermia
  Mild chest radiographic changes
  Mild arterial blood gas abnormalities

Category B: Blunted sensorium (moderate injury)
  Obtunded
  Stuporous
  Purposeful response to painful stimuli
  Mild to moderate hypothermia
  Respiratory distress (frequently)
  Chest radiographs abnormal
  Arterial blood gas abnormalities

Category C: Comatose (severe anoxia)
  Patient unarousable
  Abnormal response to pain
  Abnormal respiratory pattern
  Seizures
  Shock
  Marked arterial blood gas abnormalities
  Abnormal chest radiographs
  Dysrhythmias
  Metabolic acidosis
  Hyperkalemia/hyperglycemia
  Disseminated intravascular coagulation
  Coma progression:
    Decorticate, Cheyne Stokes respirations
    Decerebrate, central hyperventilation
    Flaccid, apneustic or cluster breathing
    Flaccid, apneic, no detectable circulation

From Wong DL: *Whaley & Wong's essentials of pediatric nursing,* ed 5, St Louis, 1997, Mosby.

ABGs are required to determine the adequacy of ventilation and the extent of hypoxemia and acidosis in seriously affected children.

Other diagnostic tests are obtained to identify associated injuries and complications. Cervical spine x-rays are obtained on all comatose near-drowning victims and any conscious victim with a suspected neck injury. Baseline electrolytes, BUN, creatinine, cardiac isoenzymes, and hemoglobin are obtained to determine complications such as electrolyte abnormalities or ischemic damage to the heart and kidneys. Toxicology screens, alcohol levels, and C-spine x-rays are indicated for adolescent near-drowning victims. Drug levels should be measured on children who are taking anticonvulsants.

Treatment. Because outcomes cannot be accurately predicted, aggressive resuscitation is initiated for virtually all pediatric near-drowning victims. The major goals of near-drowning treatment include the restoration of adequate ventilation and perfusion and the prevention of anoxic brain damage. Emergent care for unconscious near-drowning victims includes the assessment and stabilization of the ABCs with C-spine precautions. Endotracheal intubation is indicated if the Pao_2 is less than 60 on 50% oxygen or if the airway is compromised by an altered LOC.[72] Mechanical ventilation is required for near-drowning victims who do not regain adequate spontaneous ventilations. Persistent hypoxemia despite adequate spontaneous or mechanical ventilation with high percentages of inspired oxygen most likely results from intrapulmonary shunting. Positive end-expiratory pressure (PEEP) often improves ventilation-perfusion matching and therefore oxygenation. PEEP is typically begun at 5 mm Hg in children and 10 mm Hg in adolescents and then titrated to the desired effect. Mechanical ventilation and PEEP may decrease cardiac output, but this can be corrected by fluid resuscitation.

Circulatory management may include cardiac compressions, defibrillation, fluid resuscitation, and inotropic medications. Because severe hypothermia diminishes the ability to defibrillate patients, lidocaine or bretylium may be necessary in addition to continued CPR, defibrillation attempts, and aggressive rewarming. Once perfusion has been restored, fluids are usually restricted to prevent increased intracranial pressure (ICP).

Cerebral resuscitation. Hyperventilation, although controversial, may be used to decrease ICP (see Chapter 7). The efficacy of other methods of

recommended for most near-drowning victims. Although the initial chest x-ray is usually normal, initial films provide a comparison should later pulmonary deterioration arise. The initial ECG documents cardiac function and may rule out a rare previously existing dysrhythmia that could have precipitated the near-drowning event, such as prolonged QT. Nonspecific ST and T wave changes may be present in near-drowning victims with anoxic heart damage.

cerebral resuscitation, including barbiturate coma, sustained hypothermia, and osmotic diuresis, has not been established.[30,72]

Medications. Medications, including steroids and prophylactic antibiotics, have little role in the treatment of near-drowning victims. Diuretics may decrease pulmonary edema but worsen hypovolemia. Sodium bicarbonate is only administered for significant metabolic acidosis that is documented by ABGs, and only after adequate ventilation has been established. Anticonvulsants may be required to control seizures. Sedation with short-acting benzodiazepines and muscle relaxants may be necessary to control ventilation in the intubated child.

Disposition. Determining the disposition of the near-drowning victim is sometimes difficult, because even mildly affected children can deteriorate over the first few days. In general, children with submersions for less than 1 minute without loss of consciousness or the need for resuscitation at the scene may be observed at home. All other children are observed and monitored in the ED or an inpatient unit for at least 4 to 8 hours, or longer depending on their symptomatology. All severely compromised children require admission to an ICU.

Predictors of outcome. Aggressive resuscitation is initiated for most near-drowning victims, because outcomes cannot be accurately predicted. However, the decision to stop or prolong resuscitation efforts can be difficult. Factors associated with poor neurologic outcomes or delayed death include fixed and dilated pupils; flaccidity; decerebrate or decorticate posturing; signs of cerebral edema; the need for CPR in the ED; submersion or resuscitation for more than 25 minutes; delay in resuscitation for more than 10 minutes after rescue; and severe metabolic acidemia (pH < 7.10).[7,51] There is no significant difference in outcomes for salt vs. fresh water submersion incidents. Favorable predictors include young age, submersion time less than 10 minutes, initial core body temperature greater than 35° C, and no clinical signs of aspiration.[7] (There have been reports of survival after prolonged submersion in icy cold water.)

Nursing care and evaluation

Primary assessment and stabilization. Initial interventions depend on the child's condition upon arrival in the ED. The child with an altered level of consciousness or a respiratory arrest will require airway management, and the child with a cardiopulmonary arrest will require CPR and stabilization of the ABCs (see Chapter 8) (Box 10-8). Frequent suctioning of copious secretions is often necessary to maintain a patent airway, and maneuvers such as cricoid pressure (Sellick maneuver) with rescue breathing may be necessary to prevent aspiration.

Box 10-8 Emergency Care of the Unconscious Near-Drowning Victim
Assess and stabilize the airway, breathing, and circulation.
Initiate C-spine precautions as indicated.
Assess neurologic status:
Glasgow Coma Scale
Pupils
Response to pain
Control hypothermia:
Remove wet clothes; dry patient.
Administer warmed IV fluids and oxygen.
Active internal and external warming measures as necessary.
Place the child on a cardiac monitor and pulse oximeter.
Obtain a full set of vital signs; monitor core temperature using a rectal or esophageal probe.
Insert a Foley catheter and NG tube.
Obtain diagnostic tests as ordered (e.g., CBC, electrolytes, BUN, creatinine, glucose, liver function tests, PT, PTT, platelets, fibrin split products, urinalysis, chest x-ray, ABGs, cervical spinal series).
Maintain strict I & O:
Fluid restriction after cardiovascular stabilization to 50%–60% maintenance (in anticipation of increasing ICP).
Correct electrolyte imbalances.
Observe seizure precautions.
Continuously monitor cardiovascular, respiratory, and neurologic status.
Anticipate frequent suctioning in the child requiring ventilatory support.
Observe for increasing ICP.
Provide emotional support to the child and family.
Allow the parents to remain with the child whenever possible.

Cervical spine alignment is maintained when a neck injury is suspected. When ventilatory support is necessary, a nasogastric tube is inserted to prevent regurgitation and aspiration. Removal of gastric contents will also prevent the absorption of large amounts of hypotonic fluid.

Correction of hypothermia. Hypothermia is corrected as soon as possible. A low-reading esophageal or rectal probe is used to measure the core temperature. Passive external warming measures, such as drying the child, removing wet clothes, and applying warm blankets, may be implemented when the core temperature is greater than 35° C (95° F). Warmed IV fluids and heated humidified oxygen may also be given. If the core temperature is between 32° (89.6° F) and 35° C, active external warming with heating blankets, radiant warmers, or heat lamps is initiated. In addition to the above measures, active internal rewarming measures such as warmed peritoneal or gastric lavage, hemodialysis, or cardiopulmonary bypass are required when the child's core temperature is less than 32° C.[29,72] Children with temperatures of less than 28° C (82.4° F) are least likely to respond to resuscitative efforts such as defibrillation. Therefore aggressive rewarming interventions are required until the child is rewarmed to a core temperature of at least 32° C. Activities such as intubation can precipitate ventricular dysrhythmias, particularly ventricular fibrillation. Therefore the child must be monitored at all times during rewarming activities, and interventions must be performed with great care (also see the section on hypothermia in Chapter 27).

Ongoing care and evaluation. After stabilization of the ABCs, the child requires frequent assessments of respiratory status, cardiovascular status, neurologic status, and urinary output. Continuous ECG monitoring and pulse oximetry are required. Additional interventions that may require monitoring vary with the acuity level of the child but may include the insertion of a central venous pressure line or pulmonary artery catheter, Foley catheter, and arterial line. Strict intake and output is required on all children, and continuous evaluation of body temperature with the maintenance of normothermia is necessary.

Parental support. Submersion incidents are highly stressful for parents, who may feel a tremendous amount of guilt regarding the event. The uncertainty of the child's outcome adds to their anxiety and stress. Parents should be allowed to express their needs and

feelings in a nonjudgmental environment. They often require reassurance that everything possible is being done for their child. If the child is discharged, parents are informed of potential delayed complications.

Prevention. Most submersion incidents are preventable. Therefore educational information regarding preventive measures is important. Life-saving measures include promotion of adequate supervision of children, water safety and CPR courses, and swimming lessons for children. Alcohol abuse prevention education for older children is also helpful. Nurses may also advocate for improved legislation concerning physical barriers with closed gates around pools, well-marked hazardous swimming areas, and restriction of alcohol use on boats and in public swimming areas.

CYSTIC FIBROSIS

Etiology. Cystic fibrosis (CF) is an autosomal recessive inherited disorder of the exocrine glands and mucosal surfaces caused by a variety of mutations of the CF gene. It is a generalized disorder that affects multiple body organs, including the lungs, bowel, sweat and salivary glands, pancreas, liver, and male reproductive tract. The severity of the disease varies and is most likely due to the existence of more than 300 CF gene mutations.[10]

CF occurs in approximately 1 in 2500 live births,[17] primarily of Northern European extraction. In the past, CF was fatal by adolescence. Recent discoveries about the causality of CF have led to improved treatments that have increased the life span of children with CF to a mean survival age of 28 to 30 years.[17] With gene therapy research, there is even a reasonable hope for a cure. Respiratory complications continue to be the primary cause of morbidity and mortality. Hepatic decompensation and failure are the second most common cause of death from CF.

Pathophysiology. All CF patients have varying degrees of the following interrelated abnormalities: an abnormal concentration of inorganic ions in serous gland secretions, especially increased sodium chloride in sweat; an increase in viscosity of mucus secretions; and an increased susceptibility to chronic colonization of the respiratory tract by certain bacteria, especially *Pseudomonas aeruginosa.* The underlying CF genetic defect is responsible for the encoding of an abnormal protein that alters the channeling of chloride out of epithelial cells, with a subsequent increase in movement of sodium and water into the cell. Mucus secretions become dehydrated, resulting in thick, sticky mucus that obstructs pulmonary, gastrointestinal, and reproductive structures (Fig. 10-5).

In the lungs, thick mucus blocks bronchial airways and promotes inflammation and infection. Toxic chemicals released during the inflammatory and/or infectious response interfere with lung defenses and damage tissue, thus worsening the infection and inflammation. The bronchial walls become edematous from inflammation, which further increases bronchial obstruction and decreases the ability to clear the thick secretions from the airways. Inflammation may also cause bronchospasm.

Over time, acute and chronic airway inflammation can lead to fibrosis and/or emphysematous blebs. End-stage lung disease eventually causes ventilation-perfusion abnormalities. The resulting hypoxia leads to increased pulmonary vascular resistance, pulmonary hypertension, and cor pulmonale.

Clinical presentation.   Infants with CF are often normal at birth, although some may develop meconium ileus. Initial symptoms usually develop from abnormalities caused by the progressive accumulation of secretions. The most common presentation includes a combination of recurrent respiratory infections, greasy foul-smelling diarrhea, and failure to thrive.[46,88] The most consistent pulmonary symptom is a cough that worsens in frequency, severity, and productivity with progressive pulmonary disease. In general, signs and symptoms of CF vary with the severity of disease and may develop at any time from infancy to adulthood (Box 10-9).

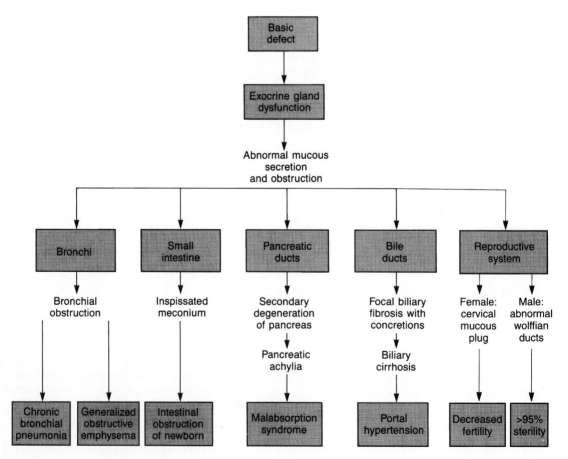

FIG. 10-5.   Effects of exocrine gland dysfunction in cystic fibrosis. (From Wong DL: *Whaley & Wong's essentials of pediatric nursing,* ed 5, St Louis, 1997, Mosby.)

Children with CF frequently present in the ED with acute respiratory or gastrointestinal complications such as pneumonia, pneumothorax, bleeding (lungs, esophagus), or intestinal obstruction. Acute respiratory illnesses are associated with exacerbation of the underlying lung disease. The severity of these pulmonary exacerbations varies. Severe exacerbations of CF are characterized by worsening physical findings, low-grade fever, weight loss, hemoptysis, and pneumothorax. Hemoptysis, which results from the erosion of bronchial arterial blood vessel walls, ranges from mild streaking to massive hemorrhage. Pneumothorax, which presents with a sudden onset of sharp chest pain, is often followed by rapid respiratory decompensation.

Emergency Department interventions

Diagnosis. The diagnosis of CF is rarely made in the ED. However, if certain diagnostic red flags are identified, the child is referred for a sweat chloride test. Chronic cough, nasal polyps in children, and *Pseudomonas* pneumonia strongly increase suspicion of CF. The diagnosis of CF can be made if typical pulmonary and/or gastrointestinal manifestations and/or a close family history of CF are present, plus a sweat CL > 60 mEq/L.[17] Genetic testing is available to confirm the diagnosis, but it does not replace the need for a sweat test because of the numerous mutations of the CF gene.

Diagnostic testing for complications of CF are tailored to the current signs and symptoms. Chest x-rays must be compared to previous films to identify respiratory infections, complications, or disease progression. In the early stages of CF, positive chest x-ray findings include hyperinflation and peribronchial thickening. With progression of the disease, airtrapping, marked pulmonary hyperexpansion, pulmonary infiltrates, and cystic lesions are often present.

Treatment. The goals of CF management include the promotion of optimal nutrition and normal growth, by pancreatic enzyme replacement, fat-soluble vitamin replacement, and a high calorie diet; the delay, or if possible the prevention, of progressive lung disease, by chest physiotherapy and infection control; and prompt recognition and aggressive treatment of complications.[17] Whatever the chief complaint in the ED, these goals should be incorporated into the plan of care.

Chest physiotherapy is an effective method of clearing lower airway secretions and thus decreasing the risk of infection. It is used in routine home management, as well as pulmonary exacerbations. Bronchodilators may be administered before chest physiotherapy to improve mucociliary clearance. Chest physiotherapy is avoided during episodes of substantial bleeding.

Medications used in the treatment of CF and its complications may include antibiotics, nasal decongestants, bronchodilators, and steroids. Mild respiratory exacerbations are treated with oral antibiotics that cover *H. influenzae* and *S. aureus* for 2 to 3 weeks,

---

Box 10-9 Signs and Symptoms of Cystic Fibrosis

Gastrointestinal
Large, bulky, loose, frothy, extremely foul-smelling stools
Voracious appetite (early in disease)
Loss of appetite (later in disease)
Weight loss or failure to grow
Marked tissue wasting
Distended abdomen
Thin extremities
Sallow skin
Evidence of deficiency of fat-soluble vitamins A, D, E, K
Anemia
Signs of meconium ileus (only occurs in 10% of neonates): abdominal distention, vomiting, dehydration, failure to pass stool

Pulmonary
Initial signs:
   Wheezy respirations
   Dry, nonproductive cough
Later signs:
   Increased dyspnea
   Paroxysmal cough
   Evidence of obstructive emphysema and patchy areas of atelectasis
Progressive involvement:
   Overinflated, barrel-shaped chest
   Cyanosis
   Clubbing of fingers and toes
   Repeated episodes of bronchitis and bronchopneumonia

Modified from Wong DL: *Whaley & Wong's essentials of pediatric nursing,* ed 5, St Louis, 1997, Mosby.

whereas moderate to severe exacerbations are treated with parenteral antibiotics or oral ciprofloxacin (in older patients) for 2 to 4 weeks.[17] If *P. aeruginosa* is suspected, a prolonged course of oral ciprofloxacin or parenteral antipseudomonal antibiotics is recommended in addition to nebulized antibiotics such as tobramycin.[10,46] Patients with CF metabolize antibiotics, especially aminoglycosides, faster than normal and therefore may require higher doses to achieve adequate serum levels.[17]

Life-threatening complications, such as profuse hemoptysis, pneumothorax, and acute respiratory distress, usually occur in children with advanced lung disease. When possible, mechanical ventilation is avoided in these children, because weaning from the ventilator can be very difficult. Carbon dioxide retention is usually associated with severe, chronic, irreversible pulmonary disease. At this stage the parents may decide to withhold various interventions such as CPR and intubation. Lung transplants may be considered for children with end-stage disease.

Several treatment methods for CF are currently under investigation. Aerosolized amiloride, a sodium channel blocker, and aerosolized rhDNase have been shown to improve lung function by decreasing the viscosity of sputum and thereby increasing mucociliary clearance.[56] Antiprotease therapy is a promising treatment that reduces the excessive protease activity, which is produced by the inflammatory response.[56,88] Protease damages the airways and is the most likely cause of bronchiectasis. However, more extensive research is required to study the safety and efficacy of antiprotease therapy. Current CF therapies merely deter the progression of the disease, but a cure may be possible through genetic research.

Nursing care and evaluation. The child with CF may present to the ED with mild symptomatology associated with the disease or with signs of advanced disease. While taking the history, one of the most important questions the nurse should ask the parents is their impression of the child's current status. Parents may relate alterations in the child's activities of daily living such as eating, elimination habits (stools), and school attendance, as well as an increase in the use of home oxygen therapy.

The child with signs of respiratory distress is treated as any other child with respiratory distress. The child's baseline oximetry is identified by asking the parents or primary health care providers. Oxygen is used to treat hypoxia, but high-concentration oxygen is administered **only** to children in severe respiratory distress.

Otherwise the oxygen concentration is titrated to maintain the child's oxygen saturation at least greater than baseline or 92%.

If significant hemoptysis is present, venous access is obtained and the amount of blood loss, as well as the circulatory and respiratory status, is monitored. If a pneumothorax occurs, high-concentration oxygen is administered by a nonrebreather mask or, if necessary, bag-valve-mask ventilation; chest tube insertion is anticipated.

The pathophysiology and management of CF are complex and best taught to parents by specialists. However, assessment of the parent's understanding of the disease and reinforcing accurate knowledge are important. The care of children with CF is highly stressful for parents, especially during exacerbations. Emotional support of the child and family fosters successful coping with this ultimately fatal disease.

BRONCHOPULMONARY DYSPLASIA (BPD)

Etiology. Bronchopulmonary dysplasia (BPD) is an acquired chronic cardiopulmonary disease characterized by respiratory distress, oxygen dependence, and abnormal chest radiographs that persist beyond 1 month of age.[1,37] Factors contributing to the development of BPD are oxygen toxicity, positive pressure ventilation, pulmonary inflammation, and nutritional deficiencies. Premature infants (especially younger than 30 weeks gestation) are at highest risk of developing BPD, because their immature lungs are more susceptible to RDS, which often requires oxygen therapy and mechanical ventilation.

The epidemiology of BPD has changed significantly in the past 20 years. The improved survival of extremely premature neonates has increased the overall incidence of BPD. However, the advent of improved therapies such as surfactant, high-frequency ventilation, and steroid administration have decreased the incidence of BPD in neonates older than 30 weeks gestation and diminished the severity of the disease in many neonates. Most of the mortality associated with BPD is due to pulmonary infections.[37]

Pathophysiology. Acute injury to the immature lungs from barotrauma, oxygen toxicity, and/or inflammation causes edema, fibrosis, and muscle hypertrophy. The resultant narrowing of the small airways obstructs air flow, increases airway resistance, and decreases lung compliance. Air becomes trapped in the lungs, resulting in overinflation and atelectasis. Airway hyperreactivity, increased mucus production, inflammation, localized infection; decreased mucociliary clearance; and dynamic obstructive lesions contribute to the airway obstruction.

The pathologic abnormalities associated with BPD lead to an increased work of breathing, ventilation-perfusion mismatching, hypoxia, and in most cases hypercapnia. Acute hypoxia exacerbates the increased airway resistance. Chronic hypoxemia may lead to increased pulmonary vascular resistance, pulmonary hypertension, and cor pulmonale. Pulmonary edema develops from damage to the alveolar capillary unit as increased pulmonary vascular permeability facilitates fluid movement into the interstitium.

The lung function of most infants with BPD returns to normal by 2 to 3 years of age.[37] It is uncertain whether this improvement is due to the repair of the damaged lung, the growth of new lung tissue, or a combination of both. Until BPD resolves, infants are particularly vulnerable to respiratory infections, respiratory failure, growth abnormalities, and developmental delays.

Clinical presentation. The severity of BPD varies from mild to severe depending on the underlying lung pathology. Pulmonary signs and symptoms, including tachypnea with shallow breathing, dyspnea, retractions, cough, paradoxical (or seesaw) respirations, and wheezing, may occur intermittently or continuously. Scattered or diffuse rales or crackles are frequently heard upon auscultation. The infant may have a barrel chest and be small for age. Infants with moderate to severe BPD are often irritable and have feeding and sleeping difficulties. Digital clubbing, if present, is a poor prognostic sign. The presence of tachycardia, tachypnea, hepatomegaly, periorbital edema, and a gallop rhythm suggest right heart failure.

Infants with BPD may present to the ED with viral respiratory infections (especially RSV), complications of the illness, or unrelated illnesses or injuries. Signs and symptoms vary with the etiology of the current problem and the severity of BPD. Unless the child is well known to the ED staff, the parents' perceptions of the child's current status compared to baseline is an important component of the history.

Emergency Department interventions. The degree of diagnostic testing performed and the treatment of the child with BPD depends on presenting signs and symptoms and the chief complaint. Tests may include chest x-rays, ABGs, or ECG if cardiac involvement is suspected. The baseline chest x-ray of the child with BPD characteristically shows scattered areas of atelectasis and patchy areas of hyperinflation. If the infant is on long-term medications such as diuretics or theophylline, serum electrolytes, bicarbonate levels, and drug levels may be required. To best interpret diagnostic test results they must be compared with previous findings to identify variations from baseline.

The treatment of the child with BPD depends on the severity of the disease and may include oxygen therapy, diuretics, and the administration of bronchodilators. Supplemental oxygen may be administered to maintain the oxygen saturation between 92% and 95% to avoid the detrimental effects of hypoxia and the possible damaging effects of hyperoxia. Intermittent or long-term furosemide may be administered to improve lung function by reducing pulmonary edema. Prolonged use of diuretics may result in hypochloremic metabolic alkalosis or renal calculi. Bronchodilators, such as beta-agonists or theophylline, decrease airway resistance and thus improve gas exchange. Theophylline also provides diuresis, respiratory center stimulation, and increased diaphragm strength.[90] The erratic pharmacokinetics of theophylline may decrease lower esophageal sphincter tone, which increases gastroesophageal reflux with potential respiratory sequelae.[37] Corticosteroids, although controversial, may improve ventilatory function in ventilator-dependent or acutely wheezing infants. Broad-spectrum antibiotics may be administered to treat possible bacterial pneumonia in the febrile infant. Mechanical ventilation is used only in the presence of apnea or respiratory failure that does not respond to medical interventions.

Nursing care and evaluation. The infant with BPD and signs of severe respiratory distress is treated emergently. Oxygenation is maximized by administering high-concentration oxygen via a face mask or oxyhood. However, because a high concentration of oxygen can produce detrimental effects in these children, oxygen saturation is maintained between 92% and 95%. Fluid balance is closely monitored and strict intake and output records maintained. Fluid intake is titrated to avoid both dehydration and pulmonary edema.

Supportive care includes interventions to minimize respiratory effort. The use of small frequent feedings prevents stomach distention, which may impair diaphragmatic excursion. Maintaining normothermia prevents the increased oxygen consumption associated with hypothermia or hyperthermia.

Because BPD is a complex disease, the parent's knowledge base is determined and discharge instructions adjusted accordingly. Parents often require emotional support and additional resources when caring for their child. Information is available from the American Lung Association.*

APNEA

Etiology. Apnea is defined as cessation of breathing for longer than 20 seconds—or less if associated with bradycardia, cyanosis, pallor, or marked hypotonia.[85] Apnea is a nonspecific response to a variety of pathologic conditions (Box 10-10). However, a cause is not identified in approximately one half of all infants with apparent life-threatening events (ALTEs).[83] It is thought that primary ventilatory defects present during sleep are the most likely etiology for idiopathic apnea.

Apnea spells are commonly referred to as ALTEs. The relationship between ALTEs and sudden infant death syndrome (SIDS) is unclear, because it is not known whether an ALTE would have progressed to a SIDS death without intervention.

There are three distinct syndromes associated with apnea in children: (1) apnea of prematurity which usually resolves by 35 to 36 weeks post conceptual age[13]; (2) apnea of infancy; and (3) obstructive apnea. Neonates and young infants are particularly susceptible to apnea because of differences in CNS maturity, respiratory reserve, and susceptibility to infectious agents. Apnea in older children more commonly results from obstruction. Obstructive apnea is frequently caused by sleep disorders; other causes may include structural airway abnormalities, such as hypertrophied tonsils and adenoids, subglottic stenosis, tracheomalacia, or craniofacial abnormalities; neuromuscular disorders, such as Down syndrome and muscular dystrophy; metabolic disorders, such as hypothyroidism or severe obesity; and infections, such as croup and epiglottitis.

Pathophysiology. Breathing control, including afferent inputs from the chemoreceptors, lung and airway receptors, and CNS, are immature at birth but develop rapidly over the first year of life. Irregular breathing patterns are common in the young infant. With hypoxemia, adults and older children typically respond with tachypnea that is maintained throughout

*American Lung Association, 1740 Broadway, New York, NY 10019 (212) 315-8700.

Box 10-10   Disorders Associated with Apneic Episodes in Infants

Infection
Sepsis
Meningitis
Respiratory (e.g., pneumonia, bronchiolitis, RSV)

CNS disorders
Seizures
Increased intracranial pressure

Metabolic disorders
Electrolyte imbalances
Hypoglycemia
Inborn errors of metabolism

Cardiovascular disorders
Congenital heart disease

Respiratory disorders
Upper airway obstruction
Aspiration of food, gastric contents, foreign body
Nasopharyngeal reflux
Asphyxia

Gastrointestinal disorders
Gastroesophageal reflux
Swallowing disorders

Other
Hypothermia
Child abuse

Modified from Wagner MH, Chesrown SE: Sudden infant death syndrome and apnea disorders. In Koff PB, Eitzman D, Neu J: *Neonatal and pediatric respiratory care*, St Louis 1993, Mosby.

---

the hypoxic period. Neonates, however, characteristically respond to hypoxemia with a brief increase in respiratory rate followed by depression of the respiratory drive that often results in apnea.[83] Hypoxemia in the neonate also decreases the response to arterial carbon dioxide tension and further depresses the respiratory drive. The infant is particularly vulnerable during sleep because of the decrease in oxygen tension.

Apnea may result from a central respiratory disorder, an obstruction of the airway, or a combination of both (mixed apnea). In central apnea there is no effort to breathe, which is caused by lack of activation of the respiratory musculature. Obstructive apnea results from unsuccessful efforts to breathe because of upper airway obstruction.

Clinical presentation. Parents describe an ALTE as a frightening event that was characterized by some combination of apnea, color change (usually cyanosis or pallor), extreme limpness, coughing, or choking. The infant usually appears completely normal on presentation to the ED, although signs and symptoms of an underlying etiology such as bronchiolitis may be present. If the ALTE was prolonged, the infant may present in respiratory failure or cardiopulmonary arrest.

Emergency Department interventions. Diagnostic testing depends on the presentation of the infant or child. If a significant life-threatening event occurred, an extensive workup is required to determine the etiology of the event, even if the infant or child is asymptomatic. It is often difficult to determine if an event was life-threatening or merely a normal variation, such as periodic breathing or breath-holding. A complete history of the event and risk factors such as prematurity or gastroesophageal reflux (GER) provides the most help in determining the significance of the event (Box 10-11). Diagnostic tests are individualized based on the initial findings and may include a septic workup, ABGs, serum bicarbonate, serum electrolytes, chest x-ray, and ECG.

If the infant is apneic on admission to the ED, immediate resuscitation is begun or continued. After stabilization, treatment is based on the child's clinical presentation and the suspected underlying etiology of the event. Infants with unexplained life-threatening apnea may be admitted for further monitoring and testing or discharged on home monitoring systems. The decision to initiate home monitoring is based on the clinical significance of the current event and the risk of recurrence.

Nursing care and evaluation. Emergent care is initiated for infants with respiratory or cardiac arrest, actual or impending respiratory failure, or a depressed level of consciousness. All infants with a significant history of an ALTE or an unclear history require cardiorespiratory and oxygen saturation monitoring in the ED. The infant's behavior and activities (e.g., sleep and feeding) are observed during the ED stay.

Box 10-11 History for ALTEs

Description of present event
Duration
Color changes, such as cyanosis or pallor
Changes in activity level, posture, and muscle tone, such as limpness or tonic-clonic movements
Other signs and symptoms such as sudden coughing or choking
Activity prior to event, such as last feeding time or sleeping
Recent changes in behavior, activity, appetite, sleep (including restlessness or snoring)
Signs and symptoms of illness, such as fever, tachypnea
Resuscitative efforts/response

Past history
Previous similar episodes
Recent trauma
Recent immunizations
Perinatal events (infants)
    Prematurity; RDS
    Labor and delivery
    Maternal health
    Resuscitative efforts
    Infection
Congenital abnormalities
Chronic illness or disorders, such as BPD or GER

Family history
Seizures
Previous infant deaths
Illness in other family members

From Torrey SB: Apnea. In Fleisher GR, Ludwig S, eds: *Textbook of pediatric emergency medicine,* Baltimore, 1993, Williams & Wilkins.

If the infant is discharged on a home monitor, parents must be well trained in the proper use of the monitor and interventions for future apnea spells (including CPR). Teaching is ideally performed by health care professionals who are specially trained to provide home monitoring education, such as pulmonary advanced practice or community health nurses. Parents are encouraged to keep a log of observations, including the infant's behavior/activity when alarms sound and feeding and sleep patterns. Twenty-four-hour-a-day access to care must be available, as well as regular follow-up care. Parents of infants with ALTEs require extensive psychosocial support and reassurance.

References

1. Abman SH, Groothius JR: Pathophysiology and treatment of bronchopulmonary dysplasia: current issues, *PCNA* 41(2):277-315, 1994.
2. Barkin RM: Cyanosis. In Barkin RM, Rosen P, eds: *Emergency pediatrics,* St Louis, 1990, Mosby.
3. Barkin RM: Respiratory distress (dyspnea). In Barkin RM, Rosen P, eds: *Emergency pediatrics,* St Louis, 1990, Mosby.
4. Barnes PJ: Effect of corticosteroids on airway hyperresponsiveness, *Am Rev Respir Dis* 141:S70-S76, 1990.
4a. Bates B: *A pocket guide to physical examination and history taking,* Philadelphia, 1991, JB Lippincott.
5. Behrman RE: Infections due to respiratory syncytial virus. In Behrman RE et al, eds: *Nelson textbook of pediatrics,* ed 14, Philadelphia, 1992, WB Saunders.
6. Bierman C, Pearlman D: Asthma. In Chernick V, Kendig EL, eds: *Disorders of the respiratory tract in children,* Philadelphia, 1990, WB Saunders.
7. Bierens J et al: Submersion in the Netherlands: prognostic indicators and results of resuscitation, *Ann Emerg Med* 19(12):1390-1395, 1990.
8. Bloomberg GR, Strunk RC: Crisis in asthma care, *PCNA* 39(6):1225-1241, 1992.
9. Boyer KM, Cherry JD: Nonbacterial pneumonia. In Feigin RD, Cherry JD: *Textbook of pediatric infectious diseases,* ed 3, Philadelphia, 1992, WB Saunders.
10. Briars G, Warner J: Cystic fibrosis, *Practitioner* 237:765-770, 1993.
11. Brilli RJ, Benzing G III, Cotecamp DH: Epiglottitis in infants less than 2 years of age, *Pediatr Emerg Care* 5:16-21, 1989.
12. Butt WW et al: Hypoxia associated with helium-oxygen therapy in neonates, *J Pediatr* 106:474-477, 1985.
13. Carroll JL, Marcus CL, Loughlin GM: Disordered control of breathing in infants and children, *Pediatr Rev* 14(2):51-66, 1993.
14. Chameides L, Hazinski MF, eds: *Textbook of pediatric advanced life support,* Dallas, 1994, American Heart Association.
15. Cimolai N, Trombley C, O'Neill D: Diagnosis of whooping cough: a new era with rapid molecular diagnostics, *Pediatr Emerg Care* 12(2):91-93, 1996.
16. Cockroft DW: Airway hyperresponsiveness: therapeutic implications, *Ann Allergy* 59:405-414, 1987.
17. Colin AA, Wohl MEB: Cystic fibrosis, *Pediatr Rev* 15(5):192-200, 1994.
18. Colley JR, Holland WW, Corkhill RT: Influence of passive smoking in parental phlegm on pneumonia and bronchitis in early childhood, *Lancet* 2:1031, 1974.
19. Committee on Infectious Disease: *1994 Red Book: Report of the Committee on Infectious Disease,* ed 23, Elk Grove Village, Ill, 1994, American Academy of Pediatrics.
20. Cooper DM: Chronic cough. In Kell VC, ed: *Practice of pediatrics,* New York, 1987, Harper and Row.
21. Cressman WR, Myer CM: Diagnosis and management of croup and epiglottitis, *PCNA* 41(2):265-276, 1994.
22. Cunningham MJ: Acute otolaryngologic surgical conditions in children, *Pediatr Ann* 235:250-256, 1994.
23. Custer JR: Croup and related disorders, *Pediatr Rev* 14(1):19-29, 1993.
24. Dagan R: Antibiotic treatment of pediatric community-acquired lower respiratory tract infections: challenges and possible solutions, *Respiration* 60(suppl 1):38-44, 1993.
25. DiGiulio GA et al: Hospital treatment of asthma: lack of benefit from theophylline given in addition to nebulized albuterol and intravenously administered corticosteroid, *J Pediatr* 122:464-469, 1993.
26. Evans R: Epidemiology of asthma in childhood, *Pediatrician* 18:250-256, 1991.
27. Ewasyshyn M, Klein M: Progress toward the development of a respiratory syncytial virus vaccine, *Pediatr Pulmonol Suppl* 11:81-83, 1995.
28. Felter RA: Infectious disorders. In Barkin RM, ed: *Pediatric emergency medicine: concepts and clinical practice,* St Louis, 1992, Mosby.
29. Fiser DH: Near-drowning, *Pediatr Rev* 14(4):148-151, 1993.
30. Gonzalez-Rothi RJ: Near drowning: consensus and controversies in pulmonary and cerebral resuscitation, *Heart Lung* 16:474-482, 1987.
31. Gorelick MH, Baker D: Epiglottitis in children, 1979 through 1992: effects of *Haemophilus influenzae* type b immunization, *Arch Pediatr Adolesc Med* 148:47-50, 1994.
32. Grad R, Taussig LM: Acute infections producing upper airway obstruction. In Chernick V, Kendig EL, eds: *Kendig's disorders of the respiratory tract in children,* Philadelphia, 1990, WB Saunders.
33. Griffin MR et al: Risk of seizures and encephalopathy after immunization with the diphtheria-tetanus-pertussis vaccine, *JAMA* 263:1641-1645, 1990.
34. Groothius JR et al: Early ribavirin treatment of respiratory syncytial virus in high risk children, *J Pediatr* 117(5):792-798, 1990.
34a. Haley K, Baker P: *Emergency nursing pediatric*

course provider manual, Chicago, 1993, Emergency Nurses Association.

35. Hall CB: Respiratory syncytial virus: what we know now, *Contemp Pediatr* Nov 1993.

36. Hazinski MF: Children are different. In Hazinski MF: *Nursing care of the critically ill child,* St Louis, 1992, Mosby.

37. Hazinski TA: Bronchopulmonary dysplasia. In Chernick V, Kendig EL, eds: *Kendig's disorders of the respiratory tract in children,* Philadelphia, 1990, WB Saunders.

38. Holinger LD: Foreign bodies of the larynx, trachea, and bronchi. In Bluestone CD, Stool SE, Scheetz MD: *Pediatric otolaryngology,* Philadelphia, 1990, WB Saunders.

39. Houck CS: Anesthetic agents, actions and toxicity. In Holbrook PR, ed: *Textbook of pediatric critical care,* Philadelphia, 1993, WB Saunders.

40. Inselman LS: Tuberculosis in children: an unsettling forecast, *Contemp Pediatr* 7:110-130, 1990.

41. Kairys SW, Olmstead EM, O'Connor GT: Steroid treatment of laryngotracheitis: a meta analysis of the evidence from randomized trials, *Pediatr* 83:683-693, 1989.

42. Kuzel RJ, Clutter DJ: Current perspectives on respiratory syncytial virus infection, *Postgrad Med* 93(1):127-141, 1993.

43. Law BJ: Pertussis. In Chernick V, Kendig EL, eds: *Kendig's disorders of the respiratory tract in children,* Philadelphia, 1990, WB Saunders.

44. Letourneau MA, Schuh S, Gausche M: Respiratory disorders. In Barkin RM, ed: *Pediatric emergency medicine: concepts and clinical practice,* St Louis, 1992, Mosby.

45. Long SS et al: Longitudinal study of adverse reactions following diphtheria-tetanus-pertussis vaccine in infancy, *Pediatr* 85:294-302, 1990.

46. Maclusky I, Levison H: Cystic fibrosis. In Chernick V, Kendig EL, eds: *Kendig's disorders of the respiratory tract in children,* Philadelphia, 1990, WB Saunders.

47. Monem GF, Kissoon N, DeNicola L: Use of magnesium sulfate in asthma in childhood, *Pediatr Ann* 25(3):136-144, 1996.

48. Morgan MJ, Martinez FD: Risk factors for developing wheezing and asthma in childhood, *PCNA* 39(6):1185-1203, 1992.

49. Murphy S, Kelly HW: Management of acute asthma, *Pediatrician* 18:287-300, 1991.

50. Myers JH, Shook JE, Ward MA: Intravenous magnesium for moderate to severe childhood asthma, *Pediatr Emerg Care* 11:5, 1995 (abstract).

51. Nagel FO, Kibel SM, Beatty DW: Childhood near-drowning—factors associated with poor outcome, *SAMJ* 78(6):422-425, 1990.

52. National Asthma Education Program, Expert Panel Report: *Executive summary: guidelines for the diagnosis and management of asthma,* Bethesda, Md, 1991, National Heart, Lung and Blood Institute; National Institutes of Health, Pub No 91-3042A.

53. Nichols DG: Emergency management of status asthmaticus in children, *Pediatr Ann* 25(7):394-400, 1996.

54. O'Brodovich HM, Haddad GG: The functional basis of respiratory pathology. In Chernick V, Kendig EL, eds: *Kendig's disorders of the respiratory tract in children,* Philadelphia, 1990, WB Saunders.

55. Ochsenschlager DW: Near-drowning. In Barkin RM, ed: *Pediatric emergency medicine: concepts and clinical practice,* St Louis, 1992, Mosby.

56. Orenstein DM: Cystic fibrosis, *Curr Prob Pediatr* 4-15, 1993.

57. Orlowski JP: Adolescent drownings: swimming, boating, diving and scuba accidents, *Pediatr Ann* 17:125, 1987.

58. Orlowski JP: Drowning, near-drowning, and ice-water submersions, *Pediatr Clin North Am* 34:75-92, 1987.

59. Orlowski JP, Abulleil MM, Phillips JM: The hemodynamic and cardiovascular effects of near-drowning in hypotonic, isotonic, or hypertonic solutions, *Ann Emerg Med* 18(10):1044-1049, 1989.

60. Ott MJ, Horn M, McLaughlin D: Pediatric TB in the 1990's, *MCN* 20(1):16-20, 1995.

61. Overall JC: Is it bacterial or viral? Laboratory differentiation, *Pediatr Rev* 14(7):251-261, 1993.

62. Pearn J: Pathophysiology of drowning, *Med J Aust* 142:586-588, 1985.

63. Pertussis surveillance: United States: 1986-88, *MMWR* 39:57-66, 1990.

64. Quackenboss JJ, Lebowitz MD, Krzyzanowski M: The normal range of diurnal changes in peak expiratory flow rates: relationship to symptoms and respiratory disease, *Am Rev Respir Dis* 143:323-330, 1991.

65. Reilly JS: Airway foreign bodies: update and analysis, *Int Anesthesiol Clin* 30(4):49-55, 1992.

66. Rice TB, Torres A: Pneumonitis and interstitial disease. In Fuhrman BP, Zimmerman JJ, eds: *Pediatric critical care,* St Louis, 1992, Mosby.

67. Robatham JL: Maturation of the respiratory system. In Shoemaker WC, Thompson WL, Holbrook PR, eds: *Textbook of critical care,* ed 2, Philadelphia, 1989, WB Saunders.

68. Rock MJ et al: Use of ketamine in asthmatic children to treat respiratory failure refractory to conventional therapy, *Crit Care Med* 14(5):514-516, 1986.

69. Schuh S et al: Efficacy of frequent nebulized ipratropium bromide added to frequent high-dose albuterol therapy in severe childhood asthma, *J Pediatr* 126:639-645, 1995.

70. Seidel HM et al: *Mosby's guide to physical examination,* ed 3, St Louis, 1995, Mosby.

70a. Semonin-Holleran R: Trauma in childhood. In Neff JA, Kidd PS: *Trauma nursing: the art and science,* St Louis, 1993, Mosby.

71. Shaw KN, Bell LM, Sherman NH: Outpatient assessment of infants with bronchiolitis, *Am J Dis Child* 145:151-155, 1991.

72. Shaw KN, Briede CA: Submersion injuries: drowning and near-drowning, *Emerg Med Clin North Am* 7(2):355-370, 1989.

73. Sheth KK, Lemanske RF: Pathogenesis of asthma, *Pediatrician* 18:257-268, 1991.

74. Shields WD et al: Relationship of pertussis immunization to the onset of neurological disorders: a retrospective epidemiologic study, *J Pediatr* 113:801-805, 1988.

75. Skinner C: The resurgence of TB, *Practitioner* 237:774-777, 1993.

76. Skolnik NS: Treatment of croup: a critical review, *AJDC* 143:1045-1049, 1989.

77. Smith DW et al: A controlled trial of aerosolized ribavirin in infants receiving mechanical ventilation for severe respiratory syncytial virus infection, *N Engl J Med* 325(1):24-29, 1991.

78. Smith M, Starke J, Marquis J: Tuberculosis and opportunistic mycobacterial infections. In Feigin RD, Cherry JD: *Textbook of pediatric infectious diseases,* Philadelphia, 1992, WB Saunders.

79. Snider DE: Recognition and elimination of tuberculosis, *Adv Intern Med* 98:169-187, 1993.

79a. Soud T: Airway, breathing, circulation, and disability: What is different about kids? *JEN* 18(2):107-116, 1992.

80. Starke JR, Jacobs RF, Jereb J: Resurgence of tuberculosis in children, *J Pediatr* 120:839-855, 1992.

81. Strube PJ, Hallam PL: Ketamine by continuous infusion in status asthmaticus, *Anaesthesia* 41:1017, 1986.

82. Thurlbeck WM: Postnatal human lung growth, *Thorax* 37:564, 1982.

83. Torrey SB: Apnea. In Fleisher GR, Ludwig S, eds: *Textbook of pediatric emergency medicine,* Baltimore, 1993, Williams & Wilkins.

84. Vogt HB: Rhinitis, *Primary Care* 17(2):309-321, 1990.

85. Wagner MH, Chesrown SE: Sudden infant death syndrome and apnea disorders. In Koff PB, Eitzman D, Neu J: *Neonatal and pediatric respiratory care,* St Louis, 1993, Mosby.

86. Walker AM et al: Neurologic events following diphtheria-tetanus-pertussis immunization, *Pediatrics* 81:345-349, 1988.

87. Welliver JR, Welliver RC: Bronchiolitis, *Pediatr Rev* 14(4):134-139, 1993.

88. Wilmott RW, Fiedler MA: Recent advances in the treatment of cystic fibrosis, *PCNA* 41(3):431-451, 1994.

89. Wong DL: *Whaley & Wong's essentials of pediatric nursing,* ed 5, St Louis, 1997, Mosby.

90. Wong DL: Whaley & Wong's nursing care of infants and children, ed 5, St Louis, 1995, Mosby.

90a. Zahr LK, Connolly M, Page DR: Assessment and management of the child with asthma, *Pediatr Nurs,* 15(2):109-114, 1989.

91. Zander J, Hazinski MF: Pulmonary disorders. In Hazinski MF: *Nursing care of the critically ill child,* St Louis, 1992, Mosby.

CHAPTER 11

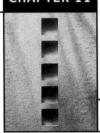

Cardiovascular System

Sharon Redfearn

INTRODUCTION

Diseases and disorders of the cardiovascular system in the neonatal and pediatric population include congenital heart defects, acquired heart diseases, and dysrhythmias. Of these cardiovascular disorders, congenital heart defects comprise the bulk of disease diagnosed and treated. Cardiovascular disorders may be hemodynamically insignificant and require little to no intervention, or the infant or child may present in a shocklike state near death. Often, infants and children with cardiovascular disorders are brought to the emergency room with nonrelated injuries and illnesses.

For the nurse in the emergency department (ED), an understanding of the most commonly occurring defects and disorders is essential to effectively triage the child and render care. This chapter describes emergency nursing care of children with common cardiovascular disorders.

CARDIAC ANATOMY AND PHYSIOLOGY

NEONATE

Embryologically, the fetal heart is formed by 8 weeks of gestational age.[54] During fetal development the placenta serves as the source for oxygenation, and the fetal lungs are filled with fluid. Most of the blood arriving at the fetal heart from the placenta is diverted away from the lungs via the foramen ovale and the ductus arteriosus. With separation of the placenta from circulation, the lungs become the source for gas exchange, and pulmonary vascular resistance declines dramatically. Blood volume to the right heart increases, which in turn increases the volume returning

to the left heart. This increase in left atrial flow closes the flap of the foramen ovale. The ductus arteriosus closes functionally via muscular constriction within 10 to 15 hours after birth.[55] With these changes the right heart acts as the low-pressure circuit, supplying desaturated blood to the lungs, and the left heart operates as the high-pressure circuit, pumping oxygenated blood to the body (Fig. 11-1).

REVIEW OF CARDIAC PHYSIOLOGY

The physiologic function of the heart is to eject blood under pressure. This action is measured in hemodynamic terms such as stroke volume (SV), blood pressure, and cardiac output (CO). CO is the volume of blood ejected by the heart in 1 minute and is the product of both heart rate (HR) and SV. SV is the volume of blood ejected by the heart with each cardiac cycle and increases by age (e.g., the stroke volume of a neonate is approximately 5 ml and of an adolescent is 85 ml).[55] Factors that can influence SV include preload, afterload, and contractility.

Cardiac output =
$$\text{Heart rate (HR)} \times \text{Stroke volume (SV)}$$

Preload, or the diastolic filling condition of the heart, is the degree of myocardial fiber stretch present before contraction. The Frank-Starling law notes the greater the heart is filled during diastole, the greater the volume or force of blood pumped from the ventricle. Factors that affect preload include systemic venous return, total blood volume, and atrial contraction.[46] Afterload is the tension that the ventricular walls must generate to overcome systemic and pulmonary vascular resistance, which oppose ventricular ejection. As a result, increases in systemic and pulmonary vascular resistance will produce an increase in

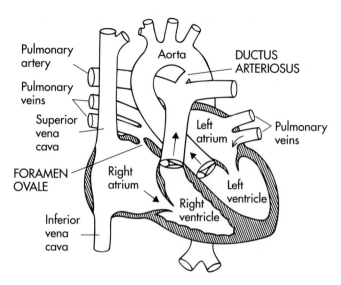

FIG. 11-1. Fetal circulation. In utero blood from placenta enters right atrium. The majority of blood is shunted across foramen ovale to left heart and out aorta. Blood that enters right ventricle and pulmonary artery is shunted across ductus arteriosus to descending aorta. After birth, blood enters right heart from vena cava and is pumped to lungs. From the lungs oxygenated blood returns to left heart via four pulmonary veins. The left ventricle then pumps oxygen-rich blood to the body.

afterload—or the tension that the ventricular walls must overcome. Increases in afterload may result in decreased stroke volume and decreased cardiac output.

Contractility describes the strength of ventricular contraction and is independent of preload, afterload, and heart rate. Sympathetic and parasympathetic stimulation, drugs, electrolyte balance, and acid-base balance affect cardiac contractility. In general, contractility is enhanced by sympathetic stimulation via catecholamines (endogenous and exogenous), digitalis, calcium, and glucagon. Hypoxia, acidosis, and drugs such as barbiturates, propranolol, procainamide, and lidocaine will decrease myocardial contractility.[46]

Although all of these factors affect cardiac output, infants and children are said to be heart-rate dependent for cardiac output. This is because of their limited stroke volume and their limited ability to increase stroke volume to compensate for volume losses. Because stroke volume is small, more rapid heart rates than found in adults are needed to maintain effective cardiac output. When the heart rate drops, cardiac output falls rapidly.

▌ NURSING HISTORY AND PHYSICAL

HISTORY OVERVIEW

When a cardiovascular disorder is suspected the history combined with the physical examination is helpful in triaging and caring for the infant or child in the emergency department. Particular areas to be assessed include the birth history, past medical history, family history, and exercise tolerance. The birth history should include prenatal and postnatal course, as well as birth weight. A comparison of birth weight to current weight will aid in assessing the adequacy of nutritional intake and growth. The past medical history may reveal significant information such as recurring hypercyanotic episodes (also called TET spells) or frequent pulmonary infections, which are often seen in children with congestive heart failure (CHF). The family history may reveal first-generation family members with hypertrophic cardiomyopathy, which can be familial; other members with congenital heart disease; or a past history of rheumatic fever within the family. A history of exercise tolerance for infants is best assessed by their ability to feed. Infants experiencing CHF are unable to take in adequate nourishment to meet the metabolic demands required for growth.

HISTORY ASSOCIATED WITH KNOWN HEART DISEASE

When an infant/child has a significant known heart defect, one of the most important components of the initial history is a comparison of the child's current status to baseline status. Parents (or caregivers) of these children are familiar with the child's normal status and can often relate important information to the nurse. Additional information that should be obtained from the caregiver includes cardiovascular diagnosis, surgical procedures (palliative vs. repair); any residual defects that are present; baseline clinical status; current medications, including dose, schedule, and time of last administration; special diet or formula; and oral vs. nasogastric feedings, including approximate volume taken with each feeding and number of feedings each day.

INITIAL EMERGENCY NURSING ASSESSMENT

The initial examination begins with a general assessment of the infant or child's degree of comfort. Indicators of the degree of comfort include color, respiratory rate and effort, and the ability to respond to the environment. If during this initial assessment the infant/child exhibits signs or symptoms of a significant congenital heart defect such as cyanosis, effortless tachypnea, labored breathing, diaphoresis, irritability, or lethargy, emergent management is required.

The onset and progression of symptoms in infants and children with significant cardiovascular disorders may be abrupt, as might occur when the ductus arteriosus closes in the neonate with a ductal dependent congenital heart defect (CHD) or progress insidiously until acute deterioration occurs, as might be exhibited in the child with supraventricular tachycardia (SVT). With these insidious symptoms, recognition of a cardiovascular disorder may occur only after cyanosis or other signs of clinical deterioration are present such as lethargy, refusal to feed, or oliguria (e.g., no wet diapers by history) (Box 11-1).

OBSERVATION

Color. Color reflects perfusion and oxygenation and is best observed in the oral mucosa, tongue, skin, and nailbeds. A cyanotic or slate-blue color occurs in the presence of at least 4 to 5 g/100 ml of deoxygenated hemoglobin in the blood. Some forms of cyanosis occur in the normal child; for example, circumoral cyanosis is common in infants and children when chilled. Acrocyanosis, which is blueness of the hands and feet, is a normal finding in newborns.

Extremities. Evaluation of the extremities for capillary refill and clubbing of the digits will provide clues as to the child's perfusion status and the presence of chronic hypoxia. Normal capillary refill in the extremities is less than 2 seconds. Greater than

---

Box 11-1 Clinical Manifestations of Congenital Heart Disease

Infants

Cyanosis—generalized; or highly vascularized areas such as the mucous membranes, lips and tongue, conjunctiva

Cyanosis peripheral or central during exertion such as crying, feeding, straining, or when immersed in water

Dyspnea, especially following physical effort such as feeding, crying, straining

Fatigue

Poor growth and development (failure to thrive)

Frequent respiratory tract infections

Feeding difficulties

Hypotonia

Excessive sweating

Syncopal attacks such as paroxysmal hyperpnea, anoxic spells

Older children

Impaired growth

Delicate, frail body build

Fatigue

Dyspnea

Orthopnea

Digital clubbing

Squatting for relief of dyspnea

Headache

Epistaxis

Leg fatigue

From Wong, DL: *Whaley & Wong's essentials of pediatric nursing,* ed 5, St. Louis, 1997, Mosby.

---

4 to 5 seconds indicates poor cardiac output. Clubbing of the nails can be found in infants and children with chronic pulmonary diseases and cyanotic congenital heart defects and is due to chronic hypoxemia and polycythemia. It is caused by thickening of the tissues at the base of the nail secondary to capillary engorgement[13] (Fig. 11-2).

Chest and abdomen. The chest and abdomen are inspected for symmetry. The apical impulse is palpated for location. If the apical impulse is hyperdynamic it may indicate volume overload, as occurs in congestive heart failure. The apical pulse

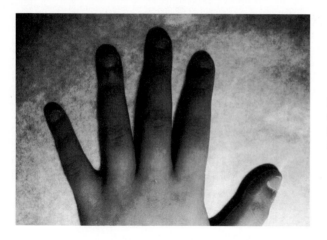

Fig. 11-2. Clubbing of the extremities observed in conditions producing chronic hypoxia such as cyanotic congenital heart defects or chronic pulmonary disorders.

and peripheral pulses are palpated for discrepancies. Children with right or combined ventricular hypertrophy may present with a bulging precordium.

Vital Signs

Tachypnea is a sensitive and reliable sign of congestive heart failure in infants and children. Tachypnea observed in congestive heart failure is typically effortless with rates as high as 80 to 100 per minute. Intercostal retractions, nasal flaring, and head bobbing are often observed.

Tachycardia in infants and children is a nonspecific finding that can be related to fever, anxiety, congestive heart failure, anemia, supraventricular tachycardia, or shock. Because parasympathetic innervation of the sinus node is dominant in the newborn, short episodes of bradycardia (HR < 90) are common in full-term infants and are usually benign.[35] In these infants, activities such as eating, nasopharyngeal suctioning, defecating, and hiccupping may contribute to a nonpathologic bradycardic event.

Blood pressure is a useful indicator of cardiac output. To obtain accurate blood pressures, the bladder of the cuff must cover two thirds of the upper arm or leg. Pressures obtained in the leg are normally higher than those in the arm. Children with known or suspected aortic arch defects, such as those with unequal pulses in the upper and lower extremities or hypertension, should have blood pressures taken in the legs and arms. A systolic pressure in the upper extremities that is more than 20 mm Hg higher than in the lower extremities is indicative of an aortic arch defect such as coarctation of the aorta.[35]

Auscultation

When auscultating the thorax for pulmonary and cardiac sounds, it is helpful to first listen to inspiratory and expiratory lung sounds and then identify abnormal sounds such as rales (crackles), wheezes, rhonchi, or stridor. Rales or crackles in infants are more commonly suggestive of pneumonia than cardiac pathology.[13] Rales associated with CHF usually represent overt pulmonary edema due to advanced myocardial failure.

When auscultating cardiac sounds, S_1 and S_2 must first be identified. Closure of the tricuspid and mitral valves is represented by S_1 and closure of the aortic and pulmonary valves is represented by S_2. There is a normal physiologic split of S_2 on inspiration, but it is a single sound on expiration.

Auscultation of a cardiac murmur may be the first sign that a cardiovascular disorder is present; however, the absence of a murmur does not always correlate with the absence of congenital heart defect. On the other hand, all murmurs heard on auscultation are not indicative of acquired or congenital heart disease. Approximately 30% to 50% of children have functionally insignificant murmurs not associated with cardiovascular disease. These innocent flow murmurs (functional murmurs) can be heard from infancy through adolescence and are easily auscultated in children because of their relatively thin chest walls. Fever, anxiety, and anemia will intensify flow murmurs.[29]

Murmurs are identified by their timing in the cardiac cycle. Thus, murmurs occurring during systole are systolic murmurs and those noted in diastole are diastolic murmurs. Most murmurs appreciated during auscultation are systolic. Diastolic murmurs may be

---

Box 11-2   Grading of Murmurs

Grade 1	Faint murmur, may be very difficult to hear
Grade 2	Soft murmur that is easily heard
Grade 3	Prominent, loud murmur
Grade 4	Loud murmur, with a palpable thrill
Grade 5	Very loud murmur, with a palpable thrill
Grade 6	Murmur that can be heard with the stethoscope off the chest

---

difficult to auscultate and when heard are indicative of significant cardiac disease. Murmurs that need further investigation include those that radiate to the axilla and back, loud murmurs with palpable thrills, murmurs that are continuous in nature (occupies diastole as well as systole), and murmurs noted in diastole[52] (Box 11-2).

PALPATION

The chest wall, liver edge, and upper and lower peripheral pulses are palpated during the examination. The chest wall is palpated for the presence of thrills by placing the hand over the anterior chest wall at the left sternal border. Thrills are significant and suggestive of an obstructive lesion such as pulmonary stenosis. The liver edge is palpated to identify the presence of hepatomegaly, which combined with tachypnea and tachycardia is suggestive of congestive heart failure. The liver edge in infants is normally 2 to 3 cm or finger-widths below the right costal margin (RCM) and by 4 to 5 years of age is 1 cm below the RCM.[13] Palpation of the upper and lower extremity pulses will identify discrepancies in strength or the absence of lower extremity pulses. These findings are suggestive of an aortic arch abnormality such as coarctation of the aorta.

CONGENITAL HEART DEFECTS (CHDs)

INCIDENCE AND ETIOLOGY

The incidence of congenital heart defects is reported as 0.8% or 8 in 1000 live births;[33] however, when a couple has an infant with a congenital heart defect, the risk of recurrence is approximately 3% or 3 in 100. The etiology of congenital heart defects is cited as multifactorial; that is, a genetic predisposition interacts with an environmental trigger resulting in cardiovascular maldevelopment.[47] Of all the causes of congenital heart defects, 8% occur in association with a syndrome and are genetic, 2% occur secondary to environmental factors, and the remaining 90% occur due to multifactorial inheritance. With recent advances in human genetics and mapping techniques, alterations in certain chromosomes are noted to occur with specific congenital heart defects (e.g., missing arm of chromosome 22, which is associated with DiGeorge syndrome and tetralogy of Fallot).[2]

HEMODYNAMICS OF CONGENITAL HEART DEFECTS

Introduction. Congenital heart defects are sometimes classified as acyanotic or cyanotic, but they can also be described by their hemodynamic properties, such as congenital heart defects that increase pulmonary blood flow—left-to-right shunts; defects that decrease pulmonary blood flow—right-to-left shunts; and defects that are obstructive. Congenital heart defects can and often do present in combinations. For some defects to be compatible with life an additional defect such as a patent ductus arteriosus, a patent foramen ovale, an atrial septal defect, or a ventricular septal defect must be present (Box 11-3).

Left-to-right shunts. Normally the ratio of pulmonary blood (Qp) flow to systemic blood (Qs) flow is 1:1 (Qp/Qs). However, in the child with a congenital heart defect this ratio will change if blood is shunted from either the left-to-right side of the heart or right-to-left side of the heart. Left-to-right shunting reflects the flow of blood from the high-pressure systemic circuit of the left heart to the low-pressure pulmonary circuit of the right heart. When left-to-right shunting occurs pulmonary blood flow increases. If the volume of blood flow is significant congestive heart failure will result. Magnitude of the shunt is determined by the size of the defect and by relative resistances of the systemic and pulmonary circuits. Hemodynamically significant left-to-right shunting is considered 2:1 or greater.[43] Because blood is shunted away from systemic circulation and back into the pulmonary circuit, resulting in an absence of cyanosis, these defects are sometimes referred to as *acyanotic*. This term is misleading, because children with acyanotic lesions can develop cyanosis. Congenital heart

---

Box 11-3 Summary of Congenital Cardiac Defects

Left-to-right shunts (acyanotic)
Patent ductus arteriosus (PDA)
Atrial septal defect (ASD)
Ventricular septal defect (VSD)
Complete atrioventricular canal defect
   (CAVCD)

Right-to-left shunts (cyanotic)
Transposition of the great arteries (TGA)
Tetralogy of Fallot (TOF)
Total anomalous pulmonary venous return
   (TAPVR)
Truncus arteriosus (TA)
Tricuspid atresia
Hypoplastic left heart syndrome (HLHS)

Obstructive lesions
Aortic stenosis (AS)
Pulmonic stenosis (PS)
Coarctation of the aorta (COA)

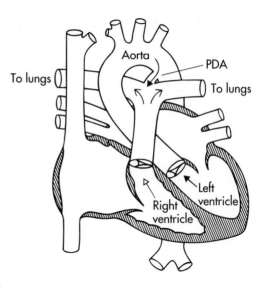

FIG. 11-3. A patent ductus arteriosus is a channel between the aorta and pulmonary artery. Blood is shunted from aorta (or high-pressure circuit) to pulmonary arteries and lungs (low-pressure circuit). The result is an increase in pulmonary blood flow.

defects commonly classified as acyanotic include patent ductus arteriosus, atrial septal defect, ventricular septal defect, and atrioventricular canal defect.

Right-to-left shunts. Defects that produce right-to-left shunts commonly produce cyanosis as oxygen-poor blood bypasses the pulmonary circuit and is mixed with systemic blood. This explains why these lesions are sometimes referred to as *cyanotic defects.*

Cyanotic congenital heart defects typically present within the first weeks of life, which coincides with the normal closure of the ductus arteriosus. In these infants the ductus arteriosus often provides the only means of pulmonary blood flow. The infant may be discharged from the nursery as a well newborn and indeed behave as any infant until closure of the ductus. Depending on the defect and any other associated defects, infants or children may manifest signs and symptoms of congestive heart failure, pulmonary edema, and/or shock. Congenital heart defects that can produce cyanosis include transposition of the great arteries, tetralogy of Fallot, total anomalous pulmonary venous return with pulmonary vein obstruction, truncus arteriosus, tricuspid atresia, and hypoplastic left heart syndrome.

Obstructive defects. Obstructive lesions may occur on the right or left side of the heart and produce an increase in afterload of the affected ventricle. Over time this leads to ventricular hypertrophy and chamber enlargement. When an obstruction is combined with another defect it will produce shunting of the blood from the area of high resistance to the area of low resistance. For example, in the child with a severe obstruction to right ventricular flow such as pulmonary stenosis and VSD, cyanosis may occur as blood is shunted away from the pulmonary circuit, through the VSD, and into systemic circulation. Defects that are classified as obstructive include pulmonary stenosis, aortic stenosis, and coarctation of the aorta.

ACYANOTIC CONGENITAL HEART DEFECTS WITH LEFT-TO-RIGHT SHUNTING

PATENT DUCTUS ARTERIOSUS (PDA)

Etiology. Patent ductus arteriosus is the persistence of a normal fetal vascular channel between the pulmonary artery and the aorta (Fig. 11-3). Failure or delay of ductal closure may occur in infants born at high altitudes; as part of the rubella syndrome; and in premature neonates. The incidence of patent ductus arteriosus is 1 in 2000 live births in full-term infants and comprises approximately 5% to 10% of all congenital heart defects.[5,22] PDAs occur with equal frequency in males and females.

Not all PDAs are isolated congenital heart defects; they may occur in conjunction with cyanotic congenital heart defects. When additional defects are present, the PDA may provide the only source of blood flow to the lungs.

Pathophysiology.   In the normal newborn closure of the PDA within the first 24 to 72 hours of life prevents shunting of blood from the area of high resistance (aorta) to the area of low resistance (pulmonary artery). If the PDA remains open, blood is shunted from the aorta to pulmonary artery (left-to-right shunting), resulting in increased blood flow to the lungs. The magnitude of the shunt and therefore the amount of pulmonary blood flow is determined by the radius of the ductus arteriosus and the resistance difference between the aorta and the pulmonary artery.[5]

Clinical presentation.   Clinical presentation depends on the age of the child; size of the PDA; and the volume of blood being shunted into the pulmonary artery. Most infants are asymptomatic and are only diagnosed when auscultatory findings reveal a continuous or "machine like" murmur days or weeks after birth.[23]

PDAs are classified as small, moderate, and large. Large shunts will produce symptoms of congestive heart failure, which include full, bounding peripheral pulses, a wide pulse pressure, hyperdynamic precordium, and a continuous murmur. Moderate shunts may produce signs of congestive heart failure, particularly when the infant is less than 3 months of age.[5] After this time, compensatory mechanisms such as myocardial hypertrophy may be present and symptoms may decrease. Typically infants with moderate shunts are tachypneic, irritable, feed poorly, and demonstrate slow weight gain. Signs of moderate shunting in the older child include easy fatigability and slightly retarded physical development. Physical examination will reveal increased heart size; full, bounding peripheral pulses; a wide pulse pressure; a hyperdynamic precordium; and a loud continuous murmur.

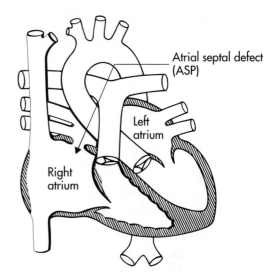

FIG. 11-4.   An atrial septal defect is characterized by an opening in the atrial septal wall. During diastole, blood shunts from left atrium to right atrium. The subsequent increase in right ventricular volume produces an increase in pulmonary blood flow.

Small shunts produce a minimal increase in pulmonary blood flow; therefore, congestive heart failure will not occur. In these children physical growth will be normal; however, on auscultation a continuous murmur will be noted.

ATRIAL SEPTAL DEFECTS (ASDs)

Etiology.   An atrial septal defect is an opening or a hole in the septum between the right and left atria that results when the atrial septum fails to form in early fetal life (Fig. 11-4). Atrial septal defects can be located anywhere in the atrial septum and may consist of single or multiple openings. ASDs are named according to their location along the atrial septum; for example, if the defect is located high in the septum it is called a *sinus venosus defect,* if it is located in the center of the septum it is called an *ostium secundum defect,* if it is low in the septum it is known as an *ostium primum defect,* and if it is found at the coronary sinus it is called a *coronary sinus ASD.* The most commonly seen ASD is of the ostium secundum type.[23] The incidence of atrial septal defects is approximately 7% of all congenital cardiac anomalies, and ASDs are more common in females than males with a 2:1 sex ratio.[33]

Pathophysiology. Atrial septal defects produce left-to-right shunting, with the exception of the coronary sinus ASD. Shunting begins once pulmonary vascular resistance falls after birth. The amount of shunting through an atrial septal defect is determined by the size of the defect and the ability of the ventricles to distend. Because the mature right ventricle is thinner and more compliant than the left, blood from the left atrium preferentially flows across the atrial septal defect to the right heart during diastole. The subsequent increase in right ventricular volume produces an increase in pulmonary blood flow. The increased flow of blood across the pulmonic valve produces physiologic pulmonic stenosis.

Clinical presentation. Few overt symptoms are associated with ASDs, and in fact most children are asymptomatic. The exceptions are infants or children with more than one CHD, such as a VSD combined with a small left ventricle, who may develop signs of congestive heart failure.[23] Generally, auscultation of a heart murmur on physical exam provides the only clue that a defect is present. Classic findings during auscultation include a systolic murmur along the left sternal border, which may also be heard in the back, and fixed splitting of S_2 (meaning that it is unaltered by respiration). Infants with large shunts may have some degree of growth retardation and an increased susceptibility to respiratory infections. Congestive heart failure rarely occurs in children with ASDs unless other cardiac anomalies are present.

VENTRICULAR SEPTAL DEFECTS (VSDs)

Etiology. A ventricular septal defect is an opening or hole in the ventricular septal wall and results from a delay in closure of the intraventricular septal wall during early fetal cardiac development (Fig. 11-5). Reasons for delays or incomplete closure are unknown. VSDs may be located anywhere along the septal wall and can consist of one hole or multiple holes of varying shapes and sizes.

Ventricular septal defects are the most common congenital heart defects found after the first week of life, accounting for approximately 20% of all congenital heart defects.[26,32] The incidence of VSD is approximately 1.5 to 2.5 per 1000 live births and it is slightly more prevalent in females than males, occurring with a frequency of 56% in females and 44% in males.[34] Approximately 50% of all VSDs undergo spontaneous closure within the first 6 months of life.[23]

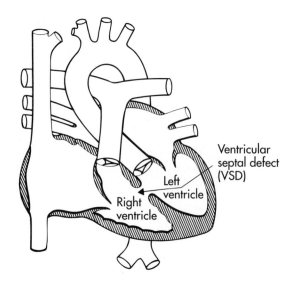

FIG. 11-5. Ventricular septal defects are characterized by an opening between the ventricular septal walls. Blood from the left ventricle (high-pressure circuit) is shunted to the right ventricle (low-pressure circuit), producing an increase in pulmonary blood flow.

Pathophysiology. The hemodynamic properties of the ventricular septal defect are determined by the size of the defect and the difference in pulmonary and systemic vascular resistance. Ventricular septal defects may be small, moderate, or large. Small VSDs produce little shunting, which is usually of no hemodynamic significance. Moderate and large VSDs, however, have moderate to large left-to-right shunts with volume overload of the pulmonary circuit, left atrium, and left ventricle. If unrepaired, large VSDs will cause irreversible pulmonary vascular disease. Once this occurs there is marked elevation of pulmonary vascular resistance, which produces right-to-left shunting. This reverse shunting through a VSD secondary to pulmonary hypertension is called *Eisenmenger's syndrome.*

Clinical presentation. Symptoms associated with VSDs are determined by the size of the shunt. Small VSDs will produce a small left-to-right shunt of no hemodynamic significance. These children, despite the presence of a systolic murmur along the left sternal border, will be otherwise asymptomatic.

Moderate and large shunts are generally identified in early infancy, as pulmonary resistance falls and a loud systolic murmur is auscultated or overt signs of congestive heart failure develop. Although infants and children with moderate defects may present in congestive heart failure, they more typically present with a history of frequent respiratory infections and tiring easily during feeding or exercise. Large defects, however, will produce signs and symptoms of congestive heart failure. On physical examination the infant will be tachypneic with a respiratory rate greater than 60 times per minute—often 80 to 100 times per minute—and hepatomegaly will be present. Feeding is a strenuous activity for these infants and they will exhibit tiring and sweating with feeds. Often they fail to thrive to the extent that they are unable to exceed their birth weight.

COMPLETE ATRIOVENTRICULAR CANAL DEFECT (CAVCD)

Etiology. A complete atrioventricular defect results when there is an interruption or deficiency during the formation of the endocardial cushions. It is characterized by a large atrioventricular septal defect and a common atrioventricular valve. This defect comprises approximately 5% of all congenital heart defects and occurs with equal frequency in both sexes.[22] Atrioventricular (AV) canal defects are present in 50% of patients with Down syndrome.[23,47]

Pathophysiology. In a complete AV canal defect the bottom portion of the atrial septum is open, and the top portion of the ventricular septum is open. Because the atria and ventricular septa are deficient, the mitral and tricuspid valves cannot attach normally to the septa. Thus there is one atrioventricular valve that extends across the open septum (Fig. 11-6). Because of the open septum, significant left-to-right shunting occurs as pulmonary vascular resistance decreases after birth. The resulting increase in pulmonary blood flow initially produces congestive heart failure. With the increase in pulmonary blood flow, these infants subsequently develop pulmonary vascular disease as pulmonary vascular resistance rises. Pulmonary blood flow will decrease and cyanosis occurs.

Clinical presentation. Complete AV canal defects are usually identified in early infancy because of the significant increase in pulmonary blood flow and the resulting symptoms of congestive heart failure. These infants are typically small and undernourished, are tachypneic, and may present to the emergency department with frequent respiratory infections. On auscultation a loud holosystolic murmur and middiastolic murmur will be heard.

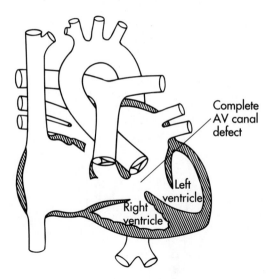

FIG. 11-6. A complete atrioventricular canal defect is characterized by the absence of the bottom portion of the atrial septum and the top portion of the ventricular septum. Mitral and tricuspid valves are one. Initially shunting is left-to-right. Over time pulmonary vascular resistance will rise, producing right-to-left shunting.

▮ OBSTRUCTIVE DEFECTS

PULMONARY STENOSIS (PS)

Etiology. Pulmonary stenosis (PS) is defined as an obstruction to outflow from the right ventricle into the pulmonary artery (Fig. 11-7). It can occur at the level of the valve, the infundibulum (area beneath the pulmonary valve), the pulmonary trunk, or the peripheral pulmonary arteries. The most frequent site of obstruction is at the valvular level and is caused by abnormal formation of the valve leaflets during fetal cardiac development. Valvular pulmonic stenosis is classified as mild, moderate, or severe depending on the degree of stenosis present. The incidence of isolated pulmonary stenosis is approximately 8% to 10% of all congenital heart defects, and it occurs more frequently in females than males.[28,51]

Pathophysiology. Pulmonary stenosis is an obstructive disorder that produces an elevation in right ventricular afterload. If the defect is classified as mild, the slight increase in pressure is generally well tolerated. When the defect is severe, the elevation in right

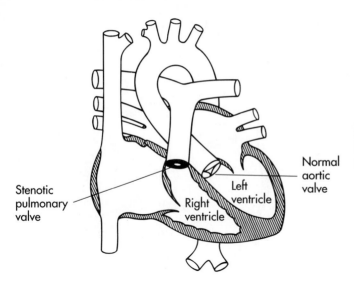

Stenotic
pulmonary
valve

Right
ventricle

Left
ventricle

Normal
aortic
valve

FIG. 11-7. Pulmonary stenosis is characterized by an obstruction to pulmonary blood flow, producing an increase in right ventricular pressure.

ventricular afterload becomes significant. Over time this increased pressure can lead to right ventricular hypertrophy. With the development of hypertrophy, diastolic compliance of the right ventricle is reduced. The right atrium must therefore contract more vigorously to fill the ventricle. This increase in right atrial pressure will ultimately produce right atrial enlargement and hypertrophy. As pressure increases in the right atrium—above pressures in the left atrium—the foramen ovale may be forced open, resulting in a right-to-left shunt. If this occurs, cyanosis and decreased pulmonary blood flow will result.

Clinical presentation. Infants and children with mild pulmonary stenosis are typically asymptomatic and are usually diagnosed when a murmur is heard on routine auscultation. The murmur associated with PS is characterized as a soft systolic murmur heard best over the second intercostal space along the left sternal border. A click may be audible, which is caused by opening of the stenotic valve.

Infants and children with moderate to severe pulmonary stenosis may be asymptomatic or may demonstrate cyanosis secondary to right-to-left shunting at the atrial level either through a stretched foramen ovale or an ASD. Because these children are limited in their ability to increase right ventricular output during exercise, exercise intolerance and even syncope may occur. The child with PS and symptoms of chest pain, dyspnea, fatigue, or syncope is treated emergently.

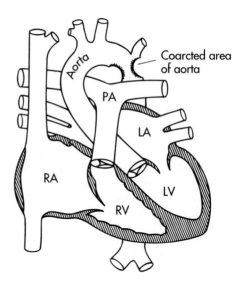

Aorta

PA

Coarcted area
of aorta

LA

RA

LV

RV

FIG. 11-8. Coarctation of the aorta characterized by a narrowing of the aorta, producing an increase in left ventricular afterload.

COARCTATION OF THE AORTA (COA)

Etiology. Coarctation of the aorta is described as a congenital narrowing of the aorta, which may be localized or significant in length (Fig. 11-8). This narrowing most frequently occurs at the junction of the ductus arteriosus and the aortic arch, just distal to the left subclavian artery.[40] The development of COA is felt to be related to changes in cardiac flow patterns in utero.[58]

Coarctation of the aorta is responsible for approximately 7% of all congenital heart defects and is the second leading cause of cardiovascular death in the first month of life.[58] There is a male predominance of 2:1, and approximately 40% of infants with COA will also have a ventricular septal defect.[23]

Pathophysiology. Coarctation of the aorta is an obstructive disorder that produces an increase in left ventricular afterload. Defects may be severe or discrete. If the defect is discrete it may not be discovered in early life. Also, collateral vessels will allow blood from the ascending aorta to circumvent the coarcted area. As left ventricular pressures increase, ventricular hypertension and hypertrophy can develop. When an isolated COA is severe it is usually discovered within days of birth as the apparently healthy neonate's ductus arteriosus closes, resulting in left ventricular failure.

Infants with both coarctation of the aorta and a VSD are rarely asymptomatic. This is because the coarctation, which obstructs systemic blood flow, forces blood to be shunted across the VSD (left-to-right shunting), increasing pulmonary blood flow. This in turn increases the amount of blood returning to the left ventricle from the lungs, contributing to further volume overload and ventricular failure.

Clinical presentation. The asymptomatic infant or child will not be diagnosed until a routine examination reveals hypertension or the presence of a murmur. The classic murmur is a systolic murmur that radiates to the back and is accompanied by a thrill. However, many times the murmur may be soft and unimpressive. On physical examination the pulses in the lower extremities will be absent or weak as compared to pulses in the upper extremities. If blood pressures in the extremities are obtained, the upper extremities will have a systolic pressure of approximately 20 mm Hg or greater than the lower extremities.[35]

Infants with severe coarctation of the aorta with or without a ventricular septal defect are tachypneic from birth and may develop congestive heart failure as early as the third or fourth day of life. Infants with the combined defects of COA and VSD usually become symptomatic between the seventh and tenth day of life. These infants often present with severe tachypnea; gross evidence of congestive heart failure, including

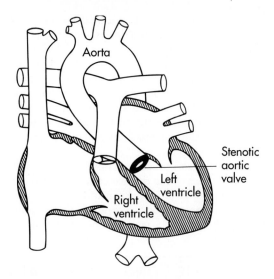

FIG. 11-9. Aortic stenosis is characterized by malformation of the aortic valve. This obstruction produces an increase in left ventricular afterload.

hepatomegaly and intercostal retractions; and the absence of peripheral pulses. A murmur may be difficult to auscultate because of the tachycardia and noisy respirations.

VALVULAR AORTIC STENOSIS (AS)

Etiology. Aortic stenosis is caused by malformation of the aortic valve during fetal cardiac development and is characterized by thickening or dysplasia of the valve leaflets or fusion of the valve leaflets (Fig. 11-9). The incidence of valvular aortic stenosis is cited as 3% to 6% of all congenital heart defects, and it occurs four times more frequently in males than females.[20,22]

Pathophysiology. Valvular aortic stenosis is classified by the degree or severity of obstruction across the stenotic valve and can be mild, moderate, or severe. In all cases the malformed aortic valve is unable to open completely, obstructing blood flow from the left ventricle. This obstruction increases left ventricular afterload and oxygen consumption. With significant increases in left ventricular afterload, hypertrophy will develop; with the associated increase in myocardial oxygen consumption, myocardial ischemia can occur.

Clinical presentation. When the infant or child is asymptomatic, normal growth and development will be observed. The child may not be diagnosed until a heart murmur is discovered during a routine physical examination. The murmur of aortic stenosis is systolic and can be appreciated best over the right upper sternal border. It is usually accompanied by both a thrill and an early systolic click, caused by opening of the stenotic valve. As cardiac output increases with age, blood flow across the aortic valve increases and aortic stenosis can progress from mild to moderate and from moderate to severe.

Infants with severe aortic stenosis develop congestive heart failure within the first couple months of life and can present in shock—ashen and pulseless. These infants may be cyanotic secondary to pulmonary edema with tachypnea, rales, and hepatomegaly.

CYANOTIC CONGENITAL HEART DEFECTS WITH RIGHT-TO-LEFT SHUNTING

TETRALOGY OF FALLOT

Etiology. Tetralogy of Fallot is the most commonly seen cyanotic congenital heart disease. It is characterized by a large and unrestricted ventricular septal defect, pulmonary stenosis and/or infundibular narrowing, an overriding aorta, and right ventricular hypertrophy (Fig. 11-10). It is among the three most common cardiac lesions requiring cardiac catheterization or surgery in the first year of life.[27] The incidence of tetralogy of Fallot is approximately 10% to 11% of all congenital heart defects,[22] with a slight predominance of males over females. The etiology of tetralogy of Fallot is unknown.

Pathophysiology. The degree or severity of pulmonary stenosis is one of the most important factors in determining the severity of the defect. The obstruction to pulmonary flow may be at the level of the valve but is more commonly located at the infundibulum, which is the muscular area beneath the pulmonary valve. With severe pulmonary stenosis, right-to-left shunting occurs and cyanosis may be observed. However, with mild or moderate pulmonary stenosis, blood will shunt from left-to-right, increasing pulmonary blood flow. These infants will be pink yet develop congestive heart failure. With growth the infundibulum may become progressively narrow, obstructing blood flow and producing hypercyanotic episodes sometimes referred to as *TET spells*.

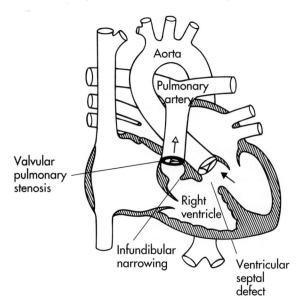

FIG. 11-10. Tetralogy of Fallot is characterized by a ventricular septal defect, overriding aorta, valvular pulmonary stenosis, and/or infundibular narrowing. The degree of pulmonary stenosis and infundibular narrowing determines the amount of unoxygenated blood shunted to the systemic circuit (right-to-left), resulting in cyanosis.

Clinical presentation. In the infant with tetralogy of Fallot, a murmur caused by pulmonary stenosis is typically present at birth. If the infant is acyanotic (blood is shunted from left-to-right via a VSD), congestive heart failure may result.

Central cyanosis associated with hyperpnea and central nervous system changes such as a loss of consciousness or seizure constitutes a TET spell or hypercyanotic episode. These spells can be self-limiting but can also result in death. They are therefore considered a medical emergency and signal the need for surgical intervention.

TRANSPOSITION OF THE GREAT ARTERIES (TGA)

Etiology. Transposition of the great arteries is the reversal of the anatomic relation of the aorta and the pulmonary artery. The aorta arises from the right ventricle and the pulmonary artery from the left ventricle. Transposition of the great arteries is the second most common cyanotic congenital heart defect encountered in early infancy. Frequency of TGA

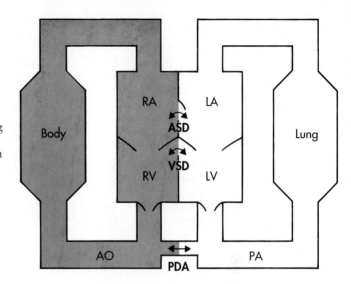

FIG. 11-11. Transposition of the great arteries is characterized by the right and left heart working as two parallel circuits. Without mixing of blood between the two circuits the infant cannot survive. Possible sites of mixing between the systemic and pulmonary circuits include a PDA, ASD, and VSD.

is approximately 5% to 7% of all congenital cardiac defects, with a strong male predominance[23] (Fig. 11-11).

Pathophysiology. In the child with transposition of the great arteries, the right and left heart work as two parallel circuits. Survival is dependent upon communication and mixing of blood between these two circuits. Mixing can occur at the level of the atria, ventricles, or great vessels—via the ductus arteriosus.

Approximately one half of the infants with transposition of the great arteries will have an intact ventricular septum, and the other half will have a ventricular septal defect.[23] Infants with an intact ventricular septum are ductal dependent. With a large atrial septal defect and ventricular septal defect there is more opportunity for mixing of blood between the two circuits. These infants may have minimal cyanosis but will demonstrate signs of congestive heart failure.

Clinical presentation. Infants with transposition of the great arteries and an intact ventricular septum present with cyanosis shortly after birth as the ductus begins to close. This cyanosis increases with crying and is not responsive to oxygen therapy. On physical examination, no audible murmur may be heard.

With a ventricular septal defect, mild cyanosis may be noted on physical examination. When a murmur is auscultated, it is typically that of a VSD murmur. Commonly these infants present with signs and symptoms of congestive heart failure, especially between

the ages of 2 and 4 weeks. Effortless tachypnea with respiratory rates of 80 per minute will often be noted. Infants with suspected TGA are considered medical emergencies.

TRUNCUS ARTERIOSUS (TA)

Etiology. Truncus arteriosus is the failure of the truncus to separate into an aorta and a pulmonary artery during fetal cardiac development. It is characterized by a single arterial vessel that originates from the heart and overrides a large ventricular septal defect (Fig. 11-12). This vessel supplies the systemic, coronary, and pulmonary circulation. The incidence of truncus arteriosus is approximately 1% to 4% of all congenital heart defects and occurs equally in both sexes.[32]

Pathophysiology. The hemodynamics of truncus arteriosus is related to the pulmonary vascular resistance, competency of the truncal valve, and presence or absence of pulmonary stenosis. For infants with relatively high pulmonary vascular resistance and no pulmonary stenosis, pulmonary blood flow may be limited. As pulmonary vascular resistance declines after birth, increased shunting of blood to the pulmonary circuit results. This increased pulmonary blood flow will produce signs and symptoms of congestive heart failure such as tachycardia, tachypnea, diaphoresis, and poor feeding. If truncal insufficiency is present, the presentation of congestive heart failure will occur early in life and will increase the volume overload.

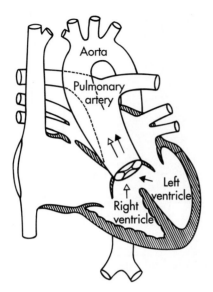

FIG. 11-12. Type I truncus arteriosus characterized by a single arterial vessel arising from the ventricles. A ventricular septal defect is present, and the truncus overrides the ventricular septum. The pulmonary, coronary, and systemic arteries arise from the arterial vessel.

Truncus arteriosus with stenosis of the pulmonary arteries diminishes blood flow to the pulmonary circuit, resulting in cyanosis that may increase as the infant grows. When pulmonary stenosis and truncal insufficiency are present, pulmonary blood flow is decreased and volume overload will result from the truncal incompetence.[42]

Clinical presentation. Depending on pulmonary vascular resistance and the presence or absence of pulmonary stenosis and/or truncal insufficiency, the infant may present with signs of congestive heart failure, cyanosis, or both. Infants and children without pulmonary stenosis will exhibit signs of congestive heart failure, bounding peripheral pulses, and a widened pulse pressure. Children with pulmonary stenosis will demonstrate varying degrees of cyanosis depending on the severity of the pulmonary stenosis.

TRICUSPID ATRESIA

Etiology. Tricuspid atresia is defined as the incomplete development of the tricuspid valve during fetal development and is associated with hypoplasia of the right ventricle. To be compatible with life, an atrial

and ventricular septal defect must be present. The incidence of tricuspid atresia is approximately 1.1% to 2.4% of all congenital heart defects, and it occurs slightly more frequently in males than females[22] (Fig. 11-13).

Pathophysiology. With tricuspid atresia there is no communication between the right atrium and right ventricle. Therefore, to sustain life, blood returning to the right heart must cross an atrial septal defect to the left heart and again cross a ventricular septal defect to enter the pulmonary circuit. In newborn infants with this defect, blood flow to the pulmonary circuit increases as pulmonary vascular resistance falls, shunting blood from the left ventricle to the hypoplastic right ventricle. As the infant grows, the ventricular septal defect becomes smaller in size, restricting the amount of blood flow shunted to the pulmonary circuit.

Transposition of the great arteries and pulmonary stenosis or atresia is often associated with tricuspid atresia. With pulmonary stenosis the obstruction to pulmonary blood flow will produce cyanosis. Transposition of the great arteries with no pulmonary stenosis may result in unrestricted pulmonary blood flow.[23]

Clinical presentation. More than 50% of infants with tricuspid atresia will present with cyanosis or murmurs in the first day of life.[53] Central cyanosis is the most frequent presenting symptom and results from the obligatory right-to-left shunting at the atrial level. The severity of cyanosis is dependent upon the degree of pulmonary blood flow. In severe cases hypoxemia and acidemia may be present. Infants with large ventricular septal defects may have minimal cyanosis because of the increase in pulmonary blood flow. This can result in signs and symptoms of congestive heart failure.

TOTAL ANOMALOUS PULMONARY VENOUS RETURN (TAPVR)

Etiology. Total anomalous pulmonary venous return is an anomaly in which the pulmonary veins do not connect with the left atrium (Fig. 11-14). Instead the pulmonary veins connect directly to the right atrium or to one of the systemic veins such as the superior vena cava or inferior vena cava. The incidence of TAPVR is approximately 1% to 2% of all congenital heart defects and occurs equally in males and females.[32,41]

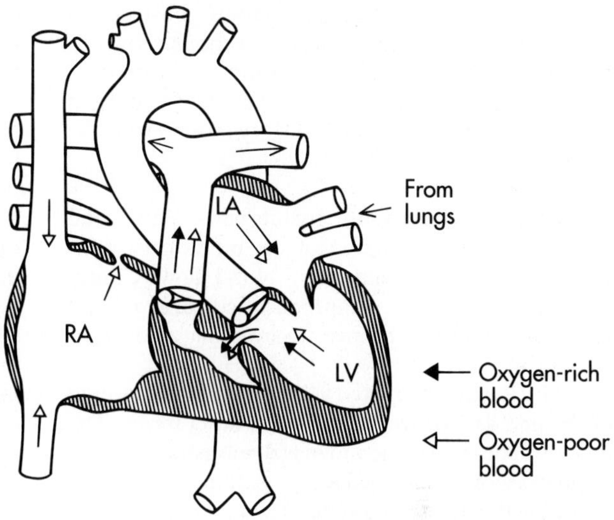

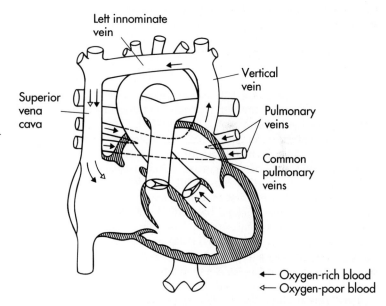

FIG. 11-13. In tricuspid atresia with hypoplastic right ventricle, systemic venous blood in the right atrium must cross an atrial septal defect or patent foramen ovale to the left atrium and into the left ventricle. From the left ventricle, blood must traverse a ventricular septal defect to enter the pulmonary circuit for oxygenation.

FIG. 11-14. In this form of TAPVR, blood returning from lungs via pulmonary veins traverses the vertical vein to the left innominate vein to the superior vena cava, where it joins blood returning to the right heart.

Pathophysiology. There are several anatomic variations of TAPVR; however, the hemodynamic properties remain the same—that of a left-to-right shunt. In TAPVR, the entire pulmonary venous blood flow returns to the right atrium where it mixes with systemic venous return. To be compatible with life, intraatrial communication (e.g., atrial septal defect or patent foramen ovale) must exist. This opening shunts blood from the right atrium to the left atrium where it moves through the left ventricle and into systemic circulation. The size of the atrial septal defect, pulmonary vascular resistance, and the presence or absence of a pulmonary venous obstruction will determine the hemodynamics and clinical presentation.

Infants with large intraatrial communications, low pulmonary vascular resistance, and no obstruction of the pulmonary veins will have increased pulmonary blood flow and a normal systemic flow.[41] Oxygen saturations may be 90% or higher depending on adequate mixing in the right atrium.

TAPVR with pulmonary venous obstruction results in a decrease in pulmonary venous return to the right atrium, pulmonary venous congestion, and pulmonary edema. With this defect oxygen saturation will be low and cyanosis will be observed.

Clinical presentation. Infants with TAPVR and minimal or no obstruction of the pulmonary veins will have increased pulmonary blood flow. Consequently, they will have symptoms of congestive heart failure, including tachypnea, tachycardia, and hepatomegaly.

TAPVR with obstructed veins is usually discovered in the first days or weeks of life due to cyanosis. The infant will be tachypneic and may demonstrate signs of respiratory distress evidenced by gasping and retractions. Further examination may yield no murmur, but hepatomegaly will be present. The more severe the obstruction, the earlier the infant presents with symptoms.

HYPOPLASTIC LEFT HEART SYNDROME (HLHS)

Etiology. Hypoplastic left heart syndrome is the underdevelopment of the left ventricle, mitral and aortic valves, and aortic arch (Fig. 11-15). This underdevelopment results in a small—hypoplastic—left ventricle and aortic and mitral valve atresia. HLHS is the leading cause of death from cardiovascular disease during the first 2 weeks of life with 95% of infants dying within the first month of life.[22] Forty percent of these infants come to medical attention within the first 2 days of life, 30% by 6 days, and 86% by 13 days.[18] The frequency of HLHS is approximately 7% of all congenital heart defects, and it occurs more frequently in males—67%—than females.[22]

Pathophysiology. In HLHS, oxygen-rich blood returning to the left atrium from the lungs is unable to enter the systemic circulation because of multiple obstructions of the left heart. This results in oxygenated blood crossing the foramen ovale and joining blood returning from the body into the right atrium. With this defect, the only way oxygenated blood can move into systemic circulation is by means of a patent ductus arteriosus—that shunts blood from the pulmonary artery to the descending aorta. The coronary arteries and myocardium also receive blood via the PDA. Because the

entire cardiac output occurs through the right ventricle, right ventricular volume overload and hypertrophy will develop.

Clinical presentation. These infants appear healthy at birth and remain asymptomatic until the ductus arteriosus begins to close, at which time an acute shocklike state will be observed. The caregiver will notice that the infant is no longer interested in feeding, the suck is no longer vigorous, and the infant is less active than normal. The most pronounced symptom is effortless tachypnea with a respiratory rate of 80 to 100 times per minute, although dyspnea may be present. Tachycardia, decreased peripheral pulses, decreased capillary refill time, and hepatomegaly will be observed. On auscultation a gallop rhythm may be present with or without a murmur.

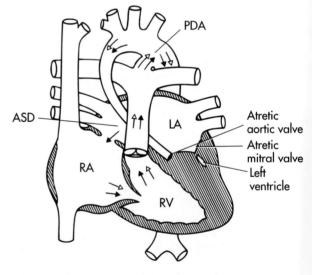

FIG. 11-15. Hypoplastic left heart syndrome is characterized by an atretic mitral valve, hypoplastic left ventricle, atretic aortic valve, and atresia of the ascending aorta. Oxygenated blood returning from the lungs must cross a patent foramen ovale or atrial septal defect to the right heart. From the pulmonary artery, blood is shunted through the ductus arteriosus to the aorta.

EMERGENCY DEPARTMENT INTERVENTIONS FOR THE CHILD WITH A CONGENITAL HEART DEFECT

DIAGNOSTIC TESTING

Numerous diagnostic tools can be used to determine the presence of a congenital heart defect. These include the chest x-ray, electrocardiogram (ECG), complete blood count, electrolytes, oxygen challenge test, and echocardiogram. Depending on the severity of symptoms, hospital admission may be necessary for ongoing evaluation and a cardiac catheterization (Table 11-1).

The chest x-ray is an important diagnostic tool in evaluating the child with a suspected congenital heart defect. Findings, however, must be correlated with the physical examination and other diagnostic studies. Anterior and posterior views can be used to assess both heart size and adequacy of pulmonary blood flow. Chest x-ray findings in infants and children with congestive heart failure will typically demonstrate an increase in heart size and increased pulmonary vascular markings. An increased heart size with no increase in pulmonary vascular markings may be seen in children with cardiac tumors or cardiomyopathy. Decreased pulmonary vascular markings and cardiomegaly are suggestive of a pulmonary obstruction.[29]

The electrocardiogram and echocardiography are also important diagnostic tools used to evaluate the child with a suspected CHD. The 12-lead ECG can evaluate heart rate and rhythm, as well as identify the presence of dysrhythmias, myocardial ischemia, hypertrophy, and chamber enlargement. The echocardiogram uses ultra–high-frequency sound waves to produce an image of intracardiac anatomy. The cardiac chambers, valves, great vessels, atrial and ventricular septa, pulmonary veins, and pericardial space can be visualized. Additionally, contractility can be assessed.

Hemoglobin and hematocrit values also contribute to the evaluation of the child with a CHD. Polycythemia in infants (beyond the newborn period) and children is often related to chronic hypoxemia produced by a cyanotic congenital lesion. Despite being polycythemic mean corpuscular hemoglobin concentration (MCHC) and/or mean corpuscular volume (MCV) may be low, requiring the child to take iron therapy.

Polycythemia increases the viscosity of the blood. Increased viscosity of the blood produces an increase in peripheral vascular resistance, which can decrease oxygen delivery to the tissues. The increased viscosity can also lead to the development of cerebral infarcts, particularly when the child is dehydrated. In contrast, severe anemia can cause congestive heart failure, because the reduced oxygen-carrying capacity of the blood stimulates a compensatory increase in the heart rate and cardiac output.

The oxygen challenge test is a useful tool to distinguish between a pulmonary and a cardiac cause in the cyanotic neonate. Initially an arterial blood gas is drawn with the infant on room air. The infant is then placed in 100% oxygen under an oxygen hood. A repeat arterial blood gas is obtained after 15 to 30 minutes. Infants with cyanotic congenital heart disease will demonstrate minimal increase in the Pao_2, whereas infants with pulmonary disease will respond with an increase in the $Pao_2 > 150$ mm Hg.[12]

TABLE 11-1	Interventional Cardiac Catheterization Procedures	
PROCEDURE	**DESCRIPTION**
Park	Opening of the atrial septum during cardiac catheterization with a bladed catheter
Pulmonary balloon valvuloplasty	Dilation of the pulmonary valve by inflation of a balloon-tipped cardiac catheter
Rashkind atrial septostomy	Opening of the atrial septum by a balloon-tipped cardiac catheter
Coils	Nonsurgical closure of PDAs
Stents	Used to maintain patency of pulmonary vessels

TREATMENT

Treatment of the child with a CHD depends on the child's clinical status and the suspected underlying defect. If the child presents with signs of congestive heart failure, digitalis and diuretics will be required (see the following section); if the neonate presents with cyanosis and signs of cardiovascular collapse as the ductus arteriosus closes, prostaglandin E_1 may be instituted; and if the infant presents with signs of a cyanotic defect, diagnostic testing may include an oxygen challenge test. Nursing care of the child with a cardiovascular disorder begins on p. 256.

CONGESTIVE HEART FAILURE (CHF)

Etiology. Congestive heart failure is a clinical syndrome that results when the heart is unable to meet the metabolic demands of the body. Although any condition or disease that increases the workload of the heart or hinders myocardial function can produce congestive heart failure, congenital heart disease is the most common cause of CHF in infants.[37] Congenital heart defects such as a ventricular septal defect, patent ductus arteriosus, atrioventricular canal, hypoplastic left heart syndrome, coarctation of the aorta, anomalous pulmonary venous return, and transposition of the great arteries are the most frequent causes of congestive heart failure in children under 1 year of age. After 1 year of age, diseases that impair myocardial function and cause heart failure include rheumatic heart disease, endocarditis, cardiomyopathy, and dysrhythmias.[56]

Pathophysiology. Congestive heart failure can be described as high output failure or low output failure. In high output failure, a congenital heart defect is usually present at the ventricular or great vessel level. The hemodynamic effect of this defect is left-to-right shunting, which increases pulmonary blood flow and volume load of the right and left heart. Severe anemia will also produce high cardiac output failure, because only high levels of cardiac output will maintain oxygen delivery.

Low output failure is seen in association with congenital heart defects that result in left heart or aortic obstruction, cardiomyopathies, and dysrhythmias. These diseases impair the ability of the heart to effectively pump blood to the systemic circuit, resulting in venous congestion. In response the body activates several compensatory mechanisms to maintain systemic perfusion, including dilation and hypertrophy of the left ventricle; vasoconstriction of the arterioles of the skin, skeletal muscles, gut, and kidneys; and retention of renal sodium and water.

Left ventricular dilation increases diastolic filling and stroke volume, whereas left ventricular hypertrophy aids in pumping against an increased afterload. Vasoconstriction is a compensatory response that redistributes blood flow. However, vasoconstriction may increase the workload—and oxygen consumption—of the already failing heart.

Clinical presentation. In infancy, one of the most important early findings indicative of a CHD that may lead to congestive heart failure is poor feeding, that is, the infant who takes a long time to feed yet may ingest less than the normal caloric requirements with each feed. In addition, the infant may become tachypneic and/or diaphoretic during these feeds. These infants are slow to gain weight and are often small for their age; in addition, the history may reveal frequent upper respiratory infections. In older children, exercise intolerance is a frequent complaint.

Signs and symptoms of congestive heart failure are related to systemic venous congestion, pulmonary venous congestion, and the adrenergic response. Signs of pulmonary venous congestion include effortless tachypnea (respiratory rates greater than 60), retractions, and nasal flaring. Signs of systemic venous congestion include hepatomegaly, edema (usually periorbital—dependent edema is rare in infants), pulmonary effusions, and ascites (also rare in children). Other findings include an S_3 gallop rhythm and diastolic rumble, which may be present with large left-to-right shunts. Jugular venous distention—common in adults—may be difficult if not impossible to appreciate in the infant because of the infant's short, fat neck. The adrenergic response includes such symptoms as sweating, decreased urine output, cool skin and extremities, weak peripheral pulses, and tachycardia.[31]

Emergency Department and nursing interventions. Diagnostic studies conducted on the child with CHF include laboratory analysis of blood and urine and a chest x-ray. The chest x-ray in the child with congestive heart failure will reveal cardiomegaly and increased pulmonary vascularity. Although an ECG may be ordered to identify the presence of a dysrhythmia, it is not considered useful in making the diagnosis of congestive heart failure.[40]

Echocardiography, when available, is an ideal diagnostic tool to evaluate intracardiac anatomy and cardiac function.

Oxygen therapy is used sparingly in children with left-to-right shunts, because oxygen is a potent vasodilator and can increase pulmonary blood flow. In these children oxygen is given when the infant or child has decreased saturations to 80% and symptoms are consistent with pulmonary edema.

Pharmacologic management. The general goal of therapy is to improve myocardial contractility and decrease the cardiac workload using pharmacologic agents. These agents include inotropic drugs that improve myocardial contractility, diuretics to reduce preload, and afterload-reducing agents to reduce ventricular afterload (Table 11-2). Other pharmacologic agents such as morphine sulfate may be used to reduce anxiety in infants and children with CHF and pulmonary edema (although its use is controversial because it can produce respiratory depression). If the neonate presents in congestive heart failure with symptoms of a shocklike state, a ductal-dependent lesion should be considered. These infants will require a continuous infusion of prostaglandin E_1.

Digoxin is the most commonly used inotropic agent in the child with congestive heart failure. Because of its inotropic effect, digoxin increases both the force and velocity of ventricular contractions while slowing the heart rate. Before administration the apical heart rate is taken for 1 full minute. Because the heart rate varies between different age children, the heart rate at which the drug should be withheld must be reviewed with the physician. Digoxin is a potent and potentially dangerous drug if improperly administered. Reviewing the dosage and method of administration with another nurse or physician cannot be overemphasized. After administration the ED nurse should monitor the child for the development of signs and symptoms of toxicity, including bradycardia, AV conduction defects, ventricular ectopy, anorexia, nausea or vomiting, diarrhea, and lethargy (Box 11-4).

Diuretics are commonly used to reduce intravascular volume and improve pulmonary edema. Among these are furosemide, bumetanide, chlorothiazide, and hydrochlorothiazide. When diuretics are administered in large doses or repeatedly, fluid depletion and electrolyte abnormalities can occur as sodium, chloride, and potassium are excreted by the kidneys. These children are monitored for signs of dehydration and electrolyte imbalances. All intake and output is recorded. Further nursing interventions can be found on pp. 256-258.

TABLE 11-2	Pharmacologic Agents Used to Treat Congestive Heart Failure
DRUG	**DOSAGE RANGE**

Digoxin	IV/PO digitalization
	    40 μg/kg/24 hr divided q6h = ½, ¼, ⅛, ⅛ *or* q8h = ½, ¼, ¼
	    Begin maintenance dose 8-12 hours after digitalization
	Maintenance
	    IV: 6-8 μg/kg/day divided q12h
	    PO: 10 μg/kg/day divided q12h

Furosemide	IV/IM/PO: 1-2 mg/kg/dose q 6, 8, or 12 h
Bumetanide	IV: 0.1-0.2 mg/kg/dose PO: 0.5-1 mg/dose
Metolazone	PO: 0.2-0.4 mg/kg/day divided every 12 hrs
Spironolactone	PO: 1.5-3 mg/kg/day divided in two to four doses
Sodium nitroprusside	IV: 0.5-8 μg/kg/min
Captopril	PO: 0.25 mg/kg/dose q8h × 2 doses; then 0.5 mg/kg/dose q8h × 2 doses; then 0.75 mg/kg/dose q8h × 2 doses; then 1 mg/kg/dose q8h

Compiled from Chemtob et al., 1989; Keeley and Bohn, 1988; Kulik, Hickey, and Lawrence, 1991.

HYPERCYANOTIC EPISODE OR "TET" SPELL

Etiology. Hypercyanotic episodes occur when the infant or child becomes acutely cyanotic, hyperpneic, and experiences central nervous system changes such as seizures or unconsciousness. These episodes are sometimes referred to as *TET spells*, because they are most commonly associated with tetralogy of Fallot; however, they can occur with any of the cyanotic congenital heart defects. The spells occur most frequently in the morning, after defecation, or after an episode of crying. However, *anything* that distresses the infant or child can precipitate a cyanotic spell, including injections, venipuncture, finger pricks, strange surroundings, and restraining of the child. Anemia and dehydration can also precipitate a spell.[17,23]

Pathophysiology. It is theorized that during a hypercyanotic episode the muscular pulmonary infundibulum spasms or narrows, causing an obstruction to pulmonary blood flow. This obstruction produces profound hypoxia and cyanosis. Cerebral perfusion can be compromised, exhibited by a loss of consciousness. Cerebral hypoxia, cerebral vascular accident, and death can result from a hypercyanotic spell.

Clinical presentation. Hypercyanotic spells are most commonly observed during the first year of life but can occur in older children. They are characterized by irritability, cyanosis that becomes profound, hyperpnea, and CNS changes—the signs usually progress in that order. Hypercyanotic spells represent a medical emergency.

Emergency Department and nursing interventions. Initial management of the child during a hypercyanotic spell requires stabilization of the ABCs and comforting and calming the child. For this reason the caregiver is allowed to remain with the child. Supplemental oxygen can be administered but only if it does not cause the infant or child to become agitated. The infant or child can be placed in the knee-chest position by pressing the legs against the chest. The knee-chest (or squatting) position increases systemic vascular resistance while the pulmonary stenosis remains the same. This results in a decrease in the right-to-left shunt and an increase in pulmonary blood flow and arterial saturation.

If comforting measures and the knee-chest position do not result in a clinical improvement or if the infant begins to seize, oxygen therapy is begun—if not begun previously. Morphine sulfate (SQ or IM: 0.1 to 0.2 mg/kg) or propranolol (Inderal) (IV: 0.01 to 0.1 mg/kg over 5 min) may be given to calm the child and reduce the spasm.[29] The use of vasodilators is avoided. Hypoxia-induced metabolic acidosis will require the administration of sodium bicarbonate (1 mEq/kg IV)—but only with documented acidosis. Intubation and ventilatory support may be required; however, intubation will not prevent future TET spells.

ACQUIRED HEART DISEASE

In adults, coronary artery disease is one of the most common forms of acquired heart disease requiring emergency intervention. In infants and children, acquired heart disease occurs secondary to an inflammatory process that affects the endocardium, myocardium, pericardium, conduction system, and coronary arteries. The clinical presentation varies from subtle signs and symptoms such as rashes and joint pain to cardiovascular collapse. Infective endocarditis, pericarditis, and myocarditis represent acquired heart diseases. Two multisystem diseases are also reviewed in this section, rheumatic fever and Kawasaki disease, because cardiac involvement is a major component of these illnesses.

INFECTIVE ENDOCARDITIS

Etiology. Infective endocarditis is an inflammation of the endocardium, which includes the valves. At one time, endocarditis most commonly occurred secondary to rheumatic heart disease. Now most cases of infective endocarditis are related to congenital heart defects and intracardiac catheters. Children with tetralogy of Fallot, aortic valve abnormalities, Blalock-Taussig shunts (BT), prosthetic valves, ventricular septal defects, patent ductus arteriosus, coarctation of the aorta, and transposition of the great arteries are considered most susceptible.[11,19] Infective organisms can be bacterial, viral, fungal, rickettsial, or chlamydial. However, *Streptococcus viridans* is responsible for 40% of the cases and staphylococci—specifically *Staphylococcus aureus*—is involved in 20% to 30% of the cases.[19]

Pathophysiology. Congenital heart defects and surgically-placed shunts and prosthetic valves produce turbulent blood flow. This turbulence damages the endothelium and results in thrombus formation. Circulating bacteria can become trapped in the thrombus, producing an endocardial infection. Unless the endocarditis is detected and treated properly, damage to the valves, embolization to other organs, renal dysfunction, and even death can occur. For this reason antibiotic prophylaxis (amoxicillin or if allergic to penicillin, erythromycin, or clindamycin) is required for all children with a congenital heart defect before undergoing surgical or dental procedures. (See Box 11-5 for precautions.)

Clinical presentation. Typically, children with infective endocarditis present with a history of low-grade fever, anorexia, weight loss, fatigue, arthralgia, arteritis, nausea, vomiting, abdominal pain, and chest pain. Infants and neonates may present with a clinical picture that is more acute and clinically resembles sepsis. On physical examination, the development of a new murmur, splenomegaly, and hepatomegaly may be present.[17]

Emergency Department interventions. Diagnostic testing performed in the child with suspected infective endocarditis includes a complete blood count (CBC) with differential, erythrocyte sedimentation

---

Box 11-5 Subacute Bacterial Endocarditis (SBE) Precautions

Infants and children at risk for SBE
- Prosthetic cardiac valves*
- Previous history of bacterial endocarditis*
- Surgically-placed systemic-to-pulmonary shunts (BT shunts) or conduits*
- Hypertrophic cardiomyopathy
- Mitral valve prolapse with regurgitation
- All congenital heart defects except isolated secundum atrial septal defects and patients who are 6 months or greater status post ASD, VSD, or PDA repair and do not have a residual defect

Procedures performed in the pediatric ER for which SBE precautions should be used
- Dental/oral surgery procedures
- Bronchoscopy with a rigid bronchoscope
- Urethral catheterization if urinary tract infection is present
- Incision and drainage of infected tissue

SBE precautions not needed for the following interventions
- Endotracheal intubation
- Spontaneous shedding of primary teeth

From Comittee on Rheumatic Fever, Endocarditis, and Kawasaki's Disease of the American Heart Association: Prevention of bacterial endocarditis, *JAMA* 22:264, 1990b.
*High risk for SBE.

---

rate (ESR), and urinalysis. In 90% of the cases the ESR will be elevated, in 40% of the cases anemia will be present, and hematuria may be present secondary to microemboli and microinfarcts in the kidneys.[19] Blood cultures are the single most important diagnostic test, with three to five sets—from different sites—being obtained over the first 24 hours.[19] Other diagnostic testing includes obtaining a chest radiograph, ECG, and echocardiogram.

Treatment requires hospital admission and intravenous antibiotic administration for 4 to 6 weeks. During this time daily blood cultures are obtained until the results indicate no growth. On discharge the parent/caregiver is reminded that antibiotic prophylaxis must be administered in the future, before any invasive procedure.

PERICARDITIS

Etiology. Pericarditis is an inflammatory process of the pericardium and the pericardial space. Enterovirus, adenovirus, and varicella are some of the most common infecting organisms; however, bacterial organisms such as *S. aureus, Streptococcus pneumoniae, Neisseria meningitidis*, and *Haemophilus influenzae* can also produce pericarditis.[17,49] Other causes of pericarditis include collagen vascular diseases, uremia, mediastinal radiation therapy, and rheumatic fever.[17]

Pathophysiology. When pericardial inflammation and/or infection is present some degree of effusion—fluid accumulation in the pericardial sac—usually results. As fluid accumulates in the pericardial sac diastolic filling and cardiac output are decreased. If the effusion progresses, cardiac tamponade can occur. Although rare in children, chronic constrictive pericarditis can occur and represents the development of a thickened, inelastic pericardium. The result is a decrease in diastolic filling of the ventricles.

Clinical presentation. Children with pericarditis often complain of a sharp precordial chest pain that radiates to the left scapula. Dyspnea is associated with the chest pain, and the child will be unable to lie flat. Other associated symptoms include cough, fever, and nasal flaring. On physical examination, a friction rub is diagnostic for pericarditis. However, the absence of a friction rub does not rule out pericarditis, because children with pericarditis and large pericardial effusions will demonstrate decreased (muffled) heart sounds and no friction rub. Distended neck veins will be present, although these may be difficult to appreciate in the infant or small child. Pulsus paradoxus, which is an inspiratory decrease in systolic blood pressure greater than 10 mm Hg, is a confirmatory finding.[50]

Emergency Department interventions. Diagnostic testing for the child with suspected pericarditis includes obtaining an ECG to detect dysrhythmias, particularly a decrease in voltage of the QRS complexes; a chest x-ray to determine heart size—the heart will be large and globular (rounded) with normal pulmonary vascular markings; and an echocardiogram to visualize the pericardial space, detect the accumulation of pericardial fluid, and assess ventricular function. Blood work includes a CBC with differential, ESR, and blood culture.

Treatment consists of the administration of a broad spectrum antibiotic because initially a bacterial etiology cannot be ruled out.[40] Depending on the clinical state of the child and the presence of cardiac tamponade, a pericardiocentesis may be required. (See Chapter 21.)

MYOCARDITIS

Etiology. Myocarditis is an inflammation of the cardiac muscle and is most commonly of viral origin. Coxsackie B accounts for approximately half of the cases of acute myocarditis, although echovirus, influenza, varicella, rubella, and gram-positive cocci can also be responsible.[19]

Pathophysiology. Inflammation of the myocardium results in depression of myocardial function. Function may be so impaired that congestive heart failure results. The heart may be dilated with little or no hypertrophy, or there may be dilation with varying degrees of left ventricular hypertrophy and endocardial thickening.

Clinical presentation. Infants and children with myocarditis often present with a recent history of a viral-type illness including fever, rhinorrhea, and diarrhea. Other early symptoms include pharyngitis, cough, malaise, dyspnea, chest pain, myalgia, and palpitations. These early symptoms can rapidly progress to more severe symptoms including lethargy, pallor, tachycardia, and respiratory distress with hepatomegaly. Tachycardia out of proportion to the fever will be present,[17] and auscultation may reveal a gallop rhythm or friction rub.

Emergency Department interventions. Diagnostic testing for the child with suspected myocarditis includes a CBC with differential, ESR, and blood culture. The white blood count and ESR are usually elevated. Because the origin is usually viral in nature, viral cultures of the blood, throat, and stool may be collected. Other diagnostic tests should include an ECG, chest x-ray, and echocardiogram. Electrocardiogram findings may include low-voltage QRS complexes or slightly inverted T waves.[19] The ECG may also demonstrate a sinus tachycardia out of proportion to the fever. The chest x-ray may reveal cardiomegaly or pericardial effusion. If congestive heart failure is present pulmonary edema will be seen. An echocardiogram is useful in assessing ventricular function, dilation of one or more of the chambers, and the absence of a structural cardiac defect.

Treatment depends on clinical presentation. Children with mild disease will require hospitalization and close monitoring to observe for signs of increasing heart failure. If left ventricular failure develops it is treated with digoxin and furosemide. Digoxin, however, should be used with caution because the acutely inflamed myocardium may be very sensitive to its use. For this reason the oral digitalizing dose of digoxin is decreased to 30 µg/kg over a 24-hour period.[19] Inotropic agents such as dopamine 2 to 10 µg/kg/minute or dobutamine 10 µg/kg/minute—or more—may be required to improve myocardial contractility and cardiac output. Afterload-reducing agents such as sodium nitroprusside may be useful in decreasing the workload of the heart but are administered only if the child is not hypovolemic. Dysrhythmias are treated to prevent further decreases in cardiac output. Antibiotics may be ordered until culture results are obtained. The use of steroids remains controversial, and their use is generally withheld in acute viral myocarditis.[40]

▌RHEUMATIC FEVER

Etiology. Rheumatic fever is a diffuse inflammatory disease of the connective tissue that involves the heart, joints, brain, blood vessels, and subcutaneous tissue. It usually follows an upper respiratory infection caused by Group A β-hemolytic streptococci that goes untreated. Cardiac involvement may include all three layers of the heart, producing rheumatic pancarditis—myocarditis, endocarditis, and pericarditis.

Rheumatic fever is rare in infants but is more common in school-age children. With the advent of penicillin and aggressive treatment of streptococcal pharyngitis, the incidence of rheumatic fever has decreased. Recently, however, there has been an increased incidence of reported cases.[14]

Pathophysiology. Rheumatic fever causes interstitial inflammation and myocardial cell damage. The acute inflammatory process can affect the cardiac conduction system and the coronary arteries. With the development of endocarditis the mitral valve and aortic valve can be affected; the tricuspid or pulmonary valves are rarely affected. As the inflammation subsides fibrosis with vascularization and contracture of the valve leaflets follows, producing a stenotic, incompetent valve. Because the valve will no longer

be able to perform efficiently, volume overload and congestive heart failure can result.

Clinical presentation. Historical information will often reveal a previous history of pharyngitis and fever. Almost 75% of children with rheumatic fever will complain of migratory polyarthritis.[38] The physical examination may reveal the presence of a fever, tachycardia out of proportion to the fever, pericardial friction rub or effusion, and a new murmur.[17] Diagnosis is made based on the modified Jones criteria (Box 11-6).

Emergency Department interventions. Diagnostic testing for determining the presence of rheumatic fever includes obtaining an ESR, C-reactive protein, CBC, and serum proteins.[14] Typically the ESR will be abnormally elevated and C-reactive proteins will be present. The CBC may yield moderate anemia with an elevated leukocyte count. Of the serum proteins, immunoglobulin A will often be elevated.[14] The antistreptolysin-O antibody test is used to assess for evidence of a recent streptococcal infection. A value of

---

Box 11-6 Modified Jones Criteria for Diagnosis of Rheumatic Fever

Major criteria
- Carditis
- Arthritis
- Chorea
- Erythema marginatum
- Subcutaneous nodules

Minor criteria
- Previous rheumatic fever
- Arthralgia
- Fever
- Acute phase reactants
- First-degree atrioventricular block

Requirements for diagnosis
- Two major criteria *or*
- One major and two minor criteria plus evidence of previous streptococcal infection
- Recent scarlet fever
- Elevated antistreptolysin-O titer
      or
- Positive throat culture

500 units is indicative of a recent streptococcal infection, and a value of 333 is borderline.[14]

Throat cultures are of little value, because there is usually a latent period of 1 to 3 weeks between the pharyngitis and the onset of rheumatic fever. A chest x-ray and electrocardiogram are obtained to assess cardiac involvement and the presence of dysrhythmias. An echocardiogram is required to assess valvular competence—particularly the aortic and mitral valves—and left ventricular function.

Treatment includes bed rest—to decrease myocardial oxygen requirements—until the acute febrile portion of the illness resolves and signs of carditis have stabilized. Salicylate therapy (90 to 120 mg/kg/day) is given every 4 hours to relieve the acute inflammatory manifestations of the disease. Benzathine penicillin 1.2 million units IM is given initially and once a month to prevent recurrence. If the child is allergic to penicillin, erythromycin 250 mg can be given orally twice a day.[14] The use of steroids is controversial; however, corticosteroids may be given if moderate carditis is present. Congestive heart failure is treated with digitalis and diuretics.

▌KAWASAKI DISEASE

Etiology. Kawasaki disease or mucocutaneous lymph node syndrome produces multisystem vasculitis with an affinity for the coronary arteries. The etiology of Kawasaki disease is unknown; therefore the diagnosis is based on clinical findings. The disease most frequently affects infants and children under 5 years of age, with a peak incidence between 18 and 24 months of age. Although Kawasaki disease is episodic and self-limiting, the most significant feature is heart disease.[1,45]

Pathophysiology. The principal feature of Kawasaki disease is systemic vasculitis of the microvessels that affects nearly every organ in the body. The heart is particularly vulnerable—specifically the coronary arteries, which can become dilated, leading to the development of coronary aneurysms. Sudden death has been reported in Kawasaki disease, not usually related to a ruptured coronary aneurysm, but instead due to thrombosis of the coronary artery.[16] Pancarditis—myocarditis, endocarditis, and pericarditis—with inflammation of the conduction system can also occur.[45]

Clinical presentation. The clinical course of Kawasaki disease is divided into three phases. The initial, or acute, phase is characterized by at least a 5-day history of fever greater than 104° F. During this time any one of a number of symptoms such as edema and redness of the hands and feet, variable rashes, conjunctival injection, strawberry tongue, fissuring and erythema of the lips, diffuse erythema of the oropharynx, and lymphadenitis may be present. This acute phase lasts approximately 8 to 15 days. The beginning of the subacute phase is marked by a decrease in the temperature and resolution of the acute physical findings. Arthritis and cardiac disease may develop during this subacute phase, which lasts for 10 to 25 days. Additionally, desquamation of the fingertips and toes occurs during this phase. The convalescent period begins when all clinical manifestations have resolved and ends when all laboratory findings have normalized—approximately 3 months from the onset of symptoms.[16,45]

Emergency Department interventions. There are no specific diagnostic tests available for determining the presence of Kawasaki disease. Laboratory studies usually performed on the child suspected of having Kawasaki disease include a CBC with differential and platelets, ESR, C-reactive protein, and urinalysis. Findings often indicate an increase in the erythrocyte sedimentation rate greater than 101 mm/hr, leukocytosis, a positive C-reactive protein, an increased platelet count, and sterile pyuria and proteinuria.[21]

A chest radiograph to assess heart size and lung fields is obtained, as well as an electrocardiogram to detect the presence of myocardial infarction or dysrhythmias. An echocardiogram is performed because aneurysm formation of the coronary arteries, myocarditis, pericarditis, pericardial effusion, and valvular incompetence may occur. Children with Kawasaki disease require hospitalization and treatment with aspirin therapy and intravenous gammaglobulin to prevent or decrease coronary artery involvement.

▌NURSING CARE OF THE CHILD WITH A CARDIOVASCULAR DISORDER (BOX 11-7)

Infants and children who exhibit signs of congestive heart failure or cyanosis require emergent management regardless of history. The first priority of care is stabilization of the airway, breathing, and circulation. At the same time, the child is placed on the cardiac monitor and pulse oximeter, venous access is achieved, and vital signs are obtained. Pulses are palpated in the upper and lower extremities. Variations in strength require blood pressures to be taken in both an upper and lower extremity.

The child with an altered neurologic status requires airway positioning to prevent the tongue from occluding the airway. If signs of respiratory failure are evident, ventilatory assistance with a bag-valve-mask device and supplemental oxygen is required. The child who is stable may be allowed to remain upright in bed and receive supplemental oxygen via face mask.

In the child with a CHD the administration of supplemental oxygen is determined by the child's clinical state. Oxygen is a potent vasodilator and can actually increase pulmonary blood flow, contributing to the development of pulmonary edema and result in blood stealing from systemic circulation. Therefore, oxygen is used only to maintain oxygen saturations of at least 95%. If the child has a defect that produces right-to-left shunting (cyanotic defect), normal oxygen saturations for that child may be as low as 75% to 85%—even with supplemental oxygen administration.

Efforts to decrease oxygen consumption such as assisting ventilation, addressing pain and fear, and limiting physical activity (e.g., bed rest in the older child or gavage feeding in the infant) may be initiated. A neutral thermal environment is also required, because hypothermia increases the metabolic rate, causing both systemic oxygen consumption and glycolysis to increase. Because the infant has limited glycogen stores, the stress of illness or the stress of hypothermia can rapidly lead to hypoglycemia. Hypoglycemia and other electrolyte imbalances such as hyponatremia, hypocalcemia, and hypokalemia will further depress myocardial function.

Inotropic support is usually indicated in children with significant *left-to-right shunts,* as is the use of diuretics such as furosemide and afterload-reducing agents such as nitroprusside. Infants with ductal-dependent lesions such as TGA, COA, or hypoplastic left heart may present with severe cardiovascular compromise and shock as the ductus arteriosus closes. In these infants prostaglandin E_1 may be required to maintain ductal patency (Table 11-3).

When the child has a *right-to-left shunt,* central cyanosis may be observed. These infants and children tolerate stress poorly and can desaturate easily. Therefore attempts at venipuncture for laboratory studies or intravenous lines should be limited and the child allowed time to calm between attempts. Crying and agitation can lead to a hypercyanotic episode. When

---

Box 11-7   Nursing Interventions for the Child with a Congenital Heart Defect (CHD)

- If awake, allow the child to maintain a position of comfort
- If the child is lethargic, establish a patent airway by positioning and clearing the airway
- Administer supplemental oxygen and observe oxygen saturations
  - High concentrations of oxygen can increase pulmonary blood flow in left-to-right shunts, worsening the pulmonary edema
  - Normal oxygen saturations may be very low in the child with a right-to-left shunt
- Assess breathing and, if required, provide ventilatory assistance with a bag-valve-mask (BVM) device
- Assess circulation and establish venous access as required
- Place the child on a cardiac monitor and pulse oximeter
- Treat dysrhythmias as identified

- Obtain vital signs, including blood pressure; if pulses are unequal obtain a blood pressure in upper and lower extremities
- Maintain a neutral thermal environment and monitor the infant/child's body temperature
- Monitor glucose level
- Monitor intake and output
- If a left-to-right shunt is suspected, anticipate diuretics and digoxin if signs of congestive heart failure are present
- If a ductal-dependent lesion is suspected in a neonate, anticipate prostaglandin
- If a right-to-left shunt is suspected, *avoid causing agitation or crying,* which will increase oxygen consumption and may stimulate a hypercyanotic episode (TET spell)
- Provide psychologic support to the family and child; keep them informed of the plan of care

TABLE 11-3	Prostaglandin E₁
To mix	0.3 mg in 100 ml of D_5W
	3 µg/ml
	1 ml/kg/hr = 0.05 µg/kg/min
Dose	0.025-0.1 µg/kg/min
Side effects	Respiratory depression and apnea
	Vasodilation
	Fever
	Seizurelike activities
Nursing actions	Place child on cardiac monitor and pulse oximeter
	Monitor respiratory rate and effort
	Place BVM device and intubation equipment at the bedside
	Monitor for seizures

Modified from Hazinski, 1992; Flynn, Engle, and Ehlers, 1992.

venous access is required extreme care must be taken to remove all air from the intravenous lines, because an air emboli may enter directly into the systemic circulation and produce a cerebral emboli.

EVALUATION

Ongoing emergency department nursing care of the child with a cardiovascular disorder requires continuous monitoring for the development of dysrhythmias. Depending on the child's clinical status and response to therapy, vital signs including temperature, pulse, respiratory rate, and blood pressure may need to be taken as often as every 5 to 10 minutes or as infrequently as every 2 to 3 hours. In addition to the above assessments the child's perfusion status (color, peripheral pulses, capillary refill) and neurologic status are continuously monitored. Respiratory status is evaluated for an increase in the work of breathing or other signs of pulmonary edema. All fluid intake (drugs and drips included) and urine output are recorded. Strictly measuring urine output is particularly important in the child receiving diuretics; therefore an indwelling urinary catheter may be required in diapered infants or critically ill children. During diuretic therapy the child is monitored for signs of dehydration and electrolyte disturbances. All parenteral fluids are administered via an infusion pump.

PSYCHOLOGIC SUPPORT

Children with cardiovascular disorders can arrive in the ED with serious life-threatening illnesses or with illnesses that are unrelated to an underlying cardiac anomaly. Parents of children with known cardiac disorders may have serious concerns regarding their child's future health. Additionally, the parent's are often quite knowledgeable about the disorder, and this knowledge can affect their confidence in the ED staff—particularly if the staff is unfamiliar with the specifics of the child's defect or the child's baseline status. Parents should be allowed to participate in the child's care, and emergency personnel should listen carefully to the family's concerns and observations. To assist personnel, the child's private physician or cardiologist may be contacted. During emergency department care the parents should be provided with continuous updates of their child's condition and allowed to stay with their child whenever possible.

The child with a cardiovascular disorder is anxious and fearful. Because some disorders can actually become worse with fear and crying, pain and anxiety should be addressed promptly. Sedatives can be administered to calm the child; however, the most effective calming procedures are to allow the parents to remain with the child; to provide a calm, quiet atmosphere; and to assign limited personnel to care for the child during the ED stay.

▌ CHEST PAIN IN CHILDREN AND ADOLESCENTS

Etiology. Chest pain in young children is a relatively uncommon presenting complaint in the ED when compared to adults. Although more common in older children and adolescents, less than 5% of these complaints are cardiac in origin.[17] In general, the most common causes of chest pain in children include musculoskeletal pain, cough, asthma, trauma, gastrointestinal problems, pneumonia, and psychologic causes.[3,29,60]

Pathophysiology. The pathophysiology of chest pain in children varies depending on the etiology. Pain may be derived from any of the structures within or surrounding the thorax, including the intercostal muscles, lungs, visceral organs, and heart. Some of the cardiac causes of chest pain in children include pericarditis, myocarditis, dysrhythmias (palpitations), hypertrophic obstructive cardiomyopathy, valvular aortic stenosis, anomalous coronary artery anatomy, past history of Kawasaki disease, and cocaine abuse.[3,29]

Clinical presentation. Clinical presentation varies depending on the cause of the chest pain. Common causes include inflammation of the chest wall—costochondritis—which is manifested by inflammation without redness at the costochondral junction. Other causes may be related to pulmonary disease or injury. For example, children with asthma often complain of chest pain associated with the increased work of breathing. Chest pain can also be of psychologic origin—from depression or anxiety—and from gastrointestinal disturbances.

Chest pain of cardiac origin is rare in children. The child at high risk is the child with chest pain on physical exertion, dyspnea, or syncope. In addition, the child with a known congenital heart defect, Kawasaki disease, or a family history of early coronary heart disease is at high risk.[40]

Emergency Department and nursing interventions. Any child arriving in the ED with a complaint of chest pain deserves a thorough history and workup. The history is valuable in determining associated symptoms, onset and description of pain, alleviating and aggravating factors, and history of drug ingestion. Family history is also important, particularly for cardiomyopathy and early coronary heart disease. Sudden death of a family member in the second, third, or fourth decade of life is suspicious for cardiomyopathy. Cardiomegaly, ST-T wave changes, or dysrhythmias should prompt a pediatric cardiology referral; these children should avoid physical activity until evaluated.[29,60]

▌ DYSRHYTHMIAS

Primary dysrhythmias are less common in infants and children than adults. However, dysrhythmias may occur secondary to electrolyte imbalances, acquired heart diseases, open-heart surgery, cardiomyopathy, and drug ingestion. Tachydysrhythmias include dysrhythmias such as supraventricular tachycardia, atrial flutter, atrial fibrillation, and ventricular tachycardia. With tachydysrhythmias ventricular filling time is compromised, resulting in decreased cardiac output and a decrease in coronary artery perfusion.

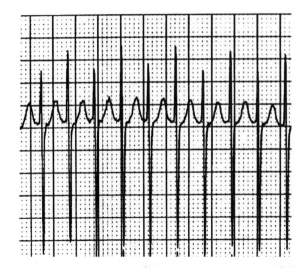

FIG. 11-16. Supraventricular tachycardia

In contrast bradydysrhythmias compromise cardiac output directly, because the compensatory response of increasing stroke volume is limited in the young child. Bradydysrhythmias may be primary or secondary in nature, although primary causes are rare. Examples of primary dysrhythmias include complete heart block and Mobitz type II. Congenital complete atrioventricular block accounts for nearly all significant primary bradycardia in infants. In the majority of children sinus bradycardia results from a variety of other problems but is most commonly the result of hypoxia.[25]

Hemodynamic assessment of the infant or child with rhythm disturbances is based on evaluation of cardiac output. Overall nursing interventions include stabilization of the ABCs of CPR and correction of hypoxemia, acidosis, hypoglycemia, and electrolyte imbalances.[4]

SUPRAVENTRICULAR TACHYCARDIA (SVT)

Supraventricular tachycardia is a narrow complex tachycardia that is often difficult to discern from sinus tachycardia. SVT accounts for 90% of dysrhythmias in children.[48] The heart rate is one of the most diagnostic parameters. Heart rates with SVT can vary between 200 and 300 beats per minute depending on the child's age and concurrent illness or underlying etiology (Fig. 11-16).

Clinical presentation. When SVT is present diastolic filling time is decreased. This leads to signs of decreased cardiac output. Depending on the duration of the dysrhythmia and the child's compensatory response, clinical evidence of SVT can vary from mild to severe. The majority of infants and children with SVT are uncomfortable and cranky but clinically stable. In contrast some children with SVT present in profound shock. Any child with sustained SVT will develop signs of congestive heart failure.

Often SVT coincides with a febrile episode. Thus temperature control over 24 to 48 hours is necessary to prevent other occurrences. Over-the-counter medications such as cold preparations can also precipitate an episode of SVT.[57]

Emergency Department and nursing interventions. The treatment for SVT depends on the severity of the clinical symptoms. If the child is clinically stable, vagal maneuvers such as placing an iced towel on the face or obtaining a rectal temperature may convert the heart rhythm to normal; massaging the eyes is contraindicated. If these maneuvers fail and venous access has been achieved, adenosine may be given by rapid IV push (Box 11-8). If adenosine is not available, digoxin may be given. Verapamil 0.1 mg/kg/bolus can be given to children over 1 year of age but is contraindicated in children less than 1 year of age, because it has been associated with cardiovascular collapse and death.[15] If all of the above measures fail, propranolol 0.1 mg/kg/dose can be administered IV every 6 hours.

In the clinically unstable child, synchronized cardioversion with 0.5 to 1 watt-sec/kg is performed. Subsequent doses may be doubled and are occasionally increased up to 10 watt-sec/kg. If the infant/child is coherent, sedation may be necessary. Cardioversion is not recommended for children who have received digoxin, because it can result in ventricular dysrhythmias or failure of the SA node to take over. Esophageal or right atrial overdrive pacing at approximately 300 beats/min may be effective.[6,25]

ATRIAL FLUTTER

Atrial flutter is characterized by rapid atrial rates of up to 300 beats/minute and flutter waves in lead II. However, this rate is rarely transmitted to the ventricles because there is often an associated AV block. Atrial flutter is associated with congenital heart disease 80% of the time (Fig. 11-17).

Box 11-8 Adenosine (Adenocard)

- 50-100 µg (0.05-0.1 mg)/kg/dose intravenously
- The dose may be increased by increments of 50 µg/kg/dose every 2 minutes until SVT is resolved.
- To administer adenosine the syringe is placed as close to the IV site as possible and 3 ml of normal saline is used as flush. The drug is pushed as rapidly as possible, and the saline flush immediately follows.
- Asystole (less than 2 seconds) will result, and a slow sinus rhythm will accelerate to a normal rate.
- Side effects include flushing, headache, and nausea.
- Children treated with adenosine can relapse back into SVT, and additional doses may be required.

Clinical presentation. The signs and symptoms of atrial flutter are similar to those of SVT (e.g., signs of delayed perfusion). Young infants may present in atrial flutter with no associated CHD; older children, however, often have an associated cardiac anomaly. Because the AV node in infants is capable of very rapid conduction, rapid ventricular rates can lead to shock or congestive heart failure. Older children tend to tolerate atrial flutter better than young infants.[7]

Emergency Department and nursing interventions. The treatment for atrial flutter depends on the severity of the symptoms. If the child is clinically stable, digitalization may be useful by producing a higher degree of AV block. When there is evidence of sinus node dysfunction, however, digoxin should be used with caution. If the child is clinically unstable, synchronized cardioversion beginning with 1 to 2 watt-sec/kg is administered. Esophageal overdrive pacing may be employed to convert to sinus rhythm. On termination of the atrial flutter, a slow junctional rhythm or asystole may occur. For this reason back-up pacing must be available.[50]

ATRIAL FIBRILLATION

Atrial fibrillation is uncommon in children and is characterized by an irregular ventricular response and

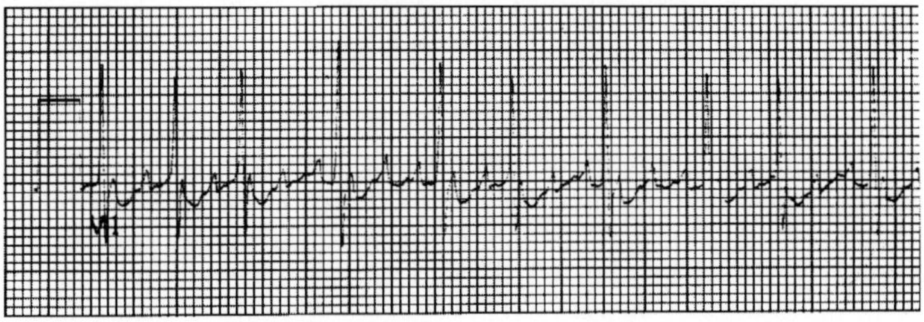

FIG. 11-17. Atrial flutter.

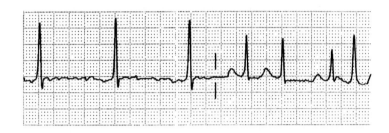

FIG. 11-18. Atrial fibrillation.

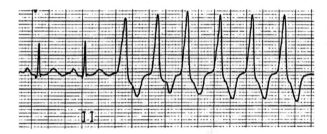

FIG. 11-19. Ventricular tachycardia.

disorganized rapid atrial activity. It is most commonly seen in older children and adolescents with a history of rheumatic heart or mitral disease, dilated cardiomyopathy, or hyperthyroidism (Fig. 11-18).[50]

Clinical presentation. Clinical presentation is similar to SVT and atrial flutter in that cardiac filling time is compromised, affecting cardiac output. The child with atrial fibrillation may present to the emergency department clinically stable or in profound shock.

Emergency Department and nursing interventions. The clinically stable child with atrial fibrillation can be digitalized.[29,50] When blood pressure and perfusion remain stable the child can be monitored for 24 hours while digoxin levels rise. If a normal sinus rhythm is not obtained within 24 to 48

hours cardioversion may be attempted. The clinically unstable child is treated with synchronized cardioversion, 1 to 2 watt-sec/kg.

VENTRICULAR TACHYCARDIA

Ventricular tachycardia is defined as three or more premature ventricular beats in a row. It can occur in children with congenital heart defects or acquired heart disease, or it can be noncardiac in origin (e.g., an electrolyte imbalance). In children with heart disease, causes include complex congenital heart disease, previous open-heart surgery, hypertrophic cardiomyopathy, intracardiac tumors, and the long QT syndrome (Fig. 11-19).

Clinical presentation. Children with ventricular tachycardia may be hemodynamically stable, exhibited by a normal blood pressure and perfusion, or clinically unstable. Clinically unstable children require emergent management.

Emergency Department and nursing interventions. Treatment is based on clinical status. If the child is clinically compromised, synchronized cardioversion is performed using 0.5 to 2 watt-sec/kg. If this is unsuccessful, propranolol 0.025 mg/kg is administered IV every 10 minutes for a total of four doses.[7] Pharmacologic therapy for both the stable and unstable child includes an initial bolus of lidocaine 1 mg/kg IV followed by a 0.5 mg/kg bolus in 10 to 15 minutes and a maintenance drip of 0.01 to 0.05 mg/kg/minute. Other pharmacologic agents used include phenytoin 15 mg/kg IV over 1 hour—used especially with digoxin toxicity, procainamide up to 15 mg/kg IV given over 20 to 60 minutes, or bretylium 5 mg/kg IV.[29,44,50]

VENTRICULAR FIBRILLATION

Ventricular fibrillation represents ineffective ventricular contractions with cessation of circulation. The approach to therapy is discussed Chapter 8.

HEART BLOCK

Heart block is classified as first degree—reflecting slowed conduction from the sinus node to the ventricle; second degree—reflecting failure of some of the impulses to transverse the AV node; and third degree—or complete AV heart block. Both Mobitz type I and Mobitz type II represent second-degree heart blocks. First-degree block may be seen in children with CHDs and acquired heart disease such as rheumatic heart disease. Mobitz type I may be a normal variant and usually requires no intervention in the child. Mobitz type II is more significant and can lead to complete heart block, syncope, and sudden death[29,50] (Fig. 11-20). Complete heart block or third-degree AV block may be congenital or secondary to myocarditis, hyperkalemia, or postoperative open-heart surgery. All three forms of heart block can be caused by digoxin toxicity (Fig. 11-21).

Clinical presentation. Children with heart block may be asymptomatic or present with vague symptoms such as easy fatiguability or shortness of breath.[7] Because of the slow heart rate, signs of decreased perfusion including pallor and delayed capillary refill may be observed, as well as a loss of consciousness—syncope.

Emergency Department and nursing interventions. Treatment depends on the type of heart block present and the underlying cause (e.g., an electrolyte imbalance). To make these determinations an ECG, chest x-ray, CBC, and serum electrolytes may be obtained. Infants who are asymptomatic with a heart

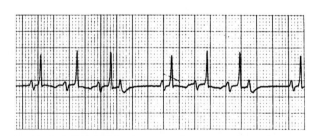

FIG. 11-20. Mobitz type II.

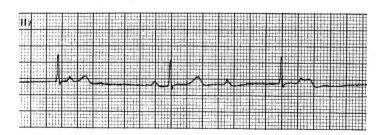

FIG. 11-21. Complete heart block.

rate of 55 or greater may be followed as outpatients. Permanent pacemaker placement is indicated for the symptomatic child, the asymptomatic infant with a heart rate of less than 55, and the child with an awake heart rate of less than 45.[50]

■ SUMMARY

Congenital heart defects comprise the bulk of cardiovascular disease in infants and children. Fortunately, however, the overall incidence of CHDs in children is low. Because of surgical advances, most children with CHDs survive to adulthood with normal life-styles. Children with complex anatomy often undergo staged operative procedures. For the pediatric emergency nurse, an understanding of the anatomy of the defect and potential hemodynamic changes is necessary to care for these children both before and between surgical procedures. Although all cardiovascular diseases are not emergencies, recognition and prompt intervention can prevent devastating consequences.

REFERENCES

1. Reference deleted in proofs.
2. Baldwin HS: What's new in cardiology: an update of current clinical practices, *Pediatr Rev* 16:443-447, 1995.
3. Bayne EJ: Chest pain in children and adolescents. In Harwood-Nuss A, ed: *The clinical practice of emergency medicine*, Philadelphia, 1991, JB Lippincott.
4. Boisvert JT, Reidy SJ, Lulu J: Overview of pediatric arrhythmias. In Hickey PA, ed: *Nurs Clin North Am* 30:365-379, 1995.
5. Brook MM, Heymann MA: Patent ductus arteriosus. In Emmanouilides GC, Reimenschneider TA, Allen, HD, Gutgesell, HP, eds: *Moss and Adams heart disease in infants, children, and adolescents including the fetus and young adult*, 5th ed, Baltimore, 1995, Williams & Wilkins.
6. Campbell RM et al: Atrial overdrive pacing for conversion of atrial flutter in children, *Pediatrics* 4:75, 1985.
7. Chameides L: Dysrhythmias. In Barkin RM, ed: *Pediatric emergency medicine: concepts and clinical practice,* St Louis, 1992, Mosby.
8. Chemtob S et al: Pharmacology of diuretics in the newborn, *Pediatr Clin North Am* 15:36, 1989.
9. Committee on Rheumatic Fever, Endocarditis, and Kawasaki's Disease of the American Heart Association: Diagnostic guidelines for Kawasaki's disease, *Am J Dis Child* 144, 1990.
10. Committee on Rheumatic Fever, Endocarditis, and Kawasaki's Disease of the American Heart Associa-

tion: Prevention of bacterial endocarditis, *JAMA* 22:264, 1990.
11. Dajani AS, Taubert KA: Infective endocarditis. In Emmanouilides GC, Reimenschneider TA, Allen, HD, Gutgesell, HP (editors): *Moss and Adams heart disease in infants, children, and adolescents including the fetus and young adult*, 5th ed, Baltimore, 1995, Williams & Wilkins.
12. Driscoll PJ: Evaluation of the cyanotic newborn. In Gillete PC, ed. *Pediatr Clin North Am* 1:37, 1990.
13. Duff DF, McNamara DG: History and physical examination of the cardiovascular system. In Garson A, Bricker JT, McNamara DG, eds: *The science and practice of pediatric cardiology*, vol 2, Philadelphia, 1990, Lea and Febiger.
14. El-Said GM, Sorour KA: Acute rheumatic fever. In Garson A, Bricker JT, McNamara DG, eds: *The science and practice of pediatric cardiology*, vol 2, Philadelphia, 1990, Lea and Febiger.
15. Epstein ML, Kiel EA, Victorica BE: Cardiac decompensation following verapamil therapy in infants with supraventricular tachycardia, *Pediatrics* 4:75, 1985.
16. Felter RA: Infectious disorders. In Barkin RM, ed: *Pediatric emergency medicine: concepts and clinical practice*, St Louis, 1992, Mosby.
17. Flynn PA, Engle MA, Ehlers KH: Cardiac issues in the pediatric emergency room. In DiMaio AM, ed: *Pediatr Clin North Am* 5:39, 1992.
18. Freedom RM & Benson, LN: Hypoplastic left heart syndrome. In Emmanouilides GC, Reimenschneider TA, Allen, HD, Gutgesell, HP (editors): *Moss and Adams heart disease in infants, children, and adolescents including the fetus and young adult*, 5th ed, Baltimore, 1995, Williams & Wilkins.
19. Friedman RA, Starke JR: Infective endocarditis. In Garson A, Bricker JT, McNamara DG, eds: *The science and practice of pediatric cardiology*, vol 2, Philadelphia, 1990, Lea and Febiger.
20. Friedman WF: Aortic Stenosis. In Emmanouilides GC, Reimenschneider TA, Allen, HD, Gutgesell, HP (editors): *Moss and Adams heart disease in infants, children, and adolescents including the fetus and young adult*, 5th ed, Baltimore, 1995, Williams & Wilkins.
21. Fukushige J, Nihill MR: Kawasaki disease. In Garsen A, Bricker JT, McNamara DG, eds: *The science and practice of pediatric cardiology*, vol 2, Philadelphia, 1990, Lea and Febiger.
22. Fyler DC: Report of the New England regional infant cardiac program, *Pediatrics* (suppl):377, 1980.
23. Fyler DC, ed: *Nadas' pediatric cardiology*, St Louis, 1992, Mosby.
24. Gillette PC et al: Neonatal cardiac arrhythmias and their potential role in sudden infant death syndrome, *Clin Perinatol* 3:15, 1988.

25. Gillette PC, Gavson A: *Pediatric arrhythmias: electrophysiology and pacing.* Philadelphia, 1990, WB Saunders Co.

26. Graham TJ, Gutgesell HP: Conotruncal abnormalities. In Long WA, ed: *Fetal and neonatal cardiology,* Philadelphia, 1990, WB Saunders.

27. Graham TP, Gutgesell HP: Ventricular septal defects. In Emmanouilides GC, Reimenschneider TA, Allen, HD, Gutgesell, HP (editors): *Moss and Adams heart disease in infants, children, and adolescents including the fetus and young adult,* 5th ed, Baltimore, 1995, Williams & Wilkins.

28. Gutgesell HP: Pulmonary valve abnormalities. In Long WA, ed: *Fetal and neonatal cardiology,* Philadelphia, 1990, WB Saunders.

29. Hakim SN, Toepper WC: Cardiac disease. In Barkin R, eds: *Emergency medicine: concepts and clinical practice,* ed 3, St Louis, 1992, Mosby.

30. Haworth SG, Bull C: Pathophysiology of congenital heart disease, *Arch Dis Child* 68:707-711, 1993.

31. Hazinski MF: Cardiovascular disorders. In Hazinski MF, ed: *Nursing care of the critically ill child,* ed 2, St Louis, 1992, Mosby.

32. Hoffman JIE: Congenital heart disease: incidence and inheritance. In Gillette PC, ed: *Pediatr Clin North Am* 1:37, 1990.

33. Hoffman JIE, Christianson MA: Congenital heart disease in a cohort of 19,502 births with long-term follow-up, *Am J Cardiol* 42:641-647, 1978.

34. Hoffman JIE, Rudolf AM: The natural history of ventricular septal defects in infancy, *Am J Cardiol* 16:634, 1965.

35. Johnson GL: Clinical examination. In Long WA, ed: *Fetal and neonatal cardiology,* Philadelphia, 1990, WB Saunders.

36. Keeley SR, Bohn DJ: The use of inotropic and after-load reducing agents in the neonates, *Clin Perinatol* 3:15, 1988.

37. Kohr LM, O'Brien P: Current management of congestive heart failure in infants and children. In Hickey PA, ed: *Nurs Clin North Am* 30:261-290, 1995.

38. Krovetz LJ, Gessner IH, Schiebler GL: *Handbook of pediatric cardiology,* ed 2, Baltimore, 1979, University Park Press.

39. Kulik LA, Hickey PA, Lawrence PR: Pharmacologic interventions for the neonate with compromised cardiac function, *J Perinat Neonat Nurs* 2:5, 1991.

40. Li MM, Klassen TP, Watters LK: In Barkin RM, ed: *Pediatric emergency medicine: concepts and clinical practice,* St Louis, 1992, Mosby.

41. Lucas RV, Krabill KA: Abnormal pulmonary venous connections. In Emmanouilides GC, Reimenschneider TA, Allen, HD, Gutgesell, HP (editors): *Moss and Adams heart disease in infants, children, and adolescents including the fetus and young adult,* 5th ed, Baltimore, 1995, Williams & Wilkins.

42. Mair DD, Edwards WD, Julsrud, PR, Seward JB, Danielson GK: Truncus arteriosus. In Emmanouilides GC, Reimenschneider TA, Allen, HD, Gutgesell, HP (editors): *Moss and Adams heart disease in infants, children, and adolescents including the fetus and young adult,* 5th ed, Baltimore, 1995, Williams & Wilkins.

43. Mas MS, Bricker JT: Clinical physiology of left-to-right shunts. In Garson A, Bricker JT, McNamara DG, eds: *The science and practice of pediatric cardiology,* vol 2, Philadelphia, 1990, Lea and Febiger.

44. Meldon SW et al: Pediatric ventricular tachycardia, *Pediatr Emerg Care* 10:294-300, 1994.

45. Melish ME, Hicks RV: Kawasaki syndrome: clinical features: pathophysiology, etiology, and therapy, *J Rheumatol* (suppl):24, 1990.

46. Milnor WR: Normal circulatory function. In Mountcastle VB, ed: *Medical physiology,* vol 2, St Louis, 1974, Mosby.

47. Nora JJ, Nora AH: The evolution of specific genetic and environmental counseling in congenital heart disease, *Circulation* 2:57, 1978.

48. O'Connor BK, Dick M: What every pediatrician should know about supraventricular tachycardia, *Pediatr Ann* 20:368-376, 1991.

49. Pinsky WW, Friedman RA: Pericarditis. In Garson A, Bricker JT, McNamara DG, eds: *The science and practice of pediatric cardiology,* vol 2, Philadelphia, 1990, Lea and Febiger.

50. Rheuban KS: Pediatric cardiac emergencies. In Schwartz GR et al, eds: *Principles and practice of emergency medicine,* ed 2, Philadelphia, 1992, Lea and Febiger.

51. Rocchini AP, Emmanouilides GC: Pulmonary stenosis. In Emmanouilides GC, Reimenschneider TA, Allen, HD, Gutgesell, HP (editors): *Moss and Adams heart disease in infants, children, and adolescents including the fetus and young adult,* 5th ed, Baltimore, 1995, Williams & Wilkins.

52. Rosenthal A: How to distinguish between innocent and pathologic murmurs in childhood, *Pediatr Clin North Am* 6:31, 1984.

53. Rosenthal A, Dick M: Tricuspid atresia. In Emmanouilides GC, Reimenshcneider TA, Allen, HD, Gutgesell, HP, editors: *Moss and Adams heart disease in infants, children, and adolescents including the fetus and young adult,* 5th ed, Baltimore, 1995, Williams & Wilkins.

54. Rudolph AM: The changes in the circulation after birth, *Circulation* 41:343-359, 1970.

55. Rudolph AM: *Congenital diseases of the heart: clinical physiologic consideration in diagnosis and management,* Chicago, 1974, Year Book Medical Publishers.

56. Talner NS: Heart failure. In Emmanouilides GC, Reimenschneider TA, Allen, HD, Gutgesell, HP, eds: *Moss and Adams heart disease in infants,*

children, and adolescents including the fetus and young adult, 5th ed, Baltimore, 1995, Williams & Wilkins.

57. Vetter VL: What every pediatrician needs to know about arrythmias in children who have had cardiac surgery, *Pediatr Ann* 20:378-385, 1991.

58. Whitley HG, Perry LW: Coarctation. In Long WA, ed: *Fetal and neonatal cardiology,* Philadelphia, 1990, WB Saunders.

59. Wong DL: *Whaley & Wong's essentials of pediatric nursing,* ed 5, St Louis, 1997, Mosby.

60. Zavaras-Angelidou KA, Weinhouse E, Nelson DB: Review of 180 episodes of chest pain in 134 children, *Pediatr Emerg Care* 8:189-192, 1992.

CHAPTER 12

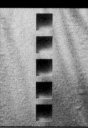

Neurologic System

Barbara Masiulis, Alison W. Schultz

INTRODUCTION

Neurologic disorders are common within the pediatric population. To effectively care for children with neurologic disorders, emergency personnel should be familiar with manifestations of the most common neurologic complaints in children and the appropriate interventions. This chapter reviews some of the more frequent diagnoses seen in this population and outlines nursing interventions. (NOTE: Head trauma is included in Chapter 22, and life-threatening neurologic emergencies are reviewed in Chapter 7.)

ANATOMY AND PHYSIOLOGY

At birth all major structures of the brain are present; however, because many of these structures are not completely developed the infant's brain is 25% of adult size.[12] Biochemical changes in neurotransmitters and myelinization of the corticospinal pathways contribute to growth and maturation of the developing brain. With development, primitive reflexes disappear, and cognition and motor functions improve.

The brain consists of three major areas, the cerebrum, the cerebellum, and the brain stem. The cerebral cortex is largely responsible for cognitive function, sensation, voluntary movement, and emotions. The brain stem is the major nerve pathway between the cerebral cortex and the spinal cord and controls many of the involuntary bodily functions, including those vital to life. The cerebellum controls spatial orientation, balance, muscle tone, and fine motor movements by processing sensory stimuli. Voluntary movement is also integrated by the cerebellum, although it can be overruled by the cerebral cortex[19] (Fig. 12-1).

At birth the cranium of the newborn is soft and malleable. The skull consists of separate bones connected by fibrous tissue referred to as *sutures*. Sutures allow for brain growth and begin to fuse around 6 to 8 months of life. The anterior and posterior fontanels are located where several bones of the skull meet. They are midline and can usually be palpated at birth, although the posterior fontanel may be closed at birth. The anterior fontanel closes between 9 and 18 months of age.

The brain and spinal column are surrounded by three vascular membranes, called the *meninges*. The tough outermost membrane (the dura mater) is separated from the middle membrane (the arachnoid) by the subdural space. The arachnoid is separated from the innermost membrane (the pia mater) by the subarachnoid space, which contains cerebrospinal fluid (see Fig. 22-2). Cerebrospinal fluid (CSF) is produced and circulated within the ventricles, the subarachnoid space, and the spinal column. CSF protects the central nervous system (CNS) from injury, and the reabsorption of CSF is one of the mechanisms by which increases in intracranial pressure (ICP) are controlled.

NURSING HISTORY AND ASSESSMENT

HISTORY

Assessing neurologic complaints in children can be complicated and time consuming because of varying developmental levels and immature verbal skills. The history provided by the parent and child (when able) is therefore an important component of the examination. The focus of the history depends on the chief complaint and presenting signs and symptoms. Im-

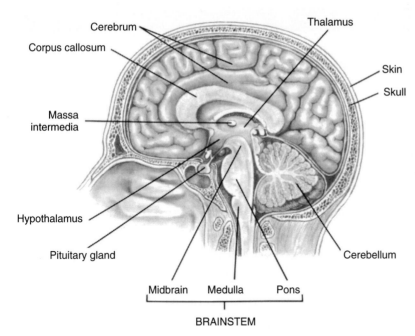

FIG. 12-1. Major structures of the brain.

Labels: Cerebrum, Corpus callosum, Massa intermedia, Hypothalamus, Pituitary gland, Thalamus, Skin, Skull, Cerebellum, Midbrain, Medulla, Pons, BRAINSTEM

portant components of the history include information regarding alterations in the child's mental state during the illness or after an injury and additional signs of illness or injury such as fever, vomiting, headaches, or visual disturbances. Other important components of the history include the infant or child's past medical history, particularly the presence of a chronic medical condition. In infants and young children the birth history may offer important information (Box 12-1).

PHYSICAL EXAMINATION

The pediatric neurologic examination consists of an evaluation of the child's level of consciousness, mental/emotional status, cranial nerve function, motor and sensory responses, and developmental level. During the examination much information can be obtained by simply observing the infant or child's activities. For example, by observing an infant's response to the environment, parents, bright lights, sounds, and touch, valuable information relating to the level of consciousness and developmental status can be obtained. Additionally, the size and shape of the head, facial characteristics, the quality of the infant's cry, and the infant's posture provide important information. In the preschooler or older child, observing the child's level of consciousness, age-appropriate response to the environment, gait, movement, and mentation offers information about neurologic integrity.

Because past or chronic neurologic or developmental disorders may affect a child's functional abilities and neurologic exam, children with neurologic disorders are evaluated in terms of their baseline physical and developmental status. In these cases the parents or caregivers are the best historians regarding their child's abilities.

In addition to observation, an assessment of reflexes provides important information regarding the infant or child's neurologic status. In the infant the presence or absence of infantile reflexes (depending on the infant's age) can identify a lesion or injury to the corticospinal tract. With development, infantile reflexes normally disappear, and their continued presence or reappearance can signal an underlying neurologic disorder (Table 12-1).

NEUROLOGIC SIGNS AND SYMPTOMS

HEADACHE

Etiology. Headache is a common complaint in the pediatric population, increasing in frequency with approaching adolescence. Although a headache may

---

Box 12-1   History and Physical Assessment for the Child with a Neurologic Complaint

History

Present illness: chief complaint, associated signs and symptoms, drug abuse or exposure, interventions

Past history: developmental, neurologic, or chronic disorders or abnormalities; medication history and allergies

Prenatal and perinatal birth history (for infants/children under 2 years of age and those with neurologic or developmental problems)

Growth and development:

Physical: growth; milestones such as sitting, walking

Cognitive: intellectual (e.g., school performance); language skills

Psychosocial: behavior; relationship with family/peers

Family history: neurologic/developmental disorders such as headaches or epilepsy

Physical assessment

Level of consciousness (LOC); mental status; developmentally appropriate behavior

Sensory-motor function

Cranial nerve function and deep tendon reflexes

Cerebellar function (e.g., coordination, gait)

Vital signs

Variations for infants and toddlers:

Head size, shape, symmetry, and facial features

Fontanels, cranial sutures

LOC: recognition of parents; eye contact; follows light/objects; responds to environment

Motor activity

Achieving milestones

Spontaneous activity; symmetry of movement

Muscle tone; posture

Reflexes—presence, absence, and symmetry

Behavior (e.g., irritability, consolability, lethargy)

Quality of cry

TABLE 12-1   Infantile Reflexes

REFLEX	TESTING
Palmar grasp	Infant will grasp a finger firmly placed against the palmar surface. Meaningful grasp occurs after 3 to 4 months of age.
Rooting	Mouth will open and face will turn to stimulated side when cheek or perioral skin is stroked. Disappears at 3 to 4 months of age when infant is awake and 7 to 8 months of age when the infant is asleep.
Vertical suspension positioning	Legs will flex at the hips and knees when the infant is supported upright with the examiner's hands under the axillae. Disappears at about 4 months of age.
Moro	Infant will stiffen extremities, index fingers and thumb will form a "C" shape, and fingers and toes will fan in response to a loud noise or extension of the infant's neck. Disappears at 4 to 6 months of age.
Tonic neck (fencing)	With the infant in the supine position the head is turned to one side and the arm and leg on that side extend. The arm and leg on the opposite side flex. Disappears at 4 to 6 months.
Sucking	Infant will suck with lips and tongue when lips are touched. Disappears at 10 to 12 months.
Placing response	Infant will flex hip and knee and place foot in stepping motion when held upright with the examiner's hands under the axillae. The age of disappearance varies but is usually around 10 to 12 months of age.

Modified from Slota MC: Neurologic assessment of the infant and toddler, *Crit Care Nurs* Sept/Oct: 91, 1983.

represent serious underlying pathology, the majority of headaches are mild and self-limited. Headaches are classified by etiology and severity.[48] They can occur acutely secondary to eye strain, pharyngitis, meningitis, viral infections, sinusitis, or traumatic injury (e.g., subarachnoid bleed), or they can be recurrent such as tension headaches and migraines. Headaches can be chronic and progressive secondary to a brain abscess, or they may be chronic and nonprogressive secondary to tension or muscle strain.

Approximately 55% of children will have experienced a headache by 15 years of age.[31] Before puberty the male to female incidence of headaches is fairly equal. After puberty more girls than boys experience headaches. Headaches in older children or adolescents are predominantly tension or migraine headaches. Headaches in children less than 5 years of age are relatively uncommon and are therefore more likely to represent an organic etiology.

Pathophysiology.   Headaches can be caused by stimulation of any of the pain-sensitive structures of the head or neck.[26] Pain may result from inflammation, displacement, traction, or dilation of pain-sensitive intracranial structures; dilation or distention of extracranial blood vessels; or spasmodic contraction of head and neck muscles.[51] The majority of headaches result from an extracranial rather than an intracranial etiology. Pain-sensitive extracranial structures include the arteries around the eyes, forehead, and temple; the sinuses and teeth; and the muscles attached to the skull, including the extraocular, neck, and jaw muscles.[13] Pain-sensitive intracranial structures include the large arteries and veins, the dura at the base of the skull, and the venous sinuses. The brain tissue, skull, and lining of the ventricles are not sensitive to pain.

Clinical presentation.   Clinical presentation varies widely depending on the etiology of the headache. Although headaches rarely present emergently, signs and symptoms associated with an emergent condition include forceful vomiting, lethargy or coma, ataxia, visual field loss, nuchal rigidity, and personality changes.

The child with a *tension headache* (muscle contraction) generally presents with a history of stress.[51] Although young children may not be able to describe the pain or relate a history of stress, older children may describe squeezing, pressing, bandlike, or dull and aching pain. Bilateral pain in the back of the head or neck is common and sleep may not provide headache relief. Tension headaches tend to be recurrent.

Migraine headaches may be "classic," "common," or "complicated." Classic migraines often present with a positive family history. They are usually preceded by an aura and are characterized by acute, unilateral throbbing or pulsating pain around the eyes, forehead, or temple; nausea and vomiting; visual changes; and photophobia. These headaches are relieved by sleep. Common migraines, which are most prevalent in children, may be preceded by visual changes but are more often preceded by mood changes, fatigue, dizziness, or nausea.[13] The headache may be described as diffuse or unilateral and often varies in intensity. Vomiting may or may not be prominent. Complicated migraines are infrequently seen in children. They are associated with transient focal neurologic deficits such as ophthalmoplegia (paralysis of one or more motor nerves of the eye) or hemiplegia and may or may not be associated with a headache. Symptoms are usually prolonged and residual neurologic deficits can last up to several weeks.

Stress and high anxiety may contribute to recurrent migraine or tension headaches. Recurrent headaches may also be associated with behavior changes such as irritability, acting out, or school problems.[35]

Emergency Department interventions.   The single most important component of the examination of the child presenting with a headache is to rule out an underlying pathologic process. Diagnostic testing such as a computed axial tomography (CT) scan, magnetic resonance imaging (MRI), or laboratory analysis of blood or CSF is only performed when an underlying illness or pathology is suspected (Box 12-2).

Box 12-2   Signs of an Organic Headache

Progression in severity and frequency over a short period of time
Awakens child during sleep
Occurs in early morning
May worsen with sneezing or coughing
Unexplained forceful vomiting
May be associated with change in gait, personality, or behavior (not associated with the headache)

Modified from Elser JM: Easing the pain of childhood headaches, *Contemp Pediatr* 11:112, 1991.

Treatment depends on the suspected diagnosis. If the headache is symptomatic of an underlying illness, the primary etiology is addressed. Once a serious underlying pathology is ruled out general interventions may include pharmacotherapy, stress management, and counseling.[16]

Recurrent tension headaches are most commonly treated with behavioral interventions such as biofeedback, behavior therapy, and physical therapy designed to reduce the pain associated with muscle contractions of the neck and shoulder. Migraine headaches are often initially treated with simple analgesics. When these are not effective in aborting the migraine, additional pharmacologic interventions may include the administration of Fiorinal (one to two tablets every 6 hours), which is a combination of acetaminophen, butalbital, and caffeine; or sumatriptan succinate. Ergotamines, which provide selective vasoconstriction of the external carotid artery and its branches[16] are not recommended in children because of serious side effects including stroke. Narcotics such as codeine or meperidine are rarely used because of their association with physical dependence and rebound headaches.[16] Prophylactic medications used to treat childhood headaches include amitriptyline (Elavil) 0.5 to 1 mg/kg/day at bedtime, cyproheptadine (Periactin) 0.25 to 0.5 mg/kg/day (bid or tid), propranolol (Inderal) 1 to 4 mg/kg/day (bid or tid), and nifedipine (Procardia) 10 to 20 mg PO tid.[52]

Antiemetics such as prochlorperazine (Compazine) and metoclopramide (Reglan) may be used in conjunction with analgesics during a migraine attack. Because vomiting and delayed gastric motility interferes with the absorption of adequate doses of analgesics, alternate routes of administration such as sublingual, rectal, or IV/IM may be necessary.

Nursing care and evaluation. Children with isolated complaints of headache rarely require emergent interventions but instead present to the emergency department (ED) for pain relief. The history and physical play important roles in the determination of the source of the headache pain. Specific historical questions will identify the characteristics of the pain, the chronologic features of the headache, the location of the pain, and associated symptoms (e.g., fever, irritability, nuchal rigidity) (Box 12-3). The child's past medical history (such as head injury, exposure to toxins, medication usage, or chronic illness) may also provide important clues to the etiology. If stress is suspected, a psychosocial assessment may be performed to explore stressors in the child's life, family and peer relationships, school performance, and signs of depression and anxiety. The physical examination requires an evaluation of the child's neurologic status, including an assessment of the level of consciousness and the child's demeanor, cranial nerves, reflexes, and motor strength. A full set of vital signs, including blood pressure, is obtained and visual acuity is tested.

Pain relief usually includes both pharmacologic and nonpharmacologic interventions. Nonpharmacologic nursing interventions include providing the child with a dark, quiet room and suggesting stress-management or relaxation techniques.

Before discharge, the headache type, potential precipitating factors, prevention, and recommended relief measures are discussed with the child and family. If recurrent headaches are present, a diary may be recommended to help the family and child identify headache frequency, severity, precipitating factors, associated symptoms, and the effectiveness of treatment. Pain medications for migraine headaches must be administered in sufficient doses and at the earliest signs of the headache to be most effective. When migraine headaches are suspected, parents should be reassured that although this problem may be life-long, effective management is available and the frequency of migraines tends to diminish with age.

SEIZURES

Etiology. Seizures are symptomatic of CNS or systemic dysfunction and may represent an acute or

---

Box 12-3 History for the Child with a Chief Complaint of Headache

Single vs. multiple
Frequency
Intensity
Location
Duration
Precipitating events (e.g., increased activity, foods, stress)
Characteristics (e.g., throbbing, pounding, dull, unilateral, diffuse)
Warning signs (e.g., aura)
Associated symptoms (e.g., nausea, ataxia, lethargy, fever)
Family history of headaches
Relief measures (e.g., medications, quiet environment)
Past medical history

chronic condition. Acute conditions that can produce seizures include fever, meningitis, encephalitis, intracranial hemorrhage, substance abuse, and metabolic imbalances. Chronic seizure disorders may be caused by CNS insult such as hypoxia or trauma, or they may be caused by congenital defects, inborn errors of metabolism, or neurocutaneous disorders (e.g., neurofibromatosis, tuberous sclerosis)[46] (Table 12-2). Recurring seizures are referred to as *epilepsy*. When the cause of the seizure disorder is unknown the child is said to have idiopathic epilepsy.

Pathophysiology. Seizure activity develops from a sudden, abnormal discharge of a group of neurons that become an epileptogenic focus.[20] This group of cells exhibits electrical excitability, firing discharges intermittently, often in bursts. These abnormal discharges result in alterations in motor function, sensation, autonomic behavior, and/or consciousness.

TABLE 12-2	Common Seizure Etiologies by Age Group
AGE GROUP	**ETIOLOGIES**
Neonatal	Perinatal hypoxia
	Birth trauma
	Intracranial hemorrhage
	Metabolic imbalances
	Hyper/hypoglycemia
	Hyper/hyponatremia
	Hypocalcemia
	Hypomagnesemia
	Inborn errors of metabolism
	Infection
	Bacterial meningitis
	Meningoencephalitis
	Congenital malformation
	Drug withdrawal
Infancy and early childhood	Febrile seizures
	Infection
	Bacterial meningitis
	Viral encephalitis
	Trauma
	Congenital malformation
	Metabolic imbalances
	Toxins
	Idiopathic
Adolescence	Idiopathic
	Trauma
	Drugs/toxins
	Metabolic

Seizures are classified as *partial* or *generalized*. Generalized seizures involve all or large parts of the cerebral cortex and are classified as *convulsive* or *nonconvulsive* (e.g., absence seizures). Partial seizures result from epileptic discharges in one area of the brain or hemisphere, but they may secondarily generalize to other areas of the brain—referred to as *partial or focal seizures with secondary generalization*. Partial seizures are further classified into those that do not alter consciousness (simple partial seizures) and those that do alter consciousness (complex partial seizures) (Table 12-3).

Seizures unique to the pediatric population include neonatal seizures, infantile spasms, and febrile seizures. *Febrile seizures* are reviewed in Chapter 26. *Neonatal seizures* occur within the first month of life and are caused by a variety of disorders, including hypoxic-ischemic encephalopathy and metabolic, infectious, toxic, structural, and maternal disturbances.[4] Neonatal seizures may be evidenced by subtle activities such as eye deviations, sucking, blinking, or pedaling movements of the legs, or they may be evidenced by tonic extension of the limbs, clonic activity in one limb—which may move to another area of the body (multifocal seizures), or flexion jerks of the upper or lower extremities (myoclonic seizures).[46]

Infantile spasms are seen in infants between 3 months and 2 years of age and may be *cryptogenic,* meaning there is no apparent cause, or *symptomatic,* meaning prenatal, perinatal, or postnatal events led to the development of the seizures.[4,20] In approximately 50% of the cases a metabolic, degenerative, or structural anomaly is present. In infants with the symptomatic form of the illness more than 80% are mentally retarded.[4,20] Tuberous sclerosis, a neurocutaneous disorder, commonly presents with infantile spasms. Infantile spasms are characterized by brief symmetric contractions of the neck, trunk, and extremities.[4] Spasms tend to occur in clusters, as many as several hundred times a day.[27]

Clinical presentation. Features of an epileptic event can include motor changes, alterations in the level of consciousness, sensory symptoms, hallucinations, and/or autonomic symptoms (e.g., loss of bowel or bladder control, sweating, salivation). The extent and site of the neural discharge determines the particular clinical manifestations (Table 12-4). Status epilepticus, which is a prolonged episode of continuous or frequent seizures between which the child does not regain consciousness, is a neurologic emergency (see Chapter 7).

TABLE 12-3	Classification of Seizures	

INTERNATIONAL CLASSIFICATION	OLD TERMINOLOGY
Partial seizures	Focal or local seizures
Simple partial seizures (consciousness not impaired)	
With motor symptoms	Jacksonian seizures
With somatosensory or special sensory symptoms	Focal sensory
With autonomic symptoms	
With psychic symptoms	
Complex partial seizures (with impairment of consciousness)	Psychomotor or temporal lobe seizures
Simple partial onset	
With impairment of consciousness at onset	
Partial seizures that secondarily generalize	
Generalized seizures (convulsive or nonconvulsive)	
Absence	Petit mal
Absence	
Atypical	
Myoclonic	Minor motor
Clonic	Grand mal
Tonic	Grand mal
Tonic-clonic	Grand mal
Atonic (astatic)	Akinetic, drop attacks

From Vining EPG, Freeman JM: Management of nonfebrile seizures, *Pediatr Rev* 8(6):186, 1986.

Emergency Department interventions. Clinical presentation and the suspected underlying etiology of the seizure(s) will determine the extent of diagnostic testing and mode of treatment (e.g., urine toxicology screen for suspected ingestion or lumbar puncture for suspected meningitis). If the child has a known seizure disorder and is on antiepileptic therapy, a serum drug level will be drawn.

Neuroimaging studies such as MRIs or CT scans are indicated in children with acute focal neurologic abnormalities or seizures that do not respond to treatment. Electroencephalograms (EEGs) are rarely performed in the emergency department, because the diffuse slowing that results after a seizure is not necessarily consistent with epilepsy.[21,49] An EEG may, however, be scheduled for several days to weeks after the event.

Treatment of the child with a history of a seizure depends on the underlying etiology. If a CNS infection such as meningitis is suspected, the child is admitted and treated with parenteral antibiotics (see p. 280). Children presenting with a single generalized tonic-clonic seizure and a normal neurologic exam are not usually treated with long-term antiepileptic therapy unless the seizures recur. Children with absence, myoclonic, akinetic, partial complex seizures, or infantile spasms are started on antiepileptics because of their high rate of recurrence. The timing of pharmacotherapy initiation depends on the acuity or intensity of seizure presentation (Table 12-5).

Nursing care and evaluation. The goals of management for an actively seizing child are to stabilize and maintain the ABCs, promptly control the seizure activity, and if possible identify and correct the cause of the event. When the child arrives with a history of seizure activity but is not currently seizing, seizure precautions are instituted, which includes padding the bed rails and placing airway equipment, suction, a bag-valve-mask device, and oxygen at the bedside. The child who begins to seize is not restrained but can be rolled onto the side. Nothing should be placed in the mouth. The airway is positioned and suctioned as needed. If the seizure does not resolve spontaneously, peripheral venous access is established to administer anticonvulsive therapy. A clear description of the seizure activity (e.g., location, duration, intensity, characteristics), the child's physiologic status during

TABLE 12-4	Clinical Manifestations of Generalized and Partial Seizures
TYPE	**DESCRIPTION**
Generalized seizures	
Absence	Brief periods of unconsciousness (5-15 seconds); child stops in middle of activity, stares, and is unresponsive. May exhibit eye fluttering, upward movement of the eyes, lip smacking, and/or hand movements (e.g., atypical absence). May be mistaken for daydreaming, inattentiveness.
Tonic-clonic	Tonic phase involves sudden loss of consciousness, followed by eyes rolling upward or outward, cessation of breathing, and falling to ground; clonic phase follows with bilateral rhythmic jerking, expiratory grunts or hyperventilation, possible bowel/bladder incontinence, profuse sweating, excessive salivation, and tongue biting. Is followed by a postictal period.
Myoclonic	Sudden, uncontrollable jerking movement of one or more of the extremities; child may be flung to the ground and sustain injuries. Usually involves momentary loss of consciousness, followed by postictal confusion.
Tonic	Loss of postural tone with flexion of upper limbs and extension of lower limbs; no evidence of clonicity. Lasts for seconds or minutes without a loss of consciousness.
Atonic	Loss of postural tone with alterations of consciousness and subsequent postictal period.
Akinetic	Sudden loss of postural muscle tone (drop attacks).
Partial seizures	
Simple partial	Seizure activity limited to one part or side of body without alterations in consciousness. Motor, sensory and/or cognitive manifestations vary with location of epileptic discharge.
Complex partial	Localized seizure activity with alteration in consciousness, which sometimes involve cognitive changes, psychomotor, or psychosensory symptoms. Frequently associated with an aura, which may be autonomic, affective, auditory, olfactory, or visual hallucination; may describe "funny feeling" at onset. A postictal period follows where the child may be disoriented and/or angry. There is no memory of the event.
Secondary generalized	Focal seizure activity that generalizes to tonic-clonic. Begins with aura, head or eye deviation, or a focal clonic activity. Postictal neurologic exam may reveal mild hemiparesis or visual field defect.

Modified from Hickey JV: *The clinical practice of neurological and neurosurgical nursing,* ed 3, Philadelphia, 1992, JB Lippincott.

the seizure (e.g., respiratory status, incontinence, level of consciousness, vital signs), and events preceding the seizures are recorded. At the conclusion of the seizure a neurologic exam is performed to determine the level of consciousness and the presence of postictal changes.

During the postictal state the airway and breathing are monitored. Continuous assessment includes ongoing evaluations of the child's neurologic status, respiratory status, and vital signs.

Seizures are frightening to both the parents and the

TABLE 12-5	Common Antiepileptic Medications		
DRUG	**INDICATIONS**	**USUAL DOSE (MG/KG/DAY)**	**THERAPEUTIC LEVELS (μG/ML)**
Carbamazepine	Partial, secondarily generalized	5-25 5-10 (monotherapy)	4-12
Phenytoin	Partial, secondarily generalized, primary generalized	5-7	10-20 (occasionally lower)
Valproic acid	Primary generalized, absence, myoclonic, akinetic, febrile, infantile spasms, some partial	10-30 20-50 (infants and polytherapy)	50-100 (150 if tolerated)
Phenobarbital	Neonatal, febrile, partial, secondarily generalized, primary generalized, akinetic	3-5 (<25 kg) 2-3 (25-50 kg) 1-2 (>50 kg)	10-40
Ethosuximide	Absence, myoclonic, akinetic	15-40	40-100
Clonazepam	Absence, primary generalized, infantile spasms	0.01-0.2	0.01-0.07
Acetazolamide	Absence, myoclonic, akinetic, partial	10-20	10-14
Felbamate*	Partial seizures in children over 12 years, Lennox-Gastaut syndrome	15-45 (max 3600)	—
Gabapentin*	Partial, secondary generalized in children over 12 years	Total daily dose 900-1800	—
Lamotrigine*	Partial, generalized	10 (monotherapy) 6 (in combination with valproate with enzyme inducing AED) 3 (if on valproic acid only)	—

Modified from Roddy and McBride, 1992.
*Additional references: Carter, 1994; Byers, 1993.

child. Often parents believe that neurologic damage will be caused by the seizure. The ED nurse can assist family members by allowing them to remain with their child whenever possible and keeping them informed of the plan of care. Parents and children should be encouraged to verbalize their concerns. If the child is to be discharged, home care instructions are given and follow-up care arranged. When a child has a known seizure disorder compliance with drug therapy is stressed. A common cause of breakthrough seizures is noncompliance with therapy or the child who has "outgrown" the current dosage of medication. Fever, infection, illness, fatigue, sleep deprivation, and emo-

tional stress may also precipitate a seizure in children with epilepsy.[14] Other potential triggers of seizures include fluid overload, loud noises, flickering lights, premenstrual changes, and alcohol consumption. Parents may also be referred to the Epilepsy Foundation of America.* (See Box 12-4 for discharge teaching.)

HYDROCEPHALUS

Etiology. Hydrocephalus is not a disease but is a clinical condition resulting from an imbalance in the

*Epilepsy Foundation of America: 1-800-EFA-1000.

Box 12-4 Discharge Teaching for Seizures

General seizure information
- Etiology of child's seizures if known
- Risk of recurrence
- Effects of seizure
- Physical/behavioral changes after seizures
- Treat child as normal as possible

Medications
- Anticonvulsants—side effects, including behavioral changes; importance of compliance; required monitoring
- Antipyretics (for febrile seizures)—alternate acetaminophen and ibuprofen every 3 hours for 48 hours

Seizure control
- Future illnesses—antipyretics immediately
- Care during a seizure—protect from injury
- Activity restrictions as indicated

Follow-up
- Appointments—scheduled
- When to call the doctor and whom to call (e.g., pediatrician or specialist)

production, absorption, or flow of CSF in the ventricular system. It can be associated with any number of acute or chronic conditions ranging from acute trauma to congenital disorders.

Hydrocephalus is classified as either communicating or noncommunicating. Communicating hydrocephalus represents an increase in the production of CSF or decreased absorption of CSF. Meningitis, subarachnoid hemorrhage, trauma, leukemia, and neoplasm are examples of conditions causing a communicating hydrocephalus. Noncommunicating hydrocephalus, which involves an obstruction in the flow of the CSF through the ventricular system, results primarily from congenital malformations, such as obstruction at the aqueduct of Sylvius between the third and fourth ventricles, Chiari II malformations—which are present in all children with myelomeningocele, and Dandy-Walker syndrome—which is failure of the development of the roof of the fourth ventricle during embryonic growth. Acquired causes of noncommunicating hydrocephalus include ventriculitis, hemorrhage, and intracranial mass lesions.

Pathophysiology. Hydrocephalus represents an accumulation of CSF in the ventricular system. With the accumulation of CSF the ventricles dilate, causing progressive compression of the brain tissue against the surrounding bony cranium. Before the cranial sutures are fused in young infants, the skull may be able to expand to accommodate *gradual* increases in volume. In very young infants one of the first signs of hydrocephalus may be an enlarging head circumference disproportionate to normal growth curve parameters. With fusion of the sutures, the skull can no longer enlarge and overt signs of increasing ICP indicate the presence of hydrocephalus.

In children with a congenital anomaly of the ventricles or permanent ventricular damage causing persistent hydrocephalus, a ventriculoperitoneal (VP) or ventriculoatrial shunt (rarely used) may be surgically implanted. The purpose of the shunt is to drain CSF from the ventricles into the peritoneal cavity or the atrium. The shunt usually consists of a ventricular catheter, flush pump, one-way valve, and distal catheter[28] (Fig. 12-2).

Clinical presentation. The clinical presentation of hydrocephalus is influenced by the etiology, acuity at onset, and the child's age. In the neonate or young infant, hydrocephalus is suspected when the head grows at an abnormal rate. The fontanels in these infants are usually open and bulging and the scalp veins dilated. As fluid continues to accumulate within the ventricles, pressure on the tectum may cause the eyes to deviate downward ("setting sun" sign). In older children, hydrocephalus is considered when signs of increasing ICP are present. In both age groups signs and symptoms of increasing ICP include alterations in the LOC (irritability, lethargy, decreased response to pain), decreased feeding or appetite, and forceful vomiting. In older children, headaches may be a complaint; in infants a high-pitched or whining cry may be heard.

Most children with hydrocephalus who are seen in the ED have already been diagnosed and treated. The child usually has had either a surgical removal of the obstruction or the placement of a ventricular shunt to divert CSF from the ventricles. Children with VP shunts may present with signs and symptoms of shunt malfunction and/or infection, both of which can be life threatening.[28] Shunts fail due to obstructions, tubing disconnections, or migration of the distal tube tip. Growth of the child or injuries may also cause shunt malfunction. Signs of shunt failure are largely related to an increasing ICP (Box 12-5). Shunt infections most commonly

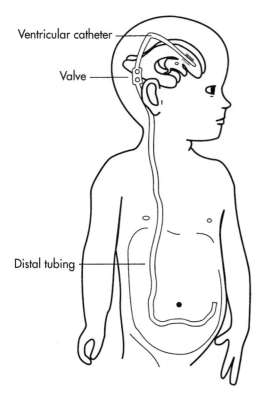

Ventricular catheter

Valve

Distal tubing

FIG. 12-2. Ventriculoperitoneal shunt. A catheter is inserted into the lateral ventricle and is threaded subcutaneously to the abdominal cavity. Small incisions are made in the scalp and the peritoneum. (From Key CB, Rothrock SG, Falk JL: Cerebral spinal fluid shunt complications: an emergency medicine perspective, *Pediatr Emerg Care* 11(5):266, 1995.)

occur in the first few months after shunt insertion. Manifestations are similar to those of other CNS infections but may be less obvious (e.g., fever and alterations in the LOC).

Emergency Department interventions. Definitive diagnostic testing for the presence of hydrocephalus is made with either a CT scan or MRI. Once identified, the treatment of hydrocephalus is dependent upon the suspected etiology and severity. In most cases consultation with neurosurgery is indicated. (For in-depth discussions of treatment based on underlying etiology, see the appropriate sections within this text. For example, subarachnoid hemorrhage is reviewed in Chapter 22, and medical management of increased ICP is reviewed in Chapter 7.)

Box 12-5   Signs and Symptoms of Shunt Malfunction
Acute Irritability Lethargy Headache Vomiting (forceful without nausea) Ataxia Strabismus Papilledema (late) Coma (late) Autonomic instability (late) Seizures **Chronic** Papilledema Altered mental functions (e.g., learning skills) Delays in developmental progress

Shunted hydrocephalus. When a shunt failure is suspected, neuroimaging studies will confirm ventricular enlargement. A "shunt series" of radiographs determines the position of the distal tube tip, integrity of the system, and availability of sufficient tubing length for growth. Pumping the palpable shunt reservoir for ease of depression and filling is an unreliable indicator of shunt function[43] and does not replace the CT scan or MRI. Repetitive pumping of the shunt is not recommended. The shunt valve may be accessed by the physician to measure CSF pressure or to obtain CSF samples for cultures and sensitivities.

Shunt malfunction is an indication for shunt revision. The timing of the surgical intervention is based on the severity of the child's condition. If the child has significantly increased ICP the neurosurgeon may manually flush the system to temporarily relieve the obstruction or may withdraw CSF until ICP levels are acceptable and surgery can be performed. Infections are usually treated with a combination of antibiotic therapy and shunt removal. Antibiotics can also be instilled intraventricularly.

Nursing care and evaluation. Children with a suspected increase in ICP are treated emergently, regardless of cause. If the child has a VP shunt with no evidence of increased ICP the triage decision is based on historical data, the chief complaint, and presenting signs and symptoms. If shunt malfunction and/or hydrocephalus is suspected the child's neurologic status, cardiorespiratory status, and vital signs are monitored continuously.

Many questions may be raised by the family; among them are concerns about the long-term effects of hydrocephalus on their child's brain and future development. The nurse should help the family identify their concerns and can facilitate communication between the health care team and the family. Providing an opportunity for parents to ventilate their concerns and giving simple, clear explanations about diagnostic procedures, the condition itself, and the treatment plan will help to allay fear and anxiety. If the child has a VP shunt, discharge teaching reinforces the signs and symptoms of increasing ICP. The National Hydrocephalus Foundation is also a source of information.*

ACUTE NEUROLOGIC CONDITIONS

MENINGITIS

Etiology. Meningitis is an acute inflammation of the meninges. It can be caused by a number of etiologies, which are classified as bacterial or aseptic (nonbacterial).

Bacterial meningitis. The incidence and etiology of bacterial meningitis varies with a child's age and the season of the year. The most common etiologies in infants include *Escherichia coli,* Group B streptococci, *Listeria monocytogenes,* and *Streptococcus pneumoniae.* Common etiologies in children include *Neisseria meningitidis, Haemophilus influenzae,* and *S. pneumoniae.* In the past *H. influenzae* type B was the predominant pathogen in preschool children, but its incidence has markedly decreased since the advent of the Hib conjugate vaccine.[9,50] In unimmunized children, however, *H. influenzae* remains the most common cause of meningitis.[55] Meningococcal meningitis, caused by *N. meningitidis,* is a particularly virulent illness that may develop at any age but is most common in school-age children.

Bacterial meningitis is associated with significant morbidity and mortality. Ninety percent of the cases of bacterial meningitis occur in children less than 5 years of age,[33] with the highest risk in the 6- to 12-month age group.[25] Despite advances in therapy, up to 35% of

*National Hydrocephalus Foundation, Route 1, River Road, Box 210A, Joliet, IL 60436; (815) 467-6548.

neonates and 10% of older children will develop long-term neurologic sequelae after bacterial meningitis.[11]

Aseptic meningitis. Aseptic meningitis is caused by both infectious and noninfectious etiologies. In contrast to bacterial meningitis, which reflects bacterial invasion of the CSF, aseptic meningitis is characterized by the absence of bacteria in the CSF. Infectious etiologies include viruses, spirochetes, fungi, rickettsiae, mycoplasma, and parasites. Aseptic meningitis may also be identified in the child with a bacterial infection that was previously treated with an antibiotic (referred to as *partially treated meningitis*). Examples of noninfectious causes include toxins, neoplasms, trauma, and collagen-vascular diseases. Viruses, particularly the enteroviruses (e.g., echovirus and coxsackievirus), are the primary cause of aseptic meningitis in children.

Aseptic meningitis is usually a benign disease with a self-limited course; however, some etiologies (e.g., herpes simplex) can produce severe neurologic sequelae or death in the host, particularly in the compromised host.[11] The incidence of aseptic meningitis varies annually from 1.5 to 4 cases per 100,000 population.[44] Most enteroviral infections occur in the summer and early fall.

Pathophysiology. Meningitis results when an infectious agent enters the CSF and causes inflammation of the vascular membranes that surround the brain and spinal cord (meninges). Infectious agents enter the CSF via blood-borne dissemination from bacteremia or sepsis or from a distant site of infection; from a local infection adjacent to the cranial structures, such as the sinuses; or from direct implantation from head trauma, skull fractures, surgical procedures, or anatomic abnormalities (e.g., meningomyelocele).

Bacterial meningitis is the most serious form of meningitis. In the majority of cases the bacteria is spread via blood-borne dissemination and may be associated with bacteremia. With bacterial invasion of the subarachnoid space, the arachnoid and pia mater become inflamed. Changes in cerebral vascular permeability and the accumulation of white blood cells and exudate result. Inflammation of pain-sensitive spinal nerves and roots produces meningeal signs. Inflammation of the cranial nerves can cause cranial neuropathies of the optic, oculomotor, facial, and auditory nerves.[4]

With inflammation of the brain, the syndrome of inappropriate antidiuretic hormone (SIADH) secretion may develop and cause fluid retention. As the blood vessels of the brain further dilate and become congested, cerebral edema and increased ICP may result. With blood vessel damage the risk of cerebral thromboses and subsequent ischemic tissue damage increases. If CSF reabsorption is obstructed by inflammatory exudate and edema, a communicating hydrocephalus may develop, further contributing to an increase in ICP. Subdural effusions can develop secondary to increased permeability of capillaries in the inner layer of the dura mater.

Cranial nerve involvement, when present, is usually temporary, although the effects can be permanent. For example, damage to the auditory nerve can cause deafness and vestibular abnormalities. Paralysis of the extraocular and facial nerves may result in ocular palsies or facial weakness. Other complications may include motor deficits, mental retardation, learning impairments, and attention deficit disorder.

Clinical presentation. The onset of meningitis may be abrupt or gradual, and clinical manifestations may be specific or nonspecific. In infants, signs and symptoms are often nonspecific but may include extreme irritability (especially in response to comfort measures); lethargy; poor feeding; vomiting; a high-pitched cry; a bulging, tense fontanel; and an increase in head circumference. Fever may be present, but hypothermia is not uncommon.

Children older than 2 years of age exhibit more typical manifestations of meningitis, including fever, anorexia, vomiting, and signs of meningeal irritation such as nuchal rigidity, irritability, back pain, headache, photophobia, changes in LOC, and positive Kernig's and Brudzinski's signs. A positive Kernig's sign is indicated by the presence of pain in the hamstring and back when the child's leg, which has been flexed at the knee and hip, is straightened. A positive Brudzinski's sign is evidenced by involuntary flexion of the knees and hips when the neck of the supine child is flexed forward (Fig. 12-3). Seizures are not uncommon in children with meningitis and occur in up to 30% of children with bacterial meningitis.[44]

Meningococcal meningitis is one of the most serious forms of bacterial meningitis. It presents

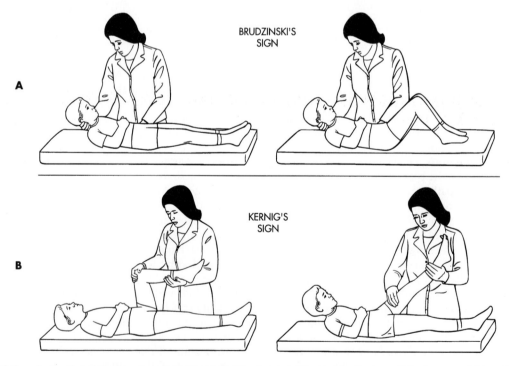

FIG. 12-3. **A,** Brudzinski's sign. A positive Brudzinski's sign is evidenced by flexion of the knees and hips when the neck of the supine child is flexed forward. **B,** Kernig's sign. A positive Kernig's sign is evidenced when the child's leg, which has been flexed at the knee and hip, is straightened causing lower back pain and resistance to straightening.

abruptly and is often accompanied by symptoms of endotoxic shock. Because a petechial, purpuric, or erythematous maculopapular rash is present in many children with meningococcal disease, the presence of high fever and rash is treated emergently. These children typically progress rapidly to profound shock, disseminated intravascular coagulation (DIC), and in many cases death despite aggressive therapy.

Emergency Department interventions

Diagnostic testing. The severity of symptoms at the time of presentation can predict outcome.[44] Therefore, early diagnosis and treatment are required to prevent morbidity and mortality. Diagnostic testing in the child with suspected meningitis includes a complete blood count (CBC) with differential, serum electrolytes, serum glucose, and a blood culture, as well as an evaluation of the CSF, a urinalysis, and urine culture. Platelet counts and clotting studies are ordered if shock is present or DIC is suspected.

A lumbar puncture (LP) is performed to obtain samples of cerebral spinal fluid. Before the LP an ophthalmoscopic exam is performed to rule out papilledema—a sign of increased ICP. If increased ICP is suspected, a head CT is indicated. During the LP, an opening pressure may be determined. Normal open-

ing pressure is less than 110 mm H_2O for a newborn and less than 200 mm H_2O for an infant or child. Samples of CSF are examined for bacteria by gram stain and culture, white blood cells with differential, glucose, and protein. The diagnosis of bacterial meningitis is confirmed by the presence of bacteria and increased leukocytes in the CSF. Aseptic meningitis is characterized by an absence of microorganisms in the CSF (negative gram stain and negative culture) in the child with meningeal signs (Table 12-6).

Treatment. The child with *viral* meningitis is treated symptomatically and may be admitted to the hospital or discharged home depending on the severity of the symptoms and the ability of the caregivers to monitor the child at home. Mild analgesics and antipyretics are usually sufficient to control headaches, other pains, and fever. Occasionally fluid management may be necessary to treat dehydration. If the child is discharged, follow-up care with a primary care provider must be ensured.

The approach to therapy in the child with *bacterial* meningitis includes fluid management, treating the underlying etiology, and preventing or ameliorating complications. In the critically ill child who exhibits signs of septic shock, broad-spectrum antibiotics are administered without waiting for laboratory results. In

TABLE 12-6	Cerebrospinal Fluid in Bacterial and Aseptic Meningitis		
CSF FINDINGS	**BACTERIAL**	**VIRAL**	**FUNGAL AND TUBERCULOUS**
Leukocytes			
Usual	>500	<500	<500
Range	0-200,000	0-2000	
Percent polymorphonuclear neutrophils, usual	>80%	<50%	<50%
Range	20%-100%	0%-100%	
Glucose			
Usual	<40 mg/dl	>40 mg/dl	<40 mg/dl
Range	0-normal	30 mg/dl–normal	
Percent CSF/blood	<30	>50	
Protein			
Usual	>100 mg/dl	<100 mg/dl	>100 mg/dl
Range	Normal–1500 mg/dl	Normal–200 mg/dl	
Stains	Gram stain	—	India ink/acid-fast

From Powell KR: Meningitis. In Hoekelman RA et al, eds: *Primary pediatric care*, St. Louis, 1992, Mosby.

the stable child with no focal neurologic signs the results of diagnostic testing may be obtained before the initiation of antibiotic therapy (Table 12-7).

In all children with bacterial meningitis fluid administration is closely monitored and fluids may be restricted to 70% of maintenance to lessen the effects of cerebral edema and/or SIADH should they develop. Conversely, sufficient fluids must be given to promote perfusion and tissue oxygenation, particularly in the presence of septic shock. During fluid therapy the development of SIADH may be reflected by a falling serum sodium (<125 mEq/L), an increase in body weight, and an increase in urine specific gravity.

Steroids may be used in the treatment of meningitis, although their use is controversial. Some studies have shown improved outcomes and fewer complications (e.g., hearing loss) in children with bacterial meningitis who received dexamethasone.[29,34,41] Steroids seem to be most effective in decreasing hearing loss with *H. influenzae* type B meningitis and when they are given early in the course of the illness (e.g., initiated concomitantly or before the first dose of antibiotics).[23] Dexamethasone given in conjunction with certain antibiotics, such as vancomycin (used to treat resistant *S. pneumococcus*), may diminish penetration of the antibiotic into the CSF.[23] Significant side effects of steroid use include the potential for gastrointestinal (GI) bleeding and a possible reduction in the immune response to viral infections.

Prophylaxis for contacts. When a child is diagnosed with *H. influenzae* type B or *N. meningitidis*, antibiotic prophylaxis is recommended for all close contacts of the child because transmission of these organisms occurs via respiratory tract secretions. In the case of *H. influenzae* type B, rifampin is administered to all household contacts and the index patient at the time of diagnosis. In cases associated with *N. meningitidis*, rifampin prophylaxis is given as soon as possible to all household contacts at the time of diagnosis, day care contacts, and anyone exposed to oral secretions of the index patient.[44] Health professionals also receive rifampin prophylaxis if contact with the child was unprotected and prolonged (e.g., mouth-to-mouth resuscitation, intubation, or suctioning) and before antibiotics were given. The dose of rifampin for children is 10 mg/kg/dose every 12 hours for four doses (2 days) or 20 mg/kg/dose once a day for 4 days (not to exceed 600 mg/dose). The dose in infants less than 1 month of age is 5 mg/kg/dose, and the dose in adults is 600 mg/dose.[9]

Nursing care and evaluation. The extent of nursing care depends on the severity of symptoms. If the child is in septic shock or is severely compromised, assessment and stabilization of the ABCs are the first priorities, followed by the administration of antibiotics. During stabilization of the ABCs a brief history is taken and a baseline physical examination is performed.

If the child is stable on arrival in the ED, a thorough history and physical are obtained and baseline data, including a head circumference (infants), vital signs, and an assessment of neurologic status, are recorded. The presence and character of rashes are also noted. If a petechial rash is present or if purpura is noted, emergent management is instituted regardless of the child's clinical presentation. Additionally, respiratory isolation precautions are instituted immediately.

TABLE 12-7	Antibiotics Used to Treat Bacterial Meningitis
PATIENTS	**ANTIBIOTIC THERAPY**
Neonates	Ampicillin or penicillin G IV IM; aminoglycoside or ampicillin and cefotaxime; appropriate dosages depend on age and weight
Children 1-3 mo	Ampicillin 200 mg/kg per day IV divided q6h and cefotaxime 200 mg/kg per day IV divided q6h
Children >3 mo	Cefotaxime 200 mg/kg per day IV divided q6h or ceftriaxone 100 mg/kg per day divided q12h
Adults	Cefotaxime 1 g IV q8h to 2 g IV q4h or ceftriaxone 1 to 2 g IV q12h

For severe penicillin allergy consider giving chloramphenicol and trimethoprim– sulfamethoxazole. If methicillin-resistant *Staphylococcus* organisms are a consideration, vancomycin 1 g IV q12h is recommended.

From Lerner AJ, ed: *The little black book of neurology*, ed 3, St. Louis, 1995, Mosby.

Vascular access is required for the administration of fluids, antibiotics, and if needed, anticonvulsants. Fluid administration is closely monitored to avoid over or underhydration. All intake and output is recorded. A decreasing urinary output may indicate the development of SIADH or shock.

Diagnostic testing is performed as ordered. During the LP, the child is held securely, but respiratory status is continuously monitored because flexion of the neck can cause respiratory compromise or aspiration. An oximeter or cardiorespiratory monitor may be useful.

Other nursing measures are instituted to provide comfort and prevent complications. Temperature management may be necessary to either reduce fever or correct hypothermia. The head of the bed may be elevated, unless contraindicated. Seizure precautions are instituted, and pain and discomfort are addressed (Box 12-6).

Meningitis is a frightening illness. The acute and sudden nature and the risk of serious morbidity or mortality lead to many concerns for the child and family. Often parents feel guilty for not seeking health care sooner for their child. To assist the parents in understanding the illness and their feelings, the disease process should be clearly explained. If the child's condition is critical and the parents are unable to remain with the child, the parents should be given continuous updates of their child's condition.

When rifampin prophylaxis is recommended the parents should be informed that the drug must be taken as ordered. They should also be told that body fluids such as urine, tears, and saliva will be red-orange in color. Contact lenses should not be worn, because they may become permanently stained. Any signs of illness must be reported to the primary health care provider immediately.

ENCEPHALITIS

Etiology. Encephalitis is an inflammation of the brain parenchyma and is often associated with meningeal involvement (meningoencephalitis). In the United States, encephalitis is most commonly caused by viruses, although bacteria, fungi, or parasites may be responsible. The following sections are specific to viral etiologies.

The majority of encephalitis cases with known causes are associated with childhood diseases (such as measles or varicella), enteroviruses (e.g., coxsackievirus, echovirus), arthropod-borne viruses (e.g., St. Louis, western equine, eastern equine, California equine), or herpes viruses. Although exceedingly rare, encephalitis can occur after childhood immunizations with live virus vaccines. Common vectors for arthropod-borne viruses (arboviruses) in the United States are mosquitoes and ticks; therefore most of these cases appear in the hot summer months. One of the most serious forms of encepha-

---

Box 12-6 Nursing Care of the Acutely Ill Child with Bacterial Meningitis

Observe strict respiratory isolation precautions
Assess and stabilize the airway and breathing
- Administer supplemental oxygen, and support ventilation and oxygenation as necessary

Assess circulatory status
- Obtain vascular access
- Administer antibiotics as ordered
- Administer fluid boluses for signs of shock, *or*
- Institute fluid restriction as ordered
- Maintain strict intake and output
- Observe for the development of SIADH

Obtain vital signs (including baseline BP)
Monitor neurologic status
- Observe baseline neurologic status
- Observe for focal neurologic signs
- Observe for signs of increased ICP
- Institute seizure precautions

Maintain normothermia
- Administer antipyretics for fever
- Provide radiant warmers or blankets for hypothermia

Obtain diagnostic tests as ordered (CBC, differential, blood culture, platelet count, clotting studies, urinalysis, urine culture)
Assist with additional diagnostic testing (e.g., lumbar puncture, CT)
Continuously monitor the child's:
- Airway and breathing
- Circulatory status (heart rate, perfusion, blood pressure, fluid intake and urine output)
- Neurologic status

Institute comfort measures
Prepare for admission
Provide psychologic support to the parents and child

litis is caused by the herpes simplex virus (HSV) which produces death or neurologic sequelae in over 70% of patients.[42]

Pathophysiology. Encephalitis results from either direct invasion of the brain by a pathogen such as HSV or rabies or indirectly as a sequela of an illness (e.g., Rocky Mountain spotted fever).[24] The pathogen can reach the brain via the blood-borne (hematogenous) route or along neuronal pathways.[24] Once the infectious agent or toxin enters the brain an inflammatory response is triggered. The result is cerebral edema that progresses to increased ICP, cellular damage, and transient neurologic dysfunction.[19] Necrotic areas can develop with or without hemorrhage, and the meninges may become inflamed.

Encephalopathy is a term used to describe conditions in which neurologic manifestations are suggestive of encephalitis, including a change in the LOC, irritability, seizures, and motor or sensory deficits.[4,19] However, with encephalopathy the brain is not inflamed.[4] An example of a condition that produces encephalopathy is Reye's syndrome.*

Clinical presentation. Encephalitis varies in severity, and the onset of symptoms may be gradual or abrupt. Initial signs and symptoms are usually nonspecific and include fever, headache, vomiting, and lethargy. Signs of meningeal irritation, such as photophobia and nuchal rigidity, may also be present. As the disease progresses, irritability, restlessness, altered behavior, confusion, disorientation, and coma may develop.[1] In severe cases death can occur. Depending on the etiologic agent and area(s) of the brain affected, focal neurologic signs may be evidenced, including speech disturbances, hemiparesis, ataxia, seizures, and cranial nerve dysfunction. Residual effects can include epilepsy, mental retardation, personality changes, dementia, paralysis, deafness, and blindness.[20] Encephalitis and viral meningitis are frequently caused by similar organisms and can be difficult to differentiate. However, unlike viral meningitis, most forms of encephalitis are associated with focal neurologic findings and an altered LOC.[1]

---

*Reye's syndrome (RS) is a multisystem disease characterized by an acute noninflammatory encephalopathy and fatty degeneration of the viscera, especially the liver. Although the exact cause of the disease remains unknown, the incidence of RS has dropped significantly since the avoidance of salicylates during flulike illnesses or varicella.

Emergency Department interventions. Because the etiologic organism is frequently not identifiable, the diagnosis of viral encephalitis is primarily determined by the clinical presentation; historical factors such as immunization status; epidemiologic factors such as age, geographic location, time of year; and results of diagnostic tests. A head CT scan rules out increased ICP before performing an LP and also detects the presence of space-occupying lesions. Focal lesions on CT scan may indicate herpes simplex encephalitis, a particularly virulent form of encephalitis. The LP can indicate the presence of bacterial meningitis or other etiologic organisms, such as fungi and mycobacteria. In viral encephalitis the cerebral spinal fluid is often clear. If leukocytes are present a predominance of polymorphonuclear cells is seen initially. Later in the course of the illness a predominance of mononuclear cells is seen.[4,42] CSF protein and glucose are usually normal.

Additional studies may include a CBC with differential and viral cultures of the blood, pharynx, urine, and stool. An EEG may be helpful in diagnosing herpes simplex encephalitis. If necessary, serologic studies are performed for evidence of syphilis, mononucleosis, and Epstein-Barr virus. Because SIADH can occur with encephalitis, serum and urine electrolytes are monitored.

Interventions for a child with possible encephalitis are similar to the management of meningitis, with the exception of antibiotic administration. In general, treatment of encephalitis is supportive and includes stabilization of the ABCs, respiratory support, control of increasing ICP, fluid and electrolyte maintenance, control of seizures as needed, and close monitoring. If herpes simplex encephalitis is suspected, acyclovir therapy is begun. Corticosteroids are controversial in the treatment of encephalitis and may reduce host defenses.[22]

Nursing care and evaluation. The child with suspected encephalitis is treated emergently. As with any child, initial assessment and stabilization of the ABCs are required. After stabilization, and while preparing for hospital admission, nursing care requires continuous assessment of the child's neurologic status to identify signs of increasing ICP and the development of seizure activity. Respiratory status is monitored for inadequate ventilatory exchange secondary to neurologic insult and airway compromise that may occur secondary to a deteriorating mental state. Fluid balance is monitored and intake and output strictly recorded. A decrease in urine output may herald the onset of SIADH or shock and requires immediate physician notification. Parents should be allowed to remain with their child whenever possible and are kept informed of the plan of care. (Also see p. 280.)

CHRONIC CONDITIONS ASSOCIATED WITH NEUROLOGIC PATHOLOGY

CEREBRAL PALSY

Etiology. Cerebral palsy (CP) is a disorder of movement and posture secondary to a nonprogressive encephalopathy.[3,56] It is not always clear whether individual factors such as prenatal, perinatal, or childhood insult to the brain actually cause CP or are merely associated with it. Contrary to popular belief, birth trauma and/or asphyxia have been demonstrated to cause only about 14% to 22% of cerebral palsy cases.[40,57] Unknown prenatal events that precipitate premature birth or difficult delivery appear to be associated with the majority of cases (Box 12-7). The incidence of congenital cerebral palsy is approximately 2 cases per 1000 live births.[56]

Pathophysiology. The pathophysiologic process in CP varies with the etiologic factor. For example, hypoxic brain injury produces necrosis of the groups of neurons most sensitive to oxygen deprivation; brain infarcts cause localized regions of damage due to ischemia; and kernicterus (the sequela of severe perinatal hyperbilirubinemia) results in damage to the basal ganglia, tectum, thalamus, and cochlea.[6]

The type, location and extent of brain injury determines neuromuscular presentation. The major categories of CP include (1) *spastic hemiplegia,* which involves the arm and leg on one side; (2) *spastic diplegia,* which involves the legs more than the arms; (3) *spastic quadriplegia,* which involves the arms and legs relatively equally; (4) *atonic/astatic* syndrome characterized by generalized hypotonia; (5) *hyperkinetic* CP, which is associated with involuntary or athetoid movements; and (6) a *cerebellar form,* which is characterized by ataxia and either spasticity or hypotonia.[36]

Infants with CP usually have an alteration in muscle tone (either hypertonia or hypotonia), delayed achievement of gross and fine motor milestones, asymmetry in the use of hands or arms, or hyperreflexia. Joint range of motion may be restricted or increased. As the infant grows, delays in muscle tone and motor development become more noticeable.

Box 12-7 Risk Factors for Cerebral Palsy

Prenatal predictors
Toxemia of pregnancy
Exposure to teratogenic drugs
Intrauterine infections (e.g., toxoplasmosis or cytomegalovirus)
Maternal malnutrition

Gestational predictors
Other birth defects
Low birth weight
Low placental weight
Abnormal fetal position
Premature separation of the placenta

Perinatal predictors
Low 10-minute Apgar score
Severe hyperbilirubinemia
Respiratory distress syndrome
Intracerebral hemorrhages
Seizures

Postnatal predictors
Head trauma
Encephalitis
Meningitis
Cerebrovascular accident
Poisonings, resulting on toxic encephalopathy
Near-drowning

Compiled from Fraley, 1992; Taft and Matthews, 1992; Torfs et al., 1990.

Neonatal reflexes usually continue beyond the expected age of disappearance.

In general, many disabilities are associated with CP. These include mental retardation, seizures, visual problems (strabismus, refractive errors), hearing impairment, dysphagia, gastroesophageal reflux (GER), joint contractures, scoliosis, hip dislocation and subluxation, oral and dental dysmorphogenesis, and perceptual deficits.[2,54,56] Secondary to these problems, children with CP are frequently delayed in cognitive, sensorimotor, language, and psychosocial development. However, some children show excellent cognitive development despite severe physical disabilities.

Clinical presentation. An ED visit for the child with CP often results from problems directly associated with CP. Falls, seizures, pain, and respiratory infections are not uncommon. Other nonspecific complaints such as inconsolability or irritability may result from a specific pathology or from the parent or caregiver being overwhelmed by the care of the special needs child.

Complaints related to falls are common in this population. Spasticity, low tone, ataxia, and uncoordinated movements, along with mental retardation, increase the child's vulnerability to falls. Head trauma, lacerations, fractures, severe bruises, and other related injuries result. Fractures are common because of the spasticity, which creates extremity paralysis and subsequent osteoporosis. Even so, child abuse must be considered in these cases because of the increased risk of maltreatment in disabled children.[58]

Children with CP are also prone to seizure disorders, particularly children with spastic quadriparesis and a very low birth weight. The clinical presentations vary depending on the child.

The child with CP may also complain of pain because spastic muscles, joint contractures, and dislocations (particularly the hip) can lead to significant discomfort. Altered sleep patterns may also contribute to the level of discomfort. Other sources of pain and discomfort may include ill-fitting braces or wheelchair seating systems, bruises from falls, and undiagnosed fractures.

Children with CP often present to the ED with signs and symptoms of respiratory distress. Because these children are relatively immobile, they are prone to the development of lower respiratory infections. The child with a feeding problem associated with oral hypersensitivity, bulbar dysphagia, or GER is prone to aspiration pneumonia.

Decubitus ulcers can occur in the child with CP because of their spasticity and immobility. Prolonged periods in wheelchairs, ill-fitting or improperly applied braces and body jackets, unequal pressure on bony prominences from scoliosis or hip dislocations, and poor nutrition[54] all contribute to the development of pressure sores.

Emergency Department interventions. The undiagnosed child with signs and symptoms of CP requires expert neurologic assessment to distinguish between CP and other conditions that cause abnormal development or muscle tone, which may be progressive and even fatal. To assist in making this determination, contact with the child's primary caregiver is required, as is consultation with a pediatric neurologist or developmental specialist.

In the diagnosed child the past medical history, including medications and a history of developmental status, is obtained to assess and manage the current problem. Common chronic interventions include antiepileptic therapy, corrective ophthalmologic surgery and lenses, hearing aids, supplemental nutrition (often via a gastrostomy tube), orthopedic surgery and bracing, and ongoing physical and occupational therapy. Because many of these children are followed by a multidisciplinary team, contact with primary or specialty caregivers regarding the child's care can often provide extremely useful information.

Signs and symptoms of illness in the child with CP vary with the chief complaint. In general the treatment of conditions associated with CP is the same as for any other child. For example, acute seizure management is the same for the child with CP and the otherwise neurologically normal child, as is the treatment of acute respiratory distress. A few exceptions follow.

When a child presents with a history of inconsolability, the presence of an acute illness or injury or feeding problem is first ruled out. Pain and discomfort related to muscle spasticity should also be considered and treated as necessary. Ibuprofen, baclofen, dantrolene, and diazepam are commonly administered.[5] If an acute etiology is not found a psychosocial assessment may be indicated. The stress of caring for a chronically ill child may have overwhelmed the caregivers, prompting an ED visit.[2]

Treatment of the child who has fallen is the same as for any other child. However, if the child wears a brace or body jacket it is left in place until spinal cord injury and fractures have been ruled out. If the cause of the fall is not apparent, seizure activity may be considered as a precipitant of the fall.

Nursing care and evaluation. Nursing care of the child with CP depends on the presenting signs and symtpoms. During assessment and stabilization, safety is a major concern because these children have a higher incidence of mental retardation, communication disorders, and seizure disorders than the general population. Crib or bedside rails are kept up at all times (except during treatments), and even older children are not left alone. Because pressure ulcers can progress rapidly in children with CP, proper initial positioning and frequent position changes are important. CP children in wheelchairs usually have special cushions and inserts to help with positioning and pressure relief. When possible, and depending on the child's clinical condition and chief complaint, the child may be allowed to remain in the chair. When venous access is required attempts should be made to place peripheral lines away from sites where contractures, spasms, or spasticity may interfere with line maintenance.

Communicating with the child who has CP can be complicated by vision and hearing impairments, articulation difficulty, or mental retardation. Parents are often masters at communicating with their child, understanding vocalizations and gestures, and are able to impart important instructions. If the parent must leave the child at any time, the nurse should attempt to learn the most essential signs or sounds (e.g., how does the child communicate elimination needs or pain and anxiety?) and calming techniques. Communication and sensory aids such as eyeglasses or hearing aids should be used whenever possible throughout the visit.

During procedures measures to reduce fear and anxiety can assist with relaxation. Parents are often extremely helpful in calming their child and may offer useful suggestions about positioning techniques. In the spastic child positioning for procedures can be difficult. The supine position often exacerbates high extensor tone, and the prone position, which usually prompts flexion, may heighten extension. When a particular position is necessary but is met with high resistance, slow, gentle, yet firm pressure with support on both sides of joints aids in the extension of spastic flexed limbs and guards against injury. Too great a force on limbs with joint contractures, however, may produce secondary trauma.

Oral medication administration is often hampered by developmental delay and dysphagia. Parental suggestions can be very helpful in facilitating the administration of fluids and medications. In general, thicker-consistency vehicles are more likely to enhance acceptance and swallowing of medications. Many younger children with significant dysphagia have gastrostomy tubes, which are used for fluid and oral medication administration (see Chapter 30).

Perhaps one of the most significant contributions the ED nurse can make when caring for the child with CP relates to providing emotional support to the child and family. Hospital visits are stressful, and the nurse can anticipate and often develop creative interventions to provide for the multiple and varied physical and psychosocial needs of the family and child with CP.

MYELOMENINGOCELE

Etiology. Myelomeningocele (spina bifida) is the most severe form of neural tube defect compatible with life. In the United States, the incidence of myelomeningocele is now less than 1:1000 live births. Individuals of Irish, English, or Welsh descent; caucasians; and females are most commonly affected.[17,38,60]

Myelomeningocele is believed to be caused by environmental factors interacting with a genetic predisposition. Recent studies implicate maternal heat exposure[39] and folate deficiency[10] as contributing causal factors. The recurrence risk for neural tube defects is approximately 3% for a couple who has previously given birth to a child with myelomeningocele.

Pathophysiology. Closure of the neural tube is normally complete by day 28 of embryonic life.[32] Failure of closure of the neural tube results in a neural tube defect. In myelomeningocele, the malformed spinal cord and nerve roots protrude through abnormal vertebral arches and soft tissue. At birth, the defect is almost always obvious at some point along the thoracic to sacral cord. Occasionally the defect protrudes anteriorly and is invisible. Defects vary in type (e.g., open or closed, amount of skin coverage), size, and placement along the cord, but all result in some degree of muscular weakness or paralysis. Higher defects generally cause greater paralysis and associated sensory impairment (Fig. 12-4).

Clinical manifestations arise from four types of problems: soft tissue malformation, vertebral body malformation, brain malformation, and spinal cord malformation.[32] Common concerns in the child with myelomeningocele include the following:

1. Hydrocephalus, which is present in approximately 80% of children with myelomeningocele.[18] Although most children with hydrocephalus receive ventriculoperitoneal or ventriculoatrial shunts, some infants are initially managed without shunts and closely monitored for rising ICP.
2. The lack of mobility in the child with myelomeningocele places the child at high risk for osteopenia, fractures, and pressure ulcers.
3. Decreased or absent sensation in the lower body places the child at high risk for burns or occult injuries; urinary tract infections secondary to a neurogenic bladder; and abdominal discomfort, rectal prolapse, hemorrhoids, or fissures due to constipation.

Clinical presentation. The clinical presentation of the child with myelomeningocele can vary widely depending on the chief complaint. The presentation

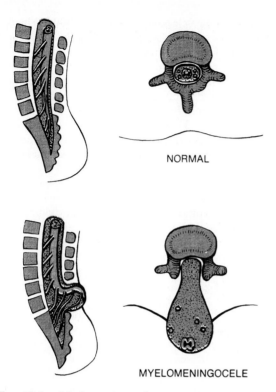

NORMAL

MYELOMENINGOCELE

FIG. 12-4. Myelomeningocele. (From Wong DL: *Whaley & Wong's essentials of pediatric nursing,* ed 5, St Louis, 1997, Mosby.)

may be directly related to the physiologic effects of the defect such as a urinary tract infection, malfunctioning VP shunt, or constipation; or complaints may be unrelated to the defect, such as the presence of a cold.

The most common clinical presentations in the child with myelomeningocele include complaints associated with a genitourinary tract infection, wound infection, shunt infection, ventriculitis, or meningitis. Other presentations that are not uncommon include burns, the presence of decubiti, allergic reactions (particularly to latex), seizures, abdominal pain, and rectal or urinary tract bleeding.

The most serious presentations relate to a possible shunt malfunction or CNS infection. Infants with a shunt malfunction may present with an increasing head circumference and/or signs of increased ICP. Older children may complain of headaches and/or exhibit signs of an increasing ICP. (See section on hydrocephalus and Box 12-5.)

Complaints of headache, fever, or malaise that cannot be traced to another source may indicate a shunt infection, ventriculitis, or meningitis. A shunt infection may closely follow shunt placement or revision of the shunt, or it may follow an unrelated systemic infection. Although rare, bowel perforation by the tip of the migrating shunt tube can produce both ventriculitis and a rigid, tender abdomen. Meningitis is caused by invasion of the CSF by any of the usual organisms.

Urinary tract infections are not uncommon in these children and may be secondary to urinary stasis or may result from the clean intermittent catheterizations necessary to periodically empty the bladder in children with neurogenic bladder. Because upper urinary tract damage is frequently associated with myelomeningocele, there is a higher probability the child will also present with signs and symptoms of pyelonephritis. Hypertension may result from the chronic renal involvement.

Paralyzed, relatively immobile extremities are at higher risk for osteopenia and fractures. The child may present with an erythematous, swollen, "hot" area on the limb but may have little to no pain due to lack of sensation. Similar symptoms may also accompany deep vein phlebitis and thrombosis.

The most frequent cause for abdominal discomfort in relation to myelomeningocele is severe constipation, caused by inadequate management of neurogenic bowel patterns of elimination. Often, constipation becomes long-standing and severe, leading to fecal impaction and paradoxical diarrhea. The neurogenic bowel is also at higher risk for intussusception and obstruction.

Emergency Department interventions. ED interventions are dependent upon the child's presenting signs and symptoms. In general the treatment of conditions associated with myelomeningocele is the same as for any other child; however, because of the wide array of conditions associated with these children the workup can often be complicated. For example, neurologic symptoms (e.g., headache, seizures, altered LOC) can reflect any number of etiologies but in the child with a VP shunt neurologic symptoms may also reflect a shunt malfunction or infection. If a shunt infection or malfunction is suspected a CT scan will be ordered. CSF may be withdrawn from the shunt by the physician for culture and sensitivity or to relieve ICP.

Treatment interventions can also sometimes differ in the child with myelomeningocele. For example, many of these children are on prophylactic antibiotics because they are prone to recurrent urinary tract infections (UTIs). When a UTI occurs, infective organisms are often resistant to the typically used agents such as amoxicillin and co-trimoxazole (i.e., Septra or Bactrim).

Constipation is confirmed by abdominal exam, rectal exam, and a flat plate radiograph of the abdomen. Severe cases can be effectively managed with a Gastrografin enema, which allows for full evacuation under controlled conditions. In less severe cases, manual disimpaction followed by a Fleets enema produces immediate evacuation of the impacted stool.

Nursing care and evaluation. Nursing care of the child with myelomeningocele ranges from providing emergent management related to such complications as neurologic compromise to providing psychosocial support to the family or child. Most children with myelomeningocele wear braces to assist with stability, help maintain alignment, and provide structural strength for mobility. If the child arrives with a suspected spinal cord injury the braces are left in place until a spinal cord injury and fractures have been ruled out.

A particularly important nursing intervention in the child with myelomeningocele is the establishment of *latex precautions.* Although children with myelomeningocele are subject to the usual range of allergies, they are at high risk for allergy to latex.[59] Even if the child has previously been nonreactive, an allergic reaction may result with additional latex exposure. Regardless of whether a latex allergy has been identified, latex exposure should be minimized during all treatments and diagnostic procedures. For example, medications are drawn up without passing a needle through a rubber stopper and administered without using latex ports. If the child requires surgery, both anesthesia and the operating room are notified. Failure to attend to this risk has been known to result in death due to anaphylactic shock* (Box 12-8).

All principles applicable to the child with special needs apply to the care of the child with myelomeningocele. In particular are the advisability of including the parents in the child's care and incorporating parental suggestions and opinions in the care planning process. Because most of these children have normal intelligence and communication abilities, they should be approached in an age-appropriate manner (see Chapter 30).

*The Spina Bifida Association of America (1-800-621-3141) offers a list of latex-containing products.

Box 12-8 Nursing Alert Regarding Latex Allergy

Because of the high risk of latex allergy in children with myelomeningocele, all interventions should be performed using nonlatex gloves and equipment. Every hospital should have policies and procedures for latex precautions that are well-known to all staff involved in patient care.

▌SUMMARY

Children arrive in emergency departments with a variety of neurologic complaints that range from simple to life threatening. The wide array of developmental abilities between infants and young children can make the neurologic assessment and interpretation of findings within the pediatric population quite difficult. Nurses caring for children should be knowledgeable of the normally occurring differences in neurologic development among different age children and should be able to identify variances from normal.

REFERENCES

1. Adler SP, Toor S, Kerkering TM: Central nervous system infections. In Pellock JM, Myer EC, eds: *Neurologic emergencies in infancy and childhood,* ed 2, Boston, 1993, Butterworth-Heinemann.
2. Barabas G, Matthews W, Zumoff P: Care-load for children and young adults with severe cerebral palsy, *Dev Med Child Neurol* 34:979-984, 1992.
3. Bax M: Terminology and classification of cerebral palsy, *Dev Med Child Neurol* 6:295-297, 1964.
4. Behrman RE, ed: *Nelson textbook of pediatrics,* ed 14, Philadelphia, 1992, WB Saunders.
5. Blackman JA, Reed MD, Roberts CD: Muscle relaxant drugs for children with cerebral palsy. In Sussman MD, ed: *The diplegic child: evaluation and management,* Rosemont, Ill, 1992, American Academy of Orthopedic Surgeons.
6. Blasco PA: Pathology of cerebral palsy. In Sussman MD (ed): *The diplegic child: evaluation and management,* Rosemont, IL, 1992, American Academy of Orthopedic Surgeons.
7. Byers VL: Novel antiepileptic drugs: nursing implications, *J Neurosci Nurs* 25(6):375-379, 1993.
8. Carter JR: The use of new antiepileptic medications in pediatric patients with epilepsy, *J Pediatr Health Care* 8(6):277-281, 1994.

9. Committee on Infectious Diseases, American Academy of Pediatrics: *1994 Red Book: Report of the Committee on Infectious Diseases,* ed 23, Elk Grove Village, Ill, 1994, American Academy of Pediatrics.

10. Czeizel AE, Dudas I: Prevention of the first occurrence of neural tube defects by preconceptional vitamin supplementation, *N Engl J Med* 327:1832-1835, 1992.

11. Dashefsky B: Life threatening infections, *Pediatr Emerg Care* 7(4):244-252, 1991.

12. Dobbing J, Sands J: Quantitative growth and development of human brain, *Arch Dis Child* 48:757, 1973.

13. Fenichel GM: Headache. In Fenichel GM, ed: *Clinical pediatric neurology: a signs and symptoms approach,* Philadelphia, 1993, WB Saunders.

14. Ferry P, Banner W, Wolf R: *Seizure disorders in children,* New York, 1986, JB Lippincott.

15. Fraley AM: *Nursing and the disabled,* Boston, 1992, Jones & Bartlett.

16. Graf WD, Riback PS: Pharmacologic treatment of recurrent pediatric headache, *Pediatr Ann* 24(9):469-474, 1995.

17. Greene WB et al: Effect of race and gender on neurological level in myelomeningocele, *Dev Med Child Neurol* 33(2):110-117, 1991.

18. Guertin SR: Cerebrospinal fluid shunts: evaluation, complications, and crisis management, *Pediatr Clin North Am* 34(1):203-217, 1987.

19. Hazinski MF: Neurologic disorders. In Hazinski MF, ed: *Nursing care of the critically ill child,* St Louis, 1992, Mosby.

20. Hickey JV: *The clinical practice of neurological and neurosurgical nursing,* ed 3, Philadelphia, 1992, JB Lippincott.

21. Hirtz DG: Generalized tonic-clonic and febrile seizures, *Pediatr Clin North Am* 36:365, 1989.

22. Ikeda M, Young R: Meningoencephalitis. In Hoekelman RA et al, eds, *Primary pediatric care,* ed 3, St Louis, 1996, Mosby.

23. Jafari HS, McCracken GH: Dexamethasone therapy in bacterial meningitis, *Pediatr Ann* 23(2):82-88, 1994.

24. Jantausch BA: Intracranial infections. In Holbrook PR, ed: *Textbook of pediatric critical care,* Philadelphia, 1993, WB Saunders.

25. Kacica MA, Lepow ML: Meningitis: clinical presentation and workup, *Pediatr Ann* 23(2):69-75, 1994.

26. Karasic RB: Headache. In Barkin RM, ed: *Pediatric emergency medicine: concepts and clinical practice,* St Louis, 1992, Mosby.

27. Kelly S: *Pediatric emergency nursing,* ed 2, Norwalk, Conn, 1994, Appleton & Lange.

28. Key CB, Rothrock SG, Falk JL: Cerebral spinal fluid shunt complications: an emergency medicine perspective, *Pediatr Emerg Care* 11(5):265-273, 1995.

29. Lebel MH et al: Dexamethasone therapy for bacterial meningitis: results of two double-blind, placebo-controlled trials, *N Engl J Med* 319:964-971, 1988.

30. Lerner AJ, ed: *The little black book of neurology,* ed 3, St Louis, 1995, Mosby.

31. Linet MS et al: An epidemiologic study of headache among adolescents and young adults, *JAMA* 261: 2211-2216, 1989.

32. Liptak GS: Spina bifida. In Hoekelman RA, ed: *Primary pediatric care,* ed. 3, St Louis, 1996, Mosby.

33. Lipton JD: Evolving concepts in pediatric bacterial meningitis—Part I: Pathophysiology and diagnosis, *Ann Emerg Med* 22(10):1602-1615, 1993.

34. Lipton JD, Schafermeyer RW: Evolving concepts in pediatric bacterial meningitis—Part II: Current management and therapeutic research, *Ann Emerg Med* 22(10):1616-1629, 1993.

35. Martin SE, Smith MS: Psychosocial factors in recurrent pediatric headache, *Pediatr Ann* 24(9):469-474, 1995.

36. Mashilov C, Kogan B: The biologic basis of cerebral palsy. In Sussman MD, ed: *The diplegic child: evaluation and management,* Rosemont, Ill, 1992, American Academy of Orthopedic Surgeons.

37. Mayo ME: Lower urinary tract dysfunction in cerebral palsy, *J Urol* 147(2):419-420, 1992.

38. McLaurin RL, Warkany J: Management of spina bifida and associated anomalies, *Compr Ther* 12(2): 60-65, 1986.

39. Milunsky A et al: Maternal heat exposure and neural tube defects, *JAMA* 268(7):882-885, 1992.

40. Naeye RL et al: Origins of cerebral palsy, *Am J Dis Child* 143(10):1154-1161, 1989.

41. Odio CM et al: The beneficial effects of early dexamethasone administration in infants and children with bacterial meningitis, *N Engl J Med* 324: 1525-1531, 1991.

42. Packer RJ, Berman PH: Neurologic emergencies. In Fleisher GR, Ludwig S, eds: *Textbook of pediatric emergency medicine,* ed 2, Baltimore, Md, 1988, Williams & Wilkins.

43. Piatt JH: Physical examination of patients with cerebrospinal fluid shunts: is there useful information in pumping the shunt? *Pediatrics* 89(3):470-473, 1992.

44. Powell KR: Meningitis. In Hoekelman RA et al, eds: *Primary pediatric care,* ed 3, St Louis, 1996, Mosby.

45. Reyes AL et al: Gastroesophageal reflux in children with cerebral palsy, *Child Care Health Dev* 19(2): 109-118, 1993.

46. Roddy S, McBride M: Seizure disorders. In Hoekelman RA et al, eds: *Primary pediatric care,* ed 3, St Louis, 1996, Mosby.

47. Reference deleted in proofs.

48. Rothner AD: A practical approach to headaches in adolescents, *Pediatr Ann* 20(4):200-205, 1991.

49. Scheuer ML, Pedley TA: The evaluation and treatment of seizures, *N Engl J Med* 323:1468, 1990.
50. Schoendorf KC et al: National trends in *Haemophilus influenzae* meningitis mortality and hospitalization among children, 1980-1991, *Pediatrics* 93(4): 663, 1994.
51. Seidel HM: Headache. In Hoekelman RA et al, eds: *Primary pediatric care,* ed 3, St Louis, 1996, Mosby.
52. Silberstein S: Forty questions about headache in the child and adolescent, *J Headache* 30:716-724, 1990.
53. Slota MC: Neurologic assessment of the infant and toddler, *Critic Care Nurs* Sept/Oct: 91, 1983.
54. Stallings VA et al: Nutrition related growth failure of children with quadriplegic cerebral palsy, *Dev Med Child Neurol* 35(2):126-138, 1993.
55. Stewart G, Burke SR, Rosenberg N: *Haemophilus influenzae* meningitis in twins, *Pediatr Emerg Care* 9(3):151-152, 1993.
56. Taft LT, Matthews WS: Cerebral palsy. In Levine M, Carey W, Crocker A, eds: *Developmental-behavioral pediatrics,* ed 2, Philadelphia, 1992, WB Saunders.
57. Torfs CP et al: Prenatal and perinatal factors in the etiology of cerebral palsy, *J Pediatr* 116(4):615-619, 1990.
58. Westcott H: The abuse of disabled children: a review of the literature, *Child Care Health Dev* 17(4):243-258, 1991.
59. Yassin S et al: Evaluation of latex allergy in patients with myelomeningocele, *Ann Allergy* 69(3):207-211, 1992.
60. Yen IH et al: The changing epidemiology of neural tube defects. United States, 1968-1989, *Am J Dis Child* 146(7):857-861, 1992.

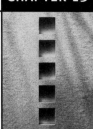

CHAPTER 13

Musculoskeletal System

Bernadette Mazurek Melnyk, Alison W. Schultz

INTRODUCTION

Children present to the emergency department (ED) with a wide variety of congenital, developmental, inflammatory, and traumatic disorders that affect the growing musculoskeletal system. Accurate assessment and early intervention of musculoskeletal problems require a basic understanding of the characteristics of the growing child's musculoskeletal system and are essential to initiate appropriate treatment and prevent permanent disability. This chapter describes anatomic and physiologic differences that predispose children to certain musculoskeletal problems and common disorders. Traumatic musculoskeletal disorders are discussed in Chapter 23.

ANATOMY AND PHYSIOLOGY

Whereas the muscular system is almost completely formed at birth, the growth and maturation of the skeletal system continue until the end of puberty. Development of skeletal contours is dependent upon the normal functioning of muscles. Growth disturbances and bone deformities can result from both muscular and skeletal abnormalities.[18]

Most epiphyses are cartilaginous at birth and are therefore invisible to radiography. With maturation, epiphyses ossify in an orderly fashion. The number and composition of ossification centers correlate with the child's age.[19] As active sites of growth, epiphyseal plates do not begin to ossify until puberty. When skeletal injuries involve nonossified or incompletely ossified sites, radiographs may be normal or unable to reveal the full extent of injury (see Chapter 23).

Blood flow tends to be sluggish in vascular beds surrounding growing metaphyses, placing children at risk for thrombosis and hematogenous osteomyelitis during periods of bacteremia. The growth plate creates a mechanical barrier preventing the spread of infection to the epiphysis, because its blood supply is separate from the metaphysis after approximately 8 months of age.[18]

NURSING ASSESSMENT

HISTORY

Assessment of a child with a suspected musculoskeletal disorder begins with a comprehensive history. Components of the history are described in Box 13-1. Common presenting musculoskeletal complaints include limp, deformity, localized or generalized weakness, swelling, pain, and stiffness of joints.

PHYSICAL EXAMINATION

The physical assessment of a child with a musculoskeletal disorder or complaint must be systematic and comprehensive (Box 13-2). Although abnormalities are often obvious, subtle signs of illness or injury can be easily overlooked. Physical manifestations can also be misleading. For example, children who present with knee pain may actually have a hip problem. Therefore, thorough assessment of a child with knee pain must include an examination of the hip.

Comparison of affected and unaffected extremities identifies the degree of deviation from normal. Functional ability often indicates the presence and/or severity of a disorder. For example, decreased use of a limb, limps, and circulatory impairment all warrant further investigation.

Limps. Limps are common presenting complaints in the emergency department (Table 13-1).

Box 13-1   History of Musculoskeletal Complaints

Present illness
Date of onset
Severity
Extent of disability
Precipitating or aggravating factors
Associated signs and symptoms of illness, such
    as cough, runny nose, fever, weight loss,
    and rash
Previous treatment and its effects
Recent trauma
Current medications
New, increased, or repetitive activities
Recent exposure to infections

Past history
Prenatal and birth history
Growth and development
Similar signs and symptoms
Previous orthopedic injuries
Chronic conditions
Recent immunizations

Family history
Congenital problems, such as musculoskeletal
    or endocrine disorders

Box 13-2   Physical Assessment of the Child with a Musculoskeletal Complaint

Observation/inspection
Posture/position
Gait/symmetry of motion
Balance
Range of motion of joints
Muscle tone
Abnormalities
    Trunk or limb deformities
    Differences in length of extremities or
        muscle wasting
    Joint swelling and erythema
    Use of orthopedic appliances, such as
        braces

Palpation
Bones
    Shape and outline
    Deformities
    Thickening
    Abnormal prominence or indentations
Joints
    Passive range of motion, including exten-
        sion, flexion, and rotation (e.g., supina-
        tion or pronation of the hands)
    Flexibility
    Temperature
    Tenderness or pain
Extremities
    Muscle strength and power during resis-
        tance maneuvers
    Circulation, including pulses, capillary re-
        fill, color, temperature, sensitivity

The patient's age and the presence or absence of pain help differentiate the cause of the limp. For children with a *painful* limp, the following conditions must be considered: trauma; infection; inflammatory disorders, such as toxic synovitis and juvenile rheumatoid arthritis; degenerative disorders, such as Legg-Perthes or Osgood-Schlatter disease; intraabdominal processes, such as appendicitis; neoplasms; and hematologic disorders, such as sickle cell disease or hemophilia with hemarthrosis. Infection, such as osteomyelitis or septic joint, must be suspected and ruled out in the older infant or toddler who presents with a limp or inability to walk.[12] Children with a *painless* limp are likely to have neurologic problems, including spinal masses or herniated discs; muscle disease, such as muscular dystrophy; joint disorders, such as congenital dislocation of the hip; bone disorders, such as spondylolisthesis; or mimicry or hysteria.[16] Definitive diagnosis relies on the clinical picture, laboratory tests, and radiologic studies. (For a complete discussion of limp, see Chapter 23.)

COMMON CONDITIONS

OSTEOMYELITIS

Etiology.   Acute osteomyelitis is a common bone infection in children. Although it can occur at any age, the peak incidence is 2 through 5 years.[9] Predisposing factors include recent orthopedic surgical procedures, open fractures, poor nutrition, chronic debilitating diseases, intravenous (IV) drug abuse, and immunocompromise.

TABLE 13-1	Differential Diagnosis of Limp	
Condition	**Diagnostic findings**	**Ancillary data**
Traumatic		
Sprains/strains	History of trauma, tenderness, erythema, restricted range of motion	X-ray studies: no fractures, soft tissue injury
Fracture	History of trauma, tenderness, erythema, edema, restricted range of motion	X-ray studies: positive/negative for fracture; if negative, then serial x-ray films, bone scan, or CT/MRI scans
Foreign body/splinter in foot	Acute onset, site of injury	X-ray studies: needed at times to localize foreign body
Infection/inflammation		
Osteomyelitis	Fever, local tenderness, edema, monoarticular	ESR/WBC elevated; x-ray studies: increased fluid or lytic lesion in bone scan positive, bone/joint aspirate positive for bacteria
Arthritis, bacterial	Febrile, monoarticular, local edema and erythema	X-ray studies: effusion; elevated WBC and ESR, positive bacteria on joint aspiration, positive bone scan
Toxic synovitis of hip	Preceding viral illness, limited range of motion	WBC positive, ESR variable; x-ray studies: positive/ negative effusion, aspirate if necessary
Juvenile rheumatoid arthritis	Abdominal symptoms, *stooped over* gait, fever	WBC elevated
Appendicitis or pelvic inflammatory disease	Abdominal, pelvic symptoms	
Neoplasm		
Osteogenic or Ewing's sarcoma	Painful limb	X-ray studies: lytic or cortical lesions
Metastatic involvement of bone marrow	Migratory pain	X-ray studies: lytic lesions, abnormal blood tests
Degenerative		
Slipped capital femoral epiphysis	Acute or chronic pain, obese child, pain in anterior groin	X-ray studies: slipped femoral head
Osgood-Schlatter disease	Tender over anterior tibia, active child	X-ray studies: usually normal may show elevation of tibial tuberosity
Chondromalacia of patella	Tender over knee, resolves with rest	X-ray studies: normal
Congenital		
Hemophilia	Variable history of trauma, history bleeding and bruising	Blood factor tests

TABLE 13-1	Differential Diagnosis of Limp—cont'd	
CONDITION	DIAGNOSTIC FINDINGS	ANCILLARY DATA
Congenital—cont'd		
Sickle cell anemia	Bone pain diffuse	Sickle screen
Scoliosis	Limp in adolescents after exercise	X-ray studies: scoliosis
Leg length discrepancy	Chronic limp	Physical findings
Vascular		
Legg-Calvé-Perthes disease	Tender hip, chronic pain	X-ray studies: bulging capsule, bone scan positive uptake

From Fink PC et al: Orthopedic disorders. In Barkin RM: *Pediatric emergency medicine: Concepts and clinical practice,* St. Louis, 1992, Mosby.

Osteomyelitis most frequently results from hematogenous (blood-borne) spread of bacteria from a distal site of infection such as otitis media or tonsillitis. Bacterial contamination can also occur directly through penetrating wounds or open fractures or indirectly by extension from adjacent wounds, abscesses, or burns (exogenous osteomyelitis). The long bones of the lower extremity are the most commonly infected, followed by the long bones of the upper extremities. Other bones, such as the vertebrae or skull, are rarely affected. Chronic osteomyelitis occurring in less than 4% of cases can develop from either inadequate or delayed treatment of the acute form or unusually resistant organisms.[23]

Staphylococcus aureus is responsible for approximately 80% of hematogenous infections. Other causes include Group A streptococcus, *Haemophilus influenzae,* Group B streptococcus, and Enterobacteriaceae in newborns.[9,15,22] Salmonella is the most common infecting organism in children with sickle hemoglobinopathies.[17] Puncture wounds through sneakers most often result in *Pseudomonas* infections. Fungi are rarely involved.

Pathophysiology. Hematogenous osteomyelitis results when bacteria travel from the distal site of infection to the small end arteries in the metaphysis (Fig. 13-1). An inflammatory reaction with exudation subsequently occurs, causing increased pressure within the bone marrow space of the rigid bone. If effective treatment is not administered, the infection spreads through the cortical bone and subperiosteal space. The periosteum can rupture, releasing pus into the soft tissue or adjacent joints. Septic thrombosis of surrounding vessels may eventually occur with ischemic infarction of the bone. Epiphyseal involvement can occur in early infancy, because blood vessels cross the growth plate before 8 months of age.[18]

Complications of osteomyelitis include septic arthritis, growth disturbances, and chronic osteomyelitis. Permanent disability and deformity are common once osteomyelitis has progressed to the chronic stage.[23]

Clinical presentation. The initial presentation of acute hematogenous osteomyelitis is variable, but in most cases the onset is abrupt. The initial phase of bacteremia may be characterized by vague symptomatology including low-grade fever, headache, and malaise or by signs of acute toxicity such as high fever, irritability, restlessness, and tachycardia. Neonates and younger infants may only exhibit failure to use the affected extremity, whereas older children may present with isolated local pain. The presence of localized swelling, tenderness, redness, and heat indicates extension of the infection through the cortical bone, resulting from pressure and inflammation within the bone marrow space. Children are usually unwilling to bear weight or use the affected limb. The extremity is often held in a semiflexed position with evidence of tense surrounding muscles. Unlike children with septic arthritis, passive range of motion of the extremity is possible, although it may be somewhat resisted and slightly limited.

Acute osteomyelitis must be suspected in any child with an acute onset of bone pain associated with fever, leukocytosis, or other signs of inflammation. Differential diagnoses include septic joint, cellulitis, fracture,

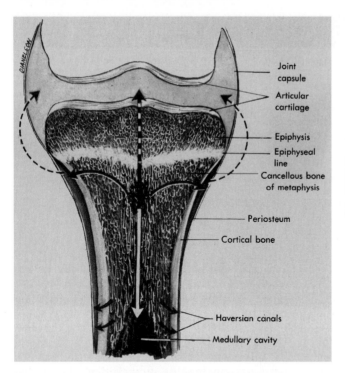

Joint
capsule

Articular
cartilage

Epiphysis

Epiphyseal
line

Cancellous bone
of metaphysis

Periosteum

Cortical bone

Haversian canals

Medullary cavity

FIG. 13-1. Diagram showing spread of acute hematogenous osteomyelitis. The interrupted lines are rare routes. (From Tachdjian MO: *Pediatric orthopedics,* ed 2, Philadelphia, 1990, WB Saunders.)

Box 13-3 Diagnostic Tests for Suspected Osteomyelitis
Laboratory specimens
CBC with differential
Erythrocyte sedimentation rate
Blood culture
Culture of wound drainage or bone aspirate
Radiologic studies
Plain x-rays
Bone scan

rheumatoid arthritis, acute rheumatic fever, leukemia, bone tumor, and soft tissue injury secondary to trauma.

Emergency Department interventions

Diagnostic tests. The most common diagnostic tests for suspected osteomyelitis are listed in Box 13-3. A marked leukocytosis with an increase in neutrophils and band cells may be present. The erythrocyte sedimentation rate (ESR), which is a sensitive indica-

tor of bone infection, is usually elevated.[22] Blood cultures are positive in approximately half of all children with osteomyelitis.[5]

Diagnosis of osteomyelitis is confirmed by the presence of two of the following criteria: (1) pus aspirated from the bone; (2) positive blood culture; (3) local signs of inflammation; or (4) radiographic changes such as bone lysis (usually not evident until at least 10 days after the onset of symptoms) or positive bone scan.[9] Bone scanning can usually detect the infectious process within 48 to 72 hours after onset.[22] Radiographs are obtained within the first 2 weeks of the disease process only to rule out malignancy or fracture.

Treatment. After completion of diagnostic tests, antibiotic therapy is initiated (Table 13-2) and continued for at least 3 to 6 weeks. If the infection responds well to a 5- to 10-day course of parenteral antibiotics, the remainder may be continued orally at home.[5,13] Surgical debridement of infected necrotic bone may be necessary if antibiotic therapy is not fully effective.

Nursing care and evaluation. Because many children with osteomyelitis have concurrent bacteremia, assessment and monitoring for septicemia

TABLE 13-2	Antibiotic Therapy of Osteomyelitis	
ANTIBIOTIC	**IV DOSE**	**INDICATION**
Nafcillin	100-200 mg/kg/day q6h	Drug of choice; treats streptococci and penicillinase-resistant staphylococcus
Cefazolin or cephalothin	100 mg/kg/day q6h	If allergic to penicillin
Carbenicillin and	400-600 mg/kg/day q4-6h	Treats pseudomonas, for example, in a puncture wound of the foot or drug abuser
Gentamicin *or*	5-7.5 mg/kg/day q8h	
Ceftazidime	100-150 mg/kg/day q8h	
Ampicillin and	200 mg/kg/day q4h	For neonates or sickle cell patient
Gentamicin and	5-7.5 mg/kg/day q8h	
Nafcillin	100-200 mg/kg/day q6h	

From Dufort and Smith-Wright, 1992.

and septic shock are important components of nursing care. Early signs of septic shock include tachycardia, disproportionate to fever, and poor peripheral perfusion (see Chapter 6). If any alterations in the ABCs exist, stabilization is the first priority of nursing care.

Evaluation of suspected osteomyelitis begins with a thorough history and physical examination. Historical questions include the character and duration of the bone or limb pain; previous similar symptoms; history of trauma or recent infection; associated signs and symptoms of illness; the presence of an underlying or chronic disorder; and current medications, including antibiotics.

The physical examination focuses on the assessment of the affected limb and evaluation for a distal or contiguous site of infection. Orthopedic consultation is usually obtained. Age-appropriate pain assessment in regard to location, intensity, and duration is important, along with evaluation of hydration and nutritional status.

Wound and skin precautions are necessary to protect staff and other patients, particularly if wound drainage is present, or during diagnostic testing and therapeutic interventions. The child's room and used equipment must be thoroughly cleaned after discharge.

Because movement or weight bearing may foster the systemic spread of infection or other complications, the affected extremity is immobilized. If a lower extremity is involved, weight bearing is not permitted.

Pain-relief measures, including positioning and supporting the affected limb on pillows, enhance the child's comfort and well-being. If analgesia or sedation is administered, its effectiveness should be periodically evaluated. Preparation of the child and parents for diagnostic tests and interventions helps to alleviate anxiety and enhance coping.

SEPTIC ARTHRITIS

Etiology. Septic arthritis is an infection of the joint that constitutes an acute medical emergency because it can cause irreversible damage to the articular cartilage, epiphysis, and growth plate.[17] Although it can occur at any age, septic arthritis usually affects infants and children less than 5 years of age. Predisposing factors include trauma, skin and soft tissue infections, IV drug abuse, femoral venipuncture in neonates, chronic debilitating diseases, and immunosuppression.

Similar to osteomyelitis, septic arthritis usually results from hematogenous (blood-borne) spread of bacteria from a distal site of infection, such as otitis media or upper respiratory infection. It may also occur directly from contamination of a puncture wound or indirectly by extension from an overlying cellulitis or underlying osteomyelitis. In children over 5 years of age, septic arthritis is frequently associated with skin infection or trauma.[16] Large joints, including the hip, knee, and shoulder, are most commonly affected. In more than 90% of children affected by septic arthritis, only one joint is involved.[22]

The etiologic agents causing septic arthritis are similar to those of osteomyelitis, with *S. aureus* being the leading offender.[17] *H. influenzae,* type B, and various strains of streptococci are typical etiologic agents in children under 6 years of age. Gonococcal arthritis may occur in sexually active or abused children and adolescents, although it is rare. Meningococcal arthritis is also rare and occurs without meningitis.

Pathophysiology. An inflammatory response is initiated when bacteria seeds the affected joint space, resulting in purulent effusion and vascular congestion. The subsequent rise in intraarticular pressure can obstruct blood flow and lead to necrosis of the epiphysis and growth plate.[17] Enzymes released by polymorphonuclear leukocytes and synovial cells destroy cartilage and collagen. If effective treatment is not implemented, destruction of the ligaments of the joint capsule may occur, resulting in joint instability and/or dislocation. This is particularly devastating when septic arthritis involves the hip joint, which can create leg length discrepancies of up to several inches.

Clinical presentation. Septic arthritis typically presents with an abrupt onset of pain in the affected extremity, fever, and rapid progression to systemic illness. Unlike children with osteomyelitis who tolerate gentle, passive range of motion, children with septic arthritis do not tolerate any active or passive attempts to manipulate the affected joint. Lower extremity involvement is accompanied by a limp. Decreased use occurs with other affected joints. Warmth, tenderness, and swelling of the joint are common but may be harder to detect in a deep joint such as the hip.

When the hip is involved, the child frequently holds it rigidly in mild flexion, abduction, and external rotation. Some children with hip involvement present with referred knee pain.[22] Attempts at weight bearing are usually very painful. With shoulder involvement, the preferred position is adduction against the trunk. Children with a septic knee joint are most comfortable when the joint is slightly flexed.

Differential diagnoses include osteomyelitis, juvenile rheumatoid arthritis, toxic synovitis, Legg-Perthes disease, and slipped capital femoral epiphysis.

Rheumatic fever most commonly presents with polyarthritis—unlike septic arthritis, which usually involves one joint.[22] The possibility of more than one disease process occurring concurrently should be considered.

Emergency Department interventions

Diagnostic tests. Septic arthritis is a clinical diagnosis, although lab work and radiographic studies are helpful to the diagnostic process. The white blood cell count may be normal or elevated with increased neutrophils and band cells. The ESR tends to be elevated. Blood cultures reveal the offending organism approximately 50% of the time.[16] X-rays may show a subtle increase in the joint space or soft tissue changes such as swelling; however, radiography is unlikely to be helpful in the early stages of infection. Dependence on imaging studies for definitive diagnosis can therefore cause a disastrous delay in diagnosis and treatment. Prompt orthopedic consultation is usually obtained.

Definitive diagnosis requires joint aspiration under fluoroscopy to obtain fluid for cultures and white blood cell count. Joint aspiration is indicated in any child who presents with arthritis and fever. A fluid sample that contains more than 100,000 white blood cells with greater than 75% neutrophils is diagnostic of septic arthritis.[17]

Treatment. Antibiotic therapy is begun as soon as the diagnosis is established and cultures are obtained. Delays in treatment may result in permanent disabling joint deformity and instability and marked limb length discrepancy. Initial antimicrobial therapy for children over the age of 5 years consists of an antistaphylococcal penicillin alone. Because *H. influenzae* is a common cause of septic arthritis in young children and approximately 40% of *H. influenzae* strains are ampicillin resistant, additional coverage with an aminoglycoside is recommended. For suspected gonococcal arthritis, ceftriaxone is the antibiotic of choice.

Hospital admission of the child with septic arthritis is mandatory. Effective treatment includes parenteral antibiotic administration for 2 to 3 weeks and wound drainage by needle aspiration of the joint or surgically by arthrotomy or arthroscopy.[22]

Nursing care and evaluation. Nursing care of the child with suspected septic arthritis includes a thorough history and physical examination, both to assist the physician in making the diagnosis and to determine the degree of systemic and local involvement. Previous trauma or recent respiratory tract infection in a child presenting with a warm, tender, swollen joint is highly suggestive of septic arthritis.

During the initial assessment the emergency nurse should evaluate the child's vital signs, perfusion, and hydration status, because septic shock is a serious complication of septic arthritis. When signs of shock are observed emergent management is indicated.

If the child is stable on arrival in the ED or during initial stabilization, the source of the infection, either contiguous or distant, must be identified. Particular attention should be directed to the ears, nose, throat, and skin.

Localized assessment of the affected joint includes inspection, palpation, and active and passive range of motion. Palpation and movement of the joint causes intense pain.

Comfort measures include immobilizing the joint and the administration of analgesics. Immobilizing the joint both decreases the degree of pain and decreases the risk of spreading the infection. Continuous monitoring includes the evaluation of pain-management interventions and observation for signs of shock and impaired perfusion of the extremity. The child and parents should be kept informed of the plan of care, including diagnostic testing, and provided with accurate information about the child's condition.

Juvenile Rheumatoid Arthritis

Etiology. Juvenile rheumatoid arthritis (JRA) is the most common rheumatic disease in the pediatric population. At any given time it affects between 40,000–100,000 children in the United States.[8] The incidence of JRA is higher in females than males. Onset primarily occurs between the ages of 1 to 3 years and 8 to 12 years.[1a]

JRA is identified clinically. It is diagnosed in any child under 16 years of age with arthritis lasting more than 6 weeks in one or more joints, and after other diagnoses have been excluded.[8,16] There are three subtypes of JRA: (1) systemic onset; (2) pauciarticular (involving fewer than five joints); and (3) polyarticular (involving five or more joints).

Although the exact cause of JRA is unknown, some evidence indicates a genetic predisposition for the disease, which is triggered by trauma, stress, or infection.[8] Autoimmune processes have also been implicated.

Pathophysiology. JRA is characterized by chronic inflammation of the synovial membrane, joint effusion, and vasculitis. With progression of the disease process, fibrin is deposited and hyperplasia and hypertrophy of the synovial lining occur. In chronic arthritis, thickened synovial membranes typically spread from the edges of the joint, causing destruction of cartilage. Eventually, adhesions between joint surfaces and ankylosis (immobility) of the joints result.

Clinical presentation. JRA is a multisystem disorder. Clinical manifestations, course, and prognosis vary widely depending on the subtype (Table 13-3). Arthritic joints are usually associated with a constellation of other signs and symptoms, such as prolonged intermittent fever, rash, or uveitis. Alternating periods of acute exacerbations and remissions are characteristic.

Most children with JRA are not diagnosed in the ED but may commonly present with acute exacerbations, complications, or additional injuries or illnesses (Box 13-4). Exacerbations involve acute inflammation of one or more joints that are swollen, warm, painful, and limited in motion.[16] Because rheumatic joints are susceptible to infection, acute exacerbations must be carefully differentiated from a superimposed septic arthritis or osteomyelitis.

Complications of JRA include cardiac, pulmonary, ophthalmic, and infectious disorders. The incidence of pericarditis is highest in children with systemic JRA. Pericarditis may be asymptomatic or present with chest pain, dyspnea, and an inability to lie flat in bed. A pericardial friction rub is typically heard, unless obscured by a pericardial effusion. Weak pulses, distant heart sounds, and signs of congestive heart failure may be present with a pericardial effusion.

Pulmonary complications include pleural effusions, pneumonitis, and diffuse interstitial disease. Classic signs of pleural effusion include chest pain, dyspnea, cough, and diminished breath sounds over the affected area. Although very rare, children with polyarticular arthritis may develop cricoarytenoid arthritis manifested by hoarseness, stridor, throat pain when swallowing, ear pain, and respiratory distress. Because of the potential for acute airway obstruction, this is an emergent complication.

Chronic uveitis, an inflammation of the vascular structure of the inner eye, occurs in approximately 25% of children with pauciarticular JRA, even after the arthritis has resolved. Classic signs of uveitis include red eye, decreased visual acuity, pain, photophobia, and unequal pupils. Chronic uveitis may result

TABLE 13-3	Clinical Manifestations of Juvenile Rheumatoid Arthritis			
		PAUCIARTICULAR		
	SYSTEMIC	EARLY-ONSET TYPE 1	LATE-ONSET TYPE 2	POLYARTICULAR
Common age group	<5 years of age	<6 years of age	>8 years of age	3-8 years—tend to have negative RF* >8 years—positive RF
Sex distribution	Girls ≈ boys	Girls > boys	Boys > girls	Girls > boys
Percentage of patients	20%	25%	15%-20%	30%-35%
Presentation	Involves multiple large and small joints May have nonpruritic, salmon-colored macular or papular rash with areas of central clearing; mostly in areas of increased heat (e.g., axilla) Fever spikes (≥ 39° C or 102° F) in the afternoon; normal at night Lymph, liver, and spleen enlargement Myalgias, arthralgias	Asymmetric arthritis involving fewer than five large joints (knees, elbows, ankles); often only one joint involved Good functional status Few systemic signs Rarely complain of pain Little erosive joint damage	Asymmetric arthritis involving fewer than five large joints, especially lower extremities (knees, ankles, toes); often only one joint involved Tendinitis may intensify joint pain Sacroiliitis in approximately 90%	Symmetric arthritis involving five or more small or large joints in any part of the body, including the temporomandibular joint and cervical spine Insidious onset with morning stiffness, low-grade fever, anorexia, fatigue, weight loss, and arthritis of both small and large joints
Potential complications	Pericarditis Pleural effusion, pneumonitis, or diffuse interstitial disease Growth retardation	Long-term problems, such as muscle atrophy and leg-length discrepancies Chronic uveitis (in approximately 25%)	Acute iritis (in approximately 10%)	Chronic uveitis occurs in a small percentage Cricoarytenoid arthritis (rare)
Course	Systemic manifestations are self-limited May develop chronic arthritis; 25% severe destructive arthritis	Arthritis mild Some ocular problems	Variable course May develop ankylosing spondylitis pattern (immobilization and pain between the articular processes, costovertebral joints, and sacroiliac joints)	If RF negative, good prognosis; 10% develop severe sequelae, especially hip and temporomandibular joint problems If RF positive, childhood course resembles adult rheumatoid disease; 50% have severe destructive arthritis

Compiled from Betz and Sowden, 1996; Faries and Johnston, 1992; Gewanter, 1992; Rosenstein and Fosarelli, 1993.
*RF = Rheumatoid factor.

Box 13-4   Symptoms of JRA Likely to Result in Visits to the Emergency Department

Acute manifestations of chronic disease
  Fever
  Joint pain
  Rash
Pericarditis
C-spine pain or injury
  Neurologic complaints
Injury to an involved joint

From Faries G, Johnston C: Allergic and immunologic diseases. In Barkin RM, ed: *Pediatric emergency medicine,* St Louis, 1992, Mosby.

---

in cataracts, glaucoma, visual loss and eventual blindness.[1a,8]

Cervical spine involvement is more common in adults than children with rheumatoid arthritis. However, the risk of atlantoaxial subluxation is increased in these children; cervical spine precautions should be initiated for any child with JRA who is involved in any traumatic incident.[6]

Emergency Department interventions

Diagnostic tests. Because there is no definitive test for JRA, diagnosis is based on clinical findings after other diagnoses such as septic arthritis, lyme disease, osteomyelitis, musculoskeletal trauma, Osgood-Schlatter disease, and leukemia are ruled out. Misdiagnosis is common in children who have monarticular disease (involvement of only one joint).[16]

The child who presents with arthritis requires laboratory studies, including a complete blood count (CBC) with differential and an ESR, and radiographs of the affected joint(s). Other tests, such as rheumatoid factor (RF) and antinuclear antibodies, if positive, are helpful in making the diagnosis. However, these tests are not very sensitive.[16]

The CBC often reveals leukocytosis and mild anemia, particularly with systemic JRA. Significant alterations in the CBC, however, suggest other problems such as infection or malignancy. The ESR is useful in differentiating inflammatory vs. noninflammatory causes of arthritis, but it can also be normal. Platelet counts and complement levels are often elevated due to the inflammatory process.

The earliest radiographic signs of JRA are nonspe-

cific soft tissue swelling of affected joints and widening of joint spaces.[21] Later in the disease process, narrowing of the joint space due to articular destruction occurs, followed by bone erosion and fusion of the joint.[18] Subluxation of the cervical spine may also be evident.

A high index of suspicion must be maintained for an underlying systemic illness in the child with JRA. Other tests are indicated if complications or underlying illness are suspected. An ECG, echocardiogram, and chest x-ray will diagnose pericarditis. Typical ECG changes include tachycardia, elevated S-T segment, and inverted T waves. A chest x-ray is indicated for any child with suspected pleural effusion.

Treatment. Children with JRA are typically treated at home, except in the event of severe exacerbations or complications. The goals of treatment are to prevent and/or correct contractural deformities of joints and growth deformities of bones[18] and to relieve pain.

Pharmacologic therapy is used to control inflammation, suppress fever, and treat complications (Table 13-4). Nonsteroidal antiinflammatory drugs (NSAIDs), especially cost-effective acetylsalicylic acid (ASA), are commonly given to control inflammation in children with JRA. Because hepatotoxicity is a complication of consistent ASA usage, especially during the first 3 months of administration, serum SGOT and SGPT levels are monitored. Other NSAIDs can be used in children who do not tolerate ASA. If NSAIDs do not produce an effective response, a slow-acting antirheumatic drug may be used. Because of the side effects with prolonged administration, corticosteroids are typically reserved for children with high fever and severe joint disease who are unresponsive to NSAIDs or those with severe pulmonary, cardiac, or ophthalmic complications. Intraarticular injections of steroids may provide temporary relief of inflammation in a large joint, allowing functional range of motion.

Children with pericarditis are admitted to the hospital for treatment with ASA, or corticosteroids if severe, and bed rest. If cardiac tamponade results from pericarditis, pericardiocentesis is indicated. Children with pulmonary complications are also typically admitted to the hospital. Thoracentesis may be necessary to relieve the respiratory distress associated with a pleural effusion. Cricoarytenoid arthritis with respiratory distress is treated with large doses of corticosteroids to decrease inflammation and airway edema. If airway obstruction is severe enough to cause increas-

TABLE 13-4	Pharmacologic Treatment of JRA	
MEDICATION	**RECOMMENDED DOSE**	**COMMENTS**
NSAIDs		
Aspirin	80-90 mg/kg/q6h or q8h	Controls inflammation and fever Recommended serum level: 20-25 mg/dl
Indomethacin	0.5-2.5 mg/kg/day	Controls fever and inflammation
Tolmetin	15-30 mg/kg/day	Controls inflammation
Ibuprofen	20-40 mg/kg/day	Controls inflammation; controls fever of infectious origin
Naproxen	10-15 mg/kg/day	Controls inflammation
Slow-acting antirheumatic drugs		Antiinflammatory used if NSAIDs are not effective
Gold compound	1 mg/kg/week IM	
D-penicillinase	125-250 mg/day	
Corticosteroids		Indicated for severe joint disease or pulmonary, cardiac, or ophthalmic complications
Prednisone	2 mg/kg/day PO	Intraarticular injections used in single joint involvement

Compiled from Athreya BH, Yancey CL, Eichenfield AH: Rheumatologic emergencies. In Fleisher G, Ludwig S, eds: *Textbook of pediatric emergency medicine,* Baltimore, 1988, Williams & Wilkins; Tachdjian MO: *Pediatric orthopedics,* ed 2, Philadelphia, 1990, WB Sanuders.

ing respiratory distress and hypoxemia, intubation or a tracheostomy must be performed immediately.

Children with acute uveitis require immediate consultation with an ophthalmologist. Treatment consists of topical corticosteroids and mydriatic agents.

After limb-threatening disorders have been ruled out in the ED, the child with arthritis of unknown origin is often discharged. Because JRA cannot be diagnosed in a child with recent onset of joint pain and swelling, follow-up by a primary care or orthopedic physician is required. The child with diagnosed JRA must be monitored closely after discharge to evaluate response to therapy and identify early signs of complications.

Nursing care and evaluation. The objectives of nursing care of a child with JRA include pain relief, early identification and intervention of complications or underlying illnesses, preservation of joint functioning, and psychosocial support. Contact with the primary care provider is important to ensure consistency with the child's plan of care in the ED.

A thorough history and physical examination identify signs and symptoms of JRA; complications; con-

current illnesses, such as upper respiratory or gastrointestinal infections; and degree of pain. Nursing priorities are determined by the clinical presentation.

During an acute exacerbation of JRA, pain relief, reduction of inflammation, and prevention of further damage take precedence. Medications to control both inflammation and pain are administered. Interventions to minimize side effects of medications are instituted and taught to caregivers. For example, giving ASA with food diminishes gastric irritation. If the child has been on long-term aspirin therapy, the emergency nurse must observe for signs and symptoms of chronic salicylate toxicity, including nausea, vomiting, fever, tinnitus, hypoglycemia, oliguria, or a bleeding disorder. Reye's syndrome, which can result from salicylate usage during certain viral infections, must be suspected in any child who has been on aspirin therapy and presents to the emergency department with vomiting and an altered mental status.

Nonpharmacologic measures to control pain, decrease inflammation, and prevent further damage include bed rest and no weight bearing or pressure on the inflamed joints. Anatomic positioning of the affected limbs maintains alignment and reduces pain. Splints are often used to provide support, relieve muscle spasm, and prevent deformities. However, routine active and passive exercises are required to maintain range of motion and prevent muscle atrophy. Applying warm moist pads to the affected joints or providing warm tub baths relieves pain and stiffness in the joints.

If pericarditis or pericardial effusion is suspected, the child must be monitored closely for signs and symptoms of cardiac tamponade, including tachycardia disproportionate to fever, paradoxic pulse pressure, dyspnea, cyanosis, and decrease in arterial pressure. Signs of cardiac tamponade are reported to the physician immediately. The child with pulmonary complications is observed closely for the three earliest signs of respiratory distress: tachycardia, tachypnea, and irritability or restlessness. Early recognition and intervention may prevent rapid deterioration and subsequent respiratory arrest. Initial nursing management includes oxygen administration, frequent monitoring of vital signs, and evaluation of hemoglobin saturation using pulse oximetry. Airway management equipment and a thoracotomy tray should be immediately available at the child's bedside.

Juvenile rheumatoid arthritis is a complex, chronic disease process that places significant strain on families. The child and caregiver benefit from education, identification of resources, and emotional support. Important information to be conveyed to the caregiver includes medication side effects and signs of toxicity; signs and symptoms of serious medical complications, including Reye's syndrome; pain-relief measures such as warm baths for joint stiffness and heating pads to affected joints; preservation of joint mobility by such activities as range of motion exercises, swimming, or bicycle riding; and proper splinting and positioning when joints are acutely inflamed. Routine eye examinations to evaluate for uveitis are recommended at 3- to 6-month intervals. Because nutritional status may be quite poor in children with polyarticular disease, referral to a nutritionist for further education and management may be warranted. Communication with the primary health care provider is important to ensure coordination of services.

Effectiveness of family coping strategies and support systems should be evaluated by emergency nurses so that appropriate referrals can be made. In addition, parents should be aware that the American Juvenile Arthritis Foundation and the Arthritis Foundation provide helpful services to families of children with JRA. The prognosis of JRA is usually good, with many children experiencing permanent remission or minimal residual problems.[8]

TOXIC OR TRANSIENT SYNOVITIS

Etiology. Toxic or transient synovitis is a self-limited acute inflammation of the hip, mainly affecting children between the ages of 18 months and 12 years.[2,16] It is the most common cause of hip pain in children, with a higher incidence in males than females.[4,14] The etiology is unknown. However, because toxic synovitis commonly follows an upper respiratory infection by several days to 2 weeks, a viral inflammatory process is suspected.[16] Trauma, bacterial infection, and allergies may also be precipitating factors.

Pathophysiology. Nonspecific inflammation and hypertrophy of the synovial membrane develops in the hip joint, causing pain and limited range of motion. Exudation of sterile fluid can result in a small joint effusion.

Clinical presentation. The child with toxic synovitis typically presents with an acute, but sometimes insidious, onset of a painful limp.[10] Pain is commonly experienced in the groin or hip but may be referred to the thigh or knee due to irritation of the anterior branch of the obturator nerve, which passes close to the hip joint.[14] Because of guarding or spasm of hip muscles, the limp is characterized by a shortened stance on the affected side.[16] The hip is typically held in flexion, abduction, and external rotation.[2] Examination reveals limitation of active and passive range of motion. If the condition is severe, the child may refuse to walk. Rarely is there systemic illness. Fever, if present, is low grade (<101° F). Toxic synovitis has a benign clinical course and usually resolves in 3 to 7 days.

Emergency Department interventions

Diagnostic tests. The diagnosis of toxic synovitis primarily relies on the clinical presentation. The white blood cell (WBC) count and ESR are usually normal or slightly elevated. Hip radiography is also typically normal, although widening of the joint space or distortion of the soft tissue planes around the hip may be visible. Ultrasound may reveal a small joint effusion.

Differential diagnoses include septic arthritis, juvenile rheumatoid arthritis, osteomyelitis of the femur, tuberculosis, slipped femoral capital epiphysis, and Legg-Perthes disease.[10] Because septic arthritis can rapidly produce irreversible damage to the joint, it must be identified promptly. Signs include fever, leukocytosis, acute spasm, and severe pain. If there is any question of a septic hip, aspiration of the hip joint under fluoroscopy must be performed. In contrast to the septic hip, in which joint fluid contains WBCs and bacterial organisms, fluid from a joint affected by toxic synovitis is sterile.

Treatment.   Children with toxic synovitis are usually managed at home with bed rest and analgesics. Hospitalization and light traction may be required in severe cases. Nonsteroidal antiinflammatory medications are commonly given, although salicylates are avoided because of the association with Reye's syndrome. Because toxic synovitis may precede or mimic septic arthritis, osteomyelitis, Legg-Perthes disease, or slipped capital femoral epiphysis, response to treatment should be carefully monitored. Toxic synovitis usually resolves in 3 to 7 days; any prolongation of symptoms requires reevaluation of the diagnosis. Medical follow-up is recommended in 5 to 7 days. Hip radiographs are usually performed every 6 months for 2 years, because 5% of these patients will develop Legg-Perthes disease.[4]

Nursing care and evaluation.   Nursing care of the child with a hip or leg pain begins with a history and physical examination, including evaluation of local joint pathology, as well as systemic illness. If a serious bacterial infection such as septic arthritis is suspected, emergent interventions may be required (see p. 296). Children with true toxic synovitis generally require symptomatic treatment only.

Positioning and pain medication will usually relieve the discomfort of orthopedic pain. Teaching parents about the disease process, bed rest, and proper administration of analgesics and potential side effects facili-

tates home management. Because 3 to 5 days of bed rest is recommended, suggestions for compliance such as audio or videotapes, games, and developmentally appropriate activities are helpful to parents. Parents need to be aware of the signs and symptoms of infection and potential sequelae such as Legg-Perthes disease and have an accessible health care provider for follow-up. In addition, reassurance of the benign nature of the disease in the great majority of children will usually help to alleviate parental anxiety.

LEGG-CALVÉ-PERTHES DISEASE

Etiology.   Legg-Perthes disease, sometimes referred to as *osteochondrosis of the femoral head* or *Legg-Calvé-Perthes disease,* is a self-limiting disorder in which there is avascular necrosis of the femoral head. It can occur in children between 3 and 11 years of age but primarily affects 4- to 8-year old males.[10] The disease is rare in African-Americans.

Although the etiology is unknown, temporary interruption in the blood supply to the femoral head plays a role in the development of avascular necrosis.[4] Family history is positive in approximately 20% of children with Legg-Perthes disease[14]; however, genetic factors do not seem to play a role in the etiology.[18] Recent trauma or a stress fracture may be a precipitating factor.

Pathophysiology.   There are five stages of Legg-Perthes disease (Table 13-5). As the disease progresses, the avascular bone cannot support weight, contributing to the formation of stress fractures in the epiphyseal head.[4] Symptoms of the disease do not appear until a fracture occurs.[18] The weak structure of new bone collapses under the fracture, resulting in a

TABLE 13-5	Five Stages of Legg-Perthes Disease	
STAGE	DURATION	DESCRIPTION
Prenecrosis		Vascular compromise to the femoral capital epiphysis
Necrosis	3-6 months	Necrosis and flattening of the femoral head
		Temporary cessation of epiphyseal growth
Resorption	6-12 months	Dead bone is reabsorbed
Reossification	18-36 months	Laying down of immature new bone on the femoral head
Remodeling		Partial or complete reformation of the femoral head
		Subluxation and/or deformity may occur

Cwinn, 1992.

second episode of vascular compromise. As subsequent reossification occurs, the femoral head is remodeled. Normal configuration may be regained or joint deformity and progressive subluxation of the hip can develop.[16] Fig. 13-2 illustrates the pathogenesis of joint deformity in Legg-Perthes disease.

Clinical presentation. Initially, the child with Legg-Perthes disease develops a painless limp that occurs intermittently after activity. Eventually the limp becomes constant and may be associated with mild hip, groin, thigh, or knee pain, which is most common on arising and at the end of the day. Onset is insidious, often over a period of weeks. Hip motion, especially medial rotation and abduction, is decreased. Symptoms are usually relieved by rest.

Twelve percent of children with Legg-Perthes disease have *bilateral hip involvement*,[14] although one hip is typically in the healing phase when the disease commences in the other hip.

Affected children often have a history of low birth weight and tend to be shorter and delayed in maturation in comparison to peers.[14,16] Behavioral disorders such as hyperactivity are common in children with Legg-Perthes disease.

Emergency Department interventions

Diagnostic tests. Diagnosis is confirmed by hip radiographs, including both standing anteroposterior (AP) and frog-leg lateral positions. A bone scan identifies the degree of avascularity.[16] Joint space widening is seen very early in the disease process. The appearance of a fracture line in the femoral head heralds the onset of clinical symptoms. In later stages, the femoral head may appear small and sclerotic. With severe involvement, findings typically reveal a small capital epiphysis with a shortened femoral neck and flattened femoral head.[4]

Other diagnoses, such as infection, toxic synovitis, and JRA, must be ruled out. It is essential to differentiate Legg-Perthes disease from acute emergencies such as septic arthritis and osteomyelitis.

Treatment. The mainstay of treatment is containment of the femoral head within the acetabulum and range-of-motion exercises.[14] The methods are controversial, and orthopedic consultation is recommended. Children with minimal involvement of the femoral head or who are less than 6 years of age can usually be managed at home with routine follow-up.[16] For those children with limited range of motion,

hospitalization with bed rest and Buck's traction is usually required. Surgery is sometimes recommended to stabilize the femoral head within the acetabulum. Nonsurgical interventions, such as the use of an abduction brace for a period of 1 year, are alternative approaches.

Children less than 8 years of age tend to have better outcomes because more time is available after healing for epiphyseal remodeling.[18] The disease process may resolve in 18 months or last up to several years.

Nursing care and evaluation. Assessment focuses on the hips and lower extremities but also includes identification of associated systemic findings. A major error in the physical examination of a child who presents with thigh or knee pain is the omission of a hip assessment.[14]

Because many children with Legg-Perthes disease are treated on an out-patient basis, teaching and emotional support are a priority. Caregivers' knowledge of the disease and its management must be evaluated and misperceptions clarified. Return demonstrations of proper range-of-motion exercises and use of orthopedic appliances are helpful. In addition, it is critical to emphasize to the family the importance of adherence to care to prevent complications. For those children requiring hospital admission, nursing care should include psychologic preparation for hospitalization.

SLIPPED CAPITAL FEMORAL EPIPHYSIS

Etiology. Slipped capital femoral epiphysis is a sudden or gradual displacement of the proximal femoral epiphysis on the femoral neck. Inactive, obese, male adolescents between the ages of 13 and 15 are most commonly affected.[2] However, the disorder can also occur in rapidly growing, tall, thin youths between 10 and 16 years of age.[21] Onset is earlier in females (11 to 13 years). The incidence is higher in African-Americans and in the eastern part of the United States. Bilateral involvement occurs in about a third of cases of slipped capital femoral epiphysis, although it is rare for the involvement to occur simultaneously.

The etiology of slipped capital femoral epiphysis is unknown, but certain factors such as genetic predisposition, defective growth plate, obesity, and hormonal factors have been implicated.[16] It has also been associated with endocrine disorders and growth hormone therapy.

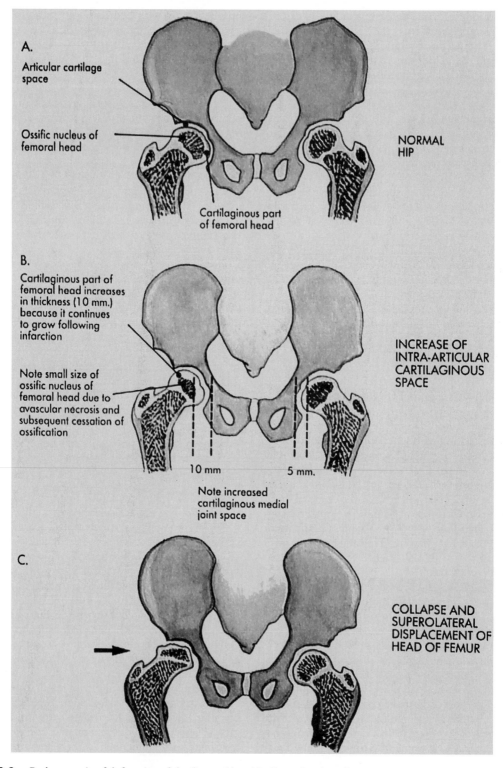

FIG. 13-2. Pathogenesis of deformity of the femoral head in Legg-Perthes disease. (From Tachdjian MO: *Pediatric orthopedics,* ed 2, Philadelphia, 1990, WB Saunders.)

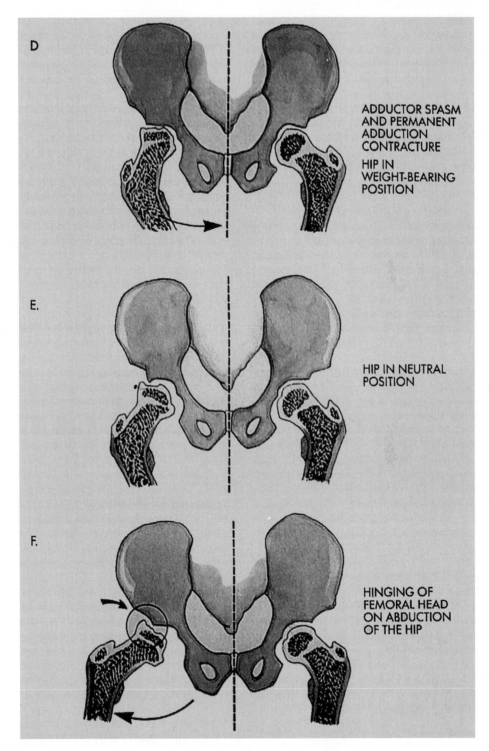

D

ADDUCTOR SPASM
AND PERMANENT
ADDUCTION
CONTRACTURE

HIP IN
WEIGHT-BEARING
POSITION

E.

HIP IN NEUTRAL
POSITION

F.

HINGING OF
FEMORAL HEAD
ON ABDUCTION
OF THE HIP

Fig. 13-2, cont'd. For legend see opposite page.

Pathophysiology. Acute slippage of the femoral epiphysis causes sudden displacement of the femoral head in relation to the femoral neck. It may be initiated by trauma or shearing stress from body weight. The chronic form starts with demineralization of the bone on the lower femoral side of the epiphysis and a widening of the growth plate. The femoral portion of the epiphysis then slides upward but remains attached by thick periosteum. Finally, the epiphysis is displaced posteriorly and inferiorly, disrupting the positional relation between the femoral head and femoral neck. An acute slippage can also occur, particularly in adolescents with chronic disease.

Clinical manifestations. In chronic slip, there is a gradual onset of dull pain in the groin, thigh, and knee with intermittent limping. Symptoms are aggravated by physical activity. The degree of limitation of hip range of motion and the extent of leg shortening depend on the severity of slip.

Acute slip presents with sudden onset of severe groin, thigh, or knee pain and inability to bear weight. Range of motion is severely limited and painful, especially hip flexion and medial rotation (Fig. 13-3). The affected leg is externally rotated and markedly shortened.

Emergency Department interventions

Diagnostic tests. Diagnosis is based on physical exam and radiography. The earliest radiographic finding in the "pre-slip" phase is widening of the growth plate. In more advanced cases, radiography will show the altered position of the femoral head on the neck (Fig. 13-4). Because nearly all displacements occur posteriorly, both AP and frog-leg views must be obtained.

Treatment. Immediate treatment must be initiated to prevent further slippage and subsequent complications such as avascular necrosis, premature degenerative arthritis, and gait deterioration. If slipped capital femoral epiphysis is suspected, all weight bearing is prohibited. With acute slippage, gentle reduction with skeletal traction is initially performed, followed by surgical pinning to fixate the hip. Orthopedic consultation is required. Prognosis varies with the severity of the slippage and the occurrence of complications.

Nursing care and evaluation. When a slipped femoral capital epiphysis is suspected, the child is immediately restricted from weight bearing. Because management of moderate to severe slippage consists of skeletal traction and surgical pinning, hospital admission is required. Psychologic preparation and emotional support are important, particularly because of the unplanned nature of admission. Finally, regular follow-up care is essential because contralateral hip involvement may occur.

OSGOOD-SCHLATTER DISEASE

Etiology. Osgood-Schlatter disease is a painful enlargement of the tibial tuberosity at the insertion of the patellar tendon. It results from repetitive pulling of the quadriceps in growing children between 10 and 16 years of age.[16] Male athletes are primarily affected. The disease is self-limiting and typically resolves in late adolescence when the epiphysis at the insertion site closes and the bone becomes stronger than the inserted ligament.[2]

Pathophysiology. Repeated contraction of the quadriceps muscle with activities such as running and jumping pulls on the patellar tendon causing detachment of cartilage fragments from the tibial tuberosity. The subsequent inflammatory and reparative process results in patellar swelling and tenderness and enlargement of the tibial tuberosity.[18] Because the patellar tendon and tubercle are extraarticular, there is no risk of permanent damage to the knee joint.

Clinical presentation. Classic presentation includes pain in the anterior aspect of the knee, which is aggravated by activity or direct pressure and is relieved by rest. Tenderness and enlargement of the tibial tuberosity is observed, especially at the point of patellar insertion to the bone. Symptoms often are first noticed when kneeling or after minor trauma.

Emergency Department interventions. Diagnosis is usually made solely by physical examination when pressure on the tibial tuberosity at the patellar tendon insertion elicits pain. If a radiograph is taken, an irregular, prominent tubercle and soft tissue swelling anterior to the knee are usually present.[16] Free bone particles may also be evident.

Osgood-Schlatter disease is typically diagnosed and treated in outpatient settings but may be seen in the ED setting as a primary or secondary complaint. Treatment includes rest, quadriceps strengthening exercises, ice packs, and nonsteroidal antiinflammatory agents such as ibuprofen. Relief of symptoms

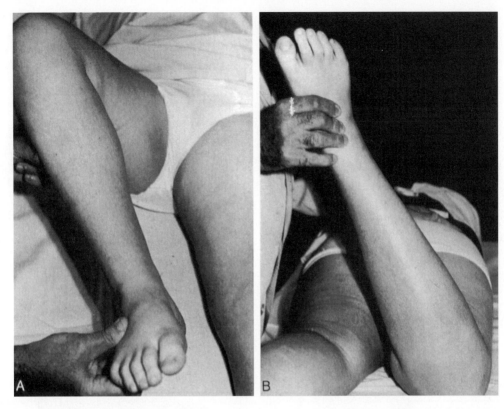

FIG. 13-3. Clinical findings in slipped capital femoral epiphysis of the right hip. (From Tachdjian MO: *Pediatric ortho-pedics,* ed 2, Philadelphia, 1990, WB Saunders.)

usually occurs in 2 to 3 weeks, after which gradual activity can be resumed. Participation in sports should be limited for 3 months. With more severe cases, immobilization with bracing or casting is sometimes necessary.

Nursing care and evaluation. Assessment of a child presenting with signs or symptoms of Osgood-Schlatter disease includes a history and a physical exam, which focuses on the affected site and lower extremity. The exam should also include evaluation of the patient for signs or symptoms of systemic illness. Once a patient is diagnosed with Osgood-Schlatter disease, nursing care focuses on educating the family regarding the disease process and appropriate care. Stretching and muscle strengthening exercises for the lower extremities are recommended and should be demonstrated before discharge. Emotional support is usually required, especially for the adolescent who must temporarily restrict sports activities.

OSTEOGENESIS IMPERFECTA

Etiology. Osteogenesis imperfecta (OI) is a connective tissue disorder and is the primary etiology of osteoporosis in children. It is characterized by fractures and skeletal deformities. The incidence of OI Type 1 is 1 in 30,000 live births.[1] Type II OI affects approximately 1 in 60,000 infants, many of which are stillborn. The remainder die soon after birth.[1] Osteoporosis results from osteopenia, which is a bone insufficiency caused by diminished production and/or excessive loss. OI comprises four distinct inherited osteoporosis syndromes. Deletions, substitutions, and mutations of collagen-formation genes are the basis for the various defects. Table 13-6 lists the types of OI with inheritance pattern, including major signs and symptoms.

Pathophysiology. OI is characterized by immature collagen formation affecting all connective tissues. The bones are primarily involved, however, due to their frequent exposure to stress. Microscopic

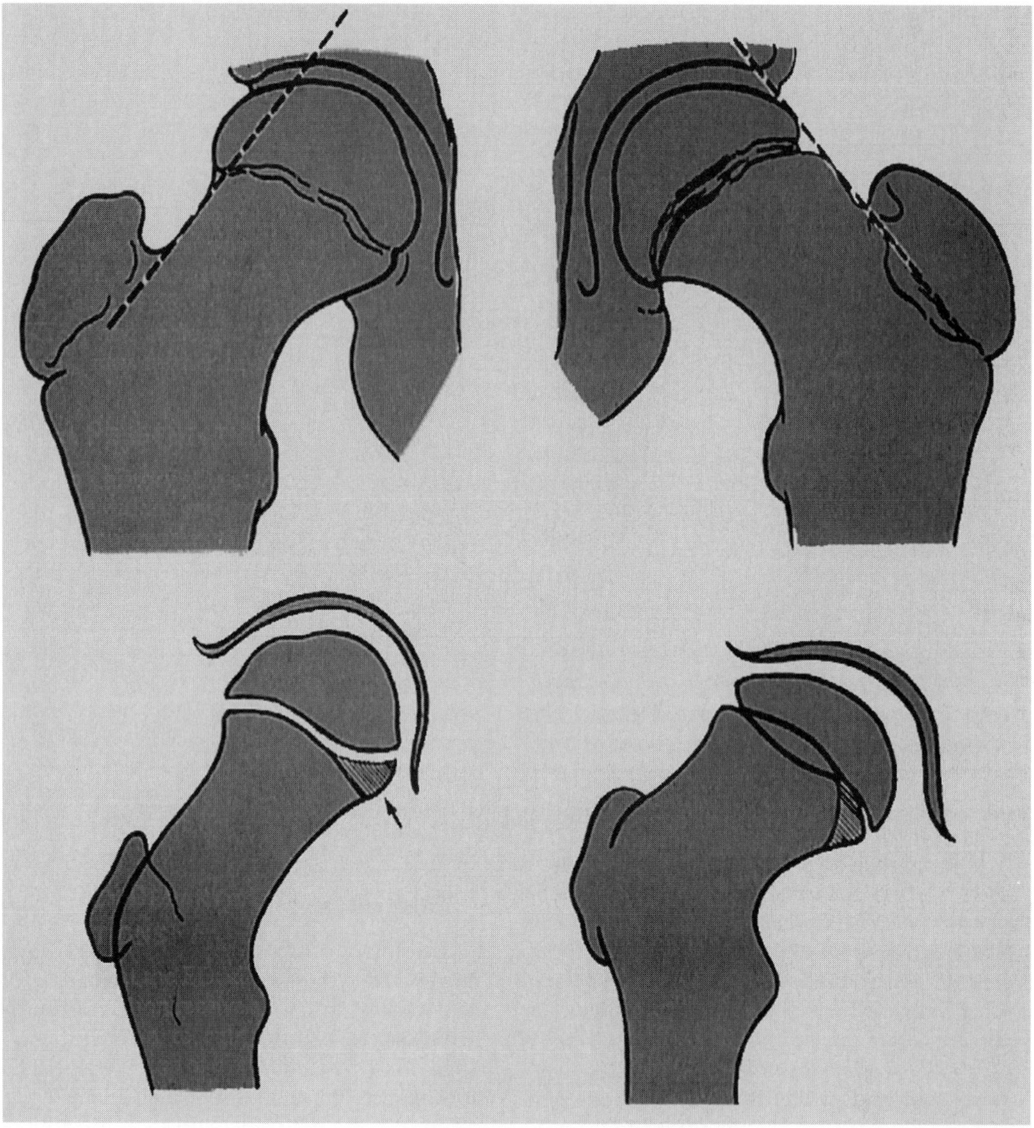

FIG. 13-4. Radiographic changes of minimal medial slip. **A,** *Normal hip:* a line along superior side of femoral neck transects overhanging ossified epiphysis; whereas, **B,** *Slipped hip:* projected neck is bared at epiphyseal plate and there is widening and irregularity of epiphyseal plate. **C,** *Normal hip:* "articular portion" of metaphysis is contained within acetabulum. **D,** *Slipped hip:* "articular portion" of metaphysis is excluded from acetabulum. (From Tachdjian MO: *Pediatric orthopedics,* ed 2, Philadelphia, 1990, WB Saunders.)

examination reveals reduced numbers of osteoblasts, disorganized and nonossified osteoid, and few bony trabeculae.[23] Children with OI who survive into adolescence usually experience some improvement attributed to increased hormone levels. Fewer fractures occur during adulthood.

Clinical presentation. In OI Type I, fractures may be present at birth but more often occur during infancy or the toddler years. Minimal trauma causes fractures in the fragile bones. Three quarters of children with OI Type I bruise easily.[23]

In OI Type II, stillbirth or perinatal death usually

TABLE 13-6	Types of Osteogenesis Imperfecta	
TYPE	**INHERITANCE**	**SIGNS AND SYMPTOMS**
I	Dominant	Frequent long-bone fractures Blue sclera Hypermobile joints, laxity of ligaments Short stature Bowed femurs and tibias Flat feet (pes planus) Kyphosis/kyphoscoliosis Brittle teeth Hearing loss
II	Dominant or recessive	Usually lethal prenatally or perinatally Low birthweight/small for gestational age Eggshell skull fractures Rib fractures Facial bone fractures Long-bone fractures Hemorrhage from damage to underlying structures
III	Recessive	Very short stature Frequent long-bone, skull, and rib fractures Kyphosis/kyphoscoliosis Normal teeth and hearing Sclera, blue in childhood; fade by adolescence
IV	Dominant	Manifests in childhood or adolescence Fewer fractures/less osteopenia Blue sclera my be present; fade by adolescence

occurs. Multiple injuries to long bones, the skull, face, and ribs are common, causing hemorrhage and damage to underlying structures. Only the rare infant, with maximum supportive care and without rib fractures, survives into childhood.

OI Type III is more severe but less common than Type I. However, it is not as uniformly lethal as OI Type II. Multiple fractures from seriously osteopenic long bones, skull, and ribs; progressive deformity; and severe growth retardation are characteristic of Type III. Rods may be inserted to stabilize the long bones. However, fractures can still occur, as can breaks in the rods.

OI Type IV is the least severe form and may not be diagnosed until later childhood or even adulthood. The child may present to the ED with frequent fractures without a history of OI.

Emergency room presentation is usually for signs and symptoms of fractures with a history of mild trauma or unknown etiology. Major trauma can cause devastating fractures and soft tissue damage. Accompanying blood loss can be life threatening. Vertebral fractures are likely, causing higher risk for spinal cord damage. Children with opalescent dentin (brittle teeth) may have many broken teeth, even after relatively minor mouth trauma.

Emergency Department intervention

Diagnostic tests. Radiographs reveal fracture(s) in osteoporotic and often deformed bones. Frequently old fractures in various stages of healing are present; therefore differentiation of OI from child abuse is very important.

Treatment. ED management is primarily concerned with the stabilization of the ABCs with cervical spinal precautions and the care of fractures (see Chapter 23). If CPR is necessary, rib and sternum fractures with potential pneumothorax or bleeding should be anticipated. Pain assessment and management is crucial. Children with OI are frequently admitted because of the complexity of the fractures/injuries.

Nursing care and evaluation. A complete examination is performed to identify all of the child's injuries and to prevent further injury. Because the child's safety is of paramount concern, particular caution must be observed when positioning or transfering the child. If the child wears protective braces or a body jacket, these should be replaced as soon as his or her condition allows. Parents can be extremely helpful with advice about positioning their child for maximum safety and comfort.

Because these children easily sustain fractures and their injuries are often more serious than ordinarily indicated by the history, the nurse must thoroughly assess the child for multiple fractures or secondary injury such as damaged nerves or blood vessels. The mouth must be carefully examined for broken teeth to reduce the risk of aspiration. Care of the child with OI is optimally managed by an experienced orthopedist.

Infants or children who present with signs and symptoms of fractures and a history of minimal trauma or inconsistent findings are evaluated for child abuse. Radiographic findings for children with OI may be similar to those of abused children, revealing multiple previous fractures. The nature of the fractures and the consistently seen osteoporosis, plus other clinical signs, such as blue sclerae, brittle teeth, and short stature, differentiate OI from child abuse.

Because of frequent injuries, ED visits, and hospitalizations, the child with OI may be more fearful or anxious or may have developed effective coping mechanisms. Because OI is an inherited condition, parental guilt related to the presence of the disorder or to feelings of inadequacy about preventing injury to their child may complicate the picture. If the diagnosis is unknown, an investigation related to possible child abuse may create additional anxiety. Children and their families need strong support and assistance to manage each crisis.

DUCHENNE'S MUSCULAR DYSTROPHY

Etiology. Duchenne's muscular dystrophy (MD) is the most severe and frequent form of the muscular dystrophies. It is a progressive myopathy resulting in increasing hypotonia and muscle weakness. An extensive evaluation is necessary to differentiate muscular dystrophy from other hypotonic conditions, such as congenital myotonic dystrophy or myasthenia gravis.[3] As an X-linked recessive disorder, Duchenne's MD almost exclusively affects male children. Mothers are typically unaffected carriers; however, the new mutation rate for this disorder is believed to be relatively high. A relatively uncommon disorder, the reported incidence is from 13 to 33 per 100,000 live born males.

Pathophysiology. The specific mechanism(s) causing muscular dystrophy are unknown, although the absence of dystrophin, a skeletal muscle protein, has been identified in children with Duchenne's MD.[11] With progressive muscle hypotonia and disuse, atrophy occurs, along with contractures and deformities of joints. Muscular hypertrophy develops, caused by fatty infiltration.[20]

Clinical presentation. Duchenne's MD usually becomes evident in affected boys by age 4, manifesting itself through delayed walking with frequent falls; early weakness of the gluteal and hip extensor muscles, causing a typical waddling gait and compensatory lumbar lordosis; and pseudohypertrophy of muscles, particularly the calves. Duchenne's dystrophy has a peculiar pattern of muscle involvement. Cranial, sphincter, and diaphragmatic muscles are spared, and clinical cardiomyopathy is uncommon. Hip and leg muscles are affected earlier than those of the trunk and arms. With increasing functional impairment, the child eventually needs braces and crutches to aid in standing and ambulation and later a wheelchair for continued mobility. As the arms weaken, greater assistance in activities of daily living becomes necessary. Weakness of back and abdominal muscles leads to kyphoscoliosis, requiring bracing with a body jacket.

Common health problems of children with MD are listed in Box 13-5. The most serious clinical condition for children with Duchenne's MD is pulmonary compromise. Even though the diaphragm is spared, weakness of other respiratory muscles causes hypoventilation and decreased pulmonary function. With

---

Box 13-5 Common Health Problems in Children with MD

Fall-related injuries
  Lacerations
  Severe contusions
  Head trauma
  Fractures
Pulmonary compromise
  Hypoventilation
  Respiratory infections
Pain/anxiety

progressive weakness, the child becomes increasingly air hungry and uncomfortable. Susceptibility to recurrent pulmonary infections is increased, with pneumonia being a serious complication. Some children receive ventilatory support to maintain pulmonary function and prevent infection.

Physical discomfort or high anxiety may result in an ED visit. Muscle pain is a frequent complaint, with joint contractures adding to the child's discomfort. In later stages, anxiety about impending death and/or signs of extreme pulmonary compromise may prompt a visit to the emergency room. With good support many parents and children are well-prepared for the child to die at home.

Emergency Department interventions

Diagnostic tests. MD may be clinically suspected in the ED in a young boy with a fall-related injury, history of frequent falls, unusual gait, and evidence of muscular weakness. Differentiation of accidental injury vs. child abuse is necessary in the undiagnosed child with multiple injuries. Findings should be communicated to the child's primary health care provider, who can arrange for a comprehensive evaluation.

The diagnosis of MD can be confirmed by muscle biopsy, serum enzyme levels, and electromyography (EMG). Degenerative changes to muscle tissue are evident on muscle biopsy. Serum creatine phosphokinase (CPK) is markedly increased early in the disease course. EMG is abnormal and may even show fibrillation in advanced disease.

Treatment. There is no effective treatment or cure for MD. Even with excellent supportive therapy, most affected boys die at about 18 years of age.[1] Management is focused on the maintenance of muscle function for as long as possible and the prevention and/or treatment of complications.

Falls. Injuries from falls must be treated with special care for the maintenance of function. Children with MD and frequent falls should be referred to their specialist for evaluation for bracing and ambulatory aids. (See Chapter 12 for diagrams of bracing.)

Hypoventilation/Respiratory Infections. Even in the presence of ventilatory support and a DNR order, the child with MD who presents with a respiratory infection requires full support and intervention, because the infection is usually treatable. Sputum culture

and sensitivities are important in the child with signs and symptoms of lower respiratory infections because of the increased probability of unusual and/or drug-resistant causative organisms. Initial antibiotics may need to be changed based on culture results and the child's response to therapy. Follow-up is required for discharged patients. Serious infections necessitate admission.

Nursing care and evaluation. Children with muscular dystrophy may present to the ED with an acute illness/injury, such as a respiratory infection or fall, or in the terminal stages of the disease. Nursing care depends on the clinical presentation of the child and, as with any child, requires the initial management of acute symptoms. Because acute illnesses such as respiratory infections are common in these children and because they are potentially more serious than in the normal healthy child, these children and their families often require psychosocial support. Consultation with a social worker or chaplain may be beneficial. Depending on the seriousness of the illness/injury, the child's primary care specialist(s) should be notified of the ED visit.

Although parents and children are aware of the progressive, terminal nature of the illness and are prepared for the child to die at home, pain, anxiety, and the fear of being alone can prompt an ED visit during the terminal stages of the disease. If this occurs nursing management is directed at providing comfort to the child and an understanding, supportive environment for the grieving family (see Chapter 9).

If a child arrives with an acute illness an assessment of the child's functional ability is necessary. Children with significant muscle weakness may need assistance with elimination and other activities, such as dressing or taking fluids. Parental input identifies the child's abilities and limitations of daily living.

Falls. Braces and other aids for ambulatory support should be removed during assessment and treatment but reapplied if the child needs to assist in transfers or if they are helpful for sitting balance. Anticipatory guidance in regard to safety is important, especially when children are young and still trying to keep up with their peers and siblings.

Respiratory infections. Selection of the form of antibiotics depends on the child's preference; for example, suspensions or syrups are given if the child has difficulty swallowing tablets or capsules. Medication instructions must be reviewed with caregivers and follow-up care encouraged. A current address and telephone number is clarified and documented for communication of culture results.

Pain/Anxiety. Even minor trauma requires pain management. Because children with MD are typically not retarded, they can be approached in an age-appropriate manner. Play and distraction, the use of security or transition objects, and keeping the parents and child together whenever possible are techniques that should be used in conjunction with appropriate pharmacologic analgesics and local anesthetics. Age-appropriate anxiety reduction strategies can be employed.

▮ SUMMARY

Without early diagnosis and treatment, many of the musculoskeletal disorders presented in this chapter can rapidly cause permanent disability in the growing child. Astute assessments and expeditious interventions may save a child from a life with physical and emotional limitations.

REFERENCES

1. Behrman RE: *Nelson textbook of pediatrics,* ed 15, Philadelphia, 1996, WB Saunders.
1a. Betz CL, Sowden L: *Mosby's pediatric nursing reference,* ed 3, St Louis, 1996, Mosby.
2. Burke MG: Extremity pain. In Hoekelman RA et al, eds: *Primary pediatric care,* ed 2, St Louis, 1992, Mosby.
3. Cole CH: Hypotonia. In Hoekelman RA et al, eds: *Primary pediatric care,* ed 2, St Louis, 1992, Mosby.
4. Cwinn AA: Musculoskeletal and soft tissue disorders. In Rosen P, Barkin RM, eds: *Emergency medicine: concepts and clinical practice,* St Louis, 1992, Mosby.
5. Dufort JE, Smith-Wright D: Osteomyelitis. In Barkin RM: *Pediatric emergency medicine: concepts and clinical practice,* St Louis, 1992, Mosby.
6. Faries G, Johnston C: Allergic and immunologic diseases. In Barkin RM, ed: *Pediatric emergency medicine: Concepts and clinical practice,* St Louis, 1992, Mosby.
7. Fink PC, Dufort JE, Smith-Wright D: Orthopedic disorders. In Barkin RM: *Pediatric emergency medicine: concepts and clinical practice,* St Louis, 1992, Mosby.
8. Gewanter HL: Juvenile arthritis. In Hoekelman RA, ed: *Primary pediatric care,* ed 2, St Louis, 1992, Mosby.
9. Gold R: Diagnosis of osteomyelitis, *Pediatr Rev* 12(10):292-297, 1991.
10. Green M: *Pediatric diagnosis. Interpretation of symptoms and signs in infants, children and adolescents,* Philadelphia, 1992, WB Saunders.
11. Hoffman EP, Brown RH Jr, Kunkel LM: Dystrophin: the protein product of the Duchenne muscular dystrophy locus, *Cell* 51:919-928, 1987.
12. Jackman KV: Acute pediatric orthopedic conditions, *Pediatr Ann* 23(5):240-249, 1994.
13. Keel TA: Bone and joint infections: guidelines to diagnosis, antibiotic therapy, and surgical indications, *Clin Rev* Sept: 49-62, 1994.
14. MacEwen GD, Dehne R: The limping child, *Pediatr Rev* 12(9):268-274, 1991.
15. Radetsky M, Davis AG: Antimicrobial use in pediatric critical care. In Fuhrman BP, Zimmerman JJ, eds: *Pediatric critical care,* St Louis, 1992, Mosby.
16. Rosenstein BJ, Fosarelli PD: *Pediatric pearls. The handbook of practical pediatrics,* ed 2, St Louis, 1993, Mosby.
17. Schwentker EP: Osteomyelitis. In Hoekelman RA, ed: *Primary pediatric care,* ed 2, St Louis, 1992, Mosby.
18. Tachdjian MO: *Pediatric orthopedics,* ed 2, Philadelphia, 1990, WB Saunders.
19. Reference deleted in proofs.
20. Wong DL: *Whaley & Wong's essentials of pediatric nursing,* ed 5, St Louis, 1997, Mosby.
21. Wong DL: *Whaley & Wong's nursing care of infants and children,* ed 5, St Louis, 1995, Mosby.
22. Zink BJ: Bone and joint infections. In Rosen P, Barkin RM, eds: *Emergency medicine: concepts and clinical practice,* St Louis, 1992, Mosby.
23. Zitelli BJ, Davis HW, eds: *Atlas of pediatric physical diagnosis,* ed 2, Philadelphia, 1992, JB Lippincott.

CHAPTER 14

Fluid and Electrolyte Imbalances

Marcy Moag Noble

INTRODUCTION

Within the body is a complex system of feedback mechanisms that regulate the volume, distribution, tonicity, and composition of body fluids.[29,30] Numerous physiologic differences between the infant, young child, and adult affect the child's ability to regulate fluid and electrolyte balance and respond effectively to illness or injury. Among these differences are variations in body fluid composition, the metabolic rate, and regulatory systems. This chapter discusses these differences and describes emergency nursing care of the child with a fluid or electrolyte disorder.

ANATOMY AND PHYSIOLOGY OF FLUID AND ELECTROLYTE BALANCE

BODY FLUID COMPOSITION

Approximately 75% of body weight is water in the full-term neonate, compared to 60% to 70% of adult weight.[28] The majority of the infant's total body water is contained in the extracellular compartment, which includes the plasma and interstitial fluid. With the higher volume of interstitial fluids, the infant has proportionately more fluid reserves to draw from with vascular fluid losses. However, the infant's large body surface area and increased metabolic rate contributes to rapid total body fluid depletion when fluid losses are excessive and/or fluid intake is inadequate. By 1 year of age the intracellular water content exceeds extracellular water content, and by 3 years of age body fluid composition in the child is the same as that of an adult (Table 14-1).

METABOLIC RATE

Infants and young children have relatively high metabolic rates and a large body surface area to volume ratio. The higher metabolic rate produces more heat, which combined with the large body surface area contributes to increased insensible water losses. Renal losses are proportionately higher both to excrete the increased waste products of metabolism and because the immature kidneys of infants, who have lower glomerular filtration rates than older children and adults, excrete large amounts of dilute urine.[4,29] The result is a daily turnover of body water that is approximately five times that of the adult.[20,23] To compensate, the infant and young child must take in proportionally larger amounts of fluid compared to the adult (Table 14-2).

REGULATORY SYSTEMS

To maintain normal body function, the volume, osmolality, and composition of body fluids are closely regulated by a complex system of feedback mechanisms. Among these systems are active transport, diffusion, and osmosis that affect the movement of water and/or electrolytes at the cellular level, as well as neurologic, renal, and endocrine feedback mechanisms that affect the intake of water and the excretion or reabsorption of water and electrolytes.

The system that regulates water intake in the body is the thirst mechanism. As fluid is normally lost through the urine, skin, lungs, and stool, rises in the osmolality of the extracellular fluid stimulate the thirst center, which is located in the hypothalamus.

Coordinated with the thirst mechanism is the hormonal regulator of water balance within the body known as the *antidiuretic hormone* (ADH), also

TABLE 14-1	Body Fluid Composition by Age		
AGE	TOTAL BODY WATER (TBW)	INTRACELLULAR WATER (ICF)	EXTRACELLULAR FLUID (ECF)
Full-term newborn	78%	33%	45%
1 Year	65%	40%	25%
3 Years	60%	40%	20%
Adult	60%	40%	20%

Modified from Barkin RM: *Pediatric emergency medicine: concepts and clinical practice,* St Louis, 1992, Mosby.

TABLE 14-2	Average Daily Water Losses in Different-Age Children Based on Body Weight*			
COMPONENT	NEWBORN TO 6 MONTHS	6 MONTHS TO 5 YEARS	5 TO 10 YEARS	ADOLESCENT
Insensible	40	30	20	10
Urinary	60	60	50	40
Fecal	20	10	—	—
TOTAL	120	100	70	50

From Boineau FG, Lewy JE: Estimation of parenteral fluid requirements, *Pediatr Clin North Am* 37:2, 1990.
*ml per kg body weight per 24 hours.

called *vasopressin* or *arginine vasopressin*.[23] ADH is produced in the hypothalamus in response to a rise in the osmolality of extracellular fluid and is then transported via axons to the posterior pituitary where it is released[27,30] ADH increases the permeability of the distal tubules and collecting ducts within the kidneys, resulting in the reabsorption of water. The elimination of urinary solutes, including sodium, continues, which results in the excretion of concentrated urine.

Another important regulatory mechanism is the renin-angiotensin-aldosterone mechanism. When decreases in extracellular fluid cause arterial pressure to drop too low, renin is released into the bloodstream from the kidneys. Renin, which is a protein enzyme, stimulates the release of angiotensin I, which has mild vasoconstrictor properties. Angiotensin I is then converted to angiotensin II almost entirely within the small vessels of the lungs.[27] As a powerful vasoconstrictor, angiotensin II immediately produces a rise in arterial pressure. It also acts on the kidneys, decreasing the excretion of both salt and water. Additionally, angiotensin II stimulates the adrenal cortex to secrete aldosterone. Aldosterone acts on the cortical and medullary collecting ducts, which reabsorb or con-

serve sodium. Increased sodium in the serum attracts water, thus increasing circulating volume.

OSMOLALITY

Despite compositional differences in water and electrolytes, the *osmolality* (or number of particles per liter of solvent) of the extracellular fluid and intracellular fluids are equal. If the osmolality in one space becomes higher than in the other, that solution is said to be hypertonic to the other. This comparison reflects *tonicity*.[6] Under normal circumstances the serum sodium reflects the osmolality of intracellular fluids and extracellular fluids as they are in a state of equilibrium regarding tonicity.[30] Normal serum osmolality is maintained between 280 and 295 mOsm/L.

ELECTROLYTES

Electrolyte balance between the intracellular and extracellular spaces plays an important role in the maintenance of body fluid balance. Sodium, potassium, and chloride are briefly reviewed in this section; however, balances between other electrolytes such as calcium,

HCO_3 (bicarbonate), HPO_4 (phosphate), and magnesium (Mg) also play important roles in fluid and electrolyte balance between the ICF and ECF spaces. These are reviewed within the appropriate sections in this chapter.

Sodium. Sodium (Na) is the principle cation in the extracellular fluid and is the most important determinant of ECF volume.[30] The renal system, mediated by hormonal influences—particularly the renin-angiotensin-aldosterone system, is primarily responsible for maintaining sodium balance within the body through excretion or reabsorption. Because young infants have a higher volume of extracellular fluid than adults, infants have a higher total body sodium.[30]

Potassium. Potassium (K) is the principle cation in the ICF. In fact, 98% of body potassium is intracellular.[41] Potassium maintains the osmolality of the ICF and helps to maintain acid-base balance; the potassium gradient between the ICF and ECF is responsible for the electrical activity of cell membranes, particularly the heart and nervous system.

Potassium homeostasis is primarily regulated by dietary intake and renal excretion, although other factors such as glucoregulatory hormones (e.g., insulin) can also affect potassium balance. Ninety percent of potassium is excreted by the kidneys, with the remaining amount eliminated in sweat and stool.[23] Infants tend to have slightly higher plasma potassium levels than older children. However, because of the higher extracellular to intracellular fluid ratio, total body potassium is lower in infants.[30,46]

Chloride. Chloride is a major anion within the extracellular compartment. It plays an important role in the reabsorption of sodium or the exchange of sodium for potassium or hydrogen ions within the kidneys. With excess chloride losses (e.g., vomiting), sodium is reabsorbed in exchange for potassium or hydrogen ions, which are excreted in excess. The result is hypokalemia and alkalosis.[1,23]

▌ DEHYDRATION

Etiology. Dehydration occurs when the total output of body fluids exceeds the total intake. The most common cause of dehydration in infants and young children is gastrointestinal losses of fluids and electrolytes that result from vomiting and/or diarrhea coupled with inadequate fluid intake. Other causes include excessive renal fluid loss (e.g., diabetes insipidus or diabetes mellitus), decreased fluid intake (starvation), and translocation of fluids (e.g., third-spacing of fluids).[47]

Pathophysiology. During periods of fluid loss or decreased fluid intake physiologic mechanisms shift fluid from the interstitial to the intravascular compartment to maintain perfusion. *Isotonic* dehydration reflects equal proportions of sodium and water losses. It is seen in 65% to 70% of children with dehydration in the United States.[23] The serum sodium concentration with isotonic dehydration remains within normal limits (130 to 150 mEq/L). *Hypotonic* (or hyponatremic) dehydration occurs when sodium losses are greater than water losses and is reflected by a serum sodium of less than 130 mEq/L. *Hypertonic* (or hypernatremic) dehydration results when free water is lost in excess of sodium and is reflected by a serum sodium of greater than 150 mEq/L. (Both hyponatremia and hypernatremia are discussed in separate sections within this chapter.)

Clinical presentation. Signs and symptoms of fluid loss depend on the severity of the losses, the serum sodium concentration, and the underlying etiology. Isotonic dehydration occurs most commonly and is measured by specific clinical parameters, as well as the degree of acute body weight loss. In infants and young children, 5% weight loss is considered mild dehydration, a 5% to 10% weight loss is considered moderate dehydration, and a 10% to 15% weight loss reflects severe dehydration. Because older children have less extracellular fluid volume, smaller percentages of weight loss represent more severe dehydration. Specific clinical findings correlate with the degree of weight loss, and these include tachycardia; changes in skin turgor, color, and temperature; a sunken fontanel (in the infant); sunken eyes; sticky or dry mucous membranes; lethargy; and a history of decreased urine output (Table 14-3).

Emergency Department interventions

Diagnostic testing. The first priority of management is the determination of the severity of fluid loss and the degree of electrolyte imbalance. In the child who is moderately to severely dehydrated, diagnostic testing usually includes serum electrolytes, glucose, hematocrit, blood urea nitrogen (BUN), creatinine, and a urinalysis. Hemoconcentration from dehydration is reflected by an increased creatinine and hemat-

TABLE 14-3	Isotonic Dehydration: Clinical Findings that Correlate with Weight Loss		
SYMPTOMS	MILD	MODERATE	SEVERE
Weight loss (infants and young children)	3%-5%	5%-10%	10%-15%
Weight loss (children >10 years of age)	3%-5%	5%-7%	7%-9%
Eyes	Normal	Sunken	Sunken, no tearing
Mucous membranes of mouth	Moist → sticky	Dry	Dry → parched
Skin color	Normal	Normal → pale	Pale, mottled
Skin turgor	Normal	Decreased	Tenting
Anterior fontanel (infants)	Normal	Sunken	Sunken
Pulse	Normal	Rapid	Rapid
Blood pressure	Normal	Normal → low	Low
Urine output	Normal	Decreased	Decreased → absent
Mental status	Normal	Normal → lethargic	Lethargic → coma

ocrit. Normal creatinine values in the infant and young child are much lower than in adults because of decreased muscle mass. Values range from 0.3 to 0.5 mg/dl in the child less than 2 years of age.[34] Higher serum creatinine values in an infant reflect a decrease in the glomerular filtration rate. An elevated BUN is helpful in evaluating renal function; however, a normal BUN in the child correlates poorly with the degree of dehydration because it is affected by other factors (e.g., a decreased dietary intake of protein will cause less of a rise in the BUN).[13]

The urinalysis is useful in interpreting the degree of dehydration and renal function. In neonates, the lack of renal concentrating ability produces relatively dilute urine; therefore in the newborn a specific gravity of greater than 1.015 is significant. In the older infant and young child a specific gravity of greater than 1.020 or 1.025 is significant.

Evaluation of serum electrolytes assists in the determination of the type of dehydration or acid-base balance. The serum sodium value is necessary to identify abnormalities in body fluid osmolality. Findings do not, however, reflect total body sodium stores. In fact, hypernatremic dehydration is often associated with mild to moderate decreases in total body sodium.[1] Because potassium is primarily found in the intracellular compartment, serum potassium levels in the dehydrated child are often normal or elevated until total body potassium is severely depleted. Additionally, serum potassium levels are affected by the acid-base balance. With metabolic acidosis, for example, circulating hydrogen ions are exchanged for intracellular potassium.

Other abnormal findings include disturbances in serum bicarbonate and chloride. Ongoing losses of bicarbonate associated with diarrhea, coupled with decreased tissue perfusion and diminished renal function, can lead to the development of metabolic acidosis. Protracted vomiting can lead to losses in sodium, hydrogen ions, potassium, and chloride and produce hypochloremic alkalosis.

Isotonic dehydration. NOTE: The management of the child in shock is presented in Chapters 6 and 8 in this text. It is therefore not reviewed in this section.

Fluid and electrolyte therapy in the volume-depleted child requires the replenishment of vascular volume, the maintenance of normal fluid and electrolyte needs, the replacement of continued abnormal losses, and the replacement of fluid and electrolyte deficits.

Initially a 20 ml/kg bolus of an isotonic crystalloid solution (normal saline [NS] or lactated Ringer's solution [LR]) is administered to expand the plasma volume and improve cardiovascular and renal function. If perfusion is impaired, the bolus is infused as rapidly as possible and repeated as needed. If the child is moderately dehydrated, the fluid bolus is infused over 20 to 30 minutes. Fluid treatment is never delayed while awaiting laboratory results.

Daily *maintenance* requirements replace normal fluid and electrolyte losses through the skin, lungs,

TABLE 14-4	Pediatric Maintenance Fluid Therapy
CHILD'S WEIGHT	**DAILY FLUID REQUIREMENTS PER KG**
First 1-10 kg	100 ml/kg/day
10-20 kg	1000 ml *plus* 50 ml/kg for each kg >10 kg
>20 kg	1500 ml *plus* 20 ml/kg for each kg >20 kg
Example: 4 month old weighing 6 kg	
6 kg	100 ml × 6 kg = 600 ml/day; 600 ml ÷ 24 hrs = 25 ml/hr
Example: 11 year old weighing 34 kg	
20 kg	1500 ml
14 kg	+ 280 ml (20 ml × 14 kg)
34 kg	1780 ml ÷ 24 hrs = 74 ml/hr

Box 14-1   Fluid Therapy for Dehydration

1. Administer bolus therapy of 20 ml/kg NS or LR as necessary to maintain perfusion
2. Calculate maintenance requirements (see Table 14-4)
3. Calculate fluid deficits
   3%–5% Body weight loss = 30–50 ml/kg
   7%–10% Body weight loss = 70–100 ml/kg
   11%–15% Body weight loss = 110–150 ml/kg
4. Calculate electrolyte requirements based on deficit and maintenance requirements
5. Estimate abnormal ongoing losses (e.g., fever, vomiting, diarrhea)
   • Fever = 10%–12% increase in maintenance water requirements for each degree (Celsius) of temperature elevation (8% increase for each degree of Fahrenheit)
   • Emesis and diarrhea = ml for ml replacement
6. Replace one half of the fluid deficit and one third of the daily maintenance requirements over the first 8 hours of therapy with $D_5\frac{1}{2}NS$
7. Add supplemental potassium to parenteral fluids once renal function has been established
8. Replace the remaining fluids (one half of the deficit and two thirds of the maintenance) over the next 16 hours

stool, and urine. Methods used to determine maintenance fluid needs in the child include body surface area (1500 to 2000 ml × m^2 ÷ 24 hours = hourly rate)[9]; estimated caloric expenditures (for each 100 calories metabolized in 24 hours the average child will require 100 to 120 ml water)[33]; and weight (Table 14-4). In addition to normal maintenance requirements, *ongoing fluid and electrolyte losses* such as those caused by vomiting, diarrhea, or fever must be replaced. Fever increases the metabolic rate and therefore increases water requirements by 10% to 12% for each degree (Celsius) of temperature elevation.[25,42] Diarrhea causes not only water loss but also sodium (10 to 90 mEq/L) and bicarbonate losses (45 mEq/L).[7]

Fluid *deficit* calculations are based on the child's clinical presentation, suspected degree and type of dehydration, and weight loss. This calculation is an approximation, because it is based on a subjective clinical assessment of the degree of dehydration. If a 10-kg child has sustained a 5% weight loss, fluid loss is estimated to be 500 ml of water (10 kg × 5% = 500 ml).

One half of the fluid deficit and one third of the daily maintenance requirements using $D_5\frac{1}{2}NS$ are replaced in the first 8 hours of treatment. The remainder deficit and maintenance fluids are replaced over the next 16 hours using oral or parenteral therapy (Box 14-1).

In the emergency department (ED), *oral rehydra-tion* with an oral electrolyte solution (OES) may be considered in the child with mild to moderate dehydration who is able to tolerate oral fluids, does not have excessive stool output, does not have a suspected surgical illness, and does not exhibit signs of shock.[16,26] Even if the child requires intravenous rehydration, discharge may be possible once urine output is adequate and the criteria listed above are met—provided close follow-up can be ensured.

Nursing care and evaluation. Initial nursing interventions for the child with dehydration depend on the history and the child's clinical presentation. The infant or child who is tolerating oral fluids, appears happy or playful, and has no significant present history (e.g., 10 to 15 stools in the past several hours) or past medical history (e.g., diabetes, cystic fibrosis) can usually be treated nonurgently. Neurologically normal children with moderate dehydration can be treated on an urgent basis, provided they are monitored while awaiting care. Children with significant signs of dehydration (e.g., sunken eyes, history of decreased urination and decreased fluid intake, dry mucous membranes, lethargy, and decreased peripheral perfusion) are treated emergently.

As in all children the airway and breathing are initially assessed and stabilized. Children who are severely dehydrated or who exhibit signs of shock receive supplemental oxygen by nonrebreather face mask. Rapid venous access is achieved using a large-bore catheter in the largest vein available, and bolus therapy is begun.

During initial fluid therapy the child's vital signs and perfusion are recorded after each 20 ml/kg bolus. Once vascular volume and perfusion have improved, and once ongoing fluid therapy is begun, the child's cardiovascular and neurologic status are assessed at least hourly. Each assessment should include an evaluation of the child's heart rate, peripheral pulses, capillary refill, skin color and temperature, level of consciousness, blood pressure, and urine output. Positive clinical responses to therapy include stable vital signs, capillary refilling time less than 2 seconds, increased urine output with a simultaneous decrease in urine specific gravity, and improvement in electrolyte and acid-base status if abnormal on admission.

The recommendations regarding oral electrolyte therapy vary depending on the area of the country and physician preferences. OES may be given after parenteral fluid therapy provided the child is able to tolerate oral fluids and does not have a severe electrolyte disturbance. The child with a history of vomiting should receive only small amounts of fluid, 5 to 15 ml every 10 minutes.[26] If the child vomits, oral fluids are withheld at least 1 hour.

On discharge the child's parents are informed of the signs and symptoms of dehydration and told to return to the ED or contact their primary care provider if these symptoms appear. Fever should be treated promptly, because high fevers contribute to significant insensible fluid losses. In addition, oral fluid administration is increased in the febrile child. Depending on the cause of the dehydration (i.e., vomiting or diarrhea) and physician preference the parents of infants may be told to resume regular feedings or to give the infant an OES, then half-strength formula, then full-strength formula over the next 24 hours. Older children may initially receive clear liquids with glucose and mineral content (e.g., sports drinks) and advance to a regular diet as tolerated within the next 24 hours. (Specific treatments for vomiting and diarrhea are discussed in Chapter 15.)

▌HYPONATREMIA

Etiology. Hyponatremia reflects a serum sodium concentration of less than 130 mEq/L and may or may not be associated with dehydration. When not associated with dehydration, hyponatremia may result from water intoxication, renal failure, or the syndrome of inappropriate ADH (SIADH) secretion. Water intoxication reflects an excess intake or infusion of free water as might result from a fresh water near-drowning episode (rare finding) or more commonly in the infant who is given large amounts of plain water for rehydration. Causes of hyponatremic dehydration (sodium losses in excess of water losses) include excessive gastrointestinal losses, excessive sweating (i.e., cystic fibrosis or adrenal insufficiency), or salt depletion from diuretic therapy.

Pathophysiology. With hyponatremia water moves rapidly from the extracellular spaces into the intracellular compartment to normalize the extracellular sodium concentration. This movement of water improves the osmolality of the ECF but depletes plasma volume. The inflow of water into the intracellular compartment results in cellular swelling that affects neurologic, cardiovascular, and musculoskeletal functioning.[11] Neurologic complications of hyponatremia include cerebral edema and intracranial hemorrhage.

SIADH. SIADH can occur secondary to a CNS infection such as meningitis or encephalitis, after compression or injury of the hypothalamus or pituitary gland (i.e., hydrocephalus, malignancy, head trauma), or with sepsis. It may also occur secondary to the administration of certain medications such as chemotherapeutic agents.

With the inappropriate release of ADH the renal distal tubules conserve water, increasing plasma volume. Serum sodium levels decrease with slightly elevated renal sodium excretion (e.g., greater than 20 mEq/L); however, in the early stages total body sodium may be normal or near normal. Free water excess results in dilutional hyponatremia, which decreases serum osmolality.[3,43]

Clinical presentation. Signs and symptoms of hyponatremia depend on the etiology, the rate of fall, and the absolute value of the serum sodium.[19] In general, signs and symptoms are nonspecific and may include nausea, vomiting, disorientation, agitation, muscle cramps, and weakness. When the serum sodium falls below 120 mEq/L seizures are common. In fact, hyponatremia is the most frequent cause of nonfebrile seizures in children under 2 years of age.[42,45] With acute water intoxication, signs and symptoms may be consistent with increasing intracranial pressure associated with cerebral edema.

Signs and symptoms of *hypotonic dehydration* are more severe because the influx of fluid into the cells rapidly depletes extracellular volume. Mild fluid losses can present with signs of hypovolemia and decompensated shock. The phenomenon of fingerprinting, or fingerprint marks that remain after pressing firmly over the child's sternum, is also seen[28] (Table 14-5).

Emergency Department interventions. The initial management of hyponatremia depends on the child's condition upon arrival. The child with mild or moderate symptoms of hyponatremia is treated by *slow* correction of the sodium imbalance with D$_5$NS followed by D$_5$½NS over 24 to 48 hours.[1,11]

Children who are seizing are treated with 4 to 6 ml/kg of 3% saline, to raise the serum sodium to at least 125 mEq/L.[11] The rate of administration of sodium in the acutely ill child is controversial, because rapid increases in serum sodium have been associated with severe neurologic consequences such as brain dehydration and osmotic demyelination syndrome.[37,48-50] The acuteness or chronicity (where the brain has had time to adapt) of the onset of hyponatremia most probably contributes to the neurologic complications associated with rapid sodium administration.[45] In general, two formulas are currently recommended regarding the rapid administration of 3% sodium to the child who is seizing: administering at a rate of 1 ml/min or administering the dose over 20 minutes.[1,42]

The use of benzodiazepines for the emergent treatment of seizures in the hyponatremic child is not recommended, because it has been found to be ineffective and causes respiratory depression in a significant number of children.[35,45] Cerebral edema, evidenced by signs of increasing intracranial pressure, is treated with the usual modalities (e.g., mannitol and hyperventilation) (see Chapter 7).

The administration or restriction of fluids in the hyponatremic child depends on the fluid balance (e.g., hypovolemia, euvolemia, hypervolemia). Treatment of the hypovolemic, hyponatremic child is the same as for any child with decreased vascular volume, that is, the initiation of bolus therapy (20 ml/kg) to expand vascular volume. In this case, however, normal saline rather than lactated Ringer's solution is given. In the euvolemic child (e.g., the child with SIADH or water intoxication) fluid restriction is instituted.[28] If the child is severely symptomatic, furosemide (1 to 2 mg/kg) can be administered followed by an infusion of 3% saline (3 to 5 ml/kg).[11,28] Treatment of the hypervolemic child (e.g., renal insufficiency, water intoxication, nephrotic syndrome) is the restriction of both water and sodium. However, if the child is severely symptomatic (e.g., convulsing) supplemental sodium may be required to reverse the neurologic symptoms, followed by severe water restriction and the administration of diuretics (Table 14-6).[11]

TABLE 14-5	Clinical Manifestations of Hypertonic and Hypotonic Dehydration	
SYMPTOMS	**HYPOTONIC** NA <130 MEQ/L	**HYPERTONIC** NA >150 MEQ/L
Skin color	Grey	Grey
Skin temperature	Cold	Cold
Skin turgor	Poor	Fair
Skin texture	Clammy, "fingerprinting"	Thick, doughy
Mucous membranes	Dry	Parched
Eyes	Sunken, no tearing	Sunken, no tearing
Anterior fontanel	Sunken	Sunken
Mental status	Coma/seizure	Irritable/seizure
Blood pressure	Significantly decreased	Decreased

TABLE 14-6	Treatment of Hyponatremia	
Severe symptoms regardless of etiology (e.g., seizures)	Administer 4-6 ml/kg of 3% sodium a rate of 1 ml/min
Mildly symptomatic losses of Na greater than water losses	Calculate Na deficit and correct with D_5NS followed by $D_5\frac{1}{2}NS$ over 24-48 hours
Water intoxication or SIADH	Institute fluid restriction of 30%-75% of daily maintenance
	Monitor for a decrease in urine output, a rise in urine specific gravity, a decreasing serum sodium (dilutional), and decreasing serum osmolality; observe for clinical signs including edema and a rise in body weight
	Acute symptoms may be treated with furosemide followed by 3% sodium
	Anticipate treatment for increased intracranial pressure
Hyponatremic dehydration	Administer 20 ml/kg bolus of normal saline; administer additional fluids to maintain perfusion
	Calculate fluid and electrolyte deficit and maintenance therapy; replace slowly over 24-48 hours
Hypervolemia (e.g., renal failure, CHF, nephrotic syndrome)	Institute fluid and sodium restriction
	Acute symptoms may be treated with diuretics

Sodium deficit calculation

Na deficit (mEq) = 135 − Serum Na ×   0.6 × Weight (kg)
                           (Total body water in liters)

HYPERNATREMIA

Etiology. Hypernatremia reflects a serum sodium concentration of greater than 150 mEq/L. It may or may not be associated with dehydration; however, in children, hypernatremia is most commonly associated with hypovolemia.[42] Infants less than 3 months of age are particularly vulnerable to hypernatremia because the immature kidneys are unable to handle the high solute load and continue to excrete water, even in the presence of volume depletion. Conditions that promote the loss of free water, such as gastrointestinal losses and/or a high fever coupled with inadequate fluid intake, most commonly precipitate hypertonic dehydration in infants and young children. Other causes of hypernatremia that may not be associated with dehydration include the administration of improperly diluted formulas or rehydration solutions or the administration of boiled milk (all of which reflect the administration of a highly concentrated solution) (Box 14-2).

Pathophysiology. With hypernatremia the elevated extracellular sodium concentration causes water to shift from the intracellular to the extracellular compartment. The result is cellular dehydration. In the brain, severe neurologic damage including thrombosis, hemorrhage, and subdural effusions may occur.[1,18] Permanent neurologic deficits can result when the serum sodium level acutely exceeds 160 mEq/L. Hypocalcemia and hyperglycemia, which are commonly associated with hypernatremia, may also contribute to neurologic findings.

Clinical presentation. Signs and symptoms of hypernatremia vary depending on the etiology and the rate of rise of the serum sodium. Neurologic symptoms caused by cellular dehydration are the most common findings and include lethargy, irritability, and muscle weakness. With severe or acute rises in serum sodium concentrations, seizures and coma occur.

In *hypertonic dehydration* plasma volume is preserved at the expense of the intracellular volume;

| Box 14-2 | Causes of Hypernatremia |

Sodium excess
Improperly mixed formula or rehydration
  solution
Excessive sodium bicarbonate administration
  during resuscitation
Ingestion of sea water (480 mEq/L)

Water deficit
Central diabetes insipidus
Nephrogenic diabetes insipidus
Diabetes mellitus
Excessive sweating
Increased insensible water loss (e.g., newborn
  on a radiant warmer)
Inadequate access to water
Lack of thirst (adipsia)

Water deficit in excess of sodium deficit
Diarrhea
Osmotic diuretics
Diabetes mellitus
Obstructive uropathy
Renal dysplasia

Modified from Conley SB: Hypernatremia, *Pediatr Clin
North Am* 37(2):365–372, 1990.

interrupt fluid shifts, and attempts to decrease cerebral edema (e.g., hyperventilation and/or mannitol administration).[1]

Most cases of hypernatremia in the child are associated with dehydration, some degree of sodium deficit, and potassium depletion (particularly with a diarrheal illness). If the dehydration is severe, plasma volume is initially expanded with bolus therapy of 20 ml/kg of normal saline or lactated Ringer's solution. When perfusion and renal function have been established, a hypotonic solution of $D_5\frac{1}{2}NS$ with supplemental potassium (20 to 40 mEq/L) is administered based on fluid deficits, daily maintenance requirements, and the presence of abnormal ongoing losses. The fluid deficit is estimated to be approximately 50 ml/kg if the serum sodium is 150 mEq/L, 90 ml/kg if serum sodium is 160 mEq/L, and 140 ml/kg if the serum sodium is 170 mEq/L.[27a]

Although rare in pediatrics, acute salt poisoning (serum sodium level > 200 mEq/L) can occur. This condition is generally not associated with dehydration, and the administration of bolus therapy may result in hypervolemia and pulmonary edema.[18] The treatment for these children is peritoneal dialysis.[18,23]

▌HYPOKALEMIA

Etiology. Hypokalemia is defined as a serum potassium concentration of less than 3.5 mEq/L. Low potassium levels may be caused by a true deficit in total body potassium secondary to vomiting, diarrhea, excessive diuretic use, laxative abuse, or renal disease. Hypokalemia may also result from an apparent deficit such as that caused by potassium shifts from the extracellular to intracellular space.

Pathophysiology. Apparent deficits of potassium can occur with alkalosis or in association with the excretion of certain substances such as insulin or $beta_2$ catecholamines, which facilitate the uptake of potassium into the cells.[14,40] The result is a decrease in the serum potassium while total body stores remain normal. Under normal conditions insulin and catecholamines promote the cellular uptake of potassium after a dietary load, preventing a serious elevation in the plasma potassium.[40] With alkalosis, potassium shifts into the cells in exchange for hydrogen ions as a component of the acid-base buffer system. With continued alkalosis, renal wasting of potassium in response to the high cellular potassium can produce actual potassium deficits.

therefore the typical signs of dehydration are not exhibited until cellular dehydration is severe (greater than 10% to 15% fluid loss). Skin may be "doughy" due to the loss of extravascular fluid, and mucous membranes will be dry or parched. Shrinkage of brain cells and hypoperfusion are exhibited by an altered level of consciousness and increasing CNS irritability (e.g., hyperreflexia, muscle twitching, seizures).

Emergency Department interventions. Correcting hypernatremia is complicated, because the osmotic changes that result during therapy can cause water to enter the brain cells and produce cerebral edema. To prevent permanent neurologic sequelae, serum sodium levels are lowered no more than 10 to 15 mEq/L over 24 hours.[24,42] Even with appropriate treatment the development of seizure activity is not uncommon. When seizures do occur, acute management may include the use of anticonvulsants, the administration of a 3% saline infusion to temporarily

Once the serum potassium level drops below normal, the ICF/ECF potassium gradient becomes larger. Alterations of the electrical properties of the nerve and muscle fibers prevent the transmission of action potentials.[27] The result is an increase in the polarization of excitable muscle and nerve tissue and diminished cellular function.

Clinical presentation. Signs and symptoms of hypokalemia vary depending on the onset of the hypokalemia and the underlying etiology. Significant signs become evident when serum potassium falls below 3.0 mEq/L. Neuromuscular dysfunction produces muscle weakness and areflexia. Weakness is usually first noted in the lower extremities and progresses up the body as potassium levels decrease. Respiratory arrest can occur from muscle paralysis. Vomiting, diminished bowel sounds, abdominal distention, and paralytic ileus may develop. Renal concentrating ability is decreased, resulting in polyuria and polydipsia.

Hypokalemia decreases cardiac conductivity and increases automaticity, creating ventricular irritability and associated dysrhythmias. On electrocardiogram (ECG), patients with hypokalemia may have flattened T waves, S-T segment depression, and premature ventricular contractions (PVCs).

Emergency Department interventions. Before initiating treatment for hypokalemia, the child's acid-base balance should be known to distinguish apparent from actual losses. If the child has an apparent loss, correction of the pH will cause potassium ions to return to the point of origin. For every 0.1-unit change in pH, there is an inverse change in the serum potassium of 0.6 mEq/L.[19]

Example:
Normal value pH = 7.40; and K = 3.6 mEq/L
In alkalosis   pH = 7.50; and K = 3.0 mEq/L

When an actual loss of potassium has occurred, supplemental potassium therapy is begun. Because potassium is an intracellular ion, low serum potassium values associated with an actual deficit often reflect a large total body deficit.[42]

Treatment depends on severity. Actual deficits associated with mild or chronic hypokalemia can be treated with oral potassium 1 to 4 mEq/kg/day given over 2 to 3 days.[33,42] Before administration the child's renal function, urine output, and ability to tolerate oral medications are evaluated. Severely hypokalemic children are treated with parenteral therapy at a rate of 0.2 to 0.3 mEq/kg/hour with a concentration of no more than 40 mEq/L.[7,42] Occasionally, to treat life-threatening cardiac or respiratory complications, the child may receive concentrations of as high as 80 mEq/L, but this concentration must be delivered through a central line. The child receiving parenteral potassium therapy requires continuous cardiovascular monitoring.

▌HYPERKALEMIA

Etiology. Hyperkalemia is defined as a serum potassium concentration of greater than 5 mEq/L. Hyperkalemia can result from a true potassium excess or from an apparent excess. Examples of etiologies that produce true excesses include acute or chronic renal disease, congenital anomalies (e.g., hypoaldosteronism), diabetes mellitus, cellular destruction (e.g., trauma, chemotherapy, hemolysis), and certain medications (e.g., potassium-sparing diuretics, beta-blocking antihypertensives). Apparent or artificial excesses can occur with acidosis, as potassium shifts from the intracellular space to the extracellular space in exchange for hydrogen ions, and when blood is drawn for laboratory analysis (e.g., tissue trauma from prolonged tourniquet application or from the hemolyzation of blood during a heel-stick or withdrawal from a small needle).

Pathophysiology. Metabolic acidosis associated with a volume deficit is perhaps the most common presentation associated with hyperkalemia in the pediatric ED.[19,42] With metabolic acidosis, intracellular potassium is replaced by hydrogen ions in an attempt to increase the plasma pH. The result is often a transient rise in the serum potassium, even when losses from vomiting or diarrhea have depleted total body potassium stores.

True hyperkalemia is rare unless renal function is impaired; however, it may occur with severe tissue necrosis (e.g., burns, tumor necrosis) or with massive hemolysis. True excesses affect the intracellular/extracellular potassium gradient, altering the electrical properties of the nerve and muscle fibers. Muscle cells may be maintained in either a polarized or depolarized state, both of which produce a decrease in action potential.[50] The most serious effects of the altered electrical properties of the cells include reduced tissue excitability and slowed conduction velocity of the heart. These changes can rapidly lead to ventricular dysrhythmias or cardiac arrest.[50]

Clinical presentation. Signs and symptoms of hyperkalemia vary depending on severity and chronicity. With minor rises in the serum potassium the child may be relatively asymptomatic. When potassium levels exceed 5 mEq/L, significant signs become evident. Neuromuscular findings include tetany caused by polarized muscle cells and flaccidity caused by depolarized cells. In either case generalized muscle weakness and/or paralysis can result. Life-threatening cardiac abnormalities may be evidence by decreased peripheral perfusion and mentation. When the child is placed on a cardiac monitor the rhythm may show tall, peaked T waves and prolongation of the PR interval. This rhythm can deteriorate into a classic sine wave evidenced by blending of the QRS complex and P wave[28,50] (Fig. 14-1).

Emergency Department interventions. Before initiating therapy for hyperkalemia the presence of an actual deficit must be confirmed. If hyperkalemia has resulted from metabolic acidosis caused by a volume deficit, correction of the deficit will usually correct the potassium imbalance.

Treatment for the child with true hyperkalemia depends on the underlying etiology, the degree of potassium imbalance, and associated signs and symptoms. The asymptomatic child with a serum potassium level of less than 6.5 mEq/L and a normal ECG or one with only peaked T waves may simply have the sources of potassium intake or potassium-sparing medications discontinued.

Once the potassium level rises above 6.5 mEq/L and ECG changes are seen, aggressive therapy is required. To stabilize the cell membranes and counteract the cardiac toxicity of potassium, calcium gluconate is administered. To move potassium into the cells several approaches can be used, including the administration of sodium bicarbonate, the use of regular insulin and glucose, and/or the use of the beta-2 agonist albuterol.[23,42,44,50]

The elimination of potassium can be enhanced using a binding agent such as Kayexalate or a loop diuretic such as furosemide. Kayexalate removes potassium ions from the gastrointestinal tract by exchanging potassium ions for sodium ions. It may therefore increase serum sodium levels. When the hyperkalemic child fails to respond to pharmacologic treatment, or when renal function is severely impaired, hemodialysis or peritoneal dialysis may be required (Table 14-7).

DISORDERS OF CALCIUM BALANCE

Calcium is an important and abundant cation found within the body. Approximately 99% of total body calcium is found within the bones and teeth; the remaining 1% is located within the intracellular and extracellular spaces.[41] Calcium is essential for skeletal mineralization, many intracellular and intercellular processes, muscle contractility, electrical conduction at membranes (especially nerves and cardiac conduction system), and enzyme activity.[23] The calcium concentration is maintained over a narrow range and is controlled by the parathyroid hormone, vitamin D, and calcitonin.[42] Dietary intake, gastrointestinal absorption, gastrointestinal and renal excretion, and resorption or release from the bones all affect calcium balance.[19,27]

Within the plasma, calcium circulates in three forms: ionized; bound to proteins (e.g., albumin); and bound to diffusible molecules such as bicarbonate, citrate, lactate, and phosphate. Ionized calcium, the

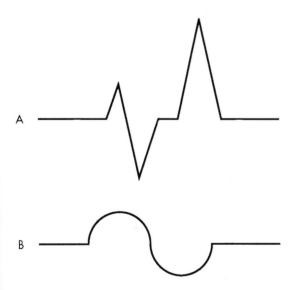

FIG. 14-1. Changes in ECG due to hyperkalemia. **A,** Loss of P wave, widening of QRS complex, tall peaked T wave. **B,** Sine-wave pattern of severe hyperkalemia.

TABLE 14-7	Treatment of Hyperkalemia

ETIOLOGY	TREATMENT
Metabolic acidosis associated with volume deficit	Administer fluid bolus therapy to expand vascular volume; reassess cardiovascular status and potassium level
Mild or asymptomatic hyper-kalemia	Decrease potassium intake and/or discontinue using potassium-sparing medications

Severe symptoms	• Place child on cardiac monitor
	• Correct cardiac manifestations: administer 10% calcium gluconate 0.5-1 ml/kg over 2-5 minutes;* continuously monitor for ECG changes, discontinue if pulse rate <100
	• Facilitate the movement of potassium into the cells
	    Sodium bicarbonate 1-2 mEq/kg over 5-10 minutes—may use in the absence of acidosis*
	    Glucose 0.5-1 g/kg and regular insulin 1 unit per 3 g of glucose—monitor blood glucose level
	    Albuterol nebulization 2.5 mg for children <25 kg, 5 mg for children >25 kg
	• Enhance the elimination of potassium
	    Administer a loop diuretic (e.g., furosemide) provided renal function is adequate
	    Administer 1-2 g/kg of sodium polystyrene sulfonate (Kayexalate) PO, via NG tube, or rectally; can be administered every 6-12 hours

Data from Cronan and Norman, 1993; Brem, 1990; Johnson, 1993; Rudzinski, Wolanyk, and Mackey, 1996.
*Calcium precipitates in bicarbonate solutions; therefore an IV line used for both agents must be thoroughly flushed.

physiologically active form, is readily available. The serum ionized calcium concentration is affected by protein binding with serum albumin, chelation with phosphate or other anions, and acid-base balance. Because of the albumin-calcium binding capacity, the serum ionized calcium decreases by 0.8 mg/dl for every 1 g/dl increase in serum albumin.[36] At the renal level, losses of phosphate tend to shift the flow of calcium from the bone to the extracellular fluid. Changes in serum pH affect the protein-calcium binding capacity. In alkalotic states, more calcium is bound to proteins and the ionized calcium level decreases. In acidotic states, calcium is released from protein-binding sites, thus increasing the availability of ionized calcium.

HYPOCALCEMIA

Etiology. Hypocalcemia is defined as a serum calcium concentration of less than 9 mg/dl.[42]

Hypocalcemia can result from many etiologies, including primary vitamin D deficiency caused by dietary deficiency or lack of sunlight exposure; secondary vitamin D deficiency caused by malabsorption diseases, chronic renal failure, or certain drugs (e.g., phenytoin, phenobarbital); reduced effect of the parathyroid hormone (e.g., hypoparathyroidism); and insensitivity or suppression of parathyroid hormone (PTH) (e.g., hypomagnesemia, burns, sepsis). Other conditions that can be associated with hypocalcemia include alkalosis, which causes increased protein-binding of calcium[5]; hyperphosphatemia; massive transfusion of anticoagulated blood products; and hypernatremia with associated potassium deficiency.[39]

Pathophysiology. When serum calcium levels fall, the parathyroid glands are stimulated to release PTH. PTH causes an immediate loss of phosphate in the urine and increases the reabsorption of calcium.

Hydrogen and magnesium ions are also reabsorbed as sodium potassium, and amino acids are lost. When phosphate is lost, calcium is mobilized from bone to plasma. Excitability of tissues in the CNS, cardiac, and muscular systems accompanies decreases in serum calcium levels.

Clinical presentation. Signs and symptoms of hypocalcemia are indicative of neuromuscular irritability. Acute findings include tetany, seizures, and laryngospasm. Early findings may include Chvostek's sign (facial muscle spasm brought on by tapping the facial nerve) and Trousseau's sign (carpal spasm brought on by pressure applied to the upper arm). Nonspecific findings include vomiting, irritability, and muscle weakness. The ECG may reveal a prolonged QT interval, bradycardia, and dysrhythmias.[42]

HYPERCALCEMIA

Etiology. Hypercalcemia is defined as a serum calcium concentration of greater than 11 mg/dl. It can result from excessive intake of calcium and vitamin D from diet, nutritional supplements, or medications; from abnormalities in regulatory mechanisms resulting in increased absorption of calcium from bone and the gastrointestinal tract; or from decreased renal excretion of calcium. Hypercalcemia is rare in the pediatric population but may be seen in patients with vitamin D toxicity, adolescents with long-term immobilization, or in children with bony malignancies. In infants an idiopathic form of hypercalcemia is associated with characteristic facies or "elfin" features and cardiac anomalies.[10]

Pathophysiology. The pathophysiology associated with an elevated serum calcium level depends on the underlying etiology. If the child has ingested excess vitamin D, then the hypercalcemia results from increased calcium absorption.[19] In hyperparathyroidism excess PTH stimulates bone resorption of calcium, which increases serum calcium levels. Other conditions that can increase bone resorption and therefore can produce hypercalcemia include prolonged immobilization and certain malignancies.[19,27]

With increases in serum calcium the renal excretion of sodium and potassium increases and the ability of the kidneys to concentrate urine is reduced. The musculoskeletal system is depressed, reflex activities are sluggish, and the QT interval of the heart is decreased.

Clinical presentation. Signs and symptoms of mild hypercalcemia (11 to 13 mg/dl) are often nonspecific and are mostly neurologic in nature. Headache, fatigue, irritability, poor feeding, and GI upset are common complaints. Severe hypercalcemia (>15 mg/dl) may present with a wide range of symptoms, including severe vomiting, hypertension, polyuric dehydration, acute renal failure, shortened QT interval on ECG, and coma.

Emergency Department interventions for the child with a calcium imbalance. Laboratory studies for the child with a suspected calcium imbalance include serum calcium, ionized calcium, serum electrolytes and magnesium, total protein, albumin, parathormone levels, and evaluation of acid-base balance. Urinalysis and urine electrolytes for calcium, phosphorus, and creatinine are also obtained. Depending on the suspected etiology an electrocardiogram, skull x-ray, chest x-ray, and skeletal survey may be valuable.

Hypocalcemia. Treatment of hypocalcemia depends on the underlying cause, the severity of the symptoms, and confounding factors. For example, if the child is alkalotic, correction of the alkalotic state may release ionized calcium into the serum. Hypomagnesemia affects hypocalcemia because it impairs the release of the PTH.

Symptomatic hypocalcemia is treated with an infusion of 10% calcium gluconate (which contains 90 mg of elemental calcium per 10 ml) 0.5 to 1 ml/kg over 3 to 5 minutes with cardiac monitoring.[7,19] If the child becomes bradycardic the infusion is discontinued. Atropine (to treat severe bradycardia) should be at the bedside. The asymptomatic child or the child whose symptoms are relieved may be treated with oral therapy, or 100 mg of elemental calcium/kg/24 hours may be added to the intravenous solution.[19]

Hypercalcemia. Treatment of hypercalcemia depends on the etiology, clinical presentation, and the child's renal function. When renal function is adequate in the symptomatic child, normal saline is infused at two times maintenance fluid requirements, and furosemide (Lasix) 1 to 2 mg/kg is administered every 6 to 8 hours, producing calciuresis.[2,7] After initial therapy, normal saline at two times maintenance is infused until serum calcium concentrations return to the normal range. Vitamin D toxicity may be treated with phosphate or sulfate infusions followed by oral pred-nisone (1 to 2 mg/kg/day).[24] Magnesium deficiency is treated with an IM dose of 50% magnesium 0.5 mEq/kg (6 mg/kg) or 0.125 ml/kg.[19] Children with acute renal failure are treated with peritoneal dialysis or hemodialysis.

ACID-BASE DISORDERS

ACID-BASE BALANCE

Acid-base balance refers to the homeostasis of hydrogen ion (H^+) concentration in the body, which is clinically reflected by the pH ($\downarrow$ pH = $\uparrow$ hydrogen ions; $\uparrow$ pH = $\downarrow$ hydrogen ions). Hydrogen ions in the form of acids (e.g., carbonic acid, sulfuric acid, phosphoric acid, ketoacids, lactic acid) are contin-ually produced and excreted to maintain the pH between 7.35 and 7.45. Intricate compensatory mechanisms including extracellular and intracellu-lar buffers and respiratory and metabolic buffers resist even transient changes in hydrogen ion con-centration.[15]

The bicarbonate-carbonic acid system is the most important of the body's buffers, because

rapid pH adjustments can occur within the extra-cellular fluid.

$$H^+ + HCO_3^- \leftrightarrow H_2CO_3 \leftrightarrow CO_2 + H_2O$$

Hydrogen ion   Bicarbonate   Carbonic acid   Carbon dioxide   Water

The acid component of the buffer (carbonic acid) is regulated by the respiratory system, which can rapidly alter the amount of carbon dioxide available for forming carbonic acid. Thus if the respiratory rate and depth increases, the amount of CO_2 available to form carbonic acid decreases and the pH rises. The base component of the system is regulated by the renal system, which can reabsorb bicarbonate ions, produce new bicarbonate ions, produce urinary buffers such as HPO_4 (phosphate) and NH_3 (ammonia), and excrete hydrogen ions.[30] Infants less than approximately 1½ years of age have a lower threshold for bicarbonate reabsorption and a decreased ability to excrete in-creased H^+ ion loads.[21,28,29] This, coupled with the infant's poorly developed respiratory musculature, limits the ability to compensate for acid-base imbal-ances, particularly metabolic acidosis.

The bicarbonate-carbonic acid buffer system can be

TABLE 14-8	Blood Gas Interpretation	
pH: Normal 7.35-7.45	Negative logarithm of hydrogen ion concentra-tion $\uparrow H^+ \rightarrow \downarrow$ pH (acidosis) $\downarrow H^+ \rightarrow \uparrow$ pH (alkalosis)
Pao_2: Normal 80-100 mm Hg	Partial pressure of dissolved oxygen in arterial blood
$Paco_2$: Normal 35-45 mm Hg	Partial pressure of carbon dioxide gas in arterial blood
HCO_3^-: Children <2 yrs = 20-25 Children >2 yrs = 22-26	Bicarbonate ion concentration; is the major blood base and is regulated by the kidneys
Base excess/deficit: Normal range +2/−2	Calculated number that is a nonrespiratory reflec-tion of acid-base balance. Positive values indi-cate increased base or a deficit of acid (metabolic alkalosis); negative values indicated decreased base or an excess of acid (metabolic acidosis)
Anion gap: Normal = 12 +/− 2 mEq/L[33] Anion gap = Na − (Cl + HCO_3)	Provides information regarding possible causes of metabolic acidosis (see text)

clinically assessed by the arterial blood pH and P_{CO_2} and the serum bicarbonate concentration or total CO_2 content. The P_{CO_2} is a measure of the acid component of the buffer system and can be converted to mM of carbonic acid (H_2CO_3) by multiplying by 0.03 (Table 14-8).[30]

METABOLIC ACIDOSIS

Etiology. Metabolic acidosis results when there is a net gain in the hydrogen ion concentration or a net loss of bicarbonate ions in the extracellular fluid, which causes the pH to fall below normal.[15,19,38] In children, metabolic acidosis most commonly results when diarrhea causes a net loss of bicarbonate. When dehydration or other conditions that decrease tissue perfusion are present, increased hydrogen ion production and lactic acidosis result, further contributing to the metabolic acidosis. Other etiologies of metabolic acidosis include ketoacidosis from diabetes or starvation; renal tubular acidosis or renal failure; or the ingestion of salicylates, methanol, or ethylene glycol. Rapid dilution of the extracellular fluid can also produce metabolic acidosis.

Pathophysiology. With metabolic acidosis numerous buffering systems are stimulated. One of the first noticeable compensatory responses is hyperventilation, which decreases the P_{CO_2}, returning the pH toward normal.[19,38] At the tissue level, positively charged hydrogen ions shift into the intracellular space in exchange for negatively charged intracellular potassium ions to maintain cell membrane electrical neutrality. Thus the serum potassium may be normal even though total body potassium is depleted. In the healthy kidneys hydrogen ions are excreted in exchange for bicarbonate ions, and new bicarbonate ions are produced.[32]

Because metabolic acidosis has many etiologies, one of the most useful classification methods is the use of the anion gap (AG), which represents an estimation of the difference between the unmeasured serum anions and "unmeasured" serum cations.[15,51]

$$AG = Na + (Cl + HCO_3)$$

A normal anion gap (12 +/− 2 mEq/L) in the acidotic child indicates a loss of bicarbonate via the kidneys or gastrointestinal tract or by rapid dilution of the extracellular fluid.[15] Most commonly, metabolic acidosis with a normal anion gap in children is associated with hyperchloremia from diarrheal fluid

losses of bicarbonate but not chloride. An increased anion gap points to acid or increased hydrogen ion concentration from tissue hypoxia associated with diarrheal dehydration or diabetic ketoacidosis, or it may be associated with the ingestion of alcohols such as ethylene glycol or methanol.[15,51] Although rare, it is also associated with inborn errors of metabolism.[38] Mild increases may be seen with decreased serum potassium, calcium, or magnesium concentrations.[15] A decreased anion gap is not helpful in determining the cause of an acid-base imbalance but may indicate an increased serum concentration of potassium, calcium, or magnesium.[15]

Clinical presentation. Signs and symptoms of metabolic acidosis vary depending on the etiology of the disorder. Tachypnea, pallor, headache, abdominal pain, vomiting, restlessness, or lethargy may be exhibited. More ominously, bradycardia, hypotension, and cardiac dysrhythmias may result from decreased myocardial contractility, myocardial irritability, decreased peripheral vascular resistance, and decreased adrenergic-receptor sensitivity.[31]

Emergency Department interventions. The treatment of metabolic acidosis is dependent on the underlying etiology. The volume-depleted child is initially treated with fluids; the ketotic child (DKA) is treated with fluids, electrolytes, and insulin; and the hypoxic child is treated with oxygen and/or ventilatory assistance.

The administration of alkalotic solutions to the child with metabolic acidosis is controversial; several alternatives to sodium bicarbonate ($NaHCO_3$) have been studied, including dichloroacetate (DCA), tromethamine (Tham), sodium carbonate (Na_2CO_3), and carbicarb.[32] In general, sodium bicarbonate 1 mEq/kg remains the treatment of choice in the emergency department for those children in whom the initial etiology of the illness has been addressed and cardiac arrest from severe acidosis has occurred or is imminent.[23] This initial dose replaces no more than one fourth to one half of the calculated bicarbonate deficit.[17,24]

$$\text{Total } HCO_3^- \text{ deficit} = \text{Base deficit} \times \text{Weight} \times 0.3$$
$$(\text{mEq/L}) \qquad (\text{kg})$$

Sodium bicarbonate administration may be detrimental to the child if ventilatory status is inadequate, hypernatremia exists, or hypovolemia and potassium imbalances are not corrected before administration.

METABOLIC ALKALOSIS

Etiology. Metabolic alkalosis results when there is a net gain in the bicarbonate ion concentration or a net loss of hydrogen ion concentration. The result is an increase in the pH above normal values. Although not common in children, metabolic alkalosis may be caused by persistent vomiting, as in pyloric stenosis or bulimia nervosa; diuretic use; or ingestion/infusion of alkali substances (e.g., sodium bicarbonate).

Pathophysiology. The pathophysiology of metabolic alkalosis depends on the underlying etiology. In infants with excessive losses of gastric contents caused by persistent vomiting (e.g., pyloric stenosis), hypochloremic metabolic alkalosis can develop from hydrogen ion and chloride losses. In children with cystic fibrosis, excessive cutaneous sodium and chloride losses not counterbalanced by dietary intake can also produce metabolic alkalosis. The aggressive administration of alkali solutions (e.g., bicarbonate) can produce metabolic alkalosis; however, this finding is usually transient unless renal function is compromised.[15]

Metabolic alkalosis also results when there is a reduction in the glomerular filtration rate, which prevents the excretion of bicarbonate (e.g., volume depletion or renal failure). Excessive volume depletion will stimulate the renin-aldosterone system, which promotes the reabsorption of sodium and the excretion of hydrogen and potassium, further contributing to the metabolic alkalosis.[15,32]

Clinical presentation. Most commonly metabolic alkalosis is an incidental finding in the child with vomiting and does not produce significant signs and symptoms. With severe metabolic alkalosis signs and symptoms are similar to those of hypocalcemia and include muscle cramps, weakness, tetany, seizures with apnea, and cardiac dysrhythmias. Hypoventilation, a compensatory response to alkalosis, will produce a rise in the P_{CO_2} and a drop in the P_{O_2}, which can affect the respiratory drive and may precipitate respiratory arrest.[23]

Emergency Department interventions. The treatment for metabolic alkalosis depends on the underlying etiology (e.g., vomiting, diuretic use) and the presence of additional findings such as volume depletion and electrolyte deficits. If the cause of the alkalosis is volume depletion from gastrointestinal losses of hydrogen ions and chloride, fluid replacement with sodium chloride will usually correct the pH.[32] Hypokalemia, which may be associated with volume depletion, must also be addressed for this approach to be effective. On rare occasions, severe metabolic alkalosis, which produces myocardial depression, may be treated with hydrochloric acid.[31]

RESPIRATORY ALKALOSIS

Etiology. Respiratory alkalosis is caused by a primary decrease in serum carbon dioxide concentration that increases the pH above 7.45. The etiology is hyperventilation. In the emergency setting, hyperventilation usually results from anxiety, fever, sepsis, salicylate poisoning, or trauma. Hyperventilation to compensate for metabolic acidosis is also common.

Pathophysiology. Respiratory alkalosis results when carbon dioxide excretion exceeds carbon dioxide production. The result is a reduction in carbonic acid, which causes the hydrogen ion concentration to fall.[23] With the rise in pH, metabolic components of the buffer system are activated, including intracellular buffers that increase the production of carbon dioxide and renal buffers that cause hydrogen ions to be retained and bicarbonate ions to be excreted.[15,23]

Clinical presentation. Classically, hyperventilating patients present with tachypnea, dizziness, syncope, and numbness and tingling of the facial muscles. As respiratory alkalosis progresses, signs and symptoms include twitching of facial muscles, carpopedal spasm (palmar flexion of hands, plantar flexion of feet), altered mental status, seizures, and cardiac dysrhythmias.

Emergency Department interventions. Treatment of the hyperventilating child requires the identification of the underlying etiology. Treatment may be as simple as having the child breathe into a paper bag to inhale CO_2 or giving antipyretics to reduce fever. Treatment of hyperventilation caused by sepsis or trauma may require rapid sequence intubation and mechanical ventilation to control the rate and depth of respirations and to decrease oxygen consumption.

RESPIRATORY ACIDOSIS

Respiratory acidosis results when alveolar ventilation is ineffective, causing a primary increase in P_{CO_2} and a decrease in arterial pH. Causes of respiratory acidosis include acute or chronic lung diseases (e.g., asthma, croup, cystic fibrosis, bronchopulmonary dysplasia), traumatic injuries that impair ventilatory function (e.g., pneumothorax or thoracic cage injuries), or conditions affecting CNS or neuromuscular function (e.g., muscular dystrophy, CNS depressant drugs). (For a complete discussion of respiratory acidosis, see Chapter 6.)

NURSING CARE AND EVALUATION OF THE CHILD WITH AN ELECTROLYTE DISTURBANCE OR ACID-BASE IMBALANCE

Initial nursing care of the child with an electrolyte or acid-base imbalance requires stabilization of the airway and breathing. If the child exhibits signs of shock or hypoxia, supplemental oxygen is administered via a nonrebreather face mask. Signs of respiratory failure or impending arrest require assistance with bag-valve-mask ventilation and ultimately endotracheal intubation.

Venous access is obtained in the largest vein available, and the site is checked frequently during the administration of fluids and electrolytes. Certain solutions such as 3% sodium, sodium bicarbonate, high-concentration potassium, calcium, and glucose are highly osmolar and can cause burning and necrosis of the veins and surrounding tissue. Both before and after the administration of any of these solutions the IV lines are flushed to prevent precipitation or other interactions with the medications that may be given.

All fluids and electrolytes are administered via an infusion pump. During therapy for sodium imbalances and during the administration of calcium, seizure precautions are instituted and the child's neurologic status is continuously monitored for signs of seizure activity and increasing intracranial pressure (e.g., irritability, confusion, decreased response to pain, hypertension, tachycardia or bradycardia, apnea). All children are placed on a pulse oximeter and cardiac monitor. In addition, cardiovascular status is closely watched for signs of decreased peripheral perfusion or shock or for the development of dysrhythmias and bradycardia.

A full set of vital signs, including blood pressure (to monitor for the development of hypotension), is taken at least hourly—more often when highly concentrated electrolyte solutions are being administered or if the child is unstable. All intake and output is monitored to assess renal function. The placement of a urinary catheter will assist in evaluating output. Serial electrolyte measurements and/or blood gases should be anticipated.

The child and family will require continuous com-

Box 14-3 Nursing Care of the Child with an Electrolyte Disturbance or Acid-Base Imbalance

Stabilize the airway and breathing
- Administer supplemental oxygen via nonrebreather face mask for respiratory distress or signs of shock
- Provide ventilatory support for respiratory arrest or signs of failure
- Obtain blood gases as indicated

Stabilize circulatory status
- Place child on a heart rate monitor and pulse oximeter
- Obtain vascular access in largest available vein
- Administer all fluid and electrolyte solutions via an infusion pump
- Monitor cardiac rhythm and peripheral perfusion during electrolyte therapy
- Closely observe the IV site for signs of burning or necrosis

Monitor neurologic status
- Evaluate baseline neurologic status
- Institute seizure precautions (for sodium imbalances and during calcium therapy)
- Observe for signs of increasing intracranial pressure (sodium imbalances)

Obtain hourly vital signs, including blood pressure—more often in the unstable child

Monitor all intake and output
- Consider the placement of a urinary catheter

Anticipate serial electrolyte and/or blood gas measurements

Provide support to the parents and child
- Communicate frequently with the parents and allow them to remain with their child whenever possible

Prepare for hospital admission

munication regarding plans for care. Even young children deserve to know when a procedure (e.g., venous access) is to be performed. When possible the parents should be allowed to remain with and comfort the child. If admission to the hospital is imminent the parents should be informed and the child prepared. If the child is to be discharged the parents are provided with information describing the etiology of the illness, how to prevent future occurrences, serious signs and symptoms that may require a trip to the ED or their private physician, and when to seek follow-up care (Box 14-3).

▎ SUMMARY

Fluid and electrolyte balance in the child is maintained in a delicate equilibrium that is sometimes altered by illness and injury. Understanding the physiology of the child's growing body provides insight into the unique responses that can result from hemodynamic imbalances. Early recognition and appropriate interventions are essential components in emergency nursing care of children with fluid and electrolyte imbalances.

REFERENCES

1. Adelman RD, Solhung MJ: Pathophysiology of body fluids and fluid therapy. In Behrman RE, Kliegman RM, Arvin AM, eds: *Nelson textbook of pediatrics,* ed 15, Philadelphia, 1996, WB Saunders.
2. Allen DB: Disorders of the endocrine system relevant to pediatric critical illness. In Fuhrman BP, Zimmerman JJ, eds: *Pediatric critical care,* St Louis, 1992, Mosby.
3. Arieff A, Llach F, Massry S: Neurologic manifestations and morbidity of hyponatremia: correlation with brain water and electrolytes, *Medicine* 55(2): 121, 1976.
4. Avner ED et al: Normal neonates and the maturational development of homeostatic mechanisms. In Ichikawa I, ed: *Pediatric textbook of fluids and electrolytes,* Baltimore, 1990, Williams & Wilkins.
5. Bacon G et al: *A practical approach to pediatric endocrinology,* ed 2, Chicago, 1990, Year Book Medical Publishers.
6. Baer CL: Fluid and electrolyte balance. In Kinney MR, Packa DR, Dunbar SB, eds: *AACN's clinical reference for critical care nursing,* St Louis, 1993, Mosby.
7. Barkin RM: Fluid and electrolyte balance. In Barkin RM, ed: *Pediatric emergency medicine: concepts and clinical practice,* St Louis, 1992, Mosby.
8. Barkin RM, Rosen P: *Emergency pediatrics: a guide to ambulatory care,* St Louis, 1994, Mosby.
9. Barnard JA, Hazinski MF: Pediatric gastrointestinal disorders. In Hazinski MF, ed: *Nursing care of the critically ill child,* ed 2, St Louis, 1992, Mosby.
10. Behrman RE, et al: *Nelson textbook of pediatrics,* 15th ed, Philadelphia, 1996, WB Saunders.
11. Berry PL, Belsha CW: Hyponatremia, *Pediatr Clin North Am* 37(2):351-364, 1990.
12. Boineau FG, Lewy JE: Estimation of parenteral fluid requirements, *Pediatr Clin North Am* 37:2, 1990.
13. Bonadio WA et al: Efficacy of measuring BUN in assessing children with dehydration due to gastroenteritis, *Ann Emerg Med* 18:755, 1989.
14. Brem A: Disorders of potassium balance, *Pediatr Clin North Am* 37(2):419-428, 1990.
15. Brewer E: Disorders of acid-base balance, *Pediatr Clin North Am* 37(2):427-448, 1990.
16. Casteel HB, Feidorek SC: Oral rehydration, *Pediatr Clin North Am* 37(2):295-311, 1990.
17. Chameides L, Hazinski MF: *Textbook of pediatric advanced life support,* Dallas, 1994, American Heart Association.
18. Conley SB: Hypernatremia, *Pediatr Clin North Am* 37(2):365-372, 1990.
19. Cronan CM, Norman ME: Renal and electrolyte emergencies. In Fleisher GR, Ludwig S, eds: *Textbook of pediatric emergency medicine,* ed 3, Baltimore, 1993, Williams & Wilkins.
20. Darrow DC: The significance of body size, *Am J Dis Child* 98:416, 1959.
21. Edelman CM Jr, Barnett HL, Troupka V: Renal concentrating mechanisms in newborn infants, *J Clin Invest* 39:1062, 1960.
22. Reference deleted in proofs.
23. Finberg L, Karavath RE, Hellerstern S, eds: *Water and electrolytes in pediatrics,* ed 2, Philadelphia, 1993, WB Saunders.
24. Fleisher GR, Ludwig S: *Textbook of pediatric emergency medicine,* ed 2, Baltimore, 1992, William & Wilkins.
25. Glaeseman PC: Pediatric fluid and electrolyte requirements, *Dimen Crit Care Nurs* 2(5):280-284, 1983.
26. Grisanti KA, Jaffe DM: Dehydration syndromes: oral rehydration and fluid placement, *Emerg Med Clin North Am* 9(3):565-588, 1991.
27. Guyton AC: *Textbook of medical physiology,* ed 8, Philadelphia, 1991, WB Saunders.
27a. Harrison HE: Parenteral fluid therapy. In Erlich F, Heldrich FJ, Tepas JJ, eds: *Pediatric Emergency Medicine,* Rockville, MD, 1987, Aspen Publishers.
28. Hazinski MF: Children are different. In Hazinski MF, ed: *Nursing care of the critically ill child,* ed 2, St Louis, 1992, Mosby.
29. Hellerstern S: Fluids and electrolytes: physiology, *Pediatr Rev* 14(2):70-79, 1993.

30. Hill LL: Body composition, normal electrolyte concentrations, and the maintenance of normal volume, tonicity and acid-base metabolism, *Pediatr Clin North Am* 37(2):241-256, 1990.
31. Holbrook PR: Acid-base disorders. In Holbrook PR, ed: *Textbook of pediatric critical care,* Philadelphia, 1993, WB Saunders.
32. Jefferson LS, Bricker JT: Acid-base balance and disorders. In Fuhrman BP, Zimmerman JJ, eds: *Pediatric critical care,* St Louis, 1992, Mosby.
33. Johnson K: *Harriet Lane handbook,* St Louis, 1993, Mosby.
34. Kallen RJ: The managment of diarrheal dehydration in infants using parenteral fluids, *Pediatr Clin North Am* 37(2):265-286, 1990.
35. Keating JP, Schears GJ, Dodge PR: Oral water intoxication in infants, *Am J Dis Child* 145:985-990, 1991.
36. Kennedy J: Renal disorders. In Hazinski MF: *Nursing care of the critically ill child,* ed 2, St Louis, 1992, Mosby.
37. Laureno R, Karp BI: Pontine and extrapontine myelinolysis following rapid correction of hyponatremia, *Lancet* i:1439, 1988.
38. Lewis M: Metabolic acidosis. In Strange GR et al, eds: *Pediatric emergency medicine: a comprehensive study guide,* New York, 1996, McGraw-Hill.
39. Lynch RE: Ionized calcium: pediatric perspective, *Pediatr Clin North Am* 37(2):373-390, 1991.
40. McDonald RA: Disorders of potassium balance, *Pediatr Ann* 24(1):31-37, 1995.
41. Metheny NM: *Fluid and electrolyte imbalances: nursing considerations,* Philadelphia, 1987, JB Lippincott.
42. Rudzinski JP, Wolanyk D, Mackey M: Fluids and electrolytes. In Strange GR et al, eds: *Pediatric emergency medicine: a comprehensive study guide,* New York, 1996, McGraw-Hill.
43. Saladino RA: Endocrine and metabolic disorders. In Barkin RM, ed: *Pediatric emergency medicine: concepts and clinical practice,* St Louis, 1992, Mosby.
44. Santensonio F et al: Evidence for a role of endogenous insulin and glucagon in the regulation of potassium homeostasis, *J Lab Clin Med* 81:809, 1973.
45. Sarnaik AP et al: Management of hyponatremic seizures in children with hypertonic saline: a safe and effective strategy, *Crit Care Med* 19(6):758-762, 1991.
46. Satlin LM, Schwartz GJ: Metabolism of potassium. In Ichikawa I, ed: *Pediatric textbook of fluids and electrolytes,* Baltimore, 1990, Williams & Wilkins.
47. Shaw KN: Dehydration. In Fleisher GR, Ludwig S, eds: *Textbook of pediatric emergency medicine,* ed 3, Baltimore, 1993, Williams & Wilkins.
48. Sterns RH: Severe symptomatic hyponatremia: treatment and outcome. A study of 64 cases, *Ann Intern Med* 107:656, 1987.
49. Sterns RH, Riggs JE, Schochet SS: Osmotic demyelination syndrome following correction of hyponatremia, *N Engl J Med* 314:1535, 1986.
50. Wood EG, Lynch RE: Fluid and electrolyte balance. In Fuhrman BP, Zimmerman JJ, eds: *Pediatric critical care,* St Louis, 1992, Mosby.
51. Wrenn K: The delta gap: an approach to mixed acid-base disorders, *Ann Emerg Med* 19(11):1310-1313, 1990.

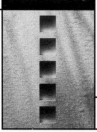

CHAPTER 15

Gastrointestinal System

Marilyn Horton, Treesa Soud, Connie Inman, Patricia Standifer

INTRODUCTION

Gastrointestinal (GI) disorders are common in children and comprise one of the largest categories of illnesses. These conditions range from acute disturbances of the GI tract to chronic pathologic states that may alter the child's life-style.

Many gastroenterologic diseases in children are similar to those of adults; however, presenting symptoms, diagnosis, and treatment may be significantly different. In addition, children have less functional reserve than adults do, and therefore common GI symptoms such as vomiting and diarrhea are poorly tolerated by children.

ANATOMY AND PHYSIOLOGY

ESOPHAGUS

The esophagus is a conduit for food and liquid to be transported from the mouth to the stomach by means of peristaltic waves. Once the food reaches the stomach, constriction of the lower esophageal sphincter prevents reflux of acidic gastric contents back into the esophagus. In the first month of life this lax-functioning sphincter contributes to frequent regurgitation, or gastroesophageal reflux, after feedings. However, gastroesophageal reflux may be observed in healthy infants as old as 9 to 12 months.[8] Reflux is normal in infants when intraabdominal pressure increases, for example, during crying, coughing, moving about, or defecating (Fig. 15-1).

STOMACH

The stomach receives ingested material and serves as a temporary reservoir during the initial phase of diges-

tion. Gastric mucus and bicarbonate ions are secreted to protect the lining of the stomach as pepsinogen, hydrochloric acid, and intrinsic factor are released.

Stomach capacity of the neonate is 10 to 20 ml of fluid, compared to 100 to 200 ml in the 2-month-old infant and 1500 ml in the adolescent.[8] Gastric motility is reduced in the neonate, but gastric emptying time is increased. Because of the infant's limited stomach capacity and propensity to swallow air during feeding, small, frequent feedings are required to maintain nutritional requirements adequately and prevent gastroesophageal reflux.

PYLORIC SPHINCTER

The distal opening of the stomach is the pylorus, which allows fluids to move from the stomach to the duodenum almost all the time. The pyloric sphincter is the circular muscle that acts much like a purse string, restricting the passage of large food particles until they have been digested to an almost fluid substance called chyme. Factors affecting delay in gastric emptying include prolonged sleep, inactivity, and the administration of sedatives. In addition, the type of ingested material can affect the rate of emptying. Liquids empty faster than solids, and carbohydrates empty faster than proteins. Fatty substances require the longest transit time. Acidic substances and hypertonic solutions empty slowly.

SMALL INTESTINE

The structures of the small intestine include the duodenum, the jejunum, and the ileum. The entire internal surface of the intestines consists of absorptive epithelial cells attached to microscopic structures called villi, which absorb electrolytes, nutrients, and fluids. In children villi tend to be leaflike, with a surface that is less functional than the fingerlike projections found in the adult (Fig. 15-2).

When damaged, the epithelial cells in the small intestine rapidly regenerate, maintaining maximum absorption; however, in very young infants regeneration takes longer. Some of the conditions that can affect the mucosal lining of the intestines and regeneration of the epithelial cells include infection, malnutrition, or injury. When these conditions occur, the resulting malabsorption can produce signs of malnutrition, which, if untreated, can lead to death.

LARGE INTESTINE

The large intestine is divided into sections—the ascending colon, the transverse colon, the descending colon, and the sigmoid colon. The primary functions of the large intestine are reabsorption of water and electrolytes and storage of feces before defecation.

The large intestine or colon begins in the lower right portion of the abdominal cavity, where the colon is separated from the small intestine by the ileocecal valve. At this junction is a blind, wormlike pouch called the appendix. In the neonate the appendix forms a small diverticulum extending from the inferior border of the cecum. Appendicitis is rare in infants and young children because of the scarcity of lymphatic tissue.[41] As the child matures and the appendix and lymphatic tissue develop, appendicitis becomes more common.

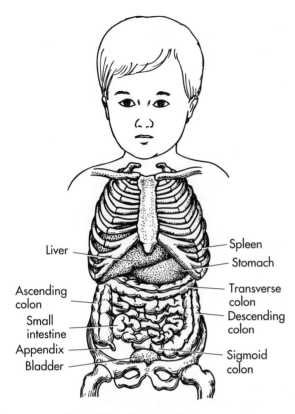

Liver
Spleen
Stomach
Ascending colon
Transverse colon
Small intestine
Descending colon
Appendix
Sigmoid colon
Bladder

FIG. 15-1. Abdominal structures.

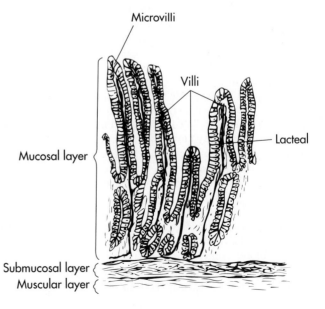

Microvilli
Villi
Mucosal layer
Lacteal
Submucosal layer
Muscular layer

FIG. 15-2. Microscopic anatomy of the intestinal wall. (From Harvey MA: *Study guide to core curriculum for critical care nursing,* ed 2, Philadelphia, 1992, WB Saunders.)

CIRCULATION

The splanchnic circulation includes three major vessels that branch from the aorta and supply blood to the stomach, small intestine, and colon. They are the inferior mesenteric artery, the superior mesenteric artery, and the celiac artery. The celiac artery is short and divides into three branches, supplying the stomach, spleen, liver, and part of the duodenum and pancreas. The superior mesenteric artery provides the rest of the blood to the small bowel and to the first half of the large bowel. The inferior mesenteric artery supplies the remaining part of the large intestine.

The portal system is a network of veins that unite to form the portal vein. The portal vein receives the venous supply from the stomach, pancreas, small intestine, and colon. It then perfuses the liver and returns to the heart by way of the hepatic vein and the inferior vena cava.

PANCREAS

The head of the pancreas fits into the concave shape of the duodenum, with its body and tail extending toward the left side of the abdominal cavity. Because of the child's relatively small abdominal cavity, compared to that of the adult, the pancreas is more easily palpated in young children.

During digestion the pancreas secretes enzymes that are responsible for the breakdown and absorption of fats, carbohydrates, and protein. To help reduce duodenal irritation, the pancreas secretes bicarbonate. Insulin, which is necessary for the utilization of glucose, is both synthesized and secreted by the pancreas.

LIVER

The liver metabolizes protein, fat, and carbohydrates. It is the primary synthesizer of plasma protein, clotting factors, and albumin. The liver is also a major storage site of fat, fat-soluble vitamins, and glycogen. Another necessary function of the liver is the breakdown and deactivation of medication and waste products, which can be delayed during infancy because of liver immaturity.

Both the hepatic artery and the portal vein supply blood to the liver. Although most oxygenated blood is supplied by the hepatic artery, approximately 80% of hepatic blood comes from the portal vein, which supplies venous blood from the GI tract, spleen, and pancreas. The liver then extracts needed substances, removes and detoxifies substances, and releases newly synthesized compounds into the blood.[22]

In the neonate the liver span ranges from 4.5 to 5 cm; in the mature adolescent it is approximately 7 to 12 cm.[1] Because of the relatively small abdominal cavity of the young child as compared to the adult, the liver is easily palpable 2 to 3 cm below the right costal margin.

GALLBLADDER

The gallbladder stores bile, which is produced by the liver and assists in the digestion and absorption of fat. The left and right hepatic ducts combine to form the common hepatic duct, which, along with the common bile duct, serves as a conduit for bile flow from the liver to the duodenum.

▌ NURSING HISTORY AND ASSESSMENT

HISTORY

Initially a focused history, based on the child's chief complaint and symptoms, is obtained. Although in most instances it is best to obtain the history from the child, very young infants and children who are nonverbal may be impossible to interview. In such situations it is necessary to rely on parental observations. Questions should be used to determine (1) the chronology of events surrounding the illness; (2) the symptoms associated with the illness; (3) any changes in patterns, such as feeding or elimination; (4) the character and location of pain associated with the illness; (5) any changes in the infant's/child's playfulness or level of consciousness; and (6) significant medical history.

Pain. Children with signs of abdominal pain require a thorough examination to rule out the presence of a surgical condition. Because identifying pain in the infant or young child is difficult, if not impossible, observational findings are important. Signs of pain in the infant range from frequent crying or irritability to disinterest in the bottle and frank lethargy. In the preschool child pain assessment is often complicated by the child's fear of the emergency department (ED) surroundings and unwillingness to cooperate during the examination. In these children parental report of pain is important. Older children are easier to assess because they are better able to communicate. Any child who is unable to walk due to pain, is bent over in severe pain, or cries out in pain is seen urgently.

Specific questions related to abdominal pain need to focus on (1) type or characteristics of the pain, (2) location of the pain, (3) severity of the pain, (4) duration of the pain, and (5) factors influencing the pain. For a complete discussion of pain assessment, see Chapter 29.

PHYSICAL ASSESSMENT

The physical examination of the pediatric patient can prove to be challenging. Although crying can produce straining, thus aiding in demonstrating the presence of a hernia or localized bulging in the abdomen, it can also complicate the interpretation of auscultatory or palpatory findings. The nurse may find it necessary to return at quiet intervals to complete the assessment. In young infants the abdomen occasionally can be examined during bottle-feeding or while the infant sucks a pacifier.

Inspection.   The initial focus of the examination is inspection. In general, the infant/child is observed for activity level and signs of a serious illness. The nurse first notes how the child arrived in the triage or examination area (e.g., wheelchair, carried, or ambulatory) and whether the child is able to climb onto the examination table without signs of pain.

Inspection of the abdomen includes observation for dilated veins, fullness or distention, movement on respiration, general contour, and gastric or intestinal peristaltic activity. The umbilicus of young infants is examined for the presence of hernias, ulceration, discharge, and excessive granulation tissue.

Auscultation.   The abdomen is auscultated for bowel sounds, which are normally heard every 10 to 13 seconds. Bowel sounds provide valuable information about peristaltic activity. In addition to abdominal auscultation, breath sounds are auscultated to rule out the presence of pneumonia or reactive airway disease, since young children with respiratory disorders may have abdominal pain as a presenting symptom.

Palpation.   The abdomen is palpated next; however, the child is first asked to point to the area that is most painful. Palpation of this area is reserved for last. The ideal position for examining the child's abdomen is with the child's head placed on a pillow and with the knees flexed. If the child will not cooperate, the examination can be performed with the child lying supine on the bed or on the parent's lap. Before deep palpation the abdomen is gently palpated at the end of expiration to identify tenderness or rigidity. Deep palpation then follows to determine the position, relative size, consistency, and contour of the liver, spleen, kidneys, and any masses. The border of the liver and spleen is also palpated. The liver is normally felt 2 to 3 cm below the right costal margin in infants and children. The spleen may be felt at the left costal margin. Tenderness of either organ is abnormal.

During the examination, crying, changes in facial expressions, or variations in the pitch of the cry may indicate pain or tenderness. Throughout the examination the child's attention can be distracted by asking questions about siblings, birthday parties, or vacations. This approach is particularly helpful in the presence of pain, tenderness, or ticklishness.

Percussion.   Percussion is performed by lightly but sharply tapping the abdomen to emit a sound. This procedure is used to determine the presence of tympany and to detect free fluid, hepatic and splenic borders, a distended bladder, or other masses.

Although not generally performed by the nurse, the last portion of the examination includes a rectal examination. The nurse should prepare the child and the parent for the examination and instruct the child to take slow, deep breaths during the examination. Stool on the examiner's glove is tested for the presence of blood.

▌ GASTROINTESTINAL SIGNS AND SYMPTOMS

Each year many outpatient visits and hospital admissions are the result of gastroenteritis. Dehydration, secondary to gastroenteritis, occurs more rapidly in small children than in adults, and it can be life-threatening. Seventy-five percent of a full-term infant's weight is water, compared to 60% to 70% in an adolescent or adult. This fluid can be quickly lost during episodes of vomiting and/or diarrhea. Because of the child's increased metabolic rate and fluid loss with evaporation, higher maintenance fluids are required per kilogram of body weight.

VOMITING

Etiology.   Vomiting is a common complaint in the pediatric population. It can be caused by numerous problems in diverse organ systems. For example, vomiting can be caused by (1) infectious processes such as gastroenteritis, upper respiratory infections (URIs), or sepsis; (2) congenital or anatomic disorders such as pyloric stenosis, gastroesophageal reflux, intussusception, or volvulus; (3) metabolic disorders such as diabetes; (4) central nervous system (CNS) dysfunction caused by head trauma, hydrocephalus, or tumors; and (5) other conditions or illnesses such as milk allergies, toxic ingestions, or appendicitis.

Pathophysiology. Vomiting is defined as the forceful act of expelling gastric contents through the mouth. It is a highly coordinated act involving closure of the gastric pylorus and the glottis, relaxation of the stomach and the esophagus, and vigorous muscle contraction of the abdominal wall. It is important to differentiate vomiting from normal physiologic spitting up in young infants, which is caused by lax functioning of the lower esophageal sphincter. Spitting up is defined as the nonforceful reflux of milk into the mouth. It is often caused by overfeeding and is usually of little consequence.

Clinical presentation. Because of the myriad of conditions that produce vomiting in the infant or child, a complete history, based on the child's age and presenting symptoms, is required. Some of the most common conditions that produce vomiting include gastroenteritis, urinary tract infections, otitis media, and pneumonia. Other examples of causes include sepsis, meningitis, hepatitis, volvulus, and intussusception.

When vomiting is the chief complaint, one important factor to note is the differentiation between vomiting and spitting up. Although swallowing is well coordinated at birth, it is common for parents to mistake regurgitation, or spitting up, of gastric contents for vomiting. Questions pertinent to all children should relate to the frequency of emesis; pattern, color, and consistency of vomitus; and other associated symptoms such as fever or diarrhea. Specific findings are discussed under each diagnostic entity in this chapter. (Emergency Department and Nursing Interventions are discussed in the section on gastroenteritis later in this chapter.)

DIARRHEA

Etiology. Diarrhea is defined as the malabsorption of water and electrolytes in the intestines. Clinically diarrhea is evidenced by frequent loose, watery stools. It is a leading cause of hospital admissions

during the first year of life, and worldwide it is the leading cause of childhood morbidity and mortality. Children who live in crowded, substandard conditions are at greatest risk of contracting illnesses that may produce diarrhea. In addition, younger children and those with chronic disease or physical impairment are likely to suffer more severe physiologic consequences when diarrhea occurs.[47]

Diarrhea is a symptom of a myriad of illnesses or disorders, with the most common cause being viral in origin (e.g., viral gastroenteritis). Other common causes include bacteria such as *Salmonella*, *Shigella*, or *Campylobacter;* antibiotic therapy, which reduces the normal flora in the intestinal tract; dietary indiscretion such as overfeeding or inappropriate mixing of formulas; toxic ingestions; and respiratory tract or urinary tract infections (Box 15-1).

Diarrhea is classified as acute or chronic and inflammatory or noninflammatory. Acute diarrhea represents a change in both the frequency and the consistency of stools. Depending on the cause, acute diarrhea often subsides without specific treatment in a relatively short period. Chronic diarrhea lasts for more than 2 weeks with a noticeable increase in frequency. Disorders such as malabsorption, abnormal bowel motility, allergic reaction, anatomic defects, or inflammatory response can be associated with chronic diarrhea.

Pathophysiology. Diarrhea results from any disruption of absorption or secretion within the digestive tract (stomach, small intestines, or colon). Three major mechanisms can contribute to the symptom of diarrhea, and they usually occur in combination. These mechanisms include (1) osmotic slowing of water absorption (the amount of water entering the gut lumen exceeds its capacity to absorb); (2) transit disorders, which increase transit time (gastric motility) and send more unabsorbed fluid into the colon; and (3) impaired electrolyte and water transport, caused by injury to the intestinal epithelial cells decreasing the total surface area available for absorption.[4] Because the child has little colonic reserve (the amount of fluid that the colon can handle at any given time), increases in water entering the colon from any of the mechanisms noted here can produce diarrhea.[26]

Clinical presentation. Because of the varied causes of diarrhea, presenting signs and symptoms can range from mild to severe (see the discussion of gastroenteritis later in this chapter). A complete history of the illness is required, including (1) onset;

> ## Box 15-1   Etiology of Diarrhea
>
> Viral agents
> > Rotavirus
> > Adenovirus
> > Cytomegalovirus
> > Norwalk virus
> > Enterovirus
>
> Bacterial agents
> > *Escherichia coli*
> > *Salmonella*
> > *Yersinia enterocolitica*
> > *Campylobacter jejuni*
> > *Shigella*
>
> Parasites
> > *Giardia lamblia*
> > *Entamoeba histolytica*
> > *Cryptosporidium*
>
> Drug therapy
> > Antibiotics (e.g., amoxicillin, amoxicillin/
> >   clavulanate potassium)
> > Laxatives
> > Ipecac
>
> Malabsorption or secretory syndromes
> > Lactase deficiency
> > Cystic fibrosis
> > Short bowel syndrome
>
> Diet
> > Overfeeding
> > Introduction of new foods
> > Improper mixing of formula
>
> Allergies
> > Milk allergy
>
> Indirectly related illness
> > Otitis media
> > Upper respiratory infection
> > Urinary tract infection

days, has a bacterial infection, or has a secondary lactase deficiency.

Consequences of diarrhea (and/or vomiting) include dehydration and electrolyte disturbances. All children with a history of diarrhea are evaluated for signs of dehydration, including decreased urination, weak peripheral pulses, mottled skin color, decreased skin turgor, delayed capillary refill, dry mucous membranes, absence of tearing, sunken eyes, sunken fontanelles (in the infant), increased respiratory rate (as compensation for metabolic acidosis), and lethargy (see Chapter 14). (Emergency Department and Nursing Interventions are discussed in the section on gastroenteritis later in this chapter.)

CONSTIPATION

Etiology.   Constipation is defined as the passage of hard or firm stools at infrequent intervals or the inability to expel stool, whether hard or soft. There are numerous causes of constipation; among them are physiologic disorders such as Hirschsprung's disease, psychogenic problems such as emotional disturbances or mental retardation, and changes in developmental patterns such as the healthy child who would rather play than develop normal elimination habits. In addition, the child's diet, gastric motility, and activity level can all affect normal elimination patterns.

Pathophysiology.   The sensation to defecate occurs when a critical volume of stool stimulates normal internal anal sphincter relaxation. When this involuntary reflex occurs, the external anal sphincter constricts to permit timely defecation. In infancy both sphincters relax at the same time, allowing spontaneous passage of stool.[27]

If stool remains in the large bowel, water and sodium continue to be absorbed. Prolonged transit time or stool retention results in hardening of the stool. When the hardened stool remains in the colon, diarrhea may occur as frequent soft or liquid stools pass around the mass.

Clinical presentation.   Diagnosing constipation and its cause is sometimes difficult, particularly in the young infant and the child who is "potty training." Parents often mistake an infant's irregular bowel habits, particularly with breast-fed babies, and the infant's apparent grunting, turning red, and even crying during bowel movements as signs of constipation. These signs alone, however, are not diagnostic of constipation. The older child who is "potty training"

(2) stool frequency, color, and consistency and presence or absence of blood in the stools; (3) amount and type of fluid intake; and (4) associated symptoms such as fever, vomiting, or weight loss. If the child has a history of acute diarrhea, the severity can be determined by asking about the number of loose or watery stools that have occurred in the past 24 hours. Chronic diarrhea is seen less frequently in the ED. It is usually caused by starvation. In other instances the affected child has been having a clear-liquid diet for several

may choose to ignore the physiologic sensation of bowel fullness and may hold the stool until abdominal pain occurs. Constipation in these children is generally not due to abnormal physiology.

Children who are constipated usually arrive in the emergency department with complaints of abdominal pain, cramps, and nausea or vomiting. The child is afebrile, and bowel sounds can be heard. When asked to point with one finger to the area of pain, the child may point to the umbilical area or indicate that the pain is all over the abdomen. The abdomen may be soft or firm with some distention, but the child will not exhibit signs of rebound tenderness or guarding. The rectal examination may reveal a large fecal mass; however, an empty rectal vault does not rule out the diagnosis of constipation.

RECTAL BLEEDING

Etiology. The causes of bloody stools in infants and children vary from benign to surgical emergencies. In the neonatal population the most common causes of rectal bleeding are anal or rectal lesions and local trauma. In the premature infant necrotizing enterocolitis can occur. As the child matures, common causes include infectious diarrhea of bacterial or viral origin; intussusception, volvulus, anal fissures, and polyps (Box 15-2).

Pathophysiology. Causes of bloody stools may reflect either an upper GI or a lower GI hemorrhage. An upper GI hemorrhage is usually represented by a black tarry stool (melena), whereas gross blood (hematochezia) is the usual finding in a lower GI hemorrhage. The associated pathophysiologic condition is dependent on the cause of the illness or injury. These conditions are discussed separately under each of the clinical entities.

Clinical presentation. Although rectal bleeding most commonly represents a benign illness in the child, any infant or child who arrives in the ED with a chief complaint of rectal bleeding is evaluated for general appearance and activity level. If the child has a history of significant bleeding and/or an altered level of consciousness, immediate attention is required. Additional associated symptoms may be important, including the presence of abdominal distention, abdominal pain, vomiting, or fever.

Questions are used to determine the amount of bleeding—how much is on the diaper or toilet paper? How often does the blood appear? Is it brown, black,

---

Box 15-2   Causes of Rectal Bleeding

- Necrotizing enterocolitis
- Milk allergy
- Anal fissure
- Volvulus
- Intussusception
- Infectious diarrhea
- Polyps
- Hemorrhoids
- Inflammatory bowel disease
- Sexual abuse

---

or red? Is it really blood, or is it just a reflection of the child's diet (e.g., red juice drinks)? What is the consistency of the stool—loose, hard balls, or blood and mucus streaked? Last, the stool is checked for blood and, depending on the suspected cause of the illness, may be sent for culture. If massive bleeding is present (or suspected), the child is closely observed for signs of fluid volume deficit and the need for blood replacement.

ABDOMINAL PAIN

Etiology. Acute abdominal pain is a common presenting complaint in the pediatric emergency department and occurs in children of all ages. Some illnesses associated with abdominal pain are predominant in certain age groups (Table 15-1). The many causes include acute surgical conditions such as appendicitis and pyloric stenosis and medical disorders such as gastroenteritis and urinary tract infections (UTIs). Extraabdominal disorders include pneumonia, asthma, and systemic illnesses (e.g., sickle cell anemia, diabetes mellitus, viral syndrome).[38]

Pathophysiology. Abdominal pain is transmitted by three neural pathways. *Visceral pain* emanates from the intraabdominal organs, where visceral afferent nerve fibers conduct impulses to the spinal cord. This type of pain has a colicky, crampy quality and is most often diffuse, generalized, and difficult to localize.[40] Often characterized as deep pain, visceral pain can induce autonomic responses such as diaphoresis, tachycardia, hypertension, and dilated pupils.[18] Visceral pain is usually generalized in the upper midline or lower abdominal area, depending on which level of the GI system is involved.

TABLE 15-1	Illness-Associated Abdominal Pain by Age	
INFANCY	**CHILDHOOD**	**ADOLESCENCE**
Intussusception	Gastroenteritis	Ectopic pregnancy
Volvulus	Appendicitis	Pelvic inflammatory disease
Incarcerated hernia	Pancreatitis	Inflammatory bowel disease
Hirschsprung's disease	Henoch-Schönlein purpura	Biliary disease
Necrotizing enterocolitis	Hemolytic-uremic syndrome	
Colic	Ulcers	
Perforation	Constipation	
	Urinary tract infection	
	Functional causes of abdominal pain	

From Grisanti KA: Abdominal pain. In Barkin RM, Rosen P, eds: *Pediatric emergency medicine: concepts and clinical practice,* ed 2, St Louis, 1996, Mosby.

Somatic pain emanates from the abdominal wall, the base of the mesentery, or the diaphragm, transmitting impulses along the somatic afferent nerve fibers in the parietal peritoneum, muscle, and skin to the spinal nerves.[12] Somatic pain is most often sharp, intense, and well localized.

Referred pain emanates from a location distant from the involved organ. It may be described as a sharp, localized sensation (e.g., shoulder pain from diaphragmatic irritation) or as a distant ache (e.g., back pain from biliary tract disease).

Respiratory illnesses are also associated with abdominal pain. Children with an asthma exacerbation and associated muscle fatigue (from increased use of chest wall and abdominal musculature) may complain of abdominal pain. Pneumonia with muscular pain or diaphragmatic irritation caused by coughing can also cause abdominal pain (Fig. 15-3).

Clinical presentation. In children with underlying medical conditions, anorexia, nausea, vomiting, and/or a low-grade fever are symptoms often associated with abdominal pain. Complaints of abdominal pain with abnormal bowel sounds, abdominal distention, bilious vomiting, and peritoneal irritation such as guarding and tenderness are most often associated with major abdominal diseases.

MEDICAL CONDITIONS

GASTROENTERITIS

Etiology. Gastroenteritis, or acute infectious diarrhea, is an inflammation of the GI tract caused by

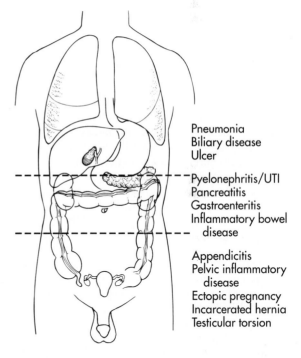

Pneumonia
Biliary disease
Ulcer

Pyelonephritis/UTI
Pancreatitis
Gastroenteritis
Inflammatory bowel disease

Appendicitis
Pelvic inflammatory disease
Ectopic pregnancy
Incarcerated hernia
Testicular torsion

FIG. 15-3. Location of abdominal pain. (From Grisanti KA: Abdominal pain. In Barkin RM, Rosen P, eds: *Pediatric emergency medicine: concepts and clinical practice,* ed 2, St Louis, 1996, Mosby.)

viral or bacterial infection or a parasitic agent. Viral diarrhea accounts for approximately 80% of all infectious diarrheas in children,[4] with the Norwalk virus and rotavirus being the most prevalent forms. Bacterial causes account for 10% to 15% of all infectious diarrhea, with *Campylobacter* being the most prevalent form.[4,9] Though all forms of gastroenteritis can be seen year round, viral diseases tend to be more common during the winter, and bacterial diseases tend to be more prevalent in the summer. Young children are those most affected by acute infectious gastroenteritis.

Pathophysiology. When an infectious agent enters the GI tract, interference with intestinal absorption produces fluid and electrolyte losses. If the agent is a virus this action is most commonly accomplished by destruction of the mucosal cells of the villi, which decreases the surface area for absorption and depresses disaccharidase levels (disaccharidase breaks down sucrose, lactose, and maltose). Bacteria may produce direct damage to the villi, but many also produce toxins that block some of the absorptive properties of the gut. The invasion of the gut by bacterial agents evokes an inflammatory response that results in leukocytosis. Subsequent mucosal ulcerations can cause erosion of the blood vessels and produce bleeding. When the organism penetrates the epithelial cells and proliferates, bacteremia can result.

Clinical presentation. Parental fear of dehydration from the limited fluid intake and excessive stooling commonly prompts an ED visit. Although the majority of children with gastroenteritis have a history of diarrhea, other complaints—such as vomiting, fever, and abdominal pain—are common. Because of the multiple etiologic factors of the illness, the signs and symptoms vary depending on the age of the child and the cause of the illness (Table 15-2).

Emergency Department interventions. All children with a history of vomiting and/or diarrhea are assessed for the presence of dehydration. If signs of severe dehydration are exhibited, parenteral fluid bolus therapy is initiated. Diagnostic testing may include a complete blood count (CBC) (to identify leukocytosis), blood urea nitrogen (BUN) to determine the degree of hydration, and electrolytes. Although the white blood count (WBC) is usually within normal limits, leukocytosis—in conjunction with clinical findings—may indicate the presence of bacteremia or sepsis. As fluid volume is lost, the degree of metabolic acidosis is exhibited by a decrease in the bicarbonate level.

The stool examination may include methylene blue stool smears for the presence of PMN leukocytes and a stool culture if the child appears to have symptoms of toxicity or is febrile. The presence of sheets of polymorphonuclear leukocytes in the stool is strongly suggestive of *Shigella*. In addition, the stool is evaluated for the presence of blood and mucus, which are suggestive of *Campylobacter, Salmonella,* or *Shigella*.

Nursing care and evaluation. The approach to the child with gastroenteritis varies depending on the age of the child and the severity and suspected cause of the illness. The emergently ill child who has signs of severe dehydration, including weak pulses, delayed capillary refill, sunken fontanel, oliguria, and absence of tearing, will require rapid volume expansion with an initial intravenous (IV) bolus of 20 ml/kg of an isotonic solution such as lactated Ringer's solution or normal saline.

Children with mild to moderate dehydration may be treated with oral rehydration or parenteral fluid therapy. If the infant/child is able to tolerate oral intake, oral glucose-electrolyte solutions such as Pedialyte or Ricelyte can be used for rehydration. Some physicians recommend stopping lactose-containing formulas or products during the acute phase of the diarrhea; instead they recommend the use of soy formula. However, this practice has not been universally accepted. If formula or breast-feeding is continued in the infant, the diarrhea may become transiently worse; however, there is usually no prolongation of the total duration of diarrhea.[35]

If oral therapy is initiated and the child is to be discharged home, the nurse must convey to the family the importance of assessing the child for signs of dehydration. Additionally, if the child is vomiting, parents frequently attempt to replace vomited fluids immediately following emesis. They should be taught to allow the child's stomach to "rest" for 1 to 2 hours following emesis and then permit the child to have 1 ounce of fluids at frequent intervals until the child is able to tolerate large amounts of fluids without emesis.

Because all forms of infectious gastroenteritis are transmitted primarily by the fecal-oral route, parents should be instructed to keep diapered children out of day care until the infectious phase of the illness has subsided. In addition, meticulous handwashing and proper disposal of diapers will prevent the spread of infection to other family members.

STOMATITIS

Etiology. Stomatitis is characterized by infectious lesions or ulcerations within the oral cavity.

TABLE 15-2	Gastroenteritis		
ETIOLOGY	**CHARACTERISTICS**	**TESTING/TREATMENT**	**TRANSMISSION**
Rotavirus	Severe prolonged diarrhea illness Most common in children 3-15 mo Occurs predominantly in winter months Typically lasts 5-7 days (incubation is 1-3 days) Usually accompanied by fever and vomiting Occasionally seen with respiratory symptoms such as cough and rhinitis	CBC, electrolytes to assess for dehydration Treatment is symptomatic Fluid therapy for dehydration as indicated Stool for rotavirus	Spread by fecal-oral route Teach frequent handwashing Requires enteric precautions
Norwalk virus (*Calicivirus*)	Rapid onset Accompanied by vomiting, fever, and headache Occurs predominantly in winter months but is seen year-round Most common in older, school-age children Typically lasts 12-60 hr	Treatment as above	Spread by fecal-oral route, airborne droplets, or contaminated food or swimming pools Child remains infective for up to 2 days after resolution of symptoms Requires enteric precautions
Adenovirus	Watery diarrhea Vomiting (usually mild) Low-grade fever Typically lasts 5-12 days (incubation is 3-10 days) Occurs predominantly in children <2 yr	Treatment as above	Spread by fecal-oral route Requires enteric precautions
Campylobacter (gram-negative bacilli)	Profuse, watery diarrhea Blood and mucus may be seen in stool Can be accompanied by fever, headache, abdominal pain, or vomiting Most commonly lasts 3-5 days Incubation is 1-7 days but can be longer	Treatment is generally supportive CBC and electrolytes may be ordered to assess for dehydration and bacteremia Stool smear for Gram stain and culture Drug of choice is erythromycin (30-50 mg/kg/24 hr for 5-7 days); use is controversial; drug is said to eradicate organism from stool in 2-3 days	Spread by fecal-oral route or pet-to-person Requires enteric precautions

Continued.

TABLE 15-2	Gastroenteritis–cont'd		
Etiology	**Characteristics**	**Testing/treatment**	**Transmission**
Salmonella *S. enteritidis* *S. choleraesuis* *S. typhi* (gram-negative bacilli)	Watery diarrhea Blood and mucus may be seen in stool Primarily affects young children <5 yr; most commonly seen in infants <1 yr Accompanied by fever, vomiting, abdominal pain Typically lasts 3-5 days Severe cases can produce bacteremia and CNS signs	Treatment is supportive CBC and electrolytes may be ordered to assess for dehydration and bacteremia Stool smear for blood, Gram stain, and culture Obtain cultures of blood, urine, stool Antibiotic therapy is controversial; generally used only if bacteremia is suspected or child is immunocompromised	Transmission is by ingestion or fecal-oral route Vectors include animals, contaminated food (e.g., chicken or eggs), water, and humans Requires enteric precautions
Shigella *S. sonnei* *S. flexneri* (gram-negative bacilli)	Signs and symptoms range from mild to severe Watery diarrhea, with as many as 10-25 stools/day Blood and mucus may be seen in stool Most common in children <5 yr Accompanied by fever, malaise, and abdominal cramps May be associated with febrile seizures Is leading cause of bacterial gastroenteritis in Southwest	CBC and electrolytes may be ordered to assess for dehydration and bacteremia Stool smear for blood, Gram stain, and culture Obtain cultures of blood, urine, stool Treat with trimethoprim (10 mg) and sulfamethoxazole 50 mg/kg/day; *or* ampicillin 200 mg/kg/day for 5 days; *or* ceftriaxone (50 mg/kg/24 hr)—is more effective than ampicillin	Transmission is fecal-oral There is high intrafamilial attack rate Requires enteric precautions
Yersinia (gram-negative bacilli)	Watery diarrhea that may contain blood and mucus Accompanied by fever, occasional vomiting, and severe abdominal pain that can mimic appendicitis (pseudoappendicitis)	Treatment is generally supportive CBC and electrolytes may be ordered to assess for dehydration and bacteremia Stool for blood, Gram stain, and culture	Transmission is fecal-oral or food-borne, particularly uncooked pork or unpasteurized milk Requires enteric precautions

TABLE 15-2	Gastroenteritis–cont'd		
ETIOLOGY	CHARACTERISTICS	TESTING/TREATMENT	TRANSMISSION
Yersinia—cont'd	Symptoms may include headaches and pharyngitis Child may develop arthritis and skin rashes Classic triad of symptoms includes fever, rash, and abdominal pain	Obtain cultures of blood, urine, and stool Persistent diarrhea may be treated with antibiotic therapy (trimethoprim and sulfamethoxazole 10-50 mg/kg/24 hr)	

Data from Boenning DA: Diarrhea and gastroenteritis. In Barkin RM, ed: *Pediatric emergency medicine: concepts and clinical practice,* ed 2, St Louis, 1992, Mosby; Committee on Infectious Diseases, American Academy of Pediatrics: *1994 Redbook: report of the Committee on Infectious Diseases,* ed 23, Elk Grove Village, Ill, 1994, The Academy; Fleisher GR: Infectious disease emergencies. In Fleisher GR, Ludwig S, eds: *Textbook of pediatric emergency medicine,* ed 3, Baltimore, 1994, Williams & Wilkins.

Common causes of stomatitis in the child include herpes simplex virus (HSV), coxsackievirus, and *Candida albicans.* Primary HSV is called gingivostomatitis and is characterized by gingival inflammation, vesicles, and ulcers.

The coxsackievirus can produce herpangina, which is characterized as severe ulcerative lesions in the oral cavity and pharynx. *Candida albicans* infections produce thrush, characterized by white patches on the oral mucosa and tongue. (Thrush is reviewed in Chapter 28.)

Pathophysiology. There are two types of HSV, type 1 and type 2. HSV type 2 usually involves the genitalia and skin below the waist. HSV type 1 usually involves the skin above the waist. In adults it typically causes "cold sores." In children, particularly neonates, both viruses can be found in either site depending on the source of the infection.[5] For example, during the birth process HSV type 2 is transmitted from the mother to the infant via the birth canal. This serious infection can cause generalized systemic infection, CNS disease, or localized infections involving the skin, eyes, and mouth. In the majority of neonates the first sign of illness is vesicular skin lesions; occasionally, however, evidence of CNS involvement occurs before the lesions appear. In the latter situation the infant requires emergent management and hospitalization for treatment with acyclovir or vidarabine. Gingivostomatitis is a common manifestation associated with a primary HSV infection in the older preschooler.

Coxsackievirus is an enterovirus that contains both group A and group B types (e.g., type A16 causes hand, foot, and mouth syndrome). Depending on the type of infection with the coxsackievirus, symptoms can range from *herpangina* (vesicles in the oral and pharyngeal cavity) to GI symptoms, CNS infections, and respiratory infections.

Clinical presentation. Signs and symptoms of herpangina include vesicles and ulcerations on the soft palate, uvula, and tonsillar pillars. Fever, headaches, muscle pain, and/or vomiting are common associated findings. Older children generally complain of a sore throat and throat pain with eating. Younger children may cry during feeding or refuse the bottle. When these symptoms are combined with abdominal pain and vesicles on the palms, soles, and/or extremities, hand, foot, and mouth disease should be suspected.

Children with gingivostomatitis are typically younger than age 5 years, usually have a high fever, and can appear quite ill. Vesicles may be seen on the tongue, gingivae, and buccal mucosa. The parent often relates a history of irritability, refusal to eat or drink, and excessive drooling.

Emergency Department and nursing interventions. Stomatitis is generally a self-limited illness, with the children at greatest risk being those who are immunocompromised. Immunocompromised children require hospitalization and viral cultures to identify the origin of the infection. Otherwise healthy children will generally not require routine diagnostic testing. However, because the refusal to eat or drink is a common complaint all children are clinically evaluated for the presence of dehydration and treated with fluid volume as appropriate.

Discharge instructions may include symptomatic treatment of the lesions with a topical anesthetic such as viscous lidocaine, which is applied to the mucous membranes with a cotton swab. Since both HSV and coxsackievirus are transmitted via the fecal-oral route and from direct contact with infected secretions, parents are instructed to use frequent handwashing and proper diaper disposal to ensure that the infection is not spread to other children in the household. The incubation period can range from 3 to 6 days for herpangina and 2 to 14 days for gingivostomatitis, children with both infections may shed the virus for several weeks (occasionally months) after the symptoms have subsided.[5]

VIRAL HEPATITIS

Etiology. Viral hepatitis is characterized by acute inflammation of the liver and can be caused by a number of viruses. Hepatitis A virus (HAV) is the most common cause of hepatitis in the child, accounting for up to one third of all hepatitis A cases occurring in the United States.[2] Other forms of hepatitis include hepatitis B (HBV), hepatitis C (HCV) (formerly known as non-A, non-B hepatitis), hepatitis D (HDV), and hepatitis E (also formerly known as non-A, non-B hepatitis). Less common causes of hepatitis include cytomegalovirus, herpesvirus, Epstein-Barr virus (EBV), varicella-zoster, rubella, and coxsackievirus B.

Depending on the etiologic basis, hepatitis can be self-limited, with complete regeneration of the liver cells; subacute or chronic, which is characterized by progressive liver destruction; or fulminant, characterized by acute liver failure and encephalopathy, which is often fatal.[47]

Fulminant hepatic failure can result from any of the viral causes of hepatitis, as well as other causes such as Reye's syndrome or acetaminophen toxicity. It is defined as severe, sudden hepatocellular injury (liver failure) and progresses rapidly.

Pathophysiology. Viral hepatitis is a progressive disorder that causes hepatic cellular necrosis. As liver damage occurs, hepatic dysfunction can result in a variety of symptoms, the most obvious of which is jaundice. Jaundice caused by hepatitis is categorized as an "obstructive" jaundice because the bilirubin formed in the blood cannot pass from the liver into the intestines for excretion. The result is that conjugated (direct) bilirubin is returned to the bloodstream. When severe obstructive jaundice occurs, the kidneys excrete significant quantities of conjugated bilirubin, causing the urine to become an intense yellow.[13] Additionally, diseases of the liver, such as hepatitis, can depress formation of clotting factors such as prothrombin because of poor vitamin K absorption in the GI tract or as a result of diseased liver cells.[13]

Clinical presentation. Presentation varies depending on the etiologic factors. During the initial phase of the illness the child may have vague symptoms of nausea or vomiting, abdominal discomfort, anorexia, malaise, and fever (which may be low grade). Because these symptoms are compatible with a flulike illness, uncomplicated or early cases of hepatitis may be missed or may resolve spontaneously (usually HAV).

The abdominal examination will reveal hepatomegaly, which may or may not be accompanied by splenomegaly. As the disease progresses, the icteric (jaundice) phase begins as evidenced by yellow skin and sclera. Urine becomes dark yellow, and stools are light or pasty in color. If coagulopathies are present, ecchymosis or purpura may be seen on the skin.

Emergency Department interventions. Initial management depends on the presenting symptoms. If the child arrives with signs of acute hepatic failure, emergent interventions are required. Most children, however, are brought to the ED with vague symptoms of illness or jaundice. To make the definitive diagnosis of hepatitis and to identify the cause, serologic testing is required (Table 15-3). Because serologic testing can take days to complete, a thorough history can often point to the source of infection, for example, a needle-stick or ingestion of raw shellfish. Additional, laboratory data include a CBC and differential, erythrocyte sedimentation rate (ESR); blood chemistries; liver function studies (no liver function study is specific for hepatitis); bilirubin; prothrombin time and partial prothrombin time (PT and PTT); and a urine test for bilirubin.

Nursing care and evaluation. Nursing care depends on the severity and cause of the disease. If the child has fulminant hepatic failure and/or coagulopa-

TABLE 15-3	Viral Hepatitis			
AGENT	TRANSMISSION	INCUBATION	SEROLOGY	TREATMENT
Hepatitis A (HAV)	Fecal-oral; food-water; spreads in day care centers and areas of poor sanitation	15-50 days; average of 25-30 days	Anti-HAV; IgM specific anti-HAV	Supportive; there is no vaccine; control measures include immune globulin (IG) 0.02 ml/kg; meticulous handwashing; proper disposal of diapers; enteric precautions
Hepatitis B (HBV)	Blood (transfusions, shared needles); body fluids (wounds, exudates, semen, saliva); can survive in dried state for 1 wk or longer	45-160 days; average of 120 days	HBsAg; anti-HBs; HBeAg; anti-HBe; anti-HBc (HBcAg); IgM anti-HBc	Supportive; can be prevented with hepatitis B vaccine (HBV); following exposure both hepatitis B vaccine and hepatitis B immune globulin (HBIG) can be administered; universal and enteric precautions
Hepatitis C (HCV)	Parenteral transmission of blood or blood products; may be sexually transmitted; in many cases no source or risk factor is found	7-9 wk; average of 2-24 wk	Anti-HCV—may be absent during acute illness; has high rate of false positivity	Supportive; alpha-interferon has been approved for use in some cases of HCV; universal precautions
Hepatitis D (delta virus) (HDV)	HDV is a "helper virus" that cannot produce infection without presence of acute or chronic HBV; transmission may be parenteral, percutaneous, or via mucous membranes (same as HBV)	HDV suprainfection, 2-8 wk; HDV coinfection with HBV 24-160 days	Anti-HDV	Supportive; universal and enteric precautions
Hepatitis E (HEV)	Fecal-oral; water; more common in adults than children	Approximately 40 days; range of 15-60 days	No serologic test available	Supportive; universal and enteric precautions

Modified from Committee on Infectious Diseases, American Academy of Pediatrics: Abstracted from Peter G: *1994 Redbook: Report of the Committee on Infectious Diseases*, ed 23, Elk Grove Village, Ill, 1994, The Academy, pp 221-241.

thies, immediate stabilization of the ABCs (airway, breathing, and circulation) and continuous monitoring are required. All fluid intake and output is measured, and the nurse should anticipate fluid restriction (usually two thirds of maintenance). Hyponatremia is a common finding, but it is usually caused by fluid retention (dilutional hyponatremia) rather than by overall sodium losses. Affected children should be transferred to a pediatric intensive care unit as soon as they are stabilized.

The majority of children with hepatitis are clinically stable, requiring only supportive nursing care and parental education. With some forms of hepatitis, such as HBV, pharmacologic agents such as hepatitis B immune globulin (HBIG) or hepatitis B vaccine may be administered. Since children may feel "ill" or tired, they generally wish to stay in bed and activities are self-limited by the illness. Parents are instructed to observe the child for signs of dehydration, frank lethargy, increasing jaundice, or bleeding problems. If any of these symptoms are observed, the parent should seek immediate medical attention. In addition, parents are informed that hepatitis is contagious and that proper handwashing and isolation can prevent the spread of the infection to other family members or friends. Depending on the cause of the hepatitis, family members may require prophylaxis.

▌ SURGICAL CONDITIONS

INTUSSUSCEPTION

Etiology. Intussusception is the telescoping of one loop of bowel into the next, more distal segment. In the majority of cases intussusception begins at or near the ileocecal valve, although it may occur at any level of the small intestine or the large intestine.

Intussusception is the most frequent surgical cause of acute intestinal obstruction in infants and young children. The majority of intussusceptions are idiopathic, occurring in otherwise healthy children between 3 months and 5 years of age. Approximately 50% of the cases are seen in infants between 3 and 12 months of age, and the condition is three times more common in males than in females.[12]

In infants predisposing factors are thought to include adenovirus or rotavirus infections. In children older than 2 years intussusception is often associated with an organic lesion in the small bowel, the most common of which is a Meckel's diverticulum. Intussusception is often preceded by an illness such as a viral

syndrome, constipation, parasites, or an ingested foreign body.

Pathophysiology. When the proximal portion of the intestine telescopes into the distal portion there is constriction of the mesentery which compromises blood supply to the intestine. Obstructed venous return produces cellular edema and inflammation. With cellular damage there is an increase in mucous production, which, when mixed with bloody fluid leaking from the engorged bowel, forms the classic "currant-jelly" stool. As the edema increases and the obstruction worsens, impaired mesenteric arterial supply results in necrosis of the intestine and eventual perforation and peritonitis (Fig. 15-4).

Clinical presentation. The initial symptom of intussusception is often colicky abdominal pain with a sudden cry or scream reported by the parent. Thereafter, during recurrent episodes of acute pain, screaming and drawing up of the infant's knees alternating

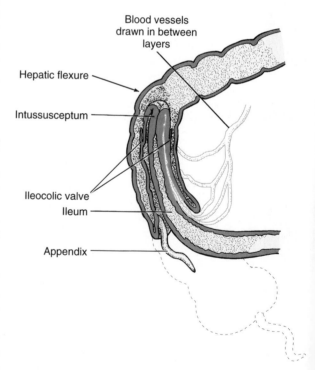

FIG. 15-4. Intussusception. (From Wong DL: *Whaley and Wong's nursing care of infants and children*, ed 5, St Louis, 1997, Mosby.)

with calm, recovery periods may be observed. Lethargy and apathy commonly occur between the episodes of pain, and cases have been documented in which lethargy is the sole feature; this condition is called painless intussusception.[7] The infant may become still and may manifest an unusual grayish type of pallor, demonstrating a shocklike state. This condition is sometimes misdiagnosed as a postictal state until the infant passes a bloody stool.[43] Lethargy and irritability are features that correlate well with the degree of bowel viability, fluid deficiency, electrolyte imbalance, and blood loss.[42]

Vomiting occurs in many children with intussusception; neonates usually have vomiting and irritability. As the obstruction progresses, bilious vomiting may occur along with abdominal distention. Abdominal palpation may reveal a nontender, sausage-shaped mass in the middle or upper right abdomen; bowel sounds may be absent on auscultation in the right lower quadrant (Dance's sign).

Early in the course of the obstructive process there is no passing of the classic currant-jelly stool, although blood may be revealed on the finger if a rectal examination is performed. Later, as the obstructive process continues and the mesenteric arterial supply is affected, the currant-jelly stool may be passed spontaneously. These characteristic stools are predominantly found in children younger than 1 year (Box 15-3).[29]

Emergency Department interventions. All interventions depend on the duration of symptoms and whether specific medical treatment or surgical therapy is required. Because many infants and children with intussusception do not initially demonstrate the classic triad of symptoms (colicky abdominal pain, vomiting, and rectal bleeding), the diagnosis requires a radiographic demonstration by contrast enema with barium or air as the contrast medium. Plain radiographs can reveal variable findings and may show a "coiled spring" of bowel with surrounding air fluid levels.[29]

The intussusception often can be reduced by a barium or air enema if it is performed in less than 48 hours of the onset of symptoms.[42] Emergency surgical reduction is required for children in whom the contrast enema is unsuccessful or those who have a bowel perforation. Laboratory analysis of CBC, BUN, and serum electrolytes is performed. Blood is obtained for a crossmatch, before proceeding to the radiology department.

Nursing care and evaluation. Infants and children suspected of having intussusception are treated emergently. On arrival in the ED, nursing interventions are initiated; these include obtaining a complete set of vital signs, assessing hydration status, and placing the child on a cardiac monitor. If signs of shock are present, the ABCs of care are initiated, and bolus therapy is begun.

All affected children are designated as NPO (nothing by mouth). If signs of dehydration are present, an intravenous infusion of lactated Ringer's solution or normal saline solution is begun. Depending on the degree of dehydration, an initial bolus of 10 to 20 ml/kg may be required, with additional bolus therapy based on reassessments of circulatory status. The child may require insertion of a nasogastric tube to relieve gastric distention, minimize the risk of vomiting and aspiration, and relieve pressure on the diaphragm.

Pain management is an important consideration in the nursing care of infants and children with intussusception. An IV dose of morphine 0.1 mg/kg or the use of another appropriate analgesic offers the child pain relief and affords enough relaxation for radiography.[40]

Parents and the affected child are often fearful and feel helpless. Simple explanations or drawing a picture may help both the child and family members understand the procedures. A bear or doll used in play therapy or diversional activity can also serve to demonstrate IV therapy, nasogastric suction, vital sign monitoring, and preoperative routines such as identification bands and NPO status.

Box 15-3   Clinical Manifestations of Intussusception

- Sudden, acute abdominal pain
- Recurrent, colicky abdominal pain (may alternate with periods of lethargy)
- Tender, distended abdomen
- Vomiting
- Bloody stools mixed with mucus, or "currant jelly" appearance (late sign)
- Lethargy
- Absent bowel sounds in lower right quadrant (Dance's sign)
- Nontender sausage-shaped mass in middle or upper right abdomen

APPENDICITIS

Etiology. Appendicitis is an inflammation of the veriform appendix. It may be classified as simple (the appendix is inflamed and intact), gangrenous (the appendix has focal or extensive necrosis with microscopic perforations), or perforated (the appendix is grossly disrupted).[44] Appendicitis is caused by an obstruction of the lumen of the appendix followed by inflammation and compromise in blood flow. Etiologic factors include a fecalith (hard lump of feces), parasites, and edema of the lymphoid tissue in response to a viral or bacterial infection or, rarely, by a kinking of the appendix.

Acute appendicitis is the most common surgical emergency in childhood. Its peak incidence occurs from 9 to 12 years of age, and the condition is characterized by a male predominance. There is an increased incidence of perforation in infants and children younger than 4 years, with a corresponding higher risk of mortality and morbidity. Delays of more than 36 hours after the onset of pain correlate with the highest rate of perforation.[23,32]

Pathophysiology. In appendicitis, inflammation disrupts the arterial blood supply, causing mucosal ulceration, which allows bacteria to invade the wall of the appendix. Ischemia and infarction result as the infection and edema further impede blood flow. The appendix becomes necrotic and gangrenous and may then perforate, causing the release of bowel bacteria into the abdominal cavity. Perforation is thought to occur more often in children than in adults because the wall of the appendix in a child is very thin. In addition, the immature omentum may not provide protection against the development of peritonitis.[21,32]

Pain associated with appendicitis is one of the first signs of inflammatory swelling. Pain signals are transmitted by stretch receptors located in the small vessels of the appendix along mesenteric nerve fibers. Periumbilical pain that becomes localized and intense, moving to the right lower quadrant results from irritation of the parietal peritoneum by small quantities of leaking inflammatory fluid. When the gangrenous or perforated appendix leaks luminal contents through the appendiceal wall, the child may feel abrupt yet temporary pain relief as intraluminal pressure is relieved. The pain will recur and intensify as localized, and then generalized peritonitis develops.

Clinical presentation. The degree of progression of the disease determines the clinical findings in the child. Classically, the older child has presenting symptoms of a sudden onset of crampy abdominal pain in the epigastric or periumbilical area that peaks and then subsides in a few hours. The pain may then reappear in the right lower quadrant, becoming progressively severe as signs of peritoneal irritation are observed (Box 15-4).

Vomiting is a symptom of great significance in children. Therefore appendicitis should be suspected in any patient who is 2 to 16 years of age with any two of the following signs and symptoms: vomiting, guarding, abdominal tenderness, and right lower quadrant pain.[33] Anorexia, diarrhea, constipation, urinary frequency, and urinary urgency also may be present. The child may walk with an exaggerated lumbar lordosis and a slightly flexed hip. Respirations are often rapid and shallow. The child with pain of peritoneal origin may grunt at the start of each expiration in an attempt to splint the diaphragm. This can result in hypoventilation and subsequent atelectasis in the lung bases.

Signs of perforation include progressively increasing fever, tachycardia, and flushed or excessively pale skin. Young children are difficult to evaluate because crying produces abdominal rigidity and such children are unable to verbalize, express, or localize pain.

Emergency Department interventions. Because the diagnosis of appendicitis is not always evident, a complete workup is usually indicated.

Box 15-4 Signs and Symptoms of Appendicitis

- Pain increasing with any movement
- Voluntary then involuntary guarding (abdominal wall contraction) whenever child's abdomen is approached
- Tenderness to palpation
- Rebound tenderness (pain following release of firm pressure placed on abdominal wall by palms of hand)
- Right lower quadrant pain with McBurney's point being location of maximum tenderness (midway between iliac crest and umbilicus)

Such a workup generally includes a CBC and differential; serum electrolytes; abdominal x-ray films, both upright and flat plate (may reveal calcified fecalith, perforation [if it has occurred], or free air in the abdominal cavity); chest x-ray films to rule out pneumonia; and urinalysis to rule out UTI. Abdominal ultrasonography may be considered when appendicitis is suspected in clinically atypical presentations because it may enable earlier diagnosis and thereby reduce complications. The WBC is not generally useful in making the diagnosis, since it is often normal or only slightly elevated. However, polymorphonuclear leukocytes and bands may be elevated on the differential. Treatment is not delayed when a child is suspected of having appendicitis because a high risk of appendiceal perforation is involved.

Nursing care and evaluation. Appendicitis can be difficult to identify because the classic clinical findings are not uniformly present. The nurse should therefore repeatedly observe and evaluate the child and inform the physician of changes in the child's clinical status. Because appendicitis is a progressive illness, manifestations will increase as time passes. The degree of progression of the disease determines the urgency of the care required[16] (Fig. 15-5).

Since many children with appendicitis come to the ED with complaints of vomiting, diarrhea, and/or decreased fluid intake, they are evaluated for the presence of dehydration and/or signs and symptoms of shock.

Infants and children with suspected appendiceal perforation and/or generalized peritonitis require venous access and parenteral fluid therapy to maintain fluid and electrolyte balance and to correct fluid losses. Strict monitoring of intake and output is required. Before surgery the child is continuously observed for the development of signs of shock. Antibiotic therapy with cefoxitin or triple antibiotics (ampicillin, gentamicin, and clindamycin) is generally initiated before surgery to cover the most common intestinal organisms. Preoperative antibiotic administration is particularly indicated when peritonitis is suspected.

All children are assessed for pain. This assessment includes a description of the type of pain, duration, and changes in location. Not only is this information useful in determining the diagnosis of appendicitis and peritonitis; it is also used as a guide in pain management.

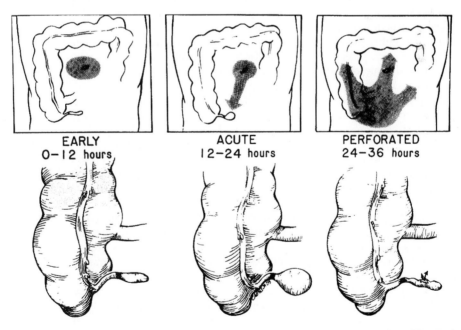

FIG. 15-5. Acute abdomen in children. (From Hatch EI: The acute abdomen in the child, *Pediatr Clin North Am* 32[5]:1153, 1985.)

When surgery is imminent, the ED nurse may help to alleviate fear by providing simple explanations and/or drawing pictures of the condition for the child and parent. Explanations to children should be made in age-appropriate language. Doll play, complete with a surgical scar, is helpful in demonstrating to a child that nothing will "fall out" of the location of the surgery. It is also beneficial in explaining IV therapy and other preoperative interventions in a nonthreatening manner.

MALROTATION OF THE BOWEL WITH VOLVULUS

Etiology. Malrotation of the bowel is a congenital anomaly associated with abnormal fixation of the intestines around the mesentery during the 10th week of gestation. Malrotation most often appears in the first month of life, but it can go unrecognized until childhood.

Pathophysiology. Classic malrotation of the intestine results from failure of the fetal bowel to rotate around the superior mesenteric artery. This results in varying degrees of obstruction of the duodenum at the points of abnormal fixation. Volvulus, which is twisting of the small intestine, results in strangulation of the superior mesenteric artery and leads to intestinal obstruction, vascular compromise, and intestinal loss. Midgut volvulus compromises the blood supply to the entire small intestine and the ascending colon, producing complete obstruction that leads to necrosis (Fig. 15-6). If this condition is not immediately treated, bowel perforation with peritonitis coupled with severe fluid and electrolyte disturbances will result, producing hypovolemic and septic shock.[4]

Clinical presentation. In the neonate volvulus usually is signaled by severe intestinal obstruction exhibited by sudden and constant abdominal pain, visible peristalsis, and bilious vomiting. Heme-positive or bloody stools may then appear, indicating vascular compromise of the bowel. Progressive abdominal distention may be observed as the obstructive process continues.

Although older children may initially have acute attacks of abdominal pain, bilious vomiting, and shock, they may also first have mild attacks of recurrent abdominal pain and episodic vomiting. Symptoms may persist for months until a more severe attack leads to evaluation and diagnosis.

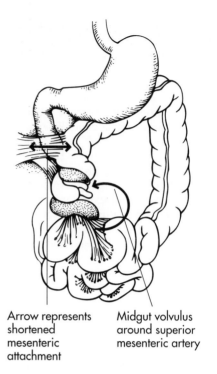

Arrow represents shortened mesenteric attachment

Midgut volvulus around superior mesenteric artery

FIG. 15-6. Volvulus. (Redrawn from Fleisher G. Ludwig S, eds: *Textbook of pediatric emergency medicine,* ed 3, Baltimore, 1993, Williams & Wilkins.

Emergency Department interventions. Complete volvulus of the bowel is an extremely serious condition in which bowel loss becomes eminent after 1 to 2 hours of total obstruction of the blood supply. The incidence of perforation, peritonitis, and extensive intestinal necrosis makes the neonate's prognosis guarded.[17] Rapid cardiovascular stabilization, IV fluid management, and nasogastric decompression are required. Surgical intervention is the top priority.

Blood is drawn for a CBC, electrolytes, and BUN, and a urinalysis is obtained. In addition, blood is held for typing and crossmatch. Abdominal x-ray films, such as a flat plate of the abdomen and a cross-table lateral plate, are usually ordered. Other testing may include an air contrast study, an upper GI with barium swallow, and/or an ultrasound of the abdomen.

Nursing care and evaluation. Infants and children with suspected volvulus are treated emergently. They require stabilization of the ABCs and constant monitoring. Venous access is indicated. If signs of shock are present, the child will require volume resuscitation with 20 ml/kg boluses of an isotonic

---

| Box 15-5 | Nursing Care of the Child with Suspected Bowel Obstruction or Perforation |

- Stabilize airway and breathing
- Observe for signs of shock; if shock is present, administer supplemental oxygen; obtain vascular access
- Place child on heart rate monitor and pulse oximeter; obtain vital signs (including blood pressure)
- Administer parenteral fluid therapy as required; if shock is present, isotonic fluid boluses will be required; prepare to correct electrolyte disturbances
- Observe mental status: infant/child may be irritable or frankly lethargic
- Maintain normothermia: infants and young children may become hypothermic rapidly
- Insert nasogastric tube and connect to low suction for gastric decompression
- Obtain laboratory work for CBC, electrolytes, BUN, glucose, and hold clot for type and cross match
- Anticipate antibiotic therapy
- Prepare child and family for surgery
- Continuously monitor vital signs, mental status, hydration status, and intake and output while child is in ED

---

solution such as normal saline or lactated Ringer's solution. A nasogastric tube is inserted and attached to constant low-pressure suction for gastric decompression (Box 15-5).

The nurse should anticipate that the infant/child will require surgery (or be transferred to a pediatric center) and make the appropriate arrangements. Because this is a rapidly progressive illness, the nurse (and when possible the physician) accompanies the child during all radiographic testing. When bowel perforation is suspected or surgery is anticipated, parenteral antibiotic therapy is initiated.

The infant/child awaiting surgical correction is maintained on a heart rate monitor and pulse oximeter and is continuously monitored for signs of shock. All fluid intake and output is measured and recorded.

Because this illness progresses rapidly, parents are often upset and confused by the aggressive pace with which interventions take place. The ED nurse should make every effort to keep the parents informed of all

treatments and allow the parents to remain with the infant/child whenever possible.

INCARCERATED HERNIAS

Etiology. A hernia is a congenital anomaly that allows the protrusion of an organ through an abnormal opening in the musculature. The small bowel, cecum, ovary, fallopian tube, or appendix may be caught inside the hernial sac. Incarcerated hernias result when a portion of bowel becomes entrapped in the hernial sac and cannot be reduced. They may develop in children with inguinal, femoral, scrotal, or umbilical hernias, although inguinal hernias are the most common cause of incarceration. Incarcerated hernias threaten the loss of testis, ovary, or a portion of bowel.

The risk of incarceration of an inguinal hernia is about 30% in infants younger than 1 year. Boys are six times more likely than girls to have an inguinal hernia. However, the incidence of incarceration in childhood is 12% to 15%, with the higher risk in females as compared with males, regardless of age.[39]

Pathophysiology. Incarcerated or strangulated hernias develop when a portion of bowel or other organ becomes entrapped in the hernial sac. As the blood supply is diminished, edema develops with a decrease in venous return. Intestinal obstruction results. If this condition is left untreated, the bowel or other entrapped organs become gangrenous.

Clinical presentation. Initially parents may notice a bulging mass in the groin or umbilicus when the infant cries or strains. In the early stages these hernias may be reducible. When the mass is associated with irritability, abdominal pain, and/or vomiting, incarceration may have occurred. As symptoms progress, localized tenderness and swelling over the mass increase, the skin over the mass becomes erythematous and discolored, and abdominal distention worsens.

Emergency Department interventions. ED treatment is dependent on the severity of illness. If the infant or child has signs of incarceration, emergent management is required. Fortunately, however, most children are clinically stable initially, and the majority of hernias can be manually reduced in the ED.

Before operative intervention the surgeon may attempt to reduce the hernia manually. Sedation with a short-acting narcotic, benzodiazapine, or both aids in reduction attempts in the tense, crying infant or child.[40] After sedation the child may be placed in the Trendelenburg position, with a cold pack placed over the groin, to let gravity aid in reduction of the hernia; or gentle manual reduction may be attempted. When manual reduction of the incarceriatied hernia is successful, the child (particularly the infant) is occasionally admitted for elective surgical repair.[36] If manual reduction is unsuccessful, emergent operative intervention is indicated.

Nursing care and evaluation. When sedation is used to facilitate the manual reduction of an incarcerated hernia, cardiac monitoring and pulse oximetry are required. Emergency airway equipment must be readily available. If an obstruction is suspected, the infant or child is designated as NPO and monitored continuously for signs of shock, which may result secondary to the gangrenous or perforated bowel. Intravenous therapy and insertion of a nasogastric tube are indicated.

PYLORIC STENOSIS

Etiology. Pyloric stenosis is a gastric outlet obstruction at the pyloric sphincter that results from a hypertrophied pyloric muscle. The cause remains controversial. Although the cause was previously viewed as congenital, it is now thought to be a developmental sequence that begins in utero and is completed in the early neonatal period. Theories regarding environmental factors such as maternal drug use and maternal anxiety also have been implicated in the incidence of the disease[19] as have peptide abnormalities in nerve fibers and cells.[45]

Pyloric stenosis is more likely to develop in siblings of children with this condition, and it occurs four times more often in children of mothers who had the disease as infants than in those whose fathers had the condition.[11] The disorder occurs most often in firstborn males, with a 5:1 male/female incidence. The age of onset is usually 2 to 5 weeks. Rarely are symptoms observed at birth or after the fourth month of life.[31]

Pathophysiology. The inner circular muscle layer of the stomach spreads out in the pyloric canal in two layers known as the right and left canalis loops. It is the hypertrophy and hyperplasia of these circular and longitudinal muscle layers that obstruct the lumen by compressing the mucosa. In the first few weeks of life the whole pylorus thickens, assuming an olive shape with a narrowing of the pyloric lumen. Initially partial obstruction occurs; this is followed by almost total obstruction. The constant peristaltic effort to move the gastric contents through the narrowed pyloric channel results in marked stomach dilation with hypertrophied musculature. Gastritis with mucosal bleeding may occur with the persistent vomiting from the luminal obstruction.

Clinical presentation. The infant with pyloric stenosis most often has presenting symptoms in the fourth to sixth week of life, with the parent complaining of forceful projectile vomiting. During the first to second week of life, there may have been only minimal regurgitation after feedings. However, as the degree of luminal obstruction increases, forceful vomiting occurs with every feeding (Box 15-6).

Vomiting associated with pyloric stenosis is nonbilious, and the amount is usually consistent with the most recent feeding. If gastritis occurs or if the gastric mucosal capillaries rupture during forceful vomiting, emesis will contain frank blood or coffee-ground type of material. The classic symptom of projectile vomiting is usually seen in the later stages of the illness.

Following an episode of vomiting, infants with pyloric stenosis are hungry and suck eagerly, yet they will continue to vomit after each feeding. Parents often report that the infant's stools have decreased in amount and frequency because only small amounts of material have passed through the pylorus. Peristaltic waves may be seen moving from the left to the right upper quadrant of the abdomen. On physical assessment an olive-sized mass, the hypertrophied pylorus, often can be palpated in the upper right quadrant (to the right of the midline, just above the umbilicus). Initial weight loss is due to dehydration, and about one

---

Box 15-6   Clinical Presentation of Pyloric Stenosis

- History of minimal vomiting following birth that progresses to projectile vomiting by 4 to 6 weeks of life
- Later history of vomiting with every feeding, even though infant appears hungry
- History of weight loss
- History of decreased stooling
- Signs of dehydration (e.g. decreased urination, sunken eyes)
- Presence of peristaltic waves of abdomen
- Palpation of olive-sized mass in abdomen

third of infants with pyloric stenosis have severe dehydration as a presenting symptom.[11] Dehydration with metabolic alkalosis, hypochloremia, and hypokalemia occurs as a result of hydrogen ion and chloride losses resulting from the persistent vomiting.

Emergency Department interventions. Pyloric stenosis is a clinical diagnosis based on the history and physical examination. In atypical cases measurement of the length of the pyloric canal may be performed with ultrasonography. If ultrasonography is unavailable, the barium swallow method is used; the presence of a narrow pylorus or the "string sign" is diagnostic of the condition. Because vomiting and aspiration may occur in the child with pyloric stenosis, a surgical consultation is usually obtained before any upper GI radiologic studies are considered.[10]

ED management depends on the severity of the illness. If the child has presenting signs of dehydration or shock, emergent management is indicated. Blood is drawn for a CBC, electrolytes, and BUN, and a urinalysis is obtained. The persistent vomiting associated with pyloric stenosis can lead to hypochloremic alkalosis because chloride is lost and the pH level rises. Additional laboratory findings include deficits in both sodium and potassium.

Treatment requires correction of electrolyte imbalances and surgical repair of the pyloris. Following successful repair, infants are usually discharged from the hospital after 3 days. The pyloric diameter, length, and muscle thickness return to the normal range within 2 to 3 months.

Nursing care and evaluation. The initial goal of therapy is to correct dehydration and electrolyte abnormalities. Because of deficits in sodium, potassium, and chloride, 5% dextrose in normal saline (sodium chloride) solution with supplemental potassium (up to 30–50 mEq/L) may be ordered. Before potassium is administered, renal function must be confirmed (the child must void). High-dose potassium administration requires the use of an IV pump and continuous cardiovascular monitoring. Surgery may be delayed until the child's hydration status is improved and electrolyte values have been corrected.

Gastric decompression with a nasogastric tube is required before surgery and will prevent postoperative vomiting.

The infant is continuously monitored; this monitoring includes frequent measurement of vital signs, assessment of respiratory rate and character, and cardiovascular status. All fluid intake and output is recorded, with attention given to the type of vomiting and the character of stools. Because affected infants may become hypothermic, a normal body temperature can be maintained by wrapping the infant and covering the head or by providing overbed warming (Box 15-7).

The infant's parents may be upset and confused by the diagnosis. The ED nurse should make every effort to keep the parents informed and should allow them to stay with their infant whenever possible.

HIRSCHSPRUNG'S DISEASE

Etiology. Hirschsprung's disease (congenital aganglionic megacolon) is a disorder of the peristaltic activity of the large intestine that interferes with the normal mechanism of defecation. It is caused by the absence of ganglionic cells in the submucosal and muscular layers of the colon.

Hirschsprung's disease is the most common cause of intestinal obstruction in the neonate; failure to pass meconium accounts for 33% of all neonatal obstruc-

---

Box 15-7   Nursing Interventions for the Child with Pyloric Stenosis

- Assess and stabilize ABCs
- Place child on cardiac monitor and pulse oximeter
- Obtain venous access
- Anticipate fluid administration
- Anticipate administration of high-dose (30–50 mEq/kg) potassium
  Potassium should not be given until renal function has been established (child has voided)
  Must be administered with IV pump
  Child must be on a cardiac monitor
- Insert nasogastric tube, as ordered
- Maintain strict monitoring of input and output
- Maintain normothermia: overbed warmer, warm blankets
- Communicate with family often, keeping them informed of treatment plans
- Allow family to remain with child as much as possible
- Reassess child's status frequently: vital signs, neurologic status, and perfusion

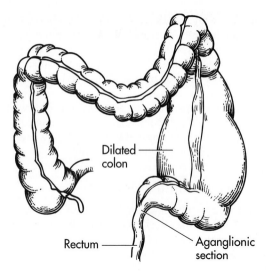

FIG. 15-7. Hirschsprung's disease.

tions.[12] The incidence is approximately 1 in 500 live births with 4:1 male predominance.[23] Approximately 10% to 15% of the affected infants have Down syndrome.[6]

Pathophysiology. The aganglionic segment may involve only a few centimeters of colon at the rectum, or it may involve the entire colon, producing a functional obstruction. Obstruction occurs because the affected bowel lacks the normal propulsive waves and contracts as a whole in response to distention.[6] The denervated segment is narrowed, with dilation and enlargement of the proximal uninvolved colon (Fig. 15-7).

Clinical presentation. The clinical presentation of Hirschsprung's disease is variable. It can appear in the neonatal period with failure to pass meconium in the first 48 hours of life or it may be associated with vomiting, abdominal distention, and shock. In childhood, if the disease persists untreated, it may be associated with chronic or intermittent constipation and abdominal enlargement.[30]

The classic symptom is failure to pass meconium in the first 48 hours of life. If the condition is undiagnosed during the early neonatal period, symptoms appear later as abdominal distention and constipation, with a bowel movement occurring only in response to suppositories or formula changes. Later-appearing symptoms of partial intestinal obstruction include abdominal distention and bilious vomiting.

The infant may develop acute episodes of enterocolitis manifested by fever and explosive diarrhea, (reported in about 50% of neonates with Hirschsprung's disease).[6]

Later in infancy the child will have alternating constipation and diarrhea as presenting symptoms, whereas the older child will initially have chronic constipation. Stools are described as foul smelling, thin, and ribbonlike and are associated with abdominal distention and palpable fecal masses. On rectal examination the rectum may feel narrowed and little or no fecal matter may be felt.

Emergency Department interventions. Children with Hirschsprung's disease may come to the ED with mild to severe signs of illness. If symptoms such as explosive bloody diarrhea or signs of peritonitis and shock are present, emergent management is required. Fortunately, the most common presenting complaint is persistent constipation. Children with this complaint are given supportive care and laboratory and radiographic studies are ordered. Blood for a CBC and electrolytes may be required to evaluate for fluid and electrolyte imbalances. Abdominal x-ray examination may reveal largely dilated loops of intestines and the absence of gas in the pelvic colon. A barium enema will reveal dilation of the bowel proximal to the narrow segment of the colon. Definitive diagnosis is made by suction rectal biopsy, with the patient under anesthesia, and microscopic demonstration of the absence of intramural ganglion cells.

Treatment depends on the child's age and general condition. Rectal irrigations are indicated to decompress the colon of the neonate, to treat enterocolitis, and to remove fecal impactions in older children.

Definitive treatment may include the surgical insertion of a temporary colostomy, which is performed if the child has enterocolitis; in younger children, when irrigations fail; and in older children, when a largely distended colon and malnourishment are involved. Resection of the bowel is performed later. In infants resection is delayed until at least 6 months of age. In older children resection is performed when good nutritional status has been achieved.

Nursing care and evaluation. As with any child, stabilization of the ABCs is required, with particular attention given to the child's hydration status and potential for shock. If the infant/child is stable, the bowel may be emptied and cleansed with colonic irrigations (Table 15-4). Isotonic solutions

		TABLE 15-4 Procedure for Rectal Irrigation	

AGE	FLUID AMOUNT (ML)	TUBE INSERTION (INCHES)
Newborn	15-20	1
Infant	120-240	1-1½
2-4 yr	240-360	2-3
4-10 yr	360-480	2-3
≥11 yr	480-720	3-4

Procedure
- Positioning:
  - Child or infant—left side with right leg flexed 45 degrees or both knees drawn up to chest
  - Infant or toddler—on back with legs flexed upward
- Use warmed saline solution (do not use tap water or soapsuds)
- Use 16 Fr (for newborn) or 20-28 Fr (older child) catheter with lubricated tip for fluid delivery
- Use gravity drain to deliver fluid after air has been expelled from tubing (do not use pressure)
- Elimination:
  - Infant or toddler—hold child's buttocks together for several minutes and place large diaper or bedpan under child
  - Older child—allow child to sit on bed pan or assist child to potty chair
- Repeat procedure until fluid expelled is clear of stool
- Monitor infant/child throughout procedure

Modified from Raffensperger, 1990; Wong, 1997.

are used for rectal irrigations in infants and children because soapsuds enemas and tap-water enemas can cause water intoxication.[6]

When fluid and electrolyte abnormalities are identified, parenteral IV therapy is initiated. If signs and symptoms of shock are present, particularly in the child with abdominal distention and suspected peritonitis or perforation, fluid resuscitation is required. A nasogastric tube is indicated to decompress the stomach and to prevent vomiting and possible aspiration. Before surgery an antibiotic bowel preparation is required.

▌LIVER TRANSPLANTS

ETIOLOGY

Since the first liver transplant was performed in 1963, liver transplantation has become a viable option in the treatment of liver failure in both adults and children. In the early days of this approach to treatment, mortality rates were high. However, with advances in immunosuppressive drug therapy survival rates have increased. Currently short-term survival rates are as high as 70% to 80%.[46]

At least one half of the children in the United States who require liver transplants have biliary atresia. These children represent one third of all patients, both adults and children, who require liver transplants.[48] Other indications for liver transplant in the child include inborn errors of metabolism, familial cholestasis (arrested flow of bile), fulminant hepatic failure, neonatal hepatitis, congenital hepatic fibrosis, toxic hepatitis, and trauma.

PATHOPHYSIOLOGY

The liver performs a variety of functions, and it affects every other organ and system within the body. Therefore when irreversible liver failure occurs, the child's only chance for survival is transplantation. Although suitably sized cadaver donors are ideal, the lack of available donors, particularly for children, has led to the development of several different proposals. These include the (1) split-liver transplant in which the right lobe and the left lobe are transplanted from a cadaver donor to two recipients; (2) reduced-size orthotopic liver transplant; and (3) living-related hepatic donation in which the left lobe or the lateral segment of the left lobe is used for transplantation in the child.[28]

Children requiring liver transplant are maintained on a strict regimen of immunosuppressive therapy. Although regimens vary from center to center and patient to patient, in general, immunosuppressive protocols include the administration of cyclosporin, prednisone, and azathioprine. Newer drugs, such as antibiotics (e.g., FK506), monoclonal antibodies (e.g., OKT3), and analogs of cyclosporin (e.g., cyclosporin G), may further improve survival rates.[28]

CLINICAL PRESENTATION

Children with a history of liver transplant are at risk of liver failure, rejection, and recurrent infections—all from the immunosuppressive therapy. In addition, the child may become hypertensive and oliguric. Hepatic coma is usually caused by liver failure or rejection following the surgery, but it may also indicate intracranial hemorrhage or infarction. Physical findings may include abdominal pain; weight gain; edema of the hands, feet, legs, or face and around the eyes (periorbital); and red patches (urticaria), blisters, rashes, or petechiae on the skin. Other signs include changes in the child's level of consciousness, such as confusion, lethargy, irritability, or memory loss.

EMERGENCY DEPARTMENT AND NURSING INTERVENTIONS

When they arrive at the ED, all children with a history of liver transplantation receive a thorough history and physical examination to rule out the possibility of overwhelming infection or liver failure. These children are placed in a private room and seen urgently. If the child demonstrates signs of liver failure or rejection, emergent managment and stabilization of the ABCs is required, including constant monitoring and continuous evaluation.

Diagnostic studies are ordered as dictated by history and physical findings. For example, if the child is febrile but otherwise clinically stable, a CBC, differential, and ESR may be ordered. If signs of liver failure are present, a CBC, electrolytes, ionized calcium, phosphorus, ammonia, serum creatinine, BUN, PT and PTT, and liver function tests are ordered.

The parents of children undergoing liver transplant are usually frightened and upset. When possible, the parents should be allowed to remain with the child. If the parent and child have been followed up regularly by a physician, nurse specialist, or social worker from a transplant team, that professional should be notified to provide support to the family.

▌ INTESTINAL PARASITES

ETIOLOGY

Intestinal parasites infect humans worldwide. However, some are more prevalent in Third World countries and are rarely seen in the United States. In general, intestinal parasites are classified as protozoa or helminths. Protozoa are unicellular organisms that multiply within the host; helminths, or worms, are multicellular and usually do not divide. Examples of protozoa include ameba and giardiasis. Examples of helminths include ascaris, pinworms, and hookworms.

AMEBIASIS

Pathophysiology. When the parasite *Entamoeba histolytica* enters the intestinal mucosa, it causes localized tissue destruction and ulceration with very little local inflammatory response. As the organisms multiply, ulcerations spread throughout the intestinal tract. If the parasite reaches the liver, it can produce liver abscesses. Because the local inflammatory response is limited, early symptoms may be absent. Definitive diagnosis is made by obtaining at least three stool samples. If there is a high index of suspicion yet the stool samples are negative, endoscopy may be performed to identify the presence of ulcers on the intestinal mucosa.

Clinical presentation. With amebiasis, the infection may be evidenced within 2 weeks of exposure or a few months following exposure. Initially few symptoms may be exhibited; however, as time passes, colicky abdominal pain and an increase in bowel movements may be seen. Occasionally, fever, chills, and severe diarrhea are observed. Children with these symptoms are at risk of rapid dehydration and severe electrolyte disturbances (Table 15-5).

GIARDIASIS

Pathophysiology. *Giardia lamblia* is more prevalent in children than in adults and is most commonly seen in Third World countries, day care settings, and residential institutions. Children with

TABLE 15-5	Overview of Gastrointestinal Parasitic Diseases			
INFECTION/AGENT	**ORGANISM**	**TRANSMISSION**	**SIGNS AND SYMPTOMS**	**TREATMENT**
Amebiasis	*Entamoeba histolytica*	Ingestion of parasite cysts by fecal-oral or water-food route Incubation may range from 2-4 wk to months or years	Gradual onset Colicky abdominal pain Frequent bowel movements Diarrhea; may contain blood and mucus Infants and young children are prone to rapid dehydration	Diloxanide furoate 10 mg/kg/24 hr × 10 days If invasive amebiasis is present, metronidazole 50 mg/kg × 10 days Enteric precautions are required
Ascariasis	*Ascaris lumbricoides*	Ingestion of parasite eggs following 2-3 wk of incubation in soil contaminated by feces Common in tropics, areas of poor sanitation, and areas where human feces is used for fertilizer	Infection is most common in preschool and school-age children Light infestation may be asymptomatic Heavy infestation can cause pulmonary symptoms (e.g., cough, blood in sputum); GI obstruction; peritonitis; common bile duct obstruction (jaundice)	Children >2 yr: mebendazole 100 mg bid × 3 days; *or* pyrantel pamoate 11 mg/kg × 1 dose; *or* piperazine 50-75 mg/kg/day × 2 days
Cryptosporidiosis	*Cryptosporidium*	Ingestion of parasite oocytes contained in feces of humans and animals Common in day care centers and immunocompromised children Incubation is 2-14 days	Commonly seen in children, particularly those <2 yr Acute onset Watery diarrhea Low-grade fever Abdominal pain Anorexia and weight loss	No specific treatment; care is supportive May require fluid and electrolyte therapy Requires enteric precautions during acute phase of illness

Continued.

Compiled from Boenning, 1996; Committee on Infectious Diseases, 1994; Kazura, 1992; Wong, 1997.

TABLE 15-5	Overview of Gastrointestinal Parasitic Diseases—cont'd			
INFECTION/AGENT	**ORGANISM**	**TRANSMISSION**	**SIGNS AND SYMPTOMS**	**TREATMENT**
Enterobiasis (pinworms)	*Enterobius vermicularis*	Eggs are deposited on perianal skin, where they are carried on contaminated clothing, bedding, or fingernails and ingested Eggs hatch in stomach and mature as they pass through intestines Mature worms deposit eggs on perianal skin, where reinfestation occurs by autoinfection	Rectal itching, especially at night Restlessness and irritability Inability to sleep In rare instances: vaginitis, salpingitis, or pelvic peritonitis	Mebendazole 100 mg × 1 dose (may be repeated in 1 wk) Linens and clothes should be washed in hot water All family members should observe meticulous hand-washing Reinfestation, even with precautionary measure, is common All family members may require treatment
Giardiasis	*Giardia lamblia*	Ingestion of parasite cysts by fecal-oral or water-food route Cysts may remain viable in water for >3 mo Common in day care centers and in immuno-compromised children Incubation is 1-4 wk	Diarrhea Weight loss Crampy abdominal pain Failure to thrive	Furazolidone 8 mg/kg/24 hr × 10 days; *or* tinidazole 50 mg/kg × 1 dose; *or* quinacrine 6 mg/kg/24 hr × 7 days Enteric precautions should be observed
Hookworms	*Ancylostoma duodenale* *Necator americanus* *Ancylostoma ceylanicum*	Ingestion of water containing eggs and larva found in fecally contaminated soil or direct penetration of skin Larvae migrate to lungs via circulatory system and are swallowed Larvae then mature into worms in small intestine Incubation is 4-6 wk	Infestations may be asymptomatic Skin reactions may occur at site of penetration Abdominal pain, anorexia, and diarrhea are all nonspecific findings Long-term effects can produce anemia, hypoalbuminemia, and edema	If severe anemia is present, it should be treated with iron before other drug therapy is instituted Drug therapy is same as for ascariasis

immunodeficiencies are predisposed to chronic symptomatic *Giardia* infections.[5]

The infection is caused when the mature cyst is ingested and enters the small intestine. There trophozoites colonize the lumen of the duodenum and proximal jejunum, attaching themselves to the intestinal epithelial cells with a large sucking disk. The diagnosis is made when either trophozoites or cysts are identified on examination of a stool smear. However, a single stool smear will not identify all cases; therefore three specimens, collected on 3 consecutive days, may be required. When the specimens remain normal, other testing, such as enzyme-linked immunosorbent assay (ELISA), counterimmune electrophoresis assay, or the string test (a string is attached to a capsule that is swallowed and later removed for examination), may be required.[4,47]

Clinical presentation. The onset of illness may be acute or chronic with a broad spectrum of manifestations. Symptoms may include acute watery diarrhea and abdominal pain or a protracted illness that includes the passage of foul-smelling stools and gas, abdominal distention, and weight loss. If the condition progresses, the child will exhibit signs of failure to thrive and anemia.

ASCARIASIS

Pathophysiology. *Ascaris lumbricoides,* or roundworms, is a helminth found exclusively in humans. Transmission occurs when the mature larva-containing eggs (ova) are excreted in the stool and remain in the soil to incubate for 2 to 3 weeks; they are then ingested via the contaminated soil. As the larva hatch in the small intestine, they move through the mucosa and migrate to the lungs and the liver. In the lungs they penetrate the alveolar spaces and ascend the tracheobronchial tree, where they are swallowed and mature into egg-laying adults. The development of mature egg-laying adults in the small intestines—from initial ingestion to migration and maturation—takes about 8 weeks. *Ascaris* organisms can be detected when ova are identified on stool examination and, occasionally, when adult worms are passed with stool or in emesis.

Clinical presentation. Signs and symptoms of infection vary from nonspecific GI symptoms to pneumonitis or acute intestinal obstruction and are associated with the degree of infestation. Pulmonary ascariasis is characterized by cough, blood-stained sputum,

eosinophilia, and transient pulmonary infiltrates.[20] Intestinal obstruction, although rare, may be evidenced by severe abdominal pain, distention, and vomiting.

ENTEROBIASIS (PINWORMS)

Pathophysiology. Pinworm infestations are found exclusively in humans and are most commonly seen in children of school age or preschool age. Infection is transmitted when eggs from the infected host are transmitted to others via clothing, linens, or dust particles and are ingested. Once ingested, the eggs hatch in the stomach and mature into small white worms as they progress through the intestinal tract. At night these worms migrate to the perianal region to lay eggs and then die. Reinfestation of the host occurs by autoinfection via the mechanisms described here. The period of communicability continues as long as the cycle of reinfestation continues and the mature female worms continue to lay eggs.

The diagnosis is made by visualizing the worms or applying a small piece of transparent tape to the perianal skin first thing in the morning, before bathing or defecating, to pick up eggs. The specimen is then placed on a glass slide and examined microscopically.

Clinical presentation. Although the clinical manifestations vary, the most common complaints in children are perianal itching and inability to sleep. Other symptoms include irritability, restlessness, and bed-wetting. Rarely seen symptoms include vaginitis, salpingitis, and pelvic peritonitis.

TAPEWORMS

Pathophysiology. There are three giant tapeworms that may cause infections in humans. These include the beef tapeworm (*Taenia saginata*), the pork tapeworm (*Taenia solium*), and the fish tapeworm (*Diphyllobothrium latum*). Fortunately, these infestations are rare in the United States. They are usually associated with the importation of food products from other areas of the world (e.g., Mexico, South America, Africa).

Other tapeworm infections that are more common in the United States include the dwarf tapeworm (*Hymenolepis nana*) and *Dipylidium caninum*. Dwarf tapeworms are transmitted person-to-person by the ingestion of eggs passed in the feces. *Dipylidium caninum* organisms are transmitted by fleas, which act as intermediate carriers. Once ingested, the ova hatch in the intestines and mature into adult worms. These worms usually reside within the ileum, where they begin producing eggs, which are then excreted in the feces. The diagnosis of tapeworm infestation is made when the eggs or tapeworm segments are identified in the stool.

Clinical presentation. Signs and symptoms vary depending on the type and degree of infestation. Any of the three giant tapeworms can migrate from the intestines to tissues throughout the body and may lead to the development of cysts within the central nervous system. Children with infections caused by the dwarf tapeworm or *Dipylidium caninum* are often asymptomatic. With severe infestation the child may complain of nausea, abdominal pain, or diarrhea. Treatment is aimed at breaking the cycle of reinfestation through strict handwashing and pharmacologic management with niclosamide or praziquantel.

Nursing care and evaluation. Specific nursing interventions require parental education of methods to control the spread of infection. For example, all linens and the child's clothes must be washed in a hot, soapy solution and meticulous handwashing techniques need to be followed. If the child wears diapers, excluding the child from day care is recommended until treatment has been completed.

▌ FOREIGN BODY INGESTIONS

Etiology. The majority of foreign body ingestions occur in children between the ages of 6 months and 6 years. Infants and toddlers are particularly vulnerable to foreign body ingestion, primarily because of their exploratory nature and their natural curiosity of the environment. They tend to put objects that are within their reach—such as coins, buttons, and small toys or pieces of toys—into their mouths. (Foreign bodies in the airway are reviewed in Chapter 10.)

Pathophysiology. When a foreign body is ingested, it can lodge in the esophagus or pass on to the stomach, where it will usually (about 80% to 90% of the time) continue through the GI tract and be excreted within 7 to 10 days.[3] Foreign bodies lodged in the esophagus can produce a variety of problems, depending on their shape, size, and location and the length of time since ingestion. The most common locations of foreign bodies in the esophagus are the cricopharyngeal muscle, the aortic knob, and the

gastroesophageal junction (the last is the least common of the three).[43]

If an esophageal foreign body compresses the trachea, signs and symptoms of respiratory distress may be evidenced immediately. Other foreign bodies, particularly those lodged within the esophagus for a long time, can lead to localized tissue swelling, tissue erosion, and even perforation, with respiratory symptoms appearing subsequently. A particularly dangerous ingestion is that of alkaline disk batteries, which may lodge in the esophagus and rapidly produce mucosal irritation and focal caustic burns as hydroxides within the battery are released.[43] GI perforations are rare with foreign body obstructions; however, they are more common with objects lodged in the esophagus and with objects that are irregularly shaped (Fig. 15-8).

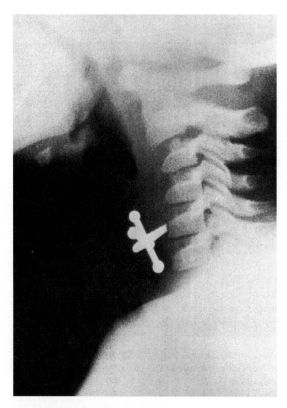

FIG. 15-8. X-ray film of foreign body in upper esophagus. Note the readily visible opaque jack in the upper esophagus of this infant. (From Swischuk LE: *Emergency imaging of the acutely ill or injured child,* Baltimore, 1994, Williams & Wilkins.)

Clinical presentation. The majority of children with a GI foreign body ingestion are asymptomatic. Commonly the only reason for the ED visit is that the parent observed the child ingesting the object or saw the child mouthing an object that subsequently disappeared. Other times, however, the history may be vague and the parent may be unaware that a foreign body was ingested. Only with careful questioning will a history of a brief period of coughing or gagging while playing, refusal to feed, increased salivation or drooling, vomiting, pain or discomfort with feeding, or abdominal pain be identified.

If the foreign body is lodged in the esophagus and is compressing the trachea, signs and symptoms of respiratory distress will be present. These include tachypnea, retractions, use of the accessory muscles of respiration (particularly the sternocleidomastoid), stridor, and wheezing. Once a foreign body remains in the esophagus for a prolonged period, local tissue ischemia can produce symptoms of respiratory disorders such as croup, asthma, or pneumonia. If esophageal perforation has occurred, the child will rapidly become febrile, will demonstrate pain on eating, and will drool.

Emergency Department interventions. ED interventions depend on the severity of symptoms associated with the ingestion. In most cases in which a child is asymptomatic, a radiograph of the GI tract is taken to identify the location of the foreign body. If the foreign body has passed into the stomach, the child may be discharged with instructions for the parent to observe the stool for passage within about 1 week. Occasionally, particularly if the child complains of abdominal pain, fever, vomiting, or diarrhea, a follow-up x-ray examination will be performed. Alkaline disk batteries that have passed into the stomach rarely cause problems, and evidence indicates that 90% of them pass through the GI tract spontaneously with no complications.[24] These children may be sent home; however, observation of the stools to document elimination is essential.

Most foreign bodies lodged within the esophagus must be removed. The exception is a small, rounded object located in the lower third of the esophagus, which may be watched for up to 12 hours for passage into the stomach. If the object is radiolucent, it may not be visible on x-ray film and therefore a barium swallow enema, CT scan, or xeroradiography may need to be done. Once the object is identified, it may be removed by endoscopy or use of a Foley catheter, depending on the size and location of the object and the length of time following the ingestion (Fig. 15-9). When esophageal edema is present, endoscopy is the method of choice; in rare instances, when the object is low in the esophagus and there is a significant risk of perforation, the object may be pushed into the stomach rather than removed.

Nursing care and evaluation. In most situations emergency nursing care of the child with a known foreign body ingestion involves supportive care and discharge teaching. If the child has ingested a foreign body that is producing respiratory symptoms such as tachypnea, retractions, or stridor, emergent airway management is indicated.

Children who are in stable condition and exhibit no signs of respiratory distress may undergo radiographic examination unaccompanied. If the foreign body is found to be in the stomach or the intestines and there are no signs of distress such as abdominal pain or vomiting, the child may be sent home. If, however, a child is demonstrating signs of respiratory distress, evidence of perforation (e.g., fever, bloody sputum), difficulty swallowing, or excessive drooling, the child needs to be monitored and accompanied by the nurse

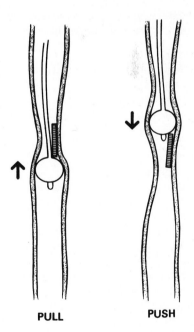

PULL   **PUSH**

FIG. 15-9. Esophageal foreign body removal with a catheter. (From Alexander et al: Catheter removal of esophageal foreign bodies: push or pull? *Am J Roentgenol* 151: 835, 1988.)

to the radiology department (or, ideally, a portable x-ray is obtained).

Whether or not respiratory distress is present, foreign bodies lodged in the esophagus are usually removed through esophagoscopy or the Foley catheter method. Although both of these techniques have been performed in the ED setting, esophagoscopy is most often performed in the operating room and the Foley catheter technique is best performed in the radiology department, where catheter insertion and removal of the object can be directly visualized. Regardless of which technique is used, venous access is usually obtained so that the child can receive sedative(s) before and during the procedure. If the Foley catheter method is used, care must be taken to prevent the child from reingesting the article once it has been moved into the oral cavity. Turning the child on the side and removing the article with forceps or a Kelly clamp helps to prevent this complication (Box 15-8). Although both the oral and the nasal route of catheter insertion can be used, the oral route tends to be more popular; however, a bite block should be used to prevent the child from biting the catheter.

Box 15-8 Nursing Considerations for Balloon Catheter Removal of a Foreign Body

- Gather equipment
  - Suction (both tonsil suction device and catheter)
  - Supplemental oxygen
  - McGill forceps, Kelly clamp, or curved forceps
  - Bag-valve-mask device
  - Laryngoscope blades and handles
  - Endotracheal tubes
  - Bite block (if oral route is used)
- Place child on heart rate monitor and pulse oximeter
- Obtain venous access and administer sedatives as ordered
- Restrain child if necessary; place the child in Trendelenburg's position; be prepared to rapidly turn child to side
- Monitor child throughout procedure; notify physician if signs of respiratory compromise are observed
- Talk softly to child and explain all procedures

Discharge instructions following the successful removal of an esophageal foreign body include reminders to the parents to observe the child for signs or symptoms of infection (e.g., fever), bleeding (in sputum or emesis), perforation, excessive drooling, or respiratory distress (including retractions and a rapid respiratory rate). Initially, on discharge, the child is started on a clear-liquid diet; if no complications are identified, the child can progress to a regular diet within the following 12 to 24 hours.

If the object has passed into the GI tract and no ED interventions were required, the parents are instructed to observe the child's stools for the next 2 weeks for the presence of the foreign body. They are also instructed to return to the ED or to their family physician if abdominal pain, bloody stools, vomiting, or fever develops.

REFERENCES

1. Athreya BH, Silverman BK, Apitzer AR: *Pediatric physical diagnosis,* Norwalk, Ct, 1985, Appleton-Century-Croft.
2. Balistreri WF: Viral hepatitis, *Pediatr Clin North Am* 35:375-407, 1988.
3. Belfer RA: Foreign body ingestions. In Barkin RM, ed: *Pediatric emergency medicine: concepts and clinical practice,* St Louis, 1992, Mosby, pp 763-765.
4. Boenning DA: Diarrhea and gastroenteritis. In Barkin RM, ed: *Pediatric emergency medicine: concepts and clinical practice,* St Louis, 1992, Mosby, pp 740-742, 765-770.
5. Committee on Infectious Diseases, American Academy of Pediatrics: *1994 Red Book: report of the Committee on Infectious Diseases,* ed 23, Elk Grove Village, Ill, 1994, The Academy.
6. De Lorimier AA, Harrison MR, Adzick NS: Pediatric surgery. In Way L, ed: *Current surgical diagnosis and treatment,* ed 9, Norwalk, Ct, 1991, Appleton & Lange, 47:1180-1190.
7. Ein SH, Stephens CA, Minor A: The painless intussusception, *J Pediatr Surg* 11:563-564, 1976.
8. Engel J: *Pocket guide to pediatric assessment,* St Louis, 1997, Mosby, p 162.
9. Fleisher GR: Infectious disease emergencies. In Fleisher GR, Ludwig S, eds: *Textbook of pediatric emergency medicine,* ed 2, Baltimore, 1994, Williams & Wilkins, pp 415-474.
10. Fuchs S, Jaffe D: Vomiting, *Pediatr Emerg Care* 6:164-169, 1990.
11. Garcia VF, Randolph JG: Pyloric stenosis: diagnosis and management, *Pediatr Rev* 11(10):293-296, 1990.

12. Grisanti KA: Abdominal pain. In Barkin RM, Rosen P, eds: *Pediatric emergency medicine: concepts and clinical practice,* St Louis, 1992, Mosby, pp 728-729.
13. Guyton AC: *Textbook of medical physiology,* ed 8, Philadelphia, 1991, WB Saunders.
14. Harvey MA: *Study guide to core curriculum for critical care nursing,* ed 2, Philadelphia, 1992, WB Saunders.
15. Reference deleted in proofs.
16. Hatch EI: The acute abdomen in children, *Pediatr Clin North Am* 32(5):1151-1156, 1985.
17. Hathaway WE et al, eds: *Current pediatric diagnosis and treatment,* ed 12, Norwalk, Ct, 1991, Appleton & Lange, pp 550-551.
18. Hickey MS, Kiernan GJ, Weaver KE: Evaluation of abdominal pain, *Emerg Med Clin North Am* 7:437-452, 1989.
19. Jedd MB et al: Factors associated with infantile hypertrophic pyloric stenosis, *Am J Dis Child* 142:334, 1988.
20. Kazura JW, Mahmoud AF: Helminths. In Behrman RE, ed: *Nelson textbook of pediatrics,* ed 14, Philadelphia, 1992, WB Saunders, pp 896-899.
21. Kottmeier PK: Appendicitis. In Welch KJ, Randolph JG, Ravitch MM: *Pediatric surgery,* ed 4, Chicago, 1986, Year Book Medical Publishers, pp 241-248.
22. Krumberger JM: *AACN's clinical reference for critical care nursing,* ed 3, St Louis, 1993, Mosby, pp 1101.
23. Leibowitz I, Grand RJ, Ziai M: The abdomen and the gastrointestinal tract. In Ziai M, ed: *Pediatrics,* ed 4, Boston, 1990, Little, Brown, pp 212-244.
24. Litovitz TL: Battery ingestions: product accessibility and clinical course, *Pediatrics* 75:469, 1985.
25. McCrory LB: A review of the second international symposium on pediatric pain, *J Pain Symptom Manage* 6:3, 1991.
26. Mohan P, Benny K: Gastrointestinal dysfunction and failure. In Holbrook PR: *Textbook of pediatric critical care,* Philadelphia, 1993, WB Saunders, pp 638-652.
27. Orenstein JB: Constipation. In Barkin RM, ed: *Pediatric emergency medicine: concepts and clinical practice,* St Louis, 1992, Mosby, pp 737-740.
28. Peters TG: Liver transplantation in 1993: selected issues, *Jacksonville Med: Duval County Med Soc* 44:4, 173-176, 1993.
29. Pollack C, Pender E: Unusual cases of intussusception, *J Emerg Med* 9:347-355, 1991.
30. Raffensperger JG: Appendicitis. In Raffensperger JG, ed: *Swenson's pediatric surgery,* ed 5, Norwalk, Ct, 1990, Appleton & Lange, pp 843-853.
31. Raffensperger JG: Hirschsprung's disease. In Raffensperger JG, ed: *Swenson's pediatric surgery,* ed 5, Norwalk, Ct, 1990, Appleton & Lange, pp 555-564.
32. Raffensperger JG: Pyloric stenosis. In Raffensperger JG, ed: *Swenson's pediatric surgery,* ed 5, Norwalk, Ct, 1990, Appleton & Lange, pp 203-219.
33. Reynolds SL, Jaffe DM: Diagnosing abdominal pain in a pediatric emergency department, *Pediatr Emerg care* 8(3):126-128, 1992.
34. Rosekrans JA: Dermatologic disorders. In Barkin RM, ed: *Pediatric emergency medicine: concepts and clinical practice,* St Louis, 1992, Mosby, pp 606-641.
35. Rosenstein BJ, Fosarelli PD: *Pediatric pearls: the handbook of practical pediatrics,* St Louis, 1993, Mosby.
36. Rowe MI et al: *Essentials of pediatric surgery,* St Louis, 1995, Mosby.
37. Rubin SZ, Martin DJ: Ultrasonography in the management of possible appendicitis in childhood, *J Pediatr Surg* 25:737-740, 1990.
38. Ruddy R: Pain—abdomen. In Fleisher GR, Ludwig S, eds: *Textbook of pediatric emergency medicine,* ed 3, Baltimore, 1993, Williams & Wilkins, pp 340-347.
39. Scherer LR, Grosfield J: Inguinal hernia and umbilical anomalies, *Pediatr Clin North Am* 40(6):1121-1131, 1993.
40. Schnaufer L, Mahboubi S: Abdominal emergencies. In Fleisher GR, Ludwig S, eds: *Textbook of pediatric emergency medicine,* ed 3, Baltimore, 1993, Williams & Wilkins, pp 1307-1335.
41. Sinclair LM: Appendicitis. In Barkin RM, ed: *Pediatric emergency medicine: concepts and clinical practice,* St Louis, 1992, Mosby, p 779.
42. Smith D et al: The role of abdominal x-rays in the diagnosis and management of intussusception, *Pediatr Emerg Care* 8:325-327, 1992.
43. Swischuk LE: *Emergency imaging of the acutely ill or injured child,* Baltimore, 1994, Williams & Wilkins.
44. Thompson JM et al: *Mosby's clinical nursing,* ed 3, St Louis, 1993, Mosby, pp 697-699.
45. Wattchow DA et al: Abnormalities of peptide-containing nerve fibers in infantile hypertrophic pyloric stenosis, *Gastroenterology* 92:443, 1987.
46. Whitington PF, Balistreri WF: Liver transplantation in pediatrics, *J Pediatr* 118:169, 1991.
47. Wong DL: *Whaley and Wong's essentials of pediatric nursing,* ed 5, St Louis, 1995, Mosby.
48. Zimmerman JJ: The pediatric critical care patient. In Fuhrman BP, Zimmerman JJ, eds: *Pediatric critical care,* St Louis, 1992, Mosby, p 3.

CHAPTER 16

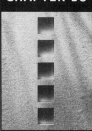

Genitourinary System

Terry Pye, Treesa Soud

INTRODUCTION

Children often come to the emergency department with complaints related to the genitourinary system. The majority of children with genitourinary complaints are successfully treated and have no long-lasting disabilities. The outcomes for a few children with repeat infections, congenital anomalies, or certain renal diseases may not be so favorable. Some of the most common disorders and those that can be life-threatening are reviewed in the section on disorders of the urinary tract later in this chapter. Certain multi-system disorders also can significantly affect renal function; these include hemolytic-uremic syndrome and Henoch-Schönlein purpura, both of which are discussed in this chapter.

Within the adolescent population, complaints related to the reproductive organs are common. Sexually transmitted diseases account for a large percentage of emergency department visits in this age group. This chapter reviews those sexually transmitted diseases that are most commonly found within this population.

ANATOMY AND PHYSIOLOGY

GENITALIA

The genitalia grow at a very slow rate during infancy and early childhood, and this growth rate does not correspond to the child's generalized growth patterns. The female genitalia consist of the vagina and the labia majora and minora (Fig. 16-1). The male genitalia consist of the scrotum, the testicles, and the penis. At birth, the male and female genitalia and the breasts may be swollen as a result of maternal estrogen withdrawal. In the female neonate maternal estrogen withdrawal also may produce a vaginal discharge, which can be bloody.

With development, physical growth may not parallel sexual awareness. Conversely, children who develop secondary sex characteristics earlier than their peers may not possess the cognitive abilities to deal with sexual maturation. As adolescence approaches, primary and secondary sex characteristics become evident with growth in the size of the genitalia and the appearance of genital and body hair.

URINARY SYSTEM

The urinary system consists of two kidneys and two ureters, the bladder, and the urethra. The kidneys are relatively large structures within the abdominal cavity of the infant and small child; they lie in the intraperitoneal space on either side of the spinal column. The right kidney is slightly lower than the left kidney. The ureters carry fluid removed from the kidneys to the bladder by way of peristaltic contractions. The bladder is a muscular organ that stores the urine. In infants it is a cylindrical abdominal organ with a capacity of 15 to 20 ml, compared to 600 to 800 ml in the adult. The bladder gradually descends into the pelvis as the child develops. Voiding in the infant is involuntary, occurring as bladder capacity is reached. As the child grows and bladder volume increases, the ability to retain urine improves. By the age of 2 to 3 years, bladder sphincter control has developed and the child is able to void voluntarily.

The kidneys are responsible for maintaining homeostasis by filtering the blood to maintain fluid and electrolyte balance and to eliminate the by-products of metabolism. Each kidney is divided into the cortex and the medulla. The cortex is the outer highly vascular portion of the kidney; it contains the glomeruli, which

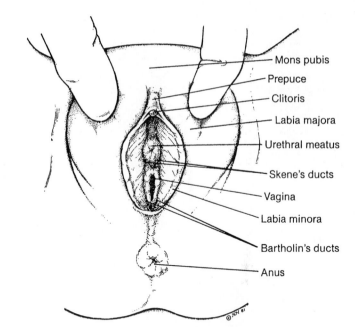

FIG. 16-1. External female genitalia. (From Whaley LF, Wong DL: *Nursing care of infants and children*, ed 5, St Louis, 1995, Mosby.)

filter water and electrolytes from the blood. Factors that can affect the glomerular filtration rate (GFR) include the permeability of the glomerular capillaries, vascular pressure, and filtration pressure. Approximately 99% of the filtered fluid is reabsorbed within the tubules.

The kidneys together contain approximately 2 million nephrons, which are formed by the 34th week of gestation. Each nephron is composed of a glomerulus and a long tubule that extends either superficially or deeply into the medulla. The tubule is composed of a proximal tubule, a loop of Henle, the distal convoluted tubule, and a collecting duct (Figs. 16-2 and 16-3). The proximal tubules are responsible for the largest percentage of glomerular filtrate and electrolyte reabsorption. Nephrons can lie close to the surface of the kidneys with short, thin loops of Henle that penetrate only the outer medulla (cortical nephrons); or deep within the cortex with long loops of Henle that extend deep into the medulla (juxtamedullary nephrons). Although all nephrons are present at birth, with development they continue to grow in size and complexity.

Both renal blood flow and GFR are low at birth. Renal blood flow in the first year of a life accounts for approximately 15% to 18% of the total cardiac output. In older children and adults renal blood-flow accounts for approximately 20% or about 1200 ml/min, through both kidneys.[10,21] In newborns the GFR is

approximately 15 to 20 ml/min/1.73 m². The rate increases to 35 to 40 ml/min/1.73 m² in the second week of life. By 6 months of age the GFR is 60 ml/min/1.73 m². It reaches adult levels of 80 to 120 ml/min/1.73 m² by 1 year of age.[2,9]

The GFR is estimated by calculating the creatinine clearance, provided that renal function is not impaired.

$$\text{GFR (clearance)} = \frac{U \ (\text{urine}) \times V \ (\text{volume of urine per minute})}{P \ (\text{plasma concentration of creatinine})}$$

Because the infant has a low GFR and the kidneys are less able to concentrate urine through tubular reabsorption than those of an adult, urinary output at birth is high and specific gravity is low (Table 16-1).

NURSING HISTORY AND ASSESSMENT

HISTORY

With a known or suspected genitourinary (GU) complaint, the investigation of symptoms should include the chief complaint, the onset and duration of symptoms, and any associated symptoms. Additional his-

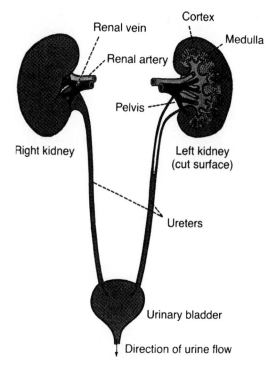

Fig. 16-2. General organizational plan of the urinary system. (From Guyton AC: *Textbook of medical physiology,* 8th ed, Philadelphia, 1991, WB Saunders.)

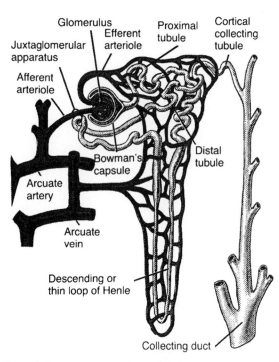

Fig. 16-3. Nephron. (From Guyton AC: *Textbook of medical physiology,* 8th ed, Philadelphia, 1991, WB Saunders.)

torical information should include the use of medications to relieve symptoms or to treat an underlying condition, and the presence of allergies. Urinary symptoms are often nonspecific in infants and young children because they are unable to relate the presence or location of pain or discomfort. In these children the nurse must first be suspicious of a urinary problem while obtaining pertinent information from the parent or caregiver. In the young febrile child with no objective symptoms, the nurse may inquire about changes in the child's voiding pattern, the presence of blood in the urine, crying with voiding, the presence of abdominal pain, and the presence of vomiting. In addition, the nurse should ask if the child's urinary output has been normal and if the child has an underlying medical condition, such as hypertension or a pulmonary, renal, or endocrine disorder.

Complaints related to the genitalia vary from the young male child with testicular torsion, to the child victim of sexual abuse, to the female adolescent with pelvic inflammatory disease. Specific historical findings are included in the clinical presentation sections within each topic. (Sexual abuse is reviewed in

Table 16-1	Normal Urine Output in the Child	
Age	**Urine output**
Infant	2 ml/kg/hr
Child	1-2 ml/kg/hr
Adolescent	0.5-1 ml/kg/hr

Modified from Hazinski MF: *Nursing care of the critically ill child,* ed 2, St Louis, 1992, Mosby.

Chapter 25). Specific questions asked of the adolescent with a complaint related to the genitalia are included in (Box 16-1).

Physical Examination

Genitalia. The physical assessment of the child with a complaint of the genitalia begins with an observation of the child's general hygiene. The child should undress completely and be placed in a hospital gown. In infants inspection of the genitalia usually can be accomplished easily. In older children,

---

Box 16-1 History of Urinary and Genital Symptoms

Urinary
History of previous problems
Urinary frequency
Urinary urgency
Dysuria
Increase or decrease in amount of urine or change in its color
Bed-wetting
Incontinence
Flank pain
Hematuria
Vomiting
Abdominal pain
Fever

Genital
History of previous problems
Sexual history
Vaginal or penile discharge
Abdominal pain
Pelvic pain
Vomiting
Fever
Genital lesions, sores, or rashes
Genital itching or burning
Menstrual history/last menstrual period

---

however, fear, anxiety, and modesty all must be considered. These children should be kept covered at all times to protect their modesty, and all procedures must be explained to them. The nurse and the physician may inspect the genitalia simultaneously to avoid subjecting the child to duplicate examinations.

The female genitalia are inspected while the child is supine with the legs in a froglike position. In the young child the mother may hold the child in this position by sitting behind the child. The labia are opened and observed for swelling, rashes, lesions, discharge, and odors. The hymen is visualized as well as the perineal area and rectum. A vaginal examination is generally not performed on young children unless sexual assault is suspected; then the examination is done to evaluate for injury and to obtain cultures and evidence (see Chapter 25). Vaginal examinations are performed on adolescents if they are sexually active or have symptoms that suggest the need for such an examination.

The male genitalia are inspected with the child in the supine position either in the bed or on the parent's lap. The penis, scrotum, and perineal area are observed for size, lesions, or unusual findings. If the child is not circumcised, the foreskin is retracted. In infants, however, the foreskin often does not retract and should not be forced. The penis is observed for discharge, and the scrotum is examined for descent of both testicles. Hypospadias or epispadias may be identified by examining the meatal opening on the ventral or dorsal surface of the penis, respectively. The abdominal and pelvic walls of both the male and the female child are palpated for the presence of masses and pain.

Urinary system. Young children and infants with urinary disorders usually arrive in the emergency department (ED) with nonspecific complaints. Often these complaints include abdominal symptoms such as vomiting and diarrhea. Older children may describe more specific symptoms, such as abdominal pain, painful urination, or hematuria. In these children an abdominal assessment is performed to rule out the presence of an illness related to the gastrointestinal system, or the urinary system.

When renal involvement is suspected, the child is evaluated for the presence of edema, which may be periorbital or generalized. Additionally, a complete set of vital signs is recorded, and the presence of hypertension is noted. Neurologic status and cardiovascular status are evaluated, both on initial presentation and throughout the ED stay.

INFECTIONS OF THE GENITAL TRACT

SEXUALLY TRANSMITTED DISEASES

Etiology. Sexually transmitted diseases (STDs) are bacterial or viral infections acquired primarily through sexual activity. Over the past decade the number of children and adolescents diagnosed with an STD has skyrocketed. In the young teen, experimentation, risk taking, and lack of knowledge are often to blame.

STDs can be transferred to the fetus during pregnancy and to the neonate during delivery and may also result from sexual abuse in young children. Sexual assault accounts for a small percentage of STDs.

Gonorrhea. *Neisseria gonorrhoea* is the most commonly reported communicable disease in the United States. It is seen in adults and children of all ages. The condition can cause a variety of infections, ranging from a form of severe conjunctivitis in the newborn to pelvic inflammatory disease. The highest rate of gonococcal infection of the genitalia is found in adolescent females and young adults.

Transmission of genital gonorrhea occurs during sexual intercourse. The incubation period is 3 to 5 days. During that time a local inflammatory response produces a purulent discharge. In the female, if the infection goes untreated and ascends the GU tract, the inflamed mucosa is replaced by fibrous tissue that can obstruct the fallopian tubes (a common cause of infertility) or the urethra. Approximately three fourths of females are symptomatic, whereas males may be asymptomatic. Females commonly have a vaginal discharge and dysuria; the external genitalia may be red and swollen. Symptomatic males will have urethritis and dysuria, and they may have a penile discharge.

Syphilis. Syphilis results when *Treponema pallidum*—a thin, motile spirochete—is contracted either through sexual contact or via transplacental transmission to the fetus from an infected mother. Syphilis acquired through sexual contact appears in three stages. The primary stage, which lasts approximately 3 to 6 weeks, is characterized by painless ulcerations (chancres) at the site of transmission; these may be internal but more commonly are external. Without treatment the ulcerations subside, leading to the second stage, which is characterized by a polymorphic rash that involves the palms of the hands and the soles of the feet. During the second stage, systemic symptoms, such as fever, malaise, splenomegaly, sore throat, headache, and arthralgia, may be manifested.[4] The third or tertiary, stage may occur 5 to 30 years later with cardiovascular disease or neurosyphilis.

Congenital syphilis causes perinatal death in approximately 40% of affected pregnancies.[1,4] In surviving infants manifestations may include low birth weight, failure to gain weight, fever, hepatitis, central nervous system (CNS) changes, and even death.

Chlamydia. *Chlamydia trachomatis* is a bacterial intracellular parasite that is transmitted through sexual contact or to the newborn during the delivery process. It is the most commonly acquired sexually transmitted infection in the United States.[4] Infections are usually asymptomatic; however, chlamydia frequently occurs in conjunction with gonorrhea, which produces a profuse vaginal discharge in females. In males it produces urethritis. In the newborn *C. trachomatis* can cause conjunctivitis and pneumonia.

Trichomonas. *Trichomonas vaginalis* is a flagellated protozoan that is primarily acquired through sexual contact, but it can also be transmitted to female neonates during delivery. Trichomonal vaginitis is most commonly identified in females, although males can be carriers. The clinical presentation includes a frothy yellow-green vaginal discharge often accompanied by itching. Dysuria and lower abdominal pain may also be present. On examination the vaginal mucosa may be edematous and the cervix may be inflamed with areas of hemorrhage (strawberry cervix).[4,20]

Genital herpes. The herpes simplex virus (HSV) can produce a wide array of illnesses ranging from generalized systemic infections to CNS diseases such as encephalitis to the localized development of "cold sores." There are two types of herpetic viruses, type 1 and type 2. Type 1 infections are commonly found on the upper body, usually the mouth or face. Type 2 infections usually involve the genitalia and are commonly transmitted via sexual contact. Both forms of the virus can be found in either site depending on the source of the infection.[4] HSV is transmitted via direct contact with a carrier, who may or may not be asymptomatic. HSV is most commonly passed to the newborn from an infected mother during the delivery process. In newborns the condition is often associated with severe symptoms such as encephalitis or sepsis, that can lead to death.

Herpes that is transmitted via sexual contact usually appears within 14 days of exposure. Presenting symptoms include painful vesicular lesions that rupture and form sores. Following the infection, HSV persists in a latent form, and lesions may reappear at any time. In young children vaginal herpes may be transmitted via direct nonsexual contact with an infected lesion on a caregiver; however, sexual abuse must always be considered.

Emergency Department and nursing interventions. ED interventions depend on the presenting symptoms. The usual complaints include painful urination, increased vaginal discharge (may be foul smelling), abdominal or pelvic pain, and occasionally fever. Diagnostic studies include a urinalysis, urine culture, and urine pregnancy test. A pelvic examination is performed, and cultures are obtained for *Neisseria* *gonorrhoeae* and *C. trachomatis.* A DNA probe may be obtained to identify the presence of *Gonococcus* or *Chlamydia* organisms. A KOH preparation is used to identify *Candida* organisms, and a wet mount is obtained to identify the *Trichomonas* organism or a yeast infection.[24] (See the discussion of pelvic inflammatory disease later in this chapter.)

Many children and adolescents have their first pelvic examination in the ED. These examinations are uncomfortable and anxiety-provoking. During the examination the ED nurse should remain with the child and explain the procedure. The parent may or may not be allowed to stay, depending on the child's preference.

Discharge instructions should include an antibiotic schedule and referrals for follow-up care. Sexually active adolescents are told to avoid sexual contact and to notify sexual partners that they need to seek medical care. Positive cultures in a young child with evidence of sexual abuse require notification of child-abuse authorities (Table 16-2).

PELVIC INFLAMMATORY DISEASE

Etiology. Pelvic inflammatory disease (PID) is an acute or chronic infection of the pelvic structures, including the urethra, cervix, uterus, fallopian tubes, and ovaries. The infection may spread into the abdominal cavity and affect the peritoneum and the intestines. Most frequently the cause is gonorrhea; the second most common cause is chlamydia (*C. trachomatis*). Secondary infections may result from the inflammatory process and can be caused by a variety of aerobic and anaerobic organisms. Among the aerobic organisms, staphylococci, streptococci, *Gardnerella vaginalis,* and *Mycoplasma hominis* have been identified.

PID is one of the most serious diseases of the sexually active female adolescent. Adolescents account for approximately 16% to 20% of all cases of PID in the United States.[20] The sexually active adolescent is up to 10 times more likely to develop PID than a sexually active adult woman.[8a]

Pathophysiology. Factors that increase the risk of contracting PID include contact with multiple sexual partners, failure to use barrier methods of contraception, the use of an intrauterine device, douching, and previous episodes of PID.[4,20] Adolescents are thought to have a predisposition to PID because of their thin, noncornified vaginal epithelium and the alkaline pH of the vaginal mucin.[1] In addition, because the cervix opens during menses, sexual activity around the time of menses allows organisms to freely pass through the os. For this reason many pelvic infections occur within days of the completion of menses. Following transmission of the organism(s), the infection ascends through the reproductive organs, beginning in the vagina and traveling upward through the cervix, uterus, fallopian tubes, and ovaries. Complications include peritonitis, recurrent infections, and chronic abdominal pain. Infertility, which results from salpingitis, occurs in 10% to 30% of patients after a single episode and depends on the severity of the infection.[4]

Clinical presentation. The most consistent presenting complaint associated with PID is lower abdominal pain. Some estimates state that as many as 95% of patients will have pain as a presenting symptom. If the pain localizes to one side, ectopic pregnancy must be ruled out. Other causes of unilateral pain include abscess formation and appendicitis. Fever and chills frequently are present. Some patients will have nausea and vomiting. Vaginal discharge is usually present, and abnormal bleeding may be experienced. The discharge, if present, is usually purulent. Urinary symptoms such as dysuria are also common; however, laboratory analysis of the urine may be negative. During the pelvic examination the child will experience increased pain with movement of the cervix and adnexa.

Emergency Department interventions. Because the primary finding in PID is lower abdominal pain, the differential diagnosis must include ectopic pregnancy, inflamed bowel, appendicitis, ruptured ovarian cyst, and spontaneous abortion. A thorough clinical examination and diagnostic testing are therefore required to rule out the presence of an emergent condition.

Laboratory tests include obtaining a complete blood count (CBC), urinalysis, urine pregnancy test (β-HCG), and erythrocyte sedimentation rate (ESR). Additional serological testing includes obtaining a Venereal Disease Research Laboratories (VDRL) test and a rapid plasma reagin (RPR) or automated reagin test (ART) to identify the presence of syphilis. The adolescent should also be offered the opportunity to be tested for human immunodeficiency virus (HIV).

During the pelvic examination cultures are obtained for *N. gonorrhoeae* and *C. trachomatis.* A DNA probe may be obtained to identify the presence of *Gonococcus* or *Chlamydia* organisms. A KOH prepa-

TABLE 16-2 Treatment of Sexually Transmitted Diseases Commonly Identified in Adolescents

Disease	Organism	Characteristics	Findings	Treatment
Chlamydia	*Chlamydia trachomatis*	Intracellular bacterial parasite	*Clinical:* in *females* may be asymptomatic or present with dysuria, urinary frequency, pelvic pain, vaginitis, or vaginal discharge; in *males* may be asymptomatic or present with urethritis or epididymitis. *Laboratory:* positive enzyme-linked immunosorbent assay (ELISA) (Chlamydiazyme); positive monoclonal antibodies; DNA probe; definitive testing requires culture	Doxycycline 100 mg bid × 7 days *or* azithromycin 1 g, one-time dose. If pregnant: erythromycin 500 mg qid for 7 days
Syphilis	*Treponema pallidum*	Thin, motile spirochete	*Clinical:* three stages of presentation: *stage 1*—painless ulcerations (chancres); *stage 2*—rash involving palms of hands and souls of feet; may also have history of fever, malaise, sore throat, headache, arthralgia; *stage 3*—5 to 30 years later includes cardiovascular disease or neurosyphilis. *Laboratory:* spirochetes identified by dark-field examination on scrapings from lesions; positive Venereal Disease Research Laboratories test (VDRL), rapid plasma reagin (RPR), or automated reagin test (ART)	Benzathine penicillin G 50,000 U/kg IM, one-time dose (not to exceed 2.4 million U); dosages and schedules vary, depending on stage of illness. If allergic: tetracycline 500 mg PO qid; *or* doxycycline 100 mg PO bid for 2 wk

Gonorrhea	*Neisseria gonor-rhoeae*	Gram-positive diplococci	*Clinical:* in *females* may be asymptomatic or present with vaginal discharge, dysuria, or red, swollen genitalia; in *males* may be asymptomatic or present with urethritis *Laboratory:* Gram's stain; culture	Ceftriaxone 125-250 mg IM If allergic: spectinomycin 2 g IM Chlamydia is usually treated also since the two organisms often coexist
Trichomonas	*Trichomonas vaginalis*	Flagellated protozoan	*Clinical:* in *females* may be asymptomatic or present with foul-smelling, yellow-green vaginal discharge, vulvovagini-tis, itching, or dysuria; in *males* may be asymptomatic or present with urethritis *Laboratory:* wet-mount prepara-tion of vaginal discharge	Metronidazole 2 g as single dose, (contraindicated in first trimes-ter of pregnancy)

Compiled from Committee on Infectious Disease, 1994; Paradise, 1993; Sirnick, 1992.

Box 16-2   Clinical Findings Diagnostic of Pelvic Inflammatory Disease

All the following must be present:
1. Lower abdominal pain by history or on physical examination
2. Cervical motion tenderness on pelvic examination
3. Adnexal tenderness

One of the following must be present:
1. Fever >38° C
2. WBC >10,500/mm^3
3. Pelvic abscess on bimanual examination or sonography
4. Purulent material from peritoneal cavity on culdocentesis or laparoscopy
5. ESR >15 mm/hr
6. Positive monoclonal antibody for *Chlamydia trachomatis* from endocervix
7. Gram's stain with gram-negative diplococci from cervix
8. WBC per oil immersion field on Gram's stain of endocervical discharge

From Barkin RM: *Pediatric emergency medicine: concepts and clinical practice,* St Louis, 1992, Mosby.

---

ration is used to identify *Candida* organisms, and a wet mount is obtained for *Trichomonas* organisms.[24] Ultrasonography of the pelvis may be performed, particularly when an ectopic pregnancy or abscess is suspected (Box 16-2).

Once the presence of PID is confirmed and after all cultures have been obtained, antibiotic therapy is begun (Table 16-3). If the adolescent has an uncomplicated infection with moderate symptoms, discharge home may be indicated if compliance with the oral antibiotic regimen can be assured. Adolescents who require admission are those who are pregnant, are HIV positive, and those with severe abdominal pain, or who appear toxic, are unable to keep down medications, or who are unrealiable to follow the treatment protocol. Adolescents with potentially surgical abdomens are also admitted.[5a,18]

Nursing care and evaluation. PID alone is not an emergent condition. However, the differential diagnosis for a female adolescent arriving in the ED with the complaint of lower abdominal pain involves a host of emergent conditions, including peritonitis,

ectopic pregnancy, spontaneous abortion, and appendicitis. For this reason the nurse who is initially evaluating the child must obtain a complete history related to the child's symptoms. Although questions about sexual history may not be appropriate to ask at a busy triage desk, inquiries regarding the date of the last menstrual period, the presence of a vaginal discharge, the degree and location of the pain, and the presence of fever, vomiting, and diarrhea are all important.

Once the child is in the privacy of a room, the nurse may inquire about sexual activity. Since adolescents usually prefer not to discuss sexual activity around their parents, the nurse should ask the parent(s) to step out of the room. If the child is sexually active and is found to have an STD; all partners should be identified. Patients with STDs are reported to the health department. If the child is young or mentally disabled, sexual abuse should be considered.

A child may be discharged if the child is not acutely ill and compliance with the discharge instructions can be ensured. The need for following the full course of antibiotic therapy must be stressed; as well as the need for follow-up care and abstinence from sexual intercourse for 2 to 3 weeks. The adolescent must be warned that failing to comply with the medication regimen and failing to seek follow-up care can result in permanent damage to the reproductive organs. Additionally, unprotected sex and sex with multiple partners places adolescents at risk for contracting HIV. Suggestions for follow-up services may include establishing a relationship with a private practitioner who specializes in adolescent services or attending a public health clinic that specializes in adolescent gynecology.

Signs and symptoms that require immediate attention include an increase in the degree of pain, an increase in fever, or any deterioration in the child's condition.

DISORDERS OF THE URINARY TRACT

URINARY TRACT INFECTION

Etiology. Urinary tract infections (UTIs) are common in childhood. They are defined as the presence of a significant number of bacteria anywhere in the urinary tract. Approximately 75% to 80% of all UTIs in children are caused by *Escherichia coli.*[12,23] Other causes include *Proteus, Klebsiella,* and occasionally *Staphylococcus saprophyticus* organisms.

TABLE 16-3	Recommended Treatment of Pelvic Inflammatory Disease	

INPATIENT TREATMENT	AMBULATORY TREATMENT*
Regimen A[†] Cefoxitin 2 g, IV, every 6 hr (or Cefotetan[‡] 2 g every 12 hr) PLUS Doxycycline[§] 100 mg, IV or PO, every 12 hr continued for at least 48 hr after clinical improvement, and followed by doxycycline[§] 100 mg, orally, 2 times a day to complete a 14-day total course OR	Cefoxitin 2 g, IM, with concurrent administration of probenecid 1 g, PO OR Equivalent cephalosporin[‡] PLUS Doxycycline[§] 100 mg, orally, 2 times a day for 14 days OR
Regimen B[†] Clindamycin 900 mg, IV, every 8 hr (15 to 40 mg/kg/day) PLUS Gentamicin[‖]: loading dose 2.0 mg/kg, IV, followed by maintenance 1.5 mg/kg, IV, every 8 hr This regimen is continued for at least 48 hr after the patient demonstrates significant clinical improvement and is followed by doxycycline[§] 100 mg, orally, 2 times a day, to complete a 14-day total course, or clindamycin 450 mg, PO, every 6 hr, to complete a 14-day total course.	For patients older than 18 yr, ofloxacin[¶] 400 mg, PO, 2 times a day for 14 days PLUS Clindamycin 450 mg, PO, 4 times a day, *or* metronidazole 500 mg, PO, 2 times a day for a total course of 14 days

From Committee on Infectious Diseases, American Academy of Pediatrics: *1995 Report of the Committee on Infectious Diseases,* ed 23, Elk Grove Village, Ill, 1995, Academy, p 354.

*Patients who do not respond to outpatient therapy within 48 hours should be hospitalized for parenteral therapy.

[†]When tuboovarian abscess is present, many clinicians use clindamycin since it provides more effective anaerobic coverage than doxycycline. Clindamycin administered intravenously appears to be effective against *C. trachomatis* infection; the effectiveness of oral clindamycin against *C. trachomatis,* however, has not been determined.

[‡]The experience with cefotetan is less than that with cefoxitin, although cefotetan provides similar antimicrobial coverage and requires frequent dosing. Clinical data are limited on other second- and third-generation cephalosporins (ceftizoxime, cefotaxime, and ceftriaxone) to replace cefoxitin or cefotetan, although many authorities believe they are also effective therapy for PID.

[§]Doxycycline administered orally has bioavailability similar to the IV formulation. Patients who do not tolerate doxycycline should receive erythromycin 500 mg, orally, 4 times a day (40 mg/kg/day) or 10 to 14 days, although this recommendation is based on limited clinical data. Use of doxycycline is ordinarily limited to patients 9 years or older because of the potential for dental staining. Doxycycline is preferred to tetracycline because of its greater bioavailability and better patient compliance.

[‖]Although short courses of aminoglycosides (≤3 days) in healthy adolescents with normal renal function do not usually necessitate monitoring of serum concentrations, some practitioners may elect to do so.

[¶]Quinolones are contraindicated for children and for adolescents younger than 18 years and for pregnant or nursing mothers.

The incidence of UTIs is higher in male infants who are younger than 3 months old than in female infants.[23] Males also tend to have a higher incidence of congenital urinary structural anomalies; however, these anomalies are rare. With development, the male-to-female ratio of UTIs dramatically reverses, and the majority of cases of UTI occur in girls.

Pathophysiology. UTIs acquired during the neonatal period are thought to originate from the bloodstream (hematogenous).[23] UTIs acquired in children and adults are usually caused by a pathogen that ascends the urethra to the bladder.

The severity of the infection and the rapidity of the development of symptoms is a reflection of the virulence of the bacteria, the susceptibility of the host, and the degree to which the organism has spread. For example, because *E. coli* can multiply rapidly, this organism tends to cause more severe symptoms than some other organisms. Urinary stasis contributes to the development of UTIs because urine is an excellent medium for bacteria. Some of the conditions that increase both the risk of stasis and of bacterial contamination include vesicoureteral reflux, urinary obstruction, poor personal hygiene, and sexual activity (Box 16-3).

Many other factors contribute to the development of UTIs among various age groups and between the sexes. The short urethra of the female is close to the anus and may be easily contaminated by stool, particularly when the infant or child is wiped from back to front. In diapered infants stool that is left in the diapers for long periods can enhance the development of an infection. In uncircumcised males the prepuce can harbor bacteria if the foreskin is not retracted and cleaned daily. Children who void infrequently (including those with decreased oral intake) or those who hold their urine are also at increased risk of developing UTIs.

Once the bacteria enters the urinary tract, it multiplies rapidly. If only the bladder is affected, the condition is called cystitis. Mucosal edema with petechiae and hemorrhage result. With inflammation the functional capacity of the bladder is affected and the detrusor muscle becomes hyperactive. The result is frequent small amounts of voided urine that contain red blood cells (RBCs) and white blood cells (WBCs). Repeated infections can produce changes in the bladder wall and the vesicoureteral junction.

When the infection ascends into the kidneys (upper UTI), it is referred to as pyelonephritis. Pyelonephritis is characterized by renal edema, which produces an enlarged kidney. Renal scarring and loss of functioning tissue can result, especially with repeat and chronic infections. Microabscess formation can occur if pyelonephritis is left untreated.

Clinical presentation. Clinical presentation varies significantly, depending on the age of the child and the severity and location of the infection. Many children with UTIs are asymptomatic; however, a variety of nonspecific symptoms usually prompt an ED visit. In neonates and infants symptoms may indicate a variety of conditions that range from gastrointestinal symptoms to sepsis. The infant may be brought to the ED because of poor appetite, failure to thrive, or irritability. Other complaints include vomiting, diarrhea, fever, or foul-smelling urine. A chronic diaper rash may also indicate the presence of a UTI. In these children the diagnosis of a UTI is based on the exclusion of other serious illnesses and a positive urine culture.

Older children and adolescents usually have more specific presenting symptoms, which may include an increase in urinary frequency, urgency, dysuria, lower abdominal pain or back pain, and hematuria. Parents may indicate that the previously potty-trained child is incontinent during the day or wets the bed at night. Fever may or may not be present. Although signs of pyelonephritis vary, common findings include fever, chills, abdominal pain, and flank pain.

Emergency Department interventions. ED management depends on the age of the child and the severity of the infection. Initially a presumptive diagnosis of UTI is made based on the symptomatology. The gold standard for diagnosing a UTI is a properly collected urine culture. A urinalysis is usually done at the same time, but it will not definitively identify the presence of an infection. A child may have an abnormal urinalysis with a negative culture or a positive urine culture with a normal urinalysis.

Urine culture results are interpreted based on colony counts and the method of collection. Specimens collected by bag are unreliable because bacteria from the perineal area can easily contaminate the urine

---

Box 16-3   Factors Contributing to Development of Urinary Tract Infection in the Child

- Poor hygiene
- Constipation
- Incomplete emptying of bladder
- Chemical irritation (e.g., bubble baths)
- Holding of urine
- Dehydration
- Tight clothes
- Diaper rash
- Sexual activity
- Obstructive lesions
- Kidney malformations
- Foreign bodies
- Urethral instrumentation

or the urine may remain in the bag for long periods before being transported to the laboratory. Urine cultures collected from the child who is voiding frequently and not allowing the urine to remain in the bladder long enough for bacteria to multiply, as well as urine collected from the child who is currently undergoing antibiotic therapy for another illness also may be unreliable.

Other than a urine culture, laboratory findings do not definitively identify the presence of a UTI or differentiate an upper UTI from a lower UTI. An elevated WBC count is often present in the child with a renal infection, but it may also indicate the presence of another infectious process. Serum creatinine may be transiently elevated, but this change is not diagnostic.

Once a presumptive diagnosis is made and the urine culture is obtained, antibiotic therapy is initiated. Depending on the severity of the symptoms, antibiotic therapy may be deferred until culture results are obtained. A variety of oral antibiotics can be prescribed for UTIs (Table 16-4). Phenazopyridine, a urinary analgesic, may be ordered, but it can be given only to children older than 6 years.[12]

The criteria for obtaining radiologic studies after a UTI are controversial. Many, children, especially males, are referred for a urologic workup after the first UTI to rule out anatomic anomalies. This workup may include a voiding cystourethrogram (VCUG), intravenous pyelogram (IVP), and renal ultrasound.

Nursing care and evaluation. Nursing care for the child with an uncomplicated UTI is primarily

TABLE 16-4	Commonly Used Oral Antibiotics for Urinary Tract Infections	
DRUG	**DOSAGE (MG/KG/24 HR)**
Amoxicillin	20-40
Amoxicillin/potassium clavulanate	40 (AMX)
Nitrofurantoin	5-7
Sulfamethizole/ trimethroprim (SMX/TMP)	8-12 TMP 40-60 SMX
Cefaclor	20-40
Cephalexin	25-50
Sulfisoxazole	120-150

From Hertz AL: Urinary tract infections. In Barkin RM: *Pediatric emergency medicine: concepts and clinical practice,* St Louis, 1992, Mosby.

supportive. One of the most important interventions is the proper collection of a urine specimen for culture. Methods of collection include obtaining a clean-catch specimen, a catheterized specimen, or a suprapubic aspiration. Bagged specimens are unreliable and should not be used (Table 16-5).

Neonates can rapidly become septic, they are therefore admitted and treated with intravenous (IV) antibiotics. Older infants and children with a high fever or other symptoms that could compromise improvement are also considered for admission. Before admission, a CBC, blood culture, and serum electrolytes may be ordered. An IV line is begun for the administration of parenteral antibiotics.

If the child is to be discharged, home management instructions should include the need for completing the antibiotic schedule as prescribed. It is also necessary to emphasize the importance of a follow-up visit after the antibiotic is completed for a repeat urine culture. Recurrent or partially treated UTIs can lead to additional problems such as hypertension, renal calculi, and chronic renal failure. Instructions should also include increasing fluid intake to dilute the urine and flush out the infection (Box 16-4). Fever and pain control can usually be achieved with acetaminophen or ibuprofen.

VESICOURETERAL REFLUX

Etiology. Vesicoureteral reflux (VUR) is a condition in which the urine is allowed to reflux into the ureter from the bladder because of an abnormality at the ureterovesical junction. Primary VUR is caused by a congenital anomaly. Secondary VUR results from an inflammatory process or from conditions that increase intravesical pressure such as neurogenic bladder.

Pathophysiology. Normally the valvular mechanism located at the ureterovesical junction allows urine to pass downward only. In the child with VUR, however, the incompetent valve allows urine to flow both out from the urethra and back up into the ureters as the child voids. After urination, urine that remains in the ureters returns to the bladder, resulting in urinary stasis. Urine remaining in the bladder acts as a reservoir for bacterial growth, which can lead to the development of urinary tract and kidney infections.

Renal damage can result from VUR because it exposes the renal pelvis to higher than normal pressures during voiding and facilitates the passage of bacteria from the bladder into the kidneys. Dilation of

TABLE 16-5	Methods of Obtaining Urine Cultures	
MODE OF COLLECTION	**PROCEDURE**	**COMMENTS**
Clean catch	Area should be cleaned with soap and water; antibacterial agents may affect reliability of culture results Child must be old enough to correctly clean self Females must keep labia spread to decrease contamination Uncircumcised males should retract foreskin and clean underneath Midstream specimen is collected	Specimens are commonly contaminated in young children but are reliable in older children
Bag specimen	Bag must be applied correctly Urine must not be allowed to remain in bag	This method is *not* recommended for collection of urine cultures; there is high rate of contamination
Catheterization	Catheter is usually inserted only long enough to obtain urine specimen Catheter size is determined by age/size of child; 5 Fr feeding tube can be used in young infants; 8 Fr feeding tube or straight catheter (or 8 Fr catheter kit) may be used in older infant or child May be difficult to perform in uncircumcised male infant Anatomic landmarks can be difficult to identify in female infant If catheter is accidentally inserted into vagina, it may be left in place to identify landmarks while additional sterile catheter is inserted into urethra	One of most reliable methods of collecting a sterile specimen; there is risk of inducing infection during catheter insertion; also there is risk of producing urethral trauma
Suprapubic bladder aspiration	Before procedure bladder should be palpable (or identified by percussion) and infant should not have voided for at least 45 to 60 minutes Area above pubic bone is cleaned with antiseptic solution, and needle attached to syringe is inserted into bladder; this procedure is performed by a physician	This method can be performed only in infants and young children (<2 yr old) (bladder is intraabdominal at this age; after this age bladder descends into pelvis) Complications are rare but include bladder hemorrhage; intestinal perforation, and hematuria

the ureter, the collecting system within the kidney, and renal scarring can result.

Clinical presentation. The most common presentation of the child with VUR is a UTI. Males with a single UTI often have a workup for the presence of VUR. Females may be evaluated after the first UTI, but more commonly they undergo a workup after repeated UTIs.

Emergency Department interventions. ED interventions are generally supportive. A urinalysis and urine culture are obtained, and a CBC and electrolyte levels are ordered if the presence of pyelonephritis is suspected (see the discussion of urinary tract infection earlier in this chapter). If reflux is suspected, the child is referred for urologic studies such as an IVP and VCUG.

Nursing care and evaluation. See the detailed discussion of urinary tract infection earlier in this chapter.

TESTICULAR TORSION

Etiology. Testicular torsion occurs when there is a twisting of the spermatic cord and vessels, inhibiting blood flow to the testicle. It can occur at any age; however, it most commonly occurs prenatally and in the prepubertal male. Prenatal or perinatal torsion is most often the result of a twist that occurs above the testis and the tunica vaginalis. It is termed extravaginal torsion. In the older child or adult, torsion is most commonly caused by twisting of the testis related to anomalous testicular suspension (bell-clapper deformity) and is termed intravaginal torsion.[22] Either form of torsion must be corrected as soon as possible to avoid death to the testicle.

Pathophysiology. Intravaginal testicular torsion is the result of an abnormality that occurs during gestational development between the 28th and 32nd weeks of life. During this period the testes move down the inguinal canal and enter the scrotum. If the tunica vaginalis, a membrane that covers the testes anteriorly, does not form correctly and covers the epididymis and the distal part of the spermatic cord, the testis is allowed to swing freely and can twist and turn, constricting the blood supply to the testicle (bell-clapper deformity)[1] (Fig. 16-4).

Clinical presentation. The most common presentation for the child with testicular torsion is the rapid onset of acute scrotal pain and swelling. Activity before onset is not contributory, since a large number of torsions occur during periods of inactivity (sleep).[25] The pain may radiate to the groin or the abdomen, and nausea and vomiting are common. The testicle appears erythematous, may be edematous, and is "high riding" in the scrotal sac. The affected side will not transilluminate. Movement or lifting of the testicle will increase the pain (Prehn's sign). The history may reveal intermittent pain before the episode, since incomplete torsion episodes can occur before an acute episode.

Emergency Department interventions. There are no specific laboratory tests that identify the presence of testicular torsion; however, a CBC and urinalysis are often obtained as a part of the routine workup. Radioisotopic scans, CT scanning, ultrasonography, and Doppler examinations have all been advocated for differentiating testicular torsion from other abnormalities. These tests, however, should not delay definitive surgical exploration. The time most recognized for salvageability of the testis is less than 6 hours. Other factors, such as a partial (incomplete) torsion, may increase the time of salvageability.

Although the definitive treatment for testicular torsion is surgery, manual detorsion may be performed

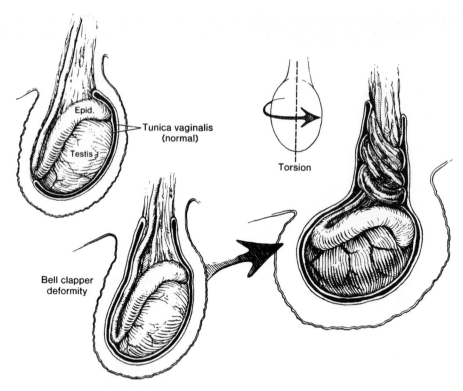

FIG. 16-4. Torsion of the testis. Bell-clapper deformity, an abnormality of testicular fixation, allows torsion of spermatic vessels with subsequent infarction of the gonad. (From Fleisher GR, Ludwig S, eds: *Textbook of pediatric emergency medicine,* ed 3, Baltimore, 1993, Williams & Wilkins.)

before surgery. If manual detorsion is attempted, the child should be adequately medicated before the procedure. The testicle is then rotated in an outward motion because most torsions occur in a medial direction. The effectiveness of manual detorsion is evaluated by relief of pain, the position of the testicle, and the presence of a pulse heard with a Doppler device.

Nursing care and evaluation. The child with suspected testicular torsion is treated emergently. Nursing care includes establishing venous access and obtaining laboratory studies in preparation for surgery. The child must remain NPO. Testicular torsion is extremely painful, and comfort measures include the prompt administration of pain medication. The prospect of surgery is frightening to both the parents and the child. They should be kept informed and given reassurance.

▍RENAL DISORDERS

ACUTE GLOMERULONEPHRITIS

Etiology. Acute glomerulonephritis (AGN) is a condition in which an immune response within the kidneys causes damage to the glomeruli, reducing glomerular filtration. It can be caused by bacterial, viral, parasitic, pharmacologic, or toxic agents. In children AGN most commonly follows an infection of the pharynx or skin caused by group A beta-hemolytic streptococci. Because only certain strains of streptococci produce glomerulonephritis, they are referred to as nephritogenic streptococci. The highest incidence of AGN occurs in children between the ages of 3 and 7 years, and males are more commonly affected than females.[15] Seasonal variations in the frequency of the illness are related to the incidence of pharyngeal

TABLE 16-6	Overview of Glomerulonephritis		
CAUSES	**PATHOPHYSIOLOGY**		**SIGNS AND SYMPTOMS**
Toxic agents In children, most commonly follows group A beta-hemolytic streptococci infection of skin or pharynx	Immune response causes damage to glomeruli Glomerular filtration is reduced; and water and salt are retained		Hematuria Periorbital edema (early finding) Malaise Headache Decreased appetite Decreased urine output Generalized edema Elevated blood pressure Encephalopathy (late finding) Congestive heart failure (late finding)

infections, which are more common in cold weather, and skin infections (impetigo) which are more common in warm weather.[1]

Pathophysiology. Glomerulonephritis is initiated by an immune response within the glomeruli. The mechanism stimulating this response is not well understood. Direct injury to the glomerular cells caused by inflammation and infection and the release of inflammatory cells mediate glomerular injury. The resulting arteriolar vasoconstriction, capillary obstruction, and endothelial cell edema impair glomerular filtration.[7] With glomerular damage, water and salt are retained and signs of renal failure become evident (see the discussion of renal failure later in this chapter).

Clinical presentation. In acute poststreptococcal glomerulonephritis symptoms usually occur 1 to 3 weeks following infection of the skin or pharynx with a nephritogenic strain of streptococcus. Presenting complaints vary considerably depending on the severity of the illness. In some cases complaints of hematuria, or "tea-colored" urine, or orbital edema are the only symptoms. In other cases the child will be febrile and complain of malaise, headache, decreased appetite, and/or decreased urine output. Blood pressure is usually elevated. In chronic or severe cases signs of renal failure will be evident, including generalized edema, oliguria, frank lethargy, encephalopathy, and congestive heart failure (Table 16-6).

Emergency Department interventions. Diagnostic testing requires obtaining a CBC, urinalysis,

serum electrolytes, antistreptolysin (ASO) titer, antideoxyribonuclease B (anti-DNAase B), serum immunoglobulin (IgG) level, and serum complement. If the child is hypertensive, a chest x-ray may be ordered to evaluate the child for the presence of congestive heart failure. The urinalysis will reveal RBCs and RBC casts, polymorphonuclear leukocytes, and proteinuria. Electrolyte imbalances include hyperkalemia, dilutional hyponatremia (because sodium and water are retained), elevated blood urea nitrogen (BUN)—azotemia, and elevated creatinine. The C3 complement is depressed and the child is often anemic.

No specific therapy is recommended for the treatment of AGN, and management is generally supportive. Fluid and salt restriction is usually required, and strict monitoring is particularly important when the child is hypertensive. Severe hypertension may be treated with diuretics, angiotensin-converting enzyme inhibitors, and vasodilators. Antibiotic therapy may be initiated; however, there is no evidence that antibiotic use affects the outcome of the illness.[1] Symptoms can last from 1 to 3 weeks, and the prognosis for full recovery in children is excellent. Complications, however, can lead to permanent kidney disease and even death.

Nursing care and evaluation. Nursing care depends on the severity of the symptoms. Rarely will children with mild cases of AGN be treated at home. In these children close follow-up and compliance with therapy must be ensured. Before discharge the importance of follow-up care must be stressed, since exacerbation of the disease can cause permanent renal damage. Water and sodium restriction, daily weights, and monitoring urine output are required. The parent should be instructed to monitor the child for signs of hypertension such as headaches, irritability, or epistaxis. Taking of daily blood pressures may be required. Signs and symptoms associated with acute renal failure, which require immediate physician notification, include changes in the child's neurologic status (e.g., increasing lethargy, confusion, seizures), difficulty breathing or an increased respiratory rate, generalized edema, significant weight gain, and decreased or absent urinary output. (Nursing care of the acutely ill child is discussed in the section on renal failure, p. 384.)

NEPHROTIC SYNDROME

Etiology. Nephrotic syndrome, sometimes referred to as nephrosis, is a form of glomerular injury that may occur idiopathically, may result from a systemic illness, or may be inherited. There is also a congenital form of the disease, which is often fatal. Primary nephrotic syndrome accounts for the majority of children with nephrotic syndrome and refers to diseases limited to the kidney. Minimal change nephrotic syndrome (MCNS) is the most common form of primary disease and accounts for approximately 80% of all cases in children.[5] The primary form mainly affects preschool children between the ages of 2 and 7 years and is twice as prevalent in males than in females until adolescence.[17] Secondary nephrotic syndrome refers to conditions in which the kidney is damaged secondary to a multisystem illness or disease, such as systemic lupus erythematosus, diabetes mellitus, or sickle-cell disease. Nephrotic syndrome may also result from an immune-mediated reaction to toxins such as heavy metals, bee venom, and certain drugs such as nonsteroidal antiinflammatory drugs, ampicillin, rifampin, and hydantoin anticonvulsants.[5,27]

Pathophysiology. Nephrotic syndrome is characterized by the loss of protein and albumin from the glomeruli into the urine. The precise mechanism that triggers this event is not well understood; however, it is probably related to a noninflammatory immunologic or metabolic process that causes an increase in the permeability of the glomerular basement membrane.[5] As hypoalbuminemia develops, a decrease in intravascular colloid osmotic pressure enhances the movement of water into the interstitial spaces and edema results. With this third-spacing of fluids, intra-

vascular volume drops. In response, aldosterone and the antidiuretic hormone are stimulated, increasing fluid and sodium reabsorption and further contributing to the edema. Depending on the progression of these events, intravascular volume may be low, normal, or high.

The synthesis of lipids is increased in the child with nephrotic syndrome and is probably stimulated by the degree of hypoproteinemia.[5] The result is an elevation in serum cholesterol and triglycerides. These changes, coupled with increased coagulation (e.g., increased platelet aggregation, decreased fibrinolytic activity, changes in coagulation factors) predispose the child to a thrombotic event, which is a serious complication of nephrotic syndrome.

Clinical presentation. The typical presentation of the child with nephrotic syndrome in the ED is edema. In early or mild cases periorbital edema may be the first sign of illness, and the child may appear otherwise healthy. In these children the edema often resolves during the day. With questioning the parents may relate a history of malaise and occasional abdominal pain. Parents may state that the child's urine output is decreased and the child's weight may be slowly increasing, even as intake is decreasing. In more severe cases the child initially has generalized edema and ascites, which can produce respiratory distress as pressure is placed on the diaphragm. Vomiting, diarrhea, and anorexia may result from pressure on the abdominal organs and edema of the intestinal wall. On examination, these children look sick. Depending on the stage of the disease, the child's blood pressure may be normal, decreased (through intravascular volume loss), or mildly elevated. Although it can occur, the child with nephrotic syndrome rarely arrives in the ED with signs of hypovolemic shock (Table 16-7).

Emergency Department interventions. Diagnostic testing requires obtaining a CBC, urinalysis, serum electrolytes, calcium, phosphorus, serum albumin, total serum protein, serum cholesterol, BUN, serum creatinine, and serum C_3 and C_4 levels. Additional laboratory studies may be ordered, such as serum antinuclear antibody and DNA binding to distinguish between primary and secondary causes of the disease. Depending on the severity of the presentation, chest x-ray and abdominal x-ray examinations may be ordered. A renal ultrasound to visualize the kidneys may also be ordered.

The urinalysis will always reveal proteinuria (>2 g/day) and may also reveal the presence of hyaline

TABLE 16-7	Overview of Nephrotic Syndrome		
CAUSES	**PATHOPHYSIOLOGY**	**SIGNS AND SYMPTOMS**
Idiopathic Triggered by systemic illness Congenital	Increased permeability of glomerular basement membrane causes protein and albumin to be lost in urine With development of hypoalbuminemia, intravascular fluid moves into interstitial spaces, resulting in edema	Periorbital edema (early sign) Generalized edema Weight gain Decreased urine output Malaise Ascites Abdominal pain, vomiting, diarrhea Respiratory distress associated with ascites or pulmonary edema Hepatomegaly

casts, a high specific gravity, and microscopic hematuria. Electrolyte imbalances may or may not be present. Mild decreases in serum sodium levels are not uncommon; however, this finding rarely requires treatment. Total serum calcium levels may be decreased because of the hypoalbuminemia (serum albumin <2 g/dl), yet serum ionized calcium is usually normal. Hyperlipidemia and hypoproteinemia will be present. Serum creatinine and BUN are usually within normal limits; however, an initial slight increase in BUN is not uncommon. If the child is volume depleted, the hematocrit level may be elevated as a result of hemoconcentration.

Treatment of the child with nephrotic syndrome depends on the severity of the symptoms. In the volume-depleted child treatment begins with the restoration of circulating volume and the stabilization of electrolyte imbalances. If the child's circulating volume is adequate, yet severe edema is compromising ventilatory status, furosemide 1 to 2 mg/kg/dose in 2 divided doses may be given. Once the serum albumin falls below 1.5 g/dl, diuretics are no longer effective. At this point the administration of albumin followed by furosemide may be required.

The primary treatment of uncomplicated cases of nephrotic syndrome is the administration of corticosteroids. Prednisone 2 mg/kg/24 hr in 2 to 3 divided doses is administered if the child is between 1 and 7 years of age and has MCNS, minimal hematuria, and a normal complement.[17] Bacterial infections are a serious complication of steroid administration in these children, and close monitoring is necessary. With the administration of prednisone, proteinuria decreases and is often gone after 2 weeks

of therapy, at which point the prednisone is tapered. If proteinuria continues after 1 month and as the prednisone is being tapered, the child may be steroid dependent.

Nursing care and evaluation. Nursing care depends on the seriousness of the child's condition on arrival in the ED. Any child with generalized edema, decreased urine output, and/or signs of respiratory distress deserves emergent care. If the child is volume depleted and is exhibiting clinical signs of shock, such as weak pulses, delayed capillary refill, and an altered mental status, volume therapy with normal saline 20 ml/kg is required to restore circulating volume. Children exhibiting signs of respiratory distress related to ascites, pressure on the diaphragm, or pulmonary edema require supplemental oxygen therapy and, depending on the severity of the distress, may be candidates for ventilatory support. These children are placed on a cardiac monitor, and their vital signs must be continuously assessed, particularly the blood pressure.

In all affected children intake and output must be strictly monitored. Urine is checked at the bedside for protein and sent to the laboratory for a complete urinalysis. If the child's condition is stable, there is minimal swelling, and the criteria for the administration of prednisone can be met (see the Emergency Department Interventions section earlier in this chapter), home management may be considered. However, maintaining follow-up care and adherence to the treatment regimen must be ensured. Parents should be instructed to place the child on a low-salt diet. This means that no salt is added to the child's food and the child is not given salty foods such as potato chips. Fluids may or may not be restricted, depending on the degree of edema, but they are also not encouraged. Parents are taught to monitor the child for increasing edema and the development of more serious complications. Measuring daily weight and monitoring urine output are simple evaluation methods. If the child develops respiratory distress, has an altered mental status, or voids infrequently or not at all, the parent must seek immediate medical care. Rest is important, but inactivity can increase the chance of a thromboembolism; therefore the child usually may continue to participate in physical activities as tolerated.

The risks of prednisone therapy are relayed to the parents by the physician; however, the nurse should reinforce to the parents that immediate follow-up care is required if the child becomes febrile. Increased appetite, gastrointestinal irritation, mood swings, weight gain, and cushingoid facies are all side effects of prednisone therapy.

Relapses of nephrotic syndrome are not uncommon during tapering of the prednisone or on completion of therapy, particularly with illness. The child should therefore avoid contact with other children who are ill. The risk of long-term renal dysfunction is minimal, however, particularly in children who respond to steroid therapy. Children usually outgrow the illness by the second decade of life; however, occasionally it progresses into adulthood.

RENAL FAILURE

Etiology.   Renal failure is categorized as acute renal failure (ARF) and chronic renal failure (CRF). ARF is defined as an acute reduction in the GFR. Multiple etiologies are responsible for ARF, including prerenal factors, primary renal causes, and postrenal factors. Although these factors are discussed separately, each can contribute to the overall impairment of renal function to varying degrees as renal failure progresses.

Prerenal factors produce a decrease in renal perfusion as occurs with hypovolemic shock caused by blood or fluid loss or third-spacing of fluids. Primary renal causes, which produce parenchymal damage, result from direct renal insult from an infectious or inflammatory process, or hypoxia. Examples include glomerulonephritis and hemolytic-uremic syndrome, which account for more than 50% of cases in children.[8] Hypoxic events can result from asphyxia (e.g., near-drowning or birth injuries) and sepsis. Postrenal causes are the result of obstructions, such as stones, strictures, or hematomas. (Box 16-5).

CRF refers to an irreversible or progressive reduc-

Box 16-5   Causes of Acute Renal Failure

I. Prerenal
  A. Decreased cardiac output (cardiogenic shock)
  B. Decreased intravascular volume (hemorrhage, dehydration, "third-spacing")
II. Renal
  A. Primary renal parenchymal disease
    1. Vascular (acute glomerulonephritis, hemolytic uremic syndrome)
    2. Interstitial (pyelonephritis, drug-induced)
  B. Acute tubular necrosis
    1. Ischemic injury (see I, B above)
    2. Nephrotoxic injury (antibiotics, uric acid)
    3. Pigmenturia (myoglobinuria, hemoglobinuria)
III. Postrenal
  A. Obstructive uropathy
    1. Posterior urethral valves
    2. Intraabdominal tumor
    3. Nephrolithiasis (rare)
  B. Renal vein thrombosis (rare outside neonatal period)

From Cronan KM and Norman ME: Renal and electrolyte emergencies. In Fleisher G, Ludwig S, eds: *Textbook of pediatric emergency medicine,* ed 3, Baltimore, 1993, Williams & Wilkins.

---

tion in GFR to below 25% of normal.[3] It may be caused by congenital lesions or malformations such as posterior urethral valves or metabolic diseases, or it may be caused by acquired diseases such as hemolytic-uremic syndrome or chronic glomerulonephritis.

Pathophysiology.   Prerenal ARF occurs when the kidney is unable to compensate for acute decreases in blood flow. Renal hypoperfusion stimulates the reabsorption of water and sodium in an attempt to restore circulating volume. Under certain conditions, where vascular volume is normal, this response may be detrimental. For example, cardiogenic shock will produce a decrease in cardiac output and therefore renal perfusion, even though circulating volume may be normal. With prerenal ARF, once renal blood flow is restored, the GFR returns to normal.

Direct insult or injury to the kidneys can produce ARF and may affect any of the normal physiologic processes within the kidney. Renal thrombosis, which can be caused by a number of etiologic complexes—from sickle cell disease to hemoconcentration—can impair renal blood flow and cause ischemic injury. Other conditions that will impair normal physiologic processes include infectious or inflammatory processes, which directly affect the arterioles and glomerular capillaries, such as AGN and pyelonephritis. Acute tubular necrosis can result from renal failure and is characterized by areas of tubular cell necrosis, which may be caused by ischemia or nephrotoxic agents. Acute tubular necrosis accounts for the majority of adult cases of ARF.[19]

With CRF, as the nephrons are damaged, glomerular capillary blood flow and pressure increase in functional nephrons. With the increased blood flow, solute load per nephron also increases. Intraglomerular hypertension and endothelial damage lead to glomerular sclerosis, which induces systemic hypertension and further aggravates hyperperfusion within the nephrons.[3]

Renal failure produces severe metabolic and physiologic derangements. Hyperkalemia, defined as a serum potassium level of greater than 6 mEq/L, results as renal potassium excretion declines. It is exacerbated with systemic tissue damage (e.g., crush injuries or cellular hypoxia from hypovolemic shock) and can produce life-threatening cardiac arrhythmias. Hypertension results as fluid and sodium are retained, with stimulation of the renin-angiotensin system and with direct renal damage such as glomerular sclerosis. With fluid retention and hypertension, congestive heart failure and pulmonary edema may occur. Seizures can result from the primary disease process, from electrolyte imbalances such as hyponatremia (water intoxication) and hypocalcemia, from hypertensive encephalopathy, or from the uremic state.[1]

Clinical presentation. The clinical presentation of the child with ARF varies depending on the cause and the progression of the disease. The one common finding is decreased or absent urinary output. In the volume-depleted child signs of dehydration or shock may be present. If parenchymal damage has occurred, hypertension, pallor, edema, activity intolerance, or lethargy may be observed. If the condition has continued for several weeks before medical care is sought, the child may have presenting signs of uremia, including an alternating mental status or seizures.

Children with CRF may initially have nonspecific symptoms such as lethargy, weakness, hypertension, and headache. Other symptoms that may be noted are abnormal bone and tooth formation, growth failure, nocturia, and salt cravings.

Emergency Department interventions. The goal of diagnostic testing is to differentiate between the various forms of renal failure. In general, a CBC, urinalysis, urine culture, serum electrolytes, calcium, phosphorus, creatinine, magnesium, and BUN are ordered. Additional laboratory studies may include serum albumin, complement, cholesterol, uric acid, SGOT, lactic dehydrogenase (LDH), or antistreptolysin-O (ASO) titer. A chest x-ray examination to evaluate heart size and pulmonary vasculature and a renal ultrasound to visualize the kidneys may also be ordered.

The urinalysis will reveal little blood or protein. Significant proteinuria may indicate the presence of nephrotic syndrome. Hematuria and proteinuria suggest the presence of glomerulonephritis. If prerenal failure is present, the specific gravity will be high; however, with acute tubular necrosis the specific gravity is often normal. Spot blood and urine studies, performed simultaneously, may be ordered to compare sodium, creatinine, and urea. Findings may be used to differentiate between prerenal failure and acute tubular necrosis.

Electrolyte imbalances are often present, the most serious of which is hyperkalemia. Hyponatremia may also be present but rarely requires treatment. Dilutional hyponatremia is not uncommon. With systemic tissue damage, metabolic acidosis results as hydrogen ion excretion and bicarbonate ion reabsorption are affected within the kidneys. Other findings may include hyperphosphatemia and hypocalcemia.

Initial management of the child in renal failure depends on the presenting symptoms and the suspected etiologic basis. If prerenal failure is present because of hypovolemic shock, volume expansion is initiated. Significant intrarenal damage that causes edema, respiratory distress, high blood pressure, and congestive heart failure requires diuretic therapy. Although furosemide is the usual drug choice, mannitol is used occasionally, particularly with myoglobinuria or hemoglobinuria.[5] Mannitol must be used judiciously, however, because if it is not excreted by the kidneys, it will remain in the vascular compartment, further contributing to extracellular volume expansion. Postrenal failure is treated on the basis of the suspected cause of the obstruction. Occasionally, emergent surgical intervention is required (Fig. 16-5).[16]

Metabolic and electrolyte disorders must also be addressed. The most important of these disorders is hyperkalemia. A mildly elevated potassium level may be treated with sodium polystyrene sulfonate (Kayexalate); however, severe hyperkalemia (potassium level >7.0 mEq/L) or symptomatic hyperkale-

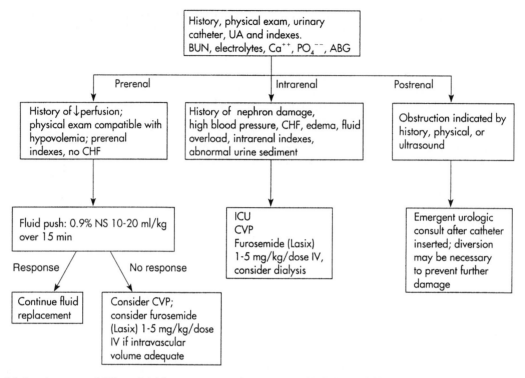

FIG. 16-5. Acute renal failure: initial assessment and treatment. *ABG,* Arterial blood gas; *BUN,* blood urea nitrogen; *Ca++,* calcium; *CHF,* congestive heart failure; *CVP,* central venous pressure; *ICU,* intensive care unit; *NS,* normal saline; *PO4--* phosphate; *UA,* urinalysis. (From Barkin RM, Rosen P: *Emergency pediatrics: a guide to ambulatory care,* ed 4, St Louis, 1994, Mosby.)

mia requires aggressive management to move potassium back into the intracellular compartment. Therapy may include the administration of sodium bicarbonate (1 to 2 mEq/kg given over 15 to 30 minutes).[14] Furosemide, along with removing excess intravascular fluid, increases the excretion of potassium. Calcium gluconate is used to modify the membrane effects of hyperkalemia and correct cardiac dysrhythmias.[14] Hyponatremia usually represents serum dilution and rarely requires treatment. In affected patients fluid and sodium restriction is often indicated. Hypocalcemia may also represent a dilutional state and does not require treatment unless the serum phosphate level is known to be high. In all children with renal failure, administration of fluid and electrolytes is judiciously calculated according to intrinsic and extrinsic fluid losses.

Nursing care and evaluation. The child arriving at the ED with a history of decreased urinary output and an alternating mental status requires emergent

management. Often, however, symptoms of ARF and CRF are nonspecific and require further exploration. For example, the combination of nausea and vomiting is a frequent complaint in the ED and can indicate any number of illnesses. When coupled with decreased urinary output, hypertension, and/or an alternating mental status, this symptom may indicate the presence of ARF. Severe dehydration evidenced by sunken eyes, decreased urine output, delayed capillary refill, and a weak, rapid pulse may also indicate the presence of ARF, as can a decreased urine output coupled with edema and signs of congestive heart failure.

Initial management of the child in renal failure depends on the severity of the symptoms. As in all patients, stabilization of the ABCs comes first. If tachypnea is present or if there is an increase in the work of breathing, supplemental oxygen administration is indicated. The child is placed on a cardiac monitor, venous access is obtained, blood for analysis is drawn, and an indwelling catheter is inserted. All fluid intake and output is scrupulously monitored. If the child is volume depleted, fluid bolus therapy with normal saline is initiated to restore renal blood flow and glomerular filtration. In the child with volume overload and edema, diuretic therapy is initiated and fluid intake is severely restricted. When a child fails to respond to fluid or diuretic therapy or if the child has a life-threatening metabolic derangement, hemodialysis or peritoneal dialysis should be anticipated. In the pediatric population peritoneal dialysis is the most frequently used mode.

Because electrolyte imbalances, particularly hyperkalemia, are common, the child's heart rate and rhythm must be observed for the development of lethal dysrhythmias. Blood pressure is monitored for the development or exacerbation of hypertension. Mental status is evaluated for neurologic findings, such as an alternating mental status, coma, or seizures, which may represent severe metabolic derangements, electrolyte disturbances, or hemolytic-uremic syndrome. The child must be continuously monitored for the development of congestive heart failure, including signs such as increasing edema, a large liver, tachypnea, an increase in the work of breathing, and rales.

The child with RF requires hospital admission. Since the child and the parents will be anxious, they will require understanding and support. They need to be kept informed of the treatment plan and provided with frequent updates (Box 16-6).

RENAL TRANSPLANTATION

Etiology. Renal transplantation was first performed during the mid-1950s. Today this procedure is considered a means to treat end-stage renal failure. There are numerous causes of end-stage renal failure, including reflux or obstructive nephropathy, renal dysplasia, and chronic glomerulonephritis.

Pathophysiology. Ideally the donor kidney comes from a close family member, but it may also be provided by an unrelated donor or come from a cadaver. Identical twins provide the best match, followed by other siblings, parents, and aunts and uncles. Cadaver kidneys have a higher rate of rejection than those of immediate family members. Rejection may occur immediately after the transplant or up to 3 to 4 years posttransplantation.

Clinical presentation. The major concern for children with a renal transplant is rejection, which can occur acutely or chronically. Although most children exhibit some of the signs of rejection, symptoms of

---

Box 16-6   Nursing Care of the Child with Acute Renal Failure

- Stabilize airway and breathing
- Stabilize circulatory status
  - Obtain full set of vital signs and child's weight
  - Place child on cardiac monitor
  - Assess distal pulses, capillary refill, skin color, and neurologic status
  - Establish peripheral venous access
  - Draw blood for analysis
  - Administer fluid volume (10-20 ml/kg) for hypovolemia
  - Administer diuretics, as ordered, for fluid retention
- Assess neurologic status
- Insert indwelling catheter
  - Measure all urine output
  - Send urine for analysis
- Continuously monitor:
  - Cardiac rhythm for development of dysrhythmias
  - Intake and output
  - Blood pressure
  - Neurologic status
  - Respiratory status (observe for development of congestive heart failure)
  - Hydration status

---

acute rejection include fever, chills, hypertension, edema, lethargy, decreased urine output, and tenderness over the graft site. Acute rejection usually occurs within 10 days of the surgery; however, it may occur up to 6 months after surgery.

Chronic rejection occurs gradually and may begin at any time after the transplant. Symptoms include hypertension and hematuria. With kidney rejection, renal function returns to the pretransplant state.

Emergency Department interventions. Renal transplant patients brought to the ED are commonly evaluated for evidence of rejection. Diagnostic studies include a CBC, serum electrolytes, calcium, phosphate, serum creatinine, urinalysis, and BUN (see the discussion of failure earlier in this chapter). Depending on the findings, the child may be admitted for supportive care, 24-hour urine collection, and a possible renal biopsy.

All postrenal transplant children must take antirejection medications such as cyclosporine and immunosuppressants such as prednisone, methylprednisolone, or azathioprine. The smallest effective dose of medications is administered because of the serious associated side effects, which include hypertension, growth failure, and infection. Rejection is treated with high-dose methylprednisolone. It also may be treated with lymphocyte monoclonal antibody.[26]

Nursing care and evaluation. Because of their immunosuppressed status, children with a history of renal transplantation, who are brought to the ED must be segregated from other children. A private or isolation room is ideal. Emergent or urgent management is warranted, depending on the child's presenting symptoms. If signs of renal failure are present, the child will require emergent interventions (see the discussion of renal failure earlier in this chapter). Nursing interventions for any child with suspected renal failure include monitoring intake and output, neurologic status, vital signs (particularly blood pressure), cardiac rhythm, and respiratory status.

▌ MULTISYSTEM DISORDERS

HEMOLYTIC-UREMIC SYNDROME

Etiology. Hemolytic-uremic syndrome (HUS) is a disease that produces renal failure, thrombocytopenia, and hemolytic anemia. The exact mechanism that leads to the development of hemolytic-uremic syndrome has not been identified; however, numerous prodromal symptoms have been associated with its development. The most common causes of HUS are bacterial or viral organisms or their toxins, which induce injury to the capillary endothelium. However,

HUS has been identified in pregnant women and has also been associated with the use of oral contraceptives and cyclosporin A.

HUS occurs predominantly in the Caucasian population on the West Coast during the summer months. It is rare in the African-American population. Outbreaks among large numbers of people have been identified, and the disease may occur in entire families. Hereditary forms of the disease have also been recognized. HUS primarily occurs in infants and young children (under the age of 5).[3]

Pathophysiology. Precisely what initiates the sequence of events that characterize HUS is unclear. Pathophysiologically a toxic agent produces multisystem compromise by damaging the endothelial cells. In children the classic prodrome of the disease is bloody diarrhea, which may be caused by *Escherichia coli*, *Shigella*, or *Salmonella* organisms. HUS can also follow an upper respiratory infection.

Once damaged, the endothelial cells swell and become occluded with fibrin deposits. Platelets adhere to the damaged sites, initiating the production of additional platelets and fibrin deposits. Normally the production of prostacyclin (PGI_2), which is a potent vasodilator and inhibits platelet aggregation, would mediate these events. However, in the patient with HUS prostacyclin production is decreased. As platelets and fibrins deposit in the glomeruli, the GFR decreases and ARF develops. RBCs are damaged as they pass through the obstructed vasculature; they may also be damaged directly by the toxin. Damaged cells are hemolyzed more easily and removed by the liver and spleen, resulting in anemia (Fig. 16-6).

Clinical presentation. Prodromal symptoms have been identified with upper respiratory infections,

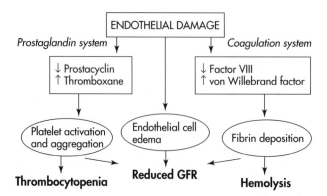

FIG. 16-6. Pathophysiology of microangiopathic disease. (From Fuhrman BP, Zimmerman JJ, eds: *Pediatric critical care,* St Louis, 1992, Mosby.)

but they are most common with gastrointestinal symptoms. Abdominal pain followed by vomiting, diarrhea, fever, and progressively worsening bloody diarrhea are the most common findings. With progression of the disease, hematuria and dehydration may occur.

After the prodromal symptoms have appeared, the patient shows signs of ARF, as evidenced by decreased urinary output, irritability, lethargy, weakness, seizures, coma, pallor, petechiae, jaundice, and/or hypertension. Other significant findings include electrolyte imbalances, pancreatic insufficiency, hepatitis, and cardiomyopathy.

Emergency Department interventions. Diagnostic testing requires obtaining a CBC, urinalysis, serum electrolytes, calcium, phosphate, BUN, serum creatinine, reticulocyte count, platelet count, prothrombin time (PT), partial thromboplastin time (PTT), fibrinogen split products, liver function tests, and a blood smear. Additional testing is based on the symptomatology.

The WBC count will be increased, and the hemoglobin and hematocrit will be decreased. The peripheral blood smear will reveal the presence of fragmented RBCs, caused by hemolysis, and the platelet count will be decreased, often below $50,000/mm^3$. The reticulocyte count is usually high. Creatinine, phosphorus, BUN, and potassium levels will be elevated, whereas sodium and calcium will be decreased. Microscopic hematuria or gross hematuria may be found in the urinalysis. Protein, WBCs, and granular and hyaline casts are also evident in the urine.

Treatment depends on the presentation. If it is early in the course of the illness, with volume depletion from severe diarrhea noted, fluid resuscitation is indicated. The child who is hypervolemic and anuric and has severe electrolyte disturbances will require dialysis. In general, treatment is supportive. It is aimed at correcting electrolyte disturbances, maintaining fluid balance, controlling hypertension, controlling bleeding secondary to thrombocytopenia, and treating anemia. Numerous approaches to therapy have been attempted, none of which has proven completely successful. Some of these therapeutic modalities include the administration of heparin, fibrinolytics, aspirin, fresh-frozen plasma, prostacyclin, vitamin E, and IgG. Plasmaphoresis also has been suggested.[5,7]

Nursing care and evaluation. The child with suspected HUS is treated emergently with stabilization of the ABCs. Because severe neurologic manifestations such as seizures or coma may occur, the child's neurologic status is constantly monitored. The child is placed on a cardiac monitor, and vital signs, including blood pressure, are recorded frequently. Vascular access is achieved, blood work is obtained, and a Foley catheter is inserted. Fluid intake and output is monitored, and fluid restriction is instituted (see the discussion of renal failure earlier in this chapter). If packed RBCs or blood products (e.g., fresh-frozen plasma and platelets) are ordered, they must be administered slowly to minimize the increase in vascular volume. Packed RBCs are administered no faster than 5 ml/kg over 4 hours and are given only for severe anemia.[3] Platelets are administered only when there is active bleeding or an extremely low platelet count because their administration can further contribute to the thrombic glomerular plugging.

Electrolyte imbalances and severe metabolic derangement can lead to the development of life-threatening dysrhythmias and encephalopathy. Fluid retention can exacerbate hypertension and lead to the development of congestive heart failure and pulmonary edema. Coagulopathies can result in active bleeding, one of the most serious consequences of which is a CNS hemorrhage. The ED nurse needs to be cognizant of the complications associated with HUS and must closely monitor the child for the development of symptoms that may indicate a deterioration in status.

Children with suspected HUS require hospital admission and may be candidates for dialysis. The child and the parents will be anxious and therefore will require support and understanding. The parents need to be kept informed of the plan of care and the child's progress. HUS is a serious, life-threatening illness. The majority of children, however, recover after 1 to 3 months of therapy and have no long-term sequelae. A few children develop CRF.

HENOCH-SCHÖNLEIN PURPURA

Etiology. Henoch-Schönlein purpura, also known as anaphylactoid purpura, is classified as a collagen-vascular disease that produces systemic vasculitis. Glomerular involvement is commonly present. The cause of the disease is unknown. However, it occurs more frequently during the winter months, when respiratory illnesses are prevalent, and has also been associated with allergic reactions and drug sensitivities. Henoch-Schönlein purpura affects more males than females, particularly between 3 and 10 years of age.[13,23]

Pathophysiology. Henoch-Schönlein purpura is a multisystem disorder that affects the smallest blood vessels and causes accumulation of WBCs in a number of organs, including the kidneys. In the kidneys there are focal and segmental increases in mesangial cells, which are an extension of connective tissue into the renal glomerulus.[1] The degree of renal involvement varies and may not develop for up to 1 month or longer after the onset of the disease. Approximately one half of children with Henoch-Schönlein purpura develop renal symptoms; however, the majority have minor manifestations, including mild hematuria and protein-uria with preserved renal function.[1] Children with severe renal involvement have poor renal function. If nephrotic syndrome develops, the prognosis is poor.

Clinical presentation. The clinical presentation of HSP varies. In some children the only presenting complaint is the presence of a maculopapular rash. This hivelike rash may cover the buttocks, lower extremities, and extensor surfaces of the arms. In males it may also cover the scrotum. The rash eventually progresses to purpura and petechiae.

Arthritic joint pain and abdominal pain are other common findings. Painful joints, particularly the knees and ankles, are common and may be accompanied by swelling. The arthritis may be migratory and transient. Abdominal pain, sometimes described as colicky, may be accompanied by diarrhea and bloody stools; it may be severe enough to mimic an acute abdomen. Hypertension is a rare finding. Hematuria represents renal involvement, which occurs in approximately one half of the patients with Henoch-Schönlein purpura.[1] Renal involvement may occur immediately, or it may be detected up to 1 month after the onset of the disease.

Emergency Department interventions. Diagnostic testing is performed to rule out the presence of an acute abdomen and to evaluate the degree of renal involvement. A CBC, platelet count, serum electrolytes, serum proteins, erythrocyte sedimentation rate, urinalysis, and serum complement are usually ordered. Depending on the presenting symptoms, additional studies may be indicated, including an abdominal x-ray examination to rule out intussusception as the cause of the severe abdominal pain.

The diagnosis of Henoch-Schönlein purpura is based on clinical findings. Diagnostic findings include a normal CBC or mild anemia. The electrolytes, complement, and platelet count will be normal. Depending on the degree of renal involvement, the urinalysis may reveal mild to moderate hematuria and proteinuria.

Treatment is supportive, and there is no one accepted approach. Steroids are useful in some children but are not given until the presence of an acute abdomen has been ruled out.

Nursing care and evaluation. Because the initial presentation of Henoch-Schönlein purpura can vary significantly, the prioritization of patient care depends on the presenting symptoms. Any child who arrives in the ED with signs of shock and decreased urine output deserves emergent care. In rare cases the child with this condition may initially have neurologic findings (e.g., coma, seizures) that are indicative of renal failure. These children also require emergent management.

The constellation of symptoms common in the child with Henoch-Schönlein purpura, including rash, polyarthralgic joint pain, and/or abdominal pain, would generally place a child in the emergent or urgent categories, depending on the severity of the symptoms. Any purpuric rash, regardless of suspected cause, requires emergent management.

Once the ABCs are assessed and stabilized, supportive care is usually all that is required. Analgesics such as acetaminophen are administered for pain, and steroids such as prednisone (1 to 2 mg/kg/24 hr bid) may be prescribed for more severe symptoms. If signs of severe renal involvement are present, the child will require emergent management and admission to the hospital (see the discussion of renal failure earlier in this chapter).

Most affected children are released home, as long as follow-up care can be ensured. Parents should be instructed to observe the child for signs of swelling and weight gain and to monitor the child's urine output. If the child has evidence of renal involvement, regardless of the degree of mildness, follow-up with a nephrologist is advised.

REFERENCES

1. Behrman RE et al: *Nelson textbook of pediatrics,* ed 14, Philadelphia, 1992, WB Saunders.
2. Brem AS: An overview of renal structure and function. In Fuhrman BP, Zimmerman JJ, eds: *Pediatric critical care,* St Louis, 1992, Mosby, pp 659-669.
3. Castillo J: Chronic renal failure. In Barkin RM, ed:

Pediatric emergency medicine: concepts and clinical practice, St Louis, 1992, Mosby, pp 1066-1068.

4. Committee on Infectious Diseases, American Academy of Pediatrics: *1994 Red book: report of the Committee on Infectious Diseases,* ed 23, Elk Grove Village, Ill, 1994, The Academy.

5. Cronan KM, Norman ME: Renal and electrolyte emergencies. In Fleisher G, Ludwig S, eds: *Textbook of pediatric emergency medicine,* ed 3, Baltimore, 1993, Williams & Wilkins, pp 690-717.

5a. Dinerman LM, Genuardi F: Pelvic inflammatory disease: evaluation, treatment, and follow-up, *Jacksonville Medicine* 47:5, 1996, pp 192-194.

6. Fleisher G: Infectious disease emergencies. In Fleisher G, Ludwig S, eds: *Textbook of pediatric emergency medicine,* ed 3, Baltimore, 1993, Williams & Wilkins, p 641.

7. Friedman AL: Acute renal disease. In Fuhrman BP, Zimmerman JJ, eds: *Pediatric critical care,* St Louis, 1992, Mosby, pp 723-739.

8. Gaudio KM, Siegel NJ: Pathogenesis and treatment of acute renal failure, *Pediatr Nephrol* 34:771, 1987.

8a. Golden N, Neuhoff H: Pelvic inflammatory disease in adolescents, *J Pediatr* 114:138-143, 1989.

9. Guignard JP et al: Glomerular filtration rate in the first three weeks of life, *J Pediatr* 87:268, 1975.

10. Guyton AC: *Textbook of medical physiology,* ed 8, Philadelphia, 1991, WB Saunders.

11. Hazinski MF: *Nursing care of the critically ill child,* ed 2, St Louis, 1992, Mosby.

12. Hertz AL: Urinary tract infections. In Barkin RM, ed: *Pediatric emergency medicine: concepts and clinical practice,* St Louis, 1992, Mosby, pp 1070-1074.

13. Hurley RM, Drummon KN: Anaphylactoid purpura nephritis: clinicopathological correlations, *J Pediatr* 81:904, 1972.

14. Jones DP, Chesney RW: Glomerular dysfunction and acute renal failure. In Fuhrman BP, Zimmerman JJ, eds: *Pediatric critical care,* St Louis, 1992, Mosby, pp 697-706.

15. Knepper JG: Poststreptococcal glomerulonephritis, acute. In Barkin RM, ed: *Pediatric emergency medicine: concepts and clinical practice,* St Louis, 1992, Mosby, pp 1068-1070.

16. Knepper JG: Renal failure. In Barkin RM, ed: *Pediatric emergency medicine: concepts and clinical practice,* St Louis, 1992, Mosby, pp 1062-1066.

17. McEnery PT, Strife CR: Nephrotic syndrome in childhood, *Pediatr Clin North Am* 89:875, 1982.

18. Melzer-Lange M: Gynecologic and obstetric emergencies. In Barkin RM, ed: *Pediatric emergency medicine: concepts and clinical practice,* St Louis, 1992, Mosby, p 796.

19. Ongkingco JRC, Bock GH: Diagnosis and management of acute renal failure in the critical care unit. In Holbrook PR, ed: *Textbook of pediatric critical care,* Philadelphia, 1993, WB Saunders, pp 585-601.

20. Paradise JE: Pediatric and adolescent gynecology. In Fleisher G, Ludwig S, eds: *Textbook of pediatric emergency medicine,* ed 3, Baltimore, 1993, Williams & Wilkins, p 932.

21. Pitts RF: *Physiology of the kidney and body fluids,* ed 3, Chicago, 1974, Year Book.

22. Rowe MI et al: *Essentials of pediatric surgery,* St Louis, 1995, Mosby.

23. Ruley EJ: *Pediatric primary care,* ed 2, St Louis, 1992, Mosby.

24. Sirnick A, Melzer-Lange M: Gynecologic and obstetric disorders. In Barkin RM, ed: *Pediatric emergency medicine: concepts and clinical practice,* St Louis, 1992, Mosby, pp 796-827.

25. Snyder HM, Caldamone AA, Duckett JW: In Fleisher GR, Ludwig S, eds: *Textbook of pediatric emergency medicine,* ed 2, Baltimore, 1988, Williams & Wilkins, p 279.

26. Stewart CL, Devarajan P, Kaskel FJ: Renal replacement therapy. In Ichikawa I, ed: *Pediatric textbook of fluids and electrolytes,* Baltimore, 1990, Williams & Wilkins.

27. Wolf TD: Pharmacological iatrogenia (adverse drug reactions). In Fuhrman BP, Zimmerman JJ, eds: *Pediatric critical care,* St Louis, 1992, Mosby, pp 1099-1105.

CHAPTER 17

Hematologic and Immune Systems

Linda Manley, Nancie Bechtel

INTRODUCTION

Hematologic and immunologic disorders arise in children who are previously healthy or those who have known or systemic diseases. To care for these children the emergency department nurse should be familiar with anatomic and physiologic considerations, history and assessment, and emergency interventions specific to each disorder. This chapter reviews the most common immunologic and hematologic disorders in children who come to an emergency department.

ANATOMY AND PHYSIOLOGY

The hematologic and immune systems are comprised of active cellular components, which include red blood cells, white blood cells, and platelets, and humoral elements, which are substances contained in body fluids, such as clotting factors. All blood cells arise from hematopoietic stem cells in the bone marrow and then differentiate into specific types of cells. Children have a number of age-dependent variances in the formation and functional capacity of these systems (Fig. 17-1 and Table 17-1).

RED BLOOD CELLS

Normal red blood cells (RBCs) are small biconcave disks with slightly depressed centers surrounded by a ringlike rim. As RBCs move through the capillaries, they have the unique ability to change into almost any shape, facilitating movement and exposing more surface area for the exchange of oxygen and carbon dioxide. In infants and young children RBCs have a shorter life span than in the older child and adult because the cells are more fragile and rupture more easily. RBCs in the neonate survive 60 to 80 days,

compared to 80 to 100 days in the child and 120 to 150 days in the adult.[21,30] Because of this increase in fragility, anemic episodes, whether physiologic or caused by a disease or illness (e.g. sickle cell disease), are usually more acute in young children than in adults (Fig. 17-2).

Primitive fetal blood cells are recognizable by the second or third week of gestation. Initially blood cells are formed in the liver; however, by 5 to 6 months of gestation the process of RBC production (erythropoiesis) primarily occurs in the bone marrow.

Throughout life RBCs are primarily produced in the bone marrow cavities, although the liver and spleen may also produce RBCs if they are in great demand. The primary bone marrow sites of RBC production change with age. In infants RBCs are produced in the bone marrow of virtually all bones. With growth, bone marrow production in the long bones gradually decreases until adulthood and is replaced with fatty tissue (yellow marrow) until adulthood, when RBC production is then limited to the ribs, sternum, vertebrae, pelvis, scapulae, skull, and proximal long bones (Fig. 17-3).

RBC production is primarily stimulated by the hormone erythropoietin, 80% of which is produced in the kidneys (the rest is produced in the liver). During periods of hypoxia, erythropoietin stimulates an increase in RBC production. Before birth erythropoiesis increases because of the relative hypoxia that is present in utero. It then declines during the first week of life as the lungs replace the placenta as the primary source of oxygenation. In children with chronic hypoxic states, such as the child with a right-to-left congenital heart defect, erythropoiesis is continuous because of the chronic hypoxia.

The process of forming mature RBCs (erythrocytes) requires multiple stages of development. It takes

BLOOD

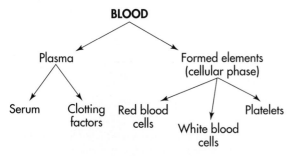

FIG. 17-1. Formed elements in the blood. (From Whitlock D et al: Hematologic and oncologic emergencies requiring critical care. In Hazinski MF: *Nursing care of the critically ill child*, ed 2, St Louis, 1992, Mosby.)

3 to 5 days and begins with a nucleated cell called a proerythroblast. This cell divides, and the subsequent cells mature and become filled with hemoglobin. Once these cells reach the reticulocyte stage, they are released into circulation where they continue to mature for 1 to 2 days before becoming erythrocytes.

RBCs primarily consist of hemoglobin (Hb), which transports oxygen to the tissues and removes carbon dioxide. The hemoglobin molecule is made up of four hemoglobin chains, including alpha, beta, gamma, and delta chains. In the adult, hemoglobin A (Hb A) is the most common form of hemoglobin and is a combination of two alpha chains and two beta chains. At birth fetal hemoglobin (Hb F) is the most common form of hemoglobin, comprising about 75% of the total hemoglobin. It is a combination of two alpha chains and two gamma chains. Hb F has a high affinity for oxygen, and because of the relative hypoxia that is present in utero, it carries 20% to 30% more oxygen than Hb A.[16] Over the first several months of life, Hb F is replaced with Hb A. (The role of oxygen transport is discussed in Chapter 6.)

WHITE BLOOD CELLS

White blood cells (WBCs) or leukocytes defend the body against invading organisms and toxic substances (Table 17-2). There are approximately 1 trillion leukocytes present in the body.[14] Production of WBCs primarily occurs in the stem cells of the bone marrow, but in some situations, especially stress, leukocytes are either formed or mature in the lymph structures (tonsils, thymus, spleen, lymph nodes). During maturation WBCs differentiate into granulocytes (neutrophils, eosinophils, basophils), also referred to as polymorphonuclear cells (PMNs) or "polys," and

TABLE 17-1	Anatomic and Physiologic Consideration in Pediatric vs. Adult Humoral Elements	
AGE GROUP	**CONSIDERATIONS**	
RBCs		
Infant	Most brittle in this age group	
	Survive 60-80 days	
	Sao_2 in polycythemic neonate is 90%	
	Sao_2 in infants is >95%	
Child	Survive 80-100 days	
	Sao_2 >95%	
Adult	Survive 120-150 days	
	Sao_2 >90%	
WBCs		
All ages*	Half-life 6-8 hr in circulating blood and 4-90 days in tissues	
Infant	Passive acquired immunity (antibacterial last 2 mo; antiviral [measles, chickenpox] lasts 6-12 mo)	
	Active acquired immunity from immunizations and from natural antigen exposure	
	Fewer circulating phagocytes	
	Immature T and B cells	
Child	Acquired immunity only	
Adult	Acquired immunity	
	More memory cells (especially B-cell lymphocytes)	
Platelets		
All ages*	Survive 7-10 days	
Infant and Child	Decreased survival time in presence of viral and/or bacterial infection	
Complement		
Infant	Lack complement-stimulating factor	

Sao₂, Arterial oxygen saturation.
*Excluding geriatric age group.

agranulocytes (lymphocytes and monocytes) (Fig. 17-4).

Each type of WBC has a specific function. *Neutrophils* are the first to respond to an invading organism; they engulf and destroy the pathogen. There are two

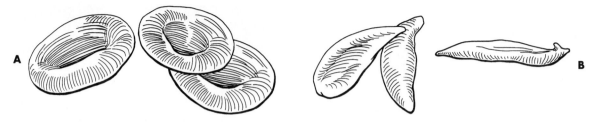

A **B**

FIG. 17-2. A, Normal red blood cells are biconcave disks with slightly depressed centers surrounded by a ringlike rim. **B,** Sickle cell–diseased red blood cells initially have a normal shape but assume an irregular S shape when stressed by hypoxia or acidosis.

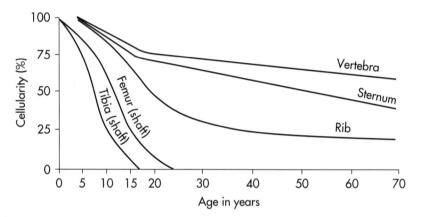

FIG. 17-3. Relative rates of red blood cell production in the different bones at different ages. (From Guyton AC: *Textbook of medical physiology,* ed 8, Philadelphia, 1991, WB Saunders.)

types of neutrophils present in the body, segmented neutrophils, which are mature cells, and bands (sometimes referred to as stabs), which are immature neutrophils. The normal life span of a neutrophil, once released into circulation, is 6 to 12 hours; however, this period is shortened when inflammation or infection is present.

Eosinophils are weakly phagocytic and therefore contribute little to the destruction of the same organisms that are susceptible to neutrophils. They are, however, attracted to sites of parasitic infections, where they attach to the parasite and release substances that kill many of them. Eosinophils also migrate to and attach to tissues involved in an allergic reaction, particularly those of the respiratory system (e.g., asthmatic attack) and the gastrointestinal tract.

Basophils are stimulated by an allergic response. During the antigen-antibody reaction they degranulate, releasing large quantities of histamine, bradykinin, serotonin, heparin, and other substances into the body.

Monocytes are immature cells that are weakly phagocytic and have very little ability to fight against infection. Once they enter the tissues, however, they differentiate into *macrophages,* which are capable of phagocytizing large foreign particles and cell fragments. Macrophages are found in many specific sites throughout the body. Tissue macrophages (histocytes) are found in the skin and subcutaneous tissue; alveolar macrophages are located in the alveolar walls of the lungs; Kupffer's cells are found in the liver sinuses; and reticulum cells are located in the spleen, bone marrow, and lymph nodes.

PLATELETS

Platelets, or thrombocytes, are necessary for clot formation. They are produced by megakaryocytes in the bone marrow at a constant rate throughout life. The life span of a platelet is 7 to 10 days. Under normal conditions, platelets are disk-shaped and do not adhere readily to each other, to circulating RBCs, or to WBCs. Platelets are activated by damage to the blood vessel wall, which initiates a series of reactions leading to the formation of a hemostatic plug. In response to

TABLE 17-2	White blood cells			
CELL TYPE	**NORMAL RELATIVE VALUE***	**FUNCTION**	**ELEVATED**	**DEPRESSED**
Neutrophils (polys)	Birth: 60% 6 mos: 30% >4 yr: 40%-55% Adult: 55%-60%	Primary defense vs. bacterial infection Phagocytize and kill bacteria	Bacterial infection Physiologic stressors Myelocytic leukemia Catecholamines Glucocorticoids Diabetic ketoacidosis Renal failure Tissue breakdown	Cancer chemotherapy Some viral infections Aplastic anemia Malnutrition
Bands	3%-5%	Immature neutrophil Phagocytize and kill bacteria	Bacterial infections	
Eosinophils	2%-3%	Respond to allergic and parasitic diseases Not bactericidal	Allergic disorders Parasitic diseases Eczema Myelogenous leukemia Autoimmune disease	May indicate elevated adrenal steroid production
Basophils	0.5%	Unknown, but do contain histamine	Granulocytic and basophilic leukemia Myeloid metaplasia	
Lymphocytes	Birth: 30% 6 mos: 60% 4-7 yr: 40%-50% 8 yr-adult: 30%-39%	Involved in antibody formation and delayed hypersensitivity	Viral infection Infectious mononucleosis Lymphocytic malignancy Chronic inflammation Autoimmune disease	Hyperthyroidism Stress Prolonged steroid therapy HIV infection Hodgkin's disease Aplastic anemia Steroid use Renal failure
Monocytes	5%-6%	Large phagocytes involved in early stage of inflammatory response	Viral, bacterial, and parasitic infections Lymphoma	Not associated with specific disorders

Compiled from Gawlikowski J: White cells at war, *Am J Nurs* 1992; *The Harriet Lane Handbook*, 1993, Mosby; Baehner RL and Miller DR, eds: *Blood diseases of infancy and childhood*, St. Louis, 1995, Mosby; Wong DL: *Whaley & Wong's nursing care of infants and children*, ed 5, St. Louis, 1995, Mosby.
*Percent of total white blood cell count.

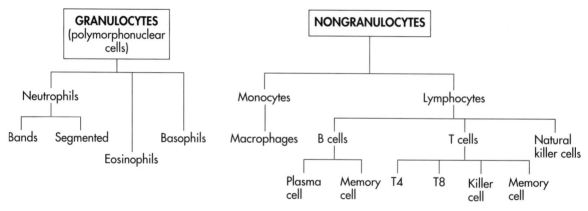

FIG. 17-4. Types of leukocytes (white blood cells). (From Kinney MR, Packa DR, Dunbar SB: *AACN's clinical reference for critical care nursing,* ed 3, St Louis, 1993, Mosby.)

injury platelets adhere to surface proteins that are expressed during inflammation or fibrin formation.

The normal platelet count is 150,000 to 400,000/mm^3. Thrombocytopenia, or low platelet count, results from inadequate production, increased destruction of platelets, or massive transfusion with bank blood. Causes of thrombocytopenia in children include bone marrow failure or suppression, idiopathic thrombocytopenic purpura, disseminated intravascular coagulation, leukemia, and acute infectious processes (Box 17-1).

IMMUNITY

Immunity is both innate and acquired (Table 17-3). Innate immunity is that which already exists in the human body. It is composed of those innate processes that normally resist inflammation or infection. Examples include the skin's resistance to invasion by pathogens, the destruction of organisms swallowed by digestive enzymes, and the phagocytosis of bacteria by the WBCs.

Acquired immunity results when certain pathogens, toxins, or foreign tissues enter the body and stimulate the formation of specific antibodies. Acquired immunity may be established in utero or throughout the life span. *Lymphocytes* are an essential component in the development of a specific immune response within the body. They promote both cell-mediated immunity (T lymphocytes) and humoral immunity (B lymphocytes).

T lymphocytes stimulate cell-mediated immunity, which protects the host from intracellular organisms (e.g., viruses, protozoa, fungi, and other nonbacterial agents), inhibit the development of abnormal cells,

---

Box 17-1   Causes of Thrombocytopenia

Decreased production
Bone-marrow failure (aplastic anemia)
Bone-marrow replacement (leukemia, other neoplasms)
Congenital amegakaryocytosis
Bone marrow suppression (chemotherapy or radiotherapy)

Increased destruction
Idiopathic thrombocytopenic purpura (ITP)
Disseminated intravascular coagulation (DIC)
Thrombotic thrombocytopenic purpura (TTP)
Collagen vascular diseases
Hemolytic-uremic syndrome (HUS)
Isoimmune neonatal thrombocytopenia
Hypersplenism
Toxins (e.g., snakebite)

From Hazinski MF: *Nursing care of the critically ill child,* ed 2, St Louis, 1992, Mosby.

---

and mediate the rejection of transplanted tissues. They account for approximately 80% of the body's lymphocytes. About one half of the T lymphocytes migrate to the thymus, where they mature and differentiate into T-cell subsets (T4 helper cells, T8 suppressor cells, cytotoxic cells, and memory cells). T4 helper cells stimulate B cells to produce antibodies and secrete interleukins that activate macrophages and other immune functions. T8 suppressor cells suppress

TABLE 17-3	Innate and Acquired Immunity
SYSTEM/STRUCTURE	**ACTION/SOURCE**
Innate immunity	
Skin	Integrity prevents pathogen entry; sweat bactericidal and fungicidal
Eyes	Blink reflex prevents pathogen entry; tears bactericidal and fungicidal
Nose	Nasal hairs trap pathogens and foreign particles; sneeze reflex ejects invading pathogens/particles; nasal secretions bactericidal
Tracheobronchial tree	Cilia trap pathogens and particles; cough reflex ejects pathogens/particles; secretions bactericidal
Gastrointestinal	Normal flora bactericidal; stomach acid bactericidal; vomiting reflex ejects pathogens/toxins
Lymphatic structures	Trap and filter pathogens
Reproductive	Vaginal secretions bactericidal; normal flora fungicidal; breast milk bactericidal
Renal	Urine bactericidal; urine flow flushes out pathogens
Blood	White blood cells, interferon, and inflammatory response
Acquired immunity	
Antibodies	Maternal (temporary)
	From natural antigen exposure
	From immunizations

Modified from Selekman, J: The multiple faces of immune deficiency in children, *Pediatr Nurs* 16(4):351-361, 1990; Thompson SW: Immune response and alterations. In Servonsky J, Opas SR, eds: *Nursing management of children*, Boston, 1987, Jones & Bartlett, pp 973-1020.

B-cell activity and prevent an overwhelming immune response. Memory cells are produced in response to an initial exposure to an antigen. They are preserved in the lymph tissue, where they are rapidly mobilized with repeated exposure to the same antigen. Cytotoxic or killer cells directly attack the invading organism or the body tissues that the invading organism has entered (e.g., viruses entering tissue cells) by inserting a toxic substance through the cell wall, which eventually destroys the cell.

B lymphocytes stimulate humoral immunity, producing antibodies, or *immunoglobins,* that recognize and aid in the destruction of a specific bacteria. There are five general classes of immunoglobins found in the body—IgM, IgG, IgA, IgE, and IgD—and they act in one of two ways. They either directly attack the pathogen or toxin, or they activate the complement system, which destroys the invader.

The complement system consists of approximately two dozen enzyme proteins that act sequentially to amplify the immune response. Complement proteins act in a variety of ways such as attracting phagocytes to the area of an antigen-antibody reaction (chemotaxis), activating phagocytosis, and directly lysing or rupturing the cell membrane of the invader. Stimulation of the complement system also contributes to the devel-opment of an inflammatory response by activating mast cells and basophils, which helps to immobilize or inactivate the invader.

Acquired immunity in the child is determined by the exposure to environmental antigens and vaccines. A variety of factors can impede the immune response in infants and children; these include major surgeries, large tissue burns, traumatic injuries, poor nutritional status, exhaustion, cold temperatures, emotional stress, sepsis, and sleep deprivation. Cigarette smoking can also suppress immunity and must be considered for children living in smoking environments. Because the infant's immune system is immature, certain antigens may hinder immune responses. For example, the measles vaccine temporarily impedes the cellular immunity response to tuberculosis.[25]

▌ NURSING ASSESSMENT

HISTORY

Because children with hematologic or immune system dysfunction are at risk of serious illness, a complete and accurate history is required when the child arrives in the emergency department (ED). Historical information should include recent illnesses and exposure to illness, allergies, past history, immunizations, and details concerning the present event. All current medications, including recent chemotherapy, antibiotics, and over-the-counter medications, must be identified. Information from the child's old chart, if available, or consultation with the child's primary or specialty health care provider will reveal important information and maintain continuity of care. The presence of implantable venous access devices, such as Broviac catheters or Port-a-caths, must be identified because these can be a source of underlying infection.

PHYSICAL EXAMINATION

As with any child who arrives at the ED, assessment begins with an initial evaluation followed by stabilization of the child's airway, breathing, and circulation (ABCs). Vital signs and the child's weight are obtained and recorded. If the child is known to be undergoing chemotherapy or has a coagulation abnormality, taking the rectal temperature is contraindicated because rectal trauma may predispose the child to hemorrhage or infection. If the child is thought to have a fever or to be hypothermic, an oral or tympanic temperature is ideal. Axillary temperatures are obtained as a last resort because they are unreliable. When recent antipyretic administration is identified through the history, the time of the last dose must be considered when temperature findings are being interpreted.

In the child with a hematologic or immune system disorder, every body system may be affected. Regardless of whether a condition has been previously diagnosed or is suspected during the ED visit, early signs and symptoms of serious illness are often subtle. Signs and symptoms that may alert the ED nurse to a potential hematologic or immune system disorder include pallor, weight loss or poor nutritional status, generalized lymphadenopathy, lack of energy, frequent infections, bleeding that is difficult to control, petechiae, and easy bruising. In children with known disorders, complaints of pain or anxiety are taken seriously. Subtle signs of pain might include restlessness, irritability, increased pulse and respiratory rate, crying, or limited mobility.

Children with a known immunologic or hematologic disorder are also assessed for evidence of neurologic dysfunction. These children are at risk for encephalopathy or intracranial hemorrhage. Subtle changes in the level of consciousness, such as irritability or lethargy, can indicate a serious underlying pathologic condition. Assessment of feeding habits, type of cry, quality of suck, and muscle tone may offer helpful clues when evaluating an infant's neurologic status. A full anterior fontanel may be consistent with increased intracranial pressure.

▌ IMMUNOLOGIC EMERGENCIES

The most common immunologic disorders in children who arrive at the ED are acquired immunodeficiency syndrome and fever and neutropenia (often caused by immunosuppressive therapy for cancer). Children with immune deficiencies are at increased risk of developing serious infection.

ACQUIRED IMMUNE DEFICIENCY SYNDROME

Etiology. Acquired immune deficiency syndrome (AIDS) is a progressively debilitating infection caused by the human immunodeficiency virus (HIV). HIV is transmitted by direct contact or transfusion of infected blood or blood products; by IV drug use from shared or dirty needles; by transmission from the mother to an infant transplacentally, perinatally, or via breast milk (rare); and by high-risk homosexual or heterosexual contact in which body secretions such as blood, semen, or vaginal secretions are exchanged. HIV is not transmitted by casual contact such as sharing glasses, coughing, or kissing.

In the past a large percentage of transmitted maternal cases were related to IV drug abuse in the mother.[5] Increasingly, such women are being infected via heterosexual transmission, rather than IV drug use.[10] As the number of women infected with HIV increases, there is a corresponding increase in the number of infected newborn infants. Transmission of HIV to older children and adolescents more commonly results from sexual activity or IV drug use.

In the decade following the report of the first pediatric AIDS case in 1982, 2,726 children in the United States under the age of thirteen were diagnosed with AIDS (1.5% of the total cases), with 1,441 related deaths.[12] AIDS is now the eighth leading cause of death in children ages 1 to 4 in the U.S. and the sixth leading cause of death in youths 15 to 24 years of age.[27] Although children of all races and socioeconomic groups are vulnerable to HIV infections, the largest percentage of known pediatric cases occurs in African-American and Hispanic children.[5,10]

It is estimated that 50% of HIV-positive children will manifest AIDS, while the others remain carriers for life.[26] Because the incubation period for HIV and the subsequent development of AIDS is highly variable, HIV infections are classified based on the presence or absence of signs and symptoms of the illness and the child's immunologic status.

Pathophysiology. HIV is a retrovirus that selectively invades white blood cells, particularly T-helper lymphocytes. HIV converts viral RNA, using reverse transcriptase, to DNA, which then integrates into the host cell DNA. The virus uses the reproductive capabilities of the host to reproduce itself. When the host cell dies, more virus is released into the body. Without T-helper cells, the immune system is significantly suppressed, predisposing the child to opportunistic infections and certain malignancies. Since infants normally have poor antibody response, decreased ability to localize infection, and less motile lymphocytes, the HIV-infected infant is at risk for the rapid development of sepsis.

The AIDS virus also affects macrophages, which can carry HIV across the blood-brain barrier into brain cells. HIV infection in infants and children results in a high incidence of neurologic disease. In children with perinatal HIV infection, clinical signs of neurologic dysfunction may appear as early as 2 months of age or as late as 5 years of age.[11] Macrophages also serve as a reservoir of infection and can contribute to the latency of the disease.[1]

Clinical presentation. The presentation of pediatric HIV infection varies by age, time of onset, and symptom complex. The course of the disease is generally more rapid in children, and all organ systems may be involved (Table 17-4). Universally, HIV-infected children exhibit signs of failure to thrive, regardless of mode of transmission or latency periods.[7] Other common presenting manifestations include persistent oral candidiasis, generalized lymphadenopathy, severe recurrent bacterial infections, protracted or recurrent diarrhea, hepatosplenomegaly, and lymphoid interstitial pneumonitis.[1] Neurologic manifestations, especially a static or progressive encephalopathy, are also common in children, although central nervous system (CNS) infections are less frequent than in adults.[13] Repetitive and rare opportunistic infections are the biggest threat to life in the child with HIV infection or AIDS.

The presentation of AIDS in the neonate may differ slightly than in the child. Newborns may be small for gestational age or premature. Failure to thrive and respiratory distress syndrome are common. Dysmorphic facial features, such as microcephaly, boxlike prominent forehead, flattened nasal bridge, and obliq-

uity of the eyes may be related to intrauterine HIV infection.[26] These findings, however, are also characteristic of fetal alcohol syndrome and may be difficult to differentiate because many HIV-positive mothers also abuse alcohol.

Emergency Department interventions. A multidisciplinary aggressive approach to the infant or child with HIV-related infection is essential in the ED. ED interventions for the HIV-infected child focus on minimizing complications, initiating antiretroviral drug therapy (if symptomatic), providing prophylaxis and/or treatment for opportunistic infections, and providing supportive care.

When an HIV infection is suspected in an infant or young child, the maternal history is reviewed to identify risk factors such as known maternal HIV infection; IV drug use; unprotected sexual contact, especially with multiple partners and/or high-risk individuals; recipient of a blood product before 1985; or past residency in a country or area with high HIV-infection rates among women.

Differential diagnoses for immunosuppression include severe combined immunodeficiency, DiGeorge syndrome, Wiskott-Aldrich syndrome, ataxia-telangiectasia (adolescents), graft-versus-host disease, neutropenia, functional neutrophil abnormality, blood dyscrasia, and hepatitis. In the newborn, differential diagnosis also includes cytomegalovirus and herpes simplex virus.

Diagnostic tests. Laboratory screening for HIV antibodies involves the enzyme-linked immunosorbent assay (ELISA) test, which, if positive, is validated by the Western blot assay. Infants born to HIV-infected mothers, however, receive HIV IgG antibodies transplacentally, which may result in a false-positive result for both assays. The polymerase chain reaction (PCR) test, is proving to be a more reliable diagnostic study. HIV-antibody testing may not be truly diagnostic until about 18 months of age, when the child's immune system is functioning adequately by itself. Cultures can also be used to detect HIV. Other clinical laboratory findings include anemia, leukopenia, hypergammaglobulinemia thrombocytopenia, altered levels of IgG and IgM, and an elevated erythrocyte sedimentation rate (ESR).[1]

Treatment. Zidovudine (ZDV; formerly AZT) and didanosine are antiretroviral agents that inhibit HIV replication. Although noncurative, these drugs minimize symptoms and may prolong life if given early

TABLE 17-4	Clinical Manifestations of AIDS	
SYSTEM/AREA	**MANIFESTATIONS**
Systemic	Failure to thrive
	Chronic fatigue
	Low-grade fever
	Increased drug hypersensitivities
Neurologic	Delayed acquisition and/or regression of normal developmental physical and cognitive abilities
	Motor dysfunctions, weakness, flaccidity, hyperreflexia, spasticity, toe-walking, shuffling gait
	Seizure disorders
	Cerebral vascular accidents
	Central nervous system lymphomas
	Aseptic meningitis
	Behavior problems
Dermatologic	Infections: skin and nail candidiasis, varicella, molluscum contagiosum
	Atrophy of hair, skin, nails
	Seborrheic dermatitis
	Papulopustular dermatitis
	Diffuse skin darkening in African-American children (thought related to zidovudine therapy)
	Drug-sensitivity rashes: pruritus, maculopapular, urticaria, or Stevens-Johnson syndrome
	Kaposi's sarcoma (rare in children)
Ocular	Blepharitis
	Conjunctivitis
	Retinitis (from cytomegalovirus and toxoplasmosis infections)
Ear, nose, throat	Chronic otitis media, hearing loss
	Chronic bacterial sinusitis
	Chronic mastoiditis
	Tonsillar and adenoidal hypertrophy, sleep apnea
	Persistent hoarseness
	Aphthous ulcers (less common in young children)
	Severe dental carries and periodontitis
	Cervical adenopathy
	Parotitis
Pulmonary	Fever, cough, exercise intolerance, dyspnea and tachypnea secondary to:
	Infectious causes
	Bacterial and viral pneumonias
	Pneumocytis carinii pneumonia
	Mycobacterium tuberculosis
	Noninfectious causes
	Reactive airway disease
	Lymphoid interstitial pneumonitis (common)
	Pulmonary fibrosis
	Pulmonary hypertension
	Aspiration pneumonitis (secondary to encephalopathy)

Modified from Church JA: Clinical aspects of HIV infection, *Pediatr Ann* 22(7):417-427, 1993; Iazzetti L: Dysrhythmias in the pediatric AIDS patient, *Pediatr Nurs* 17(1):49-51, 1991.

TABLE 17-4	Clinical Manifestations of AIDS—cont'd
SYSTEM/AREA	**MANIFESTATIONS**
Cardiac	Cardiomegaly
	Cardiomyopathy with resultant dysrhythmias and/or congestive heart failure
Gastrointestinal and hepatic	Dysphagia and painful swallowing secondary to oral and/or esophageal ulcers or candida infection
	Colitis
	Hepatomegaly, chronic hepatitis
	Cholangitis, cholecystitis
	Pancreatitis
Musculoskeletal	Short stature, delayed puberty
	Skeletal myopathies
	Malignant smooth muscle tumors
Renal and urogenital	Nephrotic syndrome with peripheral edema, proteinuria and/or hematuria
	Repeated infections with sexually transmitted diseases
	Recurrent urinary tract infections
Hematologic	Anemia, granulocytopenia, lymphopenia, and/or thrombocytopenia
	Idiopathic thrombocytopenic purpura
	Lymphoid malignancies, non-Hodgkin lymphomas, central nervous system and gastrointestinal lymphomas

in the course of HIV infection. For symptomatic episodes, oral zidovudine is given in a dose of 180 mg/m^2/dose, depending on the degree of tolerance of the child's hemoglobin and the absolute neutrophil count.[9] When children are NPO for longer than 48 hours intravenous zidovudine is administered at 120 mg/m^2/dose every 6 hours.[19] The standard of care for antiretroviral therapy of pediatric HIV infection is rapidly evolving to include newer therapies which dramatically inhibit virus replication, particularly protease inhibitors.

Pneumocystis carinii pneumonia (PCP) disease occurs in approximately one-third of infected infants and children and is the most common of the AIDS indicator diseases.[19] Unlike in adults, this infection is usually a primary infection in HIV-infected children. Signs and symptoms of PCP may be subacute or abrupt with fever, cough, tachypnea, and rales, and may be difficult to distinguish from other pulmonary infections. In the past PCP disease carried an ominous prognosis, however milder disease may occur and is consistent with long-term survival.[19] Prophylactic treatment with sulfamethoxazole and trimethoprim (SMX-TMP) is recommended for all suspected or known HIV-infected infants older than 1 month of age and all children with a previous PCP infection. Other empiric treatment in HIV-infected children

should be initiated based on specific exposure. IV immunoglobulin has been shown to prevent serious bacterial infections in symptomatic HIV-infected children and may be administered as needed or on a regular basis.[9]

Nursing care and evaluation. HIV-positive children with a fever or suspected infection will require a septic workup and a chest x-ray examination. Aggressive antibiotic therapy should be anticipated. The nurse should review the history and the chief complaint with the caregiver and determine the child's current immunization status, even though HIV-infected children may not have strong immunologic responses to vaccines.[9]

Children and families who come to the ED with HIV-related problems need strong psychologic support. A nonjudgmental approach and confidentiality are required because the social stigma associated with HIV is immense. In some cases of maternal transmission of the disease, the mother may be unaware that she is infected with HIV until the diagnosis is made in the child. There may be strong feelings of parental denial, anger, guilt, isolation, and fear regarding the disease that can frequently impede compliance with follow-up care.[28] Some pediatric tertiary care centers are now treating both children and family members simultaneously, which improves compliance and follow up. Information about local or national support groups should be provided.

Since the HIV status of most children is unknown and the signs and symptoms of HIV are nonspecific, *all* patients in the ED are considered potentially HIV-positive, and therefore universal precautions *are* observed. Handwashing is necessary after every patient contact and after removal of gloves. Gloves are worn for invasive procedures or whenever contact is likely with blood or the following body fluids: semen, vaginal secretions, and cerebrospinal, synovial, pericardial, peritoneal, pleural, and amniotic fluids.[13] Needles and other "sharps" must be promptly and properly disposed. If an occupational exposure occurs, the source patient and the exposed worker are tested for HIV and hepatitis B. Once the results are obtained, the employee is counseled regarding risk factors and the potential need for zidovudine prophylaxis. Confidentiality must be observed in accordance with state laws.

Fever with Neutropenia

Etiology. Neutropenia is characterized by an absolute neutrophil count of less than 1500 mm^3 and may result from a hereditary condition or an acquired immune deficiency. Certain infections, drugs, and chemical toxins may also cause neutropenia. Immunosuppressive therapy, which intentionally or secondarily inhibits the immune response during the treatment of a variety of pathologic conditions (including cancer and organ transplantation), frequently depresses the bone marrow sufficiently to reduce neutrophil production. Neutropenia significantly increases the risk of infection, especially with pyogenic and enteric bacteria. Secondary infections from opportunistic organisms may also occur with severe neutropenia. Fever is often the first sign of infection in the neutropenic child and should not be taken lightly.

Pathophysiology. Neutrophils are responsible for phagocytosis of bacteria in the blood. With markedly reduced neutrophils bacteria can rapidly multiply, leading to bacteremia and overwhelming sepsis (see the anatomy and physiology section earlier in this chapter). Although neutropenia is defined as an absolute neutrophil count (ANC) of less than 1500 mm^3, a significant risk of infection does not occur until the ANC is less than 500 mm^3.

Clinical presentation. On arrival in the ED, it may not be known whether the febrile child with a history of an immune deficiency disorder or immunosuppressive therapy is truly neutropenic. If risk factors are present, the child should be treated as neutropenic until proven otherwise. Other than having a fever, the child may be asymptomatic or may exhibit signs and symptoms of infection, such as irritability, lethargy, pallor, chills, dehydration, emaciation, sore throat, and general body aches. An obvious infection source, such as a large open wound, may also be found; however, neutropenic children with obvious major wound infections often lack normal inflammatory symptoms, such as erythema, edema, and purulence. If circulating WBCs are decreased, pus (an accumulation of dead WBCs) and other normal inflammatory responses may not occur. Implantable venous access devices (e.g., Broviac catheters or Port-a-caths), if present, may also be a source of infection. The absence of obvious bacterial infection does not preclude serious bacteremia.

Emergency Department interventions. The condition of neutropenic and immunosuppressed children may rapidly progress to septic shock, hypotension, and cardiovascular collapse. Management strategies focus on resuscitation, stabilizing organ function, identifying the degree of neutropenia, treating infections, and preventing further infection. Written protocols outlining care priorities are useful.

When the absolute neutrophil count (ANC) is calculated, the degree of neutropenia is determined (Box 17-2). If the ANC is less than 500 and the child is febrile, broad-spectrum parenteral antibiotics are ordered. Any delay in antibiotic administration could be fatal.

Box 17-2   Determination of Severity of Neutropenia

Absolute neutrophil count (ANC) = (% Neutrophils + % Bands) × WBC count

ANC >1000 = No increase in risk of infection
ANC 500–1000 = Moderate risk of infection
ANC <500 = Significant risk of infection
ANC <300 = Profound risk of infection

Modified from Whitlock D, Whitlock J, Coates TD: Hematologic and oncologic emergencies requiring critical care. In Hazinski MF: *Nursing care of the critically ill child,* ed 2, St Louis, 1992, Mosby, p 814.

Nursing care and evaluation. Children with fever and known or suspected neutropenia are rapidly assessed for signs of septic shock, and the ABCs of care are begun as required. Because these children are at risk of serious illness, they are immediately placed in a private room, and emergent interventions are initiated when indicated (Box 17-3). Although routine reverse isolation procedures have not been shown to be beneficial in preventing serious infection in neutropenic children,[29] a private room is often recommended to protect the neutropenic child from the multitude of infectious agents in the ED. Varicella is particularly dangerous because of its rapid dissemination. Handwashing is the single most important factor for protecting children with neutropenia.

Laboratory specimens are obtained as soon as possible with the neutropenic child. Blood cultures are drawn from each port of multilumen central lines, if present, as well as peripherally to rule out line versus systemic bacteremia. Cultures of other body fluids and wounds may also be indicated. Since a low platelet count frequently accompanies neutropenia, invasive specimens should be obtained cautiously as bleeding

may occur. Taking a rectal temperature and performing a rectal examination are contraindicated.

Many immunosuppressed children and their families have experienced repeated, and often complicated, hospital visits. The child may try to avoid a visit to the ED and may resist subsequent hospitalization, especially if the child is feeling fairly well. Allowing the child to vent his or her frustration and to express grief is important. Other strategies to provide support include offering diversional activities and allowing for periods of rest. Affected children should be given some sense of control over their environment. Allowing choices when possible and giving explanations often help these children cope with yet another hospital visit. Children with cancer can be demanding and particular about the way procedures are done (e.g., blood draws); this demonstrates their effort to maintain some semblance of control. Complying with their wishes, when feasible and safe, and supporting their individual ways of coping can be psychologically beneficial. Expediting care for these children and their families relieves some of their anxiety.

HEMATOLOGIC EMERGENCIES

Hematologic emergencies arise whenever derangements exist in any of the three active components of the blood—RBCs, WBCs, or platelets.

ANEMIA

Etiology. Anemia is caused by any condition that decreases RBC or hemoglobin production or any condition in which RBCs are destroyed or lost more rapidly than they can be produced by the body. It represents any number of pathologic conditions. Anemia may result from a primary disease, or may occur secondary to a disease, toxic substance, or immunologic response. Anemia can also result from a nutritional deficiency. Examples of conditions that produce anemia in children include sickle cell disease, in which abnormal RBCs are destroyed or sequestered by the spleen; congenitally acquired disorders of RBC production, such as Diamond-Blackfan syndrome; external blood losses resulting from trauma; and deficiencies in the enzymes and vitamins that are essential to RBC production (Box 17-4).

Pathophysiology. Classification of the anemias is based on pathophysiologic processes, such as inadequate RBC production or increased RBC destruction, and morphologic changes in RBCs, including

---

Box 17-3 Nursing Care of the Child with Fever and Suspected Neutropenia

Place child immediately in a private room.

Assess and stabilize ABCs.

Obtain history, including immunosuppression; request old chart if available.

Obtain vital signs (*no* rectal temperature) and pulse oximetry (if tachypnea or respiratory distress are observed).

Obtain laboratory specimens: CBC with differential, platelet count, blood cultures from both ports of Broviac catheter (if present) and peripherally (if requested); blood type and crossmatch; urinalysis, urine culture; other laboratory tests as indicated by patient condition.

Obtain a chest x-ray film (if requested).

Administer antipyretics as needed (*no* aspirin, *no* suppositories).

Calculate absolute neutrophil count.

If neutropenic: administer parenteral antibiotics promptly as ordered and prepare for admission.

Practice good handwashing technique.

Box 17-4 Causes of Anemia

Loss of circulating RBCs
Hemorrhage (e.g., trauma, surgery)
Bleeding disorders
Splenic sequestration

Inadequate RBC production
Congenital disorders of RBC production
  Diamond-Blackfan syndrome
Aplastic anemia (decreased functioning of
  bone marrow)
  Tumors of bone marrow
  Drugs such as chloramphenicol
  Immunosuppressive therapy
  Aplastic crisis secondary to sickle cell disease
Megaloblastic anemia (deficiencies in factors
    that produce erythroblasts in bone
    marrow)
  Vitamin B_{12} deficiency, malabsorption, or
    transport
  Folic acid deficiency or malabsorption
  Deficiency of intrinsic factor
Microcytic anemia
  Iron deficiency
  Lead poisoning
  Copper deficiency

Increased destruction of RBCs (hemolytic anemia)
Hereditary spherocytosis
Transfusion reaction
Toxins (e.g., spider bites or snake bites)
Erythroblastosis fetalis (Rh incompatibility)
Neonatal ABO incompatibility
Sickle cell anemia
Infection (e.g., malarial, clostridial)
Hemolytic-uremic syndrome
RBC enzyme abnormality (e.g., glucose-6-
  phosphate dehydrogenase deficiency)
Drug- or chemical-induced

therapy, radiation therapy, and the use of certain drugs (e.g., chloramphenicol).

Deficiencies in certain vitamins and minerals can affect the normal development of RBCs. For example, vitamin B_{12} and folic acid are important precursors to the final maturation of RBC. Deficiencies in these vitamins affect (1) the synthesis of DNA and ultimately the size and shape of the RBC, which becomes larger than normal and may be irregularly shaped (megaloblast); and (2) the cell wall of the RBC, which is fragile, causing it to have a short life span.[16]

Many conditions cause RBCs to be destroyed. Some are hereditarily acquired, such as hereditary spherocytosis, which causes the production of small, spherically shaped RBCs that are easily destroyed or damaged while passing through the spleen. Others result secondarily from a disease state such as sickle cell disease; an infection such as hemolytic-uremic syndrome; toxic substances such as spider bites, drugs, or chemicals; or an antigen-antibody response such as Rh incompatibility.

With anemia the oxygen-carrying capacity of the blood decreases and oxygen delivery to the tissues is diminished.[3,31] To compensate, stroke volume increases, as evidenced by an increase in the heart rate. To maintain vascular volume, fluid and albumin are retained and the cardiac workload is further increased by the hypervolemic state. In severe cases or in children who have an acute illness or injury (e.g., fever, acute blood loss, hemolysis), congestive heart failure can result.

Clinical presentation. The presentation of anemia varies according to the cause and the rapidity with which the anemia has occurred. When circulating RBCs are lost rapidly, as occurs with acute hemorrhage or splenic sequestration, signs of shock become evident relatively quickly. When anemia occurs over time, signs of anemia may be subtle and nonspecific (e.g., pallor, weakness, and tachycardia) as physiologic processes compensate for the decrease in oxygen-carrying capacity of the blood. With progression of the anemic state, signs may remain subtle or may become more obvious; the signs include lethargy, tachypnea, jaundice, shortness of breath on exertion, a systolic flow murmur (increased turbulence within the heart), and hepatosplenomegaly. In severe cases pulmonary edema and congestive heart failure can result.[3]

Emergency Department interventions. Initial management of the anemic child in the ED depends

size (microcytic, macrocytic, and normocytic), shape, and color.[31] The cause of the anemia can affect any of the numerous events that preclude the formation of a mature RBC, or it can affect the cells once they have been produced. Because RBC production begins in the bone marrow, any condition impairing the effective functioning of the bone marrow will impact the development of RBCs. Examples include chemo-

on the child's presentation. If the child is in hypovolemic shock from hemorrhage, splenic sequestration of blood, or a bleeding disorder, emergent interventions include stabilization of the ABCs, fluid therapy, and, possibly, blood therapy.

When a child's condition is stable and anemia is suspected, diagnostic testing is performed in an attempt to identify the cause. Laboratory testing should include a CBC (hemoglobin, hematocrit, WBC count, and platelet count), WBC differential, reticulocyte count, peripheral blood smear, and RBC distribution width. If the child has shortness of breath or signs of congestive heart failure, a chest x-ray examination may be ordered. Clinical and diagnostic findings are then evaluated to categorize the child's anemia (Fig. 17-5). If the anemia is due to a chronic process, the child is referred to the appropriate specialist or primary care physician for follow-up care (Table 17-5).

Nursing care and evaluation. The child who arrives in the ED with signs of shock is treated emergently, regardless of the suspected underlying cause. The prioritization of the care of children with vague symptoms is dependent on the history and physical findings.

If the anemic child demonstrates signs of hypoxia, respiratory distress, volume depletion, or congestive heart failure, emergent interventions must include stabilization of the ABCs. The child's airway is positioned, supplemental oxygen is delivered, venous access is achieved, and the child's heart rate, respiratory rate, and oxygen saturation level are monitored. The appropriate laboratory studies are done (e.g., CBC, reticulocyte count, blood gases), and an x-ray examination may be ordered depending on the symptomatology. When underlying hemorrhage is the suspected cause, the establishment of two large-bore IV lines is indicated and blood is obtained for typing and crossmatch. In the emergently ill child interventions are directed at identifying and treating the underlying cause.

In the anemic child with a nonemergent presentation, the history and physical examination are coupled with diagnostic studies to guide therapy. If the cause of anemia is easily treated (e.g., iron deficiency), the parent is given discharge information regarding the use of supplemental iron and referred to a private physician or a clinic. When the cause of the anemia is due to a chronic illness such as sickle cell anemia, the immediate symptoms are treated and the child is referred to the appropriate specialist (see the following discussion of sickle cell anemia).

SICKLE CELL ANEMIA

Etiology. Sickle cell disease, an autosomal recessive disorder of hemoglobin synthesis, affects approximately 1 in 500 African-Americans (50,000 in the United States) and occasionally other ethnic groups from the Mediterranean, Caribbean, Indian, African, and Middle Eastern regions.[15] Sickle cell anemia is the most common form of sickle cell disease in the United States. Approximately 8% of African-Americans carry the defective gene or sickle cell trait.[31] For a child to develop sickle cell anemia, both parents must carry the sickle cell trait.

Pathophysiology. Sickle cell–diseased erythrocytes initially have a normal round, smooth, and flexible shape and are able to glide effortlessly through capillaries. When stressed (e.g., hypoxia or acidosis), they convert to the characteristic sickle-, or S-shaped cell, which is brittle and nonflexible (see Fig. 17-2). Sickling impairs the cell's ability to move through small blood vessels and hastens the destruction of the cell. Blood viscosity is increased by the entanglement of the sickled cells, blood flow slows, and blood vessels are occluded.

Sickle cell crises are exacerbations of the pathologic condition and are therefore symptomatic of sickle cell anemia. Vasoocclusive crises are the most common type, but sequestration crises and aplastic crises can also occur. Other serious complications of sickle cell anemia include infection and acute chest syndrome.

Vasoocclusive crisis. Vasoocclusive crises occur when the sickled cells occlude the microvasculature. Local ischemia and tissue infarction can ensue, with distal perfusion severely compromised. Organs involved often include the gut, heart, liver, lungs, spleen, back, extremities, penis (resulting in priapism), or brain. A vasoocclusive crisis can be triggered by a number of stressors, including infection, overexertion, exhaustion, weather changes, cold stress, habitual drug and/or alcohol use, emotional problems, asthma exacerbation, altitude changes, anesthesia, dehydration, anemia, pregnancy, hypoxia, or acidosis.

There is a strong predisposition for anemia with sickle cell disease because of the brief life span (10 to 20 days) and the fragility of the sickled RBCs. When RBC destruction exceeds RBC production, anemia results. "Aplastic crisis" is a life-threatening anemia resulting from diminished RBC production by the bone marrow. A viral gastrointestinal or respiratory infection may trigger an aplastic crisis.

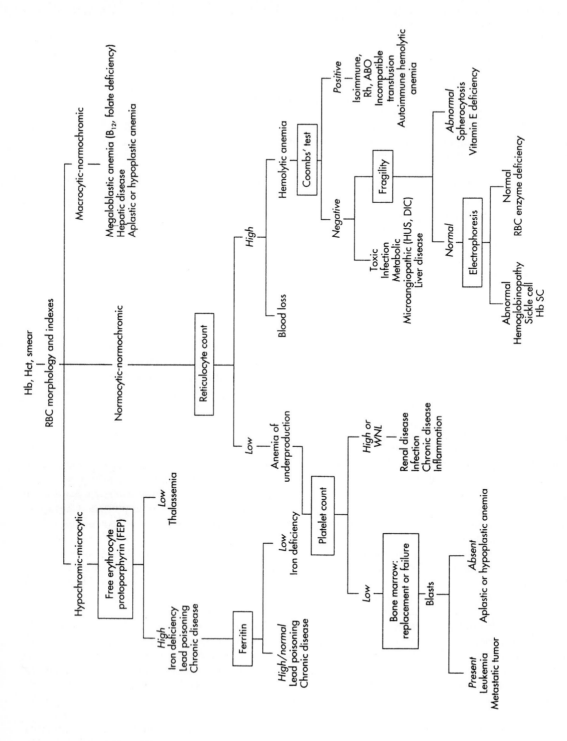

FIG. 17-5. Sample causes/differentiation of anemia. *DIC,* Disseminated intravascular coagulation; *Hb,* hemoglobin; *Hct,* hematocrit; *HUS,* hemolytic-uremic syndrome; *RBC,* red blood cell; *SC,* sickle cell; *WNL,* within normal limits. (From Barkin RM, Rosen P: *Emergency pediatrics: a guide to ambulatory care,* ed 4, St Louis, 1994, Mosby.)

TABLE 17-5	Hematologic Values in Children					
AGE	HEMOGLOBIN (gm %)	HEMATOCRIT (%)	MCV (FLUID)	MCHC (gm/% RBC)	RETICULOCYTES (%)	LEUKOCYTES (WBC/MM^3 × 1000)
1-3 days	13.7-20	45-65	110-128	29-33	1.8-4.6	18.9 (9.4-34)
1 mo	13.9-16	44-53	91-101	28-32	0.1-1.7	6-19.5
6 mo-6 yr	10.5-12.6	31-42	70-90	30-35	0.5-2.3	6-16
7-12 yr	11.5-16	33-40	77-95	31-34	0.5-1.0	4.5-13.5
Adult						
Male	14-18	42-52	80-90	31-34	0.8-2.5	4.5-11
Female	12-16	36-47	80-90	31-34	0.8-4.1	4.5-11

MCHC, Mean corpuscular hemoglobin concentration; *MCV,* mean corpuscular volume.
Data from Behrman RE, ed: *Nelson textbook of pediatrics,* ed 14, Philadelphia, 1992, WB Saunders; Green MG, ed: *The Harriet Lane Handbook,* ed 12, St Louis, 1991, Mosby; Kelly SJ: *Pediatric emergency nursing,* ed 2, Norwalk, CT, 1994, Appleton & Lange; Johnson TR, Moore WM, Jeffries JE: *Children are different: developmental physiology,* ed 2, Columbus, OH, 1978, Ross Laboratories.

Splenic sequestration. Another life-threatening complication, usually occurring in children 4 months to 3 years of age, is splenic sequestration. Massive amounts of blood pool in the spleen secondary to RBC trapping. This results in profound hypovolemic shock and anemia. Splenic sequestration may be triggered by a minor viral illness. Death can ensue unless RBCs are rapidly transfused. Once the systemic volume is replenished, the trapped splenic blood is released back into the systemic circulation.

Infection. Infection is the leading cause of childhood death in sickle cell disease.[32] Increased susceptibility to infection in children with sickle cell anemia results from a loss of splenic function. Sluggish blood flow and chronic occlusion of splenic vessels results in splenic infarction over time. Healthy spleen cells, which normally filter out bacteria and produce antibodies, are replaced with fibrotic scar tissue that hinders these normal immune processes. Initially the young child's spleen is enlarged and tender, but by approximately 6 years of age the spleen shrinks in size, becoming totally fibrous and nonfunctional, resulting in an autosplenectomy or functional asplenia. Functional asplenia leads to an increased risk of serious bacterial infection, especially from encapsulated organisms such as Pneumococcus and *Haemophilus influenzae.*

Acute chest syndrome. Acute chest syndrome is a painful crisis accompanied by respiratory distress that may progress to respiratory failure. Pulmonary infiltrates may be present. The cause of acute chest syndrome has not yet been identified, although there are some reports of bone marrow emboli with concomitant bacterial pneumonia. It may be difficult to differentiate pneumonia from an infarction of a lung segment caused by a pulmonary vasoocclusive crisis.[29]

Infarctions. In all age groups complications secondary to repeated sickle cell–induced infarctions include cerebrovascular accidents, bone necrosis (especially femoral and humoral heads), osteomyelitis, severe leg ulcerations, gallstones, renal disease, hepatosplenomegaly, cardiac myopathies, and blindness. Any body system may be chronically affected.

Clinical presentation. Sickle cell anemia rarely appears in infants less than 4 months of age because fetal hemoglobin resists sickling. As fetal hemoglobin is replaced with inherited hemoglobin S clinical manifestations may develop (Box 17-5). Anemia is often the first sign of the disease in young children.

The child with sickle cell anemia may arrive in the ED with complications of the disease or other illnesses that could precipitate a sickle cell crisis. Pallor and fatigue are often present secondary to the anemia. Fever and lethargy may herald a serious infection.

Pain is frequently the earliest sign of a vasoocclusive crisis and is the most common reason for ED visits by children with sickle cell anemia. Pain can be difficult to

Box 17-5 Clinical Manifestations of Sickle Cell Anemia

General
Growth retardation
Chronic anemia (Hb 6.5- 6.8 g/dl)
Delayed sexual maturation
Marked susceptibility to sepsis

Vasoocclusive crisis
Pain in area(s) of involvement
Manifestations related to ischemia of involved
    areas:
    Extremities: painful swelling of hands and
        feet (sickle cell dactylitis, or "hand-foot
        syndrome"), painful joints
    Abdomen: severe pain resembling acute
        surgical condition
    Cerebrum: stroke, visual disturbances
    Chest: symptoms resembling pneumonia,
        protracted episodes of pulmonary dis-
        ease
    Liver: obstructive jaundice, hepatic coma
    Kidney: hematuria

Sequestration crisis
Pooling of large amounts of blood:
    Hepatomegaly
    Splenomegaly
    Circulatory collapse

Acute chest syndrome
Tachypnea
Cough
Hypoxia
Fever
Pleuritic chest pain
Respiratory distress
Potential respiratory failure

Modified from Wong DL: *Whaley and Wong's essentials of pediatric nursing*, ed 5, St Louis, 1997, Mosby.

from sickle cell disease may be severe enough to mimic an acute surgical problem.

In infants less than 2 years of age, vasoocclusive crisis may manifest as "hand-foot syndrome," or dactylitis, in which there is painful symmetric swelling and redness of the soft tissue in the dorsal hands or feet. Dactylitis occurs secondary to vascular obstruction of the tiny bone marrow compartments of the digits and may result in bone necrosis and skin ulcerations.

Emergency Department interventions. The child who arrives in the ED with a history of sickle cell disease is rapidly and systematically assessed. In all cases the ABCs are evaluated and stabilized. Diagnostic studies are ordered according to the presenting symptoms and the suspected underlying pathologic condition. Diagnostic laboratory studies may include a complete blood count (CBC) with differential, a reticulocyte count, blood culture (if underlying infection is suspected), serum electrolytes, a hold clot for typing and crossmatch of blood, and arterial blood gases (if severe respiratory symptoms are present). Radiographic studies may include a chest x-ray if the child is in respiratory distress or a CT scan of the head, bones, or chest.

Treatment depends on the presentation. Shock is treated with fluid bolus therapy and/or volume expanders. Severe anemia or splenic sequestration is treated with fluid therapy and RBC administration. Vasoocclusive crisis is treated with fluid therapy at one and one half to two times maintenance.

The administration of narcotics should be anticipated for pain control because sickle cell disease is a chronic painful disease. Narcotics are never to be withheld in the ED for fear of drug addiction. Morphine sulfate 0.1 to 0.2 mg/kg IM or IV (maximum initial dose 10 mg) is the drug of choice for managing the pain associated with sickle cell disease. The once-popular therapy of meperidine-hydroxyzine combinations or meperidine alone is meeting with growing disfavor because of the related CNS complications, such as mood swings, irritability, and seizures.

Because infection is a major cause of death in children with sickle cell disease, children with this condition are begun on prophylactic penicillin by 4 months of age. In the ED all febrile children with known sickle cell disease are evaluated for the presence of infection and are treated with parenteral antibiotic therapy as necessary.

Nursing care and evaluation. The child with sickle cell disease may be seriously ill or may arrive with

diagnose in infants and toddlers who cannot localize and verbalize their discomfort. Crying and irritability may be nonspecific findings. Older children may be agitated or subdued and may complain of nausea and photophobia in addition to their pain. When pain can be identified by young children, it is usually present in the extremities; older children typically identify pain in their head, chest, back, or abdomen. Abdominal pain

TABLE 17-6	Hemophilia		
HEMOPHILIA A	**HEMOPHILIA B**	**VON WILLEBRAND'S DISEASE**
Factor VIII deficiency X-linked recessive trait carried in mother's genes and expressed in sons	Factor IX deficiency X-linked recessive trait carried in mother's genes and expressed in sons	Deficiency in VWD factor Many forms of VWD; most common types: type I, types IIa and IIb, and type III Types I and II are autosomal dominant; type III is autosomal recessive; VWD occurs in both males and females
Symptoms may be mild, moderate, or severe depending on baseline factor levels; severe symptoms include bleeding into muscles, joints, and organs	Symptoms same as hemophilia A	Symptoms may be mild, moderate, or severe depending on subgroup; type I, most common form of VWD, is associated with mildest symptoms

ing that mild hemophilia may be recognized in adults only after trauma or surgery, and there may be no history of bleeding.[18] Moderately affected hemophiliacs usually bleed in response to minor trauma. Seventy percent of hemophiliacs are thought to have the most severe form (0% to 1% of desired clotting factor), which manifests as spontaneous bleeding without trauma.[30] Von Willebrand's disease may approach moderate hemophilia A in severity and frequency of bleeding episodes, or it may be so mild as to be asymptomatic.

Bleeding in the joint spaces (hemarthrosis) commonly occurs in moderate to severe hemophilia, but it is rarely found in children with mild hemophilia or von Willebrand's disease. Over time frequent hemarthroses may ultimately lead to degenerative changes that limit joint function. Septic arthritis may occur, as well as compartment syndrome from muscle bleeding. Intracranial hemorrhages usually are associated with trauma.

It is estimated that 70% to 90% of hemophiliac adolescents are positive for HIV.[30] All children who received blood transfusions before 1985, when mandatory HIV testing began, and children of hemophiliacs who received blood transfusions before this date should be assessed periodically for HIV. Hepatitis is also a common complication.

Clinical presentation. Hemophilia A and hemophilia B have similar presentations, although it is important to distinguish patients with severe hemophilia from those with moderate or mild disease. The clinical hallmarks of hemophilia are joint and muscle hemorrhages, easy bruising, and prolonged (and potentially fatal) hemorrhage after surgery but not excessive bleeding after minor abrasions or cuts.[18] Hemarthrosis usually affects the knee, elbow, ankle, shoulder, or hip. Pain is often the first sign of bleeding, followed by swelling and limitation of range of motion.

A hemorrhage can occur anywhere; however, the highest morbidity and mortality are associated with hemorrhages located in the head and neck. Headache, vomiting, altered mental status, or seizures may indicate intracranial bleeding. Paralysis, weakness, and back pain may result from spinal cord hematomas. Large areas of soft tissue bleeding in the thorax can compress the trachea, causing serious airway obstruction. Gastrointestinal bleeding may appear with hematemesis, melena, abdominal pain, or shock. Laboratory findings for hemophilia A and hemophilia B reveal a prolonged partial prothrombin time (PTT), with all other bleeding factors normal.

With von Willebrand's disease hemarthroses are rare. Bleeding generally tends to be less severe and usually manifests itself with superficial bruising, epistaxis, and gum bleeding. Occasionally, epistaxis may be severe enough to compromise the airway. Prolonged oozing from cuts and marked hemorrhage after surgery or an injury may also be seen. Laboratory findings reveal a prolonged bleeding time with a normal PT and PTT.

Emergency Department interventions. In a diagnosed hemophiliac, bleeding, whether spontaneous or induced by trauma, can be a medical emergency, depending on the extent and location of bleeding. Life-threatening problems, such as airway obstruction or shock, are corrected first. Active bleeding is controlled, and rebleeding is prevented. As with all patients, universal precautions are required.

Therapeutic concentrates for factor replacement or fresh-frozen plasma are initiated as soon as possible to restore normal clotting activity. Factor concentrates include cryoprecipitate (factor VIII and fibrinogen), factor VIII, and factor IX. The required dose depends on the type and severity of hemophilia, the patient's weight, and the severity of bleeding (Box 17-7). Extremely large amounts of factor replacement may be required in major traumas or presurgery.

Rarely, hemarthroses may be so severe that aspiration is required to promote circulation. This procedure, however, carries a high risk for rebleeding. Any critical invasive procedure should be performed only after factor is administered. Since factor VIII concentrates have become more generally available, some physicians have suggested that joint disease might be prevented by regular infusions of these concentrates.[18] This approach has been used successfully in Europe,

with documentation of completely normal joints on physical examination 8 years later.[18]

An undiagnosed child with prolonged bleeding should undergo workup for a coagulation disorder. PT and PTT are determined to evaluate the extrinsic and intrinsic coagulation pathways, respectively. Other tests, which depend on the presence of a specific factor for a reaction to occur, include the thromboplastin generation test and the prothrombin consumption test. Specific factor deficiencies can be determined by assay procedures. The family history should be explored carefully.

Nursing care and evaluation. Children with hemophilia are usually seen in the ED for bleeding episodes that cannot be managed at home, trauma, or complications. Undiagnosed children with hemophilia may also come to the ED with prolonged bleeding after even minor traumatic injuries. Any child who is brought to the ED with unusual bleeding should be suspected of having hemophilia.

Nursing care of the child with known or suspected hemophilia includes continuous monitoring of hemodynamic parameters and ensuring appropriate pain management. Obtaining vital signs, a neurologic examination, and neurocirculatory checks distal to areas of bleeding are performed frequently. Any child with a change in level of consciousness or neurologic status requires an immediate head CT scan. The child is also assessed for the presence of abdominal tenderness or distention. Stools, emesis, and urine are observed and tested for blood.

Analgesics are administered as indicated. Application of ice packs, and the immobilization, and elevation of the affected joint may help arrest joint bleeding and promote patient comfort. The younger child may prefer nestling the extremity in the parent's lap. For the active child, quiet diversional activities and padded siderails may help prevent injury and a rebleeding episode.

Invasive procedures are minimized, unless they are imperative. These include intramuscular injections, rectal examinations, nasogastric tube placement, and nasotracheal suctioning. An IV catheter with the smallest diameter that can deliver the factor is used, provided that the child is hemodynamically stable. Laboratory specimens are taken when the IV catheter is inserted to minimize the number of venipunctures. If additional phlebotomy is necessary, peripheral finger-sticks are preferred over venipuncture.

Caregivers are questioned about recent medications that the child has received. Certain medications,

---

Box 17-7 Calculation of Factor Replacement

Factor VIII (Units) =
  0.5 × Weight (kg) × Desired increment (%) of factor VIII level

Factor IX (Units) =
  1 × Weight (kg) × Desired increment (%) of factor IX level

Suggested factor levels for bleeding episodes in patients with hemophilia:

Hemarthrosis	40%-50%
Muscle/Soft tissue	30%-50%
Laceration (requiring sutures)	40%-50%
Gastrointestinal	100%
Head trauma (no evidence of CNS bleeding)	50%
CNS, spinal cord injury	100%

Modified from Barkin RM: *Pediatric emergency medicine: concepts and clinical practice,* ed 2, St Louis, 1996, Mosby.

such as aspirin, ibuprofen, indomethacin, phenylbuta-zone, and guaifenesin (a common ingredient in over-the-counter expectorants), prolong bleeding times and may precipitate more severe bleeding. Parents should be cautioned about giving these substances to their hemophiliac children, and alternative drug therapies may be discussed.

Children with hemophilia are commonly given care through home management programs in which a family member administers replacement factors. If the child is discharged from the ED, clear instructions about follow-up care must be given to the family. Since factor VIII and factor IX concentrates have a half-life of 8 to 12 hours, factor replacement may be required every 12 to 24 hours until acute bleeding has resolved. If continued factor replacement is required, a saline lock may be left in place to avoid recannulating the vein. The IV line must be well secured and protected to avoid potential catheter displacement and exsanguination. Many consider the potential risks to outweigh the benefits of saline locks in children.

Additional approaches to therapy. Desmopressin (DDAVP) enhances clotting ability by increasing plasma levels of factor VIII and von Willebrand factor.[18] It is effective only in mild classic hemophilia or von Willebrand's disease and may be given to the rare child with mild hemophilia who comes to the ED. One obvious advantage of DDAVP therapy is that the risk for disease transmission is eliminated. Future administration of DDAVP may include the intranasal route, which might be available in the home setting.[18] Other drugs that may be given, in addition to factor replacement, include aminocaproic acid for oral bleeding and corticosteroids for recurrent joint bleeding or hematuria.

A recent hemophilia therapy being studied involves the cloning of the factor VIII gene for "gene therapy." Autologous cells are grown in a culture media, infected, amplified, and reimplanted. Raising the factor VIII level slightly, or above 25%, could actually cure the patient.[18]

DISSEMINATED INTRAVASCULAR COAGULATION

Etiology. Disseminated intravascular coagulation (DIC) is an acquired aberrant systemic coagulation process. Gram-negative sepsis is a major cause of DIC, but other causes include congenital heart disease, necrotizing enterocolitis, hyaline membrane disease, severe viral or rickettsial infections, acidosis, trauma (especially head injury), large burns or tissue destruction, shock, incompatible blood transfusions, malignancies, toxemic pregnancies, heat stroke, and hypothermia.

Purpura fulminans, the most severe form of DIC, usually results from a meningococcal, streptococcal, or varicella infection or from profound hypernatremia. It is characterized by the sudden onset of large ecchymoses and rapid development of gangrene of the extremities. Bleeding is partly caused by loss of vascular integrity (Table 17-7).

Pathophysiology. DIC involves an inappropriate, rapid, widespread activation of clotting factors,

TABLE 17-7	Causes of Disseminated Intravascular Coagulation in Children	
CAUSE	**EXAMPLES**
Shock	Septic, hypovolemic, cardiogenic
Infection	Gram-negative, gram-positive, viral, rickettsial, protozoal
Tissue trauma/hypoxia	Burns, crushing injuries, head injuries, extracorporeal circulation, acute hypoxia, heat stroke, hypothermia, snakebite, necrotizing enterocolitis
Malignant disease	Leukemia, solid tumors
Immunologic reactions	Incompatible transfusions, allograft rejection, immune complex disease
Cardiovascular disorders	Congenital heart disease
Pulmonary conditions	Hyaline membrane disease

Modified from Kinney MR, Packa DR, Dunbar SB: *AACN's clinical reference for critical care nursing,* ed 3, St. Louis, 1993, Mosby; Buchannan GR: Diseases of the newborn: hematopoietic diseases. In Oski FA et al: *Principles and practice of pediatrics,* Philadelphia, 1990, JB Lippincott; Emery ML: Disseminated intravascular coagulation in the neonate, *Neonat Network: J Neonat Nurs* 11(8):5-14, 1992; Wong DL: *Whaley & Wong's nursing care of infants and children,* ed 5, St. Louis, 1995, Mosby.

with aggregation and trapping of platelets. These changes result in intravascular thrombi, which plug and necrose small vessels. All available clotting factors are used at a faster rate than the body can replace them, resulting in uncontrolled hemorrhage and hemolysis. Bleeding into major organs (such as the brain) and bleeding at venipuncture sites and surgical sites can occur. Without effective treatment, end-organ failure caused by bleeding and ischemia results (Fig. 17-6).

Clinical presentation. Symptoms of DIC, generally reflect multi-organ involvement. Extremity petechiae appear first, followed by purpura, ecchymoses, extensive hematomas, and oozing from per-cutaneous IV sites. Eventually skin necrosis and gangrene may occur, as well as pulmonary emboli, stroke, or renal failure. Hematuria, guaiac-positive emesis or nasogastric secretions, guaiac-positive stools, vomiting, diarrhea, ileus, abdominal distention, respiratory distress, apnea, decreased level of consciousness, and coma are typical. Circulatory collapse and death are inevitable if untreated. Morbidity and mortality are high, even for those with full cardiovascular and respiratory support.

Emergency Department interventions. The child in DIC usually requires complex total system support. The primary focus of management is treatment of the underlying cause. Prompt and vigorous

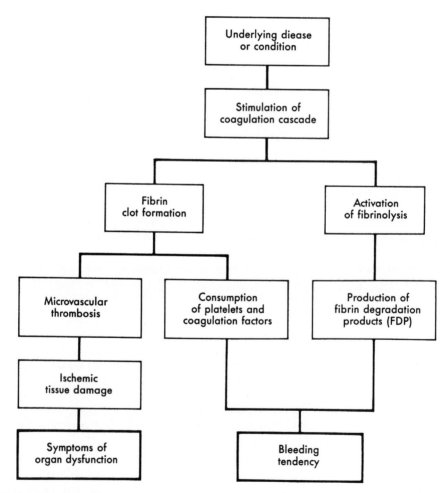

FIG. 17-6. Pathophysiology of disseminated intravascular coagulation. (From Kinney MR, Packa DR, Dunbar SB: *AACN's clinical reference for critical care nursing,* ed 3, St Louis, 1993, Mosby.)

treatment of shock, infection, acidosis, and hypoxia may eliminate the need for specific DIC therapy. Preparations for admission to a pediatric intensive care unit are required. Because multiple hematologic abnormalities are present, laboratory testing needs to include a PT, PTT, platelet count, fibrinogen level, fibrin split products, and factor V and VIII levels in addition to electrolyte and CBC values. Arterial blood gases are usually indicated, as well as both blood and urine cultures. Cerebral spinal fluid and tracheal secretion cultures also may be required.

It is likely that the child will require an artificial airway and ventilatory support. Inotropic support, with dopamine or norepinephrine, is required if severe hypotension is present. Broad-spectrum antibiotics and gram-negative specific antibiotics are initiated immediately; they are *never* delayed while diagnostic procedures are being performed. (Treatment of septic shock is reviewed in Chapter 6.)

Transfusions of platelets and fresh-frozen plasma (10 to 15 ml/kg/dose) containing several clotting factors may be beneficial. If the response to fresh-frozen plasma is poor, cryoprecipitate may be given to increase fibrinogen and factor VIII levels. Vitamin K is not helpful in treating DIC; however, it may be administered to a newborn to rule out other clotting disorders. The use of IV heparin, although controversial, is primarily indicated in purpura fulminans or in cases of widespread thrombosis or active bleeding when all other therapies have failed. An initial dose of 50 units is given parenterally, followed by a continuous drip of 10 to 15 U/kg/hr. Doses as high as 20 to 25 U/kg/hr can be administered.[2] Theoretically, heparin prevents the formation of microthrombi and blocks further consumption of clotting factors. Use of fresh-frozen plasma and platelet replacement is continued during heparin therapy.

Nursing care and evaluation. The child with suspected DIC is emergently ill and requires immediate stabilizing interventions. In some cases treating the underlying condition will reverse the DIC process; however, if signs of septic shock are present or if DIC has resulted from massive trauma or burns, immediate stabilization of the airway and breathing is required, including ventilatory support with supplemental oxygen therapy. Continuous cardiac monitoring and pulse oximetry are required, and venous access with two peripheral lines or one double-lumen line is achieved. Fluid bolus therapy is initiated if the child is hypotensive, and inotropic support, with dopamine or norepinephrine, should

be anticipated if the child does not respond to fluid therapy. An indwelling urinary catheter is inserted to evaluate fluid balance and renal function and to observe for the presence of hematuria.

The administration of fresh-frozen plasma should be anticipated. Cryoprecipitate and factor VIII may be given if the response to fresh-frozen plasma is poor. Heparin may be added to the therapeutic regimen when other clotting factors have not adequately controlled the bleeding; however the use of heparin is controversial.

While awaiting transport to a pediatric intensive care unit, the child's vital signs, respiratory status, circulatory status, neurologic status, and intake and output are monitored continuously. Analgesics and sedatives are provided to children with DIC who are intubated to minimize movement and discomfort and subsequent inadvertent dislodgment of the endotracheal tube. Reassurance and explanations are provided as appropriate for the child's developmental level. Emotional support and frequent explanations must be provided to the family regarding the illness, diagnostic evaluations, equipment, and transfer recommendations. Since the onset of DIC or the development of complications, often is fulminant, parents experience guilt feelings that they missed something critical in the child's condition at home. The ED nurse may explore these feelings with the parents. Involving ancillary support services, such as pastoral care, may also be helpful.

IDIOPATHIC THROMBOCYTOPENIC PURPURA

Etiology. Idiopathic thrombocytopenic purpura (ITP) is a common hematologic disease characterized by petechiae, purpura, and thrombocytopenia caused by platelet destruction. It is more common in children than in any other age group, with an estimated annual incidence of 4 in 100,000 children.[24] Typically, ITP occurs a few weeks after a known viral illness, such as measles, mumps, rubella, rubeola, chickenpox, mononucleosis, or a simple upper respiratory infection, but the triggering event may be unknown. ITP is usually self-limiting, with the hemorrhagic phase lasting 1 or 2 weeks and complete resolution occurring by 6 to 12 months. Occasionally, ITP becomes a chronic condition characterized by periods of remission. Chronic ITP most commonly affects females 10 years of age or older and is usually associated with another immunologic dysfunction, such as lupus erythematosus, IgA deficiency, or a malignancy (Fig. 17-7).[6,8,15]

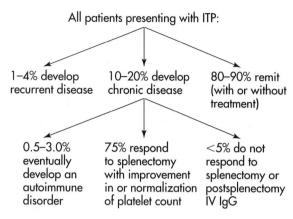

All patients presenting with ITP:

1–4% develop recurrent disease

10–20% develop chronic disease

80–90% remit (with or without treatment)

0.5–3.0% eventually develop an autoimmune disorder

75% respond to splenectomy with improvement in or normalization of platelet count

<5% do not respond to splenectomy or postsplenectomy IV IgG

FIG. 17-7. Idiopathic thrombocytopenic purpura: the natural history. (From Bray GL: Inherited and acquired disorders of hemostasis. In Holbrook PR: *Textbook of pediatric critical care*, Philadelphia, 1993, WB Saunders.)

Pathophysiology. The petechiae, purpura, and spontaneous bleeding of the skin and mucous membranes manifested by ITP result from widespread destruction of platelets caused by a probable autoimmune response. Bleeding with ITP may be mild to severe and does not correlate with the severity of the preceding viral infection. Areas that are rich in capillaries, such as the mucous membranes of the nasopharynx, gastrointestinal tract, vagina, and bladder, are the most susceptible to spontaneous bleeding.

Intracranial hemorrhage is the most serious complication of ITP and is responsible for the majority of fatalities.[24] Fortunately, this is a rare complication and the mortality rate is less than 1%. All reported cases of significant intracranial hemorrhage occurred in children with platelet counts of <20,000/μL and usually occurred within 2 to 4 weeks of onset.[8]

Clinical presentation. Many children with petechiae are referred to the ED for further testing or consultation with specialty services. The symptoms of ITP may be mild to severe. Some children appear clinically well except for asymmetrical bruising and/or petechiae on the extremities, especially over bony prominences. Bruising usually occurs with no known trauma or in unlikely places. More severe cases involve actual mucosal or organ bleeding evidenced by epistaxis, bleeding from the gums, hematuria, hematemesis, melena, hemarthrosis, and menorrhagia. Intracranial hemorrhage may appear with severe neurologic dysfunction and signs of increased intracranial pressure, such as headache or altered level of consciousness.

Emergency Department interventions. The diagnosis of ITP is based on clinical symptoms. The platelet count is generally <20,000/mm³, however the CBC is often normal.[23] Differential diagnoses for ITP include aplastic anemia or bone marrow infiltration secondary to a neoplasm. Consultation with a pediatric hematologist is recommended.

In the majority of children ITP is a relatively minor, self-limiting disorder that requires no advanced medical intervention. More severe presentations, however, may necessitate management that focuses on supporting involved body systems and correcting thrombocytopenia secondary to platelet destruction. Emergent care is indicated for profound bleeding resulting in hypovolemic shock or increased intracranial pressure. A CT scan of the brain is required for any changes in the child's neurologic status.

Packed RBCs may be necessary to support circulation and elevate the hematocrit. If the bleeding is life-threatening, platelet transfusions may have some value; plasmapheresis and an emergent splenectomy may also be considered.[2] Platelet administration is contraindicated in the treatment of non–life-threatening hemorrhage because platelet destruction continues and sensitization to foreign platelet antigens may result.[4]

IV immune globulin G (IgG) or steroids may be used to treat severe ITP.[23] IgG, 1 to 2 g/kg/day, may be administered over 1 to 4 days; then 0.5 to 1 g/kg per month is given as needed until the ITP is resolved. Steroids are suggested if the platelet count falls below 10,000/mm³ or if there is extensive bleeding.[2] Except in emergent situations, a bone marrow aspiration is absolutely essential to rule out malignancy before administration of steroids is started. Steroids do not affect the duration of ITP, but they enhance platelet production and increase capillary membrane strength, which minimizes bruising.[6,15] Immunosuppressive drug therapy, with vincristine or cyclophosphamide, has been somewhat beneficial in the treatment of chronic or severe ITP, but its use is controversial.[15]

Nursing care and evaluation. Children with petechiae are generally given a triage classification of "emergent." If the child has no symptoms other than petechiae on the extremities and/or bruising, he or she may be triaged urgently. Signs of neurologic involvement or hemorrhage warrant emergent care.

Because bleeding can occur in any body system, the child with emergent symptoms or severe manifestations of illness must be monitored closely for signs of

Box 17-8 Discharge Teaching for the Child with Idiopathic Thrombocytopenic Purpura

- Observe for signs of bleeding: coffee-ground emesis, tarry stools, central nervous system changes, abdominal distention, blood in urine.
- Administer a stool softener as required.
- Avoid high-activity or contact sports.
- Avoid medications such as aspirin, ibuprofen, and guaifenesin.
- Maintain follow-up appointments with a primary care physician or hematologist.

circulatory compromise and neurologic changes. Intake and output is recorded to evaluate hydration and renal status. Insertion of an IV line and subsequent crystalloid fluid boluses may be required to support perfusion. Noncritical invasive procedures, such as taking the rectal temperature, should be avoided, as well as procedures such as intramuscular injections. Indwelling gastric or urinary catheters may be necessary for emergent conditions, but they can irritate the delicate mucosal tissues and aggravate bleeding.

Care of the more typical patient with ITP is primarily supportive, since the disease is self-limiting. If the platelet count is <50,000, the child is admitted for evaluation and observation. Otherwise, the well-appearing child with ITP may be discharged from the ED. Parents should be instructed to seek health care if signs and symptoms of bleeding develop, especially coffee-ground emesis, tarry stools, CNS changes, or abdominal distention. A stool softener may be prescribed. Contact and high-activity sports must be avoided until the ITP is resolved and the platelet count returns to normal. Parents should be cautioned to avoid certain medications, such as aspirin, ibuprofen, and guaifenesin (common in over-the-counter expectorants), all of which may prolong bleeding. The importance of follow-up visits with the child's pediatrician or hematologist, until the ITP is completely resolved, must be stressed (Box 17-8).

▌ SUMMARY

The child with a hematologic or immunologic emergency can pose a challenge to the ED nurse and personnel. A multidisciplinary approach, including

both the child and the parent, will ensure that the highest quality of care is being provided.

REFERENCES

1. Baehner RL, Miller DR: Lymphocytes. In Miller DR, Baehner RL, eds: *Blood diseases of infancy and childhood*, St Louis, 1995, Mosby, pp 627-659.
2. Barkin RM: Hematologic disorders. In Barkin RM: *Pediatric emergency medicine: concepts and clinical practice*, St Louis, 1992, Mosby, pp 828-844.
3. Behrman RE, ed: *Nelson textbook of pediatrics*, ed 15, Philadelphia, 1994, WB Saunders.
4. Bray GL: Inherited and acquired disorders of hemostasis. In Holbrook PR: *Textbook of pediatric critical care*, Philadelphia, 1993, WB Saunders, pp 783-801.
4a. Buchannan GR: Diseases of the newborn: hematopoietic diseases. In Oski FA et al: *Principles and practice of pediatrics*, Philadelphia, 1990, JB Lippincott.
5. Caldwell MB, Rogers MF: Epidemiology of pediatric HIV infections, *Pediatr Clin North Amer* 38(1): 1-16, 1991.
6. Casella JF: Disorders of the newborn: disorders of coagulation. In Oski FA et al: *Principles and practice of pediatrics*, Philadelphia, 1990, JB Lippincott, pp 1554-1556.
7. Church JA: Clinical aspects of HIV infection, *Pediatr Ann* 22(7):417-427, 1993.
8. Corrigan JJ: Diseases of the blood. In Behrman RE, ed: *Nelson textbook of pediatrics*, Philadelphia, 1992, WB Saunders, pp. 1272-1282.
9. Cvetkovich TA, Frenkel LM: Current management of HIV infection in children, *Ped Annals* 22(7):428-435, 1993.
10. Dossett JH: Acquired immunodeficiency syndrome (AIDS) and human immunodeficiency virus infection (HIV). In Hoekelman RA et al eds: *Primary pediatric care*, ed 3, St. Louis, 1997, Mosby.
11. El Sadr W et al: Managing early HIV infection. Quick reference guide for clinicians. AHCPR Pub #94-0573, Rockville, Md, 1994, Agency for Health Care Policy and research: Public Health Service, U.S. Dept. of Health and Human Services.
11a. Emery ML: Disseminated intravascular coagulation in the neonate, *Neonat Network: J Neonat Nurs* 11(8):5-14, 1992.
12. Evans HE: Diseases of the blood. In Behrman RE, ed: *Nelson textbook of pediatrics*, Philadelphia, 1992, WB Saunders, pp 835-842.
13. Felter RA and Bower JR: Infectious disorders. In Barkin RM: *Pediatric emergency medicine: concepts and clinical practice*, ed 2, St Louis, 1996, Mosby pp. 926-971.
14. Flannery JC: Immunologic disorders. In Burrell

LO: *Adult nursing in hospital and community settings,* Norwalk, Conn, 1992, Appleton & Lange, pp 141-175.

14a. Gawlikowski J: White cells at war, *Am J Nurs,* 1992.

15. Giller RH: Hematologic disorders. In Barkin RM, Rosen P: *Emergency pediatrics: a guide to ambulatory care,* ed 4, St Louis, 1994, Mosby, pp 623-643.

15a. Green MG, ed. *The Harriet Lane Handbook,* ed 12, St. Louis, 1991, Mosby.

16. Guyton AC: *Textbook of medical physiology,* ed 8, Philadelphia, 1991, WB Saunders.

17. Hilgartner MW, Corrigan JJ: Coagulation disorders. In Miller DR, Baehner RL, eds: *Blood diseases of infancy and childhood,* St Louis, 1995, Mosby, pp 924-986.

18. Hoyer LW: Hemophilia A, *N Engl J Med* 330(1): 38-47, 1994.

18a. Iazetti L: Dysrhythmias in the pediatric AIDS patient, *Pediatr Nurs* 17(1):49-51, 1991.

19. Jenkins M: Human immunodeficiency virus type 1 infection in infants and children. In Rudolph AM, ed: *Rudolph's pediatrics,* ed 20, Stamford, 1996, Appleton & Lange, pp 655-661.

19a. Johnson TR, Moore WM, Jeffries JE: *Children are different: developmental physiology,* ed 2, Columbus, OH, 1978, Ross Laboratories.

19b. Kelly SJ: *Pediatric emergency nursing,* ed 2, Norwalk, CT, 1994, Appleton & Lange.

20. McGuire TJ, Pointer JE: Evaluation of a pulse oximeter in the prehospital setting, *Ann Emerg Med* 17(10):1058, 1988.

21. Olds SB, London ML, Ladewig PW: Physiologic response of the newborn to birth. In *Maternal newborn nursing: a family-centered approach,* ed 4, Redwood City, Calif, 1992, Addison-Wesley, pp 822-827.

22. Reference deleted in proofs.

23. Sadowitz D, Souid AK, Terndrup TE: Idiopathic thrombocytopenic purpura in children: recognition and management, *Ped Emerg Care* 12(3):222, 1996.

24. Sadowitz D, Terndrup TE: Subglottic airway hemorrhage associated with idiopathic thrombocytopenic purpura, *Ped Emerg Care* 23(3):591-595, 1994.

25. Selekman J: The multiple faces of immune deficiency in children, *Pediatr Nurs* 16(4):351-361, 1990.

25a. Thompson SW: Immune response and alterations. In Servonsky J, Opas SR, eds: Nursing management of children, Boston, 1987, Jones & Bartlett, pp 973-1020.

26. Thurber F, Berry B: Children with AIDS: issues and future directions, *J Pediatr Nurs* 5(3):168-178, 1990.

27. USDHHS 1994

28. Ward-Wimmer D: Nursing care of children with HIV infection, *Nurs Clin North Am* 23(4):719-729, 1988.

29. Whitlock D, Whitlock J, Coates TD: Hematologic and oncologic emergencies requiring critical care. In Hazinski MF: *Nursing care of the critically ill child,* ed 2, St Louis, 1992, Mosby, pp 803-827.

30. Wong DL: *Whaley and Wong's nursing care of infants and children,* ed 5, St Louis, 1995, Mosby.

31. Wong DL: *Whaley and Wong's essentials of pediatric nursing,* ed 5, St Louis, 1997, Mosby.

32. Wright L, Brown A, Davidson-Mundt A: Newborn screening: the miracle and the challenge, *J Pediatr Nurs* 7(1):26-43, 1992.

CHAPTER 18

Integumentary System

Joanne Fioravanti

INTRODUCTION

The integument is the body's largest organ. It is more exposed to microorganisms and other potentially harmful elements than any other organ system. Integumentary problems in children are common, with infections of the skin and soft tissue being responsible for 1 in every 40 visits to pediatric health care providers. Skin diseases caused by microorganisms or parasites account for 1 in 18 such visits. From 25% to 30% of children have some form of chronic or recurring skin condition. Of all pediatric office visits, 21% involve, primarily or secondarily, a skin complaint or finding.[7]

Skin problems are best treated in the primary care environment, where they can be monitored over time. Some may be sufficiently alarming to parents and uncomfortable enough to the child to prompt a visit to the emergency department. Current information about common bacterial, viral, parasitic, and fungal infections of the integument or skin, as well as inflammatory skin conditions, is discussed in this chapter.

ANATOMY AND PHYSIOLOGY

The skin, or integument, is a flexible membrane that covers the entire body surface and serves many important functions (Box 18-1). It is composed of two separate layers: the outer epidermis and the inner dermis (Figure 18-1).

EPIDERMIS

The epidermis functions as a barrier, preventing penetration of the skin from the outside and retaining substances inside. It is composed of layers of cells that are formed in the deepest layer, the stratum germina-tivum, which lies just above the dermis. Blood vessels do not extend beyond the dermis into the epidermis. Thus newly formed cells are pushed upward away from sustaining blood supply. Consequently, epidermal cells become dry and horny, which helps to make the top layer of the skin water- and trauma-resistant.

Outer cells normally flake off, or desquamate, at approximately the same rate as new cells form in the stratum germinativum. If fever or skin trauma (e.g., sunburn or laceration) occurs, desquamation accelerates. Constant pressure or irritation produces a horny layer of dead cells that form a callus (with pressure) or lichenification (with irritation).

The water content of the environment has a great impact on the epidermis. Too much water, or not enough, can cause microscopic and macroscopic breaks in the epidermal barrier, resulting in injury or insult to the skin.

Box 18-1   Functions of the Skin

• Protects against dehydration, injury, and infection
• Excretes waste products through sweat and sebaceous glands
• Assists in temperature control
    Cools body temperature by evaporation through sweat glands
    Raises body temperature via circulation of blood
• Serves as receptor of sensations—touch, pain, itch, warmth and cold—via numerous nerve endings
• Absorbs ultraviolet rays, resulting in production of vitamin D

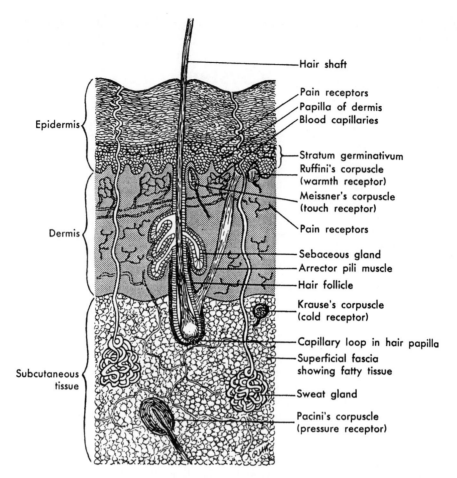

Hair shaft
Pain receptors
Papilla of dermis
Blood capillaries
Stratum germinativum
Ruffini's corpuscle (warmth receptor)
Meissner's corpuscle (touch receptor)
Pain receptors
Sebaceous gland
Arrector pili muscle
Hair follicle
Krause's corpuscle (cold receptor)
Capillary loop in hair papilla
Superficial fascia showing fatty tissue
Sweat gland
Pacini's corpuscle (pressure receptor)

Epidermis
Dermis
Subcutaneous tissue

FIG. 18-1. The skin and subcutaneous tissue. (From Hamilton MH: *Basic pediatric nursing,* ed 6, St Louis, 1991, Mosby.)

DERMIS

The dermis lies just below the epidermis. It is composed of fibrous connective tissue. This tissue is responsible for the strength and elasticity of the skin, allowing it to withstand stress yet be extensible over joints. Located in the dermis are blood vessels, hair follicles, nerve endings, mast cells, blood and lymphatic vessels, and secreting sebaceous and sweat glands. These elements are responsible for temperature regulation, host defenses, nourishment of the skin, and other regulatory functions.

Subcutaneous tissue is attached to the dermis and anchors the skin to muscle and bone. The top layer of subcutaneous tissue is called superficial fascia and is composed of connective tissue interspersed with fat, blood vessels, nerve receptors, and sebaceous and sweat glands. Superficial fascia provides nourishment

to the skin. It also cushions the skin, protecting it from trauma.

EPIDERMAL APPENDAGES

Epidermal appendages are modifications of the epithelium. These include hair, nails, and sebaceous and sweat glands.

Hair is formed from a layer of stratum germinativum cells that line small follicles embedded in the dermis and subcutaneous tissue. Hair may be cut or pulled out by the root, but as long as the stratum germinativum cells lining the follicles are alive, hair will regenerate. Growth cycles of the hair are asynchronous and vary by body site. In the scalp most of the hairs are growing (anlagen), whereas a small percentage are resting (telogen). After an acute febrile illness, hair can convert from anlagen to telogen with a period of several months of significantly thinned hair.

Nails form from modified epithelial cells. Fingernails grow approximately 1 cm in 3 months, whereas toenails grow more slowly. Damage to a nailbed is not noticeable for several weeks, until the damaged nail emerges. Total replacement of a damaged fingernail takes 3 to 4 months. Toenails require 6 to 9 months of growth. Keratin produced from the epidermal cells attaches to the top surface of the nail to form the cuticle. When the cuticle is damaged, such as with a hangnail, the seal between the cuticle and the nail is broken. This creates a pocket under the nail and fosters the development of a paronychial infection.

Sebaceous glands are present throughout the skin except on the palms of the hands and the soles and dorsa of the feet. These glands, which are located in the dermis, bud outward from the side of the hair follicle. Sebum, a semiliquid material, is formed within the sebaceous gland and travels to the surface of the skin via the hair follicle. Sebaceous glands on the face, scalp, and upper trunk are large, numerous, and very productive. Sebum production, which is androgen dependent, begins at puberty in skin areas with large numbers of sebaceous glands. When sebaceous glands become obstructed, acne can develop.

Sweat glands develop from cells in the epidermis and extend downward into the dermis. These glands open directly onto the skin via a coiled duct. Sweat glands are found over the entire surface of the skin. The autonomic nervous system governs the sweat glands on the palms of the hands, soles of the feet, axillae, and forehead. These glands play a major role in regulating body temperature and in eliminating body wastes. When body temperature rises, sweat glands produce a fluid that is 99% water, containing primarily sodium chloride and traces of potassium, urea, ammonia, and some amino acids. To maintain proper fluid balance, all lost fluids, including sweat and insensible evaporative losses through the skin, must be replaced.

NURSING HISTORY AND ASSESSMENT

A comprehensive history and physical examination are often required for the diagnosis and treatment of skin disorders in children (Box 18-2). The history is obtained from both the parent and the child. The starting point is the chief complaint and the reason for seeking medical attention at this time.

Physical assessment includes close examination of the entire skin surface and lesion(s) under adequate

---

Box 18-2 History for Child with Skin Disorder

1. Chief complaint
2. Present illness
   - When and where skin lesions first appeared
   - Initial appearance of lesions and progressive changes
   - Presence of emotional stresses
   - Recent contacts/time of exposure:
     - Persons or animals who were sick and/or had skin lesions, including childhood communicable diseases
     - Chemicals, plants, new foods, new soaps, new clothing or sheets/blankets
     - Travel
   - Associated symptoms such as fever, lethargy, cough
   - Home remedies or prescribed treatments before ED visit and their effectiveness
3. Past medical history
   - Recent or chronic illnesses/conditions, such as asthma or immunocompromise
   - Previous skin disorders
   - Allergies
   - Recent or current medications
   - Immunization history
4. Family history
   - Chronic skin disorders
   - Immunocompromise in family members

---

lighting. Vital signs, including temperature measurements, must be done on all children with skin findings.

Since skin lesions assume relatively distinct characteristics, they should be described correctly in the documentation (Box 18-3). Documentation should include the location, distribution, size, shape, color, and arrangement of lesions and should specify whether they are localized or generalized, raised or flat. Arrangements of lesions may be described as discrete (individual), clustered (close together), diffuse (scattered), or confluent (run together).

Skin lesions are classified as either primary or secondary.

In *primary lesions* skin changes are produced by a causative factor. Examples include macules, papules, nodules, vesicles, and bullae (Fig. 18-2).

Box 18-3 Definitions of Skin Lesions

Primary lesions

Macule Flat, discolored skin lesion ≦1 cm in size

Papule Elevated, discolored skin lesion ≦1 cm in size

Wheal Flat-topped, discolored lesion >1 cm in size

Cyst Elevated, thick-walled lesion containing fluid or semisolid material

Vesicle Elevated skin lesion ≦1 cm in size containing serous fluid

Bulla Vesicle >1 cm in size

Pustule Elevated lesion containing purulent fluid; variable size

Petechiae Dark-red, purplish discolorations ≦1 cm in size that do not blanch when pressed

Purpura Petechia >1 cm in size

Ecchymosis Blue, black, yellow, or red discoloration, depending on stage of healing (bruise)

Secondary lesions

Ulcer Concave lesion characterized by loss of epidermis and dermis

Excoriation Superficial abrasion

Crust Deposit of skin exudate such as blood, serum, or pus

Lichenification Rough, thickened epidermis with accentuated skin markings

In *secondary lesions* skin changes result from an alteration in the primary lesions, caused by rubbing, scratching, or healing. These lesions include excoriations, scales, ulcers, and crusts (Fig. 18-3).

▌INFECTIOUS EXANTHEMS

Infectious exanthems include a variety of communicable diseases that manifest as a rash associated with a systemic illness. Infants and young children are particularly prone to communicable diseases because of the immaturity of their immune systems. The more social interactions the child experiences outside the home, for example, daycare, the greater the risk of exposure to communicable diseases. The incidence of many childhood communicable diseases has been reduced dramatically since the advent of immunizations. Nevertheless, too many children remain under-immunized.

Children with communicable diseases frequently exhibit mild to moderate prodromal symptoms before the onset of the rash. These initial symptoms or the actual rash itself may precipitate a visit to the emergency department (ED). Since children with communicable diseases are usually contagious during the prodromal phase, all children should be screened for exposure to childhood communicable diseases at triage and isolated appropriately—especially from immunocompromised patients. The contagion check may also be helpful in diagnosing the child's illness. Diagnosis is clinically determined by the identification of a constellation of signs and symptoms, which is sometimes difficult to differentiate (Table 18-1).

ED nursing care of children with infectious exanthems focuses on (1) infection control, (2) prevention of complications, (3) provision of support and comfort measures, and (4) patient and family education.

RUBEOLA (MEASLES)

Etiology. Rubeola is a viral illness caused by a paramyxovirus. Although it occurs less frequently in countries with high immunization rates it is a common cause of preventable death worldwide. In the United States populations at risk include children younger than 15 months of age (the recommended age for immunization), nonimmunized children, and those who have received only the killed virus vaccine. Live attenuated measles virus vaccine was introduced in 1963, but the killed type of vaccine was frequently administered between 1963 and 1967. Measles outbreaks in older children and young adults immunized in early childhood have led to the American Academy of Pediatrics' recommendation for a second MMR (measles, mumps, and rubella) vaccine before entry to kindergarten or high school.

Clinical presentation. Prodromal upper respiratory symptoms and conjunctivitis precede the rash by about 3 to 4 days. Koplik's spots, which are small white spots on the oral mucosa opposite the lower molars, are diagnostic of measles. The child is most ill on the second or third day of the rash. The illness usually lasts 7 days (Figure 18-4). The characteristics of the rash vary. Early in the illness an erythematous maculopapular rash begins to appear on the face and moves downward. Initially lesions are discrete, but after several days they become confluent.

Text continued on p. 428.

Plaque—elevated, flat topped, firm, rough, superficial papule greater than 1 cm in diameter; may be coalesced papules Examples: Psoriasis; seborrheic and actinic keratoses

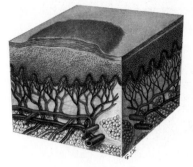

Macule—flat; nonpalpable, circumscribed; less than 1 cm in diameter; brown, red, purple, white, or tan Examples: Freckles; flat moles; rubella; rubeola

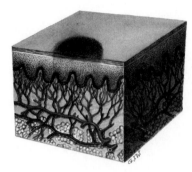

Wheal—elevated, irregular-shaped area of cutaneous edema; solid, transient, changing, variable diameter; pale pink with lighter center Examples: Urticaria; insect bites

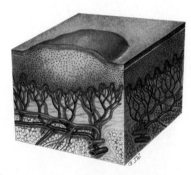

Patch—flat, nonpalpable, irregular in shape; macule that is greater than 1 cm in diameter Examples: Vitiligo; port-wine marks

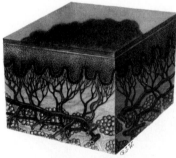

Nodule—elevated, firm, circumscribed, palpable; deeper in dermis than papule; 1 to 2 cm in diameter Examples: Erythema nodosum; lipomas

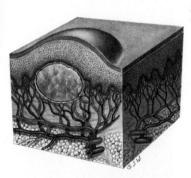

Papule—elevated, palpable, firm, circumscribed; less than 1 cm in diameter; brown, red, pink, tan, or bluish red in color Examples: Warts; drug-related eruptions; pigmented nevi

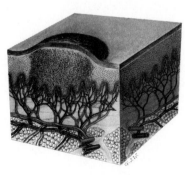

FIG. 18-2. Primary skin lesions. (From Thompson JM et al: *Mosby's clinical nursing,* ed 3, St Louis, 1993, Mosby.)

Continued.

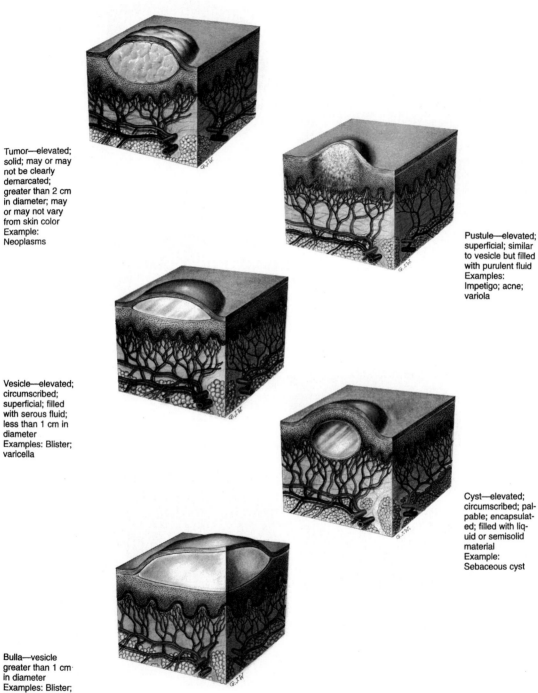

Tumor—elevated; solid; may or may not be clearly demarcated; greater than 2 cm in diameter; may or may not vary from skin color Example: Neoplasms

Pustule—elevated; superficial; similar to vesicle but filled with purulent fluid Examples: Impetigo; acne; variola

Vesicle—elevated; circumscribed; superficial; filled with serous fluid; less than 1 cm in diameter Examples: Blister; varicella

Cyst—elevated; circumscribed; palpable; encapsulated; filled with liquid or semisolid material Example: Sebaceous cyst

Bulla—vesicle greater than 1 cm in diameter Examples: Blister; pemphigus vulgaris

Fig. 18-2, cont'd. Primary skin lesions.

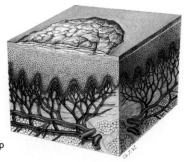

Scale—heaped-up keratinized cells; flaky exfoliation; irregular; thick or thin; dry or oily; varied size; silver, white, or tan
Examples: Psoriasis; exfoliative dermatitis

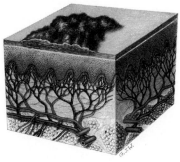

Crust—dried serum, blood, or purulent exudate; slightly elevated; size varies; brown, red, black, tan, or straw
Examples: Scab on abrasion; eczema

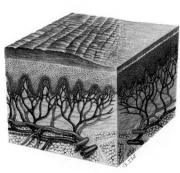

Lichenification—rough, thickened epidermis; accentuated skin markings caused by rubbing or irritation; often involves flexor aspect of extremity
Example: Chronic dermatitis

Scar—thin to thick fibrous tissue replacing injured dermis; irregular; pink, red, or white; may be atrophic or hypertrophic
Example: Healed wound or surgical incision

Keloid—irregularly shaped, elevated, progressively enlarging scar; grows beyond boundaries of wound; caused by excessive collagen formation during healing
Example: Keloid from ear piercing or burn scar

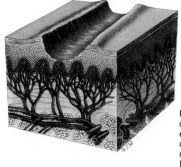

Excoriation—loss of epidermis; linear or hollowed-out crusted area; dermis exposed
Examples: Abrasion; scratch

FIG. 18-3. Secondary skin lesions. (From Thompson JM et al: *Mosby's clinical nursing*, ed 3, St Louis, 1993, Mosby.)
Continued.

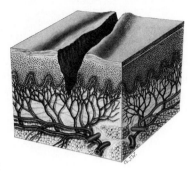

Fissure—linear crack or
break from epidermis to
dermis; small, deep, red
Examples: Athelete's foot;
cheilosis

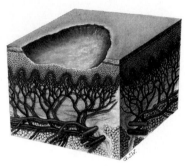

Erosion—loss of all or part
of epidermis; depressed;
moist; glistening; follows
rupture of vesicle or bulla;
larger than fissure
Examples: Varicella; variola following rupture

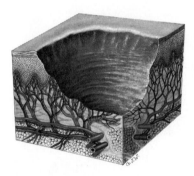

Ulcer—loss of epidermis
and dermis; concave;
varies in size; exudative;
red or reddish blue
Examples: Decubiti; stasis
ulcers

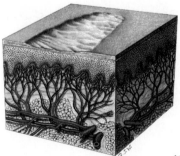

Atrophy—thinning of skin
surface and loss of skin
markings; skin translucent
and paperlike
Examples: Striae; aged
skin

FIG. 18-3, cont'd.   Secondary skin lesions.

TABLE 18-1

Summary of Infectious Exanthems

DISEASE	ETIOLOGY	PERIOD OF COMMUNCABILITY	MODE OF TRANSMISSION	INCUBATION	PRODROME	CLINICAL PRESENTATION	COMPLICATIONS
Rubeola (measles)	*Paramyxovirus*	From prodrome until 5 days after rash begins	Respiratory— airborne droplets	10-14 days	3-4 days high fever, cough, nasal congestion, conjunctivitis; Koplik's spots appear 2 days before rash	Erythematous maculopapular rash; begins on face and spreads downward; initial discrete lesions become confluent; after 3-4 days rash appears reddish-brown; fine desquamation occurs Photophobia; high fever; conjunctivitis; harsh cough	Otitis media; pneumonia; encephalitis
Mumps	*Paramyxovirus*	Immediately before and after swelling begins	Saliva of infected persons	14-21 days	Fever, headache, malaise, anorexia, earache (especially when chewing)	By day 3, parotid gland enlarges, accompanied by pain and tenderness	Deafness; arthritis; epididymoorchitis; sterility
Rubella	RNA virus; rubivirus in the *togaviridae* family	From 7 days before to 5 days after rash	Respiratory— airborne droplets; objects freshly contaminated with nasopharyngeal secretions	14-21 days	Absent in children; in adolescents low-grade fever, malaise, sore throat, cough, nasal congestion, lymphadenopathy	Discrete pink maculopapular rash with downward progression from face; rash disappears in same order as it began; usually gone in 3 days	Greatest danger is teratogenic effect on fetus Rare: arthritis, encephalitis, purpura
Varicella (chickenpox)	Varicella zoster	From 1 day before rash erupts until lesions have crusted (approximately 1 wk after rash begins)	Direct contact with infected persons via droplet spread; objects contaminated with nasopharyngeal secretions	14-21 days	Slight fever, anorexia, malaise for 24 hr	Pruritic rash rapidly progressing from macules to papules to thin vesicles that break and form crusts; all stages of rash occur simultaneously; begins centrally, spreads to face and proximal extremities Fever; lymphadenopathy	Secondary bacterial infections; varicella pneumonia; encephalitis

Continued.

TABLE
18-1

Summary of Infectious Exanthems—cont'd

Disease	Etiology	Period of Communcability	Mode of Transmission	Incubation	Prodrome	Clinical Presentation	Complications
Scarlet fever	Group A beta-hemolytic streptococci	During incubation period and clinical illness or until 24 hr after antibiotics are initiated	Close direct contact with infected person or by respiratory droplet spread; indirectly by contact with contaminated objects and food, especially dairy products	2-4 days	Acute onset of high fever, increased heart rate out of proportion to fever, headache, sore throat, stomach ache, vomiting, chills	Erythematous maculopapular "sandpaper" rash begins on neck and skinfold areas; spreads to trunk and extremities; lasts approximately 4-5 days. Petechiae in skinfolds of axillae, groin, and antecubital area (Pastia's sign). Facial flush with circumoral pallor; "strawberry tongue," generalized lymphadenopathy. Desquamation of skin lasts for 1-2 wk	Early: otitis, pneumonia, septicemia, and osteomyelitis. Late: rheumatic fever and acute glomerulonephritis
Erythema infectiosum (fifth disease)	Human parvovirus B19	Uncertain, but before onset of rash during prodrome	Unknown; most likely via contact with respiratory droplets of infected persons	4-14 days	1-4 days *mild* fever, pruritus, headache (usually not noticed by parents)	Three-stage rash: (1) Bright-red "slapped" cheeks (2) Erythematous maculopapular rash primarily on extremities, but sometimes also on trunk and buttocks (3) Fine lacy rash as maculopapular rash fades; rash may fade and reappear over next 10-14 days	Self-limited arthralgia and arthritis. Possible fetal death if mother is infected in pregnancy. Aplastic crisis in children with hemolytic disease or immune deficiency

Disease	Causative agent	Period of communicability	Incubation period	Prodromal symptoms	Rash	Complications
herpes-virus VI		Unknown	5-15 days	3-4 days high fever in otherwise well child	Temperature becomes normal when rash develops; rose-colored discrete macules or maculo-papules, nonpruritic, lasting 1-2 days	Febrile seizures
Pityriasis rosea	Unknown; probably viral	Unknown	Unknown	Sometimes malaise, headache, pharyngitis	"Herald patch," followed by small round papules that enlarge to form erythematous oval patches with scaly border; classic "Christmas tree pattern," peaks in 2-3 wk, fades over 6-12 wk	None
Hand-foot-and-mouth disease	*Coxsackie* group A enteroviruses	From 2 days before to 2 days after eruption	3-6 days	1-2 days low-grade fever, malaise, vomiting, sore throat	Small oval vesicles on hands, feet, and mucous membranes of mouth	Dehydration Rare: myocarditis, pneumonia, men-ingoencephalitis

Data from Felter, 1992; Hurwitz, 1993; Rosekrans, 1992.

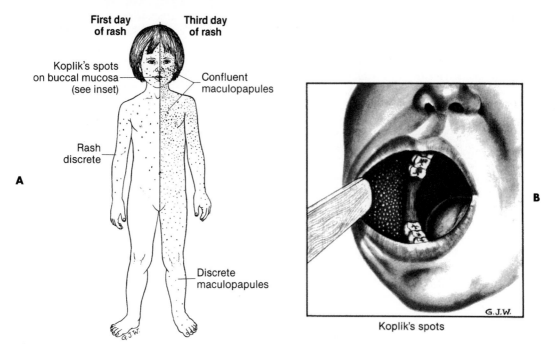

FIG. 18-4. Measles (rubeola). **A,** Distribution of rash. **B,** Koplik's spots. (From Wong DL: *Whaley and Wong's nursing care of infants and children,* ed 5, St Louis, 1995, Mosby.)

Emergency Department interventions. Prompt recognition is important to ensure that the child is evaluated, treated, and discharged from the ED with minimal exposure to others. Symptomatic support, including antipyretics and bed rest, is the primary treatment for uncomplicated measles.

Immunocompromised children and infants less than 1 year of age are most susceptible to complications of measles. Live measles vaccine that is given within 72 hours or immune serum globulin given within 6 days of exposure can prevent or moderate measles disease.[10]

Nursing care and evaluation. Respiratory isolation is required for any child suspected of having measles. If the child is diagnosed with measles, public health authorities should be informed, as well as contacts, especially schools or day care centers.

A complete history and physical examination are necessary for the diagnosis of measles and complications. Particular attention to signs and symptoms of otitis media, pneumonia, secondary bacterial skin infection, and encephalitis is warranted. Antibiotics to treat complications must be administered as pre-

scribed. If encephalitis or pneumonia is present, hospitalization is usually indicated.

In the uncomplicated case of measles, nursing care is supportive and parents should receive clear instructions on the management of their child at home. Fever spikes can be high and are treated with antipyretics (acetaminophen or ibuprofen). If the child is very uncomfortable or prone to seizures, around-the-clock administration of antipyretics is done. Sponging with cool water, which may cause chilling, is avoided. Lights should be dimmed if photophobia is present. Crusty eyelids can be cleaned with saline-saturated cotton balls. Secondary skin infections can be prevented by keeping the skin clean with tepid baths and by clipping the child's fingernails. Oatmeal or baking soda baths and antihistamines can help control itching. Using a cool-mist vaporizer and encouraging intake of clear liquids will help keep nasal secretions thin. Bed rest, although often difficult, should be encouraged. Follow-up is indicated if the child develops ear pain, cough, shortness of breath, or any change in mental status. The child can return to school or day care no sooner than 5 days after the appearance of the rash.

RUBELLA (GERMAN MEASLES)

Etiology. Rubella is a generally benign viral illness that was commonly seen before the introduction of the rubella vaccine. The greatest danger of this disease is its effect on the fetus. If a pregnant woman is infected with rubella, especially during the first trimester, her infant can be born with congenital rubella syndrome. The affected infant is usually growth-retarded, with any combination of the following: eye defects, microcephaly, seizures, mental retardation, congenital heart defects, and hearing loss.

Clinical presentation. The presentation of rubella is frequently mild and nonspecific, making diagnosis difficult. A discrete, pink maculopapular rash usually appears on the face and hairline and rapidly progresses to the neck, trunk, and extremities (Fig. 18-5). Lesions may coalesce and usually disappear by the third day. Low-grade fever is sometimes present. Lymphadenopathy in the back of the neck is characteristic of rubella, often preceding the rash by 1 to 5 days and lasting 2 to 7 days. Arthralgia may also present during the course of the illness or shortly thereafter.

Emergency Department interventions. Supportive treatment is the only treatment approach indicated for rubella. Antipyretics and analgesics are given as needed.

Nursing care and evaluation. Since rubella usually has mild and vague symptoms, the diagnosis is often made by identifying exposure and immunization status. The presence or absence of a prodrome may not be helpful, since children do not often experience signs and symptoms during this time.

Rubella is a self-limiting disease, and parents should be reassured of this fact. The child's fever and level of discomfort are assessed and treated as needed. An attempt to determine the source of the infection should be made. Parents should isolate the child from pregnant women for the period of 7 days before contagion (if known) to 1 week after appearance of the rash. If a pregnant woman is exposed, she should contact her obstetrician immediately to determine her rubella immune status.

VARICELLA (CHICKENPOX)

Etiology. Varicella is a common, highly contagious childhood illness caused by the varicella-zoster virus. Varicella vaccine has been approved by the Federal Drug Administration and is recommended for

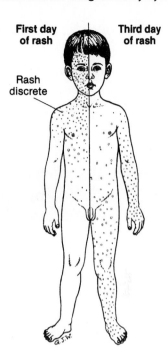

FIG. 18-5. Rubella—distribution of rash. (From Wong DL: *Whaley and Wong's nursing care of infants and children,* ed 5, St Louis, 1995, Mosby.)

high-risk patients. The virus is easily spread by respiratory droplets and contaminated objects. Young children are frequently exposed in day care and schools. Since children are contagious 24 hours before the rash appears, many are exposed without warning.

Clinical presentation. After a 24-hour prodrome of low-grade fever, anorexia, malaise, and upper respiratory symptoms, the characteristic varicella rash develops—usually on the trunk and scalp first. Small red macules quickly progress to papules and then to vesicles, which break open and form a crust (Fig. 18-6). As more vesicles develop over the next 3 to 5 days, all stages of the rash (macules, papules, vesicles and crusts) are evident simultaneously within the same vicinity. Once all lesions have formed a crust, the child is no longer infectious. Varicella lesions are intensely pruritic. Mouth lesions can interfere with the child's hydration. Fever usually occurs primarily in the first several days of the illness.

Complications of varicella include secondary bacterial infections, otitis, pneumonia, and encephalitis. Reye's syndrome has occurred in children with chickenpox who have received aspirin or other salicylates.[10]

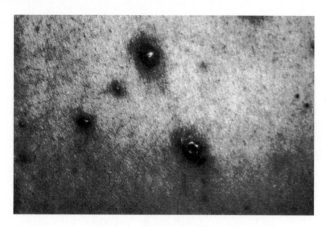

FIG. 18-6. Varicella (chickenpox). Dew-drop-on-a-rose-petal lesions in different stages of development. (From Mayo Medical Center, Department of Dermatology, Rochester, Minn.).

Children taking systemic steroids or those who are immunocompromised are at serious risk for a severe form of varicella, a higher rate of complications, and even death.[8]

Emergency Department interventions. The chickenpox rash is characteristic and therefore relatively easy to diagnose. Treatment for uncomplicated cases is primarily supportive. Acetaminophen and oral antihistamines (e.g., diphenhydramine) can provide some relief from the fever and itching. Select patients, including those taking immunosuppressant drugs, systemic corticosteroids, or long-term salicylates, may benefit from oral acyclovir if it is started within 24 hours of the exanthem. Oral acyclovir 20 mg/kg/dose four times a day for 5 days has been shown to shorten the duration and decrease the severity of varicella.[8] Acyclovir is not recommended for routine use. Intramuscular varicella-zoster immune globulin (VZIG) is recommended to prevent (or at least attenuate) chickenpox in children at high risk for severe disease or complications. VZIG must be given within 96 hours of exposure but preferably within 48 hours.[10]

Nursing care and evaluation. Strict respiratory and contact isolation is required when chickenpox is suspected in the child with fever and malaise and recent exposure to the illness. Expeditious treatment and discharge are indicated to avoid exposure to other ED patients. If a child awaiting admission is exposed, the whole pediatric inpatient unit can be unknowingly exposed. This is particularly important if a child with an altered immune status is exposed.

In the uncomplicated case parents are instructed that treatment is supportive, and they should be provided with information on comfort measures. Aspirin and other salicylates (e.g., Pepto-Bismol) should not be given to children with chickenpox because of the association of those agents with Reye's syndrome. If necessary, acetaminophen can be given for fever or discomfort. Since pruritus can be intense, fingernails should be cut short to reduce the chance of scar formation and infected lesions. Scarring generally occurs from infected lesions. Topically applied calamine lotion and oral antihistamines can be used for severe itching. Tepid baths with Aveeno or ¼ to ½ cup of baking soda or oatmeal may provide relief from itching and fever. Chilling must be avoided, however, since shivering can increase the child's temperature and make the child more uncomfortable. The child should remain isolated until the lesions are crusted. Complications are rare, but parents are instructed about the signs and symptoms of secondary skin infections, pneumonia, encephalitis, and Reye's syndrome (e.g., repetitive vomiting, change in mental status, cough). If any of these signs and symptoms occur, the primary care physician should be contacted. Steroids are withheld or tapered, if at all possible, in children exposed to chickenpox.

SCARLET FEVER

Etiology. Scarlet fever is caused by a reaction to toxins produced during a group A beta-hemolytic streptococci (GAβHS) infection. The disease usually occurs in children between the ages of 1 and 10 years during the late fall, winter, and early spring.[8] The portal of entry of GAβHS is generally the oropharynx; occasionally it is a skin wound. Only a few patients with GAβHS develop scarlet fever.

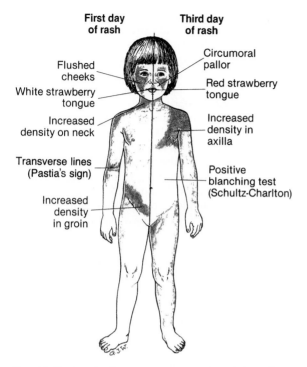

First day of rash
- Flushed cheeks
- White strawberry tongue
- Increased density on neck
- Transverse lines (Pastia's sign)
- Increased density in groin

Third day of rash
- Circumoral pallor
- Red strawberry tongue
- Increased density in axilla
- Positive blanching test (Schultz-Charlton)

FIG. 18-7. Scarlet fever. (From Wong DL: *Whaley and Wong's nursing care of infants and children,* ed 5, St Louis, 1995, Mosby.)

Clinical presentation. The child with scarlet fever usually appears and acts ill. The prodromal stage consists of an acute onset of high fever, increased heart rate out of proportion to the fever, headache, sore throat, stomach ache, vomiting, and chills. The scarlatiniform rash develops within 12 to 48 hours and lasts for approximately 4 to 5 days (Fig. 18-7). Erythematous macules and papules begin on the neck and skinfold areas and spread over the trunk and to the extremities. The rash is often described as being rough to the touch, like sandpaper. In dark-skinned children the erythematous rash may be visible only on the palms of the hands and the soles of the feet; on other parts of the body, punctate papules often resemble gooseflesh.[8] Because of increased capillary fragility, petechiae often develop in a lengthwise fashion in the skinfolds of the axillae, groin, and antecubital area (Pastia's sign). A facial flush with circumoral pallor is common.[3] A "strawberry tongue" covered with a thick white coat and hypertrophied papillae often develops. Generalized lymphadenopathy is present. As the rash fades, desquamation of the skin, especially on the fingers and toes, occurs over several weeks.

Complications of scarlet fever are related to the GAβHS infection. Early complications include otitis, pneumonia, septicemia, and osteomyelitis. Late complications include rheumatic fever and acute glomerulonephritis.

Emergency Department intervention. Children who arrive at the ED with fever, sore throat, and a scarlatiniform rash must have a throat culture performed to determine the presence of GAβHS and to differentiate the illness from viral illnesses that can cause a similar rash. The child's skin should be assessed for wounds that could be infected with GAβHS. Diagnostically, scarlet fever is differentiated from streptococcal pharyngitis only by the presence of the rash.

Scarlet fever is treated with oral or intramuscular penicillin, a cephalosporin, or oral erythromycin. Prompt treatment attenuates the rash and helps prevent most of the complications of scarlet fever, including rheumatic fever. It is questionable whether early treatment of GAβHS prevents kidney complications.[8]

Nursing care and evaluation. Respiratory isolation is indicated for the child with suspected or diagnosed scarlet fever in the prodromal or florid stage. Fever control is initiated in the ED with acetaminophen or ibuprofen. If GAβHS is identified, antibiotics are administered.

Parents should be instructed in supportive care, fever control, and medications. Rest should be encouraged. Salt-water gargles, antiseptic throat sprays, and ingestion of cool or frozen liquids often reduces the pain associated with pharyngitis. Lubricants can be applied to desquamating skin during the later stages of the illness. The child may not return to school until 24 hours after antibiotics are initiated. Follow-up should be arranged within 2 to 3 weeks of the beginning of antibiotic therapy to evaluate response to treatment and to check for complications.

FIFTH DISEASE (ERYTHEMA INFECTIOSUM)

Etiology. Fifth disease, a mild illness primarily seen in children from 3 to 12 years of age, is caused by human parvovirus B19. The illness is mildly contagious, self-limiting, and is rarely associated with complications. Infection with human parvovirus B19 during pregnancy, however, is known to be associated with a slightly increased risk of fetal death and miscarriage. Because approximately 60% of adults are not susceptible to fifth disease and only about 8% of those exposed actually develop the disease, only a few pregnant women contract the disease. Of the small number of pregnant women who become infected, the risk of fetal death is 3% to 5%.[8]

Clinical presentation. The rash of erythema infectiosum occurs in three stages.[8,12] First, the otherwise well child suddenly develops bright-red cheeks, giving the characteristic "slapped-cheek" appearance. The second stage begins approximately 1 day after the facial rash with the development of an erythematous maculopapular rash found primarily on the extremities, but sometimes also on the trunk and buttocks. The third stage begins in approximately 1 week as the rash fades, with areas of central clearing creating a fine lacy rash, which may fade and reappear over the next 10 days. Anything that irritates the skin, such as sun, heat, cold, or friction, can cause the rash to recur.

There are few, if any, symptoms besides the rash. Low-grade fever, malaise, nausea, vomiting, general aches and pains, and occasionally arthralgia may occur.

Emergency Department interventions. Diagnosis of fifth disease is based on the clinical presentation. Treatment is supportive.

Nursing care and evaluation. Isolation is not necessary because the child is not contagious when the rash appears. Children do not need to be restricted from attendance at school.

Parents should be reassured about the benign nature of the disease. Children are not usually uncomfortable, although a self-limited arthralgia and arthritis may develop. Analgesics can be prescribed. Pregnant women who have been exposed to a child with fifth disease should consult their obstetricians.

ROSEOLA INFANTUM

Etiology. Roseola infantum is one of the more common, less serious, but diagnostically problematic illnesses seen in the ED. It is caused by human herpesvirus 6 (HHV-6) and occurs in children between ages 6 months and 3 years. Roseola is sporadic, nonseasonal, and mildly contagious.

Clinical presentation. Roseola appears with sudden onset of a high fever that lasts approximately 3 to 5 days. The child is usually active and playful despite the high fever. With defervescence, a nonpru-

ritic, pink macular rash develops on the trunk and spreads to the proximal extremities. Lesions blanch with pressure. The infant often is examined in the febrile stage, before the rash appears. Without the presence of a rash it is difficult to diagnose roseola.

Emergency Department interventions. For the child who arrives at the ED with fever but no rash, the diagnosis of roseola is difficult to make. The history, including exposures, and presentation may suggest roseola, and the parents can be instructed to watch for the development of a rash. A complete physical examination is indicated. Diagnostic tests, such as complete blood count and cultures, may be performed to identify a source of infection. Treatment is supportive.

Nursing care and evaluation. Isolation precautions are not necessary. Acetaminophen or ibuprofen is administered to control the high fever, which may trigger a febrile seizure. Tepid sponge baths may facilitate defervescence. Despite attempts to keep the fever down, febrile seizures, although rare, may occur, especially with a rapid fever spike. First aid for seizures should be explained to parents. If the child has a history of febrile seizures, round-the-clock administration of antipyretics is done as a preventive measure. If the diagnosis of roseola is made in the ED, the parents should be reassured that the illness is benign.

PITYRIASIS ROSEA

Etiology. Pityriasis rosea is an innocent, self-limited disorder that can occur at any age, but it is most common in school-aged children and adolescents. Although the cause is unknown, the peak incidence is late winter and the low recurrence rate suggest an infectious, probably viral, etiologic basis.

Clinical presentation. A prodrome of malaise, headache, and pharyngitis sometimes precedes the rash. In approximately half the cases, the rash begins with the appearance of a "herald patch." This small, oval, scaly pink patch can appear anywhere on the body, but it occurs most commonly on the trunk or thighs. Central clearing produces a lesion that looks like that of tinea corporis. Within 1 to 2 weeks, many smaller lesions appear on the body concentrated on the trunk and extremities. The lesions begin as small round papules that enlarge to form erythematous oval patches with a scaly border. The patches often run

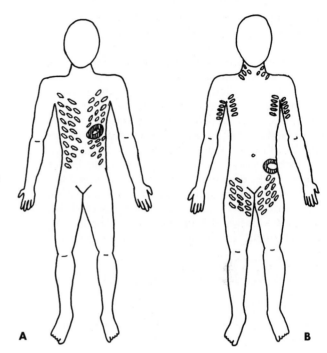

FIG. 18-8. Pityriasis rosea. Distribution in Caucasian children (**A**) and in African-American children (**B**). Herald patch is indicated by circle. (From Weston WL, Lane AT: *Color textbook of pediatric dermatology*, St. Louis, 1991, Mosby.)

parallel to the skin lines on the thorax and the back in a classic "Christmas tree" pattern (Fig. 18-8). The rash peaks in 2 to 3 weeks and slowly fades over 6 to 12 weeks. Postinflammatory hypopigmentation or hyperpigmentation is frequently noted and may persist for weeks to months after healing is complete.

Differential diagnosis includes other scaly lesions, such as tinea corporis, secondary syphilis, drug reactions, eczema, or psoriasis. The distribution of the rash in pityriasis rosea is usually the distinguishing factor.

Emergency Department interventions. Treatment is usually not required for pityriasis rosea. A serologic syphilis test is obtained for sexually active adolescents to rule out secondary syphilis.

Nursing care and evaluation. The period of communicability is unknown. However, by the time the rash breaks out, the child is probably not contagious. Parents should be informed that exposure to ultraviolet light or sunshine hastens the resolution of lesions and decreases itching. If inflammation and pruritus are severe, calamine lotion, antihistamines, and baking soda or oatmeal baths are recommended.

HAND-FOOT-MOUTH DISEASE

Etiology. Hand-foot-mouth disease is an infection caused by several of the *Coxsackie* group A enteroviruses. It occurs most commonly in the late summer and early fall. The disease is highly contagious from 2 days before to 2 days after eruption of the rash; however, the virus may be excreted in the urine for up to 2 weeks.

Clinical presentation. The rash appears abruptly and consists of small gray vesicles on an erythematous base. Lesions are characteristically located on the hands, feet, and mucous membranes of the mouth, but they may also occur on the buttocks, extremities, and face. Oral vesicles usually ulcerate and last 1 to 6 days. They can create discomfort with eating or drinking, which may lead to dehydration. Hand and foot lesions commonly occur on the dorsal aspect but also may be noted on the palms and the soles of the feet. The lesions have a distinctive oval ("football") appearance and are usually nonpruritic. Low-grade fever may last for 2 to 3 days.

Emergency Department interventions. Supportive care is the only available treatment. Antipyretics and analgesics are recommended as needed. If dehydration is present, intravenous (IV) fluids may be necessary.

Nursing care and evaluation. Fluid intake should be encouraged in whatever form the child tolerates. Acidic liquids, such as orange juice, should be avoided; cool or cold liquids are often better tolerated. Applying a 1:1 mixture of diphenhydramine (Benadryl) and Maalox to the oral lesions may alleviate some of the child's discomfort.

Parents should be reassured about the benign nature of the disease. They should be informed that the illness is not contagious after the appearance of the rash and that the lesions will resolve in several days without sequelae. Hand-foot-mouth disease may spread to other family members, including adults.

▌ BACTERIAL SKIN INFECTIONS

IMPETIGO

Etiology. Impetigo is a common, highly contagious superficial infection of the skin. The most common pathogenic organisms are *Staphylococcus aureus* and GAβHS. Impetigo occurs more frequently during warm seasons and in tropical climates. Its spread is enhanced by crowded and poor socioeconomic conditions.

Pathophysiology. Pathogenic bacteria can invade the epidermal barrier if it has been compromised. Minor skin trauma such as scratched bug bites, abrasions, or lacerations predispose the child to impetigo. Many pruritic skin conditions, such as scabies, lice, poison ivy, and atopic dermatitis, can be complicated by impetigo.

Impetigo caused by GAβHS may lead to the development of glomerulonephritis or scarlet fever. Infants colonized with *Staphylococcus aureus* can rapidly develop systemic infections such as septicemia, pneumonia, septic arthritis, or osteomyelitis.

Clinical presentation. Impetigo begins as erythematous macules that rapidly progress to thin-walled vesicles or bullae surrounded by erythema. When the vesicles break, a thin yellow fluid is released, which dries to form the thick honey-colored crusts that are characteristic of impetigo (Fig. 18-9). The area underneath the crusts is typically smooth, red, and moist. Multiple lesions are usually present, especially on the exposed areas of the face and extremities. Impetigo may also occur in a bullous form, which is

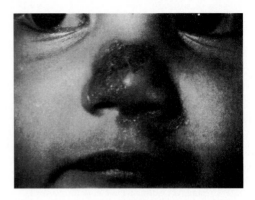

FIG. 18-9. Impetigo contagiosa. (From Weston WL, Lane AT: *Color textbook of pediatric dermatology,* St Louis, 1991, Mosby.)

caused by *S. aureus.* Lesions of bullous impetigo are characterized by clear, thin-walled blisters that break easily, leaving shiny round erosions called "coin" lesions. Bullous impetigo in neonates is especially worrisome because of the tendency toward rapid development of disseminated infection. Neonatal impetigo usually occurs around 7 to 14 days of age. Nursery-acquired infection should be suspected.

The child with impetigo is usually afebrile and does not appear ill, unless the uncommon complications of cellulitis or bacteremia occur. A history of skin erosions that have not spontaneously cleared in several days to weeks is common. Because the lesions are superficial, the risk of scarring is minimal.

Emergency Department interventions. Systemic antibiotics to eradicate staphylococci and streptococci are the treatment of choice. Dicloxacillin or cloxacillin is effective against both pathogens. However, cephalexin is also effective; it is commonly used in children because it tastes better. The use of erythromycin is equivocal because of the increasing reports of erythromycin-resistant staphylococci. If cultures are positive for streptococci, penicillin V may be used.

The topical antibiotic, mupirocin (Bactroban), has been shown to be as effective as systemic antibiotics for most cases of impetigo.[5] Many pediatric care providers recommend using mupirocin for the initial treatment of impetigo[10] and systemic antibiotics for treatment failures or extensive outbreaks on the skin.

Nursing care and evaluation. Cleansing of the impetiginous areas with antibacterial soap and gentle removal of the crusts aids in visualization of the wound and prevention of local spread. The efficacy of topical antibiotics may also be improved. Warm soaks or compresses help to soften the crusts.

The child with suspected impetigo should be isolated. Meticulous handwashing is required after contact with the child. Parents are instructed to keep the child's towels separate from those of other family members. The dosage, frequency, and side effects of prescribed medications should be explained to the parents.

CELLULITIS

Etiology. Cellulitis is a bacterial infection of the subcutaneous tissue with subsequent spread via the lymphatic system. GAβHS and *Staphylococcus aureus* are the most common bacteria causing cellulitis. Facial and periorbital cellulitis are frequently caused by *Haemophilus influenzae* in children younger than 2 years of age.

Pathophysiology. Bacteria is introduced into the subcutaneous tissue by extension from a wound (common in school-age children and adolescents), by hematogenous spread (especially in young children), or by extension from a deeper infection such as sinusitis or osteomyelitis. Wound extension occurs after a puncture or other break in the skin. Bacteria invade the wound and quickly spread to the subcutaneous tissue and possibly the dermis. Further spread occurs via the lymphatic system. Cellulitis is a serious infection that, if inappropriately treated or not treated, can lead to septicemia and death. Facial, orbital, and periorbital cellulitis, in particular, have a high rate of serious complications, such as meningitis (see Chapter 19).

Clinical presentation. Cellulitis usually results 1 to 2 days after a wound or trauma to the face or extremities. The lesions rapidly become erythematous, tender, and swollen. Fever, chills, and other systemic symptoms occur with cellulitis because of hematogenous spread or extension from underlying infections.

Certain clinical presentations lend clues to the bacterial cause. Erythematous, swollen, and painful lesions with unclear borders that spread outward from a break in the skin are usually caused by *S. aureus* organisms. GAβHS can produce a rapidly spreading cellulitis with a distinct border (erysipelas). Red lines spreading in the direction of the lymph nodes (lymphangitis) is commonly seen. A bluish hue to the lesion

may be seen particularly with *H. influenzae,* which is seen in children younger than 2 years.

Emergency Department interventions. Because of the risk of serious complications, the child with potential cellulitis is assessed and treated expeditiously. A blood culture is obtained and antibiotics that cover the organisms suspected of causing the cellulitis are administered promptly. If a streptococcal infection is presumed, IV or intramuscular (IM) penicillin is recommended. *S. aureus* cellulitis is treated with IV cephalosporins or a beta-lactamase–resistant penicillin. Oral antibiotics may be used to treat early staphylococcus or streptococcus cellulitis, but only if close follow-up and compliance can be ensured. *H. influenzae* cellulitis, because of its predominance in young children and its frequent association with septicemia, usually requires hospitalization and treatment with IV cephalosporin or ampicillin and chloramphenicol.

Nursing care and evaluation. Identifying recent bug bites, wounds, or other skin lesions by history or physical examination is helpful in determining the cause. Physical assessment focuses on the affected area and systemic signs and symptoms such as fever. The child is monitored for early signs of septic shock, which can develop rapidly particularly in infants and children who are immunocompromised.

Acetaminophen or ibuprofen can be given for fever or discomfort. Rest and immobilization of the affected area, if possible, should be encouraged. Warm compresses applied to the affected area may relieve local tenderness. Although parents should be reassured that cellulitis usually responds to antibiotics, if the child is discharged, compliance with therapy must be reinforced.

STAPHYLOCOCCAL SCALDED SKIN SYNDROME

Etiology. Staphylococcal scalded skin syndrome (SSSS) carries the greatest risk of mortality when compared to other superficial skin infections. It occurs most commonly in children younger than 5 years and results from a toxin produced by the *S. aureus* organism. The mortality rate of SSSS in children is approximately 4%, with most fatalities occurring in neonates.[8]

Pathophysiology. An exfoliative toxin produced by certain strains of the *S. aureus* organism is carried via the circulation to the skin, where it acts on the surface of epidermal cells. Insult to these cells causes separation of the intradermal cells and separation and shedding of the granular layer and stratum corneum. The original staphylococcal infection may not involve the skin, but it may be related to pharyngitis, conjunctivitis, or umbilical infection. Fluid and electrolyte imbalance and heat loss are common problems that result from the loss of protective skin. Secondary infections such as pneumonia, cellulitis, and septicemia may occur.

Clinical presentation. Initial symptoms include malaise, fever, and irritability when the skin is touched. The skin becomes generally erythematous with a "sandpaper" texture. Within 2 days or less, exudation and crusting around the mouth, nose, and eyes occurs (Fig. 18-10). The upper layer of the epidermis may become wrinkled, and thin layers of skin may be peeled off by light rubbing (Nikolsky's sign). Subsequently bullae are formed. Eventually the skin exfoliates, exposing a shiny, red, moist surface. Infants and young children usually have lesions limited to the upper portions of the body. In the newborn the entire skin surface may be involved. The initial symptoms may appear similar to those of scarlet fever, Kawasaki disease, toxic shock syndrome, or even sunburn.

Emergency Department interventions. The diagnosis is primarily based on clinical findings, but it can be verified by isolation of the *S. aureus* organism from the primary infection site, such as the conjunctiva, the nasopharynx, and occasionally the blood. The organism cannot be recovered from blisters or exfoliated areas.[8]

Aggressive treatment with IV antistaphylococcal antibiotics is required. Cefazolin or nafcillin are most commonly used. Most children, and especially infants, with SSSS are hospitalized for treatment. If close follow-up is ensured, older children, with mild involvement are occasionally managed as outpatients with oral dicloxacillin or cephalosporins.

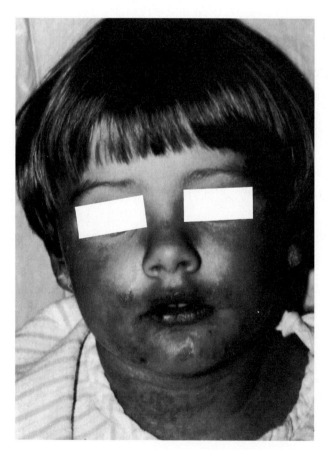

FIG. 18-10. Staphylococcal scalded skin syndrome. An exfoliative toxin elaborated by certain strains of *Staphylococcus* organisms produces bullous lesions. (Courtesy Mayo Medical Center, Department of Dermatology, Rochester, Minn.)

Nursing care and evaluation. Young children, particularly neonates or infants can be acutely ill with SSSS and should be triaged emergently. The ABCs (airway, breathing, circulation) must first be assessed and stabilized while observation is made for signs and symptoms of septic shock and dehydration. IV hydration may be necessary to replace fluid deficits and ongoing fluid loss. Administration of antibiotics should be anticipated.

Minimal handling of the skin is advised, especially in the early stages of the disease. Measures to maintain normothermia may be required because body heat is lost through the damaged tissue. Ongoing care includes frequent taking of vital signs, including body temperature, and maintaining strict intake and output measurement. Parents should be reassured that with appropriate antibiotic therapy and attention to fluid management, most children recover—without sequelae or scarring—within 2 to 3 weeks.

SUPERFICIAL FUNGAL INFECTIONS

Fungi are simple plants that feed off living or dead organic material. Superficial fungal infections invade the epidermis, hair, nails, and mucous membranes. The three common types of superficial fungal infections are the dermatophytoses (tinea), tinea versicolor,

and candidiasis. Fungal infections are common in children who live in hot, humid climates and crowded living conditions.

TINEA

Etiology. The dermatophytes, commonly referred to as tinea or ringworm, cause a variety of clinical lesions involving the skin, hair, and nails. Tinea capitis, a fungal infection of the scalp, and tinea corporis, a fungal infection of the skin, are caused by the *Trichophyton* or *Microsporum* species. *Trichophyton tonsurans* is most prevalent in crowded conditions and accounts for approximately 95% of tinea capitis in the United States.[4] *Microsporum audouinii* infrequently causes tinea infections. *Microsporum canis,* acquired from infected domestic animals, is more prevalent in suburban and rural areas. Tinea versicolor (pityriasis versicolor) is a common superficial fungal infection of the skin and is actually caused by the yeastlike organism *Malassezia furfur* (Table 18-2).

Pathophysiology. Fungal invasion of the stratum corneum (outer layer of the epidermis), the nails, or the hair is responsible for the lesions in tinea. Deeper layers of the epidermis are spared. Transmission of tinea occurs between persons or animals. The *M. canis* organism is harbored by cats and dogs and transmitted from animal to person, but not from

TABLE 18-2	Tinea Infections		
	TINEA CAPITIS	**TINEA CORPORIS**	**TINEA VERSICOLOR**
Etiology	*Trichophyton tonsurans; Microsporum audouinii; Microsporum canis*	*Microsporum canis; Trichophyton mentagrophytes*	*Pityrosporum orbiculare (Malassezia furfur)*
Epidemiology	2-10 yr; rarely occurs after puberty; boys > girls	Any age, including infants; most common in children	15-30 yr
Clinical presentation	Scaling of scalp with broken hairs and alopecia; kerion formation possible	Round or oval, with erythematous border and clear center	Oval or round scaly patches with change in skin color (usually hypopigmentation)
Treatment	Oral: griseofulvin for 6-8 wk	Topical antifungal agents for 2-3 wk	Keratolytics and topical antifungal agents for 3-4 wk; recurrences common

human to human. *T. mentagrophytes* is also generally spread from animal to person. *T. tonsurans* is transmitted from person to person. Tinea versicolor results from a proliferation of hyphal forms of *Malassezia furfur* organisms, which normally exist on the skin in a yeast form. The reason for this phenomena is unknown.

Clinical presentation. Tinea capitis is characterized by scaling of the scalp and patchy alopecia (Fig. 18-11). Lesions are usually irregular, circular, or oval patches with hairs broken off 1 to 3 mm above the scalp. In about 5% of cases of tinea capitis, short stubby hairs, broken very close to the cutaneous surface, give a "black-dot" appearance. Multiple patches are common. Kerions, which are sharply demarcated, thick, boggy, crusted inflammatory lesions covered with vesicles and pustules, occur in approximately 33% of cases of tinea capitis.[10] Kerions are thought to be associated with an allergic sensitization to the fungal infection.[8] Regional lymphadenopathy is often present.

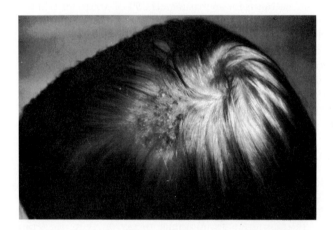

FIG. 18-11. Tinea capitis. (Courtesy Mayo Medical Center, Department of Dermatology, Rochester, Minn.)

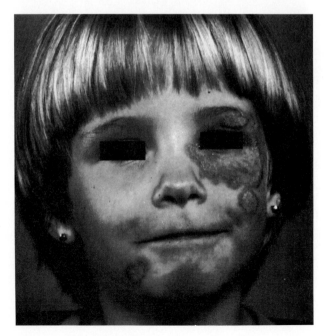

FIG. 18-12. Tinea corporis. Raised inflamed borders with scales that gradually clear in the center are characteristic. (Courtesy Mayo Medical Center, Department of Dermatology, Rochester, Minn.)

The classic tinea corporis lesion (Fig. 18-12) is a round or oval scaly patch, with a clear center, surrounded by an erythematous, vesicular, papular, or pustular border. Lesions in children commonly occur on the face but also on the trunk and limbs. Multiple lesions may coalesce. Mild pruritus is common.

Tinea versicolor is characterized by multiple oval or round scaly macular patches. Lesions tend to be hypopigmented in the summer, compared to the tanned skin, and relatively darker in the winter (Fig. 18-13). The upper trunk and arms are commonly involved, but the lesions can be more widespread.

Emergency Department interventions. Superficial fungal infections are primarily nonurgent conditions. Diagnosis of tinea is often made clinically, but it can be confirmed with a potassium hydroxide wet-mount preparation and/or a fungal culture of scrapings from the lesion. A Wood's light examination done in a completely darkened room can be helpful in identifying *M. audouinii* and *M. canis,* which fluoresce a brilliant green. However, *T. tonsurans* does not fluoresce. If the clinical presentation is typical, treatment is usually begun before the culture results are finalized.

Prolonged treatment with antifungal agents is necessary to resolve tinea infections. Topical antifungal agents are used to treat tinea corporis, but they are not effective with scalp lesions because they cannot reach the hyphae of the fungus within the hair shaft. Oral griseofulvin administered for at least 6 weeks to several months is the treatment of choice for tinea capitis. Follow-up is recommended in approximately 2 to 4 weeks to assess the efficacy of treatment. If the fungal culture is negative at this time, a total of 6 weeks of therapy is all that is required. If the culture is positive, griseofulvin therapy must be extended. A complete blood count (CBC) and liver function tests should be done to monitor for side effects of prolonged use of griseofulvin, including hepatotoxicity and agranulocytosis. Steroids may be given for treatment of kerions.

Tinea versicolor lesions should be cleansed with selenium sulfide shampoo twice a day to assist in the removal of superficial scales.[10] An alternate method is applying the shampoo overnight once a week for approximately 1 month. Topical antifungals can be used daily, but they are expensive and do not necessarily offer any advantage over the shampoo.[8]

Nursing care and evaluation. Parent education is extremely important, not only to impart knowledge but also to encourage compliance with long-term therapy. Parents should be encouraged to continue giving the medications, even if the lesions resolve, to prevent recurrence. A variety of antifungal creams are

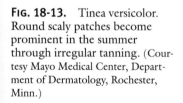

FIG. 18-13. Tinea versicolor. Round scaly patches become prominent in the summer through irregular tanning. (Courtesy Mayo Medical Center, Department of Dermatology, Rochester, Minn.)

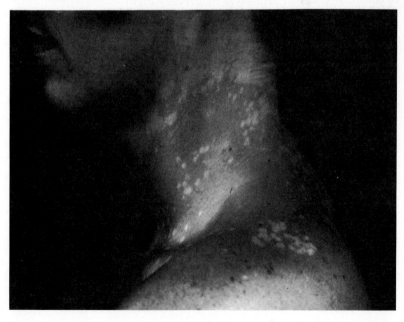

available, including clotrimazole (Lotrimin), miconazole (Micatin), and tolnaftate (Tinactin). Only small amounts should be rubbed into the lesion and the surrounding skin. If the child undergoes prolonged griseofulvin therapy, follow-up is important to monitor for side effects. Griseofulvin is better absorbed after ingestion of a fatty meal, including, for example, milk or ice cream.

Families should be instructed that good hygiene is essential when a child is diagnosed with a fungal infection. Because of the contagious nature of these infections, affected children should not exchange brushes, combs, barrettes, hats, scarves, or any other clothing that comes in contact with affected areas. Selenium sulfide shampoo, used twice a week, helps to decrease the shed of fungal spores and can decrease further spread of tinea capitis. Since tinea can be spread from animals to humans, all household pets should be examined by a veterinarian, especially if the *M. canis* organism is isolated.

Superficial fungal infections can be upsetting to children and parents. Concerns about scarring and permanent hair loss are frequently present. Hair usually regrows slowly after a tinea capitis infection, within 3 to 6 months. However, some scarring and permanent hair loss may result if a kerion is present.

Tinea versicolor has a high recurrence rate. Treatment is often seen as controlling recurrence, not necessarily curing the infection. Pigmentation does not return to normal until several months after the infection has resolved. Sunlight aids repigmentation.

THRUSH (ORAL CANDIDIASIS)

Etiology. Thrush is an infection that occurs on the tongue, palate, and buccal mucosa. It is caused by the yeastlike fungus *Candida albicans.* Although thrush is not an acute illness, it is often identified in infants or children in the ED as a secondary or incidental diagnosis. A child of any age or an adult may develop thrush, although infants are particularly susceptible. If the child is no longer using a bottle or pacifier, thrush should raise the suspicion of an immune deficiency or diabetes. Long-term glucocorticosteroid or antibiotic therapy and any alterations in host defenses, such as leukemia, seem to predispose infants and children to thrush.

Pathophysiology. The *C. albicans* organism flourishes in moist, dark, and warm places such as the mouth, the gastrointestinal tract, and the vagina. When breaks in the epidermal barrier occur in these areas the abundant fungus can invade the epidermis and cause an infection. If left untreated, thrush usually resolves spontaneously over as long as 2 months. During that time *Candida* organisms can spread to the respiratory and gastrointestinal tract.

Clinical presentation. Thrush is an inflammation of the tongue, palate, and buccal mucosa characterized by thick white patches or plaques that cannot be wiped or scraped off. The mucosa is often markedly erythematous. Thrush may be painful, but it rarely interferes with the infant's or child's ability to feed. Due to the passage of *Candida* organisms through the gastrointestinal tract, an associated diaper dermatitis is often present (see the discussion of diaper rash later in this chapter).

Emergency Department interventions. Thrush is a nonurgent problem, and there is no need for isolation of the affected child. Nystatin oral suspension, 1 ml administered in each side of the mouth four times a day, is usually prescribed. This medication is continued for 48 to 72 hours after the lesions have disappeared.

Nursing care and evaluation. Predisposing factors, such as immunologic disorders or antibiotic therapy, should be identified by history. During the physical examination, if the mouth lesions cannot be scraped off easily with a tongue blade, thrush is the likely diagnosis. The diaper area also should be examined for signs of candidal diaper dermatitis.

Parents should be instructed on how to administer antifungal agents. Nystatin is dropped onto the inside of each cheek after meals to allow the medicine to remain in contact with the lesions. If the lesions are particularly thick, the nystatin should be gently rubbed directly onto that area with a cotton-tipped swab. Nystatin is not well absorbed from the gastrointestinal tract. Bottle nipples and pacifiers should be boiled after use to kill the *Candida* organisms. If the mother suspects a yeast infection of her nipples (if breast-feeding) or vagina, she should seek treatment to prevent reinfection of the infant.

▌ DERMATITIS

Dermatitis is an inflammation of the superficial dermis and the epidermis. It is characterized by skin eruptions such as crusting, scaling, excoriation, weeping, and cracking. Dermatitis can be acute—involving vesicle formation, oozing, and crusting—or chronic—

involving epidermal thickening (lichenification) and exaggerated skin creases. Acute dermatitis is thought to result from an intense stimulus, whereas chronic dermatitis is believed to be related to a lower-grade stimulus occurring over time. Dermatitis as the chief complaint is usually a nonurgent condition. Since it is not contagious, isolation is not required. The following sections discuss diaper, atopic, contact, and seborrheic dermatitis.

DIAPER DERMATITIS

Etiology. The general term *diaper dermatitis* refers to a number of different skin problems occurring in the diaper area. The majority of children younger that 2 years of age develop some form of diaper dermatitis. About 10% of infants who wear diapers develop severe diaper rash with erythema, papules, ulcerations and/or excoriation.[10] The incidence of diaper dermatitis peaks at 9 to 12 months. It is most likely associated with dietary modifications such as an increasing variety of solid foods, decreased frequency of diaper changes, and a urine volume that exceeds the absorption capacity of diapers. Poor hygiene often leads to diaper dermatitis.

Like other skin inflammations, diaper dermatitis is caused by frequent and lengthy exposure to irritants. In the diaper area these irritants include friction, urine, feces, soaps and detergents, fabric softeners, and ointments. Containment of urine and feces by occlusive plastic-coated diapers or plastic pants increases the penetration of these alkaline substances through the skin (Fig. 18-14).

Pathophysiology. Prolonged exposure to wetness in the diaper area predisposes the skin to dermatitis. Moisture produces increased friction, with resulting maceration and abrasion damage caused by the rubbing of the diaper against the skin. Wetness also results in greater permeability of the skin and increased growth of microbes in the diaper area. The most critical element in developing diaper rash is the length of time that an infant wears a wet diaper.

Bacteria and fungi do not play a primary role in the development of diaper dermatitis. However, irritated skin is more susceptible to penetration by bacteria and fungi, thus increasing the likelihood of secondary infection. *Candida* organisms have been recovered in more than 80% of diaper rashes lasting longer than 4 days.[10]

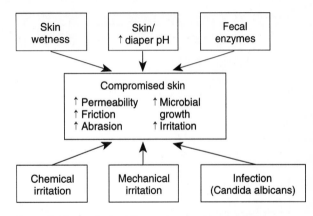

FIG. 18-14. Principal factors involved in development of diaper dermatitis. (From Wong DL: *Whaley and Wong's nursing care of infants and children*, ed 5, St Louis, 1995, Mosby.)

Clinical presentation. A number of recognizable patterns of skin eruptions can be noted in the diaper area (Table 18-3). Inflammation of the skin that is in greatest contact with the diaper (e.g., convex surfaces, mons pubis, and scrotum), with the folds spared, is consistent with chemical or mechanical irritation. *Candida* infection is characterized by a clearly demarcated widespread area of erythema on the buttocks, lower abdomen, and inner thighs. Skinfolds are affected, and the color is a distinctive beefy-red. Pinpoint pustulovesicular satellite lesions are characteristic of candidal diaper dermatitis. Whatever the clinical presentation, most forms of diaper dermatitis share a similar pathophysiology.

Emergency Department interventions. Diaper rash is commonly seen in the ED in conjunction with other problems. It is a nonurgent condition when seen as an isolated problem. The basis of treatment for all forms of diaper dermatitis is removal of the irritants and elimination of maceration by keeping the diaper area clean and dry.

If a candidal diaper rash is present, an antifungal cream is first applied 4 times a day for 2 days, then 3 times a day for 2 days, and finally 2 times a day for 10 days. For more severe infections, a low-potency topical steroid cream may be used as an additional measure. If thrush is present, oral nystatin also should be prescribed to eliminate the gastrointestinal source of *Candida* organisms.

If a harshly inflamed diaper rash does not respond to drying techniques, a 1% hydrocortisone cream can

TABLE 18-3	Skin Eruptions in Diaper Area
RASH/AREA INVOLVED	**USUAL DIAGNOSIS/CAUSE**
Convex surfaces involved; folds spared	Contact dermatitis Allergic or irritant dermatitis/chemical irritants (urine, feces, detergents, soaps)
Folds involved, sharply demarcated	Intertrigo/heat, moisture, and sweat retention Seborrheic dermatitis/inborn trait
Folds involved with satellite lesions	Seborrheic dermatitis with secondary candidiasis/inborn trait plus *Candida albicans* infection
Perianal	Chemical and mechanical irritation/chemical irritants (fecal enzymes)
Perianal with satellite lesions	Primary candidiasis/*C. albicans* infection
Band of erythema at diaper margins	"Tide mark" dermatitis/plastic or rubber border on diaper and sweat retention
Small, sterile vesicopustules	Miliaria "Heat rash," "prickly heat"/hot, humid climate in diaper area
Vesicles or bullae	Bullous impetigo/usually *Staphylococcus aureus* or combined with streptococci Herpes (less common)/herpes simplex

Modified from Jacobs AH: Eruptions in the diaper area, *Pediatr Clin North Am* 25(2):209-224, 1978.

be applied sparingly to the rash 2 to 4 times a day until the rash improves. Oral and/or topical antibiotics such as mupirocin may be prescribed if a bacterial diaper rash with vesicles or bullae is suspected.

Nursing care and evaluation. Causes of diaper rash can be indicated by the history. For example, the duration of the diaper rash, recent use of new soaps or diapers, introduction of new foods, or current or recent medications (especially antibiotics) can help to identify the probable cause of diaper dermatitis. The skin in the diaper area should be carefully examined, and the general cleanliness of the infant should be noted. The mouth should also be checked for the presence of thrush.

Parents should be taught to remove the irritants from skin surfaces and to keep the diaper area clean and dry. Diapers must be changed frequently, at least 6 times per day. Superabsorbent disposable diapers can decrease skin wetness and irritation.[9] Leaving the diaper area open to air for periods during the day is also helpful. Occlusive diaper coverings, such as plastic pants, should not be used. When contaminated with urine and feces, the diaper area should be cleansed with warm water. Soaps can be irritating and should be avoided except when fecal material cannot be removed

with water alone. Diaper "wipes" can aggravate a diaper rash because of the chemical irritants they contain.

Many parents apply occlusive ointments, such as A&D Ointment or zinc oxide, to the diaper area. These ointments may be helpful in preventing diaper rash, but when a diaper rash is present, they may trap moisture against the skin. The use of talcum powder in the diaper area poses the serious risk of accidental aspiration of talc. Ingestion of talc in large amounts has been linked to cancer. Powders that contain cornstarch are safer to use and more effective in reducing friction and moisture in the diaper area. When good hygiene is practiced and frequent diaper changes are done, neither ointments nor powders are necessary.

ATOPIC DERMATITIS

Etiology. Atopic dermatitis is one of the most common pediatric skin disorders. It occurs in approximately 10% to 15% of infants and children. The exact cause is unknown, although it appears to have a hereditary component and occurs frequently in children with asthma and allergies. Several etiologic hypotheses exist, including immunodeficiency, food allergies, and environmental allergies such as dust and mites. Atopic dermatitis is aggravated by a variety of factors, such as stress, dry skin, and contact sensitivities.

Pathophysiology. Since the etiologic basis of atopic dermatitis is unknown, its pathophysiology remains unclear.

Clinical presentation. Atopic dermatitis appears in different patterns governed by the age of the child and the distribution of lesions. Two thirds of children with atopic dermatitis develop symptoms in infancy.[10] Approximately half of these infants improve by 2 to 3 years of age.[8] Dry skin, itching, and eczematous lesions—involving erythema, scaling skin, and weeping vesicles—are characteristic of atopic dermatitis (Fig. 18-15). Lesions of atopic dermatitis usually spare the diaper area in infants, probably because of the increased hydration in this area. Lichenification (thickened, leathery hyperpigmented skin) is characteristic of chronic atopic dermatitis and occurs primarily on the wrists, ankles, and popliteal and antecubital fossae. Symptoms of atopic dermatitis are generally worse during the fall and winter and in areas of low humidity (Box 18-4).

Infants and children with atopic dermatitis are susceptibile to bacterial skin infections, with *Staphylococcus aureus* being the most common bacterial pathogen. Abscesses, cellulitis, and lymphangitis can result. Atopic dermatitis is often confused with seborrheic dermatitis, contact dermatitis, scabies, or tinea.

Emergency Department interventions. Atopic dermatitis tends to recur, but the symptoms can usually be controlled with palliative therapy. The goals of therapy are to reduce dryness, inflammation, and itching and to prevent or control bacterial infections. Skin hydration, topical corticosteroid therapy, and antihistamines are the mainstay of treatment. Bacterial infections are treated similarly to impetigo.

Nursing care and evaluation. Since atopic dermatitis is a chronic condition, its long-term treatment is best handled by the child's primary care provider. However, ED visits for atopic dermatitis may occur, especially for exacerbations and/or infections. If the child has been previously diagnosed with atopic dermatitis, the parents should be questioned about the usual therapeutic regimen. Primary care providers should be consulted to ensure coordination of care. Remissions of atopic dermatitis do occur, and the condition can be well controlled with good compli-

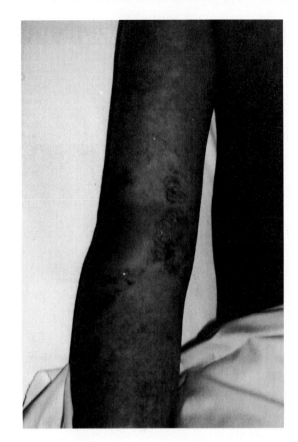

FIG. 18-15. Atopic dermatitis. Eczematous lesions in the popliteal fossa are commonly seen in childhood atopic dermatitis. (From Barkin RM: *Pediatric emergency medicine: concepts and clinical practice*, ed 2, St Louis, 1996, Mosby.)

ance to the recommended therapy. Aggravating factors should be avoided. Moisturizing dry, inflamed areas is important, as is using mild cleansing agents such as Dove, Aveeno, Basis, or Cetaphil. Moisturizing agents such as Eucerin, Vaseline, or Moisture can be applied to wet the skin, which improves absorption.

When significant weeping or crusting occurs, moisturizing treatment becomes more important. Wet compresses can be applied to affected areas 4 to 6 times per day.

Topical steroid preparations are used when significant inflammation occurs. Low- to moderate-potency nonfluorinated steroids are used (Table 18-4), except in severe cases, since prolonged application can cause systemic side effects. Ointment-based steroids mois-

Box 18-4   Clinical Manifestations of Atopic Dermatitis

Distribution of lesions
Infantile form—generalized, especially cheeks, scalp, trunk, and extensor surfaces of extremities
Childhood form—flexural areas (antecubital and popliteal fossae, neck), wrists, ankles, and feet
Preadolescent and adolescent form—face, sides of neck, hands, feet, face, and antecubital and popliteal fossae (to a lesser extent)

Appearance of lesions
Infantile form
  Erythema
  Vesicles
  Papules
  Weeping
  Oozing
  Crusting
  Scaling
  Often symmetric
Childhood form
  Symmetric involvement
  Clusters of small erythematous or flesh-colored papules or minimally scaling patches
  Dry and may be hyperpigmented
  Lichenification (thickened skin with accentuation of creases)

Keratosis pilaris (follicular hyperkeratosis) common
Adolescent/adult form
  Same as childhood manifestations
  Dry, thick lesions (lichenified plaques) common
  Confluent papules

Other manifestations
Intense itching
Unaffected skin dry and rough
Black children likely to exhibit more papular and/or follicular lesions than white children
May exhibit one or more of the following:
  Lymphadenopathy, especially near affected sites
  Increased palmar creases (many cases)
  Atopic pleats (extra line or groove of lower eyelid)
  Prone to cold hands
  Pityriasis alba (small, poorly defined areas of hypopigmentation)
  Facial pallor (especially around nose, mouth, and ears)
  Bluish discoloration beneath eyes ("allergic shiners")
  Increased susceptibility to unusual cutaneous infections (especially viral)

From Wong DL: *Whaley and Wong's essentials of pediatric nursing,* ed 5, St Louis, 1997, Mosby.

turize skin better than creams do, and they are better absorbed. Fluorinated steroids should never be used on the face because they cause permanent thinning of the skin.

Itching exacerbates the inflammation. Antihistamines such as hydroxyzine hydrochloride or diphenhydramine can be prescribed to relieve the itching; these agents are particularly useful at nighttime.

CONTACT DERMATITIS

Etiology. Contact dermatitis results from contact with an irritant, such as wet diapers, or an allergen. Common sources of contact allergens in children include metal (jewelry, buckles), shoes, topical medications (neomycin), shoes, perfumes, soaps, cosmet-

ics, poison ivy, poison oak, and poison sumac. Infants are highly susceptible to irritant contact dermatitis because of their thinner skin. However, allergic contact dermatitis is uncommon in children younger than 8 years.[10]

Pathophysiology. Contact dermatitis is manifested when the skin comes into prolonged contact with an irritant or allergen that affects skin integrity and results in local skin responses. The extent of the eruption depends on the amount and location of exposure and the strength of the irritant. Although it is not well understood, the mechanism responsible for allergic contact dermatitis is probably a genetically determined delayed hypersensitivity or a cell-mediated reaction.[2,8]

TABLE 18-4	Potency Guide for Selected Topical Steroids	
DOSE/FORM	**GENERIC NAME**	**PRODUCT NAME**
Lowest potency (antiinflammatory activity = 1)		
0.25%, 0.5%, 1.0%, and 2.5% cream; 1% ointment	Hydrocortisone	Synacort, Nutracort, Cort-Dome
0.05% cream and ointment	Desonide	Tridesilon, Desowen
0.1% cream	Dexamethasone*	Decaderm
1.0% cream	Methylprednisolone	Medrol
Moderate potency (antiinflammatory activity = 10-99)		
0.1% and 0.2% cream 0.025% ointment	Fluocinolone acetonide*	Synalar, Fluonid
0.01% cream; 0.25% lotion	Triamcinolone acetonide*	Kenalog, Aristocort
0.05% ointment	Flurandrenolide*	Cordran
0.05% cream	Desoximetasone*	Topicort LP
0.2% cream	Hydrocortisone valerate	Westcort
High potency (antiinflammatory activity = 100-499)		
0.05% cream, solution, and ointment	Fluocinonide*	Lidex
0.05% cream and ointment	Betamethasone/diproprionate*	Diprosone
0.1% cream and ointment	Halcinonide*	Halog
0.1% ointment	Amcinonide*	Cyclocort
0.25% cream and ointment	Desoximetasone*	Topicort
0.5% cream and ointment	Triamcinolone acetonide*	Kenalog, Aristocort
Highest potency (antiinflammatory activity >500)		
0.05% cream	Clobetasol proprionate*	Temovate, Dermovate
0.05% ointment	Betamethasone diproprionate*	Diprolene

From Rosekrans JA: Dermatologic disorders. In Barkin RM: *Pediatric emergency medicine: concepts and clinical practice,* ed 2, St Louis, 1997, Mosby.
*Fluorinated steroids.

Clinical presentation. The clinical presentation of contact dermatitis depends on the causative factor and is usually limited to the area exposed to the irritant or allergen. Irritant contact dermatitis causes the skin to appear erythematous and chafed. In allergic contact dermatitis lesions appear as weepy erythematous vesicles (Fig. 18-16). An urticarial reaction may occur. If exposure is prolonged, the skin takes on an erythematous lichenified appearance. The rash associated with contact dermatitis usually appears abruptly.

The distribution of the rash helps identify the cause. Contact with plant leaves or stems, such as poison ivy, produces an erythematous papulovesicular eruption that appears in a linear pattern. Environmental irritants result in an eruption on the exposed skin. Contact with metal objects produces a geometric distribution in the shape of the object (e.g., a watch).

Emergency Department interventions. Diagnosis of contact dermatitis depends on the identification of the responsible agent. This often takes extensive detective work to determine the irritant or allergen. Treatment focuses on removal of the causative agent and control of the symptoms.

Nursing care and evaluation. A history of exposure to potential irritants or allergens is important so that the source of the dermatitis, such as chemicals, soaps, or wet, dirty diapers, can be removed. In allergic dermatitis caused by poison ivy, oak, or sumac, the plant oils must be thoroughly washed from the skin with hot soapy water. Any possibly contaminated clothing or shoes should also be washed.

When inflammation is significant, mild- to moderate-potency topical steroids and antipruritics

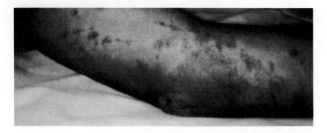

Fig. 18-16. Contact dermatitis. Linear blisters on areas of skin that are not covered by clothing are suggestive of contact with leaves or stems such as poison ivy. (From Barkin RM: *Pediatric emergency medicine: concepts and clinical practice,* ed 2, St Louis, 1997, Mosby.)

may be used to control itching (see Table 18-4). In severe allergic contact dermatitis involving more than 10% of the body surface, oral steroids may also be prescribed.

Seborrheic Dermatitis

Etiology. Seborrheic dermatitis is a scaling, crusting eruption that is thought to be related to overproduction of sebum, although the exact cause of the condition is not known. Several theories have been suggested, including food allergy, autoimmunity to the epidermis or to *Candida albicans,* or an infection with other fungal agents. There does not seem to be a genetic predisposition. Two age groups are primarily affected: infants younger than 6 months and adolescents. Seborrhea tends to appear more frequently in the spring and summer.

Pathophysiology. Since the etiologic basis is unknown, the pathophysiology of seborrhea is also not well understood.

Clinical presentation. Seborrheic dermatitis appears as waxy or greasy yellow, scalelike eruptions. Erythema may be present. Eruptions occur on the scalp (often called "cradle cap" in infants), face, midchest, postauricular areas, and the perineum—areas where sebaceous glands are most abundant. The adolescent may have erythematous, greasy scales in the nasolabial folds. Pruritus, if present, is mild.

Emergency Department interventions. Seborrheic dermatitis will generally resolve on its own if left untreated. Since resolution may take months, treatment aimed at removing the crusts is often initiated. Low-potency topical corticosteroids may be used to treat inflamed, weepy areas. The prognosis is excellent in infants, but adolescents tend to have relapses. If lesions become infected, antibiotics are prescribed.

Nursing care and evaluation. Antiseborrheic shampoos (e.g., Selsun Blue) are used to treat scalp lesions, particularly adherent crusty lesions which can first be soaked in shampoo or mineral oil for 15 minutes and then be removed with a fine-tooth comb. Topical steroids, if used, should be applied sparingly. After the lesions have cleared, adolescents may continue weekly use of antiseborrheic shampoos to prevent recurrences.

▊ Skin Parasites

The most common parasitic infestations seen in pediatric practice are scabies and pediculosis (lice). Head lice is often identified at school, and parents are often distressed that their child is infested. Parasites spread readily, especially in crowded conditions such as those that occur at home, school, day care, or camp. Often other family members have a similar condition. In the ED children with suspected parasitic infections should be isolated. Parents of children with scabies and pediculosis should be reassured that parasitic infections do not necessarily result from poor hygienic conditions but that children in day care centers and schools are often affected.

Scabies

Etiology. Scabies is a contagious disorder caused by an eight-legged mite know as *Sarcoptes scabiei.* Infants, children, and adolescents are susceptible to scabies infestation.

Pathophysiology. Scabies results when the impregnated female mite burrows into the stratum corneum layer of the skin. Eggs are laid, and fecal material is deposited in skin tunnels or burrows. These burrows form tiny, linear gray-brown lesions. The female louse dies in 30 to 40 days; her eggs reach maturity in 21 days. Individuals with scabies do not experience symptoms for 4 to 6 weeks after the initial

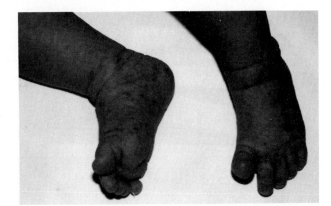

FIG. 18-17. Scabies. Infants and young children frequently have vesicles on their palms and soles. (Courtesy Mayo Medical Center, Department of Dermatology, Rochester, Minn.)

infestation, at which time a hypersensitivity reaction to mite antigens is thought to occur.[8] Thus it is often spread unknowingly. The spread of scabies requires close personal contact with an infested person or object. Since the female mite can live 2 to 3 days on the human body, clothing and bed linens can be sources of infestation.

Clinical presentation. An intensely pruritic rash is the most common chief complaint associated with scabies although the clinical presentation is variable. In older children papulovesicular and burrow-type lesions are distributed in the interdigital surfaces, axillary-cubital area, popliteal folds, and hands and wrists. The face and head are usually spared. Itching leads to punctate discrete excoriations that result from scratching.

Infants and young children develop vesicles and burrows on their palms and soles and may have lesions on their scalp, face, and trunk (Fig. 18-17). Vesicular lesions tend to be more numerous and widespread in infants. Eczematous eruptions of the face and trunk are common. Secondary bacterial infections can occur in all age groups.

Emergency Department interventions. Scabies is treated with 5% permethrin cream (Elimite) or 1% lindane lotion (Kwell). The use of lindane lotion in infants and children is controversial because of the potential for central nervous system toxicity.[10] Thus permethrin is the drug of choice for pediatric patients.

Nursing care and evaluation. Permethrin cream is applied from the neck down in the older child and adolescent. The neck and head of infants and young children should also be treated, with care taken to avoid the eyes, nose, and mouth. The cream is left on the body for 12 hours before being washed off. Because signs and symptoms of scabies may not develop for 1 to 2 months, all household members and close contacts should be treated simultaneously. If necessary, retreatment can be safely done in 2 weeks.[8] Parents must be forewarned that itching may persist for 7 to 10 days after treatment, despite elimination of the mites. They should be cautioned not to overuse the insecticide. Bed linens and clothing should be washed with hot soapy water, and carpets should be vacuumed.

PEDICULOSIS CAPITIS (HEAD LICE)

Etiology. Of the three varieties of lice that affect children—head, body, and crab (pubic) lice—head lice (pediculosis capitis) is the most common form. An estimated 6 to 10 million children are infested annually.[8] Head lice is caused by a small insect called *Pediculus humanus capitis*. The condition is more common in girls than in boys and more prevalent among Caucasians than in African-Americans most likely because of the apparent preference of head lice for fine straight hair. Crowded living conditions foster rapid transmission of head lice, which spread through person-to-person contact or via fomites such as hairbrushes, shared clothing, carpets, and linens.

Pathophysiology. Lice are parasitic insects that feed on human blood. The life cycle of the human louse begins when the female louse lays eggs (nits) on the hair shaft close to the scalp. After hatching from the eggs in about 1 week, the new lice mature over the next week and begin laying their own eggs. The adult louse lives for approximately 1 month and can survive away from the host's body for as long as 1 week, allowing transmission to occur via fomites.

Clinical presentation. Pediculosis first appears as intense itching of the scalp, caused by the crawling insect and its saliva on the skin. Small oval whitish-gray nits are visible on the hair shaft close to the scalp. Unlike dandruff, they firmly adhere to the hair and are very difficult to remove. Typical sites of involvement are the area behind the ears and the nape of the neck. Lice found in the eyebrows and eyelashes are often pubic lice; therefore, the possibility of sexual or close contact with an adult with pubic lice must be investigated. Nocturnal pruritus is often intense with pediculosis capitis. Dermatitis of the neck, shoulders, and postauricular areas and urticaria or impetigo can occur.

Emergency Department interventions. Because adult lice are difficult to see, the presence of nits on the hair shaft close to the scalp is considered diagnostic. Nits can be differentiated from dandruff or lint by attempting to pick them off the hair shaft. Nits cannot be removed easily from the hair shaft. Often nits are difficult to see, especially on children with blond hair. A Wood's light examination may be helpful, since nits fluoresce under this light.

Pediculosis can be treated with lindane (Kwell), permethrin (Nix), or pyrethrin (Rid). Permethrin is the drug of choice because of its high pediculicidal and ovicidal activities, its low toxicity, and its extended pediculicide activity, which continues for 10 to 14 days.[1] With lindane, there has been some concern about possible CNS toxicity if the agent is overused or accidentally ingested.[10] With both lindane and pyrethrin, a second application is usually recommended in 1 to 2 weeks as protection against newly hatched lice.

Nursing evaluation and care. Pediculicide shampoo or cream rinse should be applied to the hair, left on for 10 minutes, and rinsed out. Following treatment the dead nits will still be firmly attached to the hair shaft. A rinse of a 1:1 mix of white vinegar and water, left on the hair for 1 hour, facilitates nit removal with a fine-tooth comb. Although these nits are dead, many schools require the child to be nit-free before returning to class.

All family members and school contacts should be examined for nits. Clothing and bed linens should be washed in hot water and dried on a hot setting. Nonwashable items (e.g., stuffed animals) should be placed in airtight plastic bags for 2 weeks. Brushes, combs, barrettes, and hats should be washed in hot soapy water. A thorough vacuuming of carpets and furniture is usually sufficient to remove loose nits. To prevent future infestation, children should be taught not to share personal articles such as brushes, combs, and hats. It is important for parents to know that pruritus may persist for several weeks after treatment. Topical hydrocortisone cream may be helpful in alleviating the itching.

▌ MISCELLANEOUS CUTANEOUS DISORDERS

ERYTHEMA MULTIFORME

Etiology. Erythema multiforme is an acute hypersensitivity syndrome resulting from infections (usually viral) or drug reactions. There are two categories of erythema multiforme: erythema multiforme minor, in which lesions primarily occur on the skin, and erythema multiforme major (Stevens-Johnson syndrome), which also includes prodromal fever and malaise and severe mucous membrane involvement. Infections such as herpes simplex, streptococci, and mononucleosis are the most common precipitants of erythema multiforme minor in children and adolescents. *Mycoplasma* infections and drugs such as sulfonamides, penicillins, barbiturates, and phenytoin commonly cause erythema multiforme major.[8]

Pathophysiology. Although erythema multiforme appears to result from an immune response to foreign antigen, the exact mechanism of action is unknown.

Clinical presentation. Erythema multiforme minor is characterized by a sudden onset of oval or round erythematous lesions that progress over several days to marginated wheals with central vesicles or papules (Table 18-5). Central clearing of the lesions creates the erythematous rings (iris or target lesions) that are characteristic of the disease.

Erythema multiforme major is a serious disease with systemic manifestations and involvement of organ systems in addition to the skin. After the prodromal period, involvement of at least two mucosal surfaces occurs. Balanitis (inflammation of the glans penis or the glans clitoris), conjunctivitis, and stomatitis are common. Erythema, swelling, and bullae

TABLE 18-5	Summary of Erythema Multiforme	
FACTOR	**ERYTHEMA MULTIFORME MINOR**	**ERYTHEMA MULTIFORME MAJOR**
Prodrome	If present, low-grade fever and malaise	Abrupt onset of 1-14 days of high fever, malaise, sore throat, headache, upper respiratory symptoms, vomiting, diarrhea, and/or arthralgias
Cutaneous lesions	Hallmark lesions: marginated wheals with central vesicles; erythematous rings with central clearing (iris or target lesions) Symmetric distribution of erythematous macules, papules, and urticarial lesions; found especially on palms, soles, backs of hands and feet, extensor surfaces of extremities	Confluent erythema, target lesions, blisters, and often exfoliation Widespread bullae
Mucous membrane involvement	Absent or limited to one surface (usually mouth)	Severe; at least two surfaces (mouth, eyes, nose, genitalia, or rectum) Extensive bullae with grayish-white membranes, hemorrhagic crusts; and superficial erosions and ulcerations
Course of illness	Relatively benign, self-limited; may be recurrent Skin lesions erupt over 1 wk; resolve over next 1-2 wk	More prolonged (lasts up to 6 wk) and severe
Complications	Rare	Renal failure; severe eye disease
Mortality rate	Low	5%-15%

formation may be seen on the conjunctivae, and those changes can lead to corneal ulceration and partial or permanent blindness. Shortly after mucosal involvement begins, an extensive erythematous papular rash and bullae develop on any cutaneous surface, including the palms and the soles (Fig. 18-18). The lesions can progress to epidermal necrosis, with significant loss of epidermal layers. Mucosal lesions frequently interfere with the child's ability to eat or drink, causing dehydration. The course of the illness is prolonged, often lasting 3 or 4 weeks.

Emergency Department interventions. Diagnosis of erythema multiforme depends on the clinical presentation. Identification and elimination of the cause of the disorder is critical. For example, a suspected medication should be discontinued immediately; or, if an infection is present, that condition should be treated. Erythema multiforme minor resolves spontaneously and requires only symptomatic treatment.

Children with erythema multiforme major usually require hospitalization for hydration and wound management. Areas of denuded skin are treated as burns, and admission to a burn unit may be indicated. An ophthalmologic consult is obtained for any child with eye involvement.

Nursing care and evaluation. Severe disease requires immediate intervention and often hospital-

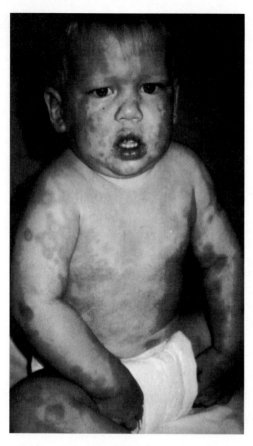

FIG. 18-18. Erythema multiforme. Diagnostic characteristics include target lesions, blistering of the mucous membranes, and a fixed eruption that does not clear with administration of epinephrine. (From Barkin RM: *Pediatric emergency medicine: concepts and clinical practice*, ed 2, St Louis, 1997, Mosby.)

ization. If the child is dehydrated, IV fluids may be necessary. Mouth sore discomfort may be relieved by half-strength hydrogen peroxide mouthwashes, a half-and-half mixture of Kaopectate or Maalox and diphenhydramine, or oral anesthetics.[8] The eyes should be cleansed frequently with warm water, and topical antibacterial ophthalmic agents should be applied to prevent infection. Mild disease requires symptomatic relief, including cool wet compresses, oatmeal baths, oral antihistamines, and oral anesthetics. The family and child will require emotional support as they cope with the serious nature of the disease. Anticipatory guidance is provided regarding the expected course of the illness and future avoidance of any causative medication.

URTICARIA (HIVES)

Etiology. Urticaria is a common benign cutaneous disorder. The cause of urticaria is not well understood, although it is thought to be a hypersensitivity reaction to a variety of agents, including foods, medications, infections, vaccines, insect bites, contact allergens, or psychogenic factors. Penicillins, cephalosporins, sulfonamides, phenytoin, and barbiturates are the most common medications that cause urticarial reactions. Causative foods include eggs, milk, peanuts, and seafood. The particular cause for an individual is frequently never identified.

Pathophysiology. Urticarial reactions are primarily caused by histamine release from the mast cells in response to antigens. Histamine and other inflammatory mediators cause vasodilation and increase vascular permeability, resulting in individual lesions.

Clinical presentation. Urticaria is characterized by transient pruritic, well-circumscribed erythematous wheals. Lesions often have blanched centers and vary in size from pinpoint papules to giant wheals (Fig. 18-19). Distribution may be localized or extensive and generalized over the entire body. Swelling (angioedema) of the distal extremities, eyelids, genitalia, and mucous membranes can occur. Individual lesions usually last for 1 to 2 hours but may persist for 24 hours. Lesions that last longer than this may indicate another skin disorder, such as erythema multiforme.

Emergency Department interventions. Diagnosis of urticaria is based on the clinical presentation. An attempt should be made to find the cause and to eliminate the causative agent. Subcutaneous epinephrine may provide short-term relief in patients with severe reactions. Long-term symptomatic treatment is achieved with oral antihistamines; the most effective agent seems to be of hydroxyzine. Topical steroids or topical antihistamines are not helpful.

Nursing evaluation and care. Parents should be reassured that urticaria resolves spontaneously; however, if a cause is not identified, resolution can take up to 1 month. Symptoms can be controlled with antihistamines, which should be tapered slowly, after the lesions disappear, to prevent recurrences. If the urticarial reaction occurred in response to nuts, seafood, or bee stings, the parents should be informed of the possibility of future anaphylactic reactions. An epinephrine administration kit should be given to the family with clear written instructions for its use. For

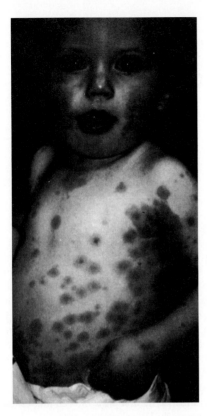

FIG. 18-19. Urticaria is the most common skin rash for which acute care is sought. (From Barkin RM: *Pediatric emergency medicine: concepts and clinical practice,* ed 2, St Louis, 1997, Mosby.)

children with severe reactions, follow-up by a pediatric primary care provider may be required, as well as a consultation with an allergist.

SUMMARY

The integument is a large and complex organ. Children are commonly affected by infectious or noninfectious skin disorders for which they are brought to the ED by concerned parents. Although many skin problems are nonacute, there are some conditions that require urgent, or even emergent, treatment. This chapter has addressed many of the common pediatric skin problems that are likely to be seen in the ED setting. Knowledge of these disorders enables the ED nurse to assess and care for children with skin problems, as well as to educate parents about home management.

REFERENCES

1. American Academy of Pediatrics, Committee on Infectious Diseases: *1994 Red book report of the Committee on Infectious Diseases,* ed. 23, Elk Grove, IL, 1994, AAP.
2. Bergstresser PR: Contact allergic dermatitis: old problems and new techniques, *Arch Dermatol* 125: 276-279, 1989.
3. Bialecki C, Feder H, Grant-Keis J: The six classic childhood exanthems: a review and update, *J Am Acad Dermatol* 21(5):891-903, 1989.
4. Cohen BA et al: Pediatric dermatology. In Zitelli BJ, Davis HW: *Atlas of pediatric physical diagnosis,* Philadelphia, 1992, JB Lippincott.
5. Dagan R: Impetigo in children: changing epidemiology and new treatments, *Pediatr Ann* 22(4):235-240, 1993.
6. Felter RA and Bower JR: Infectious disorders. In Barkin RM: *Pediatric emergency medicine: concepts and clinical practice,* ed 2, St Louis, 1997, Mosby, pp 926-971.
7. Hoekelman RH: The general pediatrician as dermatologist, *Pediatr Ann* 22(4):215-216, 1993.
8. Hurwitz S: *Clinical pediatric dermatology,* Philadelphia, 1993, WB Saunders.
9. Lane A, Render P, Helm K: Evaluation of diapers containing absorbent gelling materials with conventional disposable diapers in newborn infants, *Am J Dis Child* 144(3):315-318, 1990.
10. Rosekrans JA: Dermatologic disorders. In Barkin RM: *Pediatric emergency medicine: concepts and clinical practice,* ed 2, St Louis, 1997, Mosby, pp 672-708.
11. Weston WL: *Practical pediatric dermatology,* Boston, 1985, Little, Brown.
12. Wong DL: *Whaley and Wong's essentials of pediatric nursing,* ed. 5, St Louis, 1997, Mosby.

CHAPTER 19

Eye, Ear, Nose, and Throat Disorders

Janice S. Rogers

INTRODUCTION

Complaints related to the eyes, ears, nose, and throat (EENT) are common in pediatrics. Some are serious and may be life-threatening. Congenital, immunologic, anatomic, and mechanical problems can produce EENT conditions; however, infections and traumatic injuries are seen most commonly. The assessment of the EENT system and specific medical problems of the eye, ear, nose, and throat are outlined in this chapter.

EYE

ANATOMY AND PHYSIOLOGY

The eye is a sensory organ that performs the function of sight. Within the eye is a lens system that adjusts the amount of light that enters the eye by increasing or decreasing the size of the pupil and focuses the image on the retina (Fig. 19-1). The retina transforms the light impulses into electric impulses, which are transmitted to the optic cortex of the brain via the optic nerve (cranial nerve II).

External protection for the eyes is provided by the thin bony orbits, eyelids, eyelashes, cornea, conjunctiva, lacrimal glands, and blink reflex. Six extraocular muscles allow movement of the eye through the six cardinal directions of gaze. Cranial nerves III, IV, and VI, which are fully functional at birth, control extraocular movements. Because the oculomotor system is immature in the newborn and vision and fixation are poor, strabismus (ocular misalignment: inward—esotropia; or outward—exotropia) is common. Strabismus usually resolves by 4 to 5 months of age.[29]

The eyeball of the newborn is two thirds the size of the eye of the adult. The eyeball is less spherical than that of the adult, and the internal structures of the eye are not fully developed. The sclera is thin and translucent, the lens is more spherical, and the fundus is less pigmented. Because of the shape of the eyeball, visual acuity is estimated to be approximately 20/400 in the newborn.[4] The newborn can identify form, light, and motion. Soon after birth, the infant can fixate on an object. By 6 weeks, the infant uses coordinated movements to follow an object.[20] Response to large objects, particularly the mother's face, is one of the earliest visual responses of the infant. During the first year of life, particularly the first 4 months of life, visual acuity improves rapidly. Visual acuity continues to improve as the eye structures mature and the globe of the eye becomes more adultlike in shape.

ASSESSMENT

History. A focused history helps to determine the cause and severity of eye problems. Questions related to the onset of symptoms, signs and symptoms exhibited, exposure to toxins, or traumatic events will assist in determining the severity of the complaint. Eye complaints do not always indicate an ocular pathologic condition. For example, some neurologic disorders are accompanied by disorders of the eye or the surrounding structures (Box 19-1).

Physical examination. The physical examination provides a wealth of information about the integrity and the functioning of the eye and the neurologic system. The examination includes an assessment of both the external and the internal structures of the eye. Pathologic external findings include exophthalmos, or proptosis (forward protrusion of the eyes, which may be associated with a tumor or thyroid disease), enophthalmus (retraction of the globe, which may indicate

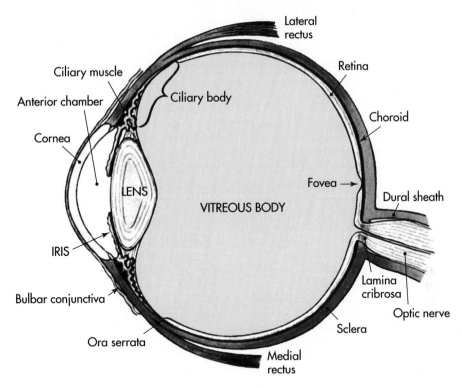

FIG. 19-1. Anatomy of the eye shown in horizontal section. (From Stein HA; Slatt BJ; Stein RM: *Ophthalmic terminology: speller and vocabulary builder,* ed 3, St Louis, 1992, Mosby.)

Box 19-1   Eye Examination: History and Physical Examination

History
- How long has the child had symptoms?
- What are the child's symptoms: redness, swelling, pain, discharge, excessive tearing, photophobia, eye rubbing?
- Has vision been affected?
- Is there a history of trauma or exposure to a toxic substance?
- Does the child have any known eye disorders or abnormalities: retinopathy, strabismus, amblyopia, nystagmus?
- Have the eye symptoms been associated with other problems: fever, sinusitis, ear infections, allergies?
- Have there been any neurologic manifestations: unsteady gait, difficulty walking, etc.?
- Is there any family history of eye problems?

Physical examination
- Observe the area surrounding the eye.
- Observe the size and symmetry of the eye, eyelid configurations, position, and function.
- Examine the conjunctiva and cornea with a flashlight.
- Assess pupil shape and size and response to light and dark.
- Assess extraocular movements by having child follow a light or a toy.
- Assist with the ophthalmoscopic examination of the internal structures of the eye.
- Assist with fluorescein and a Wood's light examination to detect abrasions or other lesions. Instill topical anesthesia before examination as ordered.

an orbital floor fracture or an anomaly), or redness of the conjunctiva and drainage (associated with conjunctivitis). Many visually or neurologically related disorders can be identified only by examining the internal structures of the eye with an ophthalmoscope. These disorders include retinal hemorrhage, cataracts, and papilledema.

Assessment of visual acuity should be attempted with all children who have eye disorders, although it is sometimes difficult to perform in the infant and young child. In infants the best indication of visual acuity is the ability to fixate and follow a small object such as a toy. Visual behavior during play or interactions with parents can also be observed. Abnormal visual behavior includes preferential staring at lights, excessive eye rubbing or poking, and photophobia. In the first year of life, nystagmus (a rhythmic oscillation of the eyes) usually indicates a loss of visual acuity.[25]

Objective testing of visual acuity may be feasible as early as 2 to 3 years of age. The Allen picture card examination, the Blackbird Preschool Vision Screening System, and the Denver Eye Screening Test can be used for the preschool population.[32,49] The Snellen symbol chart (E) can usually be successfully used in children older than 4 years, and the Snellen letter chart can be used with children older than 5 to 6 years who know their numbers and letters.[32,33] Children with eyeglasses should wear them for testing. Adult visual acuity is not achieved until approximately 6 years of age.[42] Normal visual acuity at age 3 years is 20/40; at 4 years, 20/30; and at 5-6 years is 20/20.[32]

COMMON EYE DISORDERS

Conjunctivitis

Etiology. Conjunctivitis is an inflammatory disorder of the eye caused by a variety of etiologic agents, including bacteria, viruses, environmental allergens, and chemicals. Conjunctivitis in the neonate is called ophthalmia neonatorum. In the first few days of life it usually results from the chemical irritation of postnatal eye prophylaxis or from maternal sexually transmitted diseases (STDs), which are acquired as the infant passes through the birth canal. In the past *Neisseria gonorrhoeae* was a significant cause of ophthalmia neonatorum, contributing to permanent visual disturbances and blindness. With the advent of prophylaxis, the incidence of *N. gonorrhoeae* has decreased dramatically. The most common STD now responsible for ophthalmia neonatorum is *Chlamydia* infection.

Bacterial organisms are responsible for a large number of cases in children beyond the neonatal period.[32,48] The infection may develop as a primary problem or as a superinfection in an eye that is inflamed from other causes. Pathogens include *Streptococcus pneumoniae, Haemophilus influenzae, Staphylococcus aureus,* and *Neisseria gonorrhoeae* (in sexually active adolescents or sexually abused children).

Viral conjunctivitis, especially adenovirus, is more common in older children. Allergic conjunctivitis occurs seasonally or in response to various environmental allergens. Conjunctivitis is also associated with systemic diseases, such as measles, varicella, Rocky Mountain spotted fever, and Kawasaki disease (Box 19-2).

Pathophysiology. The conjunctiva is a thin mucous membrane that lines the posterior surface of the eyelids and the eyeball (excluding the cornea). Conjunctivitis is an inflammatory disorder that causes vasodilation, migration of inflammatory cells to the affected eye, pain, and tearing.

Complications of conjunctivitis, especially gonococcal or herpetic, are severe if the cornea is infected. Corneal scarring, perforation, or necrosis may lead to

---

Box 19-2   Common Causes of Conjunctivitis in the Neonate or Child

Neonate
Chemical (silver nitrate or other eye prophylaxis)
Gonococcal *(Neisseria gonorrhoeae)*
Chlamydia *(Chlamydia trachomatis)*
Herpes simplex virus

Child
Viral causes
  Adenovirus
  Enterovirus
  Herpes simplex virus
Bacterial causes
  Haemophilus influenzae
  Staphylococcus pneumoniae
  Staphylococcus aureus
  Neisseria gonorrhoeae
Allergens
Toxins/chemicals
Systemic infections (e.g., measles, rubella, varicella, Rocky Mountain spotted fever)

permanent blindness or loss of the eye itself. Because of this risk, conjunctivitis in the neonate is considered a medical emergency. Rare complications of bacterial conjunctivitis include septicemia or meningitis.

Clinical presentation. The clinical presentation of conjunctivitis varies depending on the etiologic agent; however, the typical presentation includes a history of a "red eye," usually associated with tearing, chemosis (conjunctival edema), itching, and discharge. Pain, photophobia, and vision loss do not occur in conjunctivitis unless there is also a corneal or intraocular infection.[25]

In general, early bilateral involvement, purulent discharge, and an associated otitis media are typical of a bacterial cause. Viral conjunctivitis usually appears with a watery discharge and preauricular adenopathy, but it may resemble bacterial conjunctivitis. Allergic conjunctivitis is associated with itchy, watery eyes and injected conjunctiva. Rhinitis may or may not be present.

Emergency Department interventions. The goals of conjunctivitis therapy are to control the symptoms, to eradicate the infectious agent, and prevent complications. In the child the management of *viral conjunctivitis* is primarily supportive. Although topical antibiotics may be used to prevent bacterial superinfection, the efficacy of this practice has not been proven.[32,33] Most types of *bacterial conjunctivitis* are self-limiting. However, topical antibiotic therapy eliminates the bacteria more quickly and shortens the illness and the period of contagion.[18,32] Topical steroids are not routinely used in the child with conjunctivitis because they may induce glaucoma and worsen herpes simplex keratitis when present.[25]

Since neonates are susceptible to the damaging forms of conjunctivitis, they are treated aggressively. A Gram stain and bacterial and *Chlamydia* cultures are performed on all neonates with conjunctivitis. If herpes simplex virus is suspected, viral cultures are also done. When gonococcal or herpes conjunctivitis is suspected by history, physical examination, or Gram stain, the neonate is admitted for parenteral antibiotic or antiviral therapy. If chlamydia is suspected, the infant may be managed on an outpatient basis with both topical and systemic antibiotics.[32]

Nursing care and evaluation. To determine the seriousness of the presenting complaint, an evaluation of the onset of symptoms, known exposures, type of discharge, presence of pain or vision loss, history of trauma, and signs of systemic illness is required. Signs and symptoms of an associated illness such as an upper respiratory infection (URI), otitis media, or pharyngitis may offer clues to the cause and thus help to determine the urgency with which the child should be seen.

Nursing interventions for the child with conjunctivitis include the application of cool compresses to relieve discomfort and to moisten dried eye drainage. If a large amount of eye drainage is present, the eyes can be cleansed with warm water and cotton balls or through saline irrigation. When eye medications are ordered, these measures improve their efficacy. When the child is discharged, the parents are instructed to continue cleaning the eyes at home. Additional discharge instructions include the proper administration of eye medications. In younger children the child is held firmly (to prevent injury) while the drops or ointment is placed in the eye(s). Eye drops are applied every 2 to 4 hours by gently pulling the lower eyelid down and placing drops inside the lower lid. The uncooperative child is placed supine, and the drops are instilled in the inner corner of the eye. Eye ointments are administered 4 times a day by placing a ribbon of ointment inside the lower lid. If the child's eyes cannot be opened, a ribbon of ointment is placed on the lid margins, where it will "melt" into the eye. Parents are instructed to continue administering the eye medication until the eye is clear of drainage for 48 hours.

Conjunctivitis is easily transmitted to others by hands or fomites. Schools and day care facilities are particularly concerned about the contagiousness of conjunctivitis, and they often require the child to stay at home until the infection is resolved or well treated. Parents and children are instructed to use good handwashing technique. Towels and washcloths should not be shared.

Periorbital and orbital cellulitis

Etiology. *Periorbital cellulitis* is an infection of the superficial tissues that surround the eye. *Orbital cellulitis* is an infection of the orbit of the eye. The most common infectious agents that cause periorbital or orbital cellulitis include *Haemophilus influenzae, Streptococcus pneumoniae, Streptococcus pyogenes, Staphylococcus aureus,* and *Moraxella* (formerly *Branhamella) catarrhalis.*[11,32] Occasionally anaerobic bacteria and group A streptococcus are involved.

The peak incidence of periorbital cellulitis occurs between 2 and 4 years of age. The more serious orbital cellulitis affects older children and adolescents more commonly than younger children (Table 19-1).

Pathophysiology. In periorbital cellulitis, bacteria invade the periorbital tissues, resulting in the accumulation of inflammatory cells and fluid. The infection does not extend into the orbit. Orbital cellulitis usually results secondary to a sinus infection as sinus pressure obstructs venous and lymphatic drainage from the periorbital area, resulting in edema. Bacteria enter the orbit either directly—across the paper-thin bone that separates the ethmoid sinuses from the orbit—or through the venous system. The subsequent inflammatory response further increases the swelling and pressure in the orbit.

Serious complications can result from periorbital cellulitis,[12] but they are far more likely with orbital cellulitis. Unless treated promptly, these infections can cause abscess formation, can damage vision permanently or can lead to life-threatening conditions such as meningitis or septicemia.

Clinical presentation. Children with periorbital or orbital cellulitis often have a preceding history of an upper respiratory infection (URI), sinusitis, localized trauma, or eye surgery. Symptoms develop rapidly. They include unilateral eyelid swelling, erythema, tenderness, and warmth. Depending on the severity of the infection, the child may be febrile and/or ill appearing. If periorbital swelling with proptosis, restricted eye movements, or decreased visual acuity is present, orbital involvement has occurred.

Emergency Department interventions. The diagnosis of periorbital and orbital cellulitis is clinical. Diagnostic tests may be ordered to determine the extent of the condition and the presence of complications. Blood work may include a complete blood count (CBC) with differential and blood culture; however, blood cultures are usually negative in the non-toxic appearing child with periorbital cellulitis.[12] Topical cultures of the eye are not useful.

In the young child or neonate, and depending on the child's symptoms, a lumbar puncture may be required to rule out meningitis. A computed tomography (CT) scan is performed in children (1) with eyelid swelling and tenderness who cannot be adequately examined to rule out orbital involvement; or (2) with suspected orbital cellulitis to rule out intracranial complications or sinus involvement.[15,32]

Treatment usually consists of hospitalization and administration of parenteral antibiotics. Mild cases of

TABLE 19-1	Periorbital and Orbital Cellulitis		
	COMMON AGE GROUP	**PREDISPOSING FACTORS**	**SYMPTOMS**
Periorbital	<6 yr	Skin or eyelid infections Insect bites Trauma Upper respiratory infection, otitis, or pharyngitis Ethmoid sinusitis Nasolacrimal obstruction Herpes, adenovirus, varicella	Acute unilateral eyelid swelling, erythema, tenderness, warmth May be febrile May be conjunctival redness and swelling with or without purulent discharge
Orbital	Older children and adolescents	Sinusitis Trauma Intraorbital surgery	Acute unilateral eyelid swelling; red or purple eyelid Proptosis, decreased eye movements, pain, decreased visual acuity Fever and systemic illness common May be conjunctival redness and swelling

Compiled from Fisher MC: Conjunctivitis in children, *Pediatr Clin North Am* 34(6):1447, 1987; Maller JS: Eye disorders. In Barkin RM: *Pediatric emergency medicine: concepts and clinical practice,* ed 2, St Louis, 1997, Mosby.

periorbital cellulitis may be managed on an outpatient basis with close follow-up. The selection of antibiotic(s) depends on the age of the child and the predisposing conditions. Antibiotics commonly used for mild periorbital cellulitis include intramuscular ceftriaxone and/or an oral cephalosporin with good staphylococcal coverage, such as cephalexin. Ceftriaxone is usually given to children younger than 5 years to cover for *Haemophilus influenzae*, although this organism is decreasing in prevalence because of Hib vaccine. A penicillinase-resistant antistaphylococcal antibiotic such as nafcillin is recommended for all children with moderate to severe periorbital cellulitis and orbital cellulitis. Parenteral antibiotics for periorbital cellulitis are usually continued for approximately 3 to 5 days or until signs and symptoms resolve. Parenteral therapy for orbital cellulitis is more prolonged, often lasting up to 2 to 3 weeks.

Nursing care and evaluation. The child with periorbital or orbital cellulitis who does not appear seriously ill is treated urgently. Emergent treatment is indicated, however, if signs and symptoms of septic shock are present, if the child "looks ill" (signs of toxicity), or if the child has decreased vision or restricted eye movement.

Most children with periorbital or orbital cellulitis require an intravenous (IV) line for parenteral antibiotics. Depending on the presenting signs and symptoms, blood work, including a CBC with differential, and a blood culture may be ordered. Because of the risk of systemic spread of infection, circulatory and neurologic status are continuously monitored for signs of shock or meningitis.

If the child with mild periorbital cellulitis is discharged, the importance of compliance with antibiotic therapy and follow-up is emphasized. Clear instructions about potential signs and symptoms of deterioration, such as increasing redness and swelling, fever, or neurologic deterioration are given to the parents.

▌EAR

ANATOMY AND PHYSIOLOGY

The ear is a complex sensory organ that performs the functions of hearing, the localization and interpretation of sounds, and the maintenance of equilibrium. The ear consists of three compartments: external, middle, and inner ear. Normally, the eustachian tubes equilibrate the pressure between the middle ear and the atmosphere, protect the middle ear from nasopharyngeal secretions and sound pressures, and clear middle ear and inner ear secretions and debris into the nasopharynx. In the infant and young child the eustachian tubes are about half the length of those of the adult and fairly horizontal. Because of this difference, secretions cannot efficiently drain from the middle ear, and nasopharyngeal secretions and organisms have easier access to the middle ear. By the age of 6 years the eustachian tubes are longer and angle downward, improving their efficiency and decreasing the likelihood of middle ear infections[27] (Fig. 19-2).

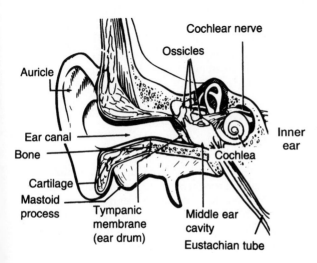

FIG. 19-2. Ear canal, middle ear, and inner ear. (From Rudy EB, Gray VR: *Handbook of health assessment,* ed 2, Norwalk, Conn, 1986, Appleton & Lange.)

The neonate's tympanic membrane is difficult to visualize with an otoscope for two reasons. First, the tympanic membrane approximates adult size at birth, but it is almost horizontal.[27] As the external auditory canal develops, the tympanic membrane becomes more vertical and therefore more easily visualized. Second, the neonate's external auditory canal is primarily cartilaginous and collapsed. Ossification of the medial two thirds of the external auditory canal is completed by age 2 years, and adult size is attained by age 9 years.[27] The lateral third of the mature ear canal remains cartilaginous throughout adulthood. Ceruminous glands, located in the cartilaginous section, secrete wax, which traps debris and thus protects the middle ear and inner ear from infection.

ASSESSMENT

History. Children may come to the emergency department (ED) with specific ear-related chief complaints or associated symptoms, such as fever, decreased appetite, or waking during the night. The history will assist in identifying the presence of an ear problem and the underlying cause. Specific information to obtain about ear complaints includes a description of present signs and symptoms, such as otalgia (ear pain), otorrhea (ear drainage), hearing loss, swelling around the ear, vertigo, tinnitus, or facial paralysis. The history may reveal frequent episodes of otitis media, tympanostomy tube insertion, or congenital malformations of the ear or the nasopharynx.

Physical examination. Nursing assessment of the child with an ear-related complaint includes an examination of the external ear, assessment of the infant/child's ability to hear, and observation of the child for associated physical findings such as eye drainage or a runny nose. During examination of the external ear, the ear canal, pinna, and the surrounding area are evaluated for evidence of trauma, inflammation, pain on movement, or drainage from the ear. An assessment of hearing in the infant may be performed by ringing a bell or snapping the fingers on either side of the infant's head and observing the infant's reaction. In an older child whispering behind the child and asking the child to repeat the words will assess gross hearing.

The tympanic membrane is assessed by pneumatic otoscopic examination. This examination is usually performed by the ED physician or nurse practitioner (NP). The ED nurse may be asked to assist with

---

Box 19-3   Procedure for Irrigating the Ear Canal

- Restrain the child as necessary.
- Place a basin and towels below the child's ear.
- Fill a 30 to 60 ml syringe with tepid water or a tepid half-strength hydrogen peroxide solution.
- Attach the syringe to tubing from a butterfly needle—where the needle has been removed about 3 cm from the hub—or to an IV catheter sheath (with the needle removed).
- If multiple irrigations are required, a dental irrigator may be used or a three-way stopcock between the syringe and the tubing can be attached to IV tubing that has been placed in a large basin of tepid water. The stopcock can then be adjusted to draw up water into the syringe, to irrigate the ear canal, and then to draw up more water—without removal of the syringe.
- Straighten the ear canal, directing a firm, but gentle stream of water against the ear canal. As fluid drains into the basin, check for wax fragments or foreign bodies.
- Repeat the procedure as necessary.

---

restraining the child or with removal of cerumen, which may impair visualization of the tympanic membrane. Cerumen can be removed with a curette (done by the physician/NP) or by irrigation or suction. Eardrops may be used to loosen the wax. The normal tympanic membrane is gray, translucent, and mobile; its bony landmarks are distinct. The light reflex, although readily visible, is not relied on to assess the tympanic membrane and middle ear function[7,35] (Box 19-3 and Fig. 19-3).

COMMON EAR DISORDERS

Otitis externa

Etiology. Otitis externa, an inflammation of the external auditory canal, is a frequent cause of ear pain in older children and adolescents. It is commonly called "swimmer's ear" because it usually occurs when the ear canal is repeatedly exposed to water. Other predisposing factors include trauma to the ear

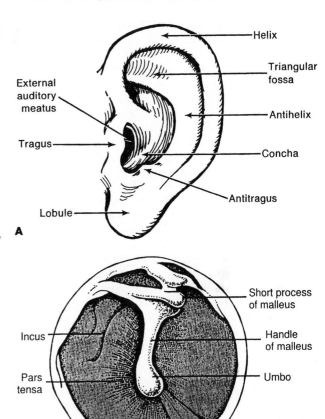

FIG. 19-3. Usual landmarks of the pinna (**A**) and tympanic membrane (**B**). (**A,** From Wong DL: *Whaley and Wong's nursing care of infants and children,* ed 5, St Louis, 1995, Mosby. **B,** From Potter PA: *Pocket guide to health assessment,* ed 3, St Louis, 1994, Mosby.)

canal by vigorous cleaning with bobby pins or other implements and the insertion of foreign bodies (Box 19-4).

A variety of pathogens cause otitis externa, however, one half to two thirds of cases are caused by *Pseudomonas aeruginosa* organisms.[5] Other etiologic organisms include *Staphylococcus aureus, Streptococcus pyogenes,* and diphtheroids. Fungal infections can cause an acute otitis externa (otomycosis); however, they occur more commonly in patients who are immunosuppressed or have uncontrolled hyperglycemia.

Pathophysiology. Repeated wetting of the ear canal alters the protective wax, and the normally bacteriostatic acidic pH becomes more alkaline. The skin in the ear canal becomes macerated, and bacteria multiply and flourish in the warm, moist environment. As the infection progresses, the ear canal fills with wet debris, which further alters the protective mechanisms

Box 19-4 Causes of Otitis Externa

- Moisture retention caused by:
  Tortuous, narrow ear canal
  Obstructive cerumen
  Foreign body
  Swimming, bathing
- Loss of acidic environment
  Decreased production of cerumen
  Increased removal of cerumen
  Alkaline exposure (soaps, bacterial degradation by-products)
- Trauma
- Dermatitis

Modified from Santamaria JP, Abrunzo TJ: Ear, nose, and throat. In Barkin RM, ed: *Pediatric emergency medicine: concepts and clinical practice,* ed 2, St Louis, 1997, Mosby, p 739.

and promotes bacterial growth. Otitis externa generally remains localized.

Clinical presentation. Otitis externa usually begins with an itchy ear canal and is followed by pain that becomes progressively worse. The classic presentation is a painful inflamed ear canal that is filled with exudate. The pain is acutely exacerbated by pressing on the tragus, pulling on the pinna, or even chewing. Discharge from the ear canal may be foul- or sour-smelling. Hearing may be muffled.

Emergency Department interventions. The diagnosis of otitis externa is based on the clinical findings. Ear cultures are occasionally performed when previous treatment has been ineffective. When systemic symptoms such as fever are present, complications (e.g., perforation) or other diagnoses (e.g., otitis media, foreign body) are considered.

Treatment consists of cleansing the ear to remove exudate and wax. This cleansing is performed to improve visualization of the ear canal and the tympanic membrane and to increase the efficacy of topical medications. Gentle suctioning of the ear canal or wiping with small cotton pledgets may be done. Irrigation with various solutions, especially alcohol or acidic solutions, is painful and therefore is avoided. Ceruminolytics are not used.

After cleansing of the ear, topical medications are instilled into the ear canal. Acetic acid otic solution is used unless edema is present, in which case acetic acid solution with hydrocortisone is prescribed. Severe infections, particularly those associated with ear discharge, also require the application of a topical antibiotic such as polymyxin B sulfate and neomycin sulfate.[39] If the tympanic membrane cannot be visualized, an otic suspension (rather than solution) is prescribed and follow-ups arranged to check the tympanic membrane once the swelling has subsided. When otitis media, lymphadenopathy, or fever is present, oral antibiotics are prescribed. Analgesics may be required to control pain.

Nursing care and evaluation. Discharge instructions include teaching caregivers how to instill otic medications (Box 19-5). No swimming is allowed until the ear has improved. Additionally, parents are instructed to protect the child's ear canal from water with ear plugs for 2 to 4 weeks. Commercial silicone ear plugs are suggested for children.

Preventive measures include thoroughly drying the ears after swimming or bathing by tilting the head to the side, fanning the ears, or using a hair dryer. The use

---

Box 19-5   Instillation of Otic Medication Drops

- Tip the child's head to the side.
- Instill enough drops to fill the otic canal—about 4 to 6 drops for adolescents; fewer for younger children.
- Keep the head to the side for several minutes to prevent the medication from draining out. Cotton may be inserted in the ear.
- A Merocel wick may be used if the ear canal is swollen. With the wick, medication enters the ear canal by capillary action. The wick should be kept moist with eardrops and removed in 24 to 48 hours.

---

of cotton swabs should be avoided. Topical agents that promote drying and acidification of the ear canals, such as aluminum acetate, isopropyl alcohol, and white vinegar can also be used.

Acute otitis media

Etiology. Acute otitis media (AOM) is any inflammation of the middle ear that has a rapid onset and lasts less than 3 weeks.[6,26] It occurs more frequently during the winter months, probably because of its association with URIs, and it is most prevalent in children younger than 3 years of age.[10,21]

AOM is usually caused by bacteria or viruses. The most common bacterial causes are *Streptococcus pneumoniae* and *Haemophilus influenzae,* which account for more than half of the cases of AOM.[26] Other causes include group B *Streptococcus, Staphylococcus aureus, Moraxella catarrhalis,* and—in infants less than 6 months of age—*Chlamydia trachomatis* organisms. Although the role of viruses in otitis media is unclear, respiratory syncytial virus, rhinovirus, adenovirus, and influenza A have been cultured from middle ear fluid.[37,38]

AOM is one of the most common conditions diagnosed in the ED, especially in febrile children. One large study showed that more than 60% of children had at least one episode of AOM by 1 year of age and 80% by age 3 years. More than 40% of the children had more than three episodes of AOM.[45]

Pathophysiology. Infants and children have short and horizontal eustachian tubes. Therefore the middle ear drains poorly and is susceptible to fluid collection. This fluid provides a medium for bacterial growth. Children at highest risk for the development of AOM are those with anatomic abnormalities such as cleft palate or those with congestion caused by conditions such as URI or allergic rhinitis.

As bacteria from the nasopharynx enters the middle ear, fluid continues to accumulate. The tympanic membrane bulges, causing pain, and the continued accumulation of fluid restricts free movement of the ossicles, causing fluctuating hearing loss. Rupture of the tympanic membrane, with subsequent drainage of middle ear fluid, usually relieves the child's pain.

Complications of acute otitis media including mastoiditis, abscess formation, and meningitis, are rare because of early recognition and treatment with antibiotics. Other sequelae are more prevalent, such as persistent or recurrent AOM or the relatively asymptomatic but chronic otitis media with effusion. When the tympanic membrane perforates, it usually heals spontaneously and without permanent damage.

Clinical presentation. AOM typically develops within the first 7 days following the onset of a URI. However, AOM may also occur in an otherwise well child. The onset is usually acute, with complaints of fever, ear pain, hearing loss, purulent ear discharge, rhinitis, cough, irritability, poor feeding, and sleep disturbances. Pulling at the ears has not been shown to be a reliable sign of otitis.[3] Because the symptoms of otitis are often subtle or nonspecific, parents may not suspect that the child has an ear infection.

Emergency Department interventions. Clinical diagnosis of AOM is based on the appearance and mobility of the tympanic membrane. The tympanic membrane in AOM is usually erythematous, devoid of bony landmarks, full or bulging, and less mobile than normal. However, all these signs do not need to be present. The most reliable indicator of the presence of otitis media is decreased mobility of the tympanic membrane in response to positive and negative pressure.[41] Tympanometry is a helpful objective adjunct to confirm tympanic membrane mobility and measure middle ear pressure. Even with these findings, however, consideration should be given to the presence of other coexisting illnesses when a child has signs of toxicity or appears seriously ill.

The treatment for acute otitis media consists of the use of an analgesic/antipyretic to treat the pain and fever and antibiotic therapy to treat the infection. Decongestants, antihistamines, and topical or oral adrenocorticosteroids have not been shown to be effective in the treatment of AOM.[6,7,39]

Oral antibiotic therapy is prescribed once the diagnosis is confirmed. Overdiagnosing AOM, particularly based on ear pain alone, can mask or only partially treat a serious underlying infection or promote the development of resistant bacteria. Amoxicillin is the most commonly recommended initial therapy. Broader-spectrum antibiotics are recommended for AOM that fails to respond to initial treatment.

If noncompliance with the dosing regimen is suspected to be a problem, a single dose of intramuscular ceftriaxone can be given. This approach has been shown to be as effective as a full course of amoxicillin.[19] Other treatment approaches, such as a shortened course of antibiotics (e.g., 3 to 5 days) or no antibiotics at all have been suggested.[13,34,40]

Nursing care and evaluation. Initial nursing care of the child with AOM includes an evaluation of the child's overall status. If the child is febrile, antipyretics are administered. If the child appears ill, further evaluation is required to determine whether a serious coexisting condition (e.g., meningitis) is present.

Most children with AOM require only supportive nursing care. At the time of discharge, instructions given to the parents include information about medication administration, side effects of the medications (e.g., diarrhea), fever and pain control, follow-up, when to call the physician, and prevention. Antibiotic administration for the whole course of therapy is stressed, even if the child begins feeling better. With the initiation of antibiotic therapy, the child's condition should begin to improve within 48 to 72 hours. If the child is not acting better in 3 days or seems worse despite the antibiotics, the parents should notify the child's pediatrician.

Although ear infections cannot be prevented completely, there are certain practices that can reduce their occurrence. Holding an infant upright during feedings and encouraging gentle nose blowing in older children deters bacteria from traveling up the eustachian tubes to the middle ear. Pinching the nose, closing the mouth, and forcing air up the eustachian tubes helps aerate the middle ear. Eliminating tobacco smoke or other irritants from the household also reduces the tendency toward nasal congestion and resulting obstruction of middle ear drainage.

FOREIGN BODIES IN EARS AND NOSE

Etiology. Foreign bodies in the ears and nose are most common in children younger than 6 years of age who self-insert small toys, button-type batteries, food, plants, or any other object that will fit into the orifice. In older children and adolescents foreign bodies are most commonly inserted inadvertently (e.g., by using a cotton-tipped applicator to remove ear wax). Another common foreign body in this age group is insects.

Pathophysiology. Once an object is inserted into the ear or nose of a young child, it tends to be retained because of the anatomic shape of the orifices. The object becomes trapped in the immature ear canal after passing the initial constriction. In the nose, the foreign body is often trapped by the turbinates.

Initial insertion of a foreign body may traumatize the tissue and cause bleeding. Depending on the size, position, movement, and antigenicity of the object, irritation continues to develop. Eventually the mucosa erodes and infection develops. Button-type batteries are particularly troublesome, since leakage of the battery contents can burn the mucosa.

Clinical presentation. Children may arrive at the ED shortly after the foreign body is inserted or later—after signs and symptoms of infection have developed. Many nasal or otic foreign bodies are not immediately discovered in young children because the incident is not reported. Sometimes foreign bodies are incidentally discovered in asymptomatic children during procedures for other health problems. The symptomatology depends on the age of the child, the type of object, and the length of time the object has been in the ear or nose. Usually the child has unilateral findings.

Otic foreign bodies. Foreign bodies in the ear can cause an alteration in hearing, foul-smelling bloody or purulent discharge, or lymphadenopathy. Ear pain is often the chief complaint. Almost half of all children with foreign bodies retained in the ear, have a concomitant otitis externa.[2]

Nasal foreign bodies. Common signs and symptoms of retained nasal foreign bodies include unilateral foul-smelling purulent discharge, pain, recurrent epistaxis, fever, alteration in olfaction, lymphadenopathy, facial swelling, and sneezing. Older children may complain of nasal plugging. A sinusitis or conjunctivitis may also be present.

Emergency Department interventions. Diagnosis depends on confirmation of the presence of a foreign body, ideally by visualizing the object. If visualization is obscured by swelling and discharge associated with an infection or by the anatomic location of the object, diagnostic x-ray films may be helpful if the object is radiopaque.

Ear. During removal of an otic foreign body, care is taken to prevent further insertion of the foreign body and to prevent perforation of the tympanic membrane by the instruments. Forceps, ear curettes, or wire loops are used to grasp or pull objects out of the ear canal. Objects that are difficult to grasp, such as hard, round, or plastic objects, may be removed by using constant wall suction. Irrigation is often successful in removing small objects that are close to the tympanic membrane. Vegetable matter is not removed by water irrigation because potential swelling of the object can increase the obstruction. In such cases isopropyl alcohol and water may be used for irrigation.[16] On discharge, and if any signs of otitis externa are present or if the ear canal was traumatized during removal of the foreign body, Cortisporin eardrops are prescribed.

Nose. The first attempt at removal of a nasal foreign body is most likely to be successful. During removal care is taken to prevent further insertion of the foreign body into the nasopharynx, which could potentially obstruct the airway or the esophagus. If the child is uncooperative or the size and shape of the object is such that it may cause an obstruction, conscious sedation or even general anesthesia should be considered. Suctioning or a variety of instruments, including curettes, wire loops, and forceps, can be used to remove nasal foreign bodies. One noninvasive method involves the child forcibly exhaling through the affected nostril while in a sitting position and manually occluding the nonaffected nostril. Following successful removal of a nasal foreign body, secondary infections are treated with antibiotics.

Live insects. The removal of a live insect poses a special problem. The insect must first be incapacitated to facilitate removal and to decrease trauma to the ear canal or the nose. In the ear, alcohol or mineral oil can be instilled, or 2% lidocaine can be instilled, to paralyze the insect. Insects or larvae in the nose are anesthetized with benzol, ether, or chloroform before removal with forceps or noseblowing.

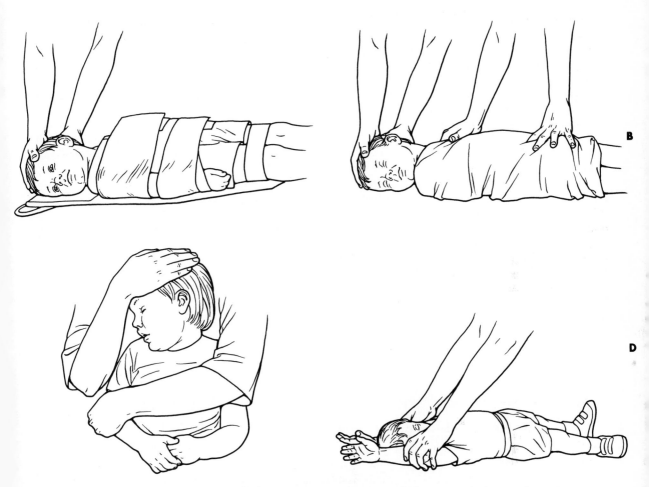

FIG. 19-4. Restraining the child for an EENT examination or removal of a foreign body. **A,** Board restraint. **B,** Sheet restraint. **C,** Child restrained while sitting in caregiver's lap. The child's legs are between the caregiver's legs. **D,** Child restrained while lying supine on the examining table. The child's arms are held above the head. (From Barkin RM: *Pediatric emergency medicine: concepts and clinical practice,* ed 2, St Louis, 1997, Mosby.)

Nursing care and evaluation. Although nasal or otic foreign bodies rarely create a medical emergency, there is always a potential for airway obstruction to occur if a nasal foreign body is aspirated either spontaneously or during removal. The ED nurse must therefore observe the child for alterations in airway patency and breathing during the procedure and must be prepared to handle the obstruction as necessary.

Before the removal of an object, an age-appropriate description is given to the child. While assisting with the procedure, the nurse can speak quietly to the child to keep him or her comfortable and calm. Since young children often protest vigorously during removal of the object, appropriate restraint is necessary (Fig. 19-4).

Discharge teaching should emphasize prevention of subsequent foreign body insertions, as well as follow-up care for the child. Potential signs of infection, such as a fever, cough, or ear pain, are explained to the parents, as well as specific information about when to call the physician regarding complications.

NOSE AND SINUSES

ANATOMY AND PHYSIOLOGY

The nose is a sensory organ that identifies odors. In addition to smell, the nose and the nasopharynx filter inspired particulate matter and humidify and warm inspired air. Immunoglobulins secreted within the nose begin to neutralize infectious organisms.

With inspiration, air enters the nares and passes through the two anterior chambers (vestibules) to the posterior openings (choanae), which lead to the nasopharynx. Several important structures within the nasal cavity are the septum, the cribriform plate, and the turbinates (or concha). The septum is membranous tissue that separates the two vestibules. The cribriform plate is located on the roof of the nose and houses the sensory endings of the olfactory nerve. The inferior, medial, and superior turbinates are plates of bone covered by a vascular mucous membrane. The turbinates greatly increase the surface area within the nasal cavity, facilitating humidification and warming of inspired air. The spaces between the turbinates make up the meatus, and both the nasolacrimal ducts and the paranasal sinuses drain into the meatus. There are four pairs of paranasal sinuses: maxillary, frontal, ethmoid, and sphenoid. These sinuses are air-filled structures in the bone that drain into the nasal passages. Any nasal obstruction that blocks drainage can decrease aeration of the sinuses, thus promoting infection. In children, sinus development varies. At birth the ethmoid and maxillary sinuses are present, but the sphenoid sinuses do not develop until between 3 and 7 years of age. The frontal sinuses do not begin to develop until approximately 7 to 12 years of age.[17] Full sinus development is not complete until adolescence (Fig. 19-5).

ASSESSMENT

History. Assessment of the child with a nasal or sinus-related complaint includes questions about past or recent trauma, suspected or known foreign bodies, prior nasal disease, surgical interventions, allergies, and breathing habits during sleep. Common symptoms associated with nasal or sinus disorders

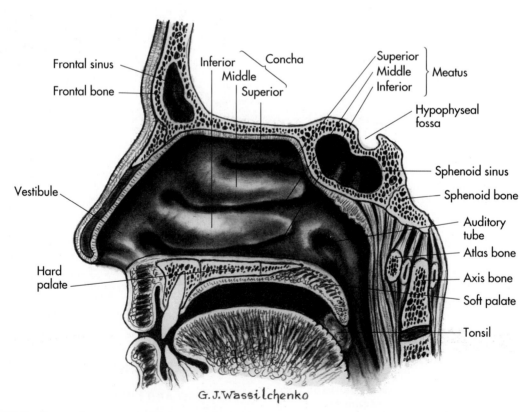

FIG. 19-5. Anatomic structures of the nose and nasopharynx. (From Seidel et al: *Mosby's guide to physical examination,* ed 3, St Louis, 1995, Mosby.)

include pain, stuffy nose, nasal discharge, and decreased ability to smell.

Physical examination. The physical examination includes inspection of the external nose for visible deformities or obstruction to airflow. Internal examination evaluates the nasal septum for position, discoloration, and bleeding; the color of the nasal mucosa; and the size and shape of the nasal turbinates. The type and location of nasal discharge often provides helpful information concerning the cause of the child's presenting complaint. For example, discharge from the middle turbinate area is consistent with infection of the anterior nasal sinuses. Sinus evaluation largely relies on palpation and gentle tapping of the supraorbital and maxillary regions to detect areas of tenderness.

COMMON NOSE AND SINUS DISORDERS

Epistaxis (nosebleeds)

Etiology. The highest incidence of epistaxis in the pediatric population occurs between the ages of 2 and 10 years.[11] Most episodes are the result of trauma, especially nose-picking. Nasal foreign bodies, URIs, or repetitive and forceful nose blowing can also traumatize the nasal passages. The majority of nosebleeds occur in the winter months, most likely resulting from breathing dry air. Other conditions that predispose the child to nosebleeds include a deviated nasal septum, infectious and allergic rhinitis, hypertension, and bleeding disorders.

Pathophysiology. Trauma to the nasal passages triggers an inflammatory response and subsequent excoriation of the nasal mucosa. The granulation tissue that forms over the injured tissues may become dislodged, especially by a child's finger or frequent forceful nose blowing, and cause bleeding. Most nosebleeds in children occur in the anterior portion of the nasal septum, which contains a rich arterial and venous network. Nosebleeds in children rarely occur posteriorly. Significant nasal trauma may result in the formation of a septal hematoma, in which the septal vessels bleed and the overlying mucous membrane stays intact. If the hematoma is untreated, a septal abscess or perforation may result.

Clinical presentation. The child with epistaxis is usually brought to the ED by an anxious caregiver who overestimates the amount and duration of the nosebleed. Severe bleeding is rare. Although bleeding from both nares is common, there is usually one side on which the bleeding started, which is suggestive of the initial bleeding point. If dizziness, pallor, or behavior changes are observed, the child may be hypovolemic.

The history may reveal recent trauma, URI, allergies, the known or suspected insertion of a foreign body, or exposure to dry air. If the child bruises easily and if there is a family history of a bleeding disorder, the presence of a hematologic disorder should be considered.

Emergency Department interventions. Diagnostic studies are rarely indicated in children with epistaxis. However, if a child is hypovolemic, a CBC, blood type and cross match, and coagulation studies are indicated.

Most nosebleeds resolve spontaneously or are controlled by firm local pressure. If bleeding persists, the site of the bleeding is identified by an internal nasal examination and appropriate treatment is initiated. Approaches to the control of epistaxis vary depending on the severity of the bleeding and the health care provider's preference. Topical thrombin, vasoconstrictors (to shrink the nasal mucosa and stop the bleeding), local anesthetics, or localized cauterization with a silver nitrate stick may be used. In rare instances nasal packing is required.

Nursing care and evaluation. Children with epistaxis rarely require emergent management. As in any child, however, if signs and symptoms of hypovolemia are present, immediate stabilization of the airway and breathing is indicated and fluid therapy is initiated. Active bleeding is controlled with substantial localized pressure to the soft parts of the nose for at least 5 to 10 minutes. The child is maintained in a sitting position with the head forward to prevent aspiration or obstruction of the airway; a basin can be provided for the child to spit out blood. Suction and airway equipment is placed at the bedside. Ongoing assessments include monitoring the child's airway, perfusion, vital signs, and degree of bleeding. Orthostatic vital signs are helpful in evaluating circulatory status. The child's response to therapy is evaluated and documented.

Since recurrences of nosebleeds are common, parents are taught to control bleeding with localized pressure. They are also instructed to notify the child's pediatrician if bleeding does not stop after

20 minutes of direct pressure or if the child feels faint or dizzy. Preventive measures are also explained (Box 19-6).

Sinusitis

Etiology. Sinusitis is a bacterial infection of one or more of the paranasal sinuses. Approximately 0.5% to 5% of sinus infections in children are secondary to URIs.[17,47] Other predisposing conditions include dental infections, allergies, or structural defects (e.g., cleft palate, septal deviation, polyps). The most common bacterial organisms responsible for producing sinusitis include *Streptococcus pneumoniae, Haemophilus influenzae,* and *Moraxella catarrhalis.* Chronic sinusitis is more often caused by anaerobic organisms.

Pathophysiology. Drainage from the paranasal sinuses into the meatus facilitates the movement of secretions and particulate matter. Any condition that obstructs drainage from the sinuses can cause secretions to stagnate, providing an optimal environment for bacterial or fungal growth. With inflammation of the sinuses, edema and purulent drainage results. In children younger than 10 years of age the ethmoids are most frequently affected.

Conditions that often occur concurrently with sinusitis include acute otitis media or laryngitis. Asthma may be triggered or exacerbated by the postnasal drainage caused by chronic sinusitis.

Complications of sinusitis are usually seen in patients with a history of chronic sinusitis following an acute exacerbation.[30] Extracranial complications include mucocele and osteomyelitis (more common in the frontal sinus); periorbital and orbital cellulitis or abscess, subperiosteal abscess, and cavernous sinus thrombosis may also occur. Intracranial complications include meningitis, cavernous vein thrombosis, and subdural and frontal lobe abscesses.

Clinical presentation. Children with sinusitis typically have a history of protracted rhinorrhea (>10 days) and a cough that is usually worse at night. Symptoms can be difficult to distinguish from a persistent URI, especially in young children. Children older than 5 years may report facial pain and headache. Adolescents tend to have the typical manifestations, including purulent nasal discharge, fever, cough, headache, facial pain, periorbital edema, fatigue, malaise, and bad breath. The most consistent findings associated with sinusitis are mucopurulent drainage from the middle meatus, periorbital swelling, or facial tenderness to light palpation (Box 19-7).

Because sinusitis is difficult to distinguish from a URI or an allergic inflammation, it is frequently overdiagnosed.[17,30] In an attempt to standardize the

---

Box 19-6 Measures to Prevent Epistaxis

- Increase the humidity in the home, for example by using a humidifier.
- Apply a small amount of petroleum jelly to the center wall inside the nose twice daily to relieve dryness and irritation.
- Trim the child's nails or cover the hands with mittens or socks to prevent nose-picking.
- Put 2 to 3 drops of warm water in each of the child's nostrils before stuffy nose is blown.
- Avoid the use of aspirin, which increases the body's tendency to bleed.
- Treat nasal allergies with antihistamines to decrease itching. If signs of a sinus infection develop, consult the child's pediatrician promptly.

Compiled from Culbertson and Manning, 1990; Santamaria and Abrunzo, 1992; Schmitt, 1992.

Box 19-7 Common Signs and Symptoms of Acute Sinusitis

- Nasal discharge, often purulent
- Cough, usually worse at night
- Fever (high with severe sinusitis)
- Headache
- Midfacial or periorbital pain or fullness
- Dental pain
- Nasal congestion or obstruction
- Periorbital swelling that is worse in morning
- Conjunctival inflammation
- Bad breath
- Sore throat from postnasal drip
- Lack of sense of smell
- Fatigue, malaise
- Decreased appetite

diagnosis of acute sinusitis; the Rhinology and Paranasal Subcommittee of the American Academy of Otolaryngology–Head and Neck Surgery developed the following criteria: (1) a history of less than 3 weeks of rhinorrhea, often purulent; (2) with some combination of midfacial or periorbital pain or fullness, nasal congestion, or obstruction; (3) intermittent fever, cheek swelling, and conjunctival inflammation.[43]

Emergency Department interventions. Sinusitis is a clinical diagnosis based on history and physical findings. Nose, throat, or nasopharyngeal cultures are usually not helpful, since they have no predictive value in determining the bacteria responsible for an acute sinusitis. They may, however, be used to rule out other potential causes such as respiratory syncytial virus or streptococcal pharyngitis. Sinus aspirate cultures yield much more reliable results, but they are obtained only when a child has failed to respond to initial antibiotic therapy, is immunosuppressed, has severe symptoms, or has life-threatening complications.[47]

Sinus x-ray films are helpful in identifying the presence of sinusitis in older children when complete sinus opacification, bone destruction, or air-fluid levels are observed.[47] Mucosal thickening is a less specific diagnostic indicator. The interpretation of x-ray films in children less than 5 years of age is more complicated because air-fluid levels are difficult to evaluate and the sinuses are difficult to appreciate, particularly if the infant or child was improperly positioned during the x-ray examination. In these children the Waters view (occipitomental) is considered the most valuable x-ray film, since it evaluates both the ethmoid and the maxillary sinuses.[44] CT scanning will definitively identify the presence of sinusitis; however, its use is primarily reserved for evaluating complications (e.g., orbital edema) and assessing chronic or recurrent sinusitis after a course of medical treatment.[30,44]

Transillumination of the frontal or maxillary sinuses may indicate the presence of sinus inflammation with fluid collection. It is only useful, however, in children older than 10 years of age because of the increased thickness of soft tissue and bone in younger children.[22,47] Normal or absent transmission of light is a useful finding, but merely diminished or dull transmission does not correlate well with clinical sinusitis.

The definitive treatment for sinusitis is the administration of antibiotics. Amoxicillin is the drug of choice for most uncomplicated cases of acute sinusitis and is generally given for 2 to 3 weeks. If the child fails to respond within 72 hours of treatment, the causative organism may be resistant and the antibiotic should be changed. The administration of other medications depends on the symptoms. This approach includes the use of topical decongestants (e.g., phenylephrine, oxymetazoline, xylometazoline), antihistamines (e.g., diphenhydramine), and intranasal steroids (e.g., beclomethasone); however, the efficacy of these drugs has not been established.[17,30,47]

Nursing care and evaluation. Nursing care of the child with sinusitis is dependent on the presenting signs and symptoms. If the child appears to have symptoms of toxicity, emergent management is indicated. For most children, however, nursing care is primarily supportive. Antipyretics, mild analgesics, and antibiotic therapy are indicated. Discharge instructions concerning medications, comfort measures, and follow-up care are communicated to parents. Parents are instructed to administer the prescribed antibiotic for the full course, even if the child is feeling better. If the child does not improve within 72 hours or if a yellow-green discharge persists after 5 days, the primary caregiver should be notified. Comfort measures include the removal of thick or dry secretions from the nares by using saline nosedrops and a bulb syringe in infants or by gentle blowing in older children. The use of a humidifier will keep secretions moist. Signs or symptoms for which the parent should seek immediate care from the primary health care provider include worsening of the child's condition or the presence of redness or swelling of the cheeks, eyelids, or forehead.

▌PHARYNX

ANATOMY AND PHYSIOLOGY

The pharynx is a passageway connecting the nasal cavity, the mouth, and the throat. It is anatomically divided into three parts: oropharynx, nasopharynx, and hypopharynx. The hypopharynx contains the laryngeal structures. The nasopharynx communicates with the nasal cavity and the eustachian tubes. On the posterior wall of the nasopharynx, opposite the nares, are the pharyngeal tonsils (also called the adenoids). Adenoidal tissue is present in infants and young children and can obstruct the eustachian tubes when inflamed. This tissue usually atrophies by puberty. The anterior portion of the oropharynx contains the teeth, tongue, and gums. Posteriorly, the uvula hangs from the soft palate. Beyond the uvula, on either side of the oropharynx, are the anterior and posterior tonsillar pillars. Immunoglobulins synthesized in the tonsillar tissue provide some defense against pathogens entering the respiratory or gastrointestinal systems (Fig. 19-6).

ASSESSMENT

History. The history plays an important role in determining the etiology of pharyngeal complaints. Historical findings may include the presence of a sore throat, lymphadenopathy, hoarse or muffled voice, trismus (inability to open the mouth because of tonic contraction of the muscles of mastication), dysphagia, and drooling. Other findings may include allergies, the presence of a chronic condition, or persistent mouth breathing.

Physical examination. The physical examination includes inspection of the oral cavity, throat, and neck. A good time to examine the mouth and throat is immediately following the ear examination, when children often open their mouths to cry. Initially, the lips, teeth, tongue, and gums are inspected. A tongue blade is used to depress the tongue to examine the posterior oropharynx. The tonsils, if present, are examined for redness, swelling, or exudate, and the integrity of the retropharyngeal wall is evaluated. The nasopharynx may be examined by using a mirror held behind the palate. This examination is often limited by the child's size and/or cooperation and the skills of the examiner.

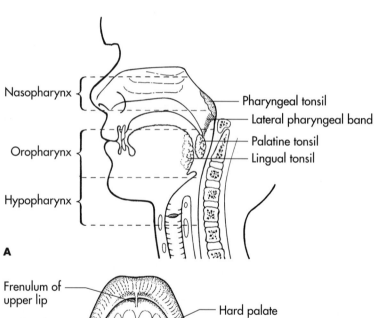

Nasopharynx

Oropharynx

Hypopharynx

Pharyngeal tonsil
Lateral pharyngeal band
Palatine tonsil
Lingual tonsil

A

FIG. 19-6. Anatomic structures of the pharynx (**A**) and oral cavity (**B**).

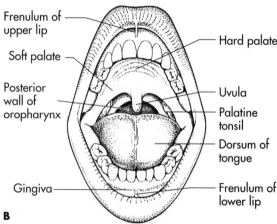

Frenulum of upper lip

Soft palate

Posterior wall of oropharynx

Gingiva

Hard palate

Uvula

Palatine tonsil

Dorsum of tongue

Frenulum of lower lip

B

PHARYNGITIS

Etiology. Pharyngitis, or a sore throat, is most commonly caused by infectious conditions; however, noninfectious causes, such as allergies and irritants, are not uncommon. Pharyngitis can also be a symptom of another illness, such as mononucleosis or varicella.

Viruses, especially respiratory viruses, are most often responsible for pharyngitis. Of the bacterial causes, group A beta-hemolytic streptococci (GAβHS) is the most common cause, accounting for 10% to 40% of all bacterial pharyngitis cases.[31] Uncommon bacterial causes of pharyngitis include *Staphylococcus aureus*, *Streptococcus pneumoniae*, *Haemophilus influenzae*, *Moraxella catarrhalis*, *Haemophilus parainfluenzae*, *Mycoplasma pneumoniae*, and *Chlamydia trachomatis* organisms. Gonococcal pharyngitis may be identified in children who have been sexually abused or in sexually active teens.

Most cases of pharyngitis occur during the colder months of the year, coinciding with peak viral incidence. GAβHS most often occurs in the late winter and early spring, but cases do appear all year long. GAβHS is most prevalent in school age children, although it can occur in younger children.[1,31]

Pathophysiology. Pharyngitis primarily results from an inflammatory or traumatic process that affects the posterior pharynx. The most concerning complications of pharyngitis are associated with GAβHS. Some strains of untreated GAβHS can result in rheumatic fever or acute poststreptococcal glomerulonephritis (APSGN). Examples of other complications of bacterial infections include peritonsillar abscess, retropharyngeal abscess, sinusitis, otitis, meningitis, and sepsis. The rate of complications with viral infections is low.

Peritonsillar abscess. A peritonsillar abscess represents an infection in the potential space between the superior constrictor muscle and the tonsil. This infection is most commonly caused by GAβHS; however, other causative agents include anaerobes, *Haemophilus influenzae, Streptococcus pneumoniae,* and *Staphylococcus aureus* organisms. The child with a peritonsillar abscess characteristically appears ill. High fever, severe throat pain, difficulty swallowing, drooling, trismus (difficulty opening the mouth caused by muscle spasm), and impaired vocal quality may be observed. Examination of the throat usually reveals unilateral tonsillar swelling and inflammation and deviation of the uvula.

Retropharyngeal abscess. A retropharyngeal abscess is an inflammation of the retropharyngeal space, which is located between the posterior pharyngeal wall and the prevertebral fascia. Before 3 to 4 years of age this space harbors a chain of lymph nodes that drain portions of the nasopharynx and the posterior nasal passages. For this reason conditions that produce increased drainage (e.g., otitis media, sinusitis, bacterial pharyngitis) increase a young child's risk of developing a retropharyngeal abscess. In fact, the majority of cases of retropharyngeal abscess occur in children younger than 6 years of age, with the highest incidence in the 6 to 12-month age group.[39,46] Another cause of retropharyngeal abscess, which can occur in any age child, is trauma to the posterior pharynx. The most common etiologies of a retropharyngeal abscess include GAβHS, oral anaerobes, and *Staphylococcus aureus* organisms.

The child with a retropharyngeal abscess appears toxic. Classic findings include a high fever, drooling, difficulting swallowing, and refusal to drink. About one fourth of patients with retropharyngeal abscess have inspiratory stridor.[11] Examination of the neck reveals cervical fullness and resistance to neck movement. Trismus may also be present. Because of the potential for airway obstruction, rupture and aspiration of drainage, or erosion of the abscess into the major blood vessels, the child with a retropharyngeal abscess is treated emergently.

Clinical presentation. Pharyngitis can be associated with a constellation of symptoms, including fever, cough, cold, vomiting, abdominal pain, and headaches. The history and presentation often assist in the differentiation of a bacterial versus viral cause, for example, known exposure to GAβHS or exposure to family members with colds or the flu. The presentation of pharyngitis with a viral cause is most commonly associated with a cough, hoarseness, and rhinorrhea. Adenovirus is often associated with conjunctivitis. Classic signs and symptoms of GAβHS include pharyngeal pain, dysphagia, fever, exudate over the tonsils and posterior pharyngeal wall, and tender anterior cervical adenopathy. Headache, malaise, and abdominal pain are also common, although these symptoms may also have other causes, such as mononucleosis or influenza. Symptoms of GAβHS in children younger than 3 years old tend to be nonspecific.

Emergency Department interventions. The goal of diagnostic testing for the child with pharyngitis is to distinguish GAβHS from a viral cause. Rapid streptococcal tests can accurately predict the presence of GAβHS; however, they are not sensitive. Therefore a throat culture is recommended if the rapid strep test is negative.

Although the treatment for viral pharyngitis is supportive, GAβHS is treated with antibiotics. If started early in the course of the illness, antibiotics shorten the course of the illness and possibly the period of contagion, and increase the child's comfort level and allow an earlier return to school or day care.[23,36] More important, if started within 9 days of onset of GAβHS pharyngitis, antibiotic therapy prevents the development of rheumatic fever.[28] Antibiotics do not significantly decrease the incidence of poststreptococcal glomerulonephritis.

Penicillin is the drug of choice for treating GAβHS. Erythromycin is recommended if the child is allergic to penicillin. When noncompliance is a concern, intramuscular penicillin is administered.

Nursing care and evaluation. The child who appears to have signs of toxicity or the child with signs and symptoms of respiratory compromise, peritonsillar abscess, or retropharyngeal abscess requires emergent management. Nursing interventions require assessment and stabilization of the ABCs (airway, breathing, circulation).

Nursing care for the child with uncomplicated pharyngitis includes supportive measures and discharge teaching. Warm salt-water gargles (¼ teaspoon per 8 ounces water), throat lozenges (for children older than 4 years of age), and analgesics can ease the discomfort of sore throats and facilitate eating and drinking. A soft diet is recommended and clear liquids are encouraged.

If the child has GAβHS, the importance of completing the course of antibiotics, even if the child feels better, is emphasized. Parents are instructed to contact the child's primary health care provider or return to the ED if the child develops severe throat pain, drooling, inability to open his or her mouth, breathing difficulty, or signs of dehydration. Any family member who develops a sore throat or other related symptoms within the next 5 days is instructed to see a physician. As always, good handwashing technique and avoidance of sharing items such as toothbrushes or drinking glasses can decrease the spread of GAβHS.

REFERENCES

1. American Academy of Pediatrics: Committee on Infectious Diseases: *1994 Red book: Report of the Committee on Infectious Disease*, Elk Grove, IL, 1994, AAP.
2. Amundson LH: Disorders of the external ear; *Prim Care* 17(2):213-231, 1990.
3. Baker RB: Is ear pulling associated with ear infection? *Pediatrics* 90:1006-1007, 1992.
4. Behrman RE, ed: *Nelson textbook of pediatrics*, ed 14, Philadelphia, 1992, WB Saunders.
5. Bergstrom L: Diseases of the external ear. In Bluestone CD, Stool WE, Scheetz MD, eds: *Pediatric otolaryngology*, Philadelphia, 1990, WB Saunders.
6. Bluestone CD: Modern management of otitis media, *Pediatr Clin North Am* 36(6):1371-1387, 1989.
7. Bluestone CD, Klein JO: Methods of examination: clinical examination. In Bluestone CD, Stool WE, Scheetz MD, eds: *Pediatric otolaryngology*, Philadelphia, 1990, WB Saunders, pp 111-124.
8. Bluestone CD, Klein JO: Otitis media, atelectasis, and eustachian tube function. In Bluestone CD, Stool WE, Scheetz MD, eds: *Pediatric otolaryngology*, Philadelphia, 1990, WB Saunders, pp 320-486.
9. Brook I, Burke P: The management of acute, serous and chronic otitis media: the role of anaerobic bacteria, *J Hosp Infect* 22 (suppl A):75-87, 1992.
10. Croteau N, Pless IB, Infante-Rivard C: Trends in medical visits and surgery for otitis media among children, *Am J Dis Child* 144:535-538, 1990.
10a. Culbertson and Manning SC: Epistaxis. In Bluestone CD, Stool WE, Scheetz MD, eds: *Pediatric otolaryngology*, Philadelphia, 1990, WB Saunders.
11. Cunningham MJ: Acute otolaryngologic surgical conditions in children, *Pediatr Ann* 23(5):250-256, 1994.
12. Dudlin A, Othman A: Acute periorbital swelling: evaluation of management protocol, *Ped Emerg Care* 12(1):16, 1996.
13. Eisen SA et al: The effect of prescribed daily dose frequency on patient medication compliance, *Arch Intern Med* 150:1881-1884, 1990.
14. Fairbanks DNF: Complications of nasal packing; *Otolaryngol Head Neck Surg* 94(3):412, 1986.
15. Fisher MC: Conjunctivitis in children, *Pediatr Clin North Am* 34(6):1447-1456, 1987.
16. Fritz S, Gabor DK, Sivertson KT: Foreign bodies of the external auditory canal, *Emerg Med Clin North Am* 5(2):183-192, 1987.
17. Giebink GS: Childhood sinusitis: pathophysiology, diagnosis and treatment, *Pediatr Infect Dis J* 13:S55-58, 1994.
18. Gigliotti F et al: Efficacy of topical antibiotic therapy in acute conjunctivitis in children, *J Pediatr* 104:623, 1984.
19. Green SM, Rothrock SG: Single-dose intramuscular ceftriaxone for acute otitis media in children, *Pediatrics* 91:23-30, 1993.

20. Gundy JH: The pediatric physical exam. In Hoekelman RA, ed: *Primary pediatric care,* ed 2, St. Louis, 1992, Mosby, pp 67-110.
21. Harrison CJ, Belhorn TH: Acute otitis media: management and prophylaxis, *Clinician Rev* 2(4):53-65, 1992.
22. Healy GB: Methods of examination. In Bluestone CD, Stool WE, Scheetz MD, eds: *Pediatric otolaryngology,* Philadelphia, 1990, WB Saunders, pp 643-646.
23. Hedges JR, Lowe RA: Approach to acute pharyngitis, *Emerg Med Clin North Am* 5(2):335-351, 1987.
24. Hendrickse WA, et al: Five vs ten days of therapy for acute otitis media, *Pediatr Infect Dis J* 7:14-23, 1988.
25. Hoyt CS, Good WV, eds: The eyes. In Rudolph AM, ed: *Rudolph's pediatrics,* ed 19, Norwalk, Conn, 1991; Appleton & Lange, pp 1889-1924.
26. Kemp ED: Otitis media, *Prim Care* 17(2):267-287, 1990.
27. Kenna M: Embryology and developmental anatomy of the ear. In Bluestone CD, Stool WE, Scheetz MD, eds: *Pediatric otolaryngology,* Philadelphia, 1990; WB Saunders, pp 77-87.
28. Kenna MA: Sore throat in children: diagnosis and management. In Bluestone CD, Stool WE, Scheetz MD, eds: *Pediatric otolaryngology,* Philadelphia, 1990, WB Saunders, pp 837-842.
29. King RA: Common ocular signs and symptoms in childhood, *Pediatr Clin North Am* 40(4):753-766, 1993.
30. Loch WE, Alleva M, Paparella MM: Sinusitis, *Prim Care* 17(2):323-334, 1990.
31. Loos GD: Pharyngitis, croup, and epiglottitis, *Prim Care* 17(2):335-345, 1990.
32. Maller JS: Eye disorders. In Barkin RM, ed: *Pediatric emergency medicine: concepts and clinical practice,* ed 2, St Louis; 1997; Mosby.
33. Nelson LB: *Pediatric ophthalmology,* Philadelphia, 1984; WB Saunders.
34. Pichichero ME: Assessing the treatment alternatives for acute otitis media, *Pediatr Infect Dis J* 13(1):S27-34, 1994.
35. Potsic WP, Handler SD, Wetmore RF: Ear, nose, throat, and mouth. In Rudolph AM, ed: *Rudolph's pediatrics,* ed 19, Norwalk, Conn, 1991, Appleton & Lange, pp 933 ff.
36. Randolph MF, et al: Effect of antibiotic therapy on the clinical course of streptococcal pharyngitis, *J Pediatr* 106:870, 1985.
37. Ruuskanen O et al: Viruses in acute otitis media: increasing evidence for clinical significance, *Pediatr Infect Dis J* 10:425-427, 1991.
38. Ruuskanen O, Heikkinen T: Otitis media: etiology and diagnosis, *Pediatr Infect Dis J* 13:S23-26, 1994.
39. Santamaria JP, Abrunzo TJ: Ear, nose, and throat. In Barkin RM, ed: *Pediatric emergency medicine: concepts and clinical practice,* ed 2, St Louis, 1997, Mosby, pp 709-754.
40. Sbarbaro JA: Strategies to improve compliance with therapy, *Am J Med* 79(suppl 6A):34-37, 1985.
41. Schwartz RH: Pneumatic otoscopy: getting the most out of the ear exam, *J Resp Dis* 4(5):82, 1983.
42. Seidel HM et al, eds: *Mosby's guide to physical examination,* ed, 3, St Louis, 1995, Mosby.
43. Stankiewicz J, Osguthorpe JD: Medical treatment of sinusitis, *Otolaryngol Head Neck Surg* 110(4):361-362, 1994.
44. Swischuk LE: *Emergency imaging of the acutely ill or injured child,* ed 3, Baltimore, 1994, Williams & Wilkins.
45. Teele DW et al: Epidemiology of otitis media during the first seven years of life in children in greater Boston: a prospective cohort study, *J Infect Dis* 160:83-94, 1989.
46. Thompson JW, Cohen SR, Reddin P: Retropharyngeal abscess in children: a retrospective and historical analysis, *Laryngoscope* 98:589-592, 1988.
47. Wald ER: Rhinitis and acute and chronic sinusitis. In Bluestone CD, Stool WE, Scheetz MD, eds: *Pediatric otolaryngology,* Philadelphia, 1990, WB Saunders, pp 729-744.
48. Weiss A et al: Acute conjunctivitis in childhood, *J Pediatr* 122:10-14, 1993.
49. Wong DL: *Whaley and Wong's essentials of pediatric nursing,* ed 5, St Louis, 1997, Mosby.

CHAPTER 20

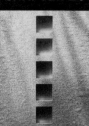

Endocrine System

Elizabeth Vaczy, Jean Mack-Fogg

Although children with endocrine disorders are generally managed as outpatients, they may come to the emergency department for diagnosis, complications, or coexisting injuries or illnesses. Complications of type I diabetes mellitus, especially diabetic ketoacidosis and hypoglycemia, are the most frequent endocrine emergencies. The other endocrine disorders discussed in this chapter are significantly less common. However, prompt recognition and management are often critical in preventing serious sequelae. Stress, including illness, injury, surgery, or emotional upset, can significantly influence the hormone levels, leading to serious abnormalities in children with endocrine disorders. In the emergency setting the effects of these stressors on the endocrine system must be assessed and the usual hormonal replacement regimens adjusted accordingly.

ANATOMY AND PHYSIOLOGY

The endocrine system is largely responsible for growth and maturation as well as the maintenance of homeostasis. Regulation of metabolism, fluid and electrolyte balance, and reproduction depend on normal endocrine functioning. Hormonal imbalances can significantly alter normal growth and development or even be life-threatening.

Hormones, which are produced and secreted into the bloodstream by various endocrine glands throughout the body, act as chemical messengers that alter cell activity (Table 20-1). The target cells or tissues are often not close to the gland. Although all tissues are exposed to the various hormones transported through the blood, only cells with receptors for a specific hormone respond. Intricate feedback mechanisms, involving the pituitary and hypothalamus, regulate hormonal balance. Endocrine disorders can result from abnormalities in any part of this feedback system.

HYPOGLYCEMIA

ETIOLOGY

Hypoglycemia is defined as a plasma glucose concentration less than 30 mg/dl in newborns younger than 3 days old or less than 40 mg/dl in the older infant or child, with or without symptoms.[4,12] These are not absolute values, however, since some children do not develop signs and symptoms until significantly lower glucose levels are reached, and others become symptomatic at higher levels, such as 50 to 70 mg/dl.

Hypoglycemia results from decreased availability or overutilization of glucose (Box 20-1). Although infants are particularly vulnerable to decreased glucose availability or diminished substrate, hypoglycemia can develop in a child of any age whenever the demand for glucose exceeds the supply. Stress, such as that associated with illnesses, injuries, fevers, or hypothermia, increases the demands for glucose. Overutilization of glucose primarily results from an excess of either endogenous or exogenous insulin. Children treated with insulin therapy for diabetes mellitus frequently encounter hypoglycemia associated with delayed or decreased food intake or with increased physical activity. Other hormonal or metabolic abnormalities, such as adrenal insufficiency or inborn errors of metabolism, can either impair glucose availability or increase the utilization of glucose.

PATHOPHYSIOLOGY

Normal blood glucose levels are maintained via intricate mechanisms that regulate glucose production and utilization. Dietary carbohydrates usually provide an adequate supply of glucose to meet the body's energy demands. Excess glucose is stored as glycogen in the liver and muscle. In the fasting state, glucose is

TABLE 20-1   Endocrine Glands and Their Function

GLAND/HORMONE	PRIMARY EFFECT
Adenohypophysis (anterior pituitary)	
Growth hormone (GH)	Promotes growth of bone and soft tissues
Thyroid-stimulating hormone (TSH)	Stimulates thyroid hormone secretion
Adrenocorticotropic hormone (ACTH)	Stimulates adrenal cortex to secrete glucocorticoids and androgens
Gonadotropins	Stimulate gonads to mature and produce sex hormones and germ cells
Follicle-stimulating hormone (FSH)	
Luteinizing hormone (LH)	
Prolactin	Stimulates milk secretion
Melanocyte-stimulating hormone (MSH)	Promotes pigmentation of skin
Neurohypophysis (posterior pituitary)	
Antidiuretic hormone (ADH)	Acts on kidney tubules to resorb water
Oxytocin	Stimulates uterine contractions
	Causes milk-ejection reflex
Thyroid gland	
Thyroid hormones	Regulate metabolic rate
	Control rate of body cell growth
Thyrocalcitonin	Influences ossification and development of bone
Parathyroid glands	
Parathyroid hormone (PTH)	Regulates calcium metabolism
Adrenal cortex	
Aldosterone	Regulates sodium retention and excretion
Sex hormones	Influence development of bones, reproductive organs, and secondary sex characteristics
Glucocorticoids	Promote metabolism
	Mobilize body defenses during stress
	Suppress inflammatory reaction
Adrenal medulla	
Catecholamines	Produce a sympathetic response
	Increase blood pressure and blood glucose levels
Islands of Langerhans of pancreas	
Insulin	Promotes utilization of glucose by cells; decreases blood glucose levels
Glucagon	Increases blood glucose levels
	Accelerates glyconeogenesis
Somatostatin	Inhibits secretion of insulin and glucagon
Ovaries	
Estrogen	Stimulates ripening of ova
	Produces female secondary sex characteristics
	Promotes epiphyseal closure of bones
Progesterone	Prepares uterus for fertilization
Testes	
Testosterone	Stimulates spermatogenesis
	Produces male secondary sex characteristics
	Promotes epiphyseal closure of bones

From Wong DL: *Whaley & Wong's essentials of pediatric nursing*, ed 5, St Louis, 1997, Mosby.

Box 20-1   Pathogenesis of Hypoglycemia in Childhood

Diminished substrate
Exogenous sources
    Decreased intake
        Fasting
        Anorexia: illness-related or psychiatric
        Chronic malnutrition
    Decreased absorption
        Infection: diarrheal illness
        Malabsorption syndromes
Endogenous sources (inborn errors of metabolism)
    Glyconeogenic enzyme deficiencies
    Glycogenolytic enzyme deficiencies
    Inadequate glycogen storage diseases
    Amino acid metabolism defects

Abnormal hormonal mediation
Hypopituitarism
Hypothyroidism
Adrenal insufficiency (congenital adrenal hyperplasia)
Inappropriate insulin
    Endogenous causes such as islet cell adenoma
    Exogenous causes such as insulin therapy and oral hypoglycemic agents

Associated disorders
Sepsis
Reye syndrome
Poisonings, such as salicylates, ethanol, and propranolol

From Saladino RA: Endocrine and metabolic disorders. In Barkin RM, ed: *Pediatric emergency medicine: concepts and clinical practice*, ed 2, St Louis, 1997, Mosby, p. 757.

Box 20-2   Symptoms of Hypoglycemia

Adrenergic
Tremors
Pallor
Sweating
Tachycardia
Tachypnea
Weakness
Hunger

CNS
Irritability
Headache
Dizziness
Visual disturbances
Confusion
Bizarre behavior
Seizures
Coma

Common symptoms during infancy
Pallor or cyanosis
Feeding difficulty
Floppiness, poor muscle tone
Temperature instability
Irritability
Lethargy
Jitteriness
Apnea

---

supplied by the breakdown of hepatic glycogen (glycogenolysis). After depletion of hepatic glycogen stores, glucose is synthesized from nonglucose substrates such as proteins and fats (glyconeogenesis). These processes are controlled by several hormonal mechanisms. Insulin, secreted by the pancreas, lowers glucose levels by increasing both glucose utilization and its storage as glycogen. The counterregulatory hormones (glucagon, epinephrine, cortisol, and growth hormone) oppose this effect and exert a glucose-raising effect by mobilizing and increasing the synthesis of glucose.

Abnormalities in any of the mechanisms regulating blood glucose concentration or diminished intake or absorption can lead to hypoglycemia. Infants, especially premature infants, are particularly prone to hypoglycemia because they have limited glycogen stores, respond slowly to glucagon, and have delayed maturation of the enzymes that promote glyconeogenesis. Infants and children have greater glucose requirements because of growth needs, a faster metabolic rate, and a proportionately larger brain when compared to adults. Since the central nervous system (CNS) depends on a continuous supply of glucose, the outcome of hypoglycemia causing most concern is permanent brain damage or death.

TABLE 20-2	Common Foods Used to Treat Hypoglycemia		
	AMOUNT (1 SERVING)	GLUCOSE (GM)	CARBOHYDRATE (GM)
Orange juice	½ cup	6.6	12.8
Apple juice	½ cup	3.1	14.5
Raisins	2 tablespoons	5.6	14.2
Regular soda	½ cup	5	13.3

CLINICAL PRESENTATION

The signs and symptoms of hypoglycemia are attributed to two causes (Box 20-2). Adrenergic symptoms, which generally occur first, result from the release of adrenaline, which mobilizes glucose and corrects hypoglycemia. If early symptoms are unrecognized or untreated, CNS symptoms develop in response to the effects of low blood sugar levels on the brain. Mild adrenergic symptoms of hypoglycemia may occur with a rapid drop in blood sugar levels despite normoglycemia. Symptoms of hypoglycemia may be confused with signs of drug or alcohol ingestion, particularly in adolescent patients. Hypoglycemia and sepsis have similar nonspecific symptoms and must be differentiated.

EMERGENCY DEPARTMENT INTERVENTIONS

Initial diagnosis requires rapid blood glucose determination via a portable blood glucose meter or glucose oxidase reagent strip. A laboratory-determined serum glucose level should be obtained as soon as possible to provide a more precise measurement. When there is a high index of suspicion for hypoglycemia, treatment should not be delayed pending laboratory results. Once hypoglycemia has been treated and the child's condition is stabilized, diagnostic tests to determine the underlying cause are necessary. These may include measurements of insulin, growth hormone, cortisol, and liver function, depending on the history and clinical presentation. Urine should be analyzed for glucose and ketones.

NURSING CARE AND EVALUATION

History. Initial management of the child with hypoglycemia depends on the clinical presentation and history. Historical information, useful in determining the etiology of the hypoglycemia, includes signs and symptoms associated with the hypoglycemia,

time of occurrence, associated activities (e.g., exercise), dietary intake (amount, type, and time of most recent meal), medications (especially insulin), and recent or current illnesses. The possibility of a toxic ingestion should also be explored, as well as a family history of endocrine or metabolic abnormalities.

Interventions. The presence of hypoglycemia is generally identified at the bedside using a meter or reagent strip. At the same time, serum glucose samples should be collected and sent to the laboratory to confirm bedside results, since blood drop size, wiping technique, or timing can affect bedside results. Treatment is never delayed while awaiting laboratory results.

Children with moderately low blood glucose levels or those who are exhibiting symptoms of hypoglycemia without altered mental status can usually be managed by giving them oral glucose containing fluids such as juice. Infants can be given oral 5% dextrose in water (D_5W) (Table 20-2).

Hypoglycemic children who are unresponsive or unable to cooperate after receiving administration of oral glucose are given a rapid intravenous bolus of 1 to 2 ml/kg (0.25 to 0.5 g/kg) of 25% dextrose in water ($D_{25}W$) solution[9a] (Fig. 20-1). Glucose boluses in neonates should be administered slowly (over 1 to 2 minutes), and a 10% dextrose ($D_{10}W$) solution should be given at 3 to 5 ml/kg.[2] The use of 50% glucose solutions is not recommended in infants or children because it is too hyperosmolar and can cause venous sclerosis. When rapid venous access cannot be achieved, oral glucose gel may be rubbed onto the gums and buccal mucosa. Once the symptoms of hypoglycemia have disappeared and the blood sugar level is normalized, a continuous intravenous (IV) infusion of 5% dextrose solution ($D_{10}W$ in neonates) is administered.

If the suspected cause of the hypoglycemia is hyperinsulinism and venous access has not been achieved, glucagon may be administered via intramus-

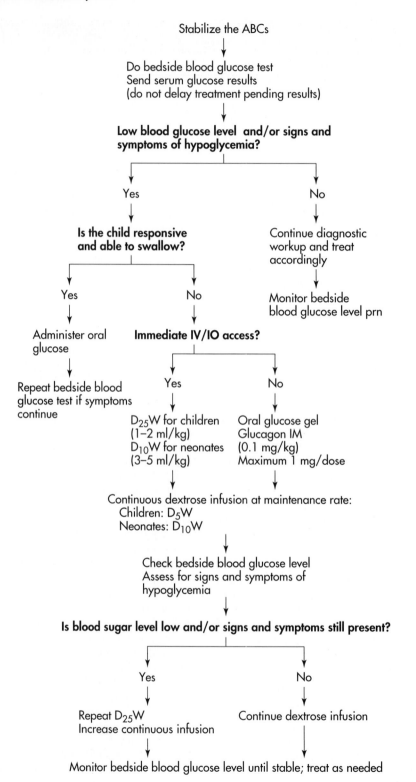

FIG. 20-1. Intervention for child with signs and symptoms of hypoglycemia or with high-risk factors. (Data from Saladino, 1992; Burchfield, 1992; Johnson, 1993.)

cular (IM) injection. Glucagon provides a transient rise in blood glucose level by promoting the breakdown of hepatic glycogen to glucose. It is only effective when glycogen stores are available, and the mobilization of glycogen can take up to 15 minutes. Side effects include nausea and vomiting. When hypopituitarism is suspected, intravenous hydrocortisone may be given to stimulate glyconeogenesis and stabilize the blood glucose level.

Evaluation. Since signs and symptoms of hypoglycemia are not always consistent with blood glucose levels, the child must be observed closely for the often subtle signs of hypoglycemia. Evaluation of the child's response to treatment includes continuous observation for signs of recurrence and obtaining bedside glucose measurements each hour.

Peripheral lines used for the administration of glucose-containing solutions must be observed for signs of extravasation. Scalp veins should never be used. If the line infiltrates, the child must be closely monitored while a new line is begun expeditiously.

Education. When appropriate, the nurse should educate the child and family regarding recognition of symptoms, prevention techniques, and treatment of hypoglycemia. Parents can be taught to prevent or minimize conditions that exacerbate hypoglycemia, such as cold stress, fever, and insufficient intake of calorie-containing fluids during vomiting. The child with diabetes should be taught to eat before exercising in order to avoid hypoglycemia. If the child has an underlying condition that predisposes him or her to hypoglycemia, the use of a medical identification bracelet should be discussed. With uncomplicated diabetic hypoglycemia, the child may be discharged when the blood glucose level has normalized after oral feedings. For an initial episode of hypoglycemia, when the etiology is unclear, hospital admission or outpatient evaluation is required.

▌ DIABETIC KETOACIDOSIS

ETIOLOGY

Diabetic ketoacidosis (DKA) is an acute, life-threatening complication of diabetes resulting from an absence or relative deficiency of insulin. Precipitating factors include illness, infection, emotional or environmental stress, surgery, trauma, or noncompliance with the diabetes regimen. DKA accounts for approximately 15% of all diabetes-related hospitalizations and is the most common cause of death in children with diabetes.[9a] A significant number of children with diabetes are in DKA at the time of diagnosis. Therefore DKA is frequently encountered in the emergency department.

PATHOPHYSIOLOGY

Hyperglycemia. DKA develops from the insulin deficiency that characterizes diabetes in combination with a stress-induced rise in the counterregulatory hormones epinephrine, cortisol, growth hormone, and glucagon. Both the insulin deficiency and the hormonal action prevent glucose from entering the cells, thus causing hyperglycemia. Serum glucose levels are further elevated by the release of glucose from the liver in response to the counterregulatory hormones (Fig. 20-2).

Metabolic acidosis. To provide glucose to the cells, fat and protein stores are broken down, resulting in increased levels of circulating amino acids and increased oxidation of free fatty acids. The free fatty acids are converted into ketone bodies by the liver, and the accumulation of their by-products (acetoacetic acid, β-hydroxybutyric acid) creates a metabolic acidosis. The pulmonary compensatory response to metabolic acidosis and ketosis is Kussmaul respirations, or an increase in the depth and rate of respirations in an attempt to "blow off" carbon dioxide. Excessive excretion of ketones produces the characteristic "fruity" acetone breath.

Dehydration and electrolyte deficiencies. As the serum glucose level rises, increased osmotic pressure in the extracellular spaces causes fluids and electrolytes to move out of the cells. The resulting intracellular dehydration further exacerbates metabolic acidosis. At the same time, the renal threshold for glucose reabsorption is exceeded and excess glucose is excreted in the urine, along with ketone bodies, sodium, and potassium. This causes an osmotic diuresis that can lead to hypovolemic shock.

Acidosis causes potassium to shift from the intracellular to the extracellular fluid in exchange for hydrogen ions. Therefore the serum potassium level may be falsely elevated, even though cellular potassium has been depleted. Once fluid therapy is initiated, serum potassium levels fall.

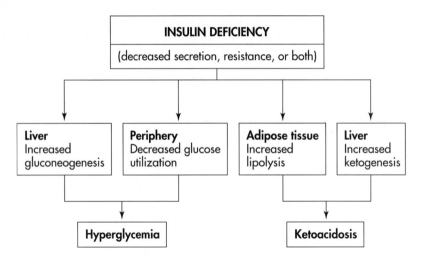

FIG. 20-2. The pathophysiologic basis of diabetic ketoacidosis. (From Siperstein MD: Diabetic ketoacidosis and hyperosmolar coma, *Endocrinol Metab Clin North Am* 21(2):416, 1992.)

CLINICAL PRESENTATION

DKA is typically gradual in onset, developing over several days. The early symptoms of hyperglycemia, including polyuria, polydipsia, anorexia or polyphagia, weight loss, and fatigue are also common presenting symptoms of the child with undiagnosed diabetes. Nausea, vomiting, lethargy, altered mental status, Kussmaul respirations, and acetone breath signal the onset of DKA.

Because of the pathophysiology of DKA, children presenting in DKA are presumed to be dehydrated regardless of presentation. Clinical signs of dehydration may be present and include tachycardia, dry mucous membranes, decreased skin turgor, delayed capillary refill, and postural changes in vital signs. Dehydration in the face of adequate urine output is indicative of DKA.

DKA can initially be confused with other diagnoses, especially in children with new-onset diabetes. Lethargy, dehydration, and acidosis may be mistaken for sepsis. Abdominal pain, frequently present with DKA, can easily be confused with appendicitis. Other possible diagnoses include shock, toxic ingestions, congenital metabolic derangements, and renal failure. Lactic acidosis and acidosis secondary to poisoning are not associated with hyperglycemia. Non-ketotic hyperosmolar coma, a syndrome also characterized by hyperglycemia, dehydration, and coma, occurs infrequently in children and is differentiated from DKA by the absence of ketonemia and ketonuria.

EMERGENCY DEPARTMENT INTERVENTIONS

DKA is a medical emergency requiring rapid assessment and diagnosis to prevent morbidity and mortality. Interventions include the restoration of fluid and electrolyte balance and the correction of hyperglycemia.

Laboratory evaluation for DKA includes measuring arterial blood gases and serum electrolytes (including creatinine and blood urea nitrogen [BUN]), doing a complete blood count (CBC) and differential count, obtaining a serum acetone determination, and doing a urinalysis. Findings diagnostic of DKA include a blood glucose level greater than 300 mg/dl, pH level less than 7.3 or serum bicarbonate level less than 15 mEq/L, and ketonemia.[9a] The urinalysis will reveal glucosuria and ketonuria. Serum hemoglobin, hematocrit, and BUN values are usually elevated secondary to hemoconcentration resulting from dehydration. An elevated white blood cell (WBC) count may indicate an underlying infection, but mild elevations are common secondary to the stress of DKA. Other causes of ketonemia or acidosis must be ruled out.

NURSING CARE AND EVALUATION

Nursing management of the child in DKA includes initial stabilization of the airway and breathing, particularly if the child has an altered level of consciousness. Once the airway is stabilized, the goals of therapy are to restore circulating volume and correct the hyperglycemia (Box 20-3).

Fluid and electrolyte replacement. Clinically stable children with mild acidosis and no vomiting may be treated with oral rehydration. However, if signs of hypovolemia are present, venous access is achieved and the child treated with 10 to 20 ml/kg of normal saline or lactated Ringer's solution administered over an hour or sooner if the child is in shock. Subsequent fluid and electrolyte deficits are replaced slowly over 36 to 48 hours with ½ normal saline solution and potassium salts.[7,9a] Fluid requirements are calculated based on estimated deficit and maintenance requirements. Once the initial correction of hypovolemia is complete *and urination has been established,* replacement of potassium losses is begun. The amount of potassium replacement per liter is based on the serum potassium level.[8] A combination of potassium chloride and potassium phosphate may be used to avoid hyperchloremia, which can exacerbate the acidosis.[7] The use of IV bicarbonate to correct acidosis is controversial and should be reserved for cases of severe acidosis with a pH less than 7.0.

This approach to fluid and electrolyte therapy provides a gradual reduction in the serum osmolality and reduces the risk of cerebral edema. As fluid and electrolyte imbalances are corrected, acidosis is reversed and serum glucose levels reduced, even before insulin therapy is initiated.

Insulin therapy. Insulin therapy reverses ketogenesis and definitively corrects hyperglycemia. Initially a bolus of 0.1 units/kg of regular insulin is given, followed by a continuous IV infusion of regular insulin mixed in normal saline solution at a rate of 0.1 units/kg/hr.[8] Although insulin can be administered intramuscularly and subcutaneously, it may be irregularly absorbed and these routes are therefore not recommended. A continuous IV infusion of insulin offers the advantage of smoother control of blood glucose level and more rapid dissipation of insulin effects.[3]

Since insulin binds to plastic, the IV tubing must be primed with approximately 50 ml of insulin solution to saturate the binding sites before infusion. An infusion pump must be used to regulate the administration rate (Box 20-4).

The goal of insulin therapy is to decrease blood sugar level by 50 to 100 mg/dl/hr. A drop in blood glucose level in excess of 100 mg/dl/hr creates

---

Box 20-3   Nursing Interventions for a Child with DKA

Stabilize airway, breathing, and circulation (ABCs)

Assess patient
  History
    Signs and symptoms of DKA
    Precipitating factors
      Infection
      Noncompliance
      Trauma
      Other factors, such as poisonings
    Medications
      Known diabetic: amount, type of insulin
    Family history
  Vital signs, including orthostatic measurements
  Physical examination
    Neurologic status
    Hydration
  Obtain laboratory results
    Bedside glucose testing
    Serum glucose electrolyte levels
    Arterial or venous blood gases
    Urinalysis
    CBC and differential count

Offer fluid resuscitation
  Obtain IV access
  Administer fluids as ordered
  Monitor infusion rate carefully

Give insulin infusion

Evaluate patient status
  Monitor for cardiac arrhythmias
  Check neurologic status for cerebral edema
  Check vital signs
  Watch for signs of hypoglycemia
  Measure bedside blood glucose test every hour
  Measure urine glucose/ketones every void
  Record intake and output
  Measure serum pH and serum chemistries

Educate child and family

> **Box 20-4   Procedure for Insulin Infusion**
>
> **Tips on insulin administration**
> - The initial dose of insulin infusion is 0.1 unit/kg/hr. If serum glucose level does not decrease at a rate of 50 to 100 mg/dl/hr, the dose may be increased to 0.2 unit/kg/hr.
> - Because insulin binds to the IV bottles, bags, and tubing, the IV tubing should be flushed with at least 50 ml of the insulin drip before patient administration. Tubing should not be changed once it has been flushed.
> - The first dose of regular subcutaneous insulin should be given 30 minutes before the termination of the drip.
>
> **Procedure**
> Mix 100 ml normal saline solution with 10 units regular insulin. In this concentration 1 ml = 0.1 unit.
>
> **Formula**
> 1 ml (0.1 unit) × weight in kg = hourly rate (ml)
>
> **Example**
> For a 20 kg child:
> 1 ml (0.1 unit) × 20 kg = 20 ml/hr

osmotic changes that may increase the risk of cerebral edema. When the blood glucose level approaches 300 mg/dl, 5% dextrose is added to the IV solution. At this point, insulin therapy is continued but the dose may be reduced to avoid hypoglycemia.

When the acidosis has resolved (pH greater than 7.3 or HCO_3 greater than 16), intravenous insulin is discontinued. Subcutaneous insulin is given 30 minutes before discontinuing IV insulin to avoid a rapid drop in insulin levels. In a known diabetic, the usual insulin regimen can be resumed. In a newly diagnosed child, insulin is generally initiated at a dose of 0.4 unit/kg in the morning (divided two-thirds NPH and one-third regular insulin) and 0.2 unit/kg in the evening (divided half NPH, half regular). Intravenous dextrose can be discontinued when food and/or fluids are well tolerated.

Although most children with DKA are admitted to the hospital, the child with mild DKA (serum pH equal to or more than 7.20 or serum bicarbonate equal to or more than 10 mmol/L) may receive initial stabilizing treatment in the emergency department and then be treated as an outpatient,[9] provided patient compliance and follow-up care are adequate. Children with moderate to severe DKA will require hospital admission, usually to an intensive care unit.

Evaluation.   Evaluation of the child's response to treatment guides ongoing management and identifies the development of complications. Monitoring includes continuous assessments of intake and output, vital signs, and neurologic status as well as periodic monitoring of blood pH and chemistries. Bedside glucose levels are checked hourly using a glucose meter or reagent strip. These measurements are periodically confirmed via the laboratory. Complications of treatment include the development of hypoglycemia or cerebral edema from fluid shifts, both of which may develop suddenly.

Education.   Children with newly diagnosed diabetes require intensive education, which can be initiated in the emergency department but must be continued by a pediatric diabetic educator and/or other appropriately trained health care provider. Admission to the hospital facilitates the education of the child and family.

Emotional support and reassurance are extremely important as the family and child learn to accept the responsibilities that accompany a chronic illness. Families can be referred to national and local diabetes agencies for additional support and information.

Reasons for noncompliance should be explored when known diabetics present in DKA and communicated to the child's primary care provider. Education regarding illness management and compliance is important for all children with diabetes and is reviewed each time the child is in DKA. Education includes emphasis on monitoring urine ketone levels during illnesses or periods of moderate elevations in blood sugar levels. The importance of continuing insulin therapy during periods of illness is emphasized as well as the potential for insulin resistance during illness.

DIABETES INSIPIDUS

ETIOLOGY

Diabetes insipidus (DI) is the inability to excrete an appropriately concentrated urine in the face of an abnormally elevated plasma osmolality. It is uncommon in children (Box 20-5). DI can be either central or nephrogenic in origin. Central DI results from a lack of antidiuretic hormone (ADH). It can be either idiopathic or acquired. Nephrogenic DI results from a lack of renal responsiveness to ADH and is extremely rare in children. In contrast to DI, the syndrome of inappropriate secretion of ADH (SIADH) results from excess secretion of ADH rather than a deficit causing water retention.

PATHOPHYSIOLOGY

ADH (vasopressin) is produced in the hypothalamus and secreted from the posterior pituitary gland. It allows reabsorption of water in the distal tubules and collecting ducts of the kidney. ADH secretion is regulated by osmoreceptors in the anterior hypothalamus. Rising plasma osmolality, as might occur with dehydration, normally causes increased ADH secretion. As water is reabsorbed, plasma osmolality decreases. A defect in the secretion or renal response to ADH results in an inappropriately dilute urine. Hypertonic dehydration can occur rapidly if the thirst mechanism or access to fluids is compromised.

CLINICAL PRESENTATION

DI is characterized by polyuria and polydipsia. The onset is usually abrupt with central DI. Enuresis is frequently the first sign. Generally, nonstressed children with an intact thirst mechanism and free access to water, do not develop significant electrolyte or fluid imbalances. These children may remain undiagnosed. However, hypertonic dehydration can occur from decreased fluid intake or increased fluid loss caused by fever, diarrhea, and vomiting. Common signs of dehydration include dry mucous membranes, lack of tears, tachycardia, and decreased skin turgor. Infants, because of their rapid metabolic rates and increased fluid requirements, are more likely to become dehydrated from a lack of free water intake. They often present with failure to thrive, lethargy, and irritability that is relieved by feedings of water.

DI should be considered in the child with head trauma when polyuria is present with maintenance or

Box 20-5	Causes of DI

Central (ADH-deficient)
Idiopathic—familial or sporadic
Secondary
- Head injury
- Infection, especially CNS related
- Neoplasm
- Intracranial surgery
- Granulomas: histiocytosis X, sarcoid
- Vascular: sickle cell disease, cerebral hemorrhage or thrombosis

Nephrogenic (ADH-resistant)
Idiopathic—familial or sporadic
Secondary
- Renal disease: polycystic kidney disease, ureteral obstruction, pyelonephritis
- Electrolyte disturbances: hypercalcemia, hypokalemia
- Toxins: alcohol, phenytoin, lithium, angiography dyes
- Granulomas: histiocytosis X, sarcoid
- Vascular: sickle cell disease

Adapted from Saladino RA: Endocrine and metabolic disorders. In Barkin RM, ed: *Pediatric emergency medicine: concepts and clinical practice,* ed 2, St Louis, 1997, Mosby.

below-maintenance fluid administration.[1] Since severe symptoms of DI can mimic sepsis, a lethargic child should always be evaluated for infection. Diabetes mellitus also presents with polyuria and polydipsia, but is easily distinguished from DI by the presence of glycosuria and an elevated serum glucose level. Other causes of hypertonic dehydration, such as diarrheal illnesses and hyperaldosteronism, should also be considered.

EMERGENCY DEPARTMENT INTERVENTIONS

Emergency department interventions for the child with DI include stabilization of the airway and breathing, particularly if the child has an altered mental status, and fluid rehydration.

The definitive diagnosis of DI is made by demonstrating an abnormally high serum osmolality in the context of a more dilute urine. In severe cases a random serum osmolality with a simultaneous urine osmolality will be diagnostic. In less severe cases a water deprivation test is necessary. The child fasts for several hours while serum and urine osmolality, specific gravity, and weight are carefully monitored. A dilute urine (<150 mOsm/L) despite a rising serum osmolality (>290 mOsm/kg) and serum sodium (>145 mEq/L) level, along with a weight loss of 3% to 5%, is considered diagnostic.[7] Nephrogenic DI can be distinguished from central DI by the lack of responsiveness to 1-desamino, 8-D-arginine vasopressin (DDAVP).

Central DI is treated with DDAVP given intranasally or subcutaneously. This requires careful titration of the dose and close monitoring of fluid and electrolyte levels. Nephrogenic DI is treated by ensuring free access to water and reducing the osmotic load through dietary manipulation. Depending on the severity of the symptoms, chlorothiazide diuretics or antiprostaglandins can be used. Both of these drugs have the net effect of promoting the proximal tubular reabsorption of glomerular filtrate.

NURSING CARE AND EVALUATION

As with any child coming to the emergency department, airway patency and respiratory status must be stabilized before definitive treatment. Once airway and breathing have been stabilized, fluid replacement therapy is begun.

Circulatory interventions include obtaining vascular access and administering rehydration fluids. If severe dehydration and decreased perfusion are present, a normal saline bolus of 20 ml/kg is indicated. Fluid replacement is based on the estimated level of free water deficit and is administered over 24 to 48 hours.[9a] Maintenance fluids and fluids to replace ongoing urinary losses are also infused. Since dehydration in DI results from free water loss, replacement fluids are hypotonic.

Ongoing care of the child with DI includes close monitoring of the child's hydration status, neurologic status, and intake and output. Urine specific gravity and osmolality and serum electrolyte levels and osmolality are evaluated frequently.

Parents should be given information regarding the disease process and how to monitor fluid intake and output at home. The need for free access to water at all times, including at school, must be emphasized. If the child is well enough to be discharged home, follow-up care by an endocrinologist or nephrologist can be arranged.

▐ HYPOCALCEMIA

ETIOLOGY

Hypocalcemia may result from a deficiency or abnormal metabolism of vitamin D, nutritional deficiencies, or malabsorption. Hypoparathyroidism and parathyroid hormone resistance (pseudohypoparathyroidism, hypomagnesemia) are rare causes of hypocalcemia. In the neonate, hypocalcemia can occur from an exacerbation of the normal postnatal drop in calcium, transient suppression of parathyroid activity secondary to maternal hyperparathyroidism, or excessive phosphorus intake from cow's milk formula. Premies and infants with birth asphyxia or diabetic mothers are more likely to become hypocalcemic.

PATHOPHYSIOLOGY

Most of the body's calcium is found in bone. The 1% to 3% of calcium found in the soft tissues and blood is necessary for nerve, muscle, and endocrine gland function. Total serum calcium concentration is tightly maintained between 8.5 and 10.5 mg/dl, but it may normally be as low as 8 mg/dl for full-term neonates and 7.5 mg/dl for premature infants. When total serum calcium level is measured, it reflects calcium that is (1) bound to protein, primarily albumin; (2) ionized; and (3) bound to other anions.

Ionized calcium, the physiologically active form of calcium, is regulated by vitamin D and the endocrine system. It is important in maintaining plasma membrane stability and permeability as well as proper neuromuscular function in cardiac, striated, and smooth muscle. Normally, ionized calcium levels are approximately half the total serum calcium level. However, a low albumin level reduces the total serum calcium level, but not the ionized form.[13] Therefore a low total calcium level does not always reflect a deficiency in ionized calcium or hypocalcemia. A low total calcium level is best evaluated by checking an ionized calcium level, which may be normal. If ionized calcium levels are not available, the total calcium level can be adjusted by adding 0.8 mg/dl to the serum calcium level for each 1 g/dl that the serum albumin level is below 4 g/dl.[10]

Normally a decrease in the ionized calcium level causes an increase in parathyroid hormone (PTH). PTH acts to restore the serum calcium level toward normal by promoting bone resorption (shifting calcium from bone to blood), increasing reabsorption of calcium in the kidney and calcium absorption from the gut. PTH also stimulates the production of active vitamin D (calcitriol), which promotes the absorption of calcium from the small intestine.

Various abnormalities in calcium metabolism, including a nutritional deficit of calcium, excessive intake of phosphorus, or intestinal malabsorption of calcium, can cause hypocalcemia. Vitamin D deficiency inhibits the intestinal absorption of calcium as well as the mobilization of calcium from bone, that helps to maintain serum calcium levels. PTH deficiency or resistance inhibits the reabsorption of calcium by the kidneys and the mobilization of calcium from bone.

CLINICAL PRESENTATION

Hypocalcemia presents with varying degrees of neuromuscular irritability. Seizures are the most common presentation in infants and young children. Jitteriness, twitching, carpopedal spasms (tetany), paresthesias, and laryngospasm are also frequently present. Although vomiting, lethargy, poor feeding, and irritability can indicate hypocalcemia in infants, it may also indicate sepsis. Two classic clinical signs associated with hypocalcemia are Chvostek's and Trousseau's signs. Chvostek's sign is positive when a facial twitch is elicited by tapping the facial nerve as it crosses the maxilla. Trousseau's sign is positive when carpal spasm is elicited by inflating a blood pressure cuff just above systolic pressure for 1 or 2 minutes.

EMERGENCY DEPARTMENT INTERVENTIONS

Symptomatic hypocalcemia requires emergency interventions, including the administration of a calcium solution. Diagnostic testing depends on the severity of the symptoms and the suspected etiology. Tests include a CBC with differential count; serum electrolyte levels, including serum phosphate, ionized calcium, magnesium, and PTH; electrocardiogram (ECG) and X-ray studies if a vitamin D deficiency or rickets is suspected. Hypocalcemia is characterized by a total serum calcium level less than 7 mg/dl, an ionized serum calcium level less than 3 mg/dl, and often an elevated serum inorganic phosphate concentration greater than 6 mg/dl. Low magnesium levels (<1 mg/dl) are sometimes present and can interfere with the response to treatment of hypocalcemia. Ideally, serum PTH levels should be drawn before treatment to distinguish between true hypoparathyroidism and pseudohypoparathyroidism, unless the etiology has previously been established.

ECG findings typically show a prolonged ST segment without alteration of the T-wave. With rickets, radiologic studies of the wrist may indicate widened distal ends of the ulna and radius and decreased bone density.

NURSING CARE AND EVALUATION

Initial nursing care requires stabilization of airway, breathing, and circulation and attaching the child to a cardiorespiratory monitor. If the child is having a seizure, seizure precautions are initiated. Tetany or seizures are treated with 0.5 to 1 ml/kg (adult: 5 to 8 ml/dose) of 10% calcium gluconate IV over no less than 5 minutes.[5,6] During its administration the child should be closely monitored for the development of dysrhythmias, particularly bradycardia, and hypotension. Once the seizure activity has dissipated, or if bradycardia develops, the infusion is discontinued.

Calcium gluconate can be administered in glucose or normal saline solution; however, it will precipitate if mixed with bicarbonate or phosphate. Extravasation can cause tissue necrosis, so the IV site must be closely monitored. Scalp veins should not be used.

If symptoms of hypocalcemia are not severe, oral therapy is preferred because of the risks of IV calcium therapy. Calcium carbonate, calcium lactate, and calcium gluconate are available in oral preparations. Hypocalcemia caused by hypoparathyroidism, pseudohypoparathyroidism, and abnormalities of vitamin D metabolism can be treated with vitamin D (calcitriol or dihydrotachysterol) in addition to calcium supplements. If the symptoms of hypocalcemia do not resolve after adequate calcium replacement, hypomagnesemia must be considered. Hypomagnesemia is treated with 25 to 50 mg/kg IV/IM of magnesium sulfate, which is repeated every 4 to 6 hours as needed.

▌ ADRENAL INSUFFICIENCY

ETIOLOGY

Adrenal insufficiency (AI) can be an acute, life-threatening condition characterized by an inadequate production of cortisol, aldosterone, or both. AI rarely occurs in children, but it can arise from a disorder anywhere within the hypothalamic-pituitary-adrenal axis (Fig. 20-3).

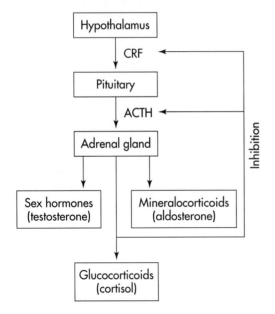

FIG. 20-3. Hypothalamic-pituitary-adrenal axis.

levels act as a negative feedback to the pituitary to inhibit ACTH release and modulate CRF release. Normally, cortisol levels increase greatly in times of stress or illness.

Aldosterone is synthesized in the adrenal glands; it promotes sodium retention and regulates blood pressure and water homeostasis. It is regulated through the renin-angiotensin system, which is responsive to volume changes and electrolyte balance.

Congenital adrenal hyperplasia. Congenital adrenal hyperplasia (CAH) is an inborn deficiency of various enzymes in the adrenal steroid synthesis pathways that results in inadequate cortisol production. Twenty-one hydroxylase deficiency is the most common defect. The pituitary responds by increasing the release of ACTH, resulting in increased adrenal androgen production (which is not dependent on the deficient enzyme). Elevated intrauterine androgen levels result in ambiguous genitalia in female newborns, but their effects are not readily apparent in boys. The production of aldosterone may or may not be decreased in CAH.

Iatrogenic AI. Iatrogenic AI occurs when exogenous glucocorticoid therapy is of sufficient dose and duration to decrease ACTH production. The degree of cortisol suppression is related to the form of glucocorticoid therapy, dose, route, and duration of therapy. Severe trauma, stress, or abrupt withdrawal of exogenous steroids leads to an acute adrenal crisis when the patient's endogenous cortisol production cannot increase sufficiently. Aldosterone production is not affected by glucocorticoid therapy because it is regulated by the renin-angiotensin system.

Hypopituitarism. Hypopituitarism results in inadequate ACTH production, leading to low cortisol levels, although there is adequate aldosterone production. Therefore electrolyte balance (sodium, potassium) is less affected.

Clinical presentation. Adrenal crisis may result from any of the disorders causing AI. Signs and symptoms vary, depending on whether or not the deficiency of cortisol is associated with aldosterone. Pure cortisol deficiency presents with hypoglycemia, weakness, and hypotension. Characteristics of aldosterone deficiency include hyponatremia, hyperkalemia, hypoglycemia, and metabolic acidosis, as well as vomiting, diarrhea, weight loss, salt craving, and circulatory failure (Box 20-6).

AI is divided into primary and secondary causes. Primary AI results from abnormalities within the adrenal gland. The most common cause of adrenal pathology in neonates is congenital adrenal hyperplasia. Other etiologies in infants and children include autoimmune processes (Addison's disease), adrenal hypoplasia, adrenal hemorrhage from trauma, adrenocorticotropin (ACTH) unresponsiveness, fulminating infections such as meningococcemia, adrenoleukodystrophy, and other enzyme defects.

Secondary AI results from problems with the hypothalamus or pituitary. It is most commonly caused by abrupt withdrawal of exogenous glucocorticoids. Hypopituitarism, which causes inadequate ACTH production and subsequently low cortisol levels, may result from CNS abnormalities, including congenital defects, trauma, tumors, infection, cranial irradiation, and surgery.

PATHOPHYSIOLOGY

Cortisol production is regulated through the hypothalamic-pituitary-adrenal axis in a negative feedback system. It stimulates glyconeogenesis and helps to maintain vascular tone. Corticotropin-releasing factor (CRF) is produced in the hypothalamus and regulates the release of ACTH from the pituitary. ACTH binds with receptors in the adrenal gland, which in turn synthesizes cortisol. Plasma cortisol

---

Box 20-6   Clinical Manifestations of Acute AI

Early symptoms
Increased irritability
Headache
Diffuse abdominal pain
Weakness
Nausea and vomiting
Diarrhea

**Generalized hemorrhagic manifestations
(Waterhouse-Friderichsen syndrome)**
Fever—increases as condition worsens
CNS signs:
    Nuchal rigidity
    Convulsions
    Stupor
    Coma

Shocklike state
Weak, rapid pulse
Decreased blood pressure
Shallow respirations
Cold, clammy skin
Cyanosis
Circulatory collapse (terminal event)

Newborn
Hyperpyrexia
Tachypnea
Cyanosis
Convulsions
Gland may be evident as palpable retroperitoneal mass (hemorrhagic)

From Wong DL: *Whaley and Wong's essentials of pediatric nursing,* ed 5, St Louis, 1997, Mosby.

---

tion in the genital region. Hyperpigmentation results from elevated ACTH production, which increases the amount of melanin present.

EMERGENCY DEPARTMENT INTERVENTIONS

Adrenal crisis can easily be confused with sepsis and hypovolemic shock. Since hormonal assays take several days to be completed, the diagnosis of AI is not readily confirmed. If AI is suspected, blood should be drawn to determine cortisol level, electrolytes, BUN, creatinine, glucose (serum and bedside blood glucose), and calcium levels. Serum cortisol levels for children normally range from 2 to 27 μg/dl and should exceed 20 μg/dl in a critically ill child or a child in shock.[5]

Stress doses of glucocorticoids are given as soon as possible after diagnostic laboratory samples are drawn and tests run. IV hydrocortisone is the usual drug of choice because it has both glucocorticoid and mineralocorticoid activity. If AI is present, one dose should produce an improvement in blood pressure and perfusion.[5] Additional hydrocortisone is then added to the IV infusion, and the dose is gradually tapered to physiologic levels over several days.

After stabilization, hospital admission is necessary. Consultation and follow-up with a pediatric endocrinologist is required for long-term management of replacement steroids.

NURSING CARE AND EVALUATION

Nursing care of the child with acute AI begins with assessment and stabilization of airway, breathing, and circulation. Children in shock or with altered mental status require oxygen therapy, cardiac monitoring, and frequent vital signs. Venous access is necessary to restore circulating volume and improve tissue perfusion. One or more boluses of 20 ml/kg of normal saline solution are administered as rapidly as possible. These are often followed by continuous infusions at an hourly rate of twice maintenance to correct the dehydration. The need for vasopressors should be anticipated.

Coexisting abnormalities or precipitating factors are treated rapidly. Hypoglycemia is corrected with 2 ml/kg of 25% dextrose, followed by a continuous infusion of 5% dextrose and saline solution. If infection is suspected, antibiotics are administered, pending the results of diagnostic tests.

Treatment of chronic AI includes oral or parenteral replacement of glucocorticoids and mineralocorti-

Female neonates with CAH have ambiguous genitalia and are usually diagnosed at birth, whereas the diagnosis in males is delayed until adrenal crisis or evidence of precocious genital development occurs. The salt-wasting form of CAH may result in adrenal crisis, with cortisol and aldosterone insufficiency in the first weeks of life, and must be treated emergently to prevent vascular collapse.

Children with chronic AI often have increased pigmentation over the entire body, particularly the pressure points, skin creases, nipples, buccal mucosa, and old scars. Infants may have increased pigmenta-

coids as needed and adequate salt and fluid intake. Glucocorticoid dosages are tripled during stressful situations, such as infections or surgery.

The child's response to fluid and cortisol replacement must be closely monitored. The nurse should observe the child for complications of overtreatment with saline solution and cortisol, such as ascending flaccid paralysis, and for signs of electrolyte abnormalities. The cardiovascular system is continuously evaluated, and seizure precautions are instituted.

The family should be encouraged to obtain a medical identification bracelet and to discuss the use of an emergency hydrocortisone kit with the pediatric endocrinologist.

▌SUMMARY

Children who come to the emergency department with an endocrine disorder may be undiagnosed or may be experiencing difficulty managing a previously diagnosed condition. These conditions can present as emergencies. Early identification, assisting with medical interventions, and performing ongoing assessment of the child's status are important nursing roles. In addition, the nurse provides emotional support and education for the child and parents and can refer them to available community resources.

REFERENCES

1. Buonocore CM, Robinson AG: The diagnosis and management of diabetes insipidus during medical emergencies, *Endocrinol Metabol Clin North Am* 22(2):411-424, 1993.
2. Burchfield DJ: Acute distress in the neonate and postnatal period. In Barkin RM, ed: *Pediatric emergency medicine: concepts and clinical practice,* St Louis, 1992, Mosby.
3. Fleckman AM: Diabetic ketoacidosis, *Endocrinol Metab Clin North Am* 22(2):181-208, 1993.
4. Haymond MW: Hypoglycemia in infants and children, *Endocrinol Metabol Clin North Am* 18:217-252, 1989.
5. Hazinski MF, Barkin RM: Shock. In Barkin RM, ed: *Pediatric emergency medicine: concepts and clinical practice,* St Louis, 1992, Mosby.
6. Johnson KB, ed: *The Harriet Lane handbook: a manual for pediatric house officers,* St Louis, 1993, Mosby.
7. Kaplan SA: *Clinical pediatric endocrinology,* Philadelphia, 1990, WB Saunders.
8. Laron Z, Karp M: Diabetes mellitus in children and adolescents. In Bertrand J, Rappaport R, Sizonenko PC, eds: *Pediatric endocrinology,* Baltimore, 1993, Williams & Wilkins.
9. Linares MY, Schunk JE, Lindsay R: Laboratory presentation in diabetic ketoacidosis and duration of therapy, *Pediatr Emerg Care* 12(5):347-351, 1996.
9a. Saladino RA: Endocrine and metabolic disorders. In Barkin RM, ed: *Pediatric emergency medicine: concepts and clinical practice,* ed 2, St Louis, 1997, Mosby.
10. Shane E: Differential diagnosis and acute management of hypocalcemic syndromes. In Favus M, ed: *Primer on the metabolic bone diseases and disorders of mineral metabolism,* Kelseyville CA, 1990, American Society for Bone and Mineral Research.
11. Siperstein MD: Diabetic ketoacidosis and hyperosmolar coma, *Endocrinol Metab Clin North Am* 21:415-432, 1992.
12. Sizonenko PC: Hypoglycemia. In Bertrand J, Rappaport R, Sizonenko PC, eds: *Pediatric endocrinology,* Baltimore, 1993, Williams & Wilkins.
13. Tohme JF, Bilezikian JP: Hypocalcemic emergencies, *Endocrinol Metab Clin North Am* 22(2):363-375, 1993.

CHAPTER 21

Multiple Trauma Management

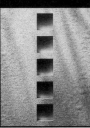

Kathy Haley

In 1993 over 12,000 children, aged 1 to 19 years, died as a result of trauma-related injuries, making trauma the leading cause of death during the childhood and adolescent years.[6,16,19] Regarded as a disease of epidemic proportion, trauma is fatal for approximately 35 American children daily.[16]

The product of pediatric trauma can be tragic and the impact on society staggering. Each year an estimated 600,000 injured children require hospitalization, accounting for almost 25% of all pediatric admissions. An estimated 30,000 children are left with permanent disability after an injury, and another 200,000 children are temporarily impaired.[4]

Pediatric trauma care is more costly than adult trauma care. The expense of hospitalization, the resources needed to mainstream a child back into society, and the years of potential work loss are staggering. The costs of unintentional pediatric injury in the United States are estimated to be between $3 and $7.5 billion annually.[11,19] By far, prevention is the most humane and cost-effective approach to care.

TRAUMA PREVENTION

Nurses play a pivotal role in injury prevention. After all, nurses who care for victims of trauma are well aware of the most common causes of traumatic injuries within their communities. As ambassadors, nurses can make a difference in injury prevention by sharing this information with community organizations, schools, and the media. Before developing a prevention activity the emergency department nurse should ask the following questions:

- How often does the injury occur?
- How much will the prevention strategy cost?
- What outcome can be expected for the money spent?
- Is the activity going to work?
- Is there an evaluation of the strategy?

PREVENTION INTERVENTIONS

There are numerous mechanisms of injury, each involving a set of factors that lead to potential injury. During the past several decades, Haddon et al. have stressed that a detailed evaluation of the events surrounding a specific injury reveals data critical for prevention efforts.[12,13] Subsequently, Haddon developed a matrix that separates the events surrounding an injury into three components, as follows: (1) primary prevention strategies, which are interventions designed to stop the injury-producing event; (2) secondary prevention strategies, which attempt to modify the seriousness of the event if it occurs; and (3) tertiary prevention mechanisms, which are designed to reduce the disability resulting from the injury such as making sure the child who is hurt is treated rapidly and appropriately (Table 21-1).

Using this approach, prevention strategies become more manageable and focused. Once a program is implemented, prevention activities should be measured for effectiveness. A discussion of several approaches follows.

Bicycle helmet use and safety. Approximately 5 million people are injured while riding bicycles each year, and of these, approximately 300 children will die.[16,25,27] Several communities have been successful in decreasing the number of head injuries associated with bicycle injures by increasing the use of helmets, and studies support these findings.[8,27,32] Prevention strategies implemented in the Seattle area used tools such as brochures, flyers, bicycle hang tags, and public service announcements and increased helmet use from 2% to 33%.[8,25]

TABLE 21-1	The Haddon Matrix				
				ENVIRONMENT	
	AGENT/VECTOR	HOST		PHYSICAL	SOCIAL
Primary prevention/ pre-event strategy	Child-proof bottle caps	Swimming lessons		Swimming pool fence	Child abuse prevention programs
Secondary prevention/ event strategy	Soft-surface playgrounds	Bicycle and motorcycle helmets		Breakaway roadside poles	Gun control laws that decrease the availability of handguns at times of disputes
Tertiary prevention/ post-event strategy	Mechanism for opening refrigerator doors from the inside	Teaching child about 911 service		Pediatric emergency medical service program	Universal insurance coverage for medical and rehabilitative services

From Eichelberger MR: *Pediatric trauma: prevention, acute care, rehabilitation,* St Louis, 1993, Mosby.

Window falls. Falls account for a significant number of pediatric emergency department visits each year. When those falls are from windows, serious injuries and possible death result. In New York City, falls from windows were a leading cause of death for children. As a result, a multifaceted prevention program was implemented and successfully lessened the number of deaths from window falls. The program included a community awareness campaign called "Children Can't Fly," legislation mandating window protection, and the installation of window guards free of charge.[23]

Safety seats/seat belts. Within the past 10 years, infant automobile safety seat and seat belt use has increased from 15% to more than 60%. This increase can be attributed to legislation for their mandatory use and increased availability of infant seats through car seat programs.[6,14] To overcome access barriers, many communities have developed loaner programs available through hospitals, clinics, and health departments to provide seats to low-income families. All 50 states have instituted legislation requiring the use of child restraint devices. Subsequently, the number of children injured in motor vehicle crashes has declined. Unfortunately, safety seat misuse rates remain high. The mandatory use of seat belts is required in all states and the District of Columbia.[29] A nationwide survey of adolescents, however, revealed that only 41% reported they wore a seat belt the last time they rode in a vehicle.[17]

Pedestrian safety. For children 5 to 9 years of age, pedestrian injuries are the single most common cause of traumatic death.[14] About 30% of all injuries occur while the child is in the crosswalk area. School safety programs for beginning school children provide an opportunity for role-playing the correct method for crossing streets. The effectiveness of such programs in producing behavior change is not overwhelming.

FUTURE INJURY PREVENTION

By far, the most cost-effective approach to trauma is prevention. The use of interventions that work must be widespread (Box 21-1). Nurses caring for injured children can teach prevention strategies by participating in patient education activities both in the community and within the emergency department.

Box 21-1   Effective Safety Strategies

- Infant car seats
- Smoke detectors
- Window guards
- Child-proof containers
- Pool enclosures
- Helmets
- Child passenger restraints

ETIOLOGY AND MECHANISMS OF PEDIATRIC TRAUMA

Pediatric trauma is not a random event, but rather a predictable sequela of potentially dangerous environments and human behavior. With the exception of mortality statistics, accurate data on the incidence of childhood injury are unavailable, since there is no single national surveillance source. Trauma centers, however, are required to maintain injury registries, and data from these sources have provided valuable information. Statistics indicate that the most common causes of childhood injury and death include falls, poisoning, motor vehicle crashes, bicycle-related injuries, firearms, burns, pedestrian injuries, drowning, and homicide.[4,6,19]

Common risk factors for childhood injury include age, behavior, and sex. Age, which reflects stages of development, is one of the most important factors and affects the patterns and frequency of injuries. Each developmental milestone is associated with specific injury risk factors (Table 21-2). Data also reveal that more males are injured than females. This is particularly true in the adolescent population, where adolescent males sustain more than two times the injuries of adolescent females.[3,6,20]

MECHANISMS OF INJURY

The mechanisms of pediatric trauma are classified as unintentional or intentional. Unintentional injuries account for about 75% of pediatric deaths, with the remaining 25% of injuries resulting from intentional trauma, usually related to violent acts such as homicide, suicide, and child maltreatment.[6]

Of all unintentional fatal injuries, which include automobile crashes, pedestrian injuries, falls, and burns,

TABLE 21-2	Developmental Age and Common Injuries	
DEVELOPMENTAL AGE GROUP	**GENERAL ANATOMIC DIFFERENCES**	**COMMON INJURIES**
Infants (0 to 12 months) Explore with mouth Increasing mobility such as rolling over, creeping, crawling; around 10 months, begin walking	Relatively large head in proportion to body Weak neck musculature and poor head control	Falls from furniture, stairs, etc. Ingestion (foreign bodies and poisons) Motor vehicle crashes
Toddlers (12 months to 3 years) Explore surroundings, curious Autonomy displayed by negative behavior Developing fine and gross motor abilities Magical thinking	Stronger neck muscles to support larger head Weak abdominal musculature and minimal body fat Compliant rib cage Pliable pelvis and protuberant bladder	Motor vehicle crashes Falls (frequently from stairs, windows, and play equipment) Burns, scalds (pulls hot items from counter) Near-drowning (pools, buckets, bathtubs) Poisonings Foreign body ingestion (peanuts, hot dogs, candy, toys)
School age (6 to 12 years) Increased gross and fine motor skills More independent Beginning risk-taking behavior Beginning sports activity	More proportionate head to torso Ribs less compliant	Pedestrian collisions Bicycle-related injuries Falls during play activities Near-drowning Violence-related injuries Sports injuries
Young adolescence (13 to 18 years) Strong peer relationship influences decision making regarding safety Experimentation with control (drugs, driving)	Physiologic and anatomic characteristics closer to adult; however, psychologic needs are different	Motor vehicle crashes Sports injuries Violence-related injuries Injuries related to drug/alcohol impairment Suicide

approximately 40% could have been prevented.[22] Therefore the use of the term *accidents* to describe the incident is discouraged, since it implies randomness and suggests that injuries are not preventable.

Motor vehicle crashes. Motor vehicle crashes are the leading cause of death in children over the age of 1 year.[16,19] Each day more than 20 children and adolescents die in motor vehicle–related incidents,

totalling approximately 8,000 children each year.[6,16] Many variables contribute to the seriousness of the injury, including use of seat belts, ejection from the vehicle, placement of impact, speed at impact, rollover, and death of another occupant. If the child is ejected from the vehicle, the risk of death is significantly greater. Side crashes are also associated with greater mortality because the occupant absorbs more direct energy.

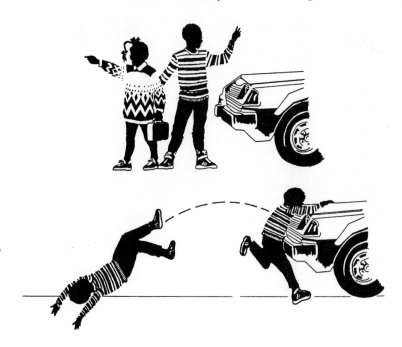

FIG. 21-1. Waddells' triad. A unique pattern of injuries results when a child is struck by a motor vehicle and is directly related to the site(s) of impact and the age and height of the child. Injuries include head trauma, lower extremity trauma, and abdominal trauma. Initially a lower extremity collides with the bumper, the torso may impact the hood or be thrown onto the vehicle, then there is contact with the front window, or the child may be thrown over the roof or to the side of the vehicle. The head usually impacts the pavement before the torso (From Hazinski MF ed: *Nursing care of the critically ill child,* ed 2, St Louis, 1992, Mosby.)

When a crash occurs, the restrained child initially collides against the restraint device. If the seat belt is worn incorrectly, the child is at risk for a pattern of injuries referred to as lap-belt injury. This combination of injuries includes laceration of solid or hollow organs and a lumbar fracture. When the child is unrestrained, the head usually comes in contact with the interior of the vehicle before the thorax or abdomen, resulting in significant head trauma.

Pedestrian/motor vehicle collisions. Pedestrian versus motor vehicle injuries are common in the pediatric population and accounted for the deaths of 1070 children and adolescents in 1994.[18] Children between the ages of 1 and 9 years are at highest risk of death or injury.[6,19]

Variables affecting the seriousness of the injuries include the speed of the vehicle, the site of impact, and the age and height of the child. A unique pattern of injuries called Waddell's triad is usually observed after a child versus motor vehicle collision; it includes head trauma, lower extremity trauma, and abdominal trauma. Initially a lower extremity collides with the bumper; the torso may impact the hood or be thrown onto the vehicle, followed by contact with the front window; or the child may be thrown over the roof or to the side of

the vehicle. The head usually impacts the pavement before the torso (Fig. 21-1).

Falls. Falls are a leading cause of nonfatal injury in the United States and a significant cause of unintentional death. Among children who fall from a distance greater than 10 to 15 feet, the most common body regions injured are the head and extremities. Injury to the extremities results when the arms and hands are extended to break a fall. Most head injuries occur as the body impacts the ground, head first.[15]

Infants and children who fall from heights less than 10 feet are unlikely to receive serious injury. There have been reports of children who sustained serious injury and death from falls of less than 5 feet. However, these cases were associated with an uncorroborated history and suspected child maltreatment.[31]

Farm machinery. Although the literature is replete with descriptions of urban injuries, there is little mention of rural or farm-related mechanisms. Farming is the only occupation where children are permitted to work with sophisticated heavy equipment at young ages. The single most dangerous activity on the farm is riding a tractor either alone or as a passenger. Most tractors weigh between 10,000 and 30,000

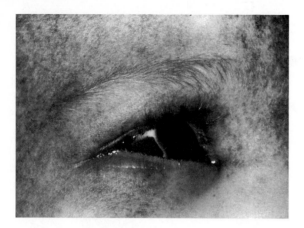

FIG. 21-2. Traumatic asphyxia with subconjunctival hemorrhage and facial petechiae after being run over by a tractor.

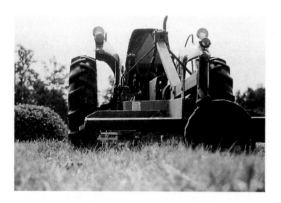

FIG. 21-3. Tractor with bush hog.

pounds. A child who falls from a tractor not only receives injuries from the fall of several feet, but he or she is often run over by the tractor's large wheels, which can result in traumatic asphyxia. This potentially fatal injury occurs exclusively in children. Other injuries can include pulmonary or cardiac contusion and laceration of the liver or spleen. The child may also be run over by equipment in tow, such as a mowing device, which can result in major tissue avulsion or death.

The child with traumatic asphyxia will be disoriented and exhibit varying symptoms of respiratory compromise immediately after the event. Later, symptoms include massive petechiae of the face, head, chest, and neck, and, most notably, subconjunctival hemorrhage (Figs. 21-2 and 21-3).

PREHOSPITAL CARE OF THE CHILD

PEDIATRIC TRAUMA TRAINING

Throughout the United States there are varying levels of trained prehospital care providers ranging from basic life support providers, usually referred to as emergency medical technicians (EMTs), to advanced life support providers, often referred to as emergency medical technicians-paramedics (EMT-Ps). Although titles and training vary, depending on area of the country, few generic programs offer comprehensive pediatric prehospital education. For example, the basic EMT course often devotes fewer than 10 hours of training to the care of ill or injured children, and the advanced EMT student may obtain 6 to 10 hours of pediatric training.[22] Recent initiatives have begun to address this issue as federally funded, emergency medical services for children (EMS-C) projects have developed numerous pediatric prehospital continuing education curriculas (see Chapter 1, The EMS System).

PREHOSPITAL ASSESSMENT

On arrival at the scene, and after the scene is secure for entry, a primary and secondary assessment is performed by the prehospital care provider. The priorities of field stabilization focus on identifying and treating immediate threats to life. The primary assessment begins with an evaluation of airway, breathing, and circulation with simultaneous immobilization of the cervical spine (Table 21-3). On completion of the primary survey, a secondary survey (head-to-toe assessment), including a full set of vital signs, is performed. If a historian/parent is available, a more detailed history is obtained. During transport, frequent reassessments for changes in status are required. When possible, a parent/caregiver should accompany the child to provide comfort and security.

ACCESS TO PEDIATRIC TRAUMA CARE

There are a limited number of pediatric trauma centers in the United States and their locations are often geographically disproportionate. Where time and distance factors preclude the child from being trans-

TABLE 21-3	Prehospital Initial Management of the Injured Child (Primary Survey)	
ABCs	**INTERVENTIONS**	**PEDIATRIC CONSIDERATIONS**
Airway (A)	Position child (neutral, in-line position with jaw thrust) Clear airway; suction debris Consider an oral airway for the unconscious child Apply pulse oximetry (optional) and cardiac monitor Apply a cervical collar (>1 year of age), towel rolls for the side of head, tape, straps, and backboard	Children have large tongues and small airways. Large occiput causes flexion of the head. Deciduous, or "baby teeth" are poorly anchored. Oral airway insertion can traumatize mucous membranes, induce bleeding, and further obstruct the airway when rotated on insertion.
Breathing (B)	Administer 100% oxygen via non-rebreather mask Ventilate using a bag-valve-mask device using 100% oxygen if respiratory effort is inadequate Intubate endotracheally when ongoing airway control is required	Oxygen is administered to all victims of pediatric trauma. When using a bag-valve-mask device, choose a small mask that fits securely to provide the least dead space and best seal. Oral intubation is preferred over nasal intubation; uncuffed tubes are used in children <8 years of age Proper endotracheal tube depth in children older than 2 yr can be estimated as follows: $$\frac{\text{Age (yr)}}{2} + 12$$
Circulation (C, control of shock)	Cricothyrotomy is rarely indicated—only for severe facial trauma, when an airway cannot be secured by any other means Apply pressure to external bleeding (control of ongoing hemorrhage) Establish venous access—2 routes, usually in the upper extremities or by intraosseous line in the tibia Monitor perfusion (capillary refill, central and peripheral pulses, skin temperature and color) Apply military antishock trousers (MAST) per protocol. (NOTE: these are not of proven benefit in children.)	Oxygen administration may be possible through the cricothyrotomy but ventilation is limited. Total circulating blood volume is significantly less for the child than the adult; therefore intravascular volume is rapidly lost with hemorrhage. The intraosseous route may be used in the unconscious child, but it is not indicated if the scene is within less than 5 minutes of the hospital (spend time with airway management); an infusion device may be required with an intraosseous line.

Continued.

TABLE 21-3	Prehospital Initial Management of the Injured Child (Primary Survey)—cont'd	
ABCs	**INTERVENTIONS**	**PEDIATRIC CONSIDERATIONS**
Circulation, *cont'd*		Signs of hypovolemia include capillary refill more than 2 seconds (unless the child is cold), tachycardia, weak or absent peripheral pulses, altered mental status.
		Treat hemorrhagic shock with 20 ml/kg boluses of lactated Ringer's or normal saline solution; additional boluses may be required.
Disability (D, neurologic status)	Assess neurologic status using AVPU or Glasgow Coma Scale; if increased ICP is suspected: hyperventilate per protocol	For signs of increased intracranial pressure, ventilate at 10 breaths per minute above normal for age.
		If coma score is less than 8 or decreases by more than 2 points, consider intubation.
Exposure (E)	Observe for hidden injuries Keep warm	Minimize heat loss by using blankets and warmed transport vehicle. Cover the child's head.

ported directly to a pediatric center, injured children may first be transported to an adult center for stabilization and later transferred to a pediatric tertiary care center. Alternatively, they may be sent to an adult trauma center with a commitment for pediatric intensive care monitoring and rehabilitation. Within these regions, standards defining triage criteria and interfacility transport are important components of the trauma system.

Although research continues to indicate that the care of the injured child differs from that of the adult—and the child should therefore be treated in a facility specializing in pediatric care—the definition of "child" varies from system to system. Age, size, and physiologic characteristics have all been used to define the pediatric patient; however, consensus among adult and pediatric physicians regarding a specific definition has not been reached. Suggested definitions include (1) the injured child 14 years of age or younger or (2) the injured child who is in the development cycle of birth through adolescence (birth to 18 years of age).

■ TRAUMA SCORING

Trauma scoring systems have been developed to provide both field and hospital personnel with a tool for evaluating the severity of injuries and facilitating primary or secondary transport of the injured child to the most appropriate facility. Although a number of injury severity scoring methods have been developed, few are specific to the pediatric patient (see Chapter 1).

Commonly used field scoring tools include the Trauma Score (TS) and the Revised Trauma Score (RTS), which requires the calculation of a Glasgow Coma Score (GCS). Because many hospital care providers lack experience in deriving a GCS for the nonverbal child, calculating the RTS score within a few seconds can be problematic. Consequently, other scoring methods such as the Pediatric Trauma Score (PTS) have been advocated for both field and hospital triage.

Other commonly used scores include the Abbrevi-

TABLE 21-4	Sample Scoring Systems		
SCORE	**DESCRIPTION**		**APPLICATION**
Abbreviated Injury Scale (AIS)	Based on anatomic injury using six body regions. Each injury receives a score of 1 to 6, with 6 usually representing fatal injury.		Scores are used to derive an ISS score. Used in both pediatric and adult trauma research.
Injury Severity Score (ISS)	Score is derived from the three highest AIS values, each squared (only one per body region). The sum score is the ISS. Scores range from 1 (least injury) to 75 (greatest injury). A score of more than 15 signifies significant pediatric trauma.		Scoring requires knowledge of AIS score. Used frequently in pediatric and adult trauma research.
Revised Trauma Score (RTS)	Uses three physiologic criteria to assess severity of patient's injury (respiratory rate, systolic blood pressure, GCS)		Developed for the adult patient but used for pediatric patients. Valuable for predicting survival among injured children.
Pediatric Trauma Score (PTS)	Includes six major components. The sum score is the PTS. Scores may range from −6 to +12. A lower score indicates a more serious injury and a lower predictability of survival.		Used both as an emergency department and a prehospital triage tool. A reliable predictor of outcome. The PTS can also be useful in mode of transport decisions. A score of less than 8 indicates need for trauma center.

ated Injury Scale (AIS) and the Injury Severity Score (ISS), which are used only after hospitalization. The AIS score rates anatomic injuries, but does not predict physiologic derangement. The ISS can be derived from the AIS to determine the cumulative effect of injuries to several body systems (Table 21-4).

PEDIATRIC TRAUMA SCORE

The PTS uses the child's size plus five physiologic parameters to determine injury severity and potential for morbidity and mortality. Total scores range from −6, the lowest, to +12, which is the highest score. Data reveal that children with scores less than or equal to 8 are at increased risk of morbidity and mortality. These children require more specialized equipment and personnel, beyond that initially available from many emergency departments.[1] For these reasons,

children with scores of 8 or less should be triaged to a pediatric trauma center or its equivalent (see Table 1–3).[1,26] For a complete discussion of scoring instruments, refer to Chapter 1, Emergency Medical Services for Children.

HOSPITAL MANAGEMENT OF THE PEDIATRIC TRAUMA VICTIM

PEDIATRIC TRAUMA AREA/EQUIPMENT

Whether the child is in an adult institution or a specialized pediatric hospital, appropriately sized pediatric equipment must be readily available to the trauma team to resuscitate injured children. Pediatric equipment that promises "one size fits all" is often misleading and usually not appropriate for all age groups. Correctly sized equipment and accessible storage are essential components of a pediatric trauma resuscitation area (see Boxes 1-5 and 1-6, p. 12).

PEDIATRIC TRAUMA TEAM

The arrival of any trauma victim to an emergency department can result in chaos which can be further compounded if the victim is a child. Because the child's condition can deteriorate rapidly, there is little time for deliberation of care or organization of equipment. Initial management therefore requires a well-organized, well-trained team activated by a predetermined plan with clearly established roles and guidelines for management.

To meet these goals, most institutions have developed trauma teams using a tiered alert system. With this approach, a full complement of personnel is summoned to care for a seriously injured child, and a less comprehensive team is called to care for the child with less complex injuries. Criteria for team activation are determined by rapid evaluation of the child's symptoms, mechanism of injury, and other relevant historical data—usually conveyed by transport personnel. On notification of the child's impending arrival, the appropriate team is notified by a variety of methods, including beepers and/or in-house announcements. Using the tiered response system, cost-effective trauma care can be delivered by avoiding the unnecessary disruption of routine activities of key hospital personnel.

Trauma team composition varies from institution to institution, ranging from as few as three team members to as many as 20. Regardless of team size, each member is assigned clearly delineated roles that reflect the qualifications and competencies required to assess and resuscitate the injured child.

Team leader. The qualifications of the trauma team leader vary from institution to institution and depend on the level of trauma care offered and the skills of the medical staff available. Ideally, medical staff serving as team leaders must demonstrate competency in trauma procedures and should have attended pediatric continuing medical education programs, including courses such as Pediatric Advanced Life Support, Advanced Pediatric Life Support, and Advanced Trauma Life Support.

Responsibilities of the team leader include directing the resuscitation and may include performing the primary and secondary assessments. Ideally the team leader collaborates with other critical care experts, such as emergency medicine physicians, or pediatric critical care specialists during the resuscitation. Ultimately the role of the surgical team leader is to provide definitive surgical intervention and direct trauma care throughout the child's entire hospitalization.

Nursing roles. Trauma nurses play a pivotal role in accessing equipment, assisting with rapid assessment, and coordinating the team. Emergency department nurses usually fill the trauma nurse role; however, other models include nurses from pediatric intensive care units, operating rooms, or transport teams.

Usually one or two nurses function within the core area (area closest to the patient). One model advocates a nurse on the left and another on the right, each working collaboratively with a physician. Some systems place only one nurse at the bedside with a circulating nurse outside the core group.

Additional roles may include a liaison nurse, drug nurse, operating room nurse, and recorder. The role of the liaison nurse is to serve as a communication link between the emergency department and other departments. Additional responsibilities include crowd control, since pediatric trauma can draw many observers.

When surgical intervention is anticipated, the presence of an operating room nurse is useful to facilitate rapid transfer to the surgical area. Some trauma centers or emergency departments include a medication nurse on the trauma team, while others use pharmacists to draw up medication, provide saline flushes, and calculate drug dosages.

Documentation is crucial; therefore one nurse is assigned to the sole task of recording. Some trauma centers place critical care nurses in this role to facilitate continuity of care from the emergency department to a critical care unit.

NURSING CARE OF THE INJURED CHILD

In recent years the specialty of both adult and pediatric trauma nursing has evolved although pediatric trauma nursing has evolved more slowly than for adults. With this evolution has come the development of many local and national pediatric emergency nursing educational programs. The most widely recognized national program was completed by the Emergency Nurses Association in 1993 and is called the Emergency Nurse Pediatric Course (ENPC). This course is designed to teach emergency nurses core pediatric emergency nursing, including trauma. The results of these educational efforts have lead to improved nursing care for the injured child.

PARENTAL PRESENCE

The nature of a traumatic event automatically places the child and family in crisis. The child's dependency on the caregiver and the caregiver's desire to meet the child's psychologic needs further exacerbate the crisis. Because the child is part of a family unit, recovery is not only the result of trauma team assessment and interventions, but also a result of support from loved ones.

When caring for an injured child, health care professionals must recognize the family in crisis and consider the needs of both child and parent. For this reason, more and more emergency departments allow parents to remain at their child's bedside during resuscitative efforts. When parents choose to be present, they should be adequately prepared and accompanied by a team member. Ideally, they should be positioned near the child's head or near enough for the child to confirm their presence.

PRIMARY AND SECONDARY SURVEYS

Any injured child must be considered at risk of dying; thus the objective of the initial phase of care is the rapid assessment and stabilization of life-threatening injuries. This systematic, standardized approach is called the primary survey. The secondary survey follows and more completely evaluates the extent of the child's injuries and establishes baseline values such as vital signs. Although the algorithm (ABCs of the primary and secondary survey) requires a step-by-step approach, in reality the trauma team initiates many of these interventions simultaneously.

The principles of the primary and secondary surveys are the same for both children and adults. The components of the pediatric primary survey include assessment of the airway, breathing, circulation, disability, and immobilization of the cervical spine. This survey should take no more than several minutes unless interventions become complex. The secondary survey includes obtaining a more complete history, taking a complete set of vital signs, and performing a complete head-to-toe assessment (Box 21-2).

Box 21-2 Primary and Secondary Trauma Survey

Primary survey: to identify and treat immediate threats to life
Airway with cervical spine immobilization
Breathing
Circulation
Disability (neurologic status)

Secondary survey: to obtain a more thorough history and assessment
Expose
Fahrenheit (institute methods to maintain body heat)
Get vital signs
History (CIAMPEDS)
Head-to-toe assessment
Inspect the back

AIRWAY (A)

Anatomy. The first priorities of pediatric trauma care are the assessment of airway patency and immobilization of the cervical spine. Airway obstruction is the most frequent source of ventilatory insufficiency in the pediatric trauma victim and the simplest problem to correct. When not identified, an airway obstruction can be fatal.

Children are at higher risk for airway obstructions than adults because of differences in airway anatomy and physiology; these differences have implications for stabilization. Nasal and oral passages are small in children, so minimal airway edema and/or secretions, will create a disproportionately higher resistance to the flow of air. The pediatric trachea is soft and compliant, resulting in airway obstruction with excessive flexion or hyperextension of the head (as might occur with improper head-tilt positioning). The relatively large occiput of the young child can produce neck flexion and airway obstruction—as the head tilts forward—when the child is placed in a supine position. The tongue is relatively large in proportion to the small oral cavity and naturally falls back into the oropharynx when the child is unconscious, obstructing the airway. Finally, mucous membranes are delicate and easily traumatized, even by simple efforts such as airway insertion, increasing the risk of airway edema and obstruction.

Additional airway differences include the positioning of the vocal cords (glottic opening) and cricoid ring and the length of the trachea. In young children the glottic opening is relatively high and anterior, making endotracheal tube insertion through the cords more difficult. The narrowest portion of the child's airway (in children less than 8 years of age) is at the cricoid ring, below the vocal cords. This means that an adequate seal can be obtained around uncuffed endotracheal tubes. In children older than 8 years of age and in adults, the glottic opening is the narrowest portion of the airway, requiring the use of cuffed endotracheal tubes. In the child less than 8 years of age, the insertion of an endotracheal tube that is too large or inflated places that child at risk for airway trauma, which can lead to subglottic stenosis.

The shorter trachea of the child requires the endotracheal tube be passed only 2 to 3 cm below the vocal cords. Beyond this point, bronchial intubation will result. Additionally, because of the short airway, the endotracheal tube can easily become displaced with slight movements—such as transferring the child from a stretcher to a bed.

Assessment. Assessment of the injured child for airway patency includes observing the airway for obvious signs of obstruction such as blood, mucus, or foreign bodies. Airway and ventilation are evaluated for signs of respiratory distress or failure that may be caused by an airway obstruction or other etiology (e.g., increasing intracranial pressure resulting from head trauma). Signs of respiratory distress caused by injury or obstruction of the pulmonary system may include nasal flaring, tachypnea, tachycardia, retractions, use of accessory muscles with or without retractions, stridor, and extreme agitation. Signs of respiratory failure include decreasing or absent breath sounds and/or respiratory rate, decreased response to pain, poor muscle tone, and decreased level of consciousness.

Interventions. The goal of airway management in the injured child is to provide a patent airway for optimal oxygenation while maintaining cervical spine immobilization. Interventions depend on the seriousness of the child's injuries and the degree of airway impairment.

In the alert, conscious child who is able to talk with normal phonation and shows no signs of airway obstruction, the only airway intervention may be the administration of supplemental oxygen. The same is true for an infant with a normal-pitched cry or good eye contact, normal vital signs, and no signs of respiratory distress.

If the infant or child is breathing spontaneously but has an altered level of consciousness, interventions include opening the airway by means of the jaw-thrust procedure while maintaining cervical spine immobilization; suctioning the mouth for secretions; administering supplemental oxygen by nonrebreather mask; and continuously reassessing ventilatory and neurologic status. A history of head trauma with suspected increased intracranial pressure requires that the child receive bag-valve-mask (BVM) ventilation and be hyperventilated.

The infant or child with no spontaneous ventilations, signs of respiratory failure, and/or signs of increased intracranial pressure requires emergency airway interventions, including positioning the airway using the jaw-thrust maneuver, directly observing the mouth for foreign bodies or secretions, suctioning as indicated, inserting an oral or nasal airway to maintain airway patency as needed ventilating with a BVM device and 100% oxygen, and preparing for intubation. Continuous assessments of vital signs, neurologic status, and the child's response to ventilatory efforts are required. A nasogastric tube is inserted to decompress the stomach, which may become distended during BVM ventilation. If head trauma or significant facial trauma is present, an orogastric tube is indicated.

Airway adjuncts such as an oral or nasal airway (the latter sometimes referred to as a nasal trumpet) can be used to maintain airway patency. Oral airways are used to displace the tongue, allowing unobstructed ventilation during BVM ventilation in the unconscious child and after intubation. The size of the oral airway is determined by measuring from the posterior tip of the earlobe to the corner of the mouth. Unlike the insertion of an oral airway in an adult, the rigid plastic airway is inserted directly using a tongue blade to depress the tongue. Rotation of the airway can produce trauma to the teeth and soft tissues of the mouth and pharynx.

Nasopharyngeal airways are inserted through the nose into the posterior pharynx. They are made of soft rubber and used in conscious children with an intact gag reflex. The diameter of the tube should be slightly smaller than the diameter of the nares, and length should equal the distance from the nares to the tragus of the ear.

Intubation. Endotracheal intubation is indicated in any child who cannot maintain airway control and/or oxygenation and ventilation (Box 21-3). Orotracheal intubation, rather than nasotracheal intubation, is preferred in the child for several reasons.

Box 21-3 Indications for Intubation

- Respiratory arrest
- Respiratory failure (hypoventilation, hypoxia despite supplemental oxygen therapy)
- To bypass direct airway obstruction caused by airway or facial trauma
- Coma: GCS or modified Pediatric Coma Score of 8 or less
- Prolonged ventilatory support indicated
- Electively when anticipated that the sequelae of the child's injuries may potentially obstruct the airway (e.g., burns)

From Chameides L, Hazinski MF: Trauma resuscitation. In *Textbook of pediatric advanced life support,* Dallas, 1994, American Heart Association.

Box 21-4 Methods for Choosing an Endotracheal Tube Size

- Use of a Broselow Resuscitation Tape
- Diameter of the child's little finger
- Diameter of the child's nares
- Use of the formula 16 + age (years) divided by 4 = size.

NOTE: These methods only *estimate* proper tube sizes. Endotracheal tubes 0.5 mm smaller and larger than the estimated size should be readily available.

First, the unique anterior position of the glottic opening makes rapid nasotracheal intubation—with simultaneous stabilization of the cervical spine—extremely difficult and time-consuming. Second, the narrow nasal passages and fragile, vascular adenoid tissue are easily traumatized during emergency intubation attempts. Nasotracheal intubation is contraindicated in the child with craniofacial trauma.

Before intubation, all equipment is assembled, including correctly sized endotracheal tubes (Box 21-4). The child is then preoxygenated for at least 2 to 3 minutes with BVM ventilation and 100% oxygen. This procedure improves oxygen stores that are more rapidly depleted in the child than in the adult. Because of the potential for cervical spine injury, the child's neck remains in a neutral position throughout the procedure. As the child is intubated, the heart rate is continuously monitored, since hypoxia or stimulation of the airway may cause bradyarrhythmias. If bradycardia occurs (pulse less than 60 beats per minute), the intubation attempt is temporarily aborted and the child oxygenated with a bag-valve device and 100% oxygen. During the intubation, pressure on the cricoid (Sellick maneuver) can be used to decrease the risk of regurgitation and subsequent aspiration and to facilitate visualization of the laryngeal structures. Intubation of the trachea is confirmed by clinical assessment parameters, including bilateral, equal breath sounds; bilateral, equal chest rise; absent breath sounds over the stomach; condensation in the endotracheal tube; and improvement in color and perfusion—in the absence of shock. Endotracheal tube placement can also be evaluated using an end-tidal CO_2 detector in children weighing more than 2 kg.

Rapid-sequence induction. A combination of pharmacologic agents, referred to as rapid-sequence induction, may be required to facilitate the safe insertion of an endotracheal tube when the infant or child is alert or semiconscious, gagging, coughing, or clenching the teeth. Rapid-sequence induction is also indicated in the head-injured, agitated child to prevent further increases in intracranial pressure and in the child with an altered GCS who is at increased risk for aspiration secondary to a full stomach.

Pharmacologic agents include the administration of a short-acting neuromuscular relaxant and a sedative. Atropine sulfate is administered to decrease the risk of bradyarrhythmias. Rapid-sequence intubation should only be performed by personnel who are properly training and skilled in advanced airway management (see Chapter 6, Respiratory Failure and Shock, which outlines the technique for rapid-sequence induction, p. 111).

Cricothyroidotomy. Although rarely indicated in pediatric trauma victims, a needle cricothyroidotomy may be performed when intubation is unsuccessful. Since anatomic landmarks for this procedure are difficult to identify in the short, thick necks of infants and young children, this procedure is difficult to perform. Needle cricothyroidotomy is considered a temporary measure, since maintaining normocarbia is difficult because of the small diameter of the needle (Fig. 21-4). Surgical cricothyroidotomy is rarely required, and should only be performed by medical personnel with experience in the technique.

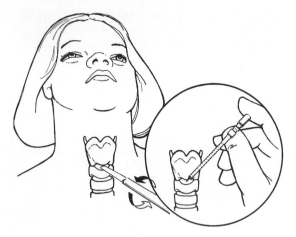

FIG. 21-4. Emergency cricothyroidotomy techniques with either a scalpel or a plastic cannula needle.

CERVICAL SPINE IMMOBILIZATION

Anatomy. Cervical spine injuries are less common in children than adults; however, any pediatric trauma patient has the potential for a cervical spine injury. Several anatomic differences impact the type of cervical spine injuries children sustain. For example, relatively weak neck musculature, a disproportionately large head, and greater cervical ligamentous flexibility result in greater stress, allowing increased neck motion when exposed to acceleration-deceleration forces. For these reasons, the most common spinal cord injuries include the cervical spine, usually through C3. Other common injuries include spinal cord injury without radiographic abnormality (SCIWORA) and ligamentous dislocation injuries. Although anatomic and physiologic features of injuries begin to change around 8 years of age, adult characteristics of injuries are usually not manifested until the age of 15 years (see Chapter 22, Trauma Selected Systems).

Assessment. Any victim of pediatric trauma who has a suspected neck injury, head injury, or history suspicious of head and/or neck injury is at risk of having a cervical spine injury. During the primary survey, both airway management and manual in-line cervical immobilization are performed simultaneously. A more thorough assessment for cervical spine injury is included in the secondary survey.

Stabilization. Immobilizing the conscious uncooperative child can be difficult even for the most skilled pediatric care provider. Younger children have short attention spans, do not like to be held down or immobilized, and cannot be relied on to hold their head still on command. For these reasons, spinal immobilization devices, towels and tape, and adequate personnel are essential. The position of the child's head for cervical spine immobilization is neutral and in-line.

Correctly sizing spinal immobilization equipment for the child is frequently difficult because of the child's unique anatomy. When placed on a backboard in the prone position, the young child's large occiput naturally produces neck flexion, placing the child at risk of further injury. To avoid this flexion, padding is placed under the child's shoulders, facilitating neutral alignment. Cervical collars, even though they are available in various sizes, including "no neck" options, must be sized correctly. Collars that are too small or too large may allow flexion or extension of the neck, causing further cervical spine injury. Collar size is determined by measuring the width from the top of the shoulder to the chin when the head is in the neutral position. A correctly sized collar rests on the shoulders while the chin is held in alignment. In addition to the cervical collar, towel rolls or commercially available devices are usually required to prevent movement of the head from side to side (Fig. 21-5).

Since movement above the waist can jeopardize in-line immobilization of the cervical spine, the child should be secured to a backboard with tape and/or transport straps placed at the shoulders, hips, and above the knees. The cervical collar is left in place until the physician has thoroughly evaluated the patient and cleared the cervical spine.

BREATHING

Anatomy. Once the airway is secured, ventilatory effectiveness is assessed. The ribs of the child are more compliant than those of the adult, and fractures are less common. Significant underlying injuries, for example, a pulmonary contusion, may be present, however, because the elastic thorax more readily transmits kinetic energy to underlying structures. In addition, the child's relatively mobile mediastinum predisposes him or her to rapid cardiovascular and ventilatory compromise when the lungs are compressed and the heart is displaced, as occurs with a tension pneumothorax.

The metabolic rate of the child is higher than that of the adult, and oxygen demands are two to three times greater. Increased respiratory effort associated

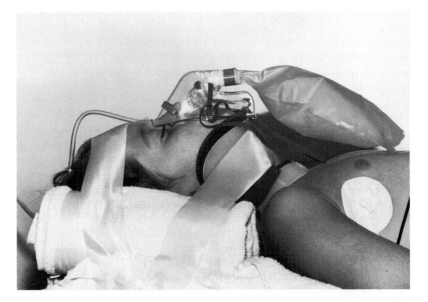

FIG. 21-5. Cervical spine immobilization. With a hard cervical collar in place, the patient's head is taped to a backboard. Linen rolls prevent lateral movement of the head. (From Hazinski MF ed: *Nursing care with the critically ill child,* ed 2, St Louis 1992, Mosby.)

with pulmonary injuries and/or hypoxia is poorly tolerated and rapidly leads to fatigue.

The diaphragm and abdominal musculature are the primary muscles used for breathing, and pulmonary capacity is limited. When gastric distention results from air swallowing (aerophagia), as may occur in the crying child or during BVM ventilation, the upward pressure on the diaphragm can impair effective ventilation.

Assessment. Ventilatory effectiveness is assessed by evaluating the following:
- Spontaneous respirations and rate of respirations
- Respiratory effort (use of accessory muscles, retractions, grunting, nasal flaring)
- The neck veins for distention or tracheal deviation (less pronounced in young children and infants)
- Chest wall integrity and evidence of trauma
- Symmetry of chest movement
- Skin color and neurologic status for signs of hypoxia (pale, dusky, or cyanotic skin color; irritability, agitation, or decreased level of consciousness)

Respiratory failure can be present even if the child shows no signs of increasing respiratory distress (e.g., retractions). For example, the child with a serious head injury may hypoventilate as a direct result of the cerebral insult. Therefore when a child exhibits signs

of hypoxia, including pale, dusky, or mottled skin, an altered mental status, and/or a decreased response to pain, respiratory failure is imminent. Cyanosis is not relied on to make the diagnosis of respiratory failure because it is considered a late finding in the child, since infants and young children are relatively anemic, compared to adults, and cyanosis is not evident until 5 g/dl of hemoglobin is desaturated. Therefore up to 50% of the child's blood must be desaturated before cyanosis will be evident.

Next, the chest is auscultated for bilateral breath sounds at the apices and bases and palpated for crepitus. The adequacy of breath sounds may be difficult to assess because sounds are easily transmitted through the child's thin chest wall. Diminished breath sounds and unequal movement of the chest are life-threatening conditions that require immediate interventions.

Interventions. Respiratory interventions vary, depending on assessment findings. The spontaneously breathing child with no symptoms of respiratory distress requires 100% oxygen by a nonrebreather mask until completion of the secondary survey or re-evaluation indicates termination of need. Suctioning is indicated if secretions are present.

When signs of respiratory distress are present, the airway is positioned and supplemental oxygen administered. If the child continues to exhibit signs of respiratory compromise, assisted or controlled ventilation with a BVM device and reservoir delivering 100% oxygen is initiated. Masks must be appropriately sized, fitting firmly on the face so as to create a seal and lessen dead space. The mask should cover both the nose and mouth, extending from the bridge of the nose to the cleft of the chin. Clear masks are ideal because they permit the visualization of any material that can obstruct the airway, as may occur with emesis.

Two types of assisted breathing devices are used in the pediatric population: self-inflating bags and anesthesia ventilation bags. Self-inflating bags have a recoil that allows the bag to refill independent of inflow from a gas source. Some are equipped with a pop-off valve, but when they are used for resuscitation, the pop-off valve is not recommended because lung compliance may be decreased and/or airway resistance may be high, activating the pop-off valve and allowing air to escape. Insufficient tidal volume results.[5] Tidal volume administered during assisted ventilation is approximately 10 to 15 ml/kg and is evaluated by the rise and fall of the chest.[5]

Anesthesia ventilation devices require more experience and equipment. The bag requires gas flow for inflation, while the pop-off valve requires adjustment to maintain gas volume in the reservoir and permit the outflow of exhaled gases (see Chapter 8, Pediatric and Neonatal Resuscitation, p. 154).

Even with ventilatory adjuncts, effective respirations may be impaired by gastric distention caused by aerophagia, aggressive ventilation by BVM, or an intubation air leak around the endotracheal tube. A nasogastric or orogastric tube is inserted to decompress the stomach, thus decreasing the risk of aspiration and lessening the pressure on the diaphragm. An orogastric tube is used with maxillofacial trauma, if a basilar skull fracture is present, or if there is a high index of suspicion to avoid insertion of the tube into the intracranial space.

If the child has continued respiratory distress, unequal breath sounds, and signs of hypovolemic shock, a pneumothorax, hemothorax, or tension pneumothorax must be suspected. Neck veins may be distended or flat. Interventions include the delivery of oxygen, possible needle thoracostomy, and preparation for chest tube placement. A needle thoracostomy is a rapid, temporary method of relieving a tension pneumothorax. Usually a 14- or 16-gauge needle is inserted into the second intercostal space in the midclavicular line, and air or fluid is drawn back into a syringe. A chest tube is later inserted using 20 cm H_2O pressure for children and 10 cm H_2O for infants (Box 21-5).[24]

Box 21-5 Chest Tube Sizes (French)	
Infant	10 to 14
Child (age 1 to 3 years)	16 to 20
School-aged child (age 4 to 7 years)	20 to 24
School-aged child (age 8 to 12 years)	28 to 32
Teenager	28 French or larger

Box 21-6 Circulating Blood Volume	
Age	Circulating blood volume (ml/kg)
Neonate	85 to 90
Infant	75 to 80
Children	70 to 75
Adult	65 to 70

Massive hemothorax is rare in children because most pulmonary lacerations are self-sealing. If the chest is dull to percussion, the neck veins are flat, breath sounds are absent on the affected side, and signs of shock are present, immediate fluid resuscitation is indicated followed by a tube thoracostomy. A sudden drainage of the pleural space can alter pleural pressure, permit further bleeding, and lead to cardiovascular collapse. Exsanguinating hemorrhage via the tube thoracostomy may require clamping of the chest tube in an attempt to tamponade bleeding. Continued deterioration after these interventions is an indication of severe chest and/or cardiac trauma.

CIRCULATION

Anatomy. Once the airway and breathing are stabilized, circulatory status is assessed. Underlying injuries can lead to significant blood loss even though there may be no obvious bleeding. Of all of the types of shock, hypovolemic shock is the most common in the injured child.

The child's circulatory system differs from the adult in several ways. The child's circulating blood volume is small compared to the adult, and functional capacity of the heart is limited (Box 21-6). However, the child is better able to physiologically compensate for volume loss than the adult. When volume loss occurs, tachycardia and peripheral vasoconstriction maintain car-

TABLE 21-5	Classification of Hemorrhagic Shock in Pediatric Trauma Patients Based on Systemic Signs			
SYSTEM	VERY MILD HEMORRHAGE (<15% BLOOD VOLUME LOSS)	MILD HEMORRHAGE (15% TO 25% BLOOD VOLUME LOSS)	MODERATE HEMORRHAGE (25% BLOOD VOLUME LOSS)	SEVERE HEMORRHAGE (40% BLOOD VOLUME LOSS)
Cardiovascular	Heart rate normal or mildly increased	Tachycardia	Significant tachycardia	Severe tachycardia
	Normal pulses	Peripheral pulses may be diminished	Thready peripheral pulses	Thready central pulses
	Normal blood pressure	Normal blood pressure	Hypotension	Significant hypotension
	Normal pH	Normal pH	Metabolic acidosis	Significant acidosis
Respiratory	Rate normal	Tachypnea	Moderate tachypnea	Severe tachypnea
Central nervous system	Slightly anxious	Irritable, confused	Irritability or lethargy	Lethargy
		Combative	Diminished pain response	Coma
Skin	Warm, pink	Cool extremities, mottling	Cool extremities, mottling or pallor	Cold extremities, pallor or cyanosis
	Capillary refill brisk	Delayed capillary refill	Prolonged capillary refill	
Kidneys	Normal urine output	Oliguria, increased specific gravity	Oliguria, increased blood urea nitrogen	Anuria

Modified from American College of Surgeons: *Advanced trauma life support course,* Chicago, 1989, American College of Surgeons; Fleisher GR, Ludwig S: *Textbook of pediatric emergency medicine,* ed 2, Baltimore, 1988, Williams & Wilkins; Soud T, Pieper P, Hazinski MF: Pediatric trauma. In Hazinski MF: *Nursing care of the critically ill child,* ed 2, St Louis, 1992, Mosby.

diac output, and therefore blood pressure, until blood loss is significant. Cardiac output is almost completely dependent on the heart rate, not stroke volume, until the heart has reached adult proportions.

Assessment. The circulatory assessment includes observation of the child's general appearance, color, and mental status. The child with adequate circulation responds to the environment appropriately for age, recognizes his or her parents, has a capillary refill time of less than 2 seconds, and has a normal pulse for age.

Signs of circulatory compromise may be observed immediately or may evolve gradually. They include tachycardia, decrease in the intensity of peripheral pulses, delayed capillary refill, pallor, mottled skin, and an altered mental status (Table 21-5).

Although cardiac tamponade is rare in children, it can be life-threatening. Because of the limited volume within the pericardial sac, tamponade will occur with smaller accumulations of air or fluid. The classic pulsus paradoxus is difficult to measure in the child, and Beck's triad (rising venous pressure, falling arterial pressure, and a small, quiet heart) is not often evident.

Interventions. Interventions for impaired circulation depend on the degree of compromise but always include providing supplemental oxygenation as well as ventilation when indicated. Additional interventions include controlling external bleeding, establishing vascular access, and providing fluid resuscitation. Direct pressure to active bleeding sites promotes hemostasis. A common site of significant bleeding that is sometimes overlooked or considered insignificant is the scalp.

In the pulseless child or the child with an inadequate pulse, cardiac compressions are indicated. Although a child may have central pulses and an apical heart beat, peripheral pulses may be absent; therefore they should always be assessed. Chest compressions are indicated in any child with a heart rate less than 60 beats per minute associated with poor systemic perfusion.

Vascular access. Achieving vascular access in the child can be difficult even for the most skilled nurse. Rapid percutaneous catheterization is easiest at the antecubital fossa; however, other sites may be used. As vascular access is being obtained, blood is drawn for laboratory analysis. Insertion of two large-bore catheters is ideal; however, once a single line is achieved, fluid resuscitation begins immediately (Box 21-7).

Because peripheral vascular access can be difficult to obtain in the child, particularly when volume-depleted (one study indicated that vascular access took 10 minutes or more in 24% of the pediatric arrest victims studied and that intravascular access was never accomplished in 6% of these patients[21]), an alternative route to peripheral vascular access may be required. Intraosseous infusion, central venous infusion, or cut-downs may be started. Central venous access, although commonly used for adults, is more difficult, is more time-consuming, and poses a greater risk of complications in the young child. Cut-downs are time-consuming and difficult for a practitioner unskilled in the technique to perform. Therefore when peripheral vascular access cannot be obtained in the unconscious child within three attempts or in less than 90 seconds, intraosseous (IO) infusion is indicated. Using the IO route, fluid, blood, and/or drugs are infused directly into the bone marrow cavity.

IO infusion, first described as a clinical technique by Tocantins in 1940,[28] is being used for ill and injured children in the prehospital and the hospital setting.

There are few contraindications to the insertion of an IO needle. These include (1) the insertion of the needle into a recently fractured bone and (2) the insertion of the needle into a bone in which a needle has previously been inserted because fluids or medications may extravasate into the subcutaneous tissue. The presence of a bone disorder such as osteogenesis imperfecta is a relative contraindication.

The site most recommended is the anterior medial aspect of the tibia 2 to 3 cm below the proximal tibial tuberosity (Fig. 21-6). This site provides a flat, easily accessible area away from significant structures such as blood vessels and nerves. An alternate site is the distal third of the femur; however, the bone is round, making insertion more difficult, especially in the older child.

Inserting an IO line is a relatively simple, safe procedure that could mean the difference between life and death for a child. After site selection the skin is prepared with an antiseptic solution and penetrated with a disposable bone marrow aspiration needle (18-gauge for children less than 6 months of age; 15-

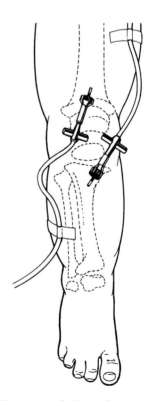

Fig. 21-6. Recommended sites for an intraosseous infusion.

Box 21-7 Suggested Catheter Size for Percutaneous Cannulation		
Infant	20 to 22 g	
Young child	18 to 20 g	
Older child	16 to 18 g	

or 16-gauge for children older than 6 months of age). The needle is directed perpendicular to the bone or at a slight 45-degree angle away from the epiphyseal plate. With firm, downward pressure the needle is turned, using a rotating boring motion. Entrance into the medullary cavity is signified by a pop and/or lack of resistance. The inner stylet is removed, and aspiration of bone marrow confirms placement. The needle should be firmly upright in the extremity. A conventional intravenous set with an infusion pump is connected and fluid resuscitation begun. The needle is taped in place, and the site is observed for extravasation of fluid or complications.

Fluid resuscitation. Fluid resuscitation begins with the administration of a 20 ml/kg fluid bolus of lactated Ringer's or normal saline solution. A syringe and stopcock placed closest to the insertion site will facilitate the rapid administration of fluids to small children. If the fluid bolus is effective, reassessment of the child's circulatory system will reveal clinical improvement evidenced by improved heart rate, mental status, peripheral pulses, and capillary refill time. If little or no improvement is evident, a second fluid bolus is indicated.

With continued signs of ongoing blood loss and impaired perfusion, blood and/or blood products are required. When the child's specific blood type is unknown or unavailable, 10 ml/kg of O-negative packed red blood cells (PRBCs) can be administered. If clinical appearance does not improve after the administration of 40 ml/kg of blood, ongoing bleeding should be suspected and surgical intervention anticipated. Fluid warming devices are used on all fluids and blood products administered to children.

Pneumatic antishock garments (PASG) have not been effective in the treatment of hypovolemic shock related to trauma except in cases involving unstable pelvic fractures.[3,5] Recent studies suggest that PASGs are not useful in the management of shock associated with pediatric blunt trauma and that they offer no survival benefit for most children with profound hypotension.[3,5,9]

DISABILITY (BRIEF NEUROLOGIC ASSESSMENT)

Anatomy. A neurologic assessment is performed in both the primary and secondary assessment to identify an alternating mental status, which may reflect shock, respiratory failure, and/or a serious head injury.

Head injuries are responsible for 70% of all traumatic deaths in children[2] and are classified as primary or secondary injuries. The primary injury results from the initial event, such as contusion, laceration, edema, and shifting of vault contents. Secondary injuries caused by hypoxia, hypercarbia, intracranial hypertension, and/or ischemia can occur minutes, hours, or even days after the initial injury.

Children are at greater risk of developing increased intracranial pressure after a head injury than adults; however, infants and young children are better able to tolerate these increases because the cranial sutures are not fused and the thin skull is more compliant. In children under 2 years of age; however, myelinization of the brain is incomplete, increasing the susceptibility of neural tissue to traumatic injury (see Chapter 22, Trauma—Selected Systems).

Assessment. The primary neurologic assessment in the child includes an evaluation of pupil size and reaction, the child's level of consciousness, and the child's activity level. The level of consciousness and activity level reflect perfusion and oxygenation of the brain, whereas pupillary changes reflect an increasing intracranial pressure.[7,30]

The AVPU mnemonic and the GCS are used to provide clear descriptions of a child's neurologic status (Box 21-8). The AVPU scale is a rapid neurologic evaluation that is useful during the initial assessment. The GCS is used during the initial assessment and for ongoing neurologic evaluation to identify changes in neurologic status. A decreasing GCS may reflect such injuries as an intracranial hemorrhage, cerebral edema, or impending herniation. The GCS, originally designed for use in adults, has been adapted for use in nonverbal infants and young children and is referred to as the Pediatric (or modified) Glasgow Coma Scale

---

Box 21-8 AVPU

A = The child is **A**lert.
V = The child responds to **V**erbal stimuli.
   (Note: This cannot be assessed in the
   nonverbal or extremely agitated child.
   If impossible to assess, use the modified
   GCS method.)
P = The child responds to **P**ainful stimuli.
U = The child does not respond to any stimuli
   (**U**nresponsive).

(PGCS) (see Chapter 7, Table 7-5, p. 137). Total scores can range from 3 to 15, with a score of 15 indicating intact neurologic function.

Interventions. Initial interventions for the child with neurologic compromise include the prevention of cerebral hypoxia and the maintenance of cerebral perfusion. When significant head injury (GCS of 8 or less) is suspected, intubation and hyperventilation are indicated to maintain a $PaCO_2$ of 25 to 30 torr. Fluid restriction is required for any child with signs of increased intracranial pressure as long as there is no evidence of shock. If shock is present, resuscitation fluids are never restricted. Once the cervical spine is determined to be clear radiographically, the child's head can be elevated to improve venous return and decrease venous pressure. If the cervical spine has not been cleared, the head may be elevated by placing a towel roll under the top of the backboard.

SECONDARY SURVEY

Once the primary survey is completed and immediate threats to life treated, the secondary survey is performed. The secondary survey includes exposing the child, obtaining vital signs, performing a head-to-toe assessment, obtaining additional historical information, inspecting the back, and continued reassessment of the components of the primary survey. Interventions are prioritized based on the severity of injuries, the potential for underlying injuries, and the child's physiologic response to the injuries.

EXPOSURE AND FAHRENHEIT

To inspect the child for hidden injuries, all clothing is removed. Exposure, however, places the child at risk for hypothermia, since significant heat loss can occur when a young child is unclothed even for a few minutes. If hypothermia develops in the traumatized child, metabolic acidosis, apnea, and cardiac dysrhythmias can result, further complicating resuscitation attempts. Because clinical signs of hypothermia such as delayed capillary refill, pallor, and cool, mottled skin can mimic shock, knowledge of the child's core temperature is important during the clinical evaluation.

Hypothermia can be prevented by frequently reassessing the child's core temperature and by providing supplemental warming measures, such as keeping the child covered, using warmed blankets, or providing radiant warmers. Additional measures include warming all resuscitation fluids before infusion and main-taining a warm ambient temperature within the resuscitation area.

VITAL SIGNS

Vital sign measurements provide valuable information about the child's response to injury and interventions. Because the child's heart rate, respiratory rate, and blood pressure vary by age, knowledge of normal pediatric values is important (see Chapter 5, Table 5-10). The first complete set of vital signs is completed and recorded within the first 5 to 10 minutes of the child's arrival in the emergency department. An apical pulse is auscultated for 1 full minute as a baseline rate, and central and peripheral pulses are compared for strength and quality. The child is next placed on a cardiorespiratory monitor—if this was not done during the primary survey. Ongoing measurements of pulse are obtained at the apical site or at the radial, brachial, carotid, or femoral arteries. Nonpathologic conditions that can produce tachycardia include pain, anxiety, or fear; however, tachycardia is also one of the earliest signs of shock. Bradycardia is always a pathologic finding and can result from late stage shock, hypothermia, or increased intracranial pressure.

Respirations are assessed for rate and depth. Determining the presence or absence of localized sounds during auscultation may be difficult because of the child's thin chest wall. Subtle changes in the pitch and quality of breath sounds may be the only clues to underlying injuries. Bradypnea reflects severe underlying pathology, whereas tachypnea may reflect fear, anxiety, or an underlying pathology.

Blood pressure is measured in both arms. Hypotension is a late sign of shock in the child. Hypertension, in combination with clinical findings, can indicate a rising intracranial pressure.

HISTORY

After the primary assessment, a member of the trauma team obtains a complete patient history, which includes a history of the traumatic event. The prehospital team, parents, witnesses, and child, when possible, can provide pertinent information that may influence the plan of care (see Table 5-5, p. 96).

HEAD-TO-TOE ASSESSMENT

Head. The secondary assessment of the head includes a reassessment of the patency of the child's airway. The head is then observed for bruising, swelling, asymmetry, or lacerations. Abnormal findings include periorbital ecchymosis (raccoon's eyes) and ecchymosis over the mastoid area (Battle's sign). Battle's sign indicates a basilar skull fracture.

Individual orifices of the face and head are inspected for evidence of injury or drainage. Clear or bloody drainage may represent leaking cerebrospinal fluid and should be tested with a chemical reagent strip. The presence of glucose is suspicious for cerebrospinal fluid. Bloody drainage can be tested by placing drops of blood on linen. Cerebrospinal fluid is present when a light outer ring forms around a dark inner circle, referred to as the halo sign.

Pupils are assessed for size, shape, reactivity, movement, and symmetry. Pupil size is described in millimeters. Abnormal eye movements include deviation of one or both pupils from the midline, constant twitching movement of the pupils, unequal pupils, or downward deviation of the eyes. Unequal or dilated pupils that do not respond to light are abnormal findings associated with increased intracranial pressure, mass lesion, or herniation.[7]

Neurologic status is reassessed using the PGCS tool. A PGCS of less than 15 is abnormal. A decrease of 2 points that cannot be explained by physiologic changes or pharmacologic interventions is associated with a significant head injury.[7]

The entire head is palpated for deformities, including lacerations, impaled objects, and depressions of the cranial vault. In the infant the fontanel and sutures are palpated to detect abnormalities such as a bulging fontanel or spreading sutures.

Depending on findings, nursing interventions include frequent reassessment of neurologic status, wound care, and preparation for diagnostic tests such as a head computed tomography (CT) and skull radiographs.

Neck. After the initial cervical spine films, the neck is observed and palpated for obvious injuries, deformities, tenderness, tracheal deviation, and jugular venous distinction. The short necks of infants and young children can make thorough examination difficult, particularly when cervical spine immobilization must be maintained. While deformity is usually obvious, tenderness is difficult to assess. Nonverbal cues of pain include facial grimacing, crying, and sudden changes in behavior with palpation. If the child is verbal, he or she should be asked if pain is felt when the area is palpated.

Interventions depend on assessment findings. These may include wound care, cervical spine radio-

graphs, and a neurosurgery consultation. A lateral radiograph of the cervical spine is not complete until all seven cervical vertebrae and T1 are visualized.

Chest. During the secondary survey the chest is reinspected for the presence of contusions, lacerations, abrasions, and penetrating wounds. The clavicles, sternum, and thorax are palpated for deformities or instability. Tenderness, swelling, crepitus, or paradoxical movement are significant findings.

Respiratory status is reassessed by auscultating breath and heart sounds and evaluating respiratory depth, rate, and effort. Breath sounds are auscultated in all quadrants, and attention is paid to differences in the pitch and quality of the sounds.

Interventions are based on findings and, in addition to those initiated during the primary survey, such as assisted ventilation and arterial blood gas analysis, may include chest radiographs (supine anteroposterior and upright posteroanterior) and chest CT.

Abdomen. The abdomen is inspected for abrasions, lacerations, distention, bruises (such as tire or lap belt marks), and abdominal breathing patterns. A rapid, shallow breathing pattern may result from an abdominal wall injury or retroperitoneal irritation. Abdominal distention may result from aerophagia or the accumulation of blood, urine, bile, pancreatic fluid, or intestinal contents. Increasing abdominal distention and tensity are among the first signs of abdominal trauma. Children with lap belt injuries may have linear bruising across the lower abdomen, creating a high index of suspicion for a jejunal or bowel injury.[10]

The child's position of comfort and degree of pain are assessed. If abdominal wall tension is present, the conscious child may flex or bend his or her knees and draw upward to relieve tension and reduce pain. Children with a splenic injury may complain of left shoulder pain or Kehr's sign, which is referred pain caused by compression of the left upper quadrant. Referred right shoulder pain may indicate hepatic injury.

The abdomen is next auscultated for bowel sounds in all four quadrants. After auscultation, the abdomen is gently palpated both anteriorly and posteriorly. Areas that are painful are palpated last. To assist the nurse in identifying those areas, the verbal, alert child can be asked to point with one finger to the area of pain. Rebound tenderness and guarding are abnormal findings indicating peritoneal irritation.

Nursing interventions depend on assessment findings; however, frequent reassessments of the child's abdomen, vital signs, and neurologic status are required to identify the progression of injuries associated with abdominal trauma. Additional nursing interventions include the insertion of a urinary catheter, if there are no signs of genitourinary trauma (e.g., blood at the urinary meatus), and the insertion of a nasogastric or orogastric tube. Children suspected to have significant abdominal injuries, not requiring emergency surgical intervention, must be accompanied by the emergency room nurse and/or physician during diagnostic imaging studies.

Operative intervention is anticipated if abdominal trauma is suspected and the child remains hemodynamically unstable after fluid resuscitation. If the child is hemodynamically stable, abdominal and pelvic x-rays, ultrasonography, and/or a CT scan may be ordered. Contrast-enhanced radiographs and/or CT scans may be performed, depending on the suspected degree of injury.

Diagnostic peritoneal lavage (DPL) to detect intraabdominal bleeding is controversial in children. It will not identify the presence of a retroperitoneal hemorrhage and may delay definitive surgical intervention in the hemodynamically unstable child. DPL is only useful when serial physical, laboratory, and diagnostic findings are unavailable or unreliable (e.g., in the comatose child)[10] (see Chapter 22, Trauma—Selected Systems).

Pelvis and genitalia.   Initially the pelvis and genitalia are inspected for ecchymosis, abrasions, lacerations, and bleeding. The urinary meatus is inspected for the presence of blood. During the assessment of the female adolescent, it should be remembered that menarche occurs at an average age of 13 years, so pregnancy is a possibility.

The pelvis is palpated for instability and pain. Integrity of the pelvis may be tested by gently pressing on the anterosuperior iliac spine to elicit signs of pain. As with any portion of the examination, the child is given an explanation before the assessment. Gentle effort is required for the younger child. An unstable pelvis and/or pain indicates a pelvic fracture. Extensive pelvic fractures are associated with a ruptured bladder. Signs of bladder injury include hematuria, inability to void, and abdominal pain. The assessment continues with a rectal examination to establish the presence of rectal tone.

Nursing interventions depend on physical findings. Normally a urinary catheter is inserted in the child with signs of significant trauma, and urinary output is monitored. However, if blood is found at the urinary meatus, catheter insertion is contraindicated until urethral injuries have been ruled out. Urine is analyzed for the presence of blood.

Extremities.   The first concern in any extremity injury is control of hemorrhage, and the second is loss of neurovascular and musculoskeletal integrity, which can lead to long-term disability. Therefore the extremities are inspected not only for obvious injuries but also for hidden injuries. Inspection may reveal obvious hemorrhage, abrasions, lacerations, contusions, deformities, or the presence of a foreign body.

Injured extremities are completely evaluated, including a complete neurovascular examination. Pallor, pain, pulselessness, paresthesia, and paralysis are signs of significant injury. Skin temperature of the extremities is compared for equality. Unequal temperatures may indicate neurovascular compromise.

If the extremity has not been splinted in the field, emergency department interventions include immobilization. The joints above and below the injury are immobilized, with evaluation of the pulse before and after the procedure. In the younger child, immobilization devices such as hare or sager traction will be too large; therefore the position of comfort is preferred until the fracture can be reduced. Armboards and air splints can be modified and used for splinting. In addition, the extremity is elevated, ice is applied, and pain and comfort measures provided.

Radiologic studies confirm the diagnosis of fracture and should include the joint above and below the fracture.

Back.   The last step in the secondary survey is inspection and palpation of the child's back and the posterior aspects of the extremities. To maintain spinal immobilization, multiple team members may be required to log-roll the child as a single unit.

The area is inspected for bleeding, lacerations, exit wounds, contusions, and presence of foreign bodies such as glass. Palpation of the back and extremities reveals deformities or tenderness.

TETANUS

Tetanus is caused by contamination of a wound by stool or dirt where *Clostridium tetani* is found. Almost any wound can be contaminated; however, deep wounds and puncture wounds particularly favor the growth of anaerobic organisms such as tetanus. Although tetanus prophylaxis is available, many children fail to receive one or all of the series of injections

TABLE 21-6	Guide to Tetanus Prophylaxis in Routine Wound Management			
HISTORY OF ADSORBED TETANUS TOXOID (DOSES)	**CLEAN, MINOR WOUNDS**		**ALL OTHER WOUNDS***	
	TD≤	**TIG≥**	**TD≤**	**TIG≥**
Unknown or <3	Yes	No	Yes	Yes
≥3§	No‖	No	No¶	No

From Peter G: 1997 *Redbook: Report of the Committee on Infectious Diseases,* ed 24, Elk Grove Village, IL, 1997, AAP.
*Such as, but not limited to, wounds contaminated with dirt, feces, soil, and saliva; puncture wounds; avulsions; and wounds resulting from missiles, crushing, burns, and frostbite.
†For children less than 7 years old; DTP or DTaP (if ≥3 doses of DTP have been previously given) is preferred to tetanus toxoid alone; if pertussis vaccine is contraindicated, DT is given. For persons 7 years of age or older, Td is preferred to tetanus toxoid alone. Td, Adult-type tetanus and diphtheria toxoids.
‡TIG, Tetanus immune globulin.
§If only three doses of fluid toxoid have been received, then a fourth dose of toxoid, preferably an adsorbed toxoid, should be given.
‖Yes, if more than 10 years since last dose.
¶Yes, if more than 5 years since last dose. (More frequent boosters are not needed and can accentuate side effects.)

necessary to achieve protective levels of circulating antibodies. The type of wound, availability of immunization records, and reliability of the parents all play a role in the decision to administer tetanus prophylaxis after a traumatic injury (Table 21-6).

SUMMARY

Traumatic injuries are a great threat to our nation's children. As caregivers who observe the devastating effects of trauma, we are in key positions to develop prevention programs both within our communities and within our institutions. In addition, once a child sustains a traumatic injury, it is our responsibility to understand childhood anatomy and physiology and convert that knowledge into effective and efficient interventions that will decrease morbidity and mortality in the pediatric population.

REFERENCES

1. Aprahamian C et al: Pediatric trauma score, *Arch Surg* 125(9):1128-1131, 1990.
2. Bruce DS: Head trauma. In Eichelberger MR, ed: *Pediatric trauma,* St Louis, 1993, Mosby.
3. Brunette DD, Fifield G, Ruiz E: Use of pneumatic antishock trousers in the management of pediatric pelvic hemorrhage, *Pediatr Emerg Care* 3:86-90, 1987.
4. Centers for Disease Control: *Childhood injuries in the United States,* Atlanta, 1990, Centers for Disease Control.
5. Chameides L, Hazinski MF, eds: *Textbook of pediatric advanced life support,* Dallas, 1994, American Heart Association.
6. Children's Safety Network: *A data book of child and adolescent injury,* Washington, DC, 1991, National Center for Education in Maternal and Child Health.
7. Dolan M: Head trauma. In Barkin RM ed: *Pediatric emergency medicine,* St Louis, 1992, Mosby.
8. DiGiuseppi CG et al: Bicycle helmet use by children: evaluation of a community-wide helmet campaign, *JAMA* 262:2256, 1989.
9. Emergency Cardiac Care Committee and Subcommittees American Heart Association: Guidelines for cardiopulmonary resuscitation and emergency cardiac care: pediatric advanced life support, *JAMA* 268:2172-2183, 1993.
10. Folton GL, Cooper A: Abdominal trauma. In Barkin RM ed: *Pediatric emergency medicine,* St Louis, 1992, Mosby.
11. Guyer B, Ellers B: Childhood injuries in the United States, *Am J Dis Child* 144:649-652, 1990.
12. Haddon W: Advances in the epidemiology of injuries as a basis for public policy, *Public Health Rep* 95: 411, 1980.
13. Haddon W: A logical framework for categorizing highway safety phenomena and activity, *J Trauma* 12:193, 1972.
14. Heppel DE, Platt LJ: Public health of children. In Eichelberger MR, ed: *Pediatric trauma,* St Louis, 1993, Mosby.
15. Musemeche CA et al: Pediatric fall from heights, *J Trauma* 31(10):1347-1349, 1991.
16. National Safety Council: *Accident facts, 1996* ed, Chicago, 1996, National Safety Council.

17. National Highway Traffic Safety Administration: *Idea sampler: buckle up America,* Washington, DC, 1991 US Department of Transportation, National Highway Traffic Safety Administration.

18. National Highway Traffic Safety Administration: *Traffic safety facts, 1994, Pedestrians,* Washington, DC, 1994, US Department of Transportation.

19. Ray LU, Yuwiler J: Child and adolescent fatal injury databook, 1994, Children's Safety Network: Injury Data Technical Assistance Center, Maternal and Child Health Bureau, US, Department of Health and Human Services, Washington, D.C.

20. *Report on the National Institute on Disability and Rehabilitation Research Pediatric Trauma Registry,* Boston, April 1993.

21. Rossetti V et al: Difficulty and delay in intravascular access in pediatric arrest, *Ann Emerg Med* 13:406, 1984.

22. Seidel JS, Henderson DP eds: *Emergency medical services for children: a report to the nation,* Washington, DC, 1991, National Center for Education in Maternal and Child Health.

22a. Soud T, Pieper P, Hazinski MF: Pediatric trauma. In Hazinski MF, ed: *Nursing care of the critically ill child,* ed 2, St Louis, 1992, Mosby.

23. Spiegal CN, Lindaman FC: Children can't fly: a program to prevent childhood morbidity and mortality from window falls, *Am J Public Health* 67: 1143, 1977.

24. Stellar J: Pediatric. In Bayley E, Turcke S eds: *A comprehensive curriculum for trauma nursing,* Boston, 1992, Jones & Bartlett.

25. Stevens CD: Injury prevention and epidemiology. In Barkin RM ed: *Pediatric emergency medicine,* St Louis, 1992, Mosby.

26. Tepas JJ III et al: The pediatric trauma score as a predictor of injury severity: an objective assessment, *J Trauma* 22:14, 1987.

27. Thompson RE, Rivara FP, Thompson DC: A case-control study of the effectiveness of bicycle safety helmets, *N Engl J Med* 320:1361, 1989.

28. Tocantins LM: Rapid absorption of substances injected into the bone marrow, *Proc Soc Exp Biol Med* 45:292-296, 1940.

29. US General Accounting Office Report: *Motor safety comprehensive state programs offer best opportunity for increased use of safety belts,* Jan 1996, # GAO-RCED 96-24.

30. Widner-Kilberg M, Moloney-Harmon P: Pediatric trauma. In: Cardonna V et al. eds: *Trauma nursing,* ed 2, Philadelphia, 1994, WB Saunders.

31. Williams RA: Injuries in infants and small children resulting from witnessed and corroborated free falls, *J Trauma* 31(10): 1350-1352, 1991.

32. Young A, Rivara FP: *Injury prevention—getting the job done,* 1992, Harborview Injury Prevention and Research Center.

CHAPTER 22

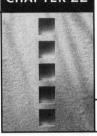

Trauma—Selected Systems

Treesa Soud, Peggy D. Saum, Scott Pikulski

■ HEAD AND NECK INJURIES

Traumatic brain injury (TBI) is the most common cause of traumatic childhood death and disability in the United States. TBI's accounts for approximately 600,000 emergency department visits each year[20] and approximately 60% of all traumatic deaths in children.[5] The incidence of TBI varies by age and gender. The younger the child, the higher is the associated mortality.[33] Children younger than 1 year of age have double the mortality associated with head trauma when compared to older children between 1 and 6 years of age, and three times the mortality of children between the ages of 6 and 12 years.[18] Males tend to have twice the incidence of head injury and four times the risk of suffering fatal head injuries when compared to females.[15,41] Although children have better recovery after TBI than adults, they may be more susceptible to long-term cognitive deficits from minor injuries.[27]

Etiology. The major cause of TBIs are motor vehicle–related incidents, which include the child as a passenger, as a pedestrian, or on a bicycle. These incidents tend to be associated with multisystem injuries and, when these multisystem injuries are combined with TBIs, produce the highest mortality figures.[32,41] Non–motor-vehicle–related head injuries result from falls, sports activities, and play. Falls are by far the most common emergency department complaint and may be accompanied by abrasions, lacerations, or hematomas. Head injuries in young, nonmobile infants are unusual, and, depending on physical findings and the mechanism of injury, may require evaluation for child maltreatment.

Anatomy and physiology. The child's unique anatomy and physiology contribute to the increased incidence of TBI during childhood and the types of injuries seen. The child's head is disproportionately large in proportion to body size and is supported by a relatively weak neck. Brain tissue is thinner, softer, and more fragile than in the adult, and cranial bones are thinner and more compliant, providing less protection. This may contribute to the increased incidence of diffuse cerebral edema that occurs more commonly in children than in adults.

Review of anatomy. The scalp is made up of five layers of tissue covering the skull. These include the skin, subcutaneous tissue, galea, loose areolar tissue, and periosteum. The skull comprises the cranial vault and the base. At birth the skull of the infant consists of separate bones connected by soft, fibrous joints known as sutures. The fontanels, anterior and posterior, are formed by the juncture of three or more of the cranial bones and are felt as soft concavities in the skull. The posterior fontanel may be closed at birth or soon thereafter. The anterior fontanel closes between ages 9 and 18 months.[3]

Three highly vascular membranes adhere to the internal surface of the skull. These membranes are collectively known as the meninges and consist of the dura mater, arachnoid, and pia mater (Figs. 22-1 and 22-2). The dura is a tough, fibrous membrane that adheres firmly to the internal surface of the skull. The subdural space is a potential space between the dura and the arachnoid layer. Hemorrhage into the subdural space usually comes from damaged veins that cross the subdural space. The epidural space is a potential space between the dura and the internal surface of the skull. Lacerations of the meningeal arteries located within this space may result in an epidural hematoma.

The arachnoid mater is the second meningeal layer and is thin and transparent. The third layer, the pia

511

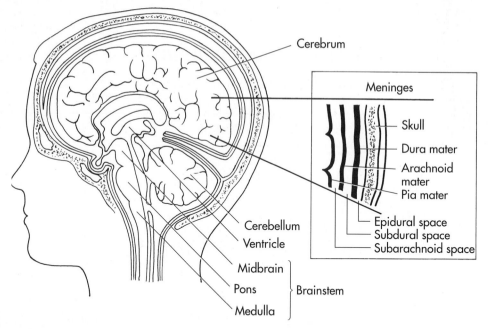

FIG. 22-1. The cranium.

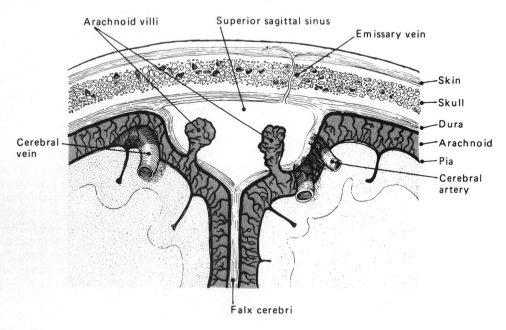

FIG. 22-2. The meninges. (From Kinney MR, Packa DR, Dunbar SB: *AACN's clinical reference for critical care nursing,* ed 3, St Louis, 1993, Mosby.)

mater, is firmly attached to the brain cortex. Between the pia mater and the arachnoid layers is the subarachnoid space, in which the cerebrospinal fluid (CSF) circulates. Bleeding into this space is classified as a subarachnoid hemorrhage.

The brain consists of the cerebrum, the cerebellum, and the brainstem. The cerebrum comprises right and left hemispheres separated by the falx. The cerebrum is further divided into frontal, occipital, parietal, and temporal lobes. It contains centers for emotions as well as motor and sensory functioning. The cerebellum controls movement, coordination, and balance and surrounds the brainstem in the posterior fossa. The brainstem, which connects the major neural pathways to and from the cerebral hemispheres, is further divided into the midbrain, pons, and medulla. The cardiorespiratory centers reside in the medulla. (For further discussion of the anatomy and physiology of the neurologic system, see Chapters 7 and 12.)

Pathophysiology. Injuries resulting from head trauma are characterized as primary or secondary injuries. Primary injuries represent the damage that is sustained at the time of the traumatic event, and the damage is not preventable. Secondary injuries result from pathophysiologic responses that follow the traumatic event. Examples of primary injuries include damage to the skin, cranium, brain tissue, and/or blood vessels. Unconsciousness immediately after an injury is also categorized as a primary injury.

Secondary injuries may occur immediately after the event or within hours or days and reflect changes in cerebral blood flow (CBF), metabolism, electrical activity, and/or CSF flow. They are often preventable with early recognition of symptoms or of injuries consistent with their presence. For example, the most common type of head trauma in children results from diffuse injury. This injury produces increased CBF, which leads to increased intracranial pressure (ICP). With early recognition, measures such as intubation and hyperventilation can be instituted to prevent the rise in ICP and any subsequent neuronal damage or herniation.

Regardless of the type of injury sustained (e.g., blunt trauma, penetrating injury, or vascular injury), increased ICP immediately after an injury is of universal concern. Within the brain there is a delicate balance of pressure between the brain tissue, CSF, and blood volume—normally when one of these substances increases, the others compensate by decreasing. Because the cranium is a fixed volume, however, significant increases in the mass of any one of these can produce increased ICP (Box 22-1).

There is conflicting evidence regarding the ability of the open sutures and fontanels of infants to expand, and therefore compensate, for increases in cerebral volume. In general, because the infant may be more tolerant of increases in ICP, early signs and symptoms may be missed. The poor outcomes reported in these infants therefore may be related to delayed recognition and treatment.

When significant increases in ICP go unrecognized and untreated, the only egress of the brain is herniation. Types of herniation syndromes include transten-

---

Box 22-1   Terms Associated with Intracranial Volume and Injuries

Intracranial volume =
   Blood volume + Brain tissue + CSF

Cerebral perfusion pressure (CPP): Defines the intravascular pressure gradient across the brain; it is equal to the difference between mean arterial pressure and ICP; measurement of ICP is an indirect means of determining CPP; normal CPP in infants and children is thought to be approximately 40 to 50 mm Hg.

   CPP = Mean arterial pressure (MAP) −
                  Intracranial pressure (ICP)

Cerebral blood flow (CBF): Reflects arterial blood flow to the brain; CBF is particularly responsive to changes in oxygen and carbon dioxide; as CO_2 decreases, CBF decreases, with the result being a decrease in ICP at the expense of cerebral perfusion; hypoxia produces an increase in CBF and a corresponding increase in ICP.

Cerebral blood volume (CBV): Reflects the total volume of intracranial blood at any given time.

Cerebral hyperemia (brain swelling): Occurs immediately after the traumatic injury and reflects an increase in CBV.

Cerebral or brain edema: Reflects an increase in the water content of the brain; is primarily the result of ischemic or hypoxic brain injury.

torial herniation—caused by lesions above the tento-rium; uncal herniation or temporal lobe herniation—caused as the temporal lobe shifts laterally across the tentorial notch; cerebellar herniation—caused by downward displacement of the cerebellum toward the foramen magnum; and brainstem herniation—caused by compression of the brainstem through the foramen magnum.

CLOSED HEAD INJURIES

Concussion. Concussions are characterized by a brief loss of neurologic function that usually causes a temporary loss of consciousness. They are most commonly associated with blunt trauma to the head but can also be caused by acceleration-deceleration forces. Temporary amnesia may occur after a concussion, although in some rare cases it can be permanent.

The child's response to a concussion is unique in that neurologic disturbances are often associated with a particular age group. In very young children and infants with a mild head injury, loss of consciousness is uncommon, yet the child may progress from a normal level of consciousness to somnolence and repeated vomiting. Children in this age range also tend to exhibit a higher incidence of postinjury seizures than older children and adults.[12]

Most children who sustain a concussion require only supportive care, and many can be observed at home with a reliable caregiver.[34] However, if the child was unconscious for longer than 5 minutes or demonstrates persistent symptoms, such as protracted vomiting or alternating levels of consciousness, a computed tomography (CT) scan and hospitalization should be anticipated.[14]

Contusion. Cerebral contusions are characterized by areas of bruising, edema, and microscopic hemorrhaging into the brain. They are most commonly associated with acceleration-deceleration injuries or blunt traumatic forces. Contusions often occur in the presence of serious concussions and are associated with longer periods of coma and mental confusion. When the contusion is located directly under the site of impact, it is called a coup injury. If the contusion is located in a remote area or opposite the site of impact, it is referred to as a contrecoup injury. In children, perhaps because of the compliant nature of the skull, coup injuries are more common.[12]

Because contusions produce areas of edema and

hemorrhage, ICP can increase. With severe intracerebral hemorrhaging, subdural, epidural, or subarachnoid hemorrhages may occur.

The neurologic deficits associated with contusions usually occur gradually and may be focal in nature. Neurologic signs are associated with the areas of the brain affected by the injury. Diagnostic testing includes a CT scan of the head to identify the presence, location, and size of the contusion. When substantial focal hemorrhage is present with concomitant severe neurologic deficits, surgical intervention should be anticipated.

Diffuse axonal injury. Diffuse axonal injury is a severe condition that results from shearing stresses caused by angular and rotational acceleration-deceleration forces. This injury produces microscopic structural damage throughout the brain that can range from minor functional disturbances of the neurons to complete disruption of the axons, producing permanent damage.[5,27] It is characterized by coma immediately after the injury with no return to consciousness. This state can last for days to weeks. Seizures are not uncommon.

The diagnosis is usually made when an emergency CT scan or magnetic resonance imaging (MRI) shows no mass lesion in the child who remains deeply comatose. Decerebrate and/or decorticate posturing is common, as is autonomic dysfunction, which produces high fever, hypertension, and diaphoresis. Although this injury does not require emergency surgical intervention, the child should be cared for in a facility equipped to manage long-term coma patients.

Intracranial hemorrhages

Epidural hematoma. Epidural hemorrhage occurs when blunt trauma to the head causes blood to accumulate between the dura and the skull. Because the dura is adherent to the skull, any separation can produce venous and/or arterial hemorrhage. Arterial tears occur most commonly and are often associated with rapidly expanding lesions that produce neurologic decompensation. These tears can be associated with linear skull fractures over the parietal or temporal areas that cross the middle meningeal artery, but they may also occur in the absence of a skull fracture (Fig. 22-3).

Epidural hematomas are more common in older children than in younger ones and may present with

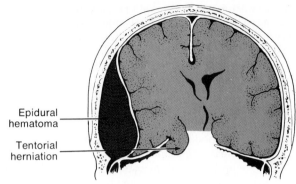

FIG. 22-3. Epidural hematoma and compression of a portion of the temporal lobe through tentorial hiatus. (From Wong DL: *Whaley & Wong's essentials of pediatric nursing,* ed 5, St Louis, 1997, Mosby.)

Epidural hematoma

Tentorial herniation

relatively mild symptoms such as sleepiness and headaches.[32] If not properly recognized and treated, a rapidly expanding lesion can quickly lead to hemiparesis on the opposite side of the injury and a dilated and fixed pupil on the side of the injury. With continued expansion of the cranial mass, and compression of cerebral contents, temporal lobe herniation and brainstem compression will result.

Children suspected to have an epidural hematoma require an immediate CT scan with constant physiologic monitoring of neurologic status. If a mass is identified, immediate surgical intervention and evacuation are indicated.

Subdural hematoma. A subdural hematoma represents an accumulation of blood in the subdural space between the dura and arachnoid membrane resulting from rupture of the bridging veins between the cerebral cortex and dura. This injury is usually associated with significant, high-velocity impacts, which produce greater cortical damage. Although subdural hematomas are rarely associated with skull fractures, they are frequently associated with brain lacerations and severe swelling (Fig. 22-4).

The occurrence and significance of subdural hematomas are age related. The most common cause of subdural hematoma in the infant is shaken impact syndrome, which is observed in victims of child abuse.[6] Additionally, subdural hemorrhage can occur as a result of birth trauma. In the older child, motor vehicle accidents and falls are the most common causes. The child with a subdural hematoma may come to the emergency department with a history of alternating mental status or without ever having regained consciousness after the injury. Infants with a subdural

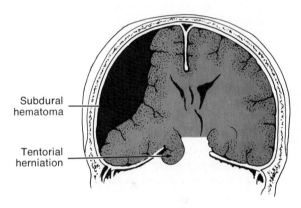

Subdural hematoma

Tentorial herniation

FIG. 22-4. Subdural hematoma. (From Wong DL: *Whaley & Wong's essentials of pediatric nursing,* ed 5, St Louis, 1997, Mosby.)

hematoma caused by shaken impact syndrome may have a bulging fontanel and separation of the sutures, vomiting, lethargy, and/or irritability (see Chapter 25, Child Maltreatment).

Diagnostic testing includes obtaining a CT scan. Skull x-rays are of little benefit, since this injury is rarely associated with a skull fracture. Surgery is indicated less often in young infants with subdural hematomas than in older children because serial subdural taps may be performed.[14] Older children are more likely to require surgery, usually because the mechanism of injury has produced severe brain injuries.[31]

Subarachnoid hemorrhage. Subarachnoid hemorrhage represents vascular injury within the ventricular and/or subarachnoid space and may be present in children with severe head injuries. Because these children can develop increased ICP rapidly, aggressive interventions for management are required. Although the need for surgical intervention is rare, hydrocephalus may occur, necessitating the surgical insertion of a ventricular drain.

Brain hemorrhages and lacerations. Brain hemorrhages and lacerations are focal injuries that can produce severe blood loss. Examples include intracerebral hematomas, impalement injuries, and bullet wounds. An intracerebral hematoma represents a direct hemorrhage within the brain and can occur in any location. Which neurologic deficits result depends on associated injuries and the area of involvement. Impalement injuries are caused by foreign bodies. Impaled objects are left in place until they can be removed by a neurosurgeon.

Firearm injuries are second only to motor vehicle accidents as the most common cause of death among adolescent males 15 to 18 years of age.[16] Of all firearm injuries, approximately 50% to 60% involve the head.[2] The outcome of firearm injuries is directly related to the degree of destruction of the cerebral contents and secondary injuries. However, even when a bullet does not penetrate the skull, significant intracranial injury can result. A high mortality is associated with the child victim of a gunshot wound to the head who is in a coma.

With any suspected brain hemorrhage or laceration a CT scan is indicated. The results will be used to determine the degree of damage to the brain and to guide the surgical approach.

Skull Fractures

Linear fractures. Linear fractures, seen as fine lines on x-ray, are the most common skull fractures observed in children. They are usually insignificant and require no specific treatment. If the fracture crosses the path of the middle meningeal artery, an epidural hemorrhage can result. Management is directed toward detecting and treating underlying brain injuries. Vomiting is relatively common with this injury.

Depressed skull fractures. A depressed skull fracture is a fracture in which a fragment or section of the skull intrudes into the cranial vault, causing pressure on the brain. Depressed skull fractures are uncommon in young children. When they do occur, they often result from an impact with a relatively small or pointed object. Fragments depressed more than the thickness of the skull usually, require operative intervention to elevate the bony fragment.

Compound fractures. Compound skull fractures are open fractures in which there is a direct communication between the cerebral surface and a scalp laceration. These fractures can be linear, depressed, or comminuted. Visible or leaking CSF is diagnostic. Early operative intervention and antimicrobial therapy are indicated when compound fractures are present.

Basilar skull fractures. Basilar skull fractures involve the basilar portion of the frontal, ethmoid, sphenoid, temporal, or occipital bones and represent severe head injury. This type of fracture is difficult, if not impossible at times, to detect and/or diagnose by x-ray studies alone. Therefore clinical findings are frequently relied on to make the diagnosis. These findings include CSF leaking from the ear or nose; raccoon eyes—periorbital ecchymosis; Battle's sign—ecchymosis behind the ears; and/or hemotympanum—blood behind the tympanic membrane. When CSF is mixed with blood, it is difficult to differentiate from blood. To differentiate the two, a drop of fluid can be placed on a piece of filter paper and observed for the formation of one or more clear rings ("ring" sign), indicating the presence of CSF.

Cervical Spine Injuries

Etiology. Cervical spine injuries (CSIs) are uncommon in young children, occurring in 0.4% of all children who come for treatment with a history of multiple trauma.[13] When these injuries do occur, however, they are most commonly associated with multiple injuries, particularly those arising from pedestrian–motor vehicle accidents and shaken impact syndrome. Other injuries that can cause cervical spine injuries in children include falls, diving accidents, and sports-related activities.

Pathophysiology. The child's cervical spine is comprised of vertebrae, the spinal cord, and blood vessels—any of which can be damaged during a traumatic event. There are seven cervical vertebrae, with the first two having a unique configuration. The axis, which is C2, has an anterior projection called the dens or odontoid process that protrudes upward into the ring of C1, also known as the atlas. They are connected by ligaments that allow full range of motion of the head on the spine (Figs. 22-5 and 22-6).

The child's unique physiology serves to protect the spine but also contributes to specific types of injuries, depending on age. Young children have dispropor-tionately large heads when compared to older children and adults, so the head—rather than the neck—takes a major portion of any impact injury. Additionally, the highly elastic neck ligaments and incompletely calci-fied synchondrosis (growth centers in the vertebral

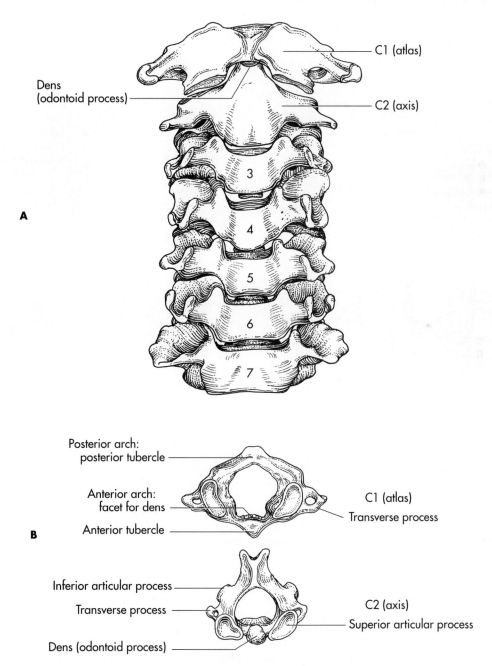

FIG. 22-5. **A,** Anterior view of the cervical vertebrae. **B,** First two cervical vertebrae viewed from above.

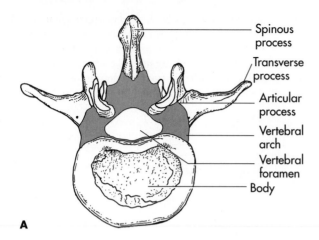

Spinous process

Transverse process

Articular process

Vertebral arch

Vertebral foramen

Body

A

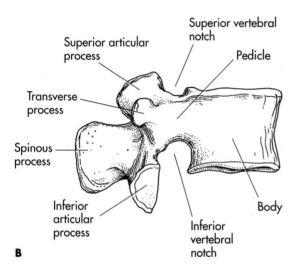

Superior articular process

Transverse process

Spinous process

Inferior articular process

Superior vertebral notch

Pedicle

Inferior vertebral notch

Body

B

FIG. 22-6. **A,** Vertebral body viewed from above. **B,** Lateral view of vertebral body.

bodies) of the child allow more movement of the neck with less likelihood of bony injuries. As the child matures, that is, by about 8 to 10 years of age, the bony cervical spine's configuration becomes similar to the adult's.[22]

These unique characteristics mean that children less than 8 years of age have a higher incidence of upper cervical spine injuries (C1 or C2) than older children or adults when exposed to acceleration/deceleration forces.[22,31,33a] In addition, fractures and vertebral dislocations are rare, with most injuries tending to involve the synchondroses, or cartilaginous portions of the vertebral body, which have not yet ossified.[22]

The anatomic variations of childhood not only contribute to the types of injuries sustained but also impact the interpretation of physical and radiographic findings. Because the child's upper cervical spine is hypermobile and the lax transverse ligament allows forward motion of the head, subluxation with or without fracture is responsible for a large number of cervical spine injuries.[46] Normal radiographic findings in the child can, however, indicate a pseudosubluxation evidenced by a 3 to 4 mm distance between the atlas and dens as compared to a less than 3 mm distance in adults.[46,47] One method used to determine whether the degree of anterior displacement of C2 on C3 is significant is the Swischuk line, in which a line is drawn from the anterior cortex of the spinous process of C1 to C3,[38] (Fig. 22-7). If the line is 2.0 mm anterior to the cortex of the spinous process of C2, a cervical pathologic condition should be suspected.[47]

Another finding that is more common in children

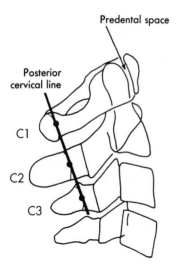

FIG. 22-7. Swischuk line. A line is drawn from the anterior cortex of the spinous process of C1 to C3. It is considered normal if it passes within 1 to 2 mm of the anterior cortex of C2. (From Rosen P et al, eds: *Emergency medicine*, ed 4, St Louis, 1997, Mosby.)

than in adults is a phenomenon known as spinal cord injury without radiographic abnormalities (SCIWORA). In this injury the child exhibits signs of spinal cord injury, such as paralysis, without evidence of injury on radiograph. Many theories have been offered regarding the etiology of the SCIWORA phenomenon. In general, it is believed that the young child's immaturely developed spinal column allows significant flexion and extension forces to be applied to the spinal cord without demonstrable vertebral damage. When SCIWORA is present, damage to the spinal cord may not be immediately evident but instead may progress insidiously over hours or days.

Finally, because the synchondroses, or growth centers, of the vertebrae are not completely calcified in infancy and early childhood, they may be mistaken for fractures after an injury. These synchondroses are evidenced by radiolucent areas on x-ray. Among the most common are the gaps between the odontoid process and the axis and the ossification centers in the spinous processes.[25]

Clinical presentation. The mechanism of injury is strongly correlated with the incidence of cervical spine injuries in children. For this reason, any child involved in a motor vehicle crash or pedestrian incident; a fall from a significant height accompanied by evidence of head trauma, or an alternating level of

consciousness or neurologic impairment; or any victim of a diving accident should be placed on a backboard with cervical spine immobilization.

Signs and symptoms of cervical spine injury are subtle and sometimes difficult to elicit in the child. Young children are often frightened and uncooperative, further complicating the examination. In general, signs of cervical spine injury included deformity; pain and/or tenderness to palpation; numbness and/or tingling of the extremities; decreased, inappropriate, or absent response to pain; decreased or absent motor responses; and/or loss of bowel or bladder control.

EMERGENCY DEPARTMENT INTERVENTIONS FOR THE CHILD WITH HEAD OR NECK INJURY

Emergency department management of head injuries requires identification of the extent of the injury(ies) and establishment of a specific diagnosis in order to treat the underlying problem. Urgency of treatment depends on the nature and severity of the injury. The goals of treatment are to protect the spinal cord and brain from further (secondary) insults by (1) preventing cord edema; (2) maintaining adequate cerebral metabolism; and (3) preventing and treating intracranial hypertension.

As with all victims of trauma, airway, breathing, and circulation (ABCs) are the first priorities of care. Because of the increased incidence of cervical spine injuries in the child with severe head trauma, cervical spine immobilization is performed and a cross-table lateral x-ray of the cervical spine obtained. Even when these x-rays initially indicate the absence of a cervical spine injury, additional studies, such as a cervical spine series or CT scan may be required. The CT scan is the diagnostic procedure of choice for children who have, or are suspected to have, a serious head injury, since it can show the exact location and size of most mass lesions.

If the child shows signs of increased ICP (such as changes in the level of consciousness, lethargy, confusion, agitation, and/or disorientation) or has an injury that predisposes him or her to the development of increased ICP, the nurse should anticipate interventions designed to decrease ICP. These include elevation of the head of the bed (only if spinal injury has been ruled out), intubation and hyperventilation, fluid restriction (unless shock is present), and the possible administration of diuretics. (For a complete discussion of the treatment of increased ICP, see Chapter 7, pp. 141-145.)

Nursing Interventions and Evaluation of the Child with Head or Neck Injury

Assessment. The initial assessment is referred to as the primary assessment and evaluates immediate threats to life using the ABC format. The secondary assessment involves a more complete evaluation and includes the head-to-toe assessment. Because the approach to the multiply injured child is covered in Chapter 21, Multiple Trauma Management, this discussion will only review the assessment and management of head or neck injuries in the child.

History. The history is important in that it guides interventions and provide clues to the extent of the injury. For example, the child with a history of significant head or neck trauma from a motor vehicle crash or pedestrian injury or a fall from a height is at high risk of sustaining a serious head or neck injury. In addition, a significant injury may be suspected in the child who was alert at the scene but lethargic or unresponsive on arrival in the emergency department (Box 22-2). Other important historical information includes the presence of allergies, the time of the child's last meal, the taking of over-the-counter or prescription medications, the child's past medical history, and his or her immunization status.

Inspection and palpation of the head and neck. Initially the head is inspected for obvious injuries, such as lacerations, abrasions, impaled objects, or depressions. Both the nares and the external ear canals are observed for signs of hemorrhage or the leakage of

CSF. The neck is also inspected for obvious signs of injury such as deformity, swelling, or ecchymosis.

The head and neck are next gently palpated to identify the presence of deformities or other abnormal findings. Palpation may reveal bony depressions in the cranium, crepitus, malalignment of the cervical spine, or abnormal mobility of the spinous processes. A bulging, tense fontanel in the infant reveals the presence of increased ICP.

Vital signs. Baseline vital signs are obtained and evaluated. Abnormal findings such as hypotension and bradycardia can indicate spinal cord injury, but these may also reflect other, concurrent conditions, such as late hemorrhagic shock caused by a liver or spleen laceration.

Other findings, characteristic of a significant pathologic condition in the adult, may be observed late in the course of the injury in a child. For example, the Cushing triad of apnea or bradypnea, bradycardia, and hypertension is a late sign of neurologic compromise in the child and is not relied on to indicate early signs of increased ICP. Pain, fear, and anxiety can also affect the interpretation of findings. All findings are therefore correlated with the child's overall status. Serially obtained vital signs provide the most important information.

Neurologic assessment. For further discussion see Chapter 12, The Neurologic System. The neurologic examination—both initially and serially—is used to evaluate the severity of the TBI and central nervous system impairment. Components of the examination include serial measurements of the child's level of consciousness, an evaluation of the cranial nerves, an evaluation of motor responses, and an assessment of the child's response to pain.

A valuable tool in assessing mental status and the potential outcome from a head injury is the Glasgow Coma Scale (GCS), which assesses eye opening, motor response, and verbal response. The difficulty with using this instrument in the young, frightened, or preverbal child resulted in the development of a Modified Glasgow Coma Scale (MGCS).[23] This tool uses the same assessment parameters as the adult scale, but the numbered criteria are more appropriate to the developmental characteristics of the child. For example, in the adult scale the best verbal response is considered orientation, whereas in the infant the best verbal response is cooing, smiling, or crying appropriately (see Chapter 7, Tables 7-4 and 7-5, p 137). Even with these modifications, interpreting MGCS findings

---

Box 22-2 Neurologic History: Pediatric Head or Neck Trauma

Mechanism of injury
Condition at the scene
Loss of consciousness after injury
Changes in mental status at the scene and during transport
Changes in behavior
Complaints of headaches
Complaints of vomiting or gagging
Seizures at the scene or during transport
Underlying neurologic illness or disease

is sometimes complicated by the child's condition. Spontaneous eye opening may be impossible to elicit in the child whose eyes are swollen shut; verbal responses are impossible to elicit in the child who is sedated or intubated. Because these conditions affect the ability to obtain an accurate score, they are documented.

Each of the three categories in the MGCS is graded separately, and the sum of the scores can range from 3 to 15 points. Morbidity and mortality are high in children with a MGCS less than 8, particularly when coupled with a history of a severe head injury.

A rapid method of assessing the child's mental status during the primary survey is denoted by AVPU, which stands for *Alert;* responds to *Verbal* stimuli; responsive only to *Painful* stimuli; and *Unresponsive* to the surroundings (see p. 505, Chapter 21). This method is especially useful in preverbal children because it provides a simple and consistent means of evaluating the child at all developmental and cognitive levels.

Another important consideration during the assessment is the presence of age-appropriate behavior. Although objective neurologic parameters are assessed by the MGCS, the age-appropriate ability to communicate, recognize parents, and respond to comforting measures also provides important clues to the child's neurologic status. It must be remembered, however, that regression is common in the frightened child; therefore the inability of the child to cooperate during the examination does not necessarily indicate the child is seriously ill.

Assessment of the cranial nerves and pupils. The pupils are assessed for equality and response to bright light. Differences in pupil diameters of more than 1 mm is abnormal unless the child has a history of normally unequal pupils (anisocoria). Abnormal pupillary responses may indicate any number of injuries, including third nerve compression or direct injury, carotid artery injury, or midbrain dysfunction.[4] Pupillary changes are late signs of increased ICP in the child.

The child's eyes are also assessed for position, and vertical and horizontal eye movements. Abnormalities of eye movement and position can indicate significant head injuries and neurologic deterioration (Table 22-1).

Because pupillary responses reflect cranial nerve function, the corneal, oculocephalic, and/or oculovestibular reflexes may be tested. The corneal reflex tests the trigeminal nerve (V) and is tested by gently stroking the cornea with a piece of cotton. The normal response should be tearing or blinking. When absent, brainstem insult or coma is present.

The oculovestibular or caloric reflex tests the trochlear (IV) and abducens (VI) cranial nerves and is

TABLE 22-1	Assessing the Eyes	
FINDING	**DESCRIPTION**	**POSSIBLE CAUSE**
Dysconjugate gaze	Eyes move independently of each other	Usually indicates injuries to pathways controlling vision
Nystagmus	Horizontal or vertical rhythmic movement of the eyes	May result from central nervous system insults, cerebellar or vestibular injuries, inner ear inflammation, drug toxicities, or blindness from infancy
Setting-sun sign	The white of the sclera can be observed between the upper eyelid and the iris, with the iris and pupil nearer the lower lid	Associated with hydrocephaly and obstructive brain lesions; most often seen in infants whose sutures have not yet closed
Isolated pupil dilation	Pupil dilates on the ipsilateral (same side) as the lesion	Compression of the oculomotor or third cranial nerve; often caused by transtentorial herniation

Adapted from Henderson DP, Seidel JS, eds: *Assessment of the pediatric patient,* Torrance, Calif, 1990, Pediatric Rural Emergency System and Education Project.

Table 22-2	The Cranial Nerves	
Number	**Name**	**Area served**
I	Olfactory	Smell
II	Optic	Vision
III, IV, VI	Oculomotor, trochlear, abducens	Ocular motility, oculocephalic reflexes; pupil size, symmetry, and reactivity
V	Trigeminal	Facial sensation and corneal reflex
VII	Facial	Facial expression and symmetry
VIII	Vestibulocochlear	Hearing and oculovestibular reflex
IX, X	Glossopharyngeal, vagus	Gag, cough, and protective airway reflexes
XI	Spinal accessory	Trapezius and sternocleidomastoid movement
XII	Hypoglossal	Tongue movement

performed by instilling a small amount of iced saline solution into the ear. Normally the eyes should deviate toward the irrigated ear; if this does not occur, brainstem injury should be suspected. Finally, the oculocephalic or dolls' eye reflex tests the oculomotor (III), trochlear (IV), and abducens (VI) cranial nerves and is performed by moving the head rapidly from side to side—*after* trauma to the cervical spine has been ruled out. Normally the eyes should move opposite the direction in which the head is turned. If the eyes remain midline during the procedure, brainstem injury has occurred (Table 22-2).

Assessment of sensory and motor function. The extremities are tested for sensory and motor function, and the deep tendon reflexes are evaluated. Movement of the extremities is observed for equality of movement, symmetry, and strength. When testing sensory and motor responses, general activity, posture, and body movement are observed.

Response to painful stimulus is evaluated and characterized as purposeful movement away from the stimulus, reflex withdrawal, rigid extension, or no response at all. Temperature, touch, and two-point discrimination are also evaluated.

Interventions. Interventions for the management of increased ICP are also discussed in Chapter 7.

Airway and positioning. The first priority of care for the victim of traumatic head injury is the establishment of a patent airway while maintaining cervical spine immobilization. The child's oropharynx is cleared of debris such as blood, mu-

cus, emesis, or broken teeth and the child is placed on a backboard and a cervical collar is applied (Box 22-3).

Because the relatively large occiput of the child can cause neck flexion when the child is placed on a backboard, a pad the length of the body may be used to maintain cervical spine alignment (Fig. 22-8). Cervical spine immobilization devices must be properly fitted to the child and should not produce hyperextension of the neck, which occurs if the collar is too large. Soft, foam collars provide no cervical spine protection, and the Philadelphia collar, which does not fit children younger than 4 years of age, immobilizes the lower cervical spine but provides little protection to the upper spine. In very young children the (Laerdal) stiff neck Baby No-neck collar can be used. Regardless of the type of collar used, the child's head should also be supported with foam blocks, Velcro straps, and towel rolls to prevent lateral movement (see Fig. 21-5, p. 501).

Supplemental oxygen is administered to all victims of head trauma, since cerebral ischemia is an important secondary complication of head injury. If respirations or respiratory effort is inadequate, bag-valve-mask (BVM) ventilation with 100% oxygen, and hyperventilation is begun. Indications for BVM ventilation and subsequent intubation include evidence of severe head and neck trauma, respiratory failure, respiratory arrest, or a GCS less than 8. The act of intubation (and suctioning) can produce a rise in ICP. Ideally, although it is not always possible, the intubation should be performed only after hyperventilation with 100% oxygen; the administration of a nondepolarizing muscle relaxant (e.g., vecuro-

> **Box 22-3   Emergency Nursing Management of the Child with Head or Neck Trauma**
>
> Position the airway and clear the airway of debris, maintaining cervical spine immobilization
> Provide assisted ventilation and hyperventilation as indicated
> >   Evidence of severe head trauma
> >   Signs of respiratory failure
> >   Respiratory arrest
> >   MGCS less than 8
>
> Place the child on a heart rate monitor and pulse oximeter
> Assist with orotracheal intubation as indicated
> Establish venous access
> >   Administer 20 ml/kg bolus of normal saline or lactated Ringer's solution if shock is present; restrict fluids if there are no signs of shock
> >   Anticipate vasoconstrictor therapy if signs of neurogenic shock are present
>
> Anticipate management of increased ICP
> >   Hyperventilation
> >   Fluid restriction and strict regulation of input & output
> >   Serial arterial blood gas measurements to monitor CO_2 and O_2 levels
> >   Elevate the head of the bed 15 to 30 degrees *only* if the blood pressure is stable and there is no evidence of vertebral or spinal damage
> >   Diuretic therapy
> >   ICP monitor or intraventricular drain
>
> Anticipate seizure control
> Anticipate surgical intervention

nium); and the administration of thiopental or a similar rapid-acting anesthetic agent—as long as the child is normotensive.[4]

Intubation is performed by the orotracheal route. Blind nasotracheal intubation is difficult, time-consuming, and not recommended in children. If the child has a basilar skull fracture, nasotracheal intubation can inadvertently penetrate the cranial vault. When neck trauma and/or edema is present, airway anatomy may be distorted, further complicating the intubation attempt. When severe facial or neck injuries prevent airway control, cricothyrotomy may be required. Only in very rare circumstances should a tracheostomy be performed and only then by someone skilled in the technique.

Circulation. Venous access is obtained and bolus therapy initiated if signs of shock are present. After the treatment of shock, fluid restriction is instituted if an intracranial lesion or cerebral edema is suspected. This is both to reduce the amount of cerebral edema that can occur secondary to the injury and to counteract the increased production of antidiuretic hormone (ADH), which contributes to fluid retention.

When shock is present, fluids are **never** withheld at the expense of tissue perfusion. Because of the child's relatively small circulating volume compared to an adult, hemorrhagic shock may occur rapidly and is evidenced by decreased pulses, delayed capillary refill, cool skin, and altered mental status. The presence of shock is treated with a 20 ml/kg bolus of normal saline or lactated Ringer's solution. Repeat boluses are administered based on the child's clinical response to therapy. Significant blood loss is treated with transfusion therapy (see Chapter 21, Multiple Trauma Management).

A relatively uncommon form of shock is neurogenic shock, which produces massive vasodilation. Signs of neurogenic shock include a wide pulse pressure, warm flushed skin, and a falling blood pressure. If neurogenic shock is identified, fluid resuscitation is required as already mentioned. Fluids containing free water such as 5% dextrose in water (D_5W) should not be used. In addition to fluid therapy, pharmacologic management with vasoconstrictor therapy may be used.

Cerebral perfusion and ICP management. Initially following a TBI there is an increase in cerebral blood flow (hyperemia), which produces increased ICP. When signs of increased ICP are present, hyperventilation is recommended to reduce $Paco_2$. When $Paco_2$ is reduced, cerebral blood flow decreases. The $Paco_2$ is maintained between 25 and 35 torr though levels less than 30 torr are used when herniation is imminent.[4,18]

In children with suspected increased ICP, serial blood gas measurements, which may be obtained through an arterial line, are required to closely monitor the child for hypocapnia, which can reduce cerebral circulation to the point where cerebral ischemia oc-

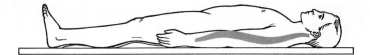

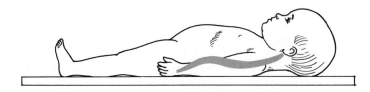

FIG. 22-8. Spinal immobilization of the child. The relatively large occiput of the child can cause the neck to flex when the child is immobilized on a backboard. The use of a pad the length of the body will produce neutral alignment.

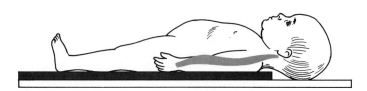

curs. In addition, respiratory alkalosis caused by hyperventilation shifts the hemoglobin-oxygen dissociation curve to the left, which impairs the unloading of oxygen to the tissues.[18]

Hypothermia (body temperature maintained between 95.0° F [35° C] and 96.8° F [36.0° C]) is a controversial method of controlling cerebral blood flow. The goal of hypothermia therapy is to decrease oxygen consumption. When hypothermia is combined with other interventions to reduce ICP, the ICP may fall below critical levels.[44] If shivering occurs, however, cerebral oxygen consumption increases.

Another method of improving ventricular drainage or cerebral venous return, and therefore treating increased ICP, is elevating the head of the bed 15 to 30 degrees. This can only be done if the blood pressure is stable and there is no evidence of vertebral or spinal cord damage. When the child is in this position, the head and neck are maintained in the midline to prevent jugular venous obstruction.[44]

Other methods of treating increased ICP include pharmacologic management and the use of ICP bolts or intraventricular catheters. These treatments are discussed in detail in Chapter 7, Life-threatening Neurologic Emergencies, pp. 144-145.

Pharmacologic management. Diuretics such as mannitol and furosemide (Lasix) may be used to control intracranial hypertension in posttraumatic comatose children (Table 22-3). Mannitol, an osmotic diuretic, rapidly reduces ICP by facilitating the diffusion of free water from the brain tissue into the serum. The usual pediatric dose is 0.25 to 1.0 g/kg[48] and may be repeated every 5 minutes as needed.[25] When mannitol is used, serum osmolality must be monitored and maintained in the 300 to 310 mOsm/L range and should not exceed 320 mOsm. Mannitol is contraindicated in the hypovolemic patient because it would further exacerbate the hypovolemic state and may produce shock.

Furosemide, which is a loop diuretic, can be given independent of or in conjunction with mannitol. The usual pediatric dose is 0.5 to 1 mg/kg.[18,25] When administered with mannitol, furosemide can potentiate mannitol's action. When any diuretic is used, the plasma sodium concentration and serum osmolarity must be frequently monitored.

Central nervous system sedatives combined with analgesics and paralytics may be useful in children who are awake enough to protest procedures such as CT scanning or are combative. Although there is no evidence that sedatives directly affect ICP, they can secondarily affect ICP by reducing muscle tension, straining, posturing, and the increased intrathoracic pressure and coughing associated with intubation.[4,44] They should be used with caution, however, since their effects can mask deteriorating neurologic status. One suggested protocol is the use of the morphine 0.1 mg/kg/hr and midazolam 0.04 mg/kg, fol-

TABLE 22-3	Pharmacologic Management of the Child with Head or Neck Injury	
DRUG	**DOSE**	**COMMENTS**
Diuretics		
Mannitol	0.25 to 1 g/kg IV	Osmotic diuretic; serum osmalality and sodium must be monitored; contraindicated in hypovolemia; monitor urine output
Furosemide (Lasix)	0.5 to 1 mg/kg IV	Loop diuretic; can potentiate the action of mannitol; monitor sodium and potassium levels; monitor urine output
Sedatives/analgesics		
Morphine	0.1 to 0.2 mg/kg IV	Used for pain control; monitor respiratory rate
Midazolam (Versed)	0.05 to 0.15 mg/kg IV or IM 0.5 to 0.75 mg/kg oral or rectal (using the IV formulation) 0.2 to 0.5 mg/kg nasal or sublingual	Used for sedation for procedures such as CT scan or intubation
Paralytic		
Vecuronium (Norcuron)	0.2 mg/kg IV	Nondepolarizing skeletal muscle relaxant used to facilitate endotracheal intubation; child must first be sedated; airway equipment must be assembled and at the bedside before administration
Barbiturate		
Pentobarbital (Nembutal sodium)	For barbiturate coma: 5 mg/kg IV loading dose; 1 to 4 mg/kg/hr continuous infusion	Use is controversial; child should have a central line, arterial line, and intraventricular monitoring device in place before use
Anticonvulsants		
Diazepam (Valium)	0.1 to 0.3 mg/kg (IV, endotracheal tube, rectal)	Used only for uncontrolled status epilepticus; monitor respiratory status
Lorazepam (Ativan)	0.03 to 0.10 mg/kg IV	Monitor respiratory status; give over 2 minutes
Phenobarbital	15 to 30 mg/kg IV	Infuse no faster than 50 mg/min or 1.5 mg/kg/min; mix only with normal saline solution
Phenytoin (Dilantin)	10-15 mg/kg IV loading dose	Infuse no faster than 1 mg/kg/min; mix only with normal saline solution; rapid administration can produce hypotension
Steroid		
Methylprednisolone (Solu-Medrol)	For spinal cord injury: 30 mg/kg IV push; followed by 5.4 mg/kg/hr for 23 hours	Indicated for spinal cord injuries; use in head-injured children is controversial

Compiled from Bruce, 1993; Cote, 1994; Ghajar and Hariri, 1992; Luerssen, 1993; Woodward, 1993.

lowed by 0.2 mg/kg/hr maintenance dose of morphine and pancuronium 0.1 mg/kg/hr.[18]

Barbiturates are occasionally used in the management of the head-injured child, although their use is controversial. Barbiturates are thought to decrease the cerebral metabolic rate and protect the brain during times of reduced cerebral perfusion, as occurs when ICP rises. When barbiturates are used the child's blood pressure, ICP, and cardiac output are continuously monitored, because high doses of barbiturates can produce hypotension and reduce cardiac output. The use of barbiturate coma is reserved for those occasions when all other methods have failed to reduce the ICP.

Steroids. There is no clear evidence that steroids are of benefit or improve the outcome of head-injured children. They have, however, proven useful in the treatment of patients with mass lesions such as brain tumors or discrete hematomas. For this reason, steroid use remains a point of controversy in the management of TBI.

In contrast, spinal cord injuries are commonly treated with steroids. In these children, intravenous methylprednisolone 30 mg/kg is given, followed by 5.4 mg/kg/hr for 23 hours.[25,47]

Seizure control. Seizures after head trauma are more likely to occur in children than in adults. They may occur within the first hour of injury or days or weeks later. A single seizure at the time of the injury generally does not require treatment, whereas a seizure occurring after the first hour following the injury may require treatment. Continuous seizures always require pharmacologic management.

Acutely, seizures may be treated with diazepam 0.1 to 0.3 mg/kg or lorazepam; however, for ongoing management phenytoin (Dilantin) or phenobarbital and occasionally carbamazepine are used. Phenytoin in a 10 to 15 mg/kg loading dose infused no faster than 1 mg/kg/min is perhaps the most widely used of the drugs, since it produces less sedation than phenobarbital. However, therapeutic blood levels of 10 to 20 mg/dl are sometimes difficult to maintain in children.[33] On the other hand, if intubation and treatment for increased ICP are required or if the child is unresponsive to phenytoin, phenobarbital may be used. The use of posttraumatic seizure prophylaxis is controversial and may be effective in preventing the early onset of seizures and seizures associated with some severe forms of head trauma, but it is not effective in preventing the development of late seizures.[39]

Ongoing care and evaluation. Regardless of the seriousness of the injury, the head-injured child is continuously monitored for changes in neurologic status, including the pupils, response to pain, level of consciousness, and motor responses (purposeful, nonpurposeful, flaccid) (Box 22-4). Vital signs include serial measurements of the child's heart rate, respiratory rate and rhythm, and blood pressure. Normothermia must be maintained as hyperthermia increases oxygen consumption.

Intake and output are monitored, but are particularly important in the child receiving diuretics. If the child does not exhibit signs of hypovolemia, fluid restriction should be expected. In addition, electrolytes and serum osmolality are monitored. Serial arterial blood gases should be anticipated.

If the child sustained a severe injury, surgery or the insertion of an ICP monitoring device is immi-

---

Box 22-4 Continuous Nursing Evaluation

Monitor child on heart rate monitor and pulse oximeter.

Obtain serial vital signs including heart rate, respiratory rate, blood pressure, and temperature.

Monitor neurologic status:
  Pupillary responses
  Response to pain
  Level of consciousness
  Motor responses

Speak softly to the child and keep the child informed, even if he or she is unconscious.

Communicate with the family often and allow them to remain with the child whenever possible.

Maintain strict intake and output records and observe for signs of hypovolemia.

Anticipate diagnostic studies:
  CT scan: child may require sedation and should be accompanied by a nurse and/or physician*
  Skull x-rays
  Serial arterial blood gas measurements

Anticipate surgical intervention*:
  Prepare the child and family

*Anticipate and prepare the child for transport to a pediatric critical care center or level I trauma center.

nent. In all cases the family should be continuously apprised of their child's status. This will facilitate further communication and establish a mechanism for them to ask questions regarding their child's care.

THORACOABDOMINAL INJURIES

Intraabdominal and/or intrathoracic trauma can be seen most commonly in the child with multisystem injuries; however, each is occasionally associated with isolated injuries. The majority of thoracoabdominal injuries in children result from blunt trauma. Data collected by the National Trauma Registry between 1985 and 1991 indicate that blunt injuries accounted for 86% of thoracic injuries and 83% of abdominal injuries.[7] Life-threatening blunt thoracic injuries are associated with a fatal outcome in 14% of all cases of childhood trauma, whereas only 9% of blunt abdomi-

nal injuries are associated with a fatal outcome. Rarely are these injuries the immediate cause of death.

Etiology. The most frequent mechanisms of injury producing blunt thoracoabdominal trauma in the child include motor vehicle–related crashes, whether as an occupant, pedestrian, or bicycle rider. Other causes include sporting activities, falls, and child abuse.[42] The most commonly injured intraabdominal organs are the spleen, liver, kidneys, and gastrointestinal tract. Injuries to major vessels and the pancreas are less common.[9] The most common injuries associated with thoracic trauma are pneumothorax or hemothorax, pulmonary contusions, and rib injuries. Less commonly seen injuries involve the heart, diaphragm, vessels, and airways/esophagus (Table 22-4).[9]

Penetrating trauma, although rarely seen in children in the past, has become more common, particu-

TABLE 22-4	National Pediatric Trauma Registry Statistics, 1985 to 1991		
	PERCENT OF TOTAL SAMPLE (N = 25,301)	DEATHS	DEATHS ATTRIBUTED TO THORACIC OR ABDOMINAL INJURIES
Thoracic injuries	6% (1553)		
Blunt	86%	195	27
Penetrating	14%	33	34
Abdominal injuries	8% (2047)		
Blunt	83%	161	35
Penetrating	17%	15	10
FREQUENCY OF INJURIES			
Thoracic injuries			
Pneumothorax/hemothorax	52%		
Lungs	49%		
Ribs	21%		
Heart	10%		
Diaphragm	4%		
Vessels	2%		
Abdominal injuries			
Liver	27%		
Spleen	27%		
Kidneys	25%		
Gastrointestinal tract	21%		
Vessels	5%		
Genitourinary tract	5%		
Pancreas	4%		

Abstracted from Cooper A et al: Mortality and truncal injury: the pediatric perspective, *J Pediatr Surg* 29:1, 33-38, 1994.

larly in adolescents in urban areas where the incidence of gunshot wounds has increased.[8,35] The mortality for children with penetrating abdominal trauma is 6%; however, the mortality associated with penetrating intrathoracic injuries is in excess of 50%.[10,35]

ANATOMY AND PHYSIOLOGY

The musculature of the child's chest and abdomen is less developed than in the adult. The ribs are flexible and located more anteriorly, affording less protection to the lungs and abdominal organs. The protuberant abdomen coupled with the thin abdominal wall places organs close to impacting forces during a traumatic event. In addition, the child's small body size causes energy that would be dissipated over a large area in an adult to be concentrated over a smaller area, predisposing the child to multiple rather than single injuries (Box 22-5).[9,37] Seemingly insignificant forces can, for these reasons, often produce significant underlying injuries.

Pathophysiology. Thoracoabdominal injuries result from either blunt or penetrating forces. Blunt trauma may cause any number of injuries within the abdominal cavity, including crushing or bursting of the solid upper abdominal organs, perforation of the hollow viscus, or shearing of the vascular supply after rapid deceleration forces.[7] In the child the most commonly injured abdominal organs are the spleen, liver, and kidneys.

Thoracic injuries are second only to head injuries as a cause of traumatic death in children.[9] The most common intrathoracic injuries resulting from blunt trauma include pneumothorax and pulmonary contusions. Although these injuries are potentially life-threatening, they are rarely the immediate cause of death in the severely injured child. Because of the child's pliable rib cage, rib fractures are uncommon; however, significant underlying injuries may be present. Conversely, because of the force required to produce rib fractures in the child, the presence of rib fractures is associated with serious underlying injuries.

In penetrating injuries the degree of damage is directly attributed to the amount of kinetic energy transferred to the surrounding tissue. Therefore, a high-velocity weapon such as a gun produces more damage to surrounding tissues than a knife wound. The degree of injury depends on the type of gun and bullets used, the bullet trajectory, and the distance of the victim from the weapon. Children with penetrating thoracic trauma are more likely to require surgical intervention than adults.

THORACIC INJURIES

Pneumothorax/tension pneumothorax. Simple or closed pneumothorax is the collection of air into the pleural space with partial or complete collapse of the lung. The most common cause of a closed pneumothorax is blunt thoracic trauma, which causes the alveoli to rupture with a resulting escape of air, collapsing the lung. Because the injury is closed, the lung seals preventing further leakage. Pneumothoraces may be small or large and may produce significant respiratory symptoms or none at all. An open pneumothorax usually results from penetrating thoracic injuries and may lead to a tension pneumothorax or hemothorax.

A tension pneumothorax may be caused by blunt or penetrating trauma and results from the progressive entry of air into the pleural space without a means of escape. The result is collapse of the lung on the affected side and progressive pressure on the opposite lung, producing a mediastinal shift away from the affected side. Subsequent compression of the heart and great vessels diminishes cardiac output.

Signs of a tension pneumothorax include marked tachypnea, tachycardia, hypotension, a tracheal shift to the opposite side (this may be difficult to appreciate

---

> **Box 22-5 Anatomic Features Contributing to Abdominal and Thoracic Injuries**
>
> **Abdomen**
> Ribs are horizontally oriented, offering less protection to the abdominal organs.
> Abdominal muscles are less developed and therefore thinner than in the adult.
> Organs are relatively large and closer to the source of impact.
>
> **Chest**
> Ribs are soft and pliable.
> Respiratory muscles are poorly developed.
> The thorax is small and less able to dissipate energy during a traumatic impact.
> The bony and cartilaginous chest wall structures are more elastic.
> The mediastinum is more mobile.

in infants and young children), absent or decreased breath sounds, and neck vein distention (also difficult to appreciate in young children). Treatment requires immediate needle or thoracostomy decompression.

Hemothorax. Hemothorax is the accumulation of blood in the pleural cavity. It can result from blunt or penetrating trauma. Signs of a hemothorax are similar to those of a pneumothorax and include tachycardia, tachypnea, and decreased breath sounds. Depending on the severity of the injury, hypovolemic shock and severe respiratory distress can result. Treatment depends on the severity of the symptoms. Hypovolemia is treated with fluid bolus therapy, and respiratory distress is treated with oxygen therapy, ventilatory support, and the insertion of a chest tube.

Pulmonary contusion. Pulmonary contusion results from a blunt parenchymal injury. It is usually caused by blunt trauma to the chest that transmits kinetic energy from the overlying chest wall to the underlying lung tissue. Pulmonary edema, alveolar hemorrhage, and desquamative alveolitis result (Fig. 22-9). Acute, life-threatening pulmonary contusions are rare; however, the increasing pulmonary capillary permeability and resultant decrease in pulmonary gas exchange can lead to the development of adult respiratory distress syndrome (ARDS). Initial management requires a strong suspicion of underlying pulmonary injuries and close monitoring for the development of respiratory symptoms. Positive pressure ventilation with oxygen support and positive end-expiratory pressure (PEEP) may be required.

Flail chest. Flail chest, although rare in children, is most commonly the result of blunt chest trauma. It is defined as rib fractures of two or more adjacent ribs at two or more sites.[40] The presence of rib fractures alone, however, does not constitute flail chest. Flail chest is characterized by the asymmetric, paradoxic inward motion of the chest during inspiration and crepitus at the fracture site.[7] Point tenderness, palpable bony deformities, and subcutaneous emphysema may also be present. Hypotension, severe respiratory distress, hypoxia, and then asphyxia can result. One or more sites may be involved, including the anterior chest, lateral chest, or posterior chest.

Because rib fractures are rarely seen in the child, flail chest is uncommon. The significant force required to produce flail chest in the child often produces severe underlying injuries of the lungs, such as pulmonary contusion and hemothorax, and abdominal organs. Other commonly associated injuries include head, pelvic, spinal, and skeletal injuries.[40] Although past treatment regimens advocated the use of mechanical ventilation, more recent approaches evaluate the extent of the child's injuries and the ability to oxygenate. Alternative methods of treating flail chest include fluid restriction and diuresis (to prevent pulmonary edema), the control of chest pain (to prevent splinting and therefore hypoventilation), providing supplemental oxygen, and encouraging coughing and deep breathing.

Pericardial tamponade. Pericardial tamponade results when a significant amount of blood, fluid, or air accumulates in the pericardial sac. It is most com-

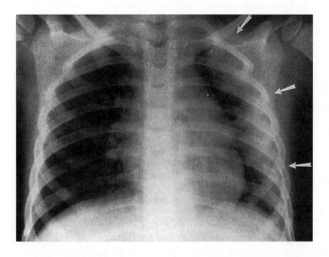

FIG. 22-9. Pulmonary contusion. (From Swischuk LE: *Emergency imaging of the acutely ill or injured child,* ed 3, Baltimore, 1994, Williams & Wilkins.)

monly associated with penetrating injuries, but can also be present after a crushing chest injury. It is rare in pediatric patients. In the child, relatively small volumes of blood or air (as little as 25 to 50 ml) can compromise venous return and ventricular function, producing signs of shock. Findings associated with pericardial tamponade include hypotension, neck vein distention, muffled heart sounds, pulsus paradoxus (a fall in arterial blood pressure of 8 to 10 mm Hg or more during inspiration), and an elevated central venous pressure. These findings, although diagnostic in the adult, may be difficult to appreciate in the child with multiple injuries who is in respiratory failure or shock; therefore a strong suspicion based on the mechanism of injury and location of the injuries is required. Other findings include air hunger, pallor, restlessness, and a rapid, thready pulse. Pericardiocentesis may be performed emergently to reduce compression of the heart and improve ventricular filling; however, definitive treatment requires direct, surgical pericardial repair.

Traumatic asphyxia. Traumatic asphyxia results when severe compressive forces suddenly increase intrathoracic pressure while the child's lungs are full of air and the glottis is closed. The sudden increase in intrathoracic pressure is transmitted to the venules of the head, neck, and upper body. Clinical findings include subconjunctival hemorrhages, petechial hemorrhages in the upper body, facial edema, cyanosis, and varying degrees of pulmonary and central nervous system dysfunction. Pulmonary contusion and intraabdominal injuries are commonly associated with traumatic asphyxia. Treatment depends on the severity of the injuries but is mostly supportive.

Traumatic diaphragmatic hernia. Traumatic diaphragmatic hernia results from severe abdominal compression from blunt or crushing forces that produce stress at both ends of the peritoneal cavity. When the diaphragm ruptures, usually on the left side (the right side is protected by the liver), abdominal contents can rapidly herniate into the chest. Signs of a right-sided herniation often develop more insidiously. Mechanisms of injury in the child include lap belt injuries, penetrating trauma, and pedestrian injuries where the child is run over by a vehicle. Treatment requires surgical intervention.

ABDOMINAL INJURIES

Splenic trauma. The spleen is one of the most commonly injured organs in the pediatric victim of blunt abdominal trauma. The spleen performs several

TABLE 22-5	CT Classification of Splenic Injury Severity
GRADE	**DESCRIPTION**
1	Capsular avulsion, superficial laceration, or subcapsular hematoma
2	Parenchymal laceration 1 to 3 cm deep and/or central/subcapsular hematoma less than 3 cm
3	Laceration greater than 3 cm deep, and/or central/subcapsular hematoma greater than 3 cm
4	Fragmentation of three or more sections, devascularization of splenic parenchyma

From Eichelberger M: *Pediatric trauma,* 1993, St. Louis, Mosby, p. 459.

important functions, including serving as a bacterial filter; performing reticuloendothelial phagocytosis, forming antibodies, and hematopoiesis. It is located on the left side of the abdomen beneath the lower ribs, close to the diaphragm, stomach, tail of the pancreas, and left kidney. Injuries to the spleen are classified according to severity and may involve the capsule, hilar vessels, and/or parenchyma (Table 22-5 and Fig. 22-10).

Clinical findings associated with splenic injuries vary and, depending on the severity of the injury, may be nonspecific. Therefore a history of the mechanism of injury is extremely important. The majority of injuries result from motor vehicle–related trauma; other common mechanisms involve play, athletic activities, and child abuse. Signs of splenic injury may include any combination of the following: abdominal bruising or ecchymosis (flank—Turner's sign; umbilical region—Cullin's sign), left abdominal or flank pain, referred pain to the left shoulder (Kehr's sign), abdominal distention, rebound tenderness, dyspnea, hypotension, or vomiting. A conservative, nonoperative approach is preferred to splenectomy with close monitoring in an intensive care unit.

Liver trauma. The incidence of liver trauma equals that of splenic trauma in the pediatric victim of abdominal trauma.[9] The majority of liver injuries in the child result from blunt trauma; however, liver lacerations are also common in victims of penetrating abdominal trauma. The liver is located in the right upper thoracoabdomen and is protected

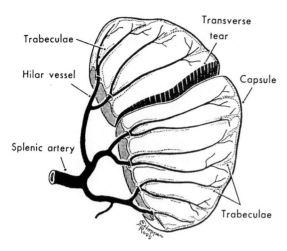

FIG. 22-10. The spleen and segmental blood supply. (From Upadhyaya P, Simpson JS: *Surg Gynecol Obstet,* 126:781, 1968. By permission of *Surgery, Gynecology & Obstetrics,* now known as the *Journal of the American College of Surgeons.*)

by the ribs. The liver in the young child is relatively large and extends slightly below the rib cage. Liver injuries are graded, depending on the severity of the injuries (e.g., laceration, hematoma, avulsion) and the location (e.g., capsular or subcapsular, parenchymal; vascular).

Clinical findings of liver damage vary, depending on the severity of the injury. Findings suggestive of liver trauma include an evaluation of the mechanism of injury, the presence of abrasions or contusions to the abdomen, abdominal tenderness and/or distention, and/or hypotension. An SGOT level of greater than 200 IU and an SGPT level greater than 100 IU correlate with the presence of hepatic injury.[43]

Kidney trauma. Renal trauma is the third most common type of intraabdominal trauma in the child. It is most commonly caused by blunt trauma associated with motor vehicle crashes. Other causes include falls from significant heights and sports-related activities. The child is more susceptible to renal injuries than the adult because of the relatively large kidneys in relation to body size, the underdeveloped abdominal wall, and the lesser protection by the rib cage. Damage may be directly related to the blunt force or may occur when acceleration-deceleration forces cause the fixed vascular pedicle to become a fulcrum, allowing the kidneys and vessels to become stretched or lacerated.[21] The

degree of renal injuries varies and may involve the parenchyma, capsule, collecting system, and/or major vessels (Fig. 22-11).

The child with kidney damage may have classic findings of flank and/or abdominal pain, ecchymosis or bruising, and/or a palpable flank mass or hematoma; be in hypovolemic shock; or be totally asymptomatic. Hematuria is considered a hallmark finding in the child with renal trauma, but the degree of hematuria does not correlate with the significance of the injury.[21]

Bowel trauma. Gastrointestinal injuries are present in approximately 21% of all significant abdominal injuries in children and may be caused by blunt or penetrating forces.[9] Children are at particular risk for gastrointestinal injuries because of their protuberant abdomens, thin abdominal wall, and propensity to swallow air (a full stomach is more prone to injury). Blunt intestinal injuries most commonly result from a direct blow to the abdomen occurring during a motor vehicle crash or as a victim of child abuse. In motor vehicle crashes, improper application of lap belt safety restraints around the abdomen can cause bowel compression, resulting in bowel laceration, perforation, or transection. In these children, bowel injuries coupled with spinal injuries are referred to as the "lap-belt complex."

Gastrointestinal injuries may affect the stomach, duodenum, small or large bowel, or mesentery. Both the mechanism of injury and the physical findings play a significant role in determining the treatment regimen. The abdomen should be examined for contusions, ecchymosis, or marks (e.g., from the seat belt). Other findings may include abdominal pain and vomiting. Significant respiratory distress may be observed in the child with pneumoperitoneum (free air in the abdomen), which is a serious complication associated with proximal bowel injuries.

EMERGENCY DEPARTMENT INTERVENTIONS

Diagnostic testing is based on physical findings, the mechanism of injury, and/or a strong suspicion of an underlying injury. Laboratory studies may include any or all of the following studies, depending on the seriousness of the child's injuries: arterial blood gases, hemoglobin and hematocrit (the spot hematocrit is of less value in determining blood loss than serial studies), liver enzymes, serum amylase (elevations may indicate injury to the pancreas or spleen), urine dipstick (blood may indicate genitourinary trauma),

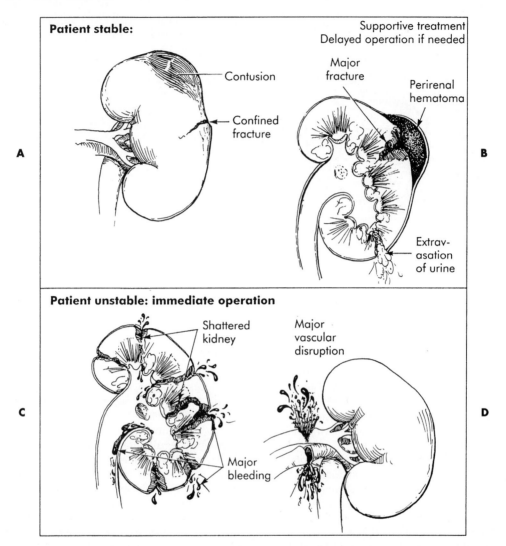

FIG. 22-11. Various types of blunt renal trauma. Types A and B often respond to nonoperative treatment. Types C and D usually require operative management. Type D requires emergency surgical intervention or loss of the kidney will result. Successful repair is rare. (From Rowe MI et al: *Essentials of pediatric surgery,* St Louis, 1995, Mosby.)

and/or urinalysis. Imaging methods used to identify underlying pathology include x-ray, CT scan, nuclear scan, or ultrasound.

Abdominal injuries. Of the tests described, the CT scan is by far the method of choice for evaluating intraabdominal injuries. It is a noninvasive procedure allowing for the examination of abdominal organs. Indications for obtaining an abdominal CT vary; however, the following criteria have been suggested: injuries from high-speed vehicular accidents and falls

from greater than two stories; significant objective findings, especially in children younger than 5 years of age and older than 11 years of age; a 10% or greater drop in the hematocrit; the presence of hematuria, gross or microscopic (more than 10 red blood cells per high power field); abnormal vital signs for age; an altered mental status; and significant head CT findings.[19]

Diagnostic peritoneal lavage (DPL) may rarely be used in the pediatric population. Although it will confirm the presence of blood or bowel contents in the

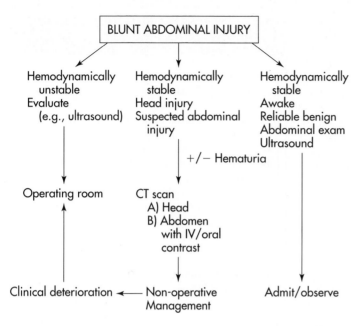

FIG. 22-12. Algorithm for blunt abdominal injuries with and without polytrauma. (From Stauffer UG: *J Pediatr Surg* 30(7):903–910, 1995.)

peritoneal space, it may miss significant injuries, such as a retroperitoneal hematoma and subcapsular liver or splenic injury.[42] It is also a painful procedure, and incisional pain may mask underlying symptoms. Despite these limitations, DPL is useful in situations where CT scanning is unavailable either because of the child's unstable condition (e.g., requiring immediate emergency department interventions or immediate surgery); or because of a lack of facilities; or in children with the "lap-belt complex" where the abdominal CT scan was normal.[42]

In general, the approach to therapy in the child victim of blunt abdominal trauma is largely conservative. Indications for surgical interventions include hemodynamic instability, diurnal instability, or the development of delayed or late complications.[37a,49] The treatment of penetrating abdominal trauma often requires surgical exploration to identify the extent of damage to the abdominal organs and to repair injuries.

Thoracic injuries. The child with chest trauma requires initial x-ray films of the chest. If significant trauma has occurred, an anteroposterior film may be taken with the child in the supine position, although this is not the ideal position for obtaining the film. Once the child's condition is stabilized and cervical spine injuries ruled out, an additional anteroposterior film may be required with the child in an upright position. CT scanning may also be used to identify

subtle injuries that may not be evident on the chest x-ray film.

Blood transfusions. Blood transfusion may be necessary; however, blood is administered only to maintain hemodynamic stability. In one study, children with hemoglobin levels as low as 6 gm% were hemodynamically stable and did not require blood transfusions. However, children with multiply injured abdominal organs were more likely to require a transfusion.[45]

Autotransfusion, or the collection and reinfusion of a patient's own blood, is used routinely in adult victims of significant trauma, particularly thoracic trauma, with large volume blood loss. Its use in children has only recently been investigated and it can be used in children with evidence of continuing blood loss and hemodynamic instability.[28]

NURSING CARE AND EVALUATION

Assessment. The primary assessment and management of the multiply injured child is reviewed in Chapter 21, Multiple Trauma Management. The purpose of this section is to review the nursing care of children with thoracoabdominal injuries.

After assessment of the ABCs, stabilization of immediate threats to life, and completion of a full set of vital signs, further assessment of the child's respiratory status is indicated. The chest is observed for respiratory effort, symmetry with inspiration and expiration, the use of accessory muscles, abdominal distention, and the presence of bruises or foreign bodies. Abdominal distention can impair the child's ability to ventilate effectively. In addition, the chest is serially auscultated for the presence of bilateral, equal breath sounds. Because of the child's thin chest wall and the close proximity of surrounding sounds to the stethoscope, the absence of air movement, as might occur with a pneumothorax, may not be appreciated. Finally, the chest wall is palpated for pain, crepitus, rib fractures, and subcutaneous emphysema.

The abdomen is observed for ecchymosis, bruising, abdominal distention, or the presence of foreign bodies. It is next auscultated for the presence of bowel sounds. If pain is present to palpation, its character, location, severity, and associated symptoms (e.g., pain referred to the shoulder) must be described. Other symptoms may include nausea, vomiting, or rebound tenderness (Box 22-6).

Interventions. With significant thoracic injuries the child's ability to ventilate effectively may be compromised. If the child is demonstrating signs of respiratory failure or airway compromise, positioning the airway and assisting ventilation with a BVM device is indicated.

Circulatory interventions are indicated in any multiply injured child where the possibility of significant underlying injuries exist. Children with signs of ongoing or significant blood loss (e.g., hemothorax, liver or spleen laceration) require the insertion of two large-bore intravenous lines for rapid fluid resuscitation.

Needle decompression and chest tube management. Needle decompression or thoracostomy of the pleural space is indicated in the child with a clinically significant pneumothorax or tension pneumothorax. To perform the needle decompression, a large-bore needle (14- to 18-gauge) with a syringe attached is inserted into the second intercostal space at the midclavicular line of the affected side or the fifth intercostal space at the anteroaxillary line. If the location of the pneumothorax is not known, the needle is inserted into the right, second intercostal space. Care must be taken to insert the needle over the rib, since the lower portion of each rib is highly vascular. Proper placement is confirmed when air is expelled or withdrawn

---

Box 22-6 Physical Findings Suggestive of Abdominal Injury

Physical signs
Rapid, shallow breathing
Abdominal tenderness
Flank or abdominal mass, contusion, or wound
Increasing abdominal girth
Blood in the urethral meatus, hematuria
Inability to void
Genital swelling or discoloration
Referred shoulder pain with upper abdominal palpation:
Right shoulder pain—hepatic injury
Left shoulder pain—splenic injury

Injuries frequently associated with abdominal injury
Fractured lower ribs
Penetrating trauma to the lower chest
Pelvic fracture
Multisystem trauma sustained during motor vehicle crash

Laboratory results
Elevated serum transaminase levels (hepatic injury)
Elevated serum amylase levels (pancreatic, small bowel injury)
Leukocytosis (may be nonspecific sign of stress or splenic trauma)

From Hazinski MF: *Nursing care of the critically ill child,* ed 2, St, Louis, 1992, Mosby.

---

into the syringe. Chest tube placement is required for ongoing care.

If the child is relatively stable, a chest tube may be rapidly inserted by personnel skilled in the technique. The area of insertion is initially cleaned and prepped with an antiseptic solution. If time permits, a local anesthetic is injected (see Box 21-5, p. 502 for chest tube sizes). The skin incision is usually made over the seventh to tenth ribs; however, the pleural space is entered one to two ribs above the incision to prevent air leakage after the tube is removed. Once the chest tube is in position, it is connected to an underwater drainage apparatus with a negative pressure of 3 to 5 cm H_2O (Fig. 22-13).

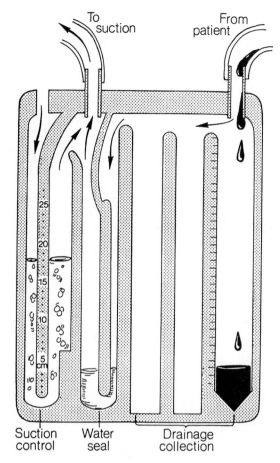

FIG. 22-13. Disposable chest drainage systems contain a collection chamber, a water seal chamber, and a suction control chamber. (From Hazinski MF: *Nursing care of the critically ill child*, ed 2, St Louis, 1992, Mosby.)

After chest tube insertion the child's ventilatory status is monitored continuously. Evaluation of respiratory rate and breath sounds and observation for the development of respiratory distress are required. If a hemothorax is present, the drainage of blood is monitored and frequent vital signs, including blood pressure, obtained. Blood loss exceeding 1 to 2 ml/kg of body weight per hour is an indication for surgical thoracotomy to control bleeding.[1]

Pericardiocentesis. Pericardiocentesis is rarely indicated in children. It is performed when blood, air, or fluid fills the pericardial sac, impairing ventricular filling and venous return to the heart. Its purpose is to rapidly decompress the pressure within the pericardial sac, and in the victim of trauma it is considered a short-term stabilizing measure. Early surgical intervention is the definitive treatment.

To perform the procedure, the left subxyphoid area is cleaned and prepped and the child attached to a cardiac monitor. A large-bore needle is slowly inserted with a large syringe (20 to 50 ml), and an alligator clip is attached.[17] This is ideally performed with echocardiography. During the procedure the nurse should monitor the child's respiratory rate, heart rate, and blood pressure and observe for the development of dysrhythmias associated with myocardial irritation. Fluid from the pericardial sac may be sent for laboratory analysis (Fig. 22-14).

After the procedure the child is continuously monitored while being prepared for surgical intervention. Complications from pericardiocentesis include arrhythmias, hemopericardium from laceration to the coronary arteries, and pneumothorax. Because pericardiocentesis may only temporarily relieve the pressure around the heart, signs of shock may redevelop.

Peritoneal lavage. Peritoneal lavage is a controversial procedure in the pediatric patient, but it has merit in some limited circumstances (see the discussion of emergency department interventions). It should only be performed by personnel skilled in the technique.

Before the procedure a urinary catheter is inserted to empty the bladder and a nasogastric (or orogastric tube) inserted to decompress the stomach. The area around the umbilicus is cleaned and prepped. A small incision is made either immediately above or just below the umbilicus. Frank blood on opening of the peritoneum is considered a positive finding. If no blood is present, a peritoneal lavage catheter is inserted into the opening and 10 to 20 ml of Ringer's lactate or normal saline solution is instilled into the abdomen. The fluid is then allowed to drain into a sterile collecting bag connected to the catheter. Fluid drained from the catheter is sent to the laboratory for red blood cell count, white blood cell count, amylase level, Gram stain, and examination for food or feces. The test is positive if the fluid contains 100 or more red blood cells per cubic millimeter.[7] The incision is closed with suture or Steri-strips.

After the test the child is continuously monitored for the development of hypovolemic shock, abdominal distention, increasing abdominal pain, fever, or any other signs that may indicate the development of peritonitis.

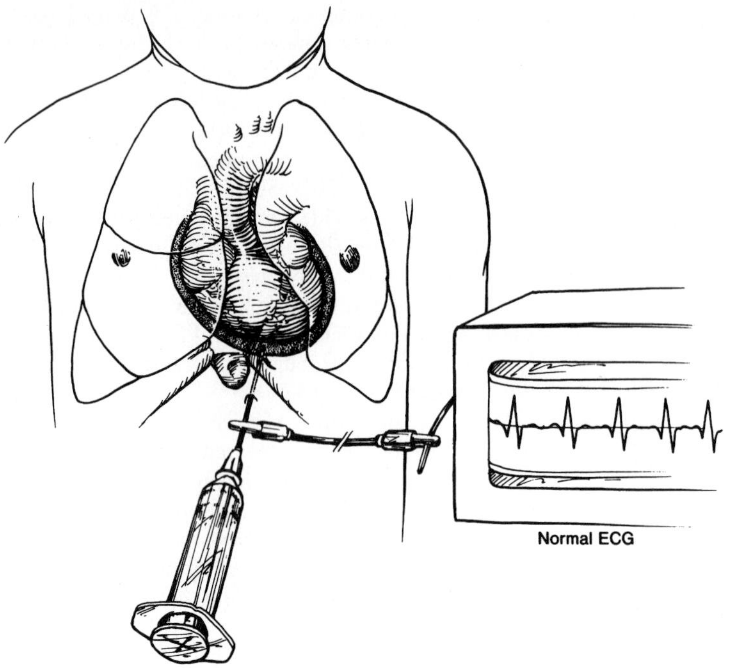

FIG. 22-14. Pericardiocentesis is performed when blood or fluid fills the pericardial sac, impairing cardiac function. A large-bore needle with a syringe and alligator clamp (for cardiac monitoring) attached is inserted into left subxiphoid area. The heart rate and rhythm are monitored continuously throughout the procedure. (From Fleisher G, Ludwig W: *Textbook of pediatric emergency medicine*, ed 3, Baltimore, 1993, Williams & Wilkins.)

Normal ECG

▌TRAUMATIC EYE INJURIES

Etiology. Children are at risk of sustaining eye injuries for various reasons. Infants and toddlers who are learning to walk and are exploring their environments can easily damage their eyes by falling on objects around them. Older children, who are more active and independent, are at risk of injuries related to play and sporting activities. Boys are at particular risk, sustaining eye injuries three to four times more often than girls.[29,36]

Pathophysiology. Eye injuries can involve any portion of the eye or the structures surrounding the eye(s). External signs and symptoms, such as lacerations, ecchymosis, or ptosis (drooping of the eyelid), may be the initial signs that an eye injury has occurred. Ocular movement can be affected by significant eye trauma, particularly trauma that involves muscle damage or entrapment. Damage to the sclera and conjunctiva is common in young children and can be caused by a laceration, foreign body, or hemorrhage.

The pupils, which are normally round and respond equally to light, may become irregularly shaped as a result of a ruptured globe or prolapse of the iris. Unequal pupils (anisocoria) may be observed with third nerve paralysis or increased intraocular pressure, as occurs with blood in the orbit. Anisocoria is, however, normal in some people; therefore, a thorough history is required when anisocoria is observed. Chapter 19 provides a complete discussion of the anatomy and physiology of the eye.)

Clinical presentation. Because eye trauma can range from a ruptured globe, to eyelid lacerations, to corneal abrasions, the clinical presentation can vary significantly. Externally the eyelids and area surrounding the eyes are observed for ecchymosis, lacerations, abrasions, or foreign bodies. Eye movements are evaluated for the absence of movement or for limited movement, and the pupils are assessed for size, response to light, and equality. Both the sclera and the conjunctiva are observed for lacerations, hemorrhages, or foreign bodies.

A high degree of suspicion that there is an underlying injury is maintained when evaluating any child with an eye injury. The presence of an apparently superficial injury may be the only clue to a more substantial underlying eye injury (Table 22-6).

Emergency Department and nursing interventions. The initial history includes a determination of

TABLE 22-6	Eye Injuries		
INJURY	**PATHOPHYSIOLOGY**	**CLINICAL PRESENTATION**	**INTERVENTIONS**
Ruptured globe	• Following the injury, the iris (or choroid) plugs the corneal wound • Crying, screaming, vomiting can increase intraocular pressure, resulting in extrusion of intraocular contents	• Iris may appear tear-drop shaped • Hyphema within the anterior chamber may be observed	• Ophthalmology consultation • Sedation for agitation; antiemetics for nausea may be required • Hard shield is required to protect the eye (no patch or pressure should be used) • Antibiotics may be required
Blowout fracture	• When pressure from a traumatic force causes the globe to "blow out" (fracture) one or more of the bones of the orbital wall	• Sunken or protruding eye(s) • Restricted eye movement • May be associated with eyeball injuries	• Ophthalomolgy consultation • CT scan of the orbit • If nerve compression is present or the eye is displaced, emergency intervention is required
Hyphema (blood in the anterior chamber)	• Caused by blood between the cornea and iris • Large hyphemas can fill the entire chamber; called a total hyphema or "eight ball" hyphema	• Blood in the anterior chamber; may be microscopic or diffuse—filling the entire chamber and obscuring the iris • Patients with bleeding disorders are at high risk for further bleeding	• Ophthalmology consultation • Strict bed rest and follow-up in the hospital or as outpatient • Sedation may be required for agitation • Patching and shielding are required
Corneal and conjunctival injuries	• Usually caused by mild surface trauma to the eye related to foreign bodies, or direct trauma from fingers or toys	• Common in children; should be suspected in "fussy" infants with no other signs of injury • Severe pain, exacerbated by blinking • Excessive tearing • Sensation of a foreign body in the eye	• Topical fluorescein (liquid or paper strips) is instilled in the eye; the eye is examined with a blue light, Wood's lamp, or Burton lamp • If corneal abrasion is present, treatment is patching (with eye closed) and antibiotics • If a corneal laceration is present, an ophthalmology consultation and strict bed rest are required; sedation for agitation may be indicated

Compiled from Fleisher GR, Ludwig SL, eds: *Textbook of pediatric emergency medicine,* ed 3, Baltimore, 1993, Williams & Wilkins; Barkin RM, ed: *Pediatric emergency medicine,* ed 2, St Louis, 1997, Mosby.

the child's normal visual acuity, whether the child wears glasses or contacts, and whether the child has ever had eye surgery or worn an eye patch. If the child is able to cooperate, a visual acuity test is performed in conjunction with the clinical examination. If the child is too young to cooperate or has sustained significant eye trauma, a thorough clinical examination is warranted. Additional historical questions determine the mechanism of injury, type of object producing the injury (e.g., blunt or sharp), and signs and symptoms following the injury (e.g., blood, fluid leakage, or photosensitivity).

When resuscitative care is required, eye injuries may be overlooked or moved down on the priority list. To prevent additional damage to the eye(s) during resuscitative efforts, an eye patch (or shield) is placed over the eye.

If a significant ocular injury is suspected, every effort is made to keep the child calm, since crying, screaming, and vomiting can increase intraocular pressure, causing intraocular contents to be expelled. Occasionally, sedation and antiemetic therapy is used.

The nurse should provide support to the parents and child who may fear the loss of sight, particularly if the injury is significant. They should be kept informed of the treatment plan and provided with frequent updates. If the child is to be discharged with a patch, the parents are given instructions for reapplying the patch if it is removed by the child. Mitts may be placed on the hands of infants to prevent them from pulling off the patch. The nurse should inform the parents of the location of the ophthalmologist or clinic that will provide the follow-up care as well as the time of the appointment. If an appointment cannot be made before the child leaves the emergency department, the parents are given the phone number and the importance of making a follow-up appointment is stressed.

REFERENCES

1. Allshouse MJ, Eichelberger MR: Patterns of thoracic injury. In Eichelberger MR, ed: *Pediatric trauma: prevention, acute care, and rehabilitation,* St Louis, 1993, Mosby.
2. Beaver BL et al: Characteristics of pediatric firearm fatalities, *J Pediatr Surg* 25:97, 1990.
3. Behrman RE et al: *Nelson textbook of pediatrics,* ed. 14, Philadelphia, 1992, WB Saunders.
4. Bruce DA: Head trauma. In Eichelberger MR, ed: *Pediatric trauma, prevention, acute care, rehabilitation,* St Louis, 1993, Mosby.
5. Bruce DA et al: Pathophysiology, treatment, and outcome following severe head injury in children, *Child's Brain* 5:174-191, 1979.
6. Bruce DA, Zimmerman RA: Shaken impact syndrome, *Pediatr Ann* 18:8, 1989.
7. Cooper A: Critical management of chest, abdomen, and extremity trauma. In Holbrook PR ed: *Textbook of pediatric critical care,* Philadelphia, 1993, WB Saunders.
8. Cooper A et al: Epidemiology of pediatric trauma; importance of population based statistics, *J Pediatr Surg* 27:149-154, 1992.
9. Cooper A et al: Mortality and thoracoabdominal injury, the pediatric perspective. Proceedings of the National Conference on Pediatric Trauma, *Pediatr Emerg Care* 9:3, 183, 1993.
10. Cooper A et al: Mortality and truncal injury: the pediatric perspective, *J Pediatr Surg* 29:1, 33-38, 1994.
11. Cote CJ: Sedation for the pediatric patient, *Pediatr Anesth* 41:1, 31-58, 1994.
12. Davis RJ et al: Head and spinal cord injury. In Rogers M, ed: *Textbook of pediatric intensive care,* Baltimore, 1987, Williams & Wilkins.
13. Di Scula C: Verbal communication regarding NPTR, 1996.
14. Dolan M: Head trauma. In Barkin RM, ed: *Pediatric emergency medicine, concepts and clinical practice,* St Louis, 1992, Mosby.
15. Duncan CC, Ment LR. In Touloukian RJ, ed: *Pediatric trauma,* St Louis, 1990, Mosby.
16. Fingerhut LA, Ingram DD, Feldman JJ: Firearm and nonfirearm homicide among persons 15-19 years of age: differences by level of urbanization, United States, 1979 through 1989, *JAMA* 267:3048, 1992.
17. Fleisher G, Ludwig S: *Textbook of pediatric emergency medicine,* ed 2, Baltimore, 1988, Williams & Wilkins.
18. Ghajar J, Hariri RJ: Management of the pediatric head injury, *Pediatr Clin North Am* 39:5, 1093-1125, 1992.
19. Hakim LS et al: Abdominal CT in pediatric blunt trauma; guidelines for appropriate utilization, proceedings of the National Conference on Pediatric Trauma, *Pediatr Emergency Care* 9:3, 1993.
20. Hennes H et al: Clinical predictors of severe head trauma in children, *Am J Dis Child* 142:1045-1047, 1988.
21. Hensle TW, Dillon P: Renal injuries. In Touloukian RJ, ed: *Pediatric trauma,* ed 2, St Louis, 1990, Mosby.
22. Herzenberg JE, Hensinger RN, Fielding JW: Fractures of the spine. In Rockwood CA, Wilkins KE, King RE, eds: *Fractures in children,* New York, 1991, JB Lippincott.
23. James HE, Anas NG, Perkin RM: *Brain insults in infants and children,* Orlando, Fla, 1985, Grune & Stratton.

24. James HE, Trauner DA: *Brain insults in infants and children,* Orlando, Fla, 1985, Grune & Stratton.
25. Johnson DL: Spinal cord injury in children. In Holbrook PR, ed: *Textbook of pediatric critical care,* Philadelphia, 1993, WB Saunders.
26. Johnson K: The Harriet Lane handbook, ed 13, St Louis, 1993, Mosby.
27. Kaufman BA, Dacey RG: Acute care management of closed head injury in childhood, *Pediatr Ann* 23:1, 18-27, 1994.
28. Kharasch SJ, Millham F, Vinci RJ: The use of autotransfusion in pediatric chest trauma, *Pediatr Emerg Care* 10:2, 109-111, 1994.
29. LaRoche GR, McIntyre L, Schertzer RM: Epidemiology of severe eye injuries in childhood, *Ophthalmology* 95:1603, 1988.
30. Levin AV: Eye trauma. In Fleisher GR, Ludwig SL, eds: *Textbook of pediatric emergency medicine,* ed 3, Baltimore, 1993, Williams & Wilkins.
31. Ludwig S, Loiselle J: Anatomy, growth, and development. In Eichelberger MR, ed, *Pediatric trauma, prevention, acute care, rehabilitation,* St Louis, 1993, Mosby.
32. Luerssen TG: General characteristics of neurologic injury. In Eichelberger MR, ed: *Pediatric trauma, prevention, acute care, rehabilitation,* St Louis, 1993, Mosby.
33. Luerssen TG, Klauber MR, Marshal LF: Outcome from head injury related to patient's age; a longitudinal prospective study of adult and pediatric head injury, *J Neurosurg* 68:409-416, 1988.
33a. Nitecki S, Moir CR: Predictive factors of the outcome of traumatic cervical spine fracture in children, *J Pediatr Surg* 29:11, 1409-1411, 1994.
34. Mitchell A Jr et al: Evaluation of minor head injury in children, *J Pediatr Surg* 29:7, 851-854, 1994.
35. Pepe P et al: The epidemiology and demography of juvenile gunshot wounds in a large municipality. Proceedings of the National Conference on Pediatric Trauma, *Pediatr Emerg Care* 9:3, 1993.
36. Rahman WM, O'Connor TJ. Facial trauma. In Barkin RM, ed: *Pediatric emergency medicine, concepts and clinical practice,* St Louis, 1992, Mosby.
37. Soud T, Pieper P, Hazinski MF: Pediatric trauma. In Hazinski MF, ed: *Nursing care of the critically ill child,* ed 2, St Louis, 1992, Mosby.
37a. Stauffer, UE: Surgical and critical care management of the child with life threatening injuries: the Swiss experience, *J Pediatr Surg* 30:7, 903-910, 1995.
38. Swischuk LE: Anterior displacement of C2 in children: physiologic or pathologic? *Radiology* 122:759, 1977.
39. Temkin NR et al: A randomized, double-blind study of phenytoin for the prevention of post-traumatic seizures, *N Engl J Med* 323:497, 1990.
40. Templeton JM: Thoracic trauma. In Fleisher GR, Ludwig S, eds: *Textbook of pediatric emergency medicine,* ed 3, Baltimore, 1993, Williams & Wilkins.
41. Tepas JJ et al: Mortality and head injury: the pediatric perspective, *J Pediatr Surg* 25:1, 92-96, 1990.
42. Thompson WR: Patterns of injury. In Eichelberger MR, ed: *Pediatric trauma: prevention, acute care, rehabilitation,* St Louis, 1993, Mosby.
43. Torres AM, Garcia VF: Hepatobiliary trauma. In Eichelberger MR, ed: *Pediatric trauma: prevention, acute care, rehabilitation,* St Louis, 1993, Mosby.
44. Tullous M, Walker ML, Wright LC: Evaluation and treatment of head injuries in children. In Fuhrman BP, Zimmerman JJ, eds: *Pediatric critical care,* St Louis, 1992, Mosby.
45. Umali E et al: Critical analysis of blood transfusion requirements as related to organ injury scaling in children with blunt abdominal trauma. Proceedings of the National Conference of Pediatric Trauma, *Pediatr Emerg Care* 9:3, 1993.
46. Venes JL, DiPietro MA: Spinal cord injury. In Touloukian RJ, ed: *Pediatric trauma,* St Louis, 1990, Mosby.
47. Woodward GA: Neck trauma. In Fleisher GR, Ludwig S, eds: *Textbook of pediatric emergency medicine,* Baltimore, 1993, Williams & Wilkins.
48. Yatsiv I: Central nervous system support techniques. In Holbrook, PR ed: *Textbook of pediatric critical care,* Philadelphia, 1993, WB Saunders.
49. Yoo SY et al: Pitfalls of nonoperative management of blunt abdominal trauma in children in Korea, *J Pediatr Surg* 31:2, 263-266, 1996.

CHAPTER 23

Musculoskeletal and Soft Tissue Injuries

Kim Schriefer, Rita Dello Stritto, Treesa Soud

Children come to emergency departments with a variety of injuries ranging from minor contusions to major trauma. Fortunately, the majority of these injuries require only ambulatory care interventions. Although major trauma accounts for relatively few visits when compared to total numbers, major trauma continues to be a significant cause of morbidity and mortality in the pediatric population (see Chapters 21 and 22). The purpose of this chapter is to review specific musculoskeletal and soft tissue injuries in children who may or may not require complex emergency department management.

Epidemiology. Children are extremely mobile and active, and they love to explore their environments. Young children, particularly toddlers learning to walk, are prone to head and facial injuries because their unsteady gait and height put them at risk for abrasions and lacerations from falls into coffee tables, fireplace grates, and corners of walls. In fact, children younger than 5 years of age suffer almost two times as many fall-related injuries as older children.[6]

Older children are more self-sufficient and therefore more mobile. They are particularly prone to injuries from playground equipment, bicycling, roller blading, or other sports-related activities. In addition, pedestrian injuries are almost twice as common in this age group when compared to younger children.[6]

Adolescents are increasingly independent. Because of this, they spend more time away from parental supervision and are vulnerable to peer pressure. Peer-related activities and risk-taking behavior contribute to the types of injuries sustained by adolescents. The most common injuries in this age group are caused by sports-related activities and motor vehicle crashes,

however, injuries associated with violence are becoming more and more common.

Another unfortunate cause of musculoskeletal and cutaneous injuries in children are non-accidental injuries resulting from child abuse. Although physical abuse can occur in a child of any age, it is most commonly recognized in children under the age of 4 years[11] (see Chapter 25, Child Maltreatment).

Prevention. Prevention requires diligent parental supervision as well as recognition of the types of injuries children are likely to sustain as they progress developmentally. The most important prevention strategy is to provide a safe environment based on the child's level of development. For example, in the infant's environment this would include removing sharp objects from reach and placing safety plugs on all electrical outlets. Older children and adolescents should be encouraged to wear protective gear such as bicycle helmets and knee and elbow pads. In addition, all children who ride bicycles, all-terrain vehicles, and other motorized vehicles should be taught to follow the rules of the road.

MUSCULOSKELETAL INJURIES

The child's musculoskeletal growth is dynamic and constantly changing. In young children and infants the bone is porous and flexible. As the child grows, bone density increases, beginning at the diaphysis. These developmental changes predispose the child to certain types of injuries at different ages. (See also Chapter 13, Musculoskeletal System.) Common skeletal injuries of childhood included cortical, buckle or torus fractures; greenstick fractures; bent or bowed bones without a visible fracture line; and epiphyseal-metaphyseal fractures.[21] Epiphyseal-metaphyseal fractures are ex-

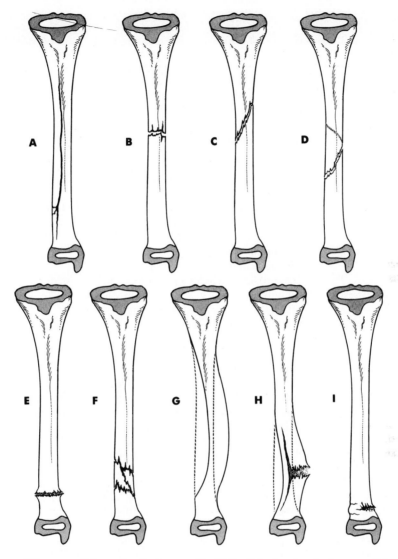

FIG. 23-1. Patterns of fractures. Schematic of a 3-year-old child's tibia showing basic types of fractures. **A,** Longitudinal; **B,** transverse; **C,** oblique; **D,** spiral; **E,** impacted; **F,** comminuted; **G,** bending/bowing; **H,** greenstick; **I,** cortical/torus. (From Barkin RM, ed: *Pediatric emergency medicine,* ed 2, St Louis, 1996, Mosby.)

tremely common in children and represent a slipping of the epiphyseal-metaphyseal surfaces caused by shearing force applied to the long bone. These injuries are also referred to as growth plate fractures (Fig. 23-1 and Table 23-1).

Bone healing in young children is more rapid than in older children and adults. This is primarily because of the abundant blood supply to the developing bone. In general, the younger the child, the more rapid is the rate of skeletal healing after traumatic injury.[14]

GROWTH PLATE INJURIES

Epidemiology. Growth plate or physeal injuries are common in children, particularly young adolescents, and are seen in up to 18% of all pediatric fractures.[1] The majority of physeal injuries occur in the radius and the ulna; however, other common areas of injury include the femur, tibia, and fibula.

Pathophysiology. Growth plate injuries involve the cartilaginous disc located between the epiphysis

TABLE 23-1	Types and Patterns of Fractures	

FRACTURES	DESCRIPTION
Types	
Diaphyseal	Involves central shaft of the bone
Metaphyseal	Involves the expanding end of the bone
Physeal	Involves the endochondral growth plate
Epiphyseal	Involves the chondro-osseous end of the long bone
Patterns	
Longitudinal	Fracture line follows the longitudinal axis
	Usually occurs in older children
Transverse	Fracture line is at a right angle to the longitudinal axis
	Common in the denser areas of the diaphysis in infants and young children
	Also common in metaphyseal fractures
Oblique	Fracture line is angled
	Common in greenstick fractures
Spiral	Fracture line encircles a portion of the bone shaft
Impacted or compression	Compression injury that usually involves the cortical and trabecular bone
Comminuted	Multiple, variably sized fragments of bone
	Uncommon in infants and young children
Bowing	Bone is deformed by bowing but no fracture is evident
	Common in infants and young children
Greenstick	Bone is bowed and incompletely fractured
	Common in infants and young children
Buckle or torus	Impaction injury primarily affects the porous metaphyseal bone
	Causes the bone to buckle (raise or bulge) rather than fracture completely
	Common in children; relatively uncommon in adolescence and adulthood
Pathologic	Occurs when the bone is abnormal
	Can be caused by tumors, infection, metabolic disorders, and hereditary disorders
Stress	Repetitive, small cortical injuries caused by relatively minor stress

Abstracted from Ogden JA: The uniqueness of growing bones. In Rockwood CA, Wilkins KE, King RF, eds: *Fractures in children,* ed 3, New York, 1991, Lippincott.

and metaphysis. These fractures can present in various forms. They are therefore described using the Salter-Harris classification[18] (Fig. 23-2).

Injuries to the growth plate include avascular necrosis, infection, or fractures and can produce significant long-term manifestations. Most injuries repair well with early recognition and treatment. Negative outcomes of significant injury can include bone growth disturbances, such as accelerated or decelerated growth to an area, a progressive angular deformity; or even arrested bone growth.

▌ LOWER EXTREMITY INJURIES

LIMP

Etiology. Limping is a common chief complaint of the musculoskeletal system in the child. Injuries, illnesses, or defects such as fractures, osteomyelitis, slipped capital femoral epiphysis, septic arthritis, or malignancies are all causes of limping. For this reason, the young child with a history of limping should always be taken seriously.

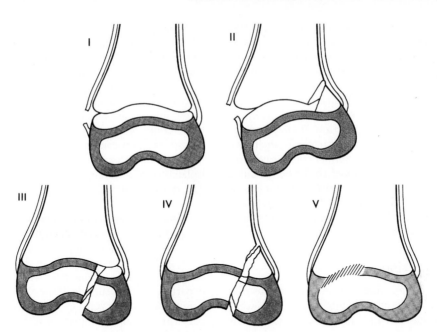

FIG. 23-2. The Salter-Harris classifications are used to describe epiphyseal injuries. *Type 1:* Fracture extends through the epiphyseal plate, resulting in displacement of the epiphysis. *Type II:* As above; additionally, a triangular segment of metaphysis is fractured. *Type III:* The fracture line runs from the joint surface through the epiphyseal plate and the epiphysis. *Type IV:* Fracture line occurs as in Type III but also passes through the adjacent metaphysis. *Type V:* Crush injury of the epiphysis; may be difficult to determine on radiograph. The prognosis for growth disturbance worsens from type I through type V. (From Barkin RM: *Pediatric emergency medicine,* ed 2, St Louis, 1996, Mosby.)

Pathophysiology. The etiology of a limp is difficult to evaluate in the very young child, since the child is unable—or unwilling—to adequately communicate with the examiner. As the child grows and becomes more cooperative, the physical examination becomes somewhat easier. Because of the wide range of etiologies, a thorough examination is warranted. Limping may represent trauma or inflammation of the pelvis, hip, or any portion of the lower leg or foot. In younger children, traumatic injury is the most common cause of a limp, particularly since the injury may not have been witnessed or may have seemed insignificant to the parent. In a child of any age, the cause of a limp can range from something as simple as an incorrectly sized shoe to something as complex as a malignant neoplasm.

Clinical presentation. Initially the child's gait should be observed, and attempts made to identify the source of the limp. While observing the child, the nurse should identify specific areas where the child may be favoring a portion of the extremity, such as not bending a knee or refusing to walk on a foot. The entire extremity, from the hip to the toes, should be examined for signs of swelling, redness, warmth to touch, pain over the bones or joints, point tenderness, and limited movement. Signs of infection may include swelling and/or warmth over the site of infection and the presence of a fever.

Emergency Department and nursing interventions. On arrival in the emergency department the nurse should initially observe the child's gait and obtain a complete history. A physical examination of the extremity should be performed and the child's vital signs obtained. A history of fever may be significant and should be reported to the physician. A neurocirculatory examination of the extremity is required, including distal pulses, skin color, capillary refill, gross and fine motor movement, and sensation. The foot should be examined for signs of calluses, foreign bodies between the toes, or ingrown toenails. Other questions that the parents may be asked include the following: Has the child received a recent intramuscular injection in the leg? Have the parents recently purchased new shoes for the child? Has the child had a history of fever, anorexia, or weight loss?

If an obvious source of the limp is not found, x-rays of the leg will be ordered to rule out traumatic injury or signs of inflammation or infection. If x-ray findings rule out a traumatic injury, laboratory tests, including a complete blood count, differential count, and sedimentation rate, may be required to further evaluate the cause of the limp. When the etiology is not found, after a full workup, the child may be sent home and asked to rest the extremity. If the limp persists, a more extensive workup is indicated.

FEMUR FRACTURES

Etiology. Femur fractures in children usually result from high-energy accidents such as significant falls, sports-related activities, motor vehicle crashes, or pedestrian or bicycle versus motor vehicle crashes. Femur fractures in children younger than 2 years of age often result from child abuse.

Pathophysiology. Femur fractures can occur at any one of a number of sites on the femur, including the neck of the femur, the trochanter, the midshaft, and the distal femur. Injuries that affect any one of the growth plates can impair blood supply, producing osseous necrosis and ultimate bone growth deformity. These injuries are rare and, when they do occur, are more commonly associated with displaced fractures. Femur fractures can produce significant hemorrhage in children, although the incidence associated with isolated injuries leading to hypovolemic shock is rare.[5] The risk is greater if the fracture is open (Fig. 23-3).

Clinical presentation. Femur fractures may be isolated injuries or occur in combination with other, sometimes significant injuries. The mechanism of injury plays an important role in the assessment and, coupled with clinical findings, will guide emergency department interventions. If the child was involved in a significant motor vehicle crash, either as a passenger or as a pedestrian, a complete head-to-toe examination should be performed to identify the presence of other serious injuries. Because femur fractures can cause significant hemorrhaging in the child and even lead to

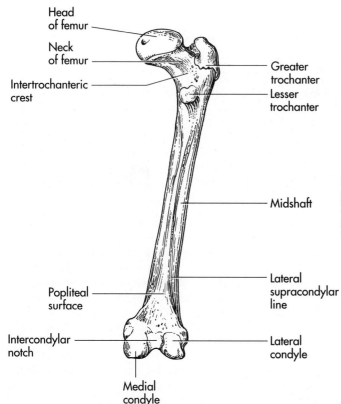

FIG. 23-3. The epiphyseal surfaces on the proximal femur include the areas between the head and neck of the femur, between the greater trochanter and the shaft, and between the lesser trochanter and shaft.

hemorrhagic shock, they should not be overlooked. Signs and symptoms of a femur fracture include severe leg pain, pain or grimacing to palpation, ecchymosis, and swelling of the thigh. Other signs include limited movement, pain on movement, and/or deformity.

Emergency Department interventions. Treatment depends on the age of the child and the type and location of the fracture. If the fracture is open, operative intervention and the possible insertion of internal fixation devices is indicated. Displaced fractures may also be treated with operative management, or the child may be placed in either skeletal or skin traction until the bones have stabilized. When the fracture is nondisplaced, a spica cast may be applied immediately. Older children, because of increased musculature in the legs, may require hospitalization and traction before application of the cast (Box 23-1).

TIBIA AND FIBULA FRACTURES

Etiology. Tibia and fibula fractures are the most common lower extremity fractures seen in young children. Fractures may include one or both bones and can affect the proximal or distal epiphysis, or the metaphysis. The mechanism of injury plays a significant role in the type of injury. Torsional or rotational forces in which the leg twists while the foot is intact produce spiral fractures of the tibial shaft while the fibula usually remains intact. This injury is most common in young children, particularly those less than 3 years of age. Fractures of both bones are most often seen in children who sustain direct trauma, such as a motor vehicle crash or sports-related injury. Tibia and fibula fractures are the most common site of stress fractures in adolescent athletes (Fig. 23-4).

Pathophysiology. Because of growth patterns within the developing bone, the types of tibia and fibula injuries sustained are often contingent on the child's age. Bone density increases in the midshaft of the tibia much more rapidly than in the fibula as the child matures. Therefore the fibula is more resilient to injury. Only approximately 30% of tibial fractures are associated with fibula fractures.[13]

Box 23-1   Nursing Care of the Child with a Fractured Femur

Immobilize the extremity.

Place ice on the injured site; if the fracture is open, place a sterile dressing on the site.

Evaluate the distal circulation (color, capillary refill, pulses) and nerve function (movement, sensation).

Closely observe the child for signs of shock from hemorrhage (capillary refill, skin color, mental status, frequent vital signs, including blood pressure).

Achieve venous access as ordered.

Administer pain medications as ordered; the child should be monitored by a pulse oximeter and/or a heart rate monitor.

Prepare for hospital admission or surgical intervention.

Prepare for skeletal or skin traction as indicated.

Provide psychologic support to both the family and child throughout the emergency department stay.

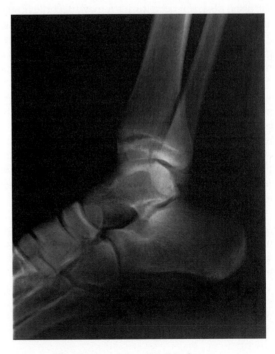

FIG. 23-4.   Salter IV tibia fracture.

Clinical presentation. Signs of a tibia and/or fibula fracture include edema, ecchymosis, pain, and deformity. If the wound is open, bleeding at the puncture site may be observed. As with all fractures, the neurovascular status of the injured extremity must be assessed, including distal pulses, capillary refill, sensation, movement of toes, and color of the extremity. One of the more severe complications of a lower leg fracture is the development of compartment syndrome.

Emergency Department interventions. Treatment of tibia and/or fibula fractures depends on the location and type of fracture. If the fracture is midshaft and nondisplaced, a long leg cast or splint may be applied to the extremity. If the fracture is displaced and cannot be reduced with a closed reduction, an open reduction will be required with possible internal pinning. All open fractures require operative intervention.

TODDLER'S FRACTURE

Etiology. Toddler's fractures are most common in children less than 3 years of age, but they can occur in children up to the age of 6 years. This fracture represents an oblique or spiral nondisplaced fracture of the distal tibia, but occasionally it may affect the fibula. The injury is usually caused by torsion of the foot (Fig. 23-5). When a midshaft spiral fracture of the tibia is present in the young child, it is most commonly caused by child abuse.

Pathophysiology. Bone growth patterns change in the maturing skeleton as the child develops. Initially, bone density increases in the midshaft and then begins to move distally down the bone shaft. In young children, particularly those learning to walk, the relatively porous bone of the distal bone shaft allows torsional forces to create oblique fractures with what may appear to be relatively minor forces.

Clinical presentation. One of the most common presentations of the child with a toddler's fracture is a history of limping or refusal to walk. The history may be insignificant; however, if the parents are questioned further, a history of minor trauma may be elicited. The ankle or lower leg may be tender to palpation and movement, particularly with passive twisting of the extremity. Swelling may be minimal or absent.

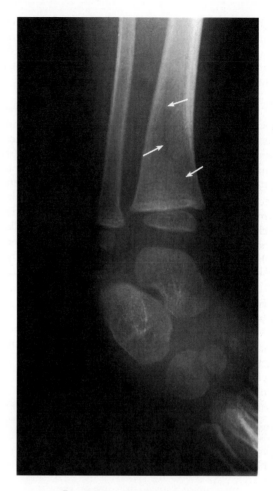

FIG. 23-5. Toddler's fracture.

Emergency Department interventions. Radiographic studies are generally indicated for the child with a history of extremity trauma or pain while walking. The diagnosis of a toddler's fracture, however, is sometimes difficult to make because the fracture may be difficult to visualize on x-ray. If a spiral fracture is identified, particularly in the midshaft, child abuse should be considered. Treatment of a toddler's fracture consists of an above-the-knee, non–weight bearing cast.

KNEE FRACTURES

Etiology. Knee injuries most commonly result from blunt trauma caused by a sports-related activity or a motor vehicle crash where the child's knee hits the dashboard. Fractures of the knee are serious injuries, since the growth plates of the distal femur, proximal tibia, and fibula are located in this area. Patellar fractures are not common in young children because of the amount of cartilage that surrounds and protects the patella.

Pathophysiology. The growth plate of the proximal tibia contributes to as much as 30% of the overall leg length. Injuries to this area, particularly those that cause posterior displacement of the shaft, may cause vascular and neural injury. Complications include recurrent deformity of the leg, arrested bone growth, and/or leg length discrepancy.[1] (Osgood-Schlatter disease, which affects the tibial tuberosity, and is seen in young adolescents, is discussed in Chapter 13, Musculoskeletal System.)

Clinical presentation. On arrival in the emergency department the child may report that a pop or tearing was felt in the knee. Edema is usually present, the child will refuse to bear weight, and a deformity may be noted. If the patella is fractured, the child will complain of knee pain, there will be an obvious deformity with edema, and the child will be unable to fully extend the knee.

Emergency Department interventions. Treatment depends on the location and type of fracture. If the fracture is displaced, an open reduction with internal fixation devices is required to immobilize the bones. If the fracture is not displaced, the knee is immobilized either with a long leg cast or a knee immobilizer. Crutches are required to prevent weight bearing.

ANKLE FRACTURES

Etiology. Ankle fractures are fairly common in the pediatric population, particularly fractures of the distal tibial physis, which is one of the weakest components of the ankle in the child.[8] Injuries to the ankle usually result from indirect trauma such as twisting or torsion of the foot.

Pathophysiology. Ankle fractures can involve the distal tibia and/or fibula, or the talus. Because tibia and fibula fractures include the lateral and medial malleolus, the growth plate will be affected. Complications of fractures of the growth plates of the distal tibia and fibula include leg length dis-

crepancies, osteoarthritis, and avascular necrosis of the distal tibial physis. Talus fractures are uncommon in young children, probably because the bone is largely cartilaginous, providing protection against forces that might cause an ossified bone to fracture.

Clinical presentation. Children under the age of 7 years with an ankle fracture may not have specific ankle pain because they have difficulty in localizing the area of pain. Other children may limp or refuse to walk. On physical examination the child may complain of point tenderness over the fracture, and the extremity may be deformed, ecchymotic, and edematous. Displaced fractures usually present with an obvious deformity and pain with any movement of the ankle.

Emergency Department interventions. Treatment varies, depending on the severity of the fracture. If the fracture is a nondisplaced talus fracture or a Salter-Harris type 1 or 2 fracture of the tibia or fibula, it is usually treated with a short leg cast to immobilize the ankle. If the fracture involves a Salter-Harris type 3 or 4 fracture, the child will require operative intervention.

FOOT FRACTURES

Etiology. With the exception of phalangeal and metatarsal injuries, injuries to the foot in young childhood are rare. When these injuries do occur, they usually result from direct trauma. Calcaneus fractures, or fractures of the heel, usually result from a fall from a height. Fractures of the navicular, cuboid, and cuneiform bones are rare and are usually caused by significant blunt or crushing trauma. For example, a heavy object may have fallen onto the top of the foot. Phalangeal and metatarsal injuries are more common in children, with phalangeal injuries most commonly occurring in the big toe (Fig. 23-6).

Pathophysiology. Foot injuries, just as any other injuries, must be evaluated for the presence of a growth plate fracture and, when such a fracture is present, these injuries should be treated appropriately. A phalangeal injury of particular concern is that of the big toe caused by a stubbing or impaction injury. Because these fractures often involve the distal physis and can cause breaks in the skin or nailbed, there is an increased incidence of osteomyelitis in these children.

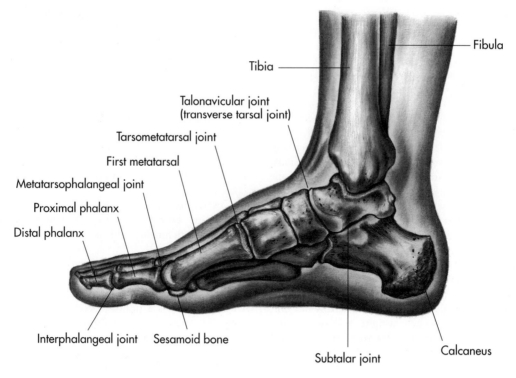

FIG. 23-6. Bones of the foot and ankle. (From Seidel HM et al: *Mosby's guide to physical examination,* ed 3, St Louis, 1995, Mosby.)

Clinical presentation. Signs and symptoms of foot injuries vary, depending on the severity and location of the fracture. In general, children with foot injuries have foot or heel pain, swelling, ecchymosis, and tenderness. The child may refuse to bear weight or walk and complain of point tenderness to palpation. Compartment syndrome is a complication of metatarsal fractures, especially if there are multiple fractures caused by a crushing type of injury.

Emergency Department interventions. Treatment of foot fractures depends on the location of the injury. If the injury involves a calcaneus fracture, the foot will require non–weight bearing immobilization. If the fracture involves a nondisplaced metatarsal fracture, the foot can be immobilized in a walking cast. Nondisplaced phalangeal fractures of the lateral four toes rarely require more than "buddy taping" of the adjacent, uninjured toes. Epiphyseal fractures of the great toe must be watched much more closely, since malalignment can alter weight-bearing of the foot.[13] These children may require prophylactic antibiotic therapy.

PELVIC FRACTURES

Etiology. Pelvic fractures in children most commonly result from high-energy accidents such as motor vehicle–related injuries where the child is a passenger or a pedestrian. Therefore there is a high risk of additional associated major injuries. Pelvic stress fractures can result from sports-related activities such as bowling and gymnastics. They are more common in adolescents than in young children.

Pathophysiology. Pelvic fractures can be subdivided into three groups: (1) avulsion fractures, (2) acetabular fractures, and (3) fractures of the pelvic ring. Avulsion fractures occur when muscular attachments to the growth plates are avulsed, usually during athletic activities. These fractures commonly involve the anterosuperior iliac spine, anteroinferior iliac spine, or iliac tuberosity. Acetabular fractures are rare in children and may be seen with posterior hip dislocations, but they are usually associated with significant trauma.

Fractures of the pelvic ring may be anterior or posterior, displaced, and/or single or multiple. Isolated nondisplaced anterior fractures are seen more often in young children than in older children and adults because of the flexibility of the pelvic structures. They are rarely associated with complications. Fractures of the pubic diastasis bone with disruption of the anterior sacroiliac joint (open book deformity) may be associated with underlying injury and, depending on the degree of displacement, may require open or closed reduction. In general, for adults and children a displaced fracture usually means there is a fracture elsewhere in the pelvic ring. Up to 80% of children with multiple fractures of the pelvic ring have associated abdominal or genitourinary injuries, although genitourinary injuries tend to be less frequent in young children than in older children and adults.[23] Approximately 40% to 60% of children with significant pelvic fractures have associated head trauma, which is usually the direct cause of death.[4]

Clinical presentation. The mechanism of injury and presenting signs and symptoms play an important role in the identification of a fractured pelvis. This is particularly true if the child has sustained significant trauma from a motor vehicle–related incident and exhibits signs of hemorrhagic shock. Physical findings of a pelvic fracture may include ecchymosis, open fractures, and/or pain and crepitus on palpation. Gentle squeezing or downward displacement of the pelvis may reveal pain on movement and pelvic instability.

Emergency Department and nursing interventions. Because pelvic fractures are commonly associated with severe multiple trauma, the principles of multiple trauma management must be followed, including stabilization of airway, breathing, and circulation (see Chapter 21, Multiple Trauma Management). All children with suspected pelvic injuries deserve continuous nursing evaluation for signs of shock that may be associated with disruption of the major pelvic vessels. In addition, fractured bones can lacerate internal viscera, producing trauma to the genitourinary tract; therefore a urinary catheter should not be inserted if there is blood at the meatus.

The diagnosis of a pelvic fracture is determined by pelvic x-ray films and computed tomography (CT) scan imaging. Additional studies can be ordered, depending on suspected underlying injuries; these may include arteriograms to identify bleeding from major pelvic vessels or urethrograms to identify the presence of urethral damage.

The treatment of pelvic fractures varies, depending on the location and severity of the fracture(s). Simple anterior pelvic fractures may be treated with strict bed rest for 4 to 6 weeks. Fractures that are displaced may require traction, open reduction and internal fixation, or a combination of approaches.[4]

UPPER EXTREMITY INJURIES

CLAVICLE FRACTURES

Etiology. The clavicle is the most commonly fractured bone in young children.[1,9,21] Greenstick or bowing injuries of the midshaft are most frequently seen in young children. These injuries usually result from lateral compression, as might occur during delivery, or from falling onto an outstretched arm. In older children, with increased ossification, displaced fractures become more common.

Pathophysiology. The age of the child and the mechanism of injury play a significant role in the type and location of the fracture. Midshaft fractures of the clavicle are most often seen in young children, since ossification begins in the center of the bone and moves outward with maturity. However, depending on the mechanism of injury, fractures at the medial physis and dislocations of the sternoclavicular joint may be observed. Because the medial physis of the clavicle is the last to fuse at around 18 years of age, clavicular growth plate injuries may be seen in adolescents and young adults.[14] Although clavicular fractures are common in children, they rarely require aggressive management and are rarely associated with long-term complications. The exception is the child who is a victim of significant trauma (e.g., motor vehicle crash) in whom a displaced clavicle fracture may damage the trachea, lungs, or mediastinum.

Clinical presentation. Children with fractures of the clavicle usually have pain, tenderness, and swelling at the site of injury. Anterior displacement of the bone may be accompanied by a protuberant mass at the sternoclavicular junction. Asymmetry of the shoulders, cradling of the injured arm, and crepitus at the site of injury may also be observed. Occasionally, particularly in infants, the initial injury will go unnoticed until callus formation at the site of the injury forms a raised, tender mass.

Emergency Department interventions. As with any victim of trauma, the child should be evaluated for the presence of other, more significant injuries. Although complications from clavicular fractures are rare, posterior displacement of clavicular bony fragments can enter the chest and damage the trachea, lungs, or mediastinum.

Definitive diagnosis is generally made with x-ray evaluation of the injured site. X-ray findings may indicate an obvious fracture or reveal callus formation indicative of a healing fracture. Because of the position of the first and second ribs, the fracture may be hidden. When clinical evidence strongly suggests a fracture, oblique or lordotic views of the area are required.[21]

Treatment depends on the age of the child and the type and location of the injury. Infants with greenstick fractures can be immobilized with a sling, whereas toddlers may require a clavicle strap. Displaced fractures may require some degree of reduction, which can usually be performed with a clavicle strap that is gradually tightened or with a figure-of-eight harness.[9,14] The child must wear the splinting device day and night for 2 to 3 weeks and should limit activity for up to 3 weeks after the splint is removed. Parents should be informed that callus formation at the site of injury will cause a bump to form that may last for up to a year after the injury.

HUMERUS FRACTURES

Etiology. Fractures of the humerus can occur proximally, distally, or midshaft. Proximal fractures are most common in older children, between 10 and 15 years of age, and are usually associated with athletic or sports injuries.[16] This fracture is usually the result of direct trauma or a fall on an outstretched arm with the shoulder extended. Shaft fractures of the humerus are rare, and the type of fracture usually reflects the mechanism of injury. For example, transverse fractures usually result from a direct blow, and oblique or comminuted fractures are caused by a fall onto the hand or elbow.

Fractures of the supracondylar (distal) humerus are common in children and account for up to 60% of elbow injuries in children between 3 and 10 years of age.[14] They typically result from a fall onto an outstretched arm, but can also be caused by a direct blow or a snapping force such as throwing a baseball too hard.[1,9]

Pathophysiology. Several growth plates on the humerus can be damaged and lead to long-term complications. For example, there are four growth plates within the distal humerus, and in the proximal humerus about 80% of the growth of the bone occurs at the humeral physis. Before adolescence the majority of proximal humeral fractures are metaphyseal. With the onset of adolescence, rapid growth makes the physeal region relatively weak and therefore more vulnerable to injury.[1] The most common proximal physeal injuries in children are type I fractures, seen most commonly in infants and toddlers, and type II

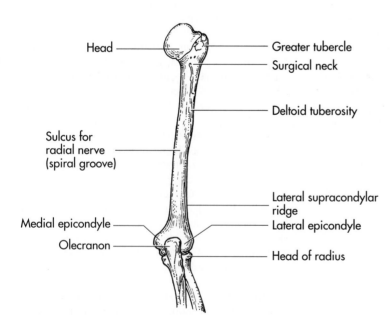

FIG. 23-7. Posterior view of the humerus and elbow.

fractures, which are more common in adolescents.[26] Of all humeral fractures observed, younger children most commonly present with supracondylar fractures (Fig. 23-7). Because the radial nerve wraps around the musculospiral groove of the humerus, neurovascular injuries with accompanying paresthesia may be present in any child with a humeral injury.[13]

Clinical presentation. Children with injuries to the humerus have complaints of pain, point tenderness, swelling, and decreased range of motion. Obvious deformities may be observed, particularly with displaced fractures. Because radial, ulnar, or medial nerves may be damaged by the injury (or the brachial

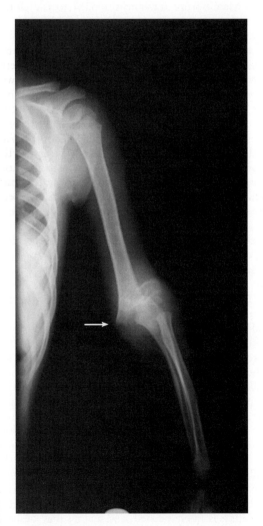

FIG. 23-8. Displaced supracondylar fracture.

artery may be compressed or spasm), neurocirculatory assessment of the distal extremity is essential. If the radial nerve has been injured, wrist drop and loss of finger extensors may occur; if the medial nerve has been affected, the child will have extension of the index finger.

Neurocirculatory damage is common with shaft fractures and supracondylar fractures, particularly those that are displaced. Displaced fractures must therefore be treated emergently with immediate immobilization and/or reduction combined with serial assessments while awaiting radiologic evaluation and possible surgical intervention. Compartment syndrome is a serious complication of this injury (Fig. 23-8).

Emergency Department interventions. Treatment depends on the location and severity of the injury. If the proximal humerus is aligned or only minimally displaced and there is no neurovascular compromise, the child is usually sent home with a sling and swathe, with directions for follow-up. Children with incomplete fractures of the shaft may also be treated with a sling and swathe; however, if the child has sustained a complete or minimally displaced fracture, a sugar-tong splint may be applied. Children with minimally displaced or nondisplaced supracondylar fractures may be placed in a long-arm posterior splint.[1] All children with fractures should be referred to an orthopedic specialist.

FOREARM FRACTURES

Etiology. Fractures of the forearm may involve the radius, the ulna, or both bones. Forearm fractures in children occur more often than all other bone fractures combined, with fractures of the distal end of the radius accounting for up to 75% of all forearm injuries.[1] Isolated ulnar fractures are extremely rare.[17] Fractures of the radius and ulna generally result from a high-energy impact such as a fall onto an outstretched arm or blunt trauma (Fig. 23-9).

Pathophysiology. Fractures of the forearm may involve the radial head and neck, the midshaft, or the distal forearm. The type of injury is usually directly related to the mechanism of injury, the age of the child, and the degree of skeletal maturation. For example, young children are more prone to greenstick injuries from a fall, whereas older children may sustain a displaced radial fracture. Because of skeletal immaturity, isolated fractures of one bone should increase the

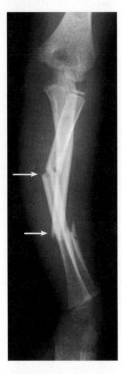

FIG. 23-9. Displaced fractures of the ulna and radius.

suspicion of a bowing injury or diaphyseal injury in the other bone.

There is a wide variety of forearm fractures and combinations of fractures, some of which include the Colles' fracture, nightstick fracture, Monteggia's fracture, Galeazzi fracture, and Smith's fracture (Table 23-2). Most of these fractures result from falls onto an outstretched hand or direct trauma.

Clinical presentation. Clinical presentation can vary from soft tissue swelling, ecchymosis, and pain and tenderness on movement, to gross deformities of the wrist and forearm. The mechanism of injury and site of injury also provide clues to the seriousness of the injury.

Emergency Department interventions. The child should initially be evaluated for the presence of other, more serious injuries. At the same time the extremity should be immobilized and evaluated for neurocirculatory status (distal pulses, color, movement, sensation). Radiographic studies will identify the type and location of the fracture(s). Treatment varies, depending on severity of the injury and ranges

from a closed reduction performed in the emergency department to an open reduction performed in the operating room. When a closed reduction is performed, a Bier block may be used (see nursing care section).

NURSEMAID'S ELBOW

Etiology. Nursemaid's elbow is one of the most common elbow injuries in children less than 5 years of age. It occurs when there is a longitudinal pull with rotation of the child's arm. The result is *subluxation of the radial head*.

Pathophysiology. Radial head subluxation occurs when abrupt traction is applied to the child's pronated or extended hand.[25] The result is partial detachment of the loosely attached annular ligament in the elbow from the radial head. This allows a portion of the radial head to sublux into the tear or allows a portion of the ligament to snap over the radial head.

Clinical presentation. The classic history on presentation in the emergency department is a report of decreased movement of the arm and pain and crying when the arm is touched or extended. Careful questioning of the parent may reveal the typical upward pull on the hand. On examination, the child will be observed holding the arm flexed, pronated, and close to the body. Occasionally, radial head subluxation occurs with falls, although this is rare. If the child reports a history of a fall, x-ray studies may be indicated.

Emergency Department and nursing interventions. Treatment is usually simple reduction of the radial head. The child's elbow should be supported with one hand, while the other hand grasps the forearm and supinates the hand, then flexes the elbow. When reduction occurs, a characteristic "pop" will be felt (Fig. 23-10). Although immediate relief of pain occurs, the child may refuse to use the arm for a brief period and should be watched until normal use is resumed. Typically, the longer the delay from injury to treatment, the longer is the return to normal use. Routine x-ray studies are not required for the child with a classic history and presentation; often if the child is sent for x-rays, the radial head will relocate when the arm is positioned for the lateral view. Splinting is rarely needed, and a sling may be used for comfort measures if needed. Again, these mea-

TABLE 23-2	Forearm Fractures and Management	
FRACTURE	**DESCRIPTION**	**MANAGEMENT**
Colles' fracture	Transverse fracture of the distal radius resulting in dorsal (posterior) angulation of the wrist; commonly accompanied by a fracture of the distal ulna. The resultant wrist deformity may resemble the profile of a fork (the dorsum of the wrist/forearm is displaced upward), so it is sometimes referred to as a "silver fork" deformity.	Because this injury often results from a fall from a high place, the child landing on his or her feet, then falling forward, the child should be evaluated for additional fractures, such as possible heel or lumbar or sacral injuries. Often reduced by closed reduction using local anesthesia. The hand is then immobilized in an anterior and posterior splint or cast for 6 to 8 weeks.
Smith's fracture	Sometimes referred to as the opposite of a Colles' fracture because it usually results from a blow to the dorsum of the wrist, causing palmar (downward) angulation of the distal radius.	Can usually be reduced by closed reduction using local anaesthesia. Because 15 degrees of flexion is required—and often difficult to maintain—an open reduction of the fracture may be necessary.[10a]
Nightstick fracture	A fracture of the ulna that results from a direct blow, such as what one might receive if hit with a nightstick.	Treatment includes splinting and eventual casting of the extremity.
Monteggia fracture	Extremely rare in children. Occurs when an isolated ulnar fracture is accompanied by a dislocated radial head. This fracture usually results from a fall onto an outstretched arm, although the exact mechanism of injury is not well understood.	Treatment requires reduction of the dislocation. Anterior dislocation requires traction be applied to an extended elbow with the elbow supinated. The arm is then casted in the flexed position. Posterior dislocation requires the elbow be placed in extension while the head of the radius is pushed forward. The arm is then casted in extension.[26]
Galeazzi fracture	A fracture of the radial shaft with an accompanying dislocation of the inferior radioulnar joint.[10a] Usually results from a fall onto an outstretched arm or from direct trauma.	Can usually be reduced by closed reduction, followed by immobilization of the extremity.

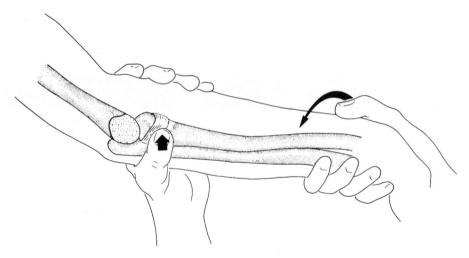

FIG. 23-10. Reduction of nursemaid's elbow. The thumb is placed over the radial head, applying direct pressure, as the forearm is rapidly supinated. A distinct "click" is often felt. (From Touloukian RJ, ed: *Pediatric trauma,* ed 2, St Louis, 1990, Mosby.)

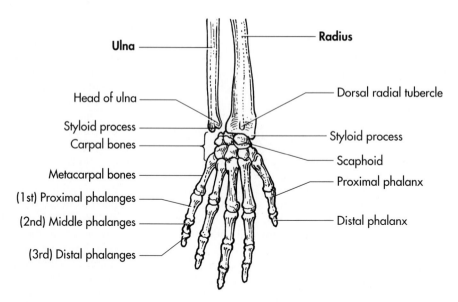

FIG. 23-11. Posterior view of the hand.

sures are usually required when there has been a delay in treatment or if the child has recurrent subluxations.

WRIST FRACTURES

Etiology. Wrist fractures involve the carpal bones of the hand and usually occur when the child falls onto a dorsiflexed or outstretched hand. Because these bones are mostly cartilaginous in the young child, carpal fractures are extremely rare. As the skeleton matures, these fractures become more common, particularly the scaphoid (navicular) bone.

Pathophysiology. The wrist contains eight small bones arranged in two transverse rows of four bones each (Fig. 23-11). In early childhood these bones are primarily made of cartilage and rarely fracture. There are three peripheral nerves that supply sensation to the hand; these include the radial nerve, the median nerve, and the ulnar nerve. Both the radial and ulnar arteries supply circulation to the hand.

Clinical presentation. The child with a wrist fracture usually has complaints of pain and tenderness over the scaphoid bone, which is located between the base of the thumb and the proximal head of the radius (also referred to as snuffbox tenderness). Additionally, both range of motion and grip will be decreased. Swelling and/or ecchymosis may be observed, depending on the severity of injury.

Emergency Department interventions. The diagnosis of scaphoid (navicular) fractures is sometimes difficult to make based on radiographic evidence alone. For this reason, the diagnosis is often based on the mechanism of injury and accompanying clinical signs and symptoms. Treatment of this injury includes immobilization of the wrist and thumb for 4 to 8 weeks. Complications or growth abnormalities are extremely rare.

HAND AND FINGER INJURIES

Etiology. Fractures of the hand and fingers may involve the metacarpal bones and/or the phalangeal bones. Metacarpal fractures are rare in young children but common in adolescent males who have been in fights or have hit a stationary object. The most frequent sites of injury are the base of the first metacarpal and the neck of the fifth metacarpal ("boxer's fracture").[26]

In older children, fractures of the proximal phalange are common and usually occur when the finger is hyperextended. Crush injuries of the distal phalanx are more common in younger children and usually result from the finger being closed in a door. Crush fractures of the fingers are often open injuries.

Pathophysiology. Depending on the degree and location of the injury, fractures of the hand and fingers can require simple treatment or complex management. Because of the complexity of the hand, even minor trauma can result in cosmetic or functional defects. For this reason, fractures of the hand should be thoroughly evaluated for the presence of rotational deformities and intraarticular injuries, which require orthopedic consultation. Epiphyseal injuries of the metacarpals are rare but may occur as a type II fracture of the proximal end of the first metacarpal. The most common fracture of the proximal phalanx is a Salter

type II at the base of the little finger. Fractures of the distal phalanx from crushing injuries, although common, rarely require complex management unless the fracture is a displaced physeal injury.

Clinical presentation. Children with hand and finger injuries usually come to the emergency department with complaints of hand pain. An assessment reveals swelling, point tenderness, limited movement, and redness or ecchymosis. Crush injuries, if closed, will be swollen and have a bluish discoloration under the fingernail. The child may complain of a throbbing pain at the site of the injury.

Emergency Department and nursing interventions. Treatment depends on the severity of the injury. Clinical and radiographic evidence is used to identify the type of injury and the potential for complications. With metacarpal fractures, only the most severe injuries require closed reduction; otherwise simple casting or splinting of the hand and forearm is indicated. Simple fractures of the middle phalanges are treated by immobilization with an adjacent finger, "buddy taping."

Crush injuries may be open or closed, and the fingernail may be partially or completely avulsed. If the nail is intact, severe bleeding under the nail (subungual hematoma) may require drainage to relieve pressure. Drainage is performed using a cautery or red-hot paper clip on the nail, directly over the hematoma. If the nail has been partially or completely avulsed and is associated with a laceration, complete removal is required for proper suturing and healing of the finger. Frequently the nail is reapplied to the fingertip after suture repair to protect the fingertip. A bulky dressing and splint should be applied to the injured finger after repair. Depending on the severity of the wound, healing may take from weeks to months; for this reason, referral to an orthopedist, hand surgeon, or plastic surgeon is recommended. Children with open wounds are treated prophylactically with antibiotics such as cephalosporin or dicloxacillin.

Crush injuries are extremely painful, and, if the injury is open or avulsed, or if a partial amputation has occurred, are frightening for both the child and parent. Often parents feel extremely guilty, blaming themselves for not preventing the injury. The emergency nurse should administer all pain medications to these children in a timely manner and be supportive of the parents. Parents should be allowed to remain with their child whenever possible, and their concerns about the long-term outcomes of the injury should be dealt with openly and honestly.

NURSING CARE AND EVALUATION OF THE CHILD WITH A FRACTURE

The child arriving in the emergency department with a suspected fracture may have sustained a single traumatic injury or be the victim of multiple trauma. For this reason the history should include the mechanism of injury and associated symptoms. The principles of multiple trauma management should be followed for any child with signs of significant trauma (see Chapter 21, Multiple Trauma).

ASSESSMENT

Fractures can present with a wide array of signs and symptoms, depending on the location, severity, and type of injury. Before palpation, the injured area should be observed for swelling, ecchymosis, deformity, symmetry (e.g., one arm longer than the other), and/or open wounds or fractures or bleeding. In addition, the child should be asked to point to the area that is most painful. Palpation of the most painful area should initially be avoided while the bones and joints proximal and distal to the extremity are examined. Using this approach the nurse is able to more accurately evaluate the presence of additional injuries in a more cooperative child. This approach is particularly useful in young children who are sometimes unable to localize pain (for example, the toddler may point to the arm as a source of pain when the fracture is really at the wrist). Additional evaluation includes pain to palpation, pain to movement, limited movement, and palpation for the presence of crepitus.

When an injury is suspected, the distal extremity is evaluated for neurovascular status, which includes palpation of the distal pulses and comparison to the unaffected extremity. Skin color, temperature, and capillary refill of the nail beds should also be assessed. Sensory-motor function is evaluated by requesting the child move the distal extremity (and fingers or toes) and by palpating the distal extremity for sensation. Tingling, burning, or the inability to move the area distal to the injury indicate neurovascular compromise.

If the child has an injury that may lead to hypovolemic shock (e.g., femur or pelvic fractures), continuous monitoring for signs and symptoms of shock is required. Some injuries are classic for child maltreatment, such as spiral fractures. Child abuse should be

Box 23-2　Guidelines for X-ray Studies of Fractures

Finger/hand injury	Evaluate all fingers, hand, and wrist.
Wrist/forearm	Evaluate wrist, hand, forearm, elbow.
Elbow	Evaluate elbow, forearm, humerus, and shoulder. NOTE: *x-ray films should not be ordered if history and physical findings indicate nursemaid's elbow (subluxed radial head).*
Humerus	Evaluate humerus, shoulder, and elbow.
Toe/foot	Evaluate all toes, foot, and ankle.
Ankle/lower leg	Evaluate foot, ankle, and upper and lower tibia.
Knee	Evaluate lower leg, femur, and knee.
Femur	Evaluate hip, knee, and entire femur. NOTE: *Although rare, children can become hypovolemic from this injury; careful assessment must rule out signs of impending shock before an x-ray film can be ordered. If in doubt, consult with the physician*

*For each suspected fracture request x-ray films based on the examination.

considered in any child when the mechanism of injury is inconsistent with the injury. All such cases should be reported to local or state authorities (see Chapter 25, Child Maltreatment).

INTERVENTIONS

On arrival in the emergency department, the injury should be immobilized and ice applied. When signs of neurovascular compromise are present, emergency management is required. If the femur is fractured, application of a traction splint may be required to stabilize the extremity and overcome muscular contraction. Once the splint is applied, the extremity should be reevaluated for improvement in circulation and sensation. If the wound is open, a sterile dressing is applied (see the discussion of open fractures).

If the neurocirculatory check of the extremity is normal and the child's condition is stable, the injury may be splinted and elevated and ice applied. Depending on emergency department protocols, the nurse may then order an x-ray film of the injury (Box 23-2). If the child is in severe pain or if x-ray evaluation is delayed, pain medication may be required before x-ray evaluation.

TABLE 23-3	Common Pain Medications	
DRUG	**DOSE**	**INDICATIONS/NURSING CONSIDERATIONS**
Morphine	0.1 to 0.2 mg/kg IV, IM, sublingual, rectal	For management of severe pain Can cause hypotension or respiratory depression Rectal administration has been associated with delayed respiratory depression
Fentanyl (Sublimaze)	0.5 to 1.0 µg/kg IV dose may be slowly increased over several minutes, maximum dose 4 to 5 µg/kg IV A transmucosal form will soon be available for oral administration	100 times more potent than morphine For management of severe pain Can cause respiratory depression, apnea, bradycardia, chest wall rigidity Child requires continuous pulse oximetry
Meperidine (Demerol)	1 to 2 mg/kg IV or IM 2 mg/kg IM or PO	For management of painful procedures lasting more than 30 minutes IV administration can produce tachycardia Can cause nervousness, tremors, disorientation, seizures Peak values are achieved 90 to 120 minutes after IM administration Child requires monitoring for respiratory depression
Codeine	1 to 2 mg/kg PO	For moderate pain management Usually administered with acetaminophen or nonsteroidal antiinflammatory drugs (NSAIDs), which increase potency Can cause nausea, vomiting, sedation

Compiled from Cote CJ: Sedation for the pediatric patient, *Pediatr Clin North Am* 41(1):21-58, 1994; Selbst SM: Pain management in the emergency department. In Schechter NL, Berde CB, Yaster M, eds: *Pain in infants, children, and adolescents,* Baltimore, 1993, Williams & Wilkins; Selbst SM, Henretig FM: The treatment of pain in the emergency department, *Pediatr Clin North Am* 48(1):131-136, 1989.

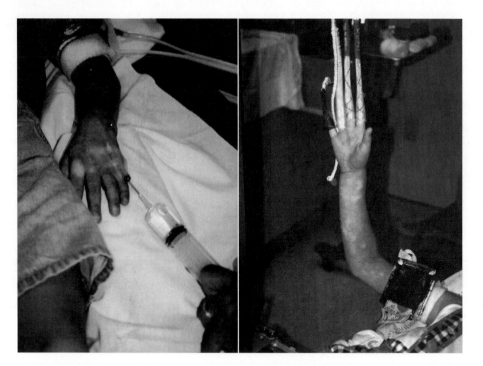

FIG. 23-12. The Bier block is used to achieve regional anesthesia for closed reductions of forearm fractures.

PAIN MANAGEMENT

Children with extremity injuries arrive in the emergency department screaming and crying, or quiet and stoic. Regardless of presentation, all children with fractures are in pain and deserve the same attention to pain management that would be afforded a more verbal, expressive adult with a fracture. Although crying children are loud and demand attention, the quietly coping child is also in pain, yet because of the child's demeanor the level of pain may not be appreciated.

Depending on the severity of the injury, pain may be controlled with oral or parenteral medications. Most commonly, intramuscular or intravenous analgesia is required with musculoskeletal trauma. The most desirable method is the intravenous route, which allows for the administration of additional medications when indicated without further invasive procedures for the child. Also, with venous access, if the child requires admission, closed reduction, or surgical intervention, further invasive pain control (e.g., intramuscular injections) can be avoided. Pain management is discussed in Chapter 29, Pain Management and Assessment (Table 23-3).

PREPARATION FOR PROCEDURES

The majority of children with fractures require simple splinting or casting with referral to an orthopedic specialist. Some children, however, require complex management while in the emergency department. All children with suspected fractures are in pain and frightened, and all respond to the stress of an emergency department visit in a variety of ways. Parents or caregivers who accompany the child may be supportive and understanding, which usually helps to calm the child, or upset, demanding, angry, or guilty. Regardless of presentation, the nurse should speak to the parent and child in a calm, reassuring voice and answer all questions honestly and openly. When pain medication is ordered, it should be administered promptly and the child allowed to rest or even sleep between physician/nurse examinations and treatments.

A number of procedures may be required for the child with a fracture, ranging from cast application to preparation for surgical intervention, any of which can demand a great deal of nursing time. Closed reductions, because they are painful and usually require the administration of sedatives and/or pain medications

---

Box 23-3   Procedure for a Bier Block

The Bier block is used to achieve regional anesthesia for closed reductions of forearm fractures.

- Explain the procedure to the child and parents.
- Place an IV catheter in the injured arm, preferably the dorsum of the hand.
- Administer analgesic agents as ordered.
- Place padding around the upper arm, and apply the blood pressure cuff from the automatic pneumatic tourniquet device.
- Inflate the cuff to 200 to 250 mm Hg.
- Prepare 1 to 2 mg/kg of lidocaine (without preservative) diluted to 0.125% (to be administered by the orthopedic surgeon).
- Wait approximately 15 minutes for adequate anesthesia to occur. The child will feel numbness and tingling. (NOTE: as the lidocaine is administered, the child's arm will become mottled.)
- After adequate anesthesia is obtained, the orthopedic surgeon will manipulate the arm to achieve reduction.
- After reduction: postreduction x-rays will be taken; the blood pressure cuff will be deflated; the IV catheter will be removed; and a cast will be placed on the arm.

Compiled from Blasier RD, White R: *Ped Emerg Care*, 1996; Bolterg R et al: *J Pediatr Orthop* 14:537–543, 1994; Juliano P et al: *J Pediatr Orthop* 12:633–635, 1992.

Box 23-4   Discharge Teaching for a Child with a Cast

Keep extremity elevated to decrease edema and improve blood flow.

Apply ice packs to decrease edema.

Check capillary refill, color, and warmth of the extremity; notify physician if abnormal.

Check distal pulses.

Assess movement of fingers or toes.

Report any tingling or numbness to physician.

Give pain medication per physician's orders; notify the physician if pain increases.

Do not put anything down inside the cast.

Do not go swimming with the cast. (NOTE: some casts are made of fiberglass and can be submerged. However, immediately after an injury the child should not be allowed to go swimming, regardless of the type of cast used.)

Notify physician of any foul odor coming from the cast.

Keep all follow-up appointments.

---

demand the greatest amount of nursing time. One such procedure, the Bier block, may be used (Fig. 23-12 and Box 23-3).

DISCHARGE TEACHING

Before discharge, the parent(s) and child (if old enough) should be given follow-up and cast and/or splint care instructions. If the child is to be cared for by an orthopedist, the parent(s) should be given the physician's name, phone number, and address. Cast care instructions should include frequent evaluation of the distal extremity, fingers, or toes for warmth, color, and sensation (Box 23-4). If the child has a splint, the

parent(s) should be informed to observe for the same symptoms as for the child with a cast; however, if there are signs that the splint is too tight, the parent(s) may be instructed to rewrap the Ace bandage more loosely and contact the physician.

SELECTED MUSCULOSKELETAL TOPICS

COMPARTMENT SYNDROME

Etiology. Compartment syndrome is a dangerous complication of extremity trauma. It is most common in the forearm or lower leg, but it can occur in any extremity. It may be seen with fractures or contusions and results when the nonelastic fascia (which encases the bone, muscle, nerves, blood vessels, and soft tissue) cannot expand to compensate for edema or bleeding. It can also occur within a casted or splinted extremity.[12]

Pathophysiology. Compartment syndrome occurs as pressure within a closed anatomic space compromises circulation and tissue function within that space. This increase in pressure can be caused by bleeding, edema, or muscle hypertrophy, or it can result from external pressure applied by casts, constricting dressings, splints, or pneumatic antishock garments (PASGs). If the pressure is not relieved, muscle ischemia, nerve damage, and occlusion of the arteries will result.

Clinical presentation. All children with significant trauma to an extremity and/or significant soft tissue swelling are continuously monitored for the development of compartment syndrome. One of the earliest signs of compartment syndrome is pain, that is usually more intense than that associated with the injury and increases when the muscle is stretched. Additional signs of compartment syndrome include a hard, tense, and swollen area; altered sensation; and numbness and tingling of the extremity. In many cases the distal pulse will be absent or weak; however, this is not always the case. In some children skin color and pulse may be normal as superficial circulation is not always affected. Late signs include pulselessness and paralysis.

Emergency Department and nursing interventions. The diagnosis of compartment syndrome is based on clinical findings. However, initial clinical findings are not always accurate, since skin color and pulses can remain normal. Therefore any child with extremity trauma requires frequent monitoring by the emergency department nurse for signs of neurovascular compromise, including skin color, capillary refill, strength of pulses, sensation, and pain to movement— particularly when the muscle is stretched. If compartment syndrome is suspected, the emergency physician must be notified immediately. Emergency interventions such as cast removal, realignment of splinting or traction, or emergency surgical fasciotomy are usually required. When treatment is delayed, necrosis and nerve damage distal to the injury can result.

Even with frequent assessments, compartment syndrome may be difficult to identify. In these cases, direct measurement of the compartment pressure may be required to confirm the diagnosis. Compartmental pressure can be measured by special commercial devices, or it may be measured using the technique described by Sherk and Black using an IV pump (Box 23-5).

OPEN FRACTURES

Etiology. Isolated open fractures are uncommon in the pediatric population. Open fractures have

---

Box 23-5   Measuring Compartment Pressure

1. Obtain an IV pump that reads pressure and set it to 20 ml/hr.
2. Attach pump tubing to a bag of normal saline solution and an 18-gauge needle.
3. Prepare the skin with betadine.
4. Read the pressure from the pump before the needle is inserted into the compartment (*initial reading*).
5. After insertion of the needle, take a pressure reading immediately from the pump (*final reading*).
6. Compartment pressure is equal to the final reading minus the initial reading.

NOTE: compartment syndrome pressure is significant if it is 10 to 30 mm Hg above the patient's diastolic pressure.

From Sherk H, Black J: Orthopedic emergencies. In Fleisher GR, Ludwig S, eds: *Textbook of pediatric emergency medicine,* ed 3, Baltimore, 1993, Williams & Wilkins.

---

been reported to occur in as many as 30% of children who have sustained multiple injuries.[22] Children are at risk of sustaining an open fracture from motor vehicle crashes and from normal, more aggressive activities and sports.

Pathophysiology. Because the mechanism of injury associated with an open fracture usually involves significant trauma, the incidence of concomitant trauma is quite high. Also, because the wound is exposed to the environment, including the skin and external contaminants such as soil, the likelihood of developing a subsequent infection is also high.

Clinical presentation. Children arriving in the emergency department with open fractures may exhibit small lacerations, abrasions, or large wounds with protruding bone. Distal pulses may be palpable and strong, or weak and thready, or absent. Regardless of presentation, the child with an open fracture requires emergent care.

Emergency Department and nursing interventions. The child with an open fracture deserves a complete head-to-toe assessment to identify the presence of other significant injuries that may require emergency management. At the same time, if the wound is bleeding, it should be controlled with a pressure dressing and the child evaluated for signs of hemorrhagic shock. In addition, the extremity should be immobilized and inline traction applied if signs of neurovascular compromise are present. If during the head-to-toe assessment no other life-threatening injuries are found, or after initial stabilization, the severity of the wound should be thoroughly evaluated, including location, length, width, and degree of damage to the soft tissue. Once the extremity has been stabilized, frequent reassessments of neurocirculatory status are required, including skin color, strength of pulses, movement, and sensation.

Medical management of an open fracture requires operative intervention after obtaining radiographic studies and a culture of the wound. Initially after the injury, the child is treated with a broad-spectrum antibiotic and tetanus prophylaxis.

▌ SOFT TISSUE INJURIES

Etiology.   Soft tissue injuries are quite common in children because of the child's exploratory nature, lack of motor coordination, and lack of judgment. Most wounds are minor cuts, scrapes, abrasions, or bruises. Lacerations are by far the most common reason for an emergency department visit by the child.

Pathophysiology.   Soft tissue wounds can range in seriousness from simple contusions to avulsions. When a wound is open, healing begins immediately as local vessels develop spasms to reduce blood flow through the injured vessel. Blood coagulation or the formation of a blood clot further decreases blood flow; platelets produce a platelet plug; and white blood cells invade the disrupted tissue to provide immediate defenses against infection. Within hours, stimulation of the platelets and fibroblasts (contained in the dermis) causes the formation of fibrous connective tissue throughout the blood clot and begins the process of regeneration.

Contusions.   A contusion is a closed wound, usually caused by a direct blow, causing the extravasation of blood into the surrounding tissue. Signs of a contusion include swelling and discoloration which may be seen immediately after an injury or several hours or days later. The most common sites of contusions in the child are bony prominences, such as the knees, shins, and forehead. Contusions over the buttocks, upper arms, back, or face are uncommon and may represent signs of child abuse. Contusions generally only require supportive care.

Abrasions.   An abrasion is the removal of the outer layer of skin (the epithelium), leaving the epidermal and dermal layers exposed. Bleeding is usually minimal, although oozing from the capillary bed can occur, particularly if the wound is large. These wounds can be painful. Abrasions should be cleaned of foreign materials such as rocks or grit by irrigation. If irrigation is not effective, the area can be abraded with a sterile surgical brush soaked in saline or povidone-iodine solution. Solutions containing detergent, such as povidone-iodine detergent, should not be used to clean the wound because they can cause damage to exposed fibroblasts.[27] After cleaning the wound, an antibiotic ointment and a sterile nonadherent dressing should be applied.

Avulsion.   An avulsion occurs when a flap of skin is torn away from the body surface; the skin may be completely torn away or remain attached to the body. There is generally a great deal of bleeding with this injury and, if so, it will require direct pressure for control of hemorrhage. Treatment of avulsion injuries varies, depending on the location and severity of the wound. Initially the wound should be cleaned and debrided to remove all foreign material. Depending on the severity of the wound, it may require loose suturing and close follow-up care. Regardless of the degree of injury, a bulky dressing should be applied over the site. Occasionally, skin grafting is required.

Puncture wounds.   Puncture wounds occur when a pointed object pierces the skin and underlying tissue. The most common items producing puncture wounds in children are pencils, nails, splinters, knives, and ice picks. Puncture wounds are classified as penetrating or perforating. Penetrating wounds have a wound entrance but no exit. Perforating wounds have both an entrance and an exit. Occasionally the object remains embedded in the child's skin. If the object is large, such as a metal spike, and deeply embedded, it should be stabilized until it can be removed surgically. Small, superficial objects such as pieces of glass may be removed in the emergency department, followed by thorough cleaning of the wound and antibiotic therapy.

Lacerations.   A laceration is a cut into the dermal layer of the skin that may be straight or jagged, superficial or deep. Lacerations may be open and gaping, exposing underlying tissues or anatomic structures. Deep lacerations with active bleeding require direct pressure to control the bleeding. The majority of lacerations require suturing but must first be cleaned and debrided. If there is any possibility of a foreign body remaining in the wound, it should be x-rayed before suturing.

Emergency Department and nursing interventions. Interventions are based on the type, location, and severity of the injury. If the injury is open, it will require irrigation and debridement. If active bleeding is present, a pressure dressing is indicated. When a foreign body is identified in the wound, or if one is suspected, an x-ray is usually indicated.

Injuries that occurred more than 24 hours before the emergency department visit deserve special attention and should be closely evaluated for signs of swelling, redness, and/or drainage. These symptoms, coupled with a systemic fever, may indicate cellulitis or bacteremia.

Laceration repair. The need for repair of lacerations is based on the degree of injury, the time delay since injury, the location of the injury, and the presence of any preexisting illnesses. The type of suture material used and the length of time until sutures are removed vary depending on the location and severity of the injury. Superficial lacerations of the face may be closed with a nylon suture or Prolene and removed within 3 to 5 days. Sutures placed in the joints of fingers are not removed for at least 10 days.

Analgesia used for pain control during wound repair ranges from topical anesthetics to central sedation (e.g., Versed, Ketamine). The choice of analgesia is based on the cooperation of the child and the expected length of the procedure. In some (although few) cases, toddlers will cooperate with topical anesthetic administration; in other cases, older children may refuse completely. In general, infants and young toddlers rarely remain still for any procedure, particularly one that is painful. In this age group, small lacerations usually require the use of a restraining device and the application of a local anesthetic, followed by rapid repair. Any child with signs of pain or with a larger laceration, which may take longer to repair, will require the use of a sedative in addition to the interventions already noted. Preschool and school-aged children, although frightened, may be "talked into" cooperating with the procedure. In these children, topical agents, such as tetracaine, adrenaline, and cocaine (TAC), may be used (see Chapter 29, Pain Assessment and Management).

Recently, Histoacryl Blue has been used for laceration repair of pediatric facial lacerations in Canada.[15] This method requires thorough cleaning of the facial wound, followed by the application of a thin layer of the tissue adhesive. The wound is then held closed for approximately 30 seconds. In a study conducted by Quinn et al (1993), the use of Histoacryl Blue was rated less painful and less time-consuming than suturing.

Regardless of the procedure used, all children are frightened of needles and therefore sutures. When suture repair is indicated, the child should be adequately prepared. Toddlers do not understand lengthy explanations and should therefore be given minimal information, but it should be honest. Preschoolers and school-aged children frequently ask many questions. Their questions should be answered honestly without causing undue fear. For example, if the child asks "Will it hurt?" an appropriate answer would be, "Yes, but only for a minute while it goes to sleep." Parents should be allowed to remain with the child, but the nurse should be alert to the fact that the parent may become queasy when looking at the wound and wound repair. If this occurs, the parent should be asked to sit in a chair rather than leave the child (Box 23-6).

Box 23-6   Preparing the Child for Suturing

Organize all equipment:
  Suture kit
  Sutures
  Lidocaine and/or TAC
  Immobilization devices
Attach the child to a heart rate monitor or pulse oximeter if sedation is given.
Explain the procedure to the child in age-appropriate language.
Explain the procedure to the parents, allowing them to stay with their child. Offer them a chair if they become queasy.
Immobilize the child and the injured area.
Speak softly to the child during the procedure using distraction techniques, as age-appropriate.
Praise the child often during the procedure, regardless of his or her cooperation.
Remove immobilization devices immediately after the procedure.

REFERENCES

1. Bachman D, Santora S: Orthopedic trauma. In Fleisher GR, Ludwig S, eds: *Textbook of pediatric emergency medicine,* ed 3, Baltimore, 1993, Williams & Wilkins.
2. Blasier RD and White R: Intravenous regional anesthesia for management of children's extremity fractures in the emergency department, *Pediatr Emerg Care* 12(6):404, 1996.
3. Bolterg R et al: Mini-dose Bier block intravenous regional anesthesia in the emergency department treatment of upper-extremity injuries, *J Pediatr Orthop* 14: 534-537, 1994.
4. Bond SJ: Pelvic fracture and retroperitoneal hematoma. In Eichelberger MR, ed: *Pediatric trauma: prevention, acute care, rehabilitation,* St Louis, 1993, Mosby.
5. Ciarello L and Fleisher G: Femoral fractures: are children at risk for significant blood loss? *Ped Emerg Care* 12(5):343-346, 1996.
6. Guyer B, Gallagher SS: An approach to epidemiology of childhood injuries, *Pediatr Clin North Am* 32:1, 5-15, 1985.
7. Hodge D: Management principles. In Barkin RM, ed: *Pediatric emergency medicine: concepts and clinical practice,* St Louis, 1992, Mosby.
8. Jackson JL, Linakis JG: Ankle and foot injuries. In Barkin RM, ed: *Pediatric emergency medicine: concepts and clinical practice,* St Louis, 1992, Mosby.
9. Joffe M: Upper extremity. In Barkin RM, ed: *Pediatric emergency medicine: concepts and clinical practice,* St Louis, 1992, Mosby.
10. Juliano P et al: Low-dose lidocaine intravenous regional anesthesia for forearm fractures in children, *J Pediatr Orthop* 12:633-635, 1992.
10a. Kearns RJ, Gartsman GM: Upper extremity fractures and dislocations. In Moore E, Feliciano D, ed: *Trauma,* ed 2, East Norwalk, CT, 1991, Appleton & Lange.
11. Marshall WN, Puls T, Davidson C: New child abuse spectrum in an era of increased awareness, *Am J Dis Child* 142:664-667, 1988.
12. Monk, HLM: Fractures are never simple, *RN* pp. 30-35, April 1993.

13. Ogden JA: Injury to the immature skeleton. In Touloukian RJ, ed: *Pediatric trauma,* ed 2, St Louis, 1990, Mosby.
14. Ogden JA: The uniqueness of growing bones. In Rockwood CA, Wilkins KE, King RE, eds: *Fractures in children* ed 3, New York, 1991, Lippincott.
15. Quinn JV et al: A randomized, controlled trial comparing a tissue adhesive with suturing in the repair of pediatric facial lacerations, *Ann Emerg Med* 22:7, 1130-1134, 1993.
16. Reed MH: Injuries. In Reed MH, ed: *Pediatric skeletal radiology,* Baltimore, 1992, Williams & Wilkins.
17. Reed MH, Genez B: Hands. In Reed MH, ed: *Pediatric skeletal radiology,* Baltimore, 1992, Williams & Wilkins.
18. Salter RB, Harris WR: Injuries involving the epiphyseal plate, *J Bone Joint Surg* 45A:587-622, 1963.
19. Seidel HM et al: *Mosby's guide to physical examination,* St Louis, 1995, Mosby.
20. Sherk H, Black J: Orthopedic emergencies. In Fleisher GR, Ludwig S, eds: *Textbook of pediatric emergency medicine,* ed 3, Baltimore, 1993, Williams & Wilkins.
21. Swischuk LE: *Emergency imaging of the acutely ill or injured child,* ed 3, Baltimore, 1994, Williams & Wilkins.
22. Thomas MD: Musculoskeletal injury. In Eichelberger MR, ed: *Pediatric trauma: prevention, acute care, rehabilitation,* St Louis, 1993, Mosby.
23. Torode I, Zieg D: Pelvic fractures in children, *J Pediatric Orthop,* pp. 76-84, 1985.
24. Torrey SB: Lower extremity and pelvis. In Barkin RM, ed: *Pediatric emergency medicine: concepts and clinical practice,* St Louis, 1992, Mosby.
25. Weiner DS: *Pediatric orthopaedics,* New York, 1993, Churchill Livingstone.
26. Williams PF, Cole WG: Fractures and dislocations. In Williams PF, Cole WG, eds: *Orthopaedic management in childhood,* ed 2, London, 1991, Chapman & Hall.
27. Zukin DD, Inaba AS, Wuerker C: In Barkin RM, ed: *Pediatric emergency medicine: concepts and clinical practice,* St Louis, 1992, Mosby.

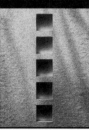

CHAPTER 24

Burn Injuries

Karen L. Winn

INTRODUCTION

Approximately 2.5 million people suffer burn injuries each year in the United States and Canada.[33] Of these, 100,000 will require hospitalization and approximately 12,000 will die as a result of their injuries.[32,35] Burn-related injuries are the leading cause of accidental death in the home for children less than 14 years of age and are the second leading cause of death in children less than 4 years of age.[21,34] In general, burn-related injuries in children account for 30% of all burn victims requiring hospitalization.[15] Seventy-five to eighty percent of burn injuries to children occur in the home, and most death-related injuries are attributed to carbon monoxide poisoning and/or smoke inhalation.[6,41]

The types of burn-related injuries children sustain vary with a child's age and development. For example, scald burns are more common in the older infant and toddler as they become mobile, begin exploring the environment, and are exposed to environmental hazards within the home (e.g., hot liquids in the kitchen, hot water in the bathroom). Children between 5 and 18 years of age are more commonly involved in burns caused by flames. In this age group, flame-related injuries account for approximately 70% of all burn injuries[9,39] (Fig. 24-1).

PREVENTION

Because the majority of burn injuries occur within the home, preventative nursing care should include public education regarding home safety measures.[15] Numerous interventions can be undertaken within the home that are directly related to the types of burn injuries children sustain.

House fires account for the largest percentage of burn-related deaths in children, with children under 5 years of age being at greatest risk.[22] House fires can be detected early by using smoke detectors. Although

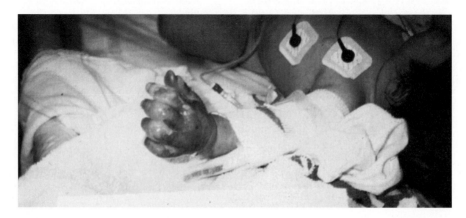

FIG. 24-1. Sixteen month old with burns to the hand after falling into a smoldering trash fire.

564

it is estimated that 75% of homes have smoke detectors, only two thirds of these units function properly. Detectors that do not function properly most commonly have dead batteries, or the batteries have been removed.[22]

Fire prevention can also be addressed with parents and children. Parents can teach children that matches and cigarette lighters are tools, not toys, and should only be used by adults. Additionally, matches, lighters, burning cigarettes, and gasoline should not be in a location where they can be reached by children. Fire drills should be held with children, and an escape route planned.

Scald injuries from tap water account for approximately one fourth of hot liquid burns, and 50% occur in children less than 5 years of age. Hot water heaters set at a temperature of 140° F to 150° F can produce a full-thickness burn in a child in 3 seconds.[22] To prevent scald injuries, hot water heaters should be set at 120° F to 125° F, and the water temperature should be tested before bathing the child.[26] Children should never be left unattended or unsupervised in the kitchen or bathroom, the rooms in which the majority of scald burns occur (Fig. 24-2).

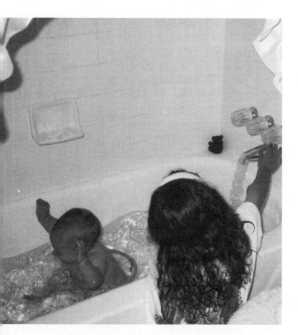

FIG. 24-2. Common bathtub scenario (with unsupervised children) that could result in a scald injury.

BURN CLASSIFICATIONS

The skin is the largest organ system in the body, and it provides many important functions. It acts as a barrier to bacterial invasion, aids in body temperature regulation, prevents the loss of fluids and electrolytes, detects sensory stimulus (hot, cold, pain), and determines an individual's appearance. The skin is comprised of an outer layer and inner layers. The outer layer, or epidermis, serves as a protective barrier. The inner layer, or dermis, contains the sweat glands, hair follicles, sebaceous glands, nerve endings, and blood vessels. A deeper inner layer, the subcutaneous tissue, contains connective tissue and adipose tissue.

SEVERITY OF THE INJURY

The severity of a burn injury is related to the source of the burn, the degree of heat, and the length of contact or exposure. Other factors that contribute to the severity of the injury include the age of the child, the anatomic location of the burn, associated injuries, and the presence of any preexisting medical conditions. Children and the elderly are at increased risk of mortality from burn injuries, because their skin is generally thinner and they have less insulating subcutaneous tissue than healthy adults.

TYPES OF BURN INJURIES

Burns are tissue injuries that have resulted from exposure to thermal, electrical, chemical, or radiation sources. Thermal injuries are caused by a flame or intense heat such as a house fire or by hot liquids such as boiling water or grease.[9] Electrical injuries, although less common, can be caused by contact with any alternating current, such as household electrical plugs, fuse boxes, or power lines, or by lightning. Chemical injuries result in varying degrees of injury and are caused by contact with an acid or alkaline chemical. The most common radiation-related burn in children results from extensive sun exposure, which produces sunburn.[16]

Configurations of burn injuries vary depending on the source and the extent of contact, and they are indicative of the cause of the injury[6] (Table 24-1 and Fig. 24-3). Identification of the source of the injury and comparison with the severity and location of the burns are particularly important when child maltreatment may have been involved. The incidence of burn abuse or neglect in children under the age of 6 varies between 20% and 50% of hospitalized cases. Because of

TABLE 24-1	Burn Configurations	
BURN INJURY	ACCIDENT	NONACCIDENT/NEGLECT/SUSPICIOUS
Scald	Nonimmersion; splash or splatter pattern (first/second degree) "Downward flow" burn—pulling down hot liquid Blisters present from quick movement into or getting out of water	Defined straight lines, forced immersion Buttocks/perineum—"donut" appearance Hands—"glove" distribution Feet—"stockings" distribution Deep partial thickness or full thickness
Flame	Second/third degree consistent with burning of clothing, spilled fuel with ignition or explosion	Children left alone in home Multiple burns at random points on the body Burns not consistent with the story
Hot object	Tips of fingers, palm, usually partial thickness (if child can freely pull away) Burn is consistent with story of injury	Actual mark on body matches size of object (e.g., cigarette, hot iron) Well-demarcated wound

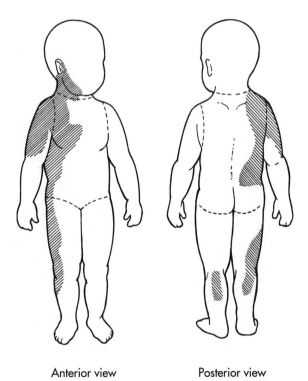

Anterior view   Posterior view

FIG. 24-3. Drawing the exact location of the injury and the pattern provides a detailed means of documenting the burn injury. This burn injury represents 20% of the child's total body surface area (TBSA).

a lack of conclusive evidence and because many cases are unreported, the true incidence may vary from the statistics.[14]

EXTENT OF INJURY

The extent and depth of the burn are important in determining care requirements and expected survival. The extent of a burn injury is determined by calculating the total body surface area (TBSA) involved. The simplest methods of calculating the TBSA of a burn are the *rule of nines* and the *palm method,* which can be used for rapid assessment and triage. The rule of nines divides the body into multiples of nine. Because the infant and young child's head equals 18% of the TBSA, compared to 9% for an adult, this method does not accurately reflect the surface area of children under 10 years of age (Fig. 24-4). The palm method is another simple, rapid method of estimating the extent of a burn in children. With this method the palmar surface of the *child's hand,* not the caregiver's hand, equals approximately 1% of the total body surface area.[28]

The most commonly used and the most accurate method of determining the extent of a burn injury in the child is the Lund and Browder chart. This method allows for growth-related differences in the body surface area of a child (Fig. 24-6). As the most time-consuming method, errors can be made. After calculating the TBSA affected by the injury, calculating the percentage of nonburned areas will double

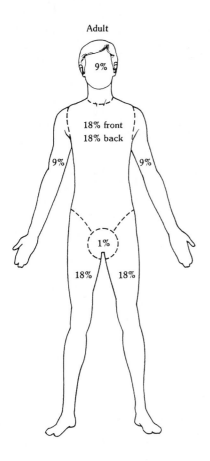

Adult

9%

18% front
18% back

9%   9%

1%

18%   18%

RULE OF NINES Changes in Body Proportions				
	1–4 Years	5–9 Years	10–14 Years	Adults
Head/Neck	19%	15%	13%	9%
Anterior trunk	16%	16%	16%	18%
One arm	9.5%	9.5%	9.5%	9%
One leg	15%	17%	18%	18%

FIG. 24-4. Rule of nines—adult and age proportion chart. The head/neck, trunk, arm, and leg are charted according to varying age-related body proportions. (From Emergency Nurses Association: *Trauma nursing core course [provider] manual,* ed 2, Chicago, 1991, Emergency Nurses Association.)

check the figures. The sum of the two calculations should approximate 100%. If a vast difference exists, the numbers should be recalculated.

DEPTH OF INJURY

Burn injuries are classified according to the depth of the injury to the skin and underlying structures. Superficial burns or first-degree burns affect only the epidermis. Second-degree burns may be *superficial* partial-thickness burns or *deep* partial-thickness burns, and they affect both the epidermis and the dermis to varying degrees. Full-thickness or third-degree burns affect all layers of the skin and the underlying subcutaneous tissue[25] (Table 24-2 and Fig. 24-7).

Initially, determining the true depth of the wound after a burn injury may be difficult because of the appearance of the wound and the body's physiologic response to the injury. This is especially true with partial-thickness involvement. Rapid edema formation compromises blood flow to the wound bed.[30] As the edema subsides, usually over 24 to 72 hours post injury, a more accurate determination of the depth of the injury can be made.

Superficial (first degree). Superficial burns involve only the epidermis. The most common cause of superficial burns in children is sunburn, which results when children play in the sunlight without a sunscreen. First-degree burns are also caused by light contact with hot objects or mild scalding by hot water or steam. Initial symptoms include erythema and local pain caused by the underlying edema. Typically, the skin is pink or light red in color and blisters are not present. The area is painful to touch and heals without scarring in 3 to 5 days. Systemic symptoms may include chills and headache. Nausea and vomiting or blistering is indicative of a deeper burn.

Extensive treatment is not usually required for first-degree injuries unless the patient is elderly or an infant.[19] Treatment measures for previously healthy children with extensive sunburn includes slight elevation if the lower extremities are involved to decrease edema, application of a water-soluble lotion, and acetaminophen every 4 hours to treat fever and pain. If systemic symptoms such as nausea and vomiting are exhibited, intravenous hydration may be initiated until the symptoms subside.[19]

Partial thickness (second degree). Partial-thickness or second-degree injuries are further classified as superficial or deep partial-thickness burns. They

Stop the Burning
A. Extinguish and remove burning clothing
B. For chemical burns — copious lavage with gallons of water
C. Avoid hypothermia — check body temperature

Examine, Establish and Maintain Airway
A. Administer humidified oxygen
B. Examine airway — laryngoscope or bronchoscope if inhalation injury suspected
C. Intubate if vocal cords are burned — check c-spine — if normal, use orotracheal intubation, if abnormal or no c-spine x-ray available do nasotracheal intubation

Resuscitate, Support Cardiopulmonary System
A. Use CPR if indicated
B. Start large bore intravenous lines in non-burned areas if possible
C. Cardiopulmonary monitor

History and Physical
A. Injury history
B. Pre-existing diseases
C. Medications
D. Allergies
E. Tetanus history
F. Examine for associated injuries

Size of Injury
A. Shade in burned areas on figures
B. Calculate size of burn by using figures and information in Fig. 24–6

Intravenous Fluids
A. Weight of patient in Kgs = _____
B. Size of burn in % total body surface area = _____

$$4 \text{ cc} \times \underset{\text{Value of A}}{\underline{\hspace{2cm}}} \times \underset{\text{Value of B}}{\underline{\hspace{2cm}}} = \underset{\text{total fluid for 24 hours}}{\underline{\hspace{3cm}}}$$

*Administer ½ 24 hour calculation in first 8 hours from time of injury using Lactated Ringers.

Accessory Tubes
A. Insert Foley catheter — urine output should be
  50cc/hour in adult,
  1cc/kg/hour in a child age (1–3)
  15–25cc/hr in a child age (3–12)
B. Insert nasogastric tube for burns > 20% TBSA and always for aerotransport

Tetanus Prophylaxis
Based on patient's immunization status

Signs of Adequate Resuscitation
A. Clear sensorium
B. Appropriate pain response
C. No nausea
D. BP normal, temp normal

Burn Wounds
A. Cover with sterile or clean sheets
B. Keep patient warm
C. Remove rings and bracelets

Call Burn Center
General guidelines for transfer—
A. Burns > 10% TBSA
B. All burns involving face, hands, feet, perineum
C. Inhalation injuries
D. Electrical injuries
E. Chemical injuries
F. Old or young people
G. Associated injuries or diseases

Fig. 24-5. Sample emergency burn protocol. (Courtesy University of South Alabama Medical Center Hospital and Clinics, Mobile, Ala.)

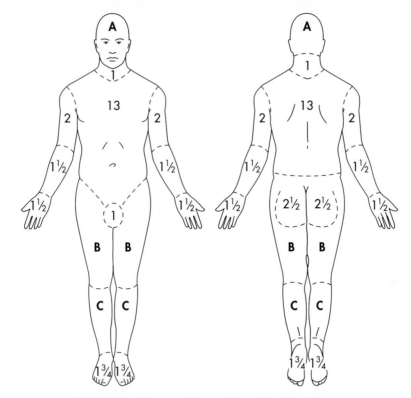

Relative Percentage of Areas Affected by Growth

	Age in Years					
	0	1	5	10	15	Adult
A—1/2 of head	9½	8½	6½	5½	4½	3½
B—1/2 of one thigh	2¾	3¼	4	4¼	4½	4¾
C—1/2 of one leg	2½	2½	2¾	3	3¼	3½

FIG. 24-6. USAMC modified Lund and Browder burn chart. The Lund and Browder chart provides a more accurate calculation of the extent of injury.

are most commonly caused by exposure to a hot liquid or object; however, flash burns from gasoline or other flammable products may also produce partial-thickness injuries of varying degrees.

Superficial partial-thickness wounds involve the epidermis and the uppermost portion of the dermis. They are usually caused by minimal exposure to a hot liquid such as splatters or splashes and are characterized by blisters and a moist red or pink skin appearance. As the blisters break, nerve endings are exposed to the air and pain is experienced. If the wound is protected from infection, superficial partial-thickness burns usually heal within 1 to 2 weeks, without scarring.

Deep partial-thickness burns involve the epidermis and the middle to lower portions of the dermis. They may appear reddish, mottled red, or whitish in color and the wound may look waxy and dry. Blisters may or may not be present. Hair follicles and nerve endings are usually present; however, pain and sensation may be dull. The healing time for deep partial-thickness wounds is 4 to 6 weeks and once healed, injured areas are prone to scarring. These wounds can convert to full-thickness wounds if uncontrolled infection occurs or if blood flow to the tissues is compromised. Deep partial-thickness burns of the hands, face, neck, or any joints can affect function.[14]

TABLE 24-2 | Depth of Injury

	DEPTH	APPEARANCE	HEALING TIME
Superficial (first degree)	Involves only the epidermis (e.g., sunburn)	Erythema, pink, red, usually dry	3-5 Days
Partial thickness (second degree)	Involves the epidermis and part of the dermis Skin blisters and/or peels	*Superficial (partial thickness)* Pink, usually moist blisters, very sensitive—painful *Deep (partial thickness)* Waxy white, some pink, less moisture, decreased sensation, minimal pain, hair follicles may or may not be intact	*Superficial* 14-21 Days *Deep* 4-6 Weeks; usually with hypertrophic scar
Full thickness (third degree)	Destroys both the epidermis and all of the dermis May extend into the subcutaneous fat, muscle, or bone	Whitish, charred (if flame), dry, leathery, brown, black, may or may not have thrombosed vessels or blisters Usually are not painful, unless mixed with some partial-thickness areas; scald injuries (hot water) often initially appear bright red/pink Bright cherry red may be due to carbon monoxide poisoning	May close as secondary healing if <3 cm^2 Usually requires skin graft for complete closure

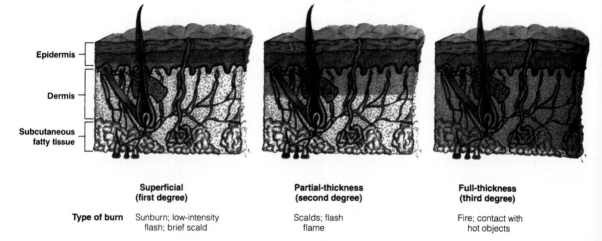

	Superficial (first degree)	Partial-thickness (second degree)	Full-thickness (third degree)
Type of burn	Sunburn; low-intensity flash; brief scald	Scalds; flash flame	Fire; contact with hot objects

FIG. 24-7. Classification of burn depth. (From Wong DL: *Whaley & Wong's nursing care of infants and children,* ed 5, St Louis, 1995, Mosby.)

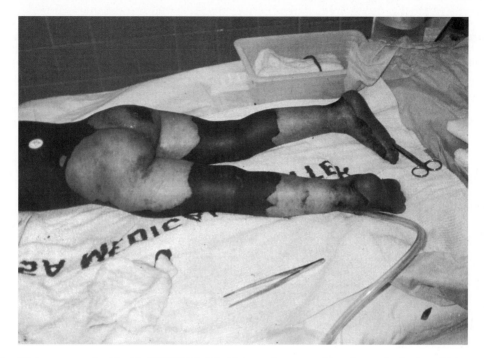

FIG. 24-8. Eighteen month old with 14% TBSA full-thickness burns resulting from a bathtub scald. Burns involve the buttocks and posterior lower legs. Circumferential burns are on the ankles.

Full thickness (third degree). Full-thickness injuries are caused by contact with concentrated chemicals or prolonged contact with liquids of high temperatures (>150° F), hot objects, flames, or ignited clothing.[14] Full-thickness injuries result when the epidermis and dermis are destroyed and extend into subcutaneous fat, muscle, or bone to varying degrees. The appearance of the wound may be charred, or it can be red, black, brown, or white in color. Typically the wound feels hard, leathery, and dry. The classic appearance is translucent with thrombosed vessels visible to the eye. Hair follicles are not intact, and nerve endings are destroyed. The child may feel pressure but not pain. Because partial- and full-thickness burns frequently present together, the report of pain may or may not be reliable in determining the depth of the injury.

Injuries involving exposed fat, muscle, tendon, or bone are sometimes referred to as *fourth-degree burns*. These injuries are typically caused by severe electrical burns or prolonged contact with flame, smoldering materials, or objects of high temperature.

Full-thickness burns are associated with high morbidity and mortality rates and therefore require emergent management. Systemic physiologic derangements, including fluid and electrolyte imbalances,

metabolic disturbances, alterations in temperature regulation, and pulmonary edema, should be expected. In most cases, treatment of the wound(s) requires surgical skin grafting.[41] Disfiguring is common, and long-term functional problems can persist for years (Fig. 24-8).

TRIAGE CRITERIA FOR PEDIATRIC PATIENTS

The American Burn Association categorizes burn injuries as minor, moderate, or major. Children with minor burns can usually be treated on an outpatient basis, with follow-up wound care and/or physical therapy.[3] Those who have sustained a moderate or major injury require treatment in a facility that specializes in burn care (Box 24-1).

NONURGENT (MINOR BURN INJURY)

Minor burn injuries are defined as those occurring on children over 2 years of age who have sustained a partial-thickness burn to less than 10% of their total body surface area with full-thickness areas of less than 2%.[15] Children with partial-thickness or full-thickness

---

Box 24-1   Burn Center Referral Criteria

- Second- and third-degree burns > 10% TBSA (in patients < 10 yrs or > 50 yrs of age)
- Second- and third-degree burns > 20% TBSA (any age group)
- Second- and third- degree burns (that involve face, hands, feet, genitalia, perineum, major joints)
- Third-degree burns > 5% TBSA (any age group)
- Significant electrical burns (include lightning)
- Significant chemical burns
- Inhalation injury
- Burns with preexisting illness affecting mortality
- Burns with concomitant trauma increasing mortality
- Children in hospitals without specialized pediatric/burn care trained personnel
- Burn injuries requiring long-term social/ emotional support (including suspected child abuse/neglect)

Data from Committee on Trauma, American College of Surgeons, *Resources for optimal care of the injured patient*, 1993.

---

burns of the hands, feet, face, or perineum are hospitalized regardless of the total body surface area involved. Individual consideration is given when small superficial (first-degree) injuries are involved. In such cases, treatment on an outpatient basis may be adequate if the parent/caregiver is reliable and follow-up care can be ensured.

URGENT (MODERATE BURN INJURY)

Urgent or moderate burns are classified as partial-thickness burns encompassing 10% to 15% of the total body surface area or full-thickness burns encompassing 2% to 10% of the total body surface area. Children less than 2 years of age with partial-thickness burns of less than 10% or full-thickness burns of less than 2% are also categorized as moderate or urgent.[3]

EMERGENT (MAJOR BURN INJURY)

Partial-thickness burn injuries that encompass greater than 15% of the total body surface area or full-

thickness burns that are greater than 10% of the total body surface area are classified as major burn injuries in children. Other burns that are classified as major include those involving the hands, feet, face, or perineal area and those caused by electrical, chemical, or inhalation injuries.[23] Burned children with a pre-existing medical condition that may complicate the injury, such as asthma or hemophilia, are also classified as major.

EMERGENCY MANAGEMENT

The management of the burn victim, from the time of injury through the recovery phase, requires a multidisciplinary team approach that begins with the emergency personnel.[36,41] Prompt and appropriate treatment can lead to a dramatic decline in mortality (Fig. 24-5).

FIELD CARE

Emergency treatment begins when the first responder renders care at the scene. To avoid further injury to the victim and to avoid injuries to the responders, the scene is initially surveyed for potential dangers such as "hot" electrical wires or burning debris and the appropriate interventions initiated (e.g., donning protective equipment). Scene treatment of the burn injury requires stopping the burning by removing the child from the burning agent or process; smothering the flames, if present; and removing loose, smoldering clothing or jewelry. The burn may briefly (no more than 5 to 10 minutes) be cooled with water, which provides comfort and limits the extent of the injury. Exposure to water for longer periods predisposes the child to hypothermia. The burn should *not* be submerged in ice or wet sheets; this practice not only contributes to the rapid development of hypothermia but also contributes to further tissue injury and necrosis. Once the burning has been halted the injured area is immediately wrapped in clean, dry dressings and the child is wrapped in blankets or sheets. One exception to the treatments listed above is the presence of chemical injuries, which require continuous irrigation.

Once the victim has been removed from the fire and the burning process halted, the primary focus of the field responder is to stabilize the airway, breathing, and circulation (ABCs). Specific burn care interventions then follow the ABCs of care. If smoke inhalation is suspected based on history (e.g., being burned in an enclosed space) or physical findings (e.g., burns to the face or nasal hairs), 100% oxygen is provided with a

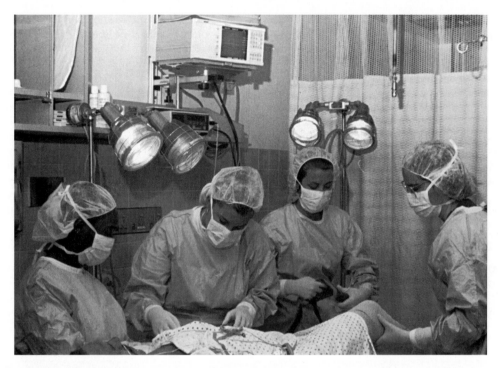

FIG. 24-9. Burn team performing assessment and wound care of a burn victim. Isolation and measures to prevent hypothermia are instituted.

nonrebreather face mask or any mechanism that is tolerated by the child. Because signs of airway or pulmonary edema may not be immediately observed, the child is continually monitored for the development of respiratory distress. In major injuries intravenous access is established; however, if the hospital is less than 30 minutes away and venous access is difficult to obtain, transportation should not be delayed.[28]

After initial stabilization and before transport, a secondary survey is performed to identify the presence of fractures and other injuries that may require stabilization. A rapid estimation of the size of the burn injury is also completed. During transport to the closest appropriate facility the child must be kept warm.[29]

EMERGENCY DEPARTMENT PREPARATIONS

Initial management of the burn victim directly affects the child's survival and degree of recovery. Therefore, time management is an important component of care. When notified of a child's impending arrival to the emergency department (ED), personnel in the receiving facility should assemble age-specific supplies and equipment necessary for airway management, fluid resuscitation, and managing associated injuries. Warm blankets, heat lamps, fluid warmers, and sterile sheets or drapes should also be readily accessible for immediate application on the child's arrival.[13] Because the burned child will require protective isolation, medical personnel should don gowns, masks, caps, and gloves.[26] Personnel assignments are also made before the child's arrival and are based on the expected degree of interventions. Initial activities of these personnel should be strictly limited to the emergent care of the burn victim (Fig. 24-9).

NURSING CARE AND EVALUATION

The initial assessment and management of the pediatric burn victim follows the same priority of care as for any pediatric victim of trauma. Burn wounds are considered secondary injuries. The priorities of care include assessment and stabilization of the airway, breathing, and circulation. After primary stabilization, the depth and extent of the wounds and/or injuries are assessed and a head-to-toe assessment is performed to identify hidden injuries. Throughout all phases of care, normothermia is maintained.

A thorough history is obtained from the child (if of age and if able), emergency response personnel, and family members or bystanders. The details and circumstances surrounding the incident (e.g., burns that occurred within a closed space), as well as the mechanism of injury (e.g., fire, chemicals, electrical), will guide treatment priorities. A history of medication usage, allergies, and immunization status is obtained, as well as the child's past medical history (Box 24-2).

FLUID RESUSCITATION

Pathophysiology. Adequate fluid resuscitation is vital to the survival of any victim of a major burn injury.[11] Even though the exact phenomenon of postburn volume shifts and vascular changes has not been determined, it is known that burn shock, or hypovolemia, occurs in injuries affecting more than 15% to 20% of total body surface area.[18] If intravascular volume loss is not replaced, systemic perfusion is compromised.

Hypovolemic shock associated with significant burn injuries results when capillary permeability increases systemically, allowing plasma fluid and proteins to leak into the interstitial spaces at the expense of vascular volume. This phenomenon is known as *third-spacing* of fluids. With the movement of protein into the extravascular space, the osmotic pressure in the interstitial tissues increase, exacerbating fluid movement.[11,18] Intravascular volume losses become apparent in the first several hours after the injury but may persist for up to 36 hours and are evidenced by the formation of edema.[11,39] The degree of fluid shift is dependent upon the severity and extent of the burn.

With the loss of fluid from the vascular compartment, blood viscosity increases. Because of hemocon-

---

Box 24-2   Emergency Department Interventions

Obtain History
- Time burn occurred, mechanism of injury (flame, chemical, electrical, hot liquid, inhalation), type of burn, percent TBSA, and location
- Past medical history (tetanus, allergies, preexisting medical conditions)
- Patient's approximate weight
- Treatment delivered before arrival

Airway/Breathing
- Determine airway patency and effectiveness of breathing
- Monitor patient for signs of suggested inhalation injury (face burns, singed hair, hoarseness, stridor)
- Observe adequacy of chest wall movement
- Maintain oxygen delivery, assist with bronchoscope and/or intubation
- Monitor oxygen saturations

Circulation
- Place on heart monitor (electrical injury—obtain 12 lead)
- Perform neurovascular checks (especially pulse checks on burned extremities)

- Establish intravenous access and administer warm IV fluids: crystalloid solution 2-4 ml/kg/% BSA burn for the first 24 hours; give half of the total in the first 8 hours of care and the remaining amount over the next 16 hours
- Avoid hypothermia (apply blankets and heat lamps); keep the child warm
- Cover burn wounds (dry, sterile towels/sheets)
- Elevate burned extremities

Other
- Insert Foley catheter (moderate or major burns or perineal burns)
- Insert a nasogastric tube (if intubated, distended abdomen, moderate or major burn)
- Obtain laboratory work (electrolytes, CBC, glucose, BUN, creatinine, urine analysis; for electrical injuries—cardiac enzymes, urine for myoglobin)
- Administer tetanus
- Administer pain medications/anxiolytics as ordered
- Provide emotional support to child and family
- Prepare for transfer to burn facility

centration, polycythemia may be evident. Movement of blood through the small blood vessels becomes sluggish, and red blood cells may become trapped or destroyed in the burned areas.

After the injury, the fluid remobilization period (fluids moving from the interstitial space back into the vascular space) usually begins approximately 24 to 36 hours after the burn, as the injured capillaries begin to heal. Intravascular fluid losses diminish and the child begins diuresis. Anemia may become evident during this period.

Fluid therapy. Children are at high risk for the development of hypovolemia after a significant burn injury because of their large body surface to volume ratio, their high metabolic rates, and their proportionately high daily turnover of body water when compared to adults. Fluid replacement calculations must therefore take these factors into consideration.

Children requiring fluid resuscitation after a burn injury include those with second- or third-degree burns covering greater than 10% to 15% of their TBSA or children with signs of shock.[16] Calculations for fluid replacement are based on the child's actual or estimated body weight, the percentage of body surface area burned, and the presence of other significant injuries (e.g., increased pulmonary capillary permeability caused by an inhalation injury).

There are numerous fluid resuscitation formulas; however, these formulas simply provide an *estimate* of the child's needs and serve as guides for initiating fluid therapy. They do not reflect the total fluids that may be required to meet the increased metabolic demands of the severely injured child or the very young infant or to treat an underlying condition such as shock. All fluid therapy is therefore based on the child's clinical condition and response to therapy. As in any emergent condition, if signs of shock are present a bolus of an isotonic crystalloid solution (e.g., normal saline or lactated Ringer's solution) in the amount of 20 ml/kg is administered and repeated as necessary.

One of the most widely used burn resuscitation formulas is the Parkland formula, which is 4 ml lactated Ringer's solution × kg of body weight × percent of TBSA burned.[24] The total amount to be administered is then divided, half is infused in the first 8 hours after the burn injury, and the other half is given over the subsequent 16 hours.

However, body weight is not the most effective means of determining fluid requirements in the child because of the large body surface to volume ratio, high metabolic rates, and high maintenance requirements. For this reason, other formulas using body surface area (BSA) rather than weight have been developed. Two such formulas are the modified Parkland formula, which adds 1500 ml × BSA (m²) to the fluid requirements obtained using the original formula,[18] and a formula recommended by Herndon, Rutan, and Rutan, which is 5000 ml/m² BSA of the burn + 2000 ml/m² total BSA (to address maintenance requirements).[12,20]

The use of colloid solutions within the first 24 hours after a burn injury is controversial, because studies have demonstrated contradictory results.[20] In general, it has been felt that if colloids are given before the reversal of the initial capillary leak, additional proteins may also leak into the tissue and produce an increase in tissue osmotic pressure, further exacerbating fluid shifting.[18] Despite these concerns, some institutions administer small amounts of colloids before the fluid mobilization period, but not until 6 to 8 hours after the injury.[21]

After the initial 24 hours following the burn injury, and after third-spacing has abated, colloid administration may enhance fluid shifting from the interstitial space back into the vascular compartment. The most commonly used colloid is albumin although some institutions use fresh frozen plasma.[21]

Electrolyte imbalances are common with major burn injuries; therefore, serum electrolytes are drawn simultaneously while obtaining vascular access to administer fluids. Hyperkalemia may be present as potassium is released into the circulation from the injured cells. Sodium, calcium, and magnesium levels may occasionally be lowered because of dilutional disturbances caused by fluid administration. Hypoalbuminemia may result from protein shifts from the intravascular to interstitial spaces, and metabolic acidosis can result with severe tissue damage and inadequate fluid resuscitation. Daily electrolyte requirements include sodium 3 to 8 mg/kg/day and potassium 2 to 4 mEq/kg/day; however, potassium levels must be monitored because supplemental potassium may not be required in the initial resuscitation fluids.[7,39]

Ongoing care. With the stabilization of the ABCs and the initiation of fluid therapy, secondary interventions include ongoing assessments of the child's pulmonary status to identify the development of pulmonary edema caused by fluid shifts. If significant fluid shifting has occurred a central venous pressure (CVP) line may be inserted to monitor preload augmentation and to protect against volume overload. Hydration status is also continuously monitored by evaluating the child's capillary refill, peripheral pulses, neurologic status, heart rate, and urine output. Once a Foley catheter has been inserted and urine output can be measured, the goal of fluid therapy is to maintain a urine output of 1 cc/kg/hr. In the child with significant burns, urine may be red-brown in color because damaged myoglobin and hemoglobin are filtered through the kidneys. Also in children with significant burns, a nasogastric tube is required to prevent gastric distention and possible aspiration, and to alleviate the potential effects of ileus associated with shock.[38a]

Complications of underresuscitation of the burn-injured child include a continuation of decreased peripheral perfusion, hypovolemic shock, decreased renal perfusion, and conversion of partial-thickness to full-thickness burns caused by the low output state.[18] Conversely, overresuscitation can lead to cardiac overload, pulmonary edema, circulatory compromise, decreased chest wall compliance due to excessive edema, and decreased oxygen tension (Box 24-3).

Tetanus prophylaxis. Burn wounds are considered contaminated; therefore all burn victims receive tetanus prophylaxis unless a booster was received within the preceding 6 months. Intramuscular administration of 0.5 ml tetanus toxoid is given if more than 5 years have elapsed since the last tetanus prophylaxis. Two hundred and fifty (250) units of tetanus immunoglobin (TIG) is given, in addition to the tetanus toxoid if the child did not receive a tetanus immunization within the previous 10 years.[10a]

Analgesia. Burn injuries produce severe pain, stress, and anxiety. Pain management is therefore an essential component of the burn treatment regimen. Nursing interventions that can assist with pain management include keeping the wound covered so it is not exposed to air (second-degree wounds are especially painful when exposed to air), slightly elevating an injured extremity, providing emotional support by allowing the parent to be with the child whenever possible, and speaking gently while informing the child about the frightening procedures that are occurring.

Pharmacologic management of pain includes the administration of analgesics, anxiolytics, and/or sedatives. Before the administration of any of these medications the child's airway, breathing, and circulation must be stabilized.[43] Once the child is hemodynamically stable and there are no injuries that would contraindicate administration (such as a head injury), pain medications can be administered. The preferred route of administration is the intravenous route, because intramuscular absorption may be compromised in burn patients. After administration the child is continuously monitored both for the relief of pain and for the development of symptoms of respiratory depression or hypotension[43] (Box 24-4).

Burn wound care. The degree of burn care interventions depends on the available supplies within

---

Box 24-3 Desirable Responses to Fluid Therapy

- Adequate peripheral circulation
- Alert, lucid level of consciousness
- Heart rate in normal/upper limits for age
- Blood pressure normal for age
- Normal cardiac output
- Urine output 1 cc/kg/hr
- Specific gravity 1.010-1.025
- Serum sodium 135-145 mEq/L
- Serum osmolarity 272-294 mOsm/L
- Hct 35%-45%

Box 24-4 Commonly Used Medications in Burn-Injured Children

- Morphine—0.1-0.2 mg/kg/dose every 1 to 2 hours prn IV push over 4 to 5 minutes (maximum 15 mg/dose)
- Demerol—1-1.5 mg/kg/dose every 3 to 4 hours prn slow IV push (maximum 100 mg every 4 hours)
- Versed—0.08 mg/kg/dose (over 20 to 30 seconds) IV push

Data from Benitz WE, Tatro DS: *The pediatric drug handbook*, ed 2, Chicago, 1988, Year Book Medical Publishers.

the emergency department, the severity of the burn(s), and the recommendations of the burn center staff—if the child is being transferred to a burn unit. After stabilization of the ABCs, initial burn care includes removing superficial debris such as soot, dirt, or grass from the burns using an antibacterial solution. Sterile burn dressings are then used to cover the burns on the body or an extremity using a topical antimicrobial ointment such as 1% silver sulfadiazine. Burns to the face may be treated with neomycin sulfate and left uncovered.

In general, extensive burn wound care, such as surgical removal of eschar, is not performed in the emergency department. If the child is being transferred to a burn unit or facility within 2 to 4 hours, interventions other than those listed below are usually not required. While providing wound care, the child's normal body temperature must be maintained using dry sterile sheets or blankets (Box 24-5).

Box 24-5 General Guidelines for Burn Wound Care in the ED

- Premedicate the child for pain.
- Gather dressing supplies (gauze, saline, antiseptic cleanser, forceps, scissors, sterile absorbent dressings).
- Cleanse the wound with an antiseptic/antibacterial solution such as chlorhexidine gluconate. Avoid the eyes.
- Shave or trim hair around ear or facial burns (except the eyebrows).
- Remove loose, necrotic tissue.
- Remove blisters except on palms and soles of feet.
- Apply antimicrobial creams/ointments such as silver sulfadiazine to body wounds and cover with a dressing; facial wounds are treated with Neomycin or Bacitracin and left uncovered.
- Apply absorbent dressing to wounds (e.g., Exudry, gauze).
- Wrap with outer dressing to secure (Kerlex, Conform).
- Dressings should be applied to facilitate movement, exercise, and antideformity positioning.

Stabilization for transport. If the decision is made to transfer the child, the burn center is contacted and transfer guidelines are established.[26] Many burn facilities provide standard transfer protocols on request to assist the referring facility when preparing for transport (see Figs. 24-5 and 24-6). Pertinent patient information, treatments provided in the ED, the name and phone number of a contact person, and the expected departure and arrival times must all be conveyed to the receiving institution.[24] Copies of the medical record should accompany the child.

Before transport the child is "packaged" with blankets or drapes to prevent hypothermia. Indwelling lines and tubes are secured thoroughly, because accidental dislodgement with progressive edema formation may make placement difficult during transport or at the receiving facility. The family should be allowed to see the child before the transfer.

Throughout resuscitative care the family should be kept informed of the child's status. As soon as possible, family members should be allowed to see the child. When the child requires transport to a burn facility, the parents/caregivers should be involved in the decision to transfer the child. Arrangements for the parents to accompany or follow their child can be made through the receiving institution, the transport team, and/or the referring facility. Many burn facilities assist parents who are from out of town in locating a place to stay while their child is hospitalized.

Discharge: Home instructions. Children with minor burns may be treated as outpatients.[12] Involvement of the child (if age appropriate) and family is essential to the success of any discharge treatment plan. Therefore, before discharge to the home setting, the reliability of the parent/caregiver to perform treatments or maintain follow-up care is assessed. Support systems available to the family should be identified (e.g., transportation for follow-up, child care) and appropriate referrals made. Definitive follow-up care (e.g., physical therapy, surgical or primary care appointment) is arranged before discharge.

Discharge information should include instructions on burn care dressing changes, the recommended degree of exercise and activity, dietary requirements, and need for compliance with outpatient wound care therapy and follow-up. Written discharge instructions are given to the parents to reinforce verbal instructions (Fig. 24-10).

UNIVERSITY OF SOUTH ALABAMA HOSPITALS AND CLINICS

BURNS
Patient Instruction Sheet

You have received a minor burn of _____.
Burns are classified according to the depth of the injury of the skin and the percent (%) of body that is burned.

Superficial (1st degree):	Redness of the outermost part of the skin.
Partial Thickness (2nd degree):	Redness of the skin with blisters. You may also have some swelling with this type of burn.
Full Thickness (3rd degree):	This involves the full thickness of the skin. This type of burn is usually not painful, but it is the most serious type of burn.

1st and 2nd degree burns are painful. They will heal if properly cared for. 3rd degree burns are not painful because the nerves have been destroyed, however they may become painful as the nerves begin to regenerate. As the burns heal, you are likely to experience itching and dryness of the skin.

HOW TO TAKE CARE OF YOUR BURN

1. Clean the burned area twice a day with soap and water.
2. If there are blisters present, **do not** break them. If they do break, keep them clean.
3. If you have 2nd or 3rd degree burns, keep them clean and covered with a sterile dressing.
4. Wear loose, non-restrictive clothing over the burned area and elevate it above the level of the heart.
5. Watch for signs of infection: (fever, foul odor, slow healing, redness or warmth around wound edges).
6. Eat well balanced meals.
7. Avoid changes in extreme heat or cold.
8. If you have been given a prescription for:
   A. Medicated cream—apply as directed and keep the area covered.
   B. Pain medication—take as directed and avoid drinking alcohol, driving, or operating heavy machinery.
9. Keep your follow-up appointment with Burn Clinic.
10. Tylenol can be taken for mild pain, if you have not received a Rx for pain medication.

1st degree burns should heal within 5–7 days. 2nd degree burns should heal within 10–21 days. 3rd degree burns may require follow-up care with a plastic surgeon.

If you have questions or problems, contact the Burn Center at _____ or the Emergency Department at _____.

USAMC 145

Fig. 24-10.   Patient instruction sheet for burns. (Courtesy University of South Alabama Hospitals and Clinics, Mobile, Ala.)

SELECTED BURN INJURIES

INHALATION INJURIES

Etiology. Inhalation injuries result from the inhalation of hot air or steam, toxins such as smoke and industrial pollutants, or chemicals such as gasoline or kerosene. The most common inhalation injuries in children result from exposure to house fires where the byproducts of combustion produce toxins such as carbon monoxide and cyanide.

Pathophysiology. Pathophysiologic effects of inhalation injuries depend on the source of the inhalation injury, degree of exposure, and degree of underlying damage. Thermal inhalation injuries are usually limited to the pharynx, because the heat is rapidly cooled before passage into the lower airways. Injuries to the upper airway can produce airway edema and obstruction. The inhalation of gases or aerosols can affect both the upper and lower airways as the toxin moves throughout the tracheobronchial tree. Damage to the pulmonary mucosa leads to capillary leak within the pulmonary bed and produces pulmonary edema. It can also contribute significantly to systemic vascular volume losses.

The most commonly inhaled toxin is smoke, which contains particulate matter and any number of toxins or gases that are related to the substance(s) burning. Evidence indicates that smoke inhalation decreases the production of surfactant, resulting in areas of atelectasis within the lungs. Mild erythema, charring, and marked congestion may also be found in the trachea and bronchi as a result of smoke inhalation.

The most common and one of the most lethal gases produced during a fire is carbon monoxide. Carbon monoxide is an odorless, colorless gas that is normally absent in the bloodstream. People who smoke heavily (and children who are exposed to passive smoke) or people who live in large urban areas where smog and factory pollutants are common may have minimal levels in their blood. When a child is exposed to smoke, serum carbon monoxide levels rapidly elevate to dangerous levels. Because carbon monoxide has an approximately 250 times greater affinity for hemoglobin than oxygen, it competes with the oxygen molecule and binds more readily to the hemoglobin.[8,41a] The inability of the hemoglobin to deliver oxygen to the tissues results in tissue hypoxia. With progressive hypoxia, organs with normally high oxygen consumption, such as the central nervous system and heart, are affected.

Clinical presentation. An inhalation injury is suspected in any child with facial burns or with any burns combined with a history of being confined within an enclosed space (Fig. 24-11). If significant thermal burns are present, particularly to the upper torso, face, and neck, pulmonary complications may be evident early after the injury. Even if the child does not demonstrate immediate signs of airway compromise, progressive edema formation can eventually lead to an airway obstruction.[10]

Classic signs of the presence of an inhalation injury include singed nasal hairs, darkened oral or nasal membranes, carbonaceous sputum, or soot on the tongue.[10] Other respiratory signs and symptoms suggestive of an inhalation injury include tachypnea, stridor, retractions, rales, or wheezing (Box 24-6).

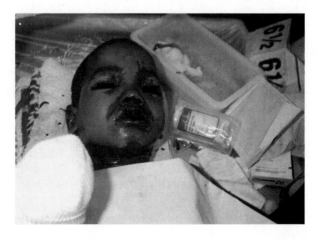

FIG. 24-11. Eight year old with facial burns and impending airway obstruction. This 6% TBSA partial-thickness injury resulted when an aerosol can exploded during a trash fire.

Effects of carbon monoxide poisoning may be exhibited by respiratory symptoms and CNS findings such as an altered level of consciousness, seizures, or coma. Effects on the cardiovascular system include diminished cardiac output evidenced by decreased peripheral perfusion and hypotension. Signs of myocardial ischemia may also be present. In children signs and symptoms of carbon monoxide poisoning are exhibited with lower carboxyhemoglobin serum concentrations than adults (Table 24-3).

Emergency Department interventions. Initial management of the child with a suspected or known inhalation injury requires stabilization of the ABCs. Supplemental oxygen is administered, and diagnostic testing is begun to determine the degree of airway and pulmonary damage.

Diagnostic testing includes obtaining a chest x-ray to observe for infiltrates indicative of pulmonary edema; however, this finding may not be evident immediately after the event. A more conclusive diagnostic procedure to determine the extent of airway damage is direct visualization of the posterior larynx and vocal cords.[28] This procedure, which is usually performed by a physician, requires the use of a laryngoscope or fiberoptic bronchoscope to view the vocal cords.

Additional testing is based on symptomatology, the degree of suspected pulmonary damage, and the presence of other injuries. A complete blood count (CBC), electrolytes, blood urea nitrogen (BUN), creatinine, and arterial blood gases are routinely ordered. If smoke inhalation has occurred or is a possibility, a serum carboxyhemoglobin (COHg) level will be obtained as soon as possible on the child's arrival in the ED. Because the COHg level begins to fall after the inhalation episode, findings may not accurately reflect the degree of hypoxic tissue damage.

Nursing care and evaluation. Treatment of an inhalation injury begins at the scene, with high-concentration oxygen administered via a nonrebreather face mask. If carbon monoxide poisoning is present it is completely reversible with oxygen administration, provided anoxic damage to the central nervous system has not already occurred. If signs of airway obstruction are present, the child's airway is positioned and cleared. Airway management including bag-mask ventilation and intubation is initiated as indicated to maintain oxygenation and ventilation.

On arrival in the emergency department most burn victims are awake and alert. High-concentration supplemental oxygen is applied by nonrebreather face mask, and the child is placed in a semi-Fowler's position. If the child/infant will not tolerate the mask, blow-by cool oxygen mist can be used. As the rest of the ABCs are evaluated and stabilized, the child is placed on a cardiorespiratory monitor and pulse oximeter. In the presence of carbon monoxide poisoning, however, pulse oximetry will not adequately reflect tissue hypoxia, because COHb is recognized as saturated hemoglobin by the oximeter.

During the emergency department stay, and if intubation has not already been performed, the child

---

Box 24-6 Signs Suggestive of Inhalation Injury

- Erythema or swelling of oropharynx/nasopharynx
- Soot or carbonaceous sputum
- Stridor, hoarseness
- Grunting, nasal flaring, sternal retractions
- Wheezes, rales
- Mechanism of injury suggesting possible inhalation (closed-space injury)
- Swelling or blistering of posterior larynx or vocal cords

TABLE 24-3 Carboxyhemoglobin Levels and Clinical Presentation

LEVEL	DEGREE OF TOXICITY	SYMPTOMS
<20%	Mild	Headache, visual changes, confusion
20%-40%	Moderate	Weakness, nausea/vomiting, dulled sensation
40%-60%	Severe	Memory loss, poor coordination
>60%	Rapid demise/fatal	Convulsions, cardiovascular collapse, neurologic collapse, coma

From D'Italia JG: Burns. In Joy C, ed: *Pediatric trauma nursing*, Rockville, Md, 1989, Aspen Publishers; Luterman A, Curreri PW: Emergency protocol for the severely burned patient, *Hosp Med* October: 131-146, 1984.

is continuously monitored for the development of airway tissue edema and pulmonary compromise. These signs may not be evident for up to 24 hours after the injury and are sometimes not exhibited until 3 to 5 days after the injury. Severe stridor, grunting, nasal flaring, sternal retractions, inability to swallow, or handling secretions (drooling) are signs of an impending respiratory failure. If these signs develop in the emergency department, endotracheal intubation is indicated. Orotracheal intubation is the preferred route in children. Because the child may initially present awake and alert, with no obvious signs of respiratory distress, a slow, insidious progression of respiratory symptoms may be difficult to appreciate. If upper airway edema is allowed to progress, however, intubation may be difficult to perform once signs of respiratory compromise develop.

If the child has significant burn injuries and requires emergent resuscitative management, consideration should be given to transferring the child to a burn facility (see Box 24-1).

ELECTRICAL INJURIES

Etiology. Electrical injuries account for a small percentage of pediatric burn injuries. The incidence of all electrical injuries by age is 1.6% in children 0 to 23 months, 2.7% in children 2 to 4 years, 2.2% in children 5 to 12 years, and 3.8% in children 13 to 18 years.[9] Because young children are curious and commonly place objects in their mouths, most electrical injuries in this age child are to the face and hands during play with unprotected household electrical sockets or while mouthing or sucking extension cords (Fig. 24-12).

Rare causes of electrical injuries in children include noninvasive infant monitoring devices (respiratory monitors, pulse oximeter, heart monitors)[5] and exposure to high-voltage electricity (transformers, electrical lines, or lightning). Most high-voltage incidences occur in males between the ages of 7 and 16 years who contact transformers or power lines. These injuries are often severe enough to result in amputations or death.

Pathophysiology. Electrical injury may result from contact with any alternating current, direct current, or lightning. The actual tissue injury from electricity depends on the type of current, the strength of the current, the duration of contact, and the path that the current travels through the body.[24] Electrical burns may appear minor, because the full extent of the injury is not externally visible. The entrance and exit sites may account for a relatively small percentage of the TBSA burned; however, underlying tissue destruction may be extensive. Thus, appearance alone should not be relied on when determining care requirements.

Electrical injuries can produce muscle damage, vascular thrombosis, fractures from muscle tetany, and internal organ damage.[27] Myoglobinuria from muscle necrosis may lead to tubular necrosis and/or renal failure. The most serious immediate problem associated with electrical injuries is ventricular fibrillation, asystole, or other dysrhythmia.

Clinical presentation. Clinical manifestations of electrical injuries range from no symptoms at all to full cardiopulmonary arrest depending on the source and degree of exposure. Dysrhythmias are common and can include bradycardia, tachycardia, PVCs, PACs,

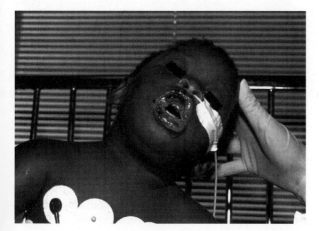

FIG. 24-12. Nine month old with an electrical injury to the mouth after sucking and gnawing on an electrical cord.

conduction defects, atrial fibrillation, or ventricular fibrillation. Immediate neurologic manifestations may include agitation, amnesia, loss of consciousness, or motor disturbances. Other disturbances include signs of renal and/or pulmonary dysfunction and solid organ or visceral damage.

Cutaneous injuries vary in severity from small necrotic areas to large eviscerated wounds. Point-of-entry wounds may appear charred, and exit wounds may appear explosive. They are usually ischemic, painless, and dry. Injuries to the oral mucosa caused by biting or chewing on electrical cords can produce necrotic tissue damage, as well as liquefaction necrosis of the oral tissues.[17]

Emergency Department interventions. In addition to the evaluation and stabilization of the ABCs, initial emergency department interventions specific to high- voltage electrical injuries include monitoring the patient for dysrhythmias by obtaining a 12-lead ECG, obtaining cardiac enzymes, and evaluating the urine for myoglobin. A complete neurologic examination is also performed.

Nursing care and evaluation. On arrival in the emergency department the ABCs are assessed and stabilized and the child is placed on a heart rate monitor and pulse oximeter. Specific interventions for the child with an electrical injury include continuous assessment of the airway, ventilation, cardiovascular status, urine output, and signs of underlying organ or tissue damage. If the electrical current passed through an extremity, the extremity is monitored for signs of compartment syndrome (pain, pallor, paresthesia, pulselessness, and paralysis).[30] If arc burns or flame injuries are present, the percent of TBSA of the burn will be increased and fluid resuscitation should be adjusted accordingly. Fluid therapy is titrat·d to maintain a urine output of 1 to 1.5 ml/kg of body weight per hour or above.[20]

CHEMICAL INJURIES

Etiology. The majority of chemical injuries are industry related. They therefore account for the smallest percentage of burn injuries in children. The distribution of all chemical injuries occurring in children less than 18 years of age is 1% in infants 0 to 23 months of age, 1% in children 2 to 4 years of age, 0.6% in children 5 to 12 years of age, and 2% in children 13 to 18 years of age.[9] Acids and alkaline agents, found in many household products such as drain cleaner, account for the highest number of chemical injuries in

children.[41] Exposure to or ingestion of miniature batteries made for watches, calculators, and cameras is also a source of chemical injuries in children because the child is exposed to the caustic components within the battery.[6]

Pathophysiology. The extent of injury from a caustic substance depends on several factors, including the type of agent (acid, alkali, liquid, or solid), concentration of the agent, quantity of the agent, duration of contact, type of contact (skin, eyes, inhalation, or ingestion), penetration and action of the agent, form of the agent (solid, liquid), and molarity of the agent.[30a,42a]

Exposure to an alkali agent tends to produce immediate damage, with deep penetration into the tissues described as liquefaction necrosis. Contact with an acidic substance causes eschar formation, which limits penetration of the toxin and tends to produce superficial necrosis.

Ingested liquid *alkali* agents such as liquid lye produce immediate tissue damage that most commonly involves the oropharynx and esophagus. Because the agent is neutralized with passage through the esophagus, damage to the stomach may not occur. Ingested *acidic* substances may not produce immediate tissue injury, as in the case of alkali ingestions, but instead tissue injury may evolve with continued exposure to the toxin as it passes through the gastrointestinal tract. Therefore, acidic ingestions are more likely to involve the stomach.

Clinical presentation. Children who arrive in the emergency department with a history of toxic exposure may be asymptomatic or present with signs of cardiorespiratory compromise. Burn injuries may range from small localized lesions to large, open wounds. If a caustic agent was ingested, the oropharynx may be red with ulcerous lesions but may also show no evidence of the ingestion—particularly if the agent was acidic. Airway symptoms may or may not correlate with the presence of burns in the oropharynx and may be seen immediately or progress as tissue edema worsens. Signs of airway compromise include stridor, tachypnea, drooling, and difficulting speaking (dysphonia). Vomiting, abdominal pain or tenderness, signs of shock, and coma are all signs of significant burns and may indicate the presence of an esophageal or gastric perforation.

Emergency Department interventions. Emergency department interventions and diagnostic testing depend on the degree of exposure to the toxin and the location of contact. Laboratory studies such as a CBC, electrolytes, BUN, creatinine, and glucose are performed when a child is exposed to surface toxins or has ingested a toxin that may produce a systemic response. A chest x-ray is ordered if signs of respiratory distress or compromise are present or to identify the location of a foreign body such as a battery. An x-ray of the abdomen is performed to rule out the presence of a perforation when the child exhibits gastrointestinal symptoms (see Chapter 15, p. 361, for the treatment of foreign body ingestions such as batteries).

Nursing care and evaluation.   On arrival in the emergency department the ABCs are assessed and stabilized. All clothing is removed, and the child's skin and oral mucosa are inspected for burn injuries.[28,30] To avoid exposure to the toxin, medical personnel should wear protective gloves, a gown, and goggles. If a dermal exposure occurred, the skin is immediately irrigated with water or saline solution for a minimum of 10 to 15 minutes. Irrigation is not delayed while searching for a specific neutralizing agent. The period of time of irrigation depends on the agent involved and the time required to return the pH of the skin to normal. Certain chemicals such as acids may require irrigation for up to 6 hours. Longer periods may be required for some alkalies.[13,41] The poison control center is accessed and reference manuals consulted to determine the recommended irrigation time and additional treatments for the specific agent. If the eyes have been exposed to a chemical, they are irrigated continuously.[9] An ophthalmology consult may be ordered depending on the toxin and the degree of suspected ocular damage.

If the toxin was ingested, immediate home care may have consisted of the oral administration of water or milk—as advised by poison control. In the hospital the child is allowed nothing by mouth. The goal of therapy is to prevent vomiting, which could produce further damage to the esophagus or airway. The placement of a gastric lavage tube or nasogastric tube is therefore contraindicated.

Airway obstruction is the most immediate threat to life after the ingestion of a caustic substance and can result immediately following the ingestion or progress as tissue edema worsens. The child's airway and breathing status are therefore continuously monitored for signs of airway compromise. Additionally, the child is evaluated for the presence of abdominal pain, vomiting, drooling, or an altered mental status. An intravenous catheter is usually indicated, and blood work can be drawn simultaneously with the insertion of the catheter. Vital signs are taken frequently, and the child

is observed for signs of shock. Depending on the substance ingested and the suspected degree of damage, the nurse may anticipate the child going to surgery to have an endoscopic evaluation of the esophagus.

CIRCUMFERENTIAL BURNS

Etiology.   Circumferential burns are described as full-thickness burns that encircle an area of the body such as the chest, abdomen, or an extremity. Flame burns to clothing are a common cause of circumferential, full-thickness injuries, as are immersion burns to the lower extremities caused when the abused child is submerged in hot water.

Pathophysiology.   Full-thickness injuries result in complete destruction of the epidermis and dermis with a loss of skin elasticity. This loss of elasticity results in a "tourniquet effect" as rapidly forming edema compromises blood flow distal to a burned extremity or compromises chest wall movement with circumferential thoracic burns. Circumferential abdominal burns can also impair ventilatory efforts as pediatric patients require adequate abdominal movement to ventilate effectively. Therefore, any full-thickness injury that encircles an extremity, the chest, or the abdomen requires special treatment.[19]

Clinical presentation.   The child with a circumferential burn may initially show no signs of circulatory compromise. However with the progression of edema, signs and symptoms of compromise become evident. If the burn is to an extremity, signs of neurovascular compromise include numbness, tightness or pain, diminished or nonpalpable pulses, delayed capillary refill, and pallor. The child with circumferential burns to the chest wall or abdomen is observed for signs of respiratory compromise, including inadequate chest expansion, rapid shallow respirations, decreased oxygenation, and an altered mental status.

Emergency Department interventions.   Surgical interventions to relieve areas where blood flow or chest expansion is compromised include an escharotomy or fasciotomy.[19] An escharotomy is an incision through eschar (dead tissue) to the subcutaneous fat layer. It is usually a painless procedure, because it is performed through the full-thickness injury. A fasciotomy is a deeper incision into the muscle compartment or through the fascia covering of the muscle. These procedures are rarely required in the emergency room setting. Exceptions include a compromised respiratory status or absent blood flow to an extremity.

Nursing care and evaluation. As with all children, stabilization of the ABCs is the primary, initial focus of care. In the child with circumferential burns, specific nursing interventions include continuous monitoring of distal pulses and perfusion in the involved extremity or continuous monitoring of ventilatory status and chest expansion in the child with chest or abdominal burns.[36] If the burn involves an extremity, the extremity is slightly elevated to decrease the formation of dependent edema. As palpable pulses become faint, an ultrasonic Doppler may be used to detect adequate blood flow. A Doppler-detected radial pulse or dorsalis pedis pulse is indicative of adequate blood flow. Intravenous lines are not placed in injured extremities with circumferential involvement.

When an escharotomy is indicated, the ED nurse should gather the necessary supplies, including a sterile instrument set (e.g., knife handle, scalpel blades, hemostats), an electrocautery unit, Betadine, sterile 4 × 4 gauzes, sterile gauze dressings, Kerlex, silver sulfadiazine cream, and elastic bandages. Although the incision is made through damaged tissue where pain may not be felt, strong consideration should be given to the administration of an analgesic or a sedative before performing the procedure. During the procedure the extremity is palpated for the return of distal pulses, or the thorax is evaluated for improvement in chest expansion. The incision site is dressed with a Betadine-soaked gauze or a calcium alginate and covered with silver sulfadiazine and a dressing. The newer dressings, calcium alginates (e.g., Kaltostat) may also be used to line the escharotomy incision to prevent oozing or bleeding as circulation is restored to the injured area. After the procedure, routine postescharotomy care involves monitoring vital signs, including blood pressure, and observing for signs of significant blood loss. If an extremity is involved, pulses and perfusion are evaluated hourly. Should bleeding occur, an elastic bandage may be applied to the extremity.

▌SUMMARY

Nursing care for the burn-injured patient is specialized, multifaceted, and can be emotionally and physically taxing. This stress is enhanced when emergency personnel infrequently treat severely burned children. To decrease stress and improve knowledge of burn care management, medical professionals should attend educational programs that address burn care issues. Additionally, stress is reduced with the development of protocols for stabilization and transport by providing management guidelines that streamline resuscitative efforts.

REFERENCES

1. American Burn Association: Hospital and prehospital resources for optimal care of patients with burn injury: guidelines for development and operation of burn centers, *J Burn Care Rehabil* 11 (2):97-104, 1990.
2. Antoon A, Remensnyder JP: Burns in children. In Baswick JA, ed: *The art and science of burn care,* Rockville, Md, 1987, Aspen Publishers.
3. Battan FK: Emergencies and accidents. In Hay WW et al, ed: *Current pediatric diagnosis and treatment,* ed 12, Norwalk, Conn, 1995, Appleton and Lange.
4. Baxter CR: Fluid volume and electrolyte changes of the early post burn period, *Clin Plast Surg* 1:693-709, 1974.
5. Baker GL, Moni MM: Infant monitoring resulting in burns—tissue damage: literature and case report, *J Burn Care Rehabil* 14(1):113-119, 1993.
6. Bernardo LM, Sullivan K: Care of the pediatric patient with burns. In Trofino RB, ed: *Nursing care of the burn injured patient,* Philadelphia, 1991, FA Davis.
7. Brown PA et al: *Quick reference to pediatric intensive care nursing,* Rockville, Md, 1989, Aspen Publishers.
8. Carvajal HF, Griffith JA: Burn and inhalation injuries. In Fuhrman BP, Zimmerman JJ, eds: *Pediatric critical care,* St. Louis, 1992, Mosby.
9. Carvajal HF, Parks DH: *Burns in children: pediatric burn management,* Chicago, 1988, Year Book Medical Publisher.
10. Church JM: Facial injuries in children with multiple trauma. In Marcus RE, ed: *Trauma in children,* Rockville, Md, 1986, Aspen Publishers.
10a. Committee on Infectious Diseases, *1994 Red Book,* Elk Grove, Ill, 1994, American Academy of Pediatrics.
11. Demling RH: Fluid resuscitation. In Boswick JA Jr, ed: *The art and science of burn care,* Rockville, Md, 1987, Aspen Publishers.
12. Desai MH, Herndon DN: Burns. In Trunkey DD, Lewis FR, eds: *Current therapy of trauma,* ed 3, St Louis, 1991, BC Decker.
13. D'Italia JG: Burns. In Joy C, ed: *Pediatric trauma nursing,* Rockville, Md, 1989, Aspen Publishers.
14. Finkelstein JL et al: Pediatric burns: an overview, *Pediatr Clin North Am* 39(5):1145-1163, 1992.
15. Foster JE, Ford EG: Burn injury. In Ford EG, Andrassy RJ, eds: *Pediatric trauma: initial assessment and management,* Philadelphia, 1994, WB Saunders.

6. Guzzetta PC, Holihan JA: Burns. In Eichelberger MR, Pratsch GL, eds: *Pediatric trauma care*, Rockville, Md, 1988, Aspen Publishers.

7. Hall ML, Sills RM: Electrical and lightning injuries. In Barkin RM, ed: *Pediatric energy medicine concepts and clinical practice*, St Louis, 1992, Mosby.

8. Heink NR: Fluid resuscitation and the role of exchange transfusion in pediatric burn shock, *Crit Care Nurs* 12(7):50-56, 1992.

9. Helvig B: Trauma to the integument: burns. In Howell E, Widra L, Hill MG: *Comprehensive trauma nursing: theory and practice*, Glenview, Ill, 1988, Scott, Foresman, and Company.

20. Herndon DN, Rutan RL, Rutan TC: Management of the pediatric patient with burns, *J Burn Care Rehabil* 14(1):3-7, 1993.

21. Herndon DN et al: Management of burn injuries. In Eichelberger MR, ed: *Pediatric trauma: prevention, acute care, rehabilitation*, St Louis, 1993, Mosby.

22. The National Committee for Injury Prevention and Control: *Injury prevention: meeting the challenge*. Oxford, 1989, Oxford University Press.

23. Joffe MD: Burns. In Fleisher G, Ludwig S, eds: *Textbook of pediatric emergency medicine*, ed 3, Baltimore, Md, 1993, Williams & Wilkins.

24. Knezevich BA: *Trauma nursing: principles and practice*, Norwalk, Conn, 1986, Appleton-Century-Crofts.

25. Kravitz M: Thermal injuries. In Cardona VD et al: *Trauma nursing: from resuscitation through rehabilitation*, Philadelphia, 1988, WB Saunders.

26. Lanros NE: *Assessment and intervention in emergency nursing*, ed 3, Norwalk, Conn, 1988, Appleton & Lange.

27. Lazear SE: Tissue integrity burns. In Neff JA, Kidd PS, eds: *Trauma nursing: the art and science*, St Louis, 1993, Mosby.

28. Luterman A, Curreri PW: Emergency protocol for the severely burned patient, *Hosp Med* October:131-146, 1984.

29. Luterman A, Talley MA: Field management of burn injuries, *Emerg Med Serv* 17(7):30, 1988.

30. Marvin JA: Burns and thermal injuries. In Sheehy SB, ed: *Emergency nursing principles and practice*, St Louis, 1992, Mosby.

30a. McManus B: Caustics. In Strange GR et al, eds: *Pediatric emergency medicine: a comprehensive study guide*, New York, 1996, McGraw-Hill.

31. Mott SR, James SR, Sperhac AM: *Nursing care of children and families*, ed 2, Redwood City, Calif, 1990, Benjamin-Cummings Publishing.

32. National Center for Health Statistics: *Hospital discharge abstract data survey*, 1989.

33. National Center for Health Statistics: *National health interview survey, 1990; stats Canada*, 1989.

34. National Center for Health Statistics: *US Bureau of the census file RESPO793*, 1995.

35. National Fire Protection Association: *Fire incident reporting system data*, 1990.

36. Parks DH: Timing of burn therapy in the pediatric patient, *Clin Plast Surg* 17(1):65-70, 1990.

37. *Resources for optimal care of the injured patient. Committee on Trauma: American College of Surgeons*, 1993, Library of Congress Cataloging-in-Publication Data.

38. Rowe MI, Arago A: Fluid in shock resuscitation, *Pediatr Clin North Am* 22(2):269-273, 1975.

38a. Rowe MI et al: *Essentials of pediatric surgery*, St Louis, 1995, Mosby.

39. Sadowski DA: Care of the child with burns. In Hazinski MF, ed: *Nursing care of the critically ill child*, ed 3, St Louis, 1992, Mosby.

40. Sheehy SB, Marvin JA, Jimmerson CL: *Manual of clinical trauma care: the first hour*, St Louis, 1989, Mosby.

41. Thelan LA et al: *Critical care nursing: diagnosis and management*, St Louis, 1994, Mosby.

41a. Turnbull T: Carbon monoxide. In Strange GR et al: *Pediatric emergency medicine: a comprehensive study guide*, New York, 1996, McGraw-Hill.

42. Walton RL, Matory WE: Wound care. In Saunders CE, Ho MI, eds: *Current emergency diagnosis and treatment*, ed 4, Norwalk, Conn, 1992, Appleton & Lange.

42a. Wasserman GS: Caustics. In Barkin RM, ed: *Pediatric emergency care: concepts and clinical practice*, St Louis, 1992, Mosby.

43. Woolley S, Drueck C: Burn injuries. In Kitt S, Kaiser J, eds: *Emergency nursing: a physiologic and clinical perspective*, Philadelphia, 1990, WB Saunders.

CHAPTER 25

Child Maltreatment

Sandra L. Elvik

INTRODUCTION

The issue of child abuse invokes many different feelings and emotions. There may be painful memories of abuse suffered in childhood. Anger is common, making it difficult to be therapeutic with a family. Some deny that an adult could abuse or molest an innocent child. Child abuse, however, is a reality of our society. In 1990, more than 1.5 million children and adolescents were victims of abuse or neglect.[5] Maltreatment occurred primarily at the hands of parents or other caregivers.

Many children die from abuse and neglect. Between 1979 and 1988, McClain et al. found that 90% of fatal abuse occurred in children less than 5 years of age; 40% of these children were infants.[24] In the United States, three children die from maltreatment every day.[25]

There has been a dramatic increase in reported cases of child abuse. A survey conducted throughout the United States in 1992 by the National Center on the Prevention of Child Abuse (NCPCA) found that approximately 3 million children were reported to Child Protective Service (CPS) agencies for alleged child abuse and neglect. This represented a 6% increase in reports from the previous year.[25] Between 1985 and 1992, the NCPCA survey identified a 50% increase in the number of cases reported to CPS agencies.

Whether the actual incidence of child abuse is rising is unclear. Reporting of child abuse may have risen due to improved public awareness and the passage of mandatory reporting laws for professionals who work with children. On the other hand, the incidence of child maltreatment may actually have increased as a result of many societal problems. Social problems identified by CPS agencies include substance abuse (especially alcohol); financial stress, due to unemployment and the struggling economy; family/domestic violence; lack of knowledge in the area of normal child growth and development; lack of parenting skills and lack of the use of appropriate discipline; and lack of social support.[25]

In many cases of maltreatment, the child is brought to the nearest emergency department (ED) by prehospital care providers or law enforcement agents who may report suspicions of abuse or neglect. Parents also bring their child to the ED with chief complaints of injuries that are suspicious of abuse or neglect. Suspicions of maltreatment may also arise during ED visits for problems not related to child maltreatment. Nurses must be alert for signs and symptoms of abuse in *all* children. Education concerning the historical and clinical indicators of abuse and appropriate interventions assists nurses in identifying potential maltreatment, providing appropriate resources for children and families, and complying with legal mandates.

DEFINITIONS

States vary in the legal definitions of child abuse and neglect. The terms *child abuse* and *child maltreatment* are often used interchangeably to describe physical, emotional, or sexual abuse or neglect. ED nurses must be aware of the legal definitions of child abuse terminology in their particular state (Box 25-1).

PHYSICAL ABUSE

Physical abuse is an act of physical injury or trauma that is inflicted by nonaccidental means. Although described historically, it was not until the 1960s that Kempe coined the phrase *the battered child syndrome* to describe the various manifestations of physical abuse.[19] Injury occurs either through *commission*, referring to a deliberate act, or *omission*, which implies negligence or failure to protect.[12] The most common types of physical abuse are bruises, burns, fractures, and head and eye trauma.

NEGLECT

Neglect entails a caregiver who is unable or unwilling to provide the most basic needs for the child. The definition of *basic needs* may differ geographically and personally but includes such things as shelter, food, clothing, medical care/immunizations, education, and emotional nurturing. Some states legally define this as *general neglect,* as opposed to *severe neglect.* In severe neglect, a caregiver willfully places the child in imminent danger of impairment. Factors contributing to neglect include poverty or illness in the family.[15] Maternal factors that are associated with neglect include lower scores on parenting skill scales, having several children under the age of 6 years in the home, and having dropped out of school before reaching the twelfth grade.[4]

SEXUAL ABUSE

Sexual abuse entails the involvement of children, adolescents, or developmentally immature adults in some kind of sexual activity that they do not fully understand. This includes fondling, inappropriate kissing on the mouth, oral-genital or oral-anal contact, exposure of the adult's genitalia to the child, penetration of the vagina or anus, and sexual exploitation, such as the involvement of the child in pornographic activities. The perpetrator of the abuse is known to the child in about 80% of cases. There is usually some form of coercion involved, such as threat of harm to the child or a loved one.[7,20] *Incest* is sexual activity between relatives, such as a daughter and a father. *Acute sexual assault* generally implies sexual contact within the past 48 to 96 hours. The victim must be assessed quickly to collect possible forensic specimens such as semen. *Chronic sexual abuse* occurs over days to years.

EMOTIONAL ABUSE

Emotional abuse is the most difficult type of abuse to prove. There are usually no injuries or severe changes in the child's physical condition. Included are unusual or bizarre forms of punishment, such as locking a child in a closet. Aggressive or belittling remarks are often made to the child. Emotional abuse results in a markedly low self-esteem, which may persist into adulthood.

Box 25-1   Definitions of Forms of Child Maltreatment*

Physical abuse
An act of physical injury or trauma that is inflicted by nonaccidental means

Neglect
Caregiver is unable or unwilling to provide the most basic needs for the child

Sexual abuse
The involvement of children, adolescents, or developmentally immature adults in sexual activity that they do not understand

Emotional abuse
Involves abnormal behaviors such as bizarre forms of punishment or aggressive or belittling remarks to the child; it is the most difficult form of abuse to prove

*The specific definitions of abuse vary from state to state. ED nurses should be aware of the child abuse laws and the definitions of maltreatment within their states.

CHARACTERISTICS/RISK FACTORS

ABUSIVE ADULTS

There is no model available to predict a child abuser. Adult perpetrators of maltreatment come from all racial, religious, educational, and socioeconomic backgrounds. However, frequently observed characteristics have been described and are listed in Table 25-1. ED nurses should be aware of these factors when assessing the child and family.

Child abuse has been thought to be intergenerational, implying that the abused child is destined to become an abusive parent. After a review of the available data on abusive parents, Kaufman and Zigler concluded that maltreatment of a child does increase the risk of perpetuating an abusive cycle but does not lead children down an inevitable pathway of abusing their own children.[18]

Abusive adults frequently have difficulty controlling aggressive impulses. They strike out at their child to relieve their own frustration and anxiety. Low

TABLE 25-1	Factors Associated With Child Maltreatment	
PARENTAL	**CHILD**	
Family stress, such as loss of a job, death of a partner, financial problems, marital discord, life changes	Prematurity	
Young/inexperienced parents with limited resources	Congenital anomalies, especially visible ones such as cleft lip or spina bifida	
History as a child of abuse/neglect	Developmental delays	
Substance abuse	Temperament—child is perceived as "different" or "difficult" (e.g., hyperactive, fussy, difficult to feed)	
Poor parenting models while growing up		
Social isolation from family/friends		
Unrealistic expectation of child's capabilities		
Domestic violence, either as victims or witnesses to violence		

self-esteem is common, as is inadequate knowledge of child rearing. It is common to regard the adult who mistreats a child as a "bad" parent or person. In fact, the parent may actually love the child but may be severely affected by stressors and limited personal and social resources. By virtue of seeking medical attention for the child in the case of abuse, the caregiver may actually be giving a cry for help. With intervention by various agencies, including child protective services, many parents can learn how to cope with stress and can develop effective parenting techniques.

ABUSED CHILDREN

Although there are no absolute predictors that indicate which children will be abused, there are characteristics that increase the likelihood of maltreatment. Abusive caregivers often describe the child as "different" from other children. The differences may be actual, such as congenital anomalies, or perceived, such as certain behavioral characteristics. Premature babies often have physical, developmental, or temperamental abnormalities. Additionally, the protracted hospital course may affect the early bonding between parent and child. Obvious congenital abnormalities, such as cleft lip, may create feelings of disgust for the child. Individual personality traits may also increase the risk of maltreatment. Children who are "hyperactive" or who refuse to follow directions can be frustrating for the parent, as can infants who are difficult to feed or excessively fussy. Parents may feel ill equipped to deal with particular temperaments or behaviors. All of these factors increase the stress on families, thus increasing the potential for abuse.

Box 25-2   Suspicious Historical Information

Major details of the incident change (e.g., time of day, location)
Historian changes story
Different historians/different history
Injury inconsistent with growth and development
History inconsistent with injury
Delay in seeking care
Long distance in traveling for care

NURSING HISTORY

The role of the nurse in a case of child abuse cannot be underestimated. Based on the initial assessment, the ED nurse identifies situations that warrant further investigation. Although certain factors raise suspicions (Box 25-2), it should be emphasized that one indicator is not diagnostic. It is a pattern or combination of historical, psychosocial, and physical indicators that corroborates the diagnosis of child maltreatment.

As other professionals such as physicians and social workers interview the family, glaring differences in the story given to various personnel are highly suspicious. Additionally, several versions of the proposed mechanism of injury may be given, or the story may change with different historians. For this reason it is best to separately interview all of the adults present.

INTERVIEWING THE CHILD

Depending on age and developmental capacity, the child can disclose how he or she was injured. Children as young as 2 years of age may be communicative enough to be interviewed. However, if the child is incapable of answering questions, the exchange is terminated. It is best if the child is questioned apart from the caregiver. Open-ended questions, rather than leading ones, are used. It is not appropriate to say, "Your parents hit you, didn't they?" It is appropriate, though, to voice concern over the injury and then ask how something like that could have happened.

Some children will not disclose physical or sexual abuse in order to protect their parent or to avoid retaliation by the abuser. Children frequently defend or protect their parent because they fear loss of their only source of love and security, little though it may be. Their fear of an unknown situation is frequently greater than that of their present situation. Silence may be maintained for years because the perpetrator threatens to severely punish or kill the child or someone to whom the child is emotionally attached. Positive incentives are also used to keep abuse secret. Sexually abused children often describe the special treats and money that they were given to keep the details of their molestation hidden. Some children refuse to disclose sexual contact because they have experienced pleasurable feelings during the molestation. Although they may not completely understand the significance of the molestation, some children enjoy the extra attention and closeness received.

PARENTAL/CAREGIVER HISTORY

Frequently, the history provided by the parent/caregiver is incompatible with the injury. Children are naturally curious and may injure themselves in unusual ways. Burns, fractures, and other forms of trauma can occur accidentally as children explore their environment or try to master new activities, such as riding a bike. However, each injury must be evaluated in light of the history to ascertain if the two are compatible. Often the injuries are much more severe than the historical information suggests, or the pattern or type of injury is not consistent with the identified mechanism.

With a nonaccidental injury, the parent/caregiver may attribute the injury to a child who is developmentally incapable of having been in a particular situation. For example, a 6-month-old baby with multiple bruises is said to "fall a lot." Even "early walkers" do not walk or climb at 6 months of age. Such a history

would be suspicious and therefore warrant further investigation.

Another concerning factor is a delay in parents seeking care for their child. Some caregivers fear that the health care system will report them to social service agencies or take away their child if they come to the hospital with an injured child. In reality, it is more likely that the family will be reported for failing to have the injury treated in a timely manner. This is especially true if such a delay results in severe morbidity or death.

The nurse should also be dubious of a family who has come a great distance from home to obtain treatment for their child's injuries. A family who is afraid of being reported to the authorities may travel to a hospital where there is no knowledge of their history or primary health care provider. Suspicion is also raised when a family seeks health care for their child at several different health care facilities. It is therefore advantageous for hospitals, and especially EDs, to have some means of communicating with each other. Computerized systems have been used in some states to access information on high-risk families. To maintain confidentiality, only selected personnel have access to the information.

PSYCHOSOCIAL ASSESSMENT

The psychosocial assessment is performed by a combination of health care providers, including nurses, physicians, and/or social workers. It includes both historical information and observation of child and caregiver behavior. All of the persons in the household and any other caregivers (e.g., babysitters, grandparents) must be clearly identified. Family stressors should be explored, as well as various cultural practices (such as cupping or coin rubbing) that may explain suspicious physical findings.

CHILD BEHAVIOR

Children respond to maltreatment in a variety of ways. Behaviors that are suggestive of abuse or neglect are described in Box 25-3. Although individual indicators are not diagnostic, their presence should raise suspicion of abuse. Patterns or combinations of these child behaviors warrant further investigation.

CAREGIVER BEHAVIOR

Caregivers also exhibit various behavioral responses to actual or alleged maltreatment of their child. Caregivers may show little concern for their child and

Box 25-3   Clinical Manifestations of Potential Child Maltreatment

Physical neglect

Suggestive physical findings
Failure to thrive

Signs of malnutrition, such as thin extremities, abdominal distention, lack of subcutaneous fat

Poor personal hygiene, especially of teeth

Unclean and/or inappropriate dress

Evidence of poor health care, such as nonimmunized status, untreated infections, frequent colds

Frequent injuries from lack of supervision

Suggestive behaviors
Dull and inactive; excessively passive or sleepy

Self-stimulatory behaviors, such as finger-sucking or rocking

Begging or stealing food

Absenteeism from school

Drug or alcohol addiction

Vandalism or shoplifting

} in older child

Emotional abuse and neglect

Suggestive physical findings
Failure to thrive

Feeding disorders, such as rumination

Enuresis

Sleep disorders

Suggestive behaviors
Self-stimulatory behaviors, such as biting, rocking, sucking

During infancy, lack of social smile and stranger anxiety

Withdrawal

Unusual fearfulness

Antisocial behavior, such as destructiveness, stealing, cruelty

Extremes of behavior, such as overcompliant and passive or aggressive and demanding

Lags in emotional and intellectual development, especially language

Suicide attempts

Physical abuse

Suggestive physical findings
Bruises and welts

On face, lips, mouth, back, buttocks, thighs, or areas of torso

Regular patterns descriptive of object used, such as belt buckle, hand, wire hanger,

Physical abuse—Cont'd
chain, wooden spoon, squeeze or pinch marks

May be present in various stages of healing

Burns

On soles of feet, palms of hands, back, or buttocks

Patterns descriptive of object used, such as round cigar or cigarette burns, "glovelike" sharply demarcated areas from immersion in scalding water, rope burns on wrists or ankles from being bound, burns in the shape of an iron, radiator, or electric stove burner

Absence of "splash" marks and presence of symmetric burns

Stun gun injury—lesions circular, fairly uniform (up to 0.5 cm), and paired about 5 cm apart.[11a]

Fractures and dislocations

Skull, nose, or facial structures

Injury may denote type of abuse, such as spiral fracture or dislocation from twisting of an extremity or whiplash from shaking the child

Multiple new or old fractures in various stages of healing

Lacerations and abrasions

On backs of arms, legs, torso, face, or external genitalia

Unusual symptoms, such as abdominal swelling, pain, and vomiting from punching

Descriptive marks such as from human bites or pulling the hair out

Chemical

Unexplained repeated poisoning, especially drug overdose

Unexplained sudden illness, such as hypoglycemia from insulin administration

Suggestive behaviors
Wary of physical contact with adults

Apparent fear of parents or going home

Lying very still while surveying environment

Inappropriate reaction to injury, such as failure to cry from pain

Lack of reaction to frightening events

Apprehensive when hearing other children cry

Indiscriminate friendliness and displays of affection

Superficial relationships

Box 25-3   Clinical Manifestations of Potential Child Maltreatment—cont'd

Acting-out behavior, such as aggression, to seek attention

Withdrawal behavior

Sexual abuse

Suggestive physical findings

Bruises, bleeding, lacerations or irritation of external genitalia, anus, mouth, or throat

Torn, stained, or bloody underclothing

Pain on urination or pain, swelling, and itching of genital area

Penile discharge

Sexually transmitted disease, nonspecific vaginitis, or venereal warts (prepubertal children)

Difficulty in walking or sitting

Unusual odor in the genital area

Recurrent urinary tract infections

Presence of sperm

Pregnancy in young adolescent

Suggestive behaviors

Sudden emergence of sexually related problems, including excessive or public masturbation, age-inappropriate sexual play, promiscuity, or overtly seductive behavior

Sexual abuse—Cont'd

Withdrawn, excessive daydreaming

Preoccupied with fantasies, especially in play

Poor relationships with peers

Sudden changes, such as anxiety, loss or gain of weight, clinging behavior

In incestuous relationships, excessive anger at mother for not protecting daughter

Regressive behavior, such as bed-wetting or thumb-sucking

Sudden onset of phobias or fears, particularly fears of the dark, men, strangers, or particular settings or situations (e.g., undue fear of leaving the house or staying at the daycare center or the baby-sitter's house)

Running away from home

Substance abuse, particularly of alcohol or mood-elevating drugs

Profound and rapid personality changes, especially extreme depression, hostility, and aggression (often accompanied by social withdrawal)

Rapidly declining school performance

Suicidal attempts or ideation

From Wong DL: *Whaley & Wong's-essentials of pediatric nursing,* ed 5, St Louis, 1997, Mosby.

---

be more preoccupied with their own needs. Basic comfort measures for their child, for example, during procedures, are frequently absent. Criticism or anger with the child for causing or provoking the events resulting in the injury may be expressed. Caregivers may deny that they or their partner had any part in causing the child's injury. Anger is commonly directed at the police, CPS workers, or ED staff. Hostility may escalate to the point of physical confrontation. Grief reactions may be exhibited when the caregiver is confronted with severe disability or death of their child secondary to the injuries sustained. Parental guilt for not protecting child may be intense.

▎PHYSICAL ASSESSMENT

Assessment of the child for physical findings suggestive of abuse includes a complete, head-to-toe evaluation. The general appearance of the child, including nutri-

tional status, mental status, cleanliness, and appropriateness of clothing, is observed. To avoid missing important information, such as subtle bruising, the child must be completely undressed, although this can be performed in stages to help the child feel more at ease. An ideal time for the nurse to begin this process is while obtaining the vital signs and child's weight.

Every part of the child's body is assessed. Evaluation of the mouth includes inspection of teeth and gums for overall health and all mouth surfaces for bruising or bleeding or tearing of the frenulum, regardless of the age of the child. The scalp is examined and palpated for the presence of masses, tenderness, or areas of alopecia. Areas that can hide inflicted trauma, such as behind the ears and infants' fleshy necks, must be inspected.

The infant's genital and anal areas can be easily assessed while taking a rectal temperature. The infant is positioned for comfort, with the supine position being more acceptable than the prone position. If any rectal trauma such as redness, bruises, or bleeding is present, the temperature should be measured with a different method, such as an axillary or tympanic thermometer. In most EDs the nurse does not perform the in-depth assessment of the anogenital area in the child. However, once the nurse identifies the particular words used by the child for the genital and anal areas, it is appropriate to ask the child if he or she has any urogenital complaints.

SIGNIFICANT CLINICAL FINDINGS

BRUISES

Bruises are the most common type of inflicted injuries. However, it is not unusual for a child to sustain accidental cutaneous injuries. A classic example is the toddler who frequently falls as he or she becomes more mobile. Several characteristics help differentiate non-accidental wounds from the "normal" bruises of childhood. Unintentional bruises are primarily over the bony prominences, such as the forehead, elbows, knees, and shins. The injuries are generally in one plane of the body and are of uniform color and shape. Unusual places for accidental bruising are the face and cheeks, behind the ears, abdomen, lower back and buttocks (Fig. 25-1), upper and inner thighs, and the genital area.

Depending on the force of the blow to the skin and the resulting capillary rupture, the wound can take on the impression of the object used. Some children have several different configurations of bruises from the same abusive episode (Fig. 25-2). Oval marks on the chest and abdomen resulting from grabbing with the fingertips may be overlooked dur-

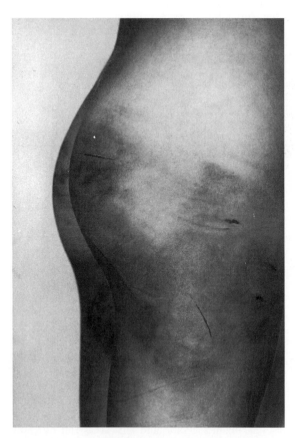

FIG. 25-1. Seven-year-old male hit with a wooden paddle on the buttocks. Abraded areas are from the skin being torn by a rough edge in the paddle.

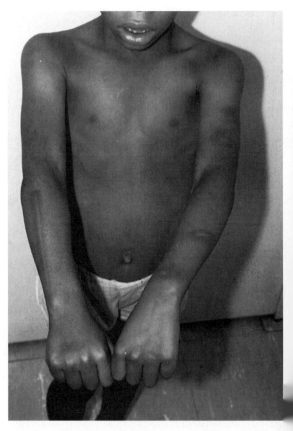

FIG. 25-2. Nine-year-old male who described being hit with a belt. Note linear bruise on right arm. Circular lesions on left arm are possible from the belt buckle.

ing the evaluation.[29] Linear bruises are caused by rulers, tree branches (a "switch"), or belts and generally follow curved body surfaces. Wounds that have a looped configuration suggest the use of cords, belts, or wire coat hangers that have been coiled in half (Fig. 25-3). Such lesions are diagnostic of nonaccidental trauma.

Multiple bruises in different stages of healing are also suspicious. In this instance, more than one episode of inflicted trauma is likely. Bruises undergo characteristic changes during the healing process (Table 25-2).

BITE MARKS

Bite marks are regularly found in physically or sexually abused children and are considered deliberate until proven otherwise. Bite marks can appear alone or with a suck mark ("hickey") (Fig. 25-4). Accidental bites can be caused by toddlers who bite other children or by animals such as dogs, cats, and rodents. Differentiating features exist between adult and animal or children's teeth. Animals tend to have smaller teeth, smaller dental arches, and more penetrating edges.[2] In humans, if the measurement between the canine teeth in the maxillary arch is 3 cm or more, the bite was caused by an adult.[29] Dental consultation is often recommended for these measurements. With the help of plaster impressions of the teeth of the suspicious parties, carbon paper, and a great deal of skill, forensic dental experts can identify the exact person who bit the child.

BURNS

Children may burn themselves accidentally. Portable floor heaters and irons are notorious for burning an inquisitive toddler. Hot liquids on the stove may be pulled onto a child who is learning to climb and reaching for objects. Pulling hot liquids off a stove or table results in a splash burn. The initial point of contact is usually the head and shoulders, followed by a cascade effect downward toward the arms, chest, abdomen, and legs.

Many burns result from neglect or abuse. With intentionally inflicted burns, the injury and the history provided by the caregiver often do not match. A common history given by the caregiver is that the child, while briefly left alone, turned on the hot water faucet in the sink or bathtub. Knowing the most common intentional burn patterns assists in determining if the burn resulted from abuse. Inflicted burns include glove and stocking burns, immersion scalds, and cigarette burns. Holding a child's hands or feet under scalding liquid causes a glove or stocking pattern. These intentional burns have a symmetrical pattern with definite lines of demarcation and an absent splash effect. Immersion burns to the buttocks and the back of the thighs has been used as punishment

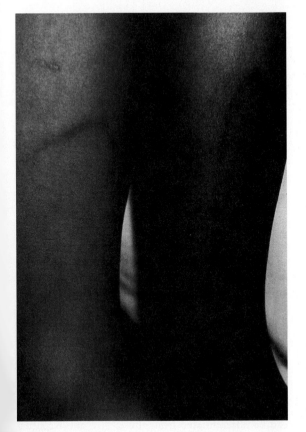

FIG. 25-3. Five-year-old male with loop marks caused by an extension cord.

TABLE 25-2	Approximate Color Changes of Bruises
COLOR	APPROXIMATE AGE
Swollen, some tenderness progressing to red	Hours to 1 day
Blue-purple	1-5 days
Green	5-7 days
Brown	7-10 days
Yellow	10-14 days
Clear	Within 1 month

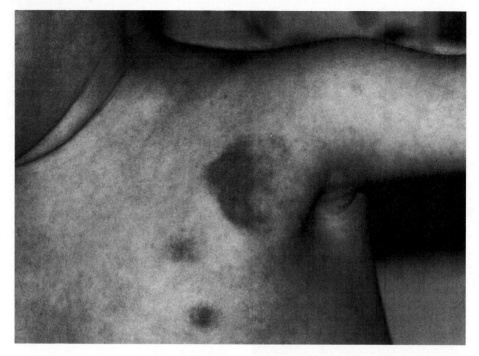

FIG. 25-4. Fifteen-month-old female with pinch and suck mark close to right axilla.

for the child who, in the process of toilet training, soils his or her pants at an inappropriate time for the parent. During forcible immersion in the hot liquid, skin areas that are in close contact with the surface of the sink, bathtub, or other skin (e.g., skin folds, creases) are typically spared. Classically, there is a doughnut-shaped burn on the buttocks, with sparing of the central buttocks and the inner gluteal fold area. Intentional cigarette burns are well-demarcated, deep, circular burns. Numerous cigarette burns may be present.

Full-thickness burns in adults develop in 6 seconds when water is 140° F (60° C), 2 seconds when water is 150° F (66° C), and 10 minutes when water is 120° F (49° C). Because of their thinner skin, children burn even more quickly. Keeping hot water heaters set at lower temperatures may prevent many burns in the home, including intentional immersions.

FRACTURES

Bone injuries in children are consistent with significant trauma. Although fractures can occur accidentally, the nurse should be suspicious of any fracture in young children, especially infants. Underlying bone diseases such as osteogenesis imperfecta, may rarely contribut to bone injuries.

Delay in seeking care for fractures may sugges abuse or neglect but is not diagnostic. Signs c fractures are sometimes subtle in the child, especiall when the causative incident was not witnessed. De creased use of the injured extremity, an unexplaine increase in crying or "whimpering," resistance t clothing or diaper changes, or a decrease in appetite o sleep may be the only symptoms. If obvious signs of fracture, such as marked swelling, bruising, or defor mity, are present in a child who was injured more tha a couple of days previously, abuse or neglect should b suspected.

Rib fractures are uncommon, especially in infants The pliable bones in young children are able t withstand a great amount of pressure. Rib fractures, present, are therefore highly suggestive of child abus in children less than 5 years of age.[17] In seriou injuries, caregivers may report that "vigorous cardio pulmonary resuscitation" (CPR) caused the rib frac tures. However, fractures from resuscitative effort can be differentiated from abuse.[10] In abusive situa tions, multiple rib fractures in various stages of healin are usually present. Intentionally inflicted rib injuries involve fractures of the posterior rib neck rather than the lateral fractures seen with CPR. Associated signs of abuse, such as unexplained bruising, are evident.

Fractures associated with abuse are usually transverse, oblique, or spiral. Twisting of an extremity results in a spiral fracture. Spiral fractures, resulting from a twisting of an extremity, are usually associated with abuse. However, accidental spiral fractures can occur. For example, a toddler who falls from a chair with a foot caught in the rungs could sustain enough twisting force to create a spiral fracture. The reported mechanism of injury must be considered carefully in relation to the injury. Transverse and oblique fractures are completely through the bone but lack the rotation of the spiral fracture.

Differentiating characteristics of inflicted long bone trauma include the following: (1) the caregiver's inability to remember an episode of falling, or a more minor episode was recalled in cases of serious injuries; (2) the presence of radius/ulna, tibia/fibula, or femur fractures in children less than 1 year of age; and (3) metaphyseal or midshaft fractures of the humerus.[21] The forces required to produce metaphyseal or epiphyseal fractures rarely occur accidentally.[17]

HEAD INJURY

Head injury is the most common manifestation of nonaccidental trauma in infants less than 1 year of age.[3] Falls are a commonly reported mechanism of injury given by the caregivers. If serious damage is present in a fall reported to be 10 feet or less, abuse should be suspected.[3,16,30] Obvious scalp hematomas may be associated with underlying trauma. Other suspicious head injuries include bilateral skull fractures in children or any skull fracture in infants, cerebral edema and retinal hemorrhages, subdural hematomas, subarachnoid bleeds, and traction alopecia and scalp swelling related to hair pulling. Unfortunately, head injuries are often missed and may not be fully appreciated until autopsy.

EMERGENCY DEPARTMENT INTERVENTIONS

After obtaining a complete history and physical exam, various laboratory tests or radiographic studies may be performed to assist in substantiating child maltreatment. Coagulation studies rule out blood dyscrasias, such as hemophilia or leukemia, as possible etiologies for multiple bruises, despite any contradicting history of organic disorders. Minimum hematologic studies include a complete blood count (CBC), platelet count, prothrombin time (PT), and partial thromboplastin time (PTT).

Radiographic studies such as simple x-rays, computerized axial tomography (CAT scan), magnetic resonance imaging (MRI), ultrasonography, or bone scans may be ordered depending on the type and severity of the injury. Total body radiographic studies ("skeletal survey" or "trauma series") are indicated in children less than 2 years of age with clinical evidence of physical abuse or in infants less than 1 year of age with evidence of significant neglect.[13] This survey focuses primarily on the long bones. Fractures in various stages of healing are consistent with abuse.

A child who has been sexually assaulted deserves special attention to minimize potential long-term physical side effects and to document findings. Cultures of the vagina or urethra, throat, and rectum for *Neisseria gonorrhoeae* and *Chlamydia trachomatis* and serologic tests for syphilis are frequently indicated. Testing for exposure to the human immunodeficiency virus (HIV) may also be performed, with strict compliance with legal and confidentiality requirements.

Medical interventions for child maltreatment include the assessment and stabilization of the child, the identification of maltreatment, and treatment of specific injuries. Social workers are usually involved to assess the home environment and family functioning. Team discussions of the potential for abuse in each individual situation are highly beneficial.

NURSING CARE AND EVALUATION

Nursing care of the maltreated child includes the management of the particular injuries, identification of abuse or neglect, protection of the child from further abuse, support of the child and family, and coordination of the various health care providers and agencies that are involved.

COMMUNICATION WITH FAMILIES

Several approaches can be used when communicating with the family of an abused or neglected child. *Active listening* is a technique in which listeners attune themselves to the speaker, without forming answers and opinions. The speaker is free to discuss personal issues, impressions, or problems. Active listeners non-verbally indicate that they hear what is being said, such as by leaning forward or head nodding.

Open-ended questions can be used to help draw a parent into a conversation by requiring more than a *yes* or *no* response. Parents may begin to provide information that helps the nurse to understand the family's needs. This information can then be shared with the health care team.

By conveying a *caring attitude,* the nurse relays to parents an understanding of the stressors in their life. Nurses can then focus interest on the health and safety of the child, which often allows the parent to relax. Hostile parents may begin to calm down.

Finally, *honest communication* is vital in dealing with abusive families. Parents should be informed about the suspicions surrounding the child's injury, concerns for the child's safety, and notification of law enforcement or social service agencies. Explaining the procedures involved in a child abuse investigation will help to allay some of the fear. Again, placing the emphasis on the well-being of the child can avoid a hostile or aggressive demeanor on the part of the caregiver. The nurse may offer to sit with the family or child during the police and social services interviews and can act as an advocate for the family.

FAMILY SUPPORT

Strong negative feelings toward the family can make the tasks of offering support and understanding to the parents very difficult. However, families should be encouraged to discuss the myriad of feelings generated by the maltreatment of their child, including anger, grief, or guilt. Genuine concern may help to motivate the family to change. In contrast, accusation and punishment will alienate the family from the health care system and potentially place the child in more danger. In addition, wrongfully accusing a caregiver of abuse will further alienate the family. It may be very difficult to determine the actual perpetrator of abuse in the busy ED environment.

PREVENTION OF FURTHER ABUSE

Nurses are mandated to report suspicions of child abuse to child protective agencies according to the laws of their state. Emergent removal of the child from the home is initiated when there is imminent danger to the child. Foster placement or admission to the hospital may be immediately arranged. If the child is admitted for medical reasons, a protective referral is still made from the ED to ensure adequate investiga-

tion of the case. If discharge is deemed safe both medically and socially, a child protective services caseworker is obligated to investigate the report within a specified time frame. Various recommendations can result from an investigation. The case may be unsubstantiated and closed, or it may be kept active. Recommendations for removal of the child from the home or assistance with the resolution of various social or medical problems depends on the outcome of the investigation.

Because stress plays a large role in child maltreatment, measures to relieve stress are supportive of the family and may prevent further abuse. Many parents have little knowledge of effective parenting techniques and frequently cannot cope with the frustrations of raising a child. Discipline commonly takes the form of physical punishment, which may be severe. Harsh discipline may even be exhibited in the ED. Role-modeling of acceptable child care and disciplinary techniques has a more positive effect than lecturing, which often alienates families who already have low self-esteem. Any positive behavior on the part of the caregiver should be praised. Referral of the family to various resources, whether for food, housing, transportation, parenting classes, daycare, or psychiatric care, can support the family and protect the child. Social workers are particularly helpful in identifying psychosocial stressors and facilitating referrals to local agencies.

Effective parent teaching involves not only patience and compassion but also knowledge of resources. Nurses must be familiar with local social service agencies, child abuse hotlines, and rape crisis centers in their area. There are also national resources for both parents and children. These agencies provide support and education in child abuse related issues. Some organizations make publications available for a small fee. The ED nurse may want to make these brochures available in the waiting area. Hospital staff may also find this information valuable.

DOCUMENTATION AND EVIDENCE COLLECTION

In the case of child abuse, appropriate documentation is critical. Findings from the interview and physical assessment must be accurately recorded, because court hearings may occur months to years from the time that the child was evaluated in the ED. Notes written in the chart are often the only means of recollecting the events that transpired.

Historical information must be detailed. Changes

in the history between various persons involved or over time should be recorded. Spontaneous statements made by caregivers or children are documented in quotations. Examples include, "My husband cannot control himself when he is drunk," or "My mom hit me in the face with her shoe."

All lesions or other abnormalities found during the physical exam are recorded, including the size of wounds, both in vertical and horizontal diameters; the shape of the lesion; the color or colors observed; and the exact location on the body where the abnormalities are seen. The face of a clock can be used to describe the location of unusual findings, especially in anogenital examinations; for example, "bruise of the hymen at 4 o'clock."

Many states have standardized reporting forms that are completed in cases of suspected child abuse. These forms often have printed shapes of the body on which the abnormalities can be drawn. Otherwise, the nurse can sketch the injured areas of the body in the nursing notes. "Rape kits" are often available for the collection of evidence in recent cases of alleged penetration but may be modified according to the child's needs. Health care providers must be extremely careful to maintain the chain of evidence so that the evidence will be admissible in court.

All visible injuries, such as bruises or burns, are photographed if at all possible. A hospital photographer is best equipped to obtain reliable and professional pictures that can be used as evidence in court. However, this service is not always available. Many EDs keep a camera on site to take pictures of injuries. While a high-quality 35-mm camera is recommended, it is reassuring to also have an instant camera that immediately produces a picture, even if the quality is not as good as 35-mm photographs. When photographing injuries, the child's name and other identifying information such as date of birth and medical record number and a ruler must be included in the photograph. A standard color chart is often included as well.

LEGAL ISSUES

MANDITORY REPORTING

All 50 states have a child abuse reporting law and a list of what constitutes a mandated report. The laws require that a report be filed based on suspicion of abuse or neglect. The nurse as a mandated reporter need not be an actual witness to the abusive episode. There is immunity from civil or criminal liability if the report was based on "reasonable suspicion." This means that a reasonable person in a similar role could draw on past experience and training and also suspect that abuse has occurred. Failure to report a suspicion can result in severe punishment, including a fine and/or imprisonment.

Names of social service agencies vary depending on the state and include the Department of Social Services, Child Protective Services, Department of Children's Services, and others. It is the responsibility of such agencies to ensure that children are in safe environments and that their basic needs are met. Most states have a "hotline" that allows for anonymous reporting of abuse or neglect. Caseworkers respond to a report within hours to days, based on the emergence of the information given to the hotline personnel. These agents have the jurisdiction in most parts of the country to remove a child from an unsafe home, at least until a court hearing can be held.

A report of child abuse and neglect can also be made to the local law enforcement agency. Police are mainly interested in capturing the perpetrator of a crime. The report should be made to the agency in the city where the alleged crime occurred, which is not necessarily where the child lives. In some states, it is preferable to notify law enforcement of the suspected abuse first. Law enforcement officers respond to the hospital, take a report from the involved parties, and notify the social service agency. Other states elect to have social services notified as the primary agency, and they in turn contact the appropriate law enforcement organization. Nurses should become familiar with their state's variations on the child abuse reporting laws.

In a case of child abuse or neglect, nurses are part of the team that includes police and social services. Statements from all of the parties involved are obtained and the nurse should ensure that his or her name is spelled correctly in the report. More importantly, the statements recorded by the officials should accurately reflect the observations of the nurse.

COURT CASES

Nurses who were involved in the care of the abused or neglected child may be subpoenaed by the court to testify. During court proceedings, nurses will be asked to describe their education and training. Inquiries are then made regarding the history and physical exam obtained during the ED visit. Answers must be honest and objective regardless of whether the questions are asked by the prosecution or defense.

There are different courts in which child abuse cases are tried, depending on the circumstances of the case. In a criminal court, there is a victim of a crime and an identified suspect. The purpose is to prove "beyond a reasonable doubt" that a *particular* person committed the crime. Some attorneys may not file a case if the victim is too young to testify. Many arbitrarily place this age at 5 years or younger. Children testifying in criminal court must relate the history of abuse, often with the perpetrator in the courtroom. Children are asked to remember exact details about the abuse or molestation, including dates and times of the day that the incidents occurred. They are expected to be clear and consistent in the testimony, even under strenuous cross examination by a defense attorney. More courts across the country are becoming "user friendly" for the sake of the child. Some of the helpful techniques utilized include allowing frequent breaks and having a trusted person seated close to the child in the witness box during testimony. A few courts allow the child to testify in a separate room, apart from the alleged perpetrator and the jury. Closed circuit television into the courtroom permits the jury to view testimony from the child. Other courts are hesitant to use this method, because many feel that it interferes with the suspect's constitutional right to face the accuser. Court preparation classes are being developed nationally for children who may become witnesses. The children visit an actual courtroom and are allowed to sit in the jury box, the witness box, and the judge's seat. The common procedures that happen in a court of law are explained, and there are often "mock trials" in which the children act out the roles of the participants in a hearing.

Juvenile Dependency Court hears testimony from children, parents, and professionals to determine if a child's environment is safe. In this court, there must be a "preponderance of evidence" for the removal of a child from parental care. The judge must decide if the home is more unsafe than not. If the child is removed, parents are usually given specific mandates, such as counseling or parenting classes, to regain custody of the child. Most judges are hesitant to permanently remove a child from the birth parents, regardless of the type of abuse that has occurred.

CUSTODY DISPUTES

In a court of family law, cases dealing with divorce and custody issues are heard. There is an overlap between the functions of the dependency and family courts in some states. Child abuse allegations occasionally arise in the course of custody hearings. In these cases, it is not uncommon for one parent to accuse the other of abusing or molesting the child. It is in the best interest of the child to complete an evaluation for the alleged episode. A study by Paradise, Rostain, and Nathanson in 1988 found a small increase in the number of unfounded child abuse cases when custody issues were in question.[26] However, more than half of these cases were later substantiated. Further, it was younger, nonverbal children who were most often involved in the unsubstantiated cases. This was explained by the inability of the professional to obtain historical information from the child regarding maltreatment. Many legal professionals look to the health care system for the definitive answer as to whether or not abuse occurred. However, because trauma, if present at all, often heals quickly and completely in a child, the medical examination is rarely helpful for either the parents or the attorneys as they search for concrete evidence of past abuse.

▌SPECIFIC CONDITIONS

SEXUAL ABUSE

The identified perpetrator of sexual abuse is commonly a male who is known to the child. Incidents involving children in pornography and prostitution may involve strangers, however, who frequently victimize runaway children. Sexual abusers come from all levels of society and frequently appear to be "normal" people.

Child victims of sexual abuse can exhibit extremes of behavior in the ED, ranging from unresponsive and apathetic to overly affectionate and outgoing. The child may appear frightened of the abusive caregiver or excessively clingy. Inappropriate reactions to patient care, from passive and accepting of discomfort to unduly uncooperative and fearful, may be expressed. Child behaviors identified by history that are suggestive of sexual abuse are described in Box 25-3.

Parental response to sexual abuse varies according to the circumstances of the abuse, the identity of the perpetrator, and personal patterns of reactions. The parent may not believe the child or be supportive. Blame and anger may be directed at the offender or the child. Parents may even threaten to punish the child. Others may feel excruciating guilt for neglecting to believe the child or prevent the abuse.

Clinical presentation. In most cases of molestation, even with a credible history from the child, the

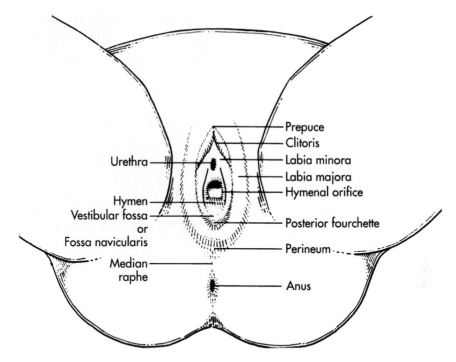

FIG. 25-5. Female genitalia as assessed in the supine position. Labia are separated to view hymen.

examination is normal. Many sexually abusive acts are not traumatic to the child's tissues and do not result in scars, hymenal tears, or other abnormalities. A normal examination in no way means that the child was fabricating the historical information of sexual abuse.

In cases of suspected molestation of a female, the greatest visualization of the genitalia occurs with the child in the supine position and the labia majora gently separated (Fig. 25-5). The child should never be physically restrained for this examination because of additional psychologic trauma. Conscious sedation or general anesthesia may be considered in cases of severe, acute genital trauma to evaluate the need for surgical intervention. Significant genital findings are listed in Box 25-4. It is important to recognize that the diagnosis of sexual abuse is not made on one finding but is based on a combination of findings, perhaps with a corroborating history from the child.

There are several normal variations in hymenal shapes. In addition, a girl may have one to two different hymenal configurations during her life, due to the fluctuations in estrogen levels during development.[23]

Chronic sexual abuse may cause defects or tears in

Box 25-4 Significant Genital Findings
Unusual erythema
Vaginal/penile discharge
Lesions
Gaping vaginal opening with loss of hymen
Defects (tears) completely through the hymen
Vaginal/penile bleeding or bruising

the hymen. Another significant finding is the loss of hymenal tissue, referred to as *attenuation,* or narrowing of the hymenal rim. This is indicative of a slow wearing away of the hymen that occurs over time with vaginal penetration.[1]

Typical normal hymens are depicted in Fig. 25-6. There are no absolute accepted diameters for the opening of the hymen. Many factors must be considered, such as the activities a child participates in and the child's size. The hymenal orifice varies in size from one girl to another. Therefore, specific introital measurements may not indicate abuse. In general, if a prepubertal child has a gaping vaginal opening,

Crescentic   Annular   Redundant

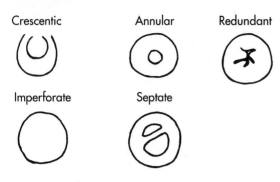

Imperforate   Septate

FIG. 25-6. Normal hymenal configurations.

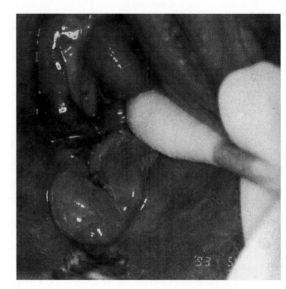

FIG. 25-7. Fourteen-year-old female who was abducted and assaulted over several hours. Hymen is swollen, and there is a fresh laceration visible below the hymen. Cotton applicator indicates darkened areas, which are fresh bruises of the hymen.

greater than 10 mm (1 cm), this constitutes a suspicious finding and should be evaluated further.

Victims of an acute assault, or "rape," usually exhibit abnormal physical findings. Although some findings may be visible for up to 2 weeks after the incident, other abnormalities are completely healed within a few days. Edema or bruises of the genital area and lacerations of the hymen and posterior fourchette may be present (Fig. 25-7). However, girls who have entered puberty, even after an alleged rape, may have no findings due to the elasticity of the estrogenized hymen.

Parents often worry that redness of the child's genital area, with or without vaginal discharge, is indicative of sexual abuse. Although it can be a sign of abuse, there are numerous benign reasons for erythematous genitalia, including use of harsh soaps, frequent bubble baths, tight-fitting clothing, or nylon underpants. Wiping from back to front after toileting or lack of cleanliness can also cause irritation.

Vaginal discharges in prepubertal girls are significant. These can be acquired nonsexually or sexually. Girls with otitis media or pharyngitis may autoinnoculate their genital areas with the bacteria responsible for the ear or throat infection. Pinworms (*Enterobius vermicularis*) may migrate from the rectum to the vagina.[8] Sexually transmitted diseases (STDs) in prepubertal children are almost always related to sexual abuse. Prepubertal girls are primarily infected in the vulvar region with secondary transmission to the vagina. Adolescents develop a cervicitis first. Before puberty, infection with either *N. gonorrhoeae* or *C. trachomatis* causes vulvar erythema, edema of the genitalia, and dysuria. A thick yellow-green purulent discharge is commonly seen with gonorrheal infections. There may be no discharge with vaginal chlamydia. Ulcerated, painless genital lesions (chancres) often indicate primary syphilis. Ulcerated genital lesions associated with pain are associated with the herpes simplex virus (HSV). *Condylomata acuminata* (venereal warts) commonly appear as thickened raised layers of warty lesions on the external genital area, cervix, penis, or anal opening. The warts resolve without treatment, then may reappear and spread. Urination and defecation can be painful. Bleeding may occur, especially with bowel movements.

Children with a discharge or genital lesions should be cultured for STDs. In cases of suspected sexual abuse, the "rapid tests" such as direct immunofluorescent antibody (DFA) and enzyme-linked immunosorbentassay (ELISA) should be avoided. Only cultures are accepted as the "gold standard."[14]

Most anal examinations are normal, regardless of the history of penetration.[7] Unusual anal findings are listed in Box 25-5. Sexual abuse may cause a loss of muscle tone. Depending on the amount of penetrating force and the size of the object used, the anus may sustain deep tears. If the rectum is full of stool, the anus can take on a gaping appearance, which is similar to the look of some children after repetitive anal penetration.[23] If a large anal opening with visible stool is present, the child should be encouraged to have a bowel movement. After 20 to 30 minutes, the area

> **Box 25-5   Unusual Anal Findings**
>
> Gaping anal opening in the absence of stool
> Rectal bleeding
> Deep tears of the sphincter muscle
> Lesions

should be reassessed. Often the passage of stool allows the anus to return to normal (Figs. 25-8 and 25-9).

Emergency Department and nursing interventions. Sexual abuse that presents after 72 hours is not considered emergent unless the child is in imminent danger. The ED, however, is the point of entry into the health care system for many children with a chief complaint of sexual abuse. After a complete assessment of the child's physical status and the safety of the home environment, the child should be referred for specialized follow-up care. Centers for the comprehensive evaluation of the sexually abused child have been developed in many areas. These facilities are staffed by multidisciplinary teams, including medical and nursing personnel, social workers, child psychologists, and often detectives and child protection workers.[1,31] Multidisciplinary team centers serve as a first site for a sexual abuse assessment or as a referral source from a variety of health care providers.

MUNCHAUSEN SYNDROME BY PROXY

Munchausen syndrome by proxy (MSP) is a cluster of symptoms in which an illness, often severe in nature, is produced by artificial means. Most often the parent or caregiver is the perpetrator, and the victim is an infant or toddler.[28] Many methods are used to simulate illness in the child, including the addition of maternal blood or sugar to the child's urine, poisoning the child, or suffocating the child to cause apnea or seizures. This disorder is difficult to prove, especially in the ED, and often the child dies before intervention occurs. The mother is usually the primary suspect and frequently has had training in nursing or another health-related field. A maternal psychiatric history and a dysfunctional family are common. Fathers are often absent from the home and usually deny that the mother could be the cause of the problem.

Clinical presentation. The child is repeatedly brought to health care facilities for fabricated illnesses.

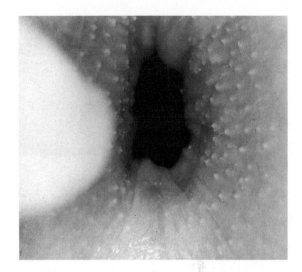

FIG. 25-8. Twelve-year-old male with a gaping appearance of anus. Note loss of normal perianal folds (rugae).

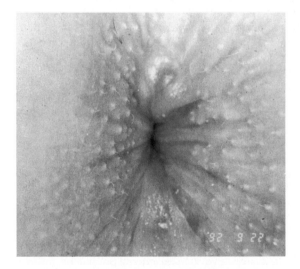

FIG. 25-9. Same view as in Fig. 25-8, taken 30 minutes after a bowel movement. Note resolution of gaping appearance. Rugal folds have returned to normal.

The child often presents with baffling, multisystem problems, necessitating consultation from numerous subspecialists, who are unable to find a cause for the strange symptoms. When confronted with the possibility that nothing is medically wrong with the child, the mother becomes irate, often removing the child from the hospital. The mother then "doctor shops"

> **Box 25-6 Warning Signs of Munchausen Syndrome by Proxy**
>
> Unexplained, prolonged, recurrent, or extremely rare illness
> Discrepancies between clinical findings and history
> Illness unresponsive to treatment
> Signs and symptoms occurring only in parent's presence
> Parent knowledgeable about illness, procedures, and treatments
> Parent very interested in interacting with the medical staff
> Parent very attentive to the child (refuses to leave the child's bedside)
>
> Modified from Wong DL: *Whaley & Wong's essentials of pediatric nursing,* ed 5, St Louis, 1997, Mosby.

until she finds someone who will perform the multitude of tests that she seeks. Interestingly, the symptoms diminish or disappear in the absence of the parent.

Several methods have been used to "catch" the parent in the act of fabricating the illness of the child. In one case, a video camera was installed in a child's hospital room. The child's mother was seen administering numerous solutions orally to her son, including mineral oil and milk of magnesia, to cause profuse diarrhea.[9] It may be difficult, though, to identify this syndrome in the ED. Patterns may be established by reviewing old charts. Warning signs of MSP are listed in Box 25-6. If the child is not in imminent danger, concerns should be shared with the primary care provider and follow-up arranged. A child protective services referral should be made if strong suspicions of MSP are present. During a thorough investigation, it is not unusual to discover that more than one child in the family has died under unusual circumstances.

SHAKEN BABY SYNDROME

The "shaken baby" or "shaken impact" syndrome is described as an acceleration-deceleration injury involving vigorous shaking of a very young child held by the upper extremities, shoulders, or thorax. There may be impact between the head and a solid object, such as a wall or the soft crib mattress. However, no external signs of trauma are usually present.

Infants have weaker neck muscles and heavier and larger heads than older children or adults. When shaken, the brain moves back and forth within the skull, causing stress and eventual shearing of the cortical veins. Tearing of these and other blood vessels results in subdural hematomas, subarachnoid hemorrhage, cerebral edema, and increased intracranial pressure. This tension can then result in the retinal hemorrhages that are commonly seen in this syndrome.[6]

Clinical presentation. Infants presenting with this syndrome are usually less than 1 year of age, with the majority being under 6 months.[6] Symptoms are vague and may be confused with sepsis, and they include vomiting, lethargy, irritability, seizures, bulging or full fontanels, and decreased appetite. Bruises or fractures may be observed in the area where the child was held during shaking episodes. Subarachnoid bleeding is usually evident on CT scan and examination of the cerebrospinal fluid.

Unfortunately many injuries from "shaken baby syndrome" result in death. Delays in seeking care are common, and the infant is often brought to the hospital with severe alteration in mental status. ED health care providers must have a high index of suspicion for this syndrome in any infant with unexplained altered mental status. The presence of a subdural hematoma on an infant's CT scan is strongly suggestive of physical abuse.

FAILURE TO THRIVE

Failure to thrive (FTT) is the slowing or cessation of normal growth. A child with FTT has a measurement of weight or height below the fifth percentile on a standardized growth chart, or the child falls two standard deviations on the growth chart between visits to the health care provider.[20,27] The numerous organic reasons for FTT, such as cardiac defects, gastrointestinal problems, or metabolic disorders, must be considered in the ED. "Nonorganic" FTT is associated with psychosocial factors, including a disturbance in maternal/child attachment, lack of parental knowledge of infant nutrition, lack of resources, or a deficiency in maternal care. In some states there is an overlap between the definitions of neglect and nonorganic FTT, as the latter may involve the intentional failure to provide adequate food and stimulation. Observation of the interactions be-

Box 25-7 Parental Maladaptive Behaviors Toward Infant

Persistent ambivalence or negative feelings about the fetus and the pregnancy during the prenatal period

Makes no plans for obtaining basic infant supplies

Appears indifferent to infant at time of delivery; may appear sad or angry; is expressionless

Makes no effort to establish eye contact with infant

Handles infant only when necessary

Does not talk to infant

Makes few or no spontaneous movements with infant

Asks few questions about care

Sees infant as ugly, fat, or unattractive

Displays disgust with infant's drooling and sucking sounds; is revolted by infant's body fluids

Annoyed by diaper changing

Perceives infant's odor as revolting

Holds infant with little support to head and body

Holds infant away from body during feeding or props bottle for feeding; seldom cuddles infant

Does not coo or talk to infant

Refers to infant in an impersonal manner

Develops inappropriate responses to infant's needs, such as leaving infant in one place for long periods, leaving child alone in room, overfeeding or underfeeding, overstimulating or understimulating infant, forcing or refusing eye contact, bouncing or tickling infant when child is fatigued

Cannot discriminate between infant's signals for hunger, comfort, rest, or body contact

Is convinced that infant has a defect or disease even when reassured to the contrary

Makes negative statements regarding parenting role

Believes infant is judging him or her and efforts as an adult

Believes infant does not love him or her

Develops paradoxical attitudes and behaviors toward infant

From Wong DL: *Whaley & Wong's: essentials of pediatric nursing,* ed 5, St Louis, 1997, Mosby.

Box 25-8 Clinical Manifestations of Nonorganic Failure to Thrive

Growth failure—below fifth percentile in weight

Developmental retardation—social, motor, adaptive, language

Apathy

Withdrawn behavior

Distressed look and/or cry

Minimal smiling

Avoidance of eye contact

"Radar gaze" (wide-eyed gaze and continual scan of the environment)

No fear of strangers (at age when stranger anxiety is normal)

Poor hygiene

Feeding or eating disorders

Hypertonic, stiff and unyielding or flaccid and unresponsive

Arching of back

Lower extremity scissoring

"Strap-hangers" position in crib

Modified from Wong DL: *Whaley & Wong's essentials of pediatric nursing,* ed 5, St Louis, 1997, Mosby.

tween the child and the caregiver may help distinguish between the two entities. Maladaptive parental behaviors are frequently displayed with nonorganic FTT (Box 25-7).

Clinical presentation. Infants with nonorganic FTT display frequent negative interactions with their caregivers. Infant needs, such as timely feeding, are often omitted. The baby learns that the world is not a place of trust. Certain behavioral characteristics are commonly displayed (Box 25-8). When held close, the hypertonic infant may arch his or her back in an attempt to pull away from the holder. When the infant is held away from the adult's body, the baby often brightens up and begins to coo and smile, while the unusual behaviors temporarily diminish.[27] Conversely, the baby may be hypotonic, especially in later stages as the infant becomes resigned to a nonnurturing environment. Changes in muscle tone may result in the "strap-hangers" position. When the infant is lying down, the arms are bent at the elbow and wrist. The baby appears to be holding the strap on a bus or subway. Infants with nonorganic FTT are typically difficult and frustrating to feed. Irritability and sleep disturbances are also common.

Emergency Department and nursing interventions. When children who have weight loss or poor weight gain are seen in the ED, numerous organic causes must be ruled out. Because the evaluation of this disorder is complex, the infant is often admitted for comprehensive testing and observation of feeding behaviors and the maternal-child relationship. In the ED, a detailed history often provides clues to the etiology of FTT. Observation of the general appearance of the child and parent-infant behaviors can yield important information. A complete physical exam is performed, including assessment of hydration status. Screening laboratory and radiologic tests may reveal organic diagnoses. Families of children with FTT benefit from a caring and supportive health care team who can address the various facets of this disorder.

PRIMARY PREVENTION

ED nurses play a significant role in both the primary prevention of child abuse and the identification of child abuse. Prevention is facilitated by evaluating the parent-child interactions while in the emergency department and role-modeling child care and disciplinary techniques. Handouts regarding the signs of child abuse, the signs of parental stress, and available support services can be provided to parents and information posted on bulletin boards and in waiting areas. Parents or caregivers must be made aware that maltreatment is frequently inflicted by persons that the child knows or trusts. Additionally, during an ED visit children can be taught to avoid situations that put them at risk for abuse.

Children learn much about their world from what is taught at school. Although nurses are often asked to present classes on topics such as nutrition and exercise, more schools are requesting that nurses teach about child abuse and neglect. Curricula on these topics are being developed nationally. Frequently there is a disclosure of abuse or neglect after such a presentation. The primary goal of this class, however, is to teach children strategies to protect them from getting into a high-risk situation before abuse or abduction occurs. Educational content also stresses that a child is in charge of his or her own body. For those children who have already been victimized, the class reinforces that the child is not at fault for the abuse.

Parent education can also be performed in a variety of ways, including discussions at PTA meetings or booths at fairs or shopping malls. Information should include behavioral warning signs of maltreatment, such as fear of leaving the house, refusal to go to school, sleep disturbances, and nightmares. Resources such as Parents Anonymous and Parents United International, Inc., can be described and phone numbers and addresses provided. Printed materials are often available from these organizations.

Professionals who regularly work with abused and neglected children find these cases to be particularly draining. It is difficult to imagine that such horror and pain could be inflicted on a child. To face this reality is to become aware of one's own potential to harm others. For this reason, the nurse must practice his or her own prevention, especially related to burnout. Regardless of the strategy used, whether it be exercise, sharing with a close friend, meditation, or other stress-relieving activities, the nurse is better able to cope with stress if it can be released in appropriate ways.

SUMMARY

Child abuse and neglect are multidimensional problems, affecting many people and agencies. Physical injuries can kill a child or cause serious lifelong deficits. Sexual abuse can affect a child's ability to have significant relationship long into adulthood. The evaluation for child maltreatment takes a great deal of time and energy to complete. This puts added stress on an already busy emergency department. In spite of these obstacles, nurses can facilitate the coordination of services to children and their families. They can provide preventative education to parents and children. Finally, as advocates for children and families, nurses can support legislation and programs that will help protect these most vulnerable members of our society.

REFERENCES

1. Berkowitz CD: Pediatric sexual abuse. In Reisdorf EJ, Roberts MR, Wienstein JG, eds: *Pediatric emergency medicine*, Philadelphia, 1993, W. Saunders.
2. Bernat JE: Dental trauma and bite mark evaluation. In Ludwig S, Kornberg AE, eds: *Child abuse—a medical reference*, ed 2, New York, 1992, Churchill Livingstone.
3. Billmire ME, Myers PA: Serious head injury i

infants: accident or abuse? *Pediatrics* 75:340-342, 1985.

4. Brayden RM et al: Antecedents of child neglect in the first two years of life, *J Pediatr* 120:426-429, 1992.
5. Christoffel KK: Violent death and injury in US children and adolescents, *Am J Dis Child* 144:697-700, 1990.
6. Coody D et al: Shaken baby syndrome: identification and prevention for nurse practitioners, *J Pediatr Health Care* 8:50-56, 1994.
7. Elvik SL: From disclosure to court: the facets of sexual abuse, *J Pediatr Health Care* 1:136-140, 1987.
8. Elvik SL: Vaginal discharge in the prepubertal girl, *J Pediatr Health Care* 4:181-185, 1990.
9. Epstein MA et al: Munchausen syndrome by proxy: considerations in diagnosis and confirmation by video surveillance, *Pediatrics* 80:220-224, 1987.
10. Feldman KW, Brewer DK: Child abuse, cardiopulmonary resuscitation, and rib fractures, *Pediatrics* 73:339-342, 1984.
11. Feldman KW et al: Tap water scald burns in children, *Pediatrics* 62:1-7, 1978.
11a. Frechette A, Rimsza ME: Stun gun injury: a new presentation of the battered child syndrome, *Pediatrics* 89(5):898-901, 1992.
12. Goodman MH: The physical abuse of children: then and now, *Nurs Pract Forum* 1:84-89, 1990.
13. Haley K: *Emergency nursing pediatric course manual,* Chicago, 1993, Emergency Nurses Association.
14. Hammerschlag MR, Rettig PJ, Shields ME: False positive results with the use of chlamydial antigen tests in the evaluation of suspected sexual abuse in children, *Pediatr Infect Dis* 7:11-14, 1983.
15. Helfer RE: The neglect of our children, *Pediatr Clin North Am* 37:923-940, 1990.
16. Helfer RE, Slovis TL, Black M: Injuries resulting when small children fall out of bed, *Pediatrics* 60:533-535, 1977.
17. Hyden PW, Gallagher TA: Child abuse intervention in the emergency room, *Pediatr Clin North Am* 39(5):1053-1081, 1992.
18. Kaufman J, Zigler E: Do abused children become abusive parents? *Am J Orthopsychiatr* 57:186-191, 1987.
19. Kempe CH et al: The battered-child syndrome, *JAMA* 181:17-24, 1962.
20. Kempe RS, Cutler C, Dean J: The infant with failure to thrive. In Kempe CH, Helfer RE, eds: *The battered child,* ed 3, Chicago, 1980, The University of Chicago Press.
21. Leventhal JM et al: Fractures in young children, *Am J Dis Child* 147:87-92, 1993.
22. McCann J et al: Genital findings in prepubertal girls selected for nonabuse: a descriptive study, *Pediatrics* 86:428-438, 1990.
23. McCann J et al: Perianal findings in prepubertal children selected for nonabuse: a descriptive study, *Child Abuse Neglect* 13:179-193, 1989.
24. McClain PW et al: Estimates of fatal child abuse and neglect, United States, 1979 through 1988, *Pediatrics* 91:338-343, 1993.
25. National Committee for the Prevention of Child Abuse: *Current trends in child abuse reporting and fatalities: the results of the 1992 annual fifty state survey,* May 1993.
26. Paradise JE, Rostain AL, Nathanson M: Substantiation of sexual abuse charges when parents dispute custody or visitation, *Pediatrics* 81:835-839, 1988.
27. Sklaren BC: Nonorganic failure to thrive in infancy: assessment and intervention, *Nurs Pract Forum* 1:18-83, 1990.
28. Turk LJ, Hanrahan KM, Weber ER: Munchausen syndrome by proxy: a nursing overview, *Issues Compr Pediatr Nurs* 13:279-288, 1990.
29. Williams JJ: Child abuse. In Reisdorff EJ, Roberts MR, Wiegenstein JG, eds: *Pediatric emergency medicine,* Philadelphia, 1993, WB Saunders.
30. Williams RA: Injuries in infants and small children resulting from witnessed and corroborated free falls, *J Trauma* 31:1350-1352, 1991.
31. Wilson EP: Multidisciplinary approach to child protection. In Ludwig S, Kornberg AE, eds: *Child abuse—a medical reference,* ed 2, New York, 1992, Churchill Livingstone.

CHAPTER 26

The Febrile Child

Treesa Soud

Fever accounts for as many as 20% to 25% of all pediatric emergency visits,[41] with the most common causes being infectious or inflammatory processes that are easily treated. Among the most common febrile illnesses seen in the pediatric emergency department are otitis media, upper respiratory infections, gastroenteritis, and urinary tract infections. One study of pediatric emergency department visits found that less than 1% of all febrile children (temperatures 101° F or higher) required a hospital admission, and only 3 of the 32 admissions were for a serious illness.[18] Although fevers in excess of 105.2° to 105.8° F (40 to 41.0° C) have been associated with an increased incidence of serious infections, such as bacteremia or meningitis,[30,31,38] *fever is not diagnostic* and therefore must be evaluated in conjunction with clinical and historical findings.

DEFINITION

Fever is defined as a temperature above the usual range of normal. However, *what is normal* is a question of some debate. The accepted temperature of 98.6° F (37° C) was derived in 1868 when Wunderlich studied the axillary temperatures of over 25,000 adults using a primitive thermometer. Although this number has been questioned many times over the years (for example, one recent study suggests 98.2° F is the mean temperature of healthy adults),[28] 98.6° F has remained the accepted, normal temperature for both adults and children.

Normal temperature ranges for children have been extrapolated from studies of adults; however, there is no universal agreement on the definition of fever in infants and children. Because infants and young children have higher body surface area-to-volume ratios and less well-developed body temperature regulating mechanisms than adults, it could be speculated there would be a greater variation in mean temperatures. One recent study suggests this to be true by finding the mean rectal temperature of healthy infants less than 3 months of age varied slightly by age[23] (Table 26-1). Although the variation is small, it could be significant when the decision to admit a young infant is based on an established body temperature.

The definition of fever in children varies among institutions, with some using a rectal temperature of 100.4° F (38° C) and others up to 100.8° F (38.2° C).

TABLE 26-1	Mean Rectal Temperature by Age Infants Less Than 3 Months Old		
AGE	NO. OF PATIENTS	MEAN (°C [°F])	FEVER = MEAN + 2 SD
≤30 days	299	37.4 (99.4)	38.0 (100.4)
31 to 60 days	211	37.5 (99.5)	38.1 (100.6)
61 to 91 days	181	37.6 (99.6)	38.2 (100.8)
Total sample	691	37.5 (99.5)	38.1 (100.6)

SD, Standard deviation.
From Herzog LW, Coyne LJ: *Clin Pediatr* 32(3):143, 1993.

The most widely used definition is a rectal temperature of 100.4° F (38° C) or higher. However, variability in the method of obtaining the temperature (rectal, oral, tympanic, axillary), the skills of the person taking the temperature, the cooperation of the child, the time of the day, and the temperature of the ambient environment can all affect the temperature reading.

ETIOLOGY

High body temperatures can be caused by any number of factors, including (1) exposure to extreme heat (e.g., heat stroke); (2) decreased heat loss (e.g., infant tightly wrapped in blankets); (3) abnormalities within the brain (e.g., tumors); (4) abnormal heat production within the body (e.g., malignant hyperthermia); or (5) an underlying infection or inflammatory process (Table 26-2). Extremely high body temperatures (greater than 107.6° F [42.2° C]) are rare in the pediatric population and usually result from heat stroke or

a central nervous system disorder. Organ damage can occur when temperatures approach this range.

PATHOPHYSIOLOGY

BODY TEMPERATURE REGULATION

Body temperature is regulated in the perioptic region of the hypothalamus and is maintained by a complex reflex loop that involves peripheral receptors located in the skin and deep organs. When impulses are sent to the hypothalamus, either by means of the reflex loop or by the temperature of circulating blood, thermally sensitive neurons within the hypothalamus, which respond to either heat or cold, stimulate the physiologic temperature regulating responses.

Body temperature is a balance between heat produced and heat lost. Heat is a by-product of metabolism, and most heat is produced in the deep organs such as the liver, brain, heart, and skeletal muscle. In the healthy individual an increase in heat production, is exhibited by vasoconstriction, shivering and chills, and piloerection (goosebumps). Young infants are unable to shiver to generate heat and instead rely almost entirely on chemical or "nonshivering" thermogenesis, which results in the oxidation of mitochondria-rich brown fat. Infants have more brown fat than adults, so 100% of their heat production may be by chemical thermogenesis, compared to 10% to 15% in adults.

Body temperature decreases (1) when heat is conducted away from the internal organs to the skin and (2) when there is a decrease in the rate of heat production. Radiation, conduction, convection, and evaporation play important roles in the dissipation of body heat. *Radiation* is the dissipation of body heat as it moves into the air or space from a warm to cool environment. But radiation can be used to warm the body, as can be seen with the use of radiant warmers or lights. *Conduction* involves the transfer of heat from matter to matter and depends on a substance's ability to conduct heat away from the body. For example, direct contact with a metal surface rapidly conducts heat away from the body, yet certain fabrics, such as wool, act as insulators to trap heat close to the body. *Convection* is a change of position of the heated particles by the movement of a liquid or air over an object. For example, a newborn infant in a draft quickly becomes hypothermic as cool air moves over the infant's skin. *Evaporation* represents the dissipation of body heat as water evaporates from the skin and lungs.

TABLE 26-2	Causes of Abnormal Increases in Body Temperature
• Exposure to extreme heat	• Heatstroke
	• Heat exhaustion
• Decreased heat loss	• Tightly bundled infant
	• Atropine poisoning
• Abnormal heat production	• Malignant hyperthermia
	• Thyrotoxic crisis
• Abnormalities within the brain	• Central nervous system (CNS) lesions in the hypothalamus
	• Prolonged seizure activity
• Infectious or inflammatory processes	• Viral illnesses
	• Bacterial illnesses
	• Fungal infections
	• Rickettsia (Rocky Mountain spotted fever)
	• Protozoa (malaria)
	• Collagen-vascular illnesses (Kawasaki disease, acute rheumatic fever)

TEMPERATURE CONTROL IN INFANTS

Temperature control in neonates is tenuous because of their (1) immature central nervous system (CNS), which can cause wide variations in body temperature; (2) lack of subcutaneous fat, which contributes to greater than normal heat loss into the environment; and (3) proportionately higher metabolic rates when compared to older children and adults. When the body temperature rises the metabolic rate increases further, approximately 10% for every 1° C rise in body temperature.[53] As the metabolic rate rises, caloric expenditures, oxygen consumption, and cardiac output increase. These physiologic effects can produce hypoxia, acidosis, and hypoglycemia.

The infant's limited ability to dissipate body heat by sweating is another factor that affects body heat. One study of newborns who were tightly bundled and exposed to a *warm ambient environment* demonstrated that body temperature may rise into the febrile range (over 100.4° F [38° C]).[5] Another study of older infants (between 2 weeks and 95 days old) who were bundled in a *normal temperate environment* maintained a rectal temperature within the normal range.[22] Therefore older infants who are bundled appear to be better able to dissipate body heat, even when bundled, whereas neonates who are bundled and exposed to a warm ambient environment (e.g., in an unairconditioned car on a hot day) are less able to compensate.

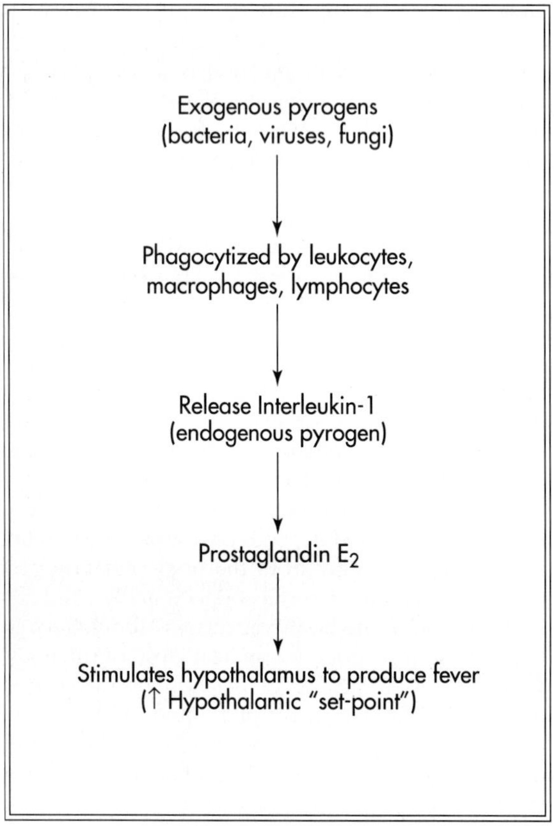

PATHOPHYSIOLOGY OF FEVER CAUSED BY AN INFECTIOUS AGENT

When an infectious agent enters the body, the production of endogenous pyrogens causes the "set point" of the temperature regulating center to move to a higher level than normal. As the set point moves upward, all of the body's mechanisms for raising body temperature are stimulated. Some pyrogens affect the set point directly; others act indirectly and may take several hours of latency, as occurs with infections caused by gram-negative bacteria (Figs. 26-1 and 26-2).

When the factor that is causing the fever is removed, the hypothalamic temperature regulating center is reset to a normal level. Because body temperature is high, the child's skin will feel hot as vasodilation and intense sweating occur to dissipate the heat. In the days before antibiotics, this "crisis" was awaited, since

Exogenous pyrogens
(bacteria, viruses, fungi)

↓

Phagocytized by leukocytes,
macrophages, lymphocytes

↓

Release Interleukin-1
(endogenous pyrogen)

↓

Prostaglandin E₂

↓

Stimulates hypothalamus to produce fever
(↑ Hypothalamic "set-point")

FIG. 26-1. Pyrogen production.

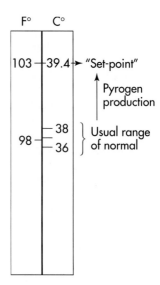

FIG. 26-2. The hypothalamic "set point."

it indicated the patient's body had either overwhelmed the toxins or lost its ability to fight the infection.

Whether or not fever plays a protective role during an infectious process is a source of debate. Although it is known that extremely high body temperatures, above 107.6° F (42.2°C), can cause tissue damage, low-grade fevers may increase mobility and activity of the white cells and stimulate antibody production, improving the immune response to illness.[27,47]

Fever can also have harmful effects, since it increases the metabolic rate and therefore caloric expenditures and oxygen consumption. When the metabolic rate increases, heart rate, respiratory rate, and insensible fluid losses increase. In the otherwise healthy child, these physiologic changes may not be dangerous; however, in the critically ill child, an elevated temperature may further deplete physiologic reserves.

ANTIPYRETICS

The use of antipyretics for the treatment of fever in children is controversial, and there is no specific degree of fever that requires treatment. Those who advocate using antipyretics note that with fever defervescence, the child's clinical appearance improves as the child begins to feel better. Additionally, the negative physiologic effects of the fever are reversed as the fever decreases (e.g., oxygen consumption, caloric expenditure).

Conversely, it is felt that treating fever in a "well-appearing" child may further contribute to "fever phobia," reinforcing to the caregiver that the child requires treatment—even though the "treatment" is an antipyretic. What is agreed on is that fever should be treated in the critically ill child and in children with chronic conditions, since body temperatures above normal contribute to the loss of physiologic reserves.

Antipyretics reduce fever by blocking the formation of prostaglandins, which act on the hypothalamus to induce the fever reaction. Acetaminophen and ibuprofen are the two most commonly used antipyretics in children. Aspirin is not recommended, particularly in the presence of chickenpox, because aspirin usage has been associated with the development of Reye syndrome. Ibuprofen and acetaminophen have been found to be equally effective in decreasing body temperature when given as initial doses of ibuprofen 10 mg/kg and acetaminophen 15 mg/kg[51] (see the discussion of nursing care).

Several theories have been suggested regarding the

child's clinical and physiologic responses to antipyretic therapy. It has been speculated that an improvement in the child's clinical appearance after antipyretic therapy is an indication the child is not seriously ill. Although this has been disputed,[6] it is known that if the fussy or difficult-to-examine child is given an antipyretic and is allowed to remain in the mother's lap until the fever subsides, the skilled examiner may be able to more readily evaluate the child and better determine the need for diagnostic testing.[29]

It has also been suggested that children who experience a significant drop in temperature after the administration of an antipyretic are less likely to be seriously ill. Several studies, however, were unable to correlate this drop in body temperature with the seriousness of the illness.[4,13,49,55] One study did indicate that the younger the infant, the more significant is the temperature drop after antipyretic administration, but this finding was *not* predictive of the seriousness of the illness.[13]

FEBRILE SEIZURES

Febrile seizures account for the majority of seizure activity seen in the pediatric population. They are brief and self-limited and are characterized by tonic-clonic movements lasting less than 15 minutes followed by a brief postictal period.[50] Febrile seizures usually occur within the first 24 hours of the onset of the illness, often within the first few hours of the onset of fever. When the child awakens, a normal level of consciousness will be observed and the child should appear nontoxic. *The true febrile seizure does not cause neurologic damage or lead to learning disabilities, nor is it predictive of the development of a lifelong seizure disorder.*[20]

From 2% to 5% of all febrile children will experience a febrile seizure. The peak incidence is between 8 to 20 months of age; however, febrile seizures may occur in children up to 5 or 6 years of age.[19] Once a child has one febrile seizure, the risk of a second febrile seizure occurring is approximately 30%.[39] Hereditary factors may play a role in the child's susceptibility to the development of febrile seizures. The child with a parent or sibling who had a febrile seizure is three to four times more likely to also have a febrile seizure.[19]

The exact cause of febrile seizures is unknown. Factors that are known to affect the seizure threshold are the height of the fever, the age of the child, and the degree of illness.[19,20] Although the height of the fever is a factor affecting the incidence of febrile seizures (febrile seizures are more commonly associated with a temperature of at least 102.2° F [39° C]), the height alone is not predictive of an impending febrile seizure. In fact, children with fevers as low 100.4° F (38° C) can exhibit seizure activity when age and hereditary disposition are factored into the equation.[3,19]

The age of the child plays a significant role in the propensity for seizures. Because of the immature cortex in the young infant, seizure activity is rarely exhibited unless significant neurologic dysfunction has occurred. When seizure activity does occur, it is rarely exhibited by classic symptoms. As the cortex develops in the young child, it becomes more excitable and therefore more prone to seizure activity. With maturation of the cortex, the likelihood of seizure activity decreases. The incidence of febrile seizures in the infant and young child coincides with the developing cerebral cortex.

Febrile seizures are most commonly the result of a nonserious illness. The presence of a potentially life-threatening CNS infection such as meningitis, however, must be considered. In addition to seizure activity, the febrile child with a serious bacterial infection will appear toxic and exhibit clinical signs of serious illness.[36] These signs include petechiae, signs of meningeal irritation (e.g., nuchal rigidity), coma, persistent drowsiness, repeated seizure activity, focal seizures, paresis, or paralysis.

▌ CLINICAL PRESENTATION

Fever is a symptom of illness and not an illness in and of itself. Yet parents and health care workers continue to place a much greater initial emphasis on the height of the fever than on the history or clinical signs of illness. Perhaps the fact that fever is an easily measured variable contributes to this phenomenon. Regardless of the degree of fever, a complete history and physical examination should be obtained to identify the presence of any serious illness.

Some febrile children, regardless of the height of the fever or clinical presentation, meet criteria that indicate an increased risk of serious illness. These include (1) infants younger than 6 to 8 weeks of age; (2) immunocompromised children such as those receiving chemotherapy or those who have human immunodeficiency virus (HIV) or sickle cell disease (SSD); (3) children younger than 2 years of age with no obvious source of infection; and (4) children with chronic illnesses such as cystic fibrosis or bronchopulmonary dysplasia.

INFANTS: BIRTH UNTIL 2 TO 3 MONTHS OF AGE

Infants younger than 2 to 3 months of age do not have the immunocompetence of older children and are reliant on maternal antibodies for protection. Febrile infants in this age range have a higher incidence of serious illness than older infants and young children and are more difficult to evaluate clinically; they therefore may require routine diagnostic testing to rule out the presence of serious underlying illness.

Although the majority of febrile young infants are not seriously ill, studies have shown that the younger the infant, the higher is the incidence of serious illness, particularly in infants younger than 28 days of age.[13,52] The degree of fever is also more closely correlated with the seriousness of the illness in infants younger than 1 month of age[11,12]; however, a lack of fever or "low-grade" fever does not rule out the presence of serious bacterial infection. In fact, septic young infants are often hypothermic.

Clinical assessment of febrile young infants is more difficult to perform than assessment of older children, since they do not manifest the same signs of serious illness as might be observed in older children (e.g., nuchal rigidity). Additionally, infants are neurologically immature and unable to perform the tasks of older children (e.g., rolling over, crawling, head control, social smile), making the assessment parameters nonspecific (e.g., fussiness, feeding patterns, elimination pattern). As infants move into the 2- to 3-month age range and progress developmentally, clinical assessment becomes somewhat easier and the guidelines for hospitalization are less stringent.

Clinical observation scales defining assessment criteria for febrile children, such as the Yale Scale, have proved useful in older children but are not reliable in infants younger than 8 weeks of age[5,33] (Table 26-3). Although these studies indicate that the skill of the examiner plays a significant role in the identification of the seriously ill child, they also suggest that even skilled practitioners have difficulty detecting seriously ill young infants.

Criteria for evaluating febrile infants includes an overall impression coupled with the history and physical examination. Specific clinical criteria include irritability, consolability, color, respiratory status, and hydration. When obvious clinical signs of illness are absent, the history becomes an essential component of the evaluation. Parental report of feeding patterns,

TABLE 26-3	Clinical Observation Scale (Yale Scale)		
OBSERVATION ITEM	**1 NORMAL**	**3 MODERATE IMPAIRMENT**	**5 SEVERE IMPAIRMENT**
Quality of cry	Strong with normal tone *or* content and not crying	Whimpering *or* sobbing	Weak *or* moaning *or* high pitched
Reaction to parent stimulation	Cries briefly then stops *or* content and not crying	Cries off and on	Continual cry *or* hardly responds
State variation	If awake → stays awake *or* if asleep and stimulated → wakes up quickly	Eyes close briefly → awake *or* awakes with prolonged stimulation	Falls asleep *or* will not rouse
Color	Pink	Pale extremities *or* acro-cyanosis	Pale *or* cyanotic *or* mottled *or* ashen
Hydration	Skin normal, eyes normal *and* mucous membranes moist	Skin, eyes—normal *and* mouth slightly dry	Skin doughy *or* tented *and* dry mucous membranes *and/or* sunken eyes
Response (talk, smile) to social overtures	Smiles *or* alerts (≤2 months)	Brief smile *or* alerts briefly (≤2 months)	No smile; face dull, expressionless *or* no alerting (≤2 months)

Scoring: The scores obtained on all six criteria should be totaled. The maximum possible score is 30, which would indicate the most serious illness; the least possible score, 6, indicates a normal clinical examination.
- Children with scores ≥16 have a higher incidence of serious illness.
- Some children with scores of 11 to 15 may be seriously ill but are most commonly not seriously ill.
- Children with scores ≤10 are most commonly not seriously ill.

Example: A 2-year-old child arrives in the emergency department with a history of fever. He is alertly observing activities and cries vigorously when the triage nurse obtains his vital signs. His lips are cracked and his mouth is slightly dry, but his mucous membranes are pink. He smiles briefly when stimulated by his mother, but he cries more often than not.
- Quality of cry   (1)   Strong
- Reaction to parent   (3)   Cries off and on
- State variation   (1)   Alertly observing emergency department activities
- Color   (1)   Mucous membranes are pink
- Hydration   (3)   Lips cracked, mucous membranes slightly dry
- Response to overtures   (3)   Smiles briefly

TOTAL SCORE   **(12)   Probably not seriously ill. Complete history and physical examination should be performed to identify source of fever.**

Data from McCarthy PL et al: Observational scales to identify serious illness in febrile children, *Pediatrics* 70(5):806, 1982.

Box 26-1   Assessment of the Febrile Young Infant

Initial impression
A Activity level
B Breathing (respiratory effort)
C Color
    Consolability
D Degree of irritability
    Degree of hydration

History
• Changes in feeding pattern
• Changes in elimination pattern (bowel and bladder)
• Changes in body temperature (highest fever measured)
• Changes in skin color and temperature
• Changes in breathing pattern
• Changes in activity level, including eye contact, sleepiness, sucking
• Changes in demeanor, including crying frequently, inconsolable crying, disinterest in the bottle or breast

elimination patterns, height of the fever, skin color, breathing patterns, and activity level all provide important clues to the infant's status (Box 26-1).

CHILDREN 2 TO 3 MONTHS UNTIL 2 YEARS OF AGE

The most common illnesses observed in children 3 months of age to 2 years of age include upper respiratory infections, otitis media, gastroenteritis, and urinary tract infections. More serious but less common illnesses include meningitis, epiglottitis, bronchiolitis, and occult bacteremia. The one diagnosis in this age range that has received the most attention in the literature is occult bacteremia, since studies have demonstrated an occurrence rate of up to 10% in both well and ill-appearing febrile children (usually defined as ≥102.2° F [39° C] or ≥102.8° F [39.3° C]).[29,34,35] Despite this fact, the degree of fever has been found to be a less sensitive indicator of the seriousness of the illness, even when these children have fevers the nurse might consider "high" (e.g., ≥103° F (39.4° C).[54] Instead, clinical and historical findings were more closely correlated with

the seriousness of the illness. One study compared temperatures as high as 106° F (41.1° C) to temperatures in the 102.4° to 104° F (39.1° to 40° C) range and found there was no increase in the frequency of serious bacterial infections or bacteremia in the children studied.[1]

Clinical assessment and history are the most important indicators of serious illness in this age group. The initial assessment should include an overall evaluation of child's activity level and awareness and interaction with the environment. Febrile children who "look well", are playful, mobile, and bright-eyed; maintain eye contact; and are easily consoled, are rarely seriously ill. Children who "look ill" may present with obvious signs of serious illness, such as nuchal rigidity and/or toxicity, or subtle signs of illness that simply indicate the child "feels bad," such as hugging the parent (Fig. 26-3).

The history will provide additional clues to the child's status and influence initial patient management. For example, parents of a child who appears to "feel bad" may report significant changes in feeding patterns, sleeping patterns, and demeanor (e.g., irritability or inconsolability), which might indicate that the child is more seriously ill than the initial impression might suggest. Additional questions should include the length of the illness, associated signs and symptoms, history of illness in the family, previous illness, and current medications. Febrile children with chronic illnesses that may compromise immune function, such as sickle cell anemia, and children receiving immunosuppressive therapy require immediate emergency department evaluation (Box 26-2) (see Chapter 17, The Hematologic and Immune Systems).

CHILDREN OVER 2 YEARS OF AGE

Children in this age range are more easily evaluated. They are usually more cooperative during the examination because neuromuscular and cognitive abilities are better developed. Although occult bacteremia may occur in children older than 2 years of age, the incidence begins to drop by 3 years of age. As in younger children, a thorough evaluation is required to identify the cause of the fever. The initial impression includes observing the child for signs of toxicity as well as evaluating airway patency, breathing effectiveness and pattern, skin for color and rashes, strength of pulses, capillary refill, and neurologic status, including assessment for signs of nuchal rigidity.

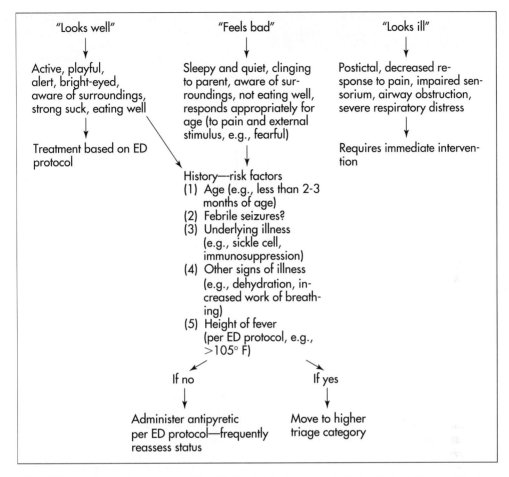

"Looks well"

↓

Active, playful, alert, bright-eyed, aware of surroundings, strong suck, eating well

↓

Treatment based on ED protocol

"Feels bad"

↓

Sleepy and quiet, clinging to parent, aware of surroundings, not eating well, responds appropriately for age (to pain and external stimulus, e.g., fearful)

↓

History—risk factors
(1) Age (e.g., less than 2-3 months of age)
(2) Febrile seizures?
(3) Underlying illness (e.g., sickle cell, immunosuppression)
(4) Other signs of illness (e.g., dehydration, increased work of breathing)
(5) Height of fever (per ED protocol, e.g., >105° F)

If no

↓

Administer antipyretic per ED protocol—frequently reassess status

If yes

↓

Move to higher triage category

"Looks ill"

↓

Postictal, decreased response to pain, impaired sensorium, airway obstruction, severe respiratory distress

↓

Requires immediate intervention

FIG. 26-3. Clinical impression of the febrile child. (From Soud T: The febrile child in the ED, *J Emerg Nurs* 19(4):356, 1993.)

Box 26-2   Nursing History

1. Length of illness
2. Signs and symptoms associated with the illness
   - Vomiting, diarrhea
   - Changes in eating and drinking patterns
   - Changes in activity level
   - Changes in voiding pattern
   - Changes in sleep pattern
   - Drowsiness
3. Exposure to illness (e.g., day care, school, home)
4. Previous illnesses (e.g., frequent ear infections)

5. Allergies and immunizations
6. Medications
   - Antipyretics and doses administered
   - Immunosuppressive drugs
   - Antibiotics
7. Significant past medical history
   - Prematurity
   - Congenital heart disease
   - Sickle cell disease
   - Cystic fibrosis
   - Bronchopulmonary dysplasia (BPD)
   - Other chronic illness

Box 26-3   The Sepsis Workup in the Febrile Neonate

- Complete blood count and differential count
- Blood culture
- Urinalysis
- Urine culture
- Chest x-ray (if respiratory symptoms are present, such as an upper respiratory tract infection and cough or congestion)
- Lumbar puncture for cerebrospinal fluid analysis
  - Culture
  - Cell count
  - Glucose
  - Protein
  - Gram stain

Box 26-4   "Low-Risk" Criteria in Febrile Infants Who Do Not Have an Apparent Source of Infection

- Previously healthy
- Do not appear clinically ill
- No focal bacterial infection on physical examination (except otitis media)
- Good social situation
- Negative laboratory screening
  - White blood cell count of 5000 to 15,000/mm^3
  - Less than 1500 bands/mm^3
  - Normal urinalysis (<5 white blood cells per high powered field)
  - Less than 3 white blood cells per high powered field in stool (if diarrhea is present)

From Baraff LJ, et al: Practice guidelines for the management of infants and children 0-36 months of age with fever without source, *Pediatrics* 92(1):4, 1993.

EMERGENCY DEPARTMENT INTERVENTIONS

Medical protocols for managing the febrile child vary significantly from institution to institution and between specialties, for example, pediatrics and emergency medicine. In general, management of the febrile child is more aggressive in the emergency department than in the private practice or clinic setting, where the medical team is more familiar with the child and family. In 1993 practice guidelines were set by a panel of experts recommending that all febrile neonates (less than 28 days of age) be hospitalized and receive a sepsis evaluation.[7] The guidelines are less strict when applied to children 2 to 3 months of age.

Emergency department interventions are determined by the initial clinical impression, age of the child, and history and physical findings. Febrile infants younger than 28 days of age usually require a full sepsis workup and admission. Some physicians routinely treat these infants with antimicrobial therapy regardless of test results; others may not treat with antimicrobial therapy, pending culture results (Box 26-3).

Older infants, between 1 and 3 months of age, who appear well and are found to have a focal sign of infection may be sent home but only after the infant has been determined to be "low risk" and if the parent is considered reliable to maintain close follow-up (Box

26-4). If the well-appearing infant has no focal signs of infection but meets the low-risk criteria, the infant may or may not receive ceftriaxone parenterally pending culture results and depending on physician preference. Regardless, close follow-up with reliable parents must be assured.[7,8] All ill-appearing young infants, regardless of body temperature, require a full sepsis workup (Fig. 26-4).

Children 3 to 24 months of age who do not appear ill and have an obvious focal source of infection (e.g., otitis media, cellulitis) are treated symptomatically, and the tests ordered are based on physical findings. When the child looks well but history and physical findings reveal no obvious focal findings, a urinalysis and white blood cell count may be ordered. A urine culture may also be ordered, since the absence of pyuria does not completely rule out a urinary tract infection; a small percentage of such infections are not associated with pyuria.[17] If the white blood cell count is greater than 15,000 cells/mm^3, a blood culture is obtained. A chest x-ray is indicated if the child shows evidence of significant respiratory tract involvement (e.g., tachypnea with signs of increased work of breathing or adventitious sounds). When these tests fail to reveal a bacterial source of infection, the child may be treated with antimicrobial therapy before

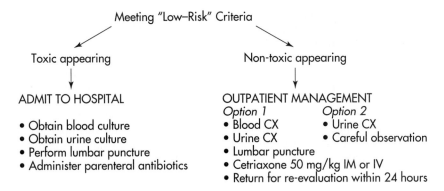

Meeting "Low–Risk" Criteria

Toxic appearing → ADMIT TO HOSPITAL
- Obtain blood culture
- Obtain urine culture
- Perform lumbar puncture
- Administer parenteral antibiotics

Non-toxic appearing → OUTPATIENT MANAGEMENT

Option 1
- Blood CX
- Urine CX
- Lumbar puncture
- Cetriaxone 50 mg/kg IM or IV
- Return for re-evaluation within 24 hours

Option 2
- Urine CX
- Careful observation

FIG. 26-4. Management of fever without a source in the infants and young children (28 to 90 days old). (From Baraff LJ et al: Practice guidelines for the management of infants and children 0-36 months of age with fever without source. *Pediatrics* 92:1, 1993.)

being discharged from the emergency department or at home until culture results are obtained. The child may also be sent home with a return visit scheduled within 24 hours. Febrile children at high risk for serious illness, such as those with a history of bronchopulmonary dysplasia, sickle cell disease, steroid administration, or those with a central venous line (e.g., Port-a-Cath or Broviac), generally require an extensive workup based on the history and presenting signs and symptoms.

Children older than 2 to 3 years of age are treated symptomatically. As in younger children, the child's history and appearance guide emergency department management.

NURSING CARE AND EVALUATION

INITIAL IMPRESSION AND TRIAGE

Triage of the febrile child varies from institution to institution. Physician preference and physical layout of the department are major influences. In general, febrile neonates, regardless of presentation, are triaged emergently. Children who look ill, regardless of body temperature, are also triaged as emergently.

Some emergency departments have established triage guidelines that use the height of the fever as the criterion for triaging a child emergently or urgently. In departments where nurses with primarily adult experience triage children, this practice may be warranted, since nurses with limited experience may lack the clinical skills necessary to identify a serious illness such

as meningitis. But in departments where experienced pediatric nurses triage children, it may prevent other children, whom the nurse clinically assesses to be more seriously ill, from being given priority care. In these settings the general appearance of the child coupled with the child's age, risk factors, history, and chief complaint should be used to prioritize care, rather than the height of the fever (see Chapter 5, Pediatric Triage).

Many infants and young children come to the emergency department with a history of fever at home, yet on arrival they are afebrile or have a low-grade temperature. In these situations the nurse should ask the caregiver how the temperature was taken and where it was taken (e.g., rectally, ear, skin temperature strips, tactile, etc.). Tactile temperatures are notoriously unreliable, and studies of young infants (less than 3 months of age) have shown that if the infant is afebrile on arrival in the emergency department and does not exhibit signs of serious illness, the infant is unlikely to have a serious illness.[10,12] Conversely, the infant who is afebrile on arrival in the emergency department but who had a documented rectal fever at home should be treated as any other febrile infant.[37]

Occasionally, infants younger than 2 to 3 months of age arrive in the emergency department with questionable fevers, that is, a fever 0.2° to 0.4° F over what is considered high (fever is defined as ≥ 100.4° F [38° C]), for example 100.6° F. Because the body temperatures of young infants tend to equalize with the environment, the nurse should note (1) how the infant was dressed (Was he bundled?); (2) the air temperature outside (Is it a hot day?); and (3) if the infant was transported to the emergency department in an un-air-conditioned environment. If the infant looks well and the history does not suggest a serious illness, the infant can be dressed loosely and the temperature retaken in 15 minutes.

ROUTES FOR TAKING THE CHILD'S TEMPERATURE

There is much debate regarding the most effective method of obtaining accurate temperatures in children. If the chief complaint is a foreign body in the eye, obtaining an accurate core body temperature is less important than if the child arrives with a 3-day history of cold symptoms, fussiness, and diarrhea or if the child is a neonate. Therefore less invasive methods of obtaining body temperatures may be used on children who are not at high risk for a serious febrile illness. These methods include axillary or auditory canal temperatures. In general, the rectal route remains the "gold standard" method of obtaining reliable temperatures in young infants[42,50] (Box 26-5).

Box 26-5	Comparison of Routes for Taking the Child's Temperature

Rectal	Rectal temperatures most closely represent the core temperature of the body and are therefore the most reliable method of determining temperature elevation in the child. Because the height of the fever may be the determining factor when deciding to admit an infant—particularly the neonate—rectal temperatures remain the "gold standard." Although there is concern that rectal perforation may occur, reports of this are rare.[21,45] Rectal temperatures are contraindicated in immunosuppressed children and in infants with anal atresia.
Oral	The oral route is another common site used to obtain the child's temperature. Accuracy associated with use of this site depends on the child's cooperation with the procedure; therefore oral temperatures are generally not recommended until the child is approximately 3 to 5 years of age. Oral temperatures are more variable than rectal temperatures, and these variations can be caused by a number of factors, including the consumption of warm or cold liquids, hyperventilation (as might occur during an asthma attack), and the positioning of the thermometer in the sublingual pocket.
Axillary	Axillary temperatures are the least reliable method of determining the child's body temperature. Because the axillary temperature relies on the temperature of the skin, it may be affected by sweating and alterations in perfusion.[42] Attempts to predict the child's oral or rectal temperature using axillary measurements have been unsuccessful.[2,14] The one exception to the axillary-versus-core-temperature variation is the neonate. Neonates have a fairly homogeneous body temperature, and the temperature gradient between the axilla and core temperature is small, particularly when the environmental temperature is controlled, as it is in a hospital newborn unit. Although this method is used in many newborn units, it has not gained wide acceptance in hospital emergency department since the infant's exposure to extreme environmental temperatures cannot be controlled.
Auditory canal (tympanic)	Auditory canal thermometers (ACT) reflect the average temperature of the tympanic membrane, which represents core temperature and the cooler skin of the auditory canal. These thermometers use built-in conversion factors to estimate either oral or rectal temperature of the child. Numerous studies have debated the efficacy of ACTs to obtain accurate temperature readings. Although findings in both adults and children have been contradictory, studies in children seem to confirm inconsistencies in measurements.[9,26] For this reason, ACT measurements should not be used when temperature measurement is critical, for example, when the decision to admit an infant will be based on the height of the body temperature.

ANTIPYRETIC ADMINISTRATION

Antipyretic therapy is often given before the child is seen by the physician, both to alleviate the child's discomfort and to decrease the body temperature. Some emergency departments administer antipyretics to all febrile children (temperature at least 101° F [38.3° C]) over the age of 3 months; others only administer antipyretic therapy when the child appears to "feel bad" or is at risk (e.g., history of febrile seizures). Acetaminophen liquid, 15 mg/kg, is used primarily; however, ibuprofen 10 mg/kg is being used with more frequency in young children. Salicylates are no longer recommended because of an association with the development of Reye's syndrome.

Before giving an antipyretic, the parents are asked if their child received a medication to reduce the fever within 4 hours of arrival in the emergency department. If the child received no acetaminophen or received less than the recommended dose, it can be administered by the nurse. If the child received acetaminophen but remains febrile and "feels bad," ibuprofen 10 mg/kg may be administered. Ibuprofen is contraindicated in children with known allergies to salicylates, liver or renal disease, bleeding disorders, or gastrointestinal disorders such as ulcers. There is some debate as to whether ibuprofen should be administered to children with chickenpox, since its chemical makeup is similar to that of aspirin; however, there is no documented evidence that the administration of ibuprofen in the presence of chickenpox increases a child's risk of developing Reye syndrome (Table 26-4).

SPONGING

Hyperpyrexic children (temperature over 105° F [40.6° C]) or children who have a history of febrile seizures are occasionally sponged while in the emergency department. Although this practice is somewhat controversial, its use as a method of temperature reduction continues.[48] One study indicated that although children who received both acetaminophen and sponging cooled more quickly than children who received acetaminophen alone, there was no difference in overall temperature change between the two groups at the end of 2 hours.[44]

When sponging is performed, lukewarm water—not cold water—is used. Alcohol is *never* indicated, since it may be absorbed into the skin, causing toxicity. Unfortunately, shivering is a common response to sponging in the emergency department, since the environmental temperature is difficult to control. Shivering represents an increase in the metabolic rate

in an attempt to maintain body temperature at the hypothalamic set point and may actually cause the temperature to rise further. For this reason, sponging should be performed only when the child is at greatest risk for serious sequelae resulting directly from the fever, such as with repeated febrile seizures.[41]

DIAGNOSTIC PROCEDURES

Diagnostic testing is performed on all children who "look sick," which usually includes a white blood cell count and urinalysis. When a urinalysis and/or culture is ordered in a very young child, urine should be collected before painful or fear-producing procedures such as a lumbar or venipuncture, since the child may urinate spontaneously during the procedure. If a urine bag is used for collecting the specimen, the surrounding skin should be thoroughly cleaned and dried before the bag is placed on the child. Urine cultures collected from a bagged specimen are generally considered unreliable. For this reason, when an accurate urine culture is required in a diapered child, urinary catheterization or suprapubic bladder aspiration should be performed. Some physicians, however, reserve these "invasive" procedures for children in whom they strongly suspect a urinary tract infection.

When blood work is obtained, an intravenous (IV) or intermittent catheter may be inserted to maintain vascular access and/or administer fluids and antibiotics. If the child appears to "feel bad" and blood work is ordered, it is helpful to ask the physician if an intermittent (heparin lock) catheter can be inserted at that time. Children tolerate venipuncture poorly, and the child who may have been cooperative for one venipuncture is not likely to cooperate for a second. Children well enough to be discharged but requiring parenteral antimicrobial therapy can then receive the drug intravenously rather than intramuscularly before discharge. Although some nurses have expressed the concern that drawing blood cultures through an IV catheter increases the risk of contamination, this is not the case as long as the site has been properly prepared.[24]

A lumbar puncture should be anticipated for all children in whom sepsis or meningitis is suspected. Many institutions require the physician obtain parental consent before performing the procedure. Depending on physician preference, the child may be placed in the lateral decubitus position or in an upright, bent-forward position. During the procedure the child's respiratory and cardiovascular status must

TABLE 26-4	Suggested Guideline for Antipyretic Administration
Infants younger than 8 weeks of age	Should not receive an antipyretic before being seen by the physician
Infants 8 weeks to 6 months of age	If rectal temperature ≥101° F (38.3° C) and infant has not received acetaminophen in the past 4 hours, administer 15 mg/kg of acetaminophen
	If infant received antipyretic therapy before arrival but the nurse determines the child was underdosed, give the appropriate balance of the dose
Children older than 6 months of age	If the oral or rectal temperature is ≥101° F and child has not received acetaminophen in the past 4 hours, administer 15 mg/kg of acetaminophen
	If the oral or rectal temperature is ≥102° F and/or child has received acetaminophen in the past 4 hours, administer 10 mg/kg of ibuprofen
	NOTE: If a child's temperature is ≥102° F the emergency nurse may administer either acetaminophen or ibuprofen depending on history, height of the fever, and antipyretic therapy given before arrival in the emergency department. Acetaminophen suppositories may be given to the child with protracted vomiting.

Acetaminophen—contraindications/exclusions
1. History of any recent overdose or toxic ingestion
2. Allergy to acetaminophen
3. History of liver disease
4. Any child less than 2 months of age—until seen by a physician
5. Isolated abdominal pain

Ibuprofen—contraindications/exclusions
1. History of any recent overdose or toxic ingestion
2. Allergy to aspirin or nonsteroidal antiinflammatory agents
3. History of kidney disease, ulcer, gastrointestinal bleeding, or severe liver disease
4. Any child <6 months of age unless approved by the emergency department physician
5. Any history of blood dyscrasias, including platelet disorders
6. Any child with chickenpox or on chemotherapy unless approved by the emergency department physician

NOTE: Any febrile child who fits the emergent criteria or appears ill should be seen immediately by an emergency department physician.

be continuously monitored, since flexion of the neck may compromise the airway.

FLUID ADMINISTRATION

Increased oral fluid intake is often recommended in the febrile child, since fever increases insensible fluid losses through the skin and respiratory tract. If the child looks well and the history is negative for serious illness, oral fluids should be encouraged. If the child is mildly to severely dehydrated and has a history of significant vomiting, parenteral fluids may be indicated. Some children with a chronic or acute illness may require fluid restriction or close monitoring of fluid intake and output (e.g., congestive heart failure, renal failure, or bacterial meningitis).

Box 26-6   Clinical Evaluation of the Febrile Infant and Child

General appearance
  *A*irway patency, audible sounds
  *B*reathing pattern, work of breathing
  *C*olor of skin, rashes
  *D*egree of responsiveness to people and the
    environment:
      Arousability
      Consolability
      Recognition of the parent(s)
      Age-appropriate response to pain
        and fear
      Playfulness
      Social smile
      Eye contact
Fontanel (infants)
Character of cry
Hydration status
Vital signs (temperature, pulse, respiratory
  rate, baseline blood pressure)
  NOTE: Pulse and respiratory rate are nor-
  mally elevated as the body temperature
  rises.
All abnormal parameters should be reassessed
  at least every 30 minutes, or more often if a
  serious illness is suspected.

EVALUATION

Febrile children should be reassessed frequently for general appearance, activity level, demeanor, and temperature reduction (Box 26-6). In the busy emergency department the child with a moderate fever on arrival may look quite ill as body temperature rises or as the illness progresses, or the child may improve in appearance as the body temperature decreases. The child who refused eye contact, was clinging to the parent, and cried continuously during the initial assessment may later be smiling, playful, and exploring the examination room. Conversely, the child may become irritable, less arousable, or unconcerned with the environment. All of these observational findings should be documented by the nurse.

One area of disagreement regarding reassessment parameters is that of retaking the child's temperature after antipyretic therapy. From a nursing perspective, all interventions are reevaluated. Therefore the degree of temperature reduction is evaluated after antipyretic therapy. However, temperature reduction alone is not a reflection of the child's clinical status, nor is there evidence that fever reduction is an indication of the seriousness of the illness. This finding then simply indicates that the child did or did not respond to the antipyretic. If the child remains febrile, what discharge parameters are then acceptable (i.e., height of the fever, degree of temperature reduction, or clinical appearance)? Nurses and physicians who argue this point believe the clinical appearance coupled with risk factors are the most important assessment parameters, not the height of the fever or the degree of temperature reduction. Using this philosophy, documentation of the child's clinical status at discharge is most important.

∎ SUMMARY

Management of the febrile child in the emergency department is a controversial topic for which there are many acceptable approaches. In the emergency department where nurses and physicians possess limited knowledge of pediatrics, strict, objective criteria may be used to guide treatment (age and height of the fever). Conversely, in emergency departments familiar with pediatric care, clinical appearance may be relied on more heavily than height of the fever, or the child's age. Regardless of the approach, the emergency department nurse should be familiar with institutional protocols for the initial assessment, acceptable interventions, and reevaluation of the febrile child.

REFERENCES

1. Alpert G, Hibbert E, Fleisher GR: Case-control study of hyperpyrexia in children, *Pediatr Infect Dis J* 9(3):160-161, 1990.
2. Anagnostakis D et al: Rectal-axillary temperature difference in febrile and afebrile infants and children, *Clin Pediatr* 32(5):268-272, 1993.
3. Applegate MS, Lo W: Febrile seizures: concepts concerning prognosis and clinical management, *J Fam Pract* 29:424-428, 1989.
4. Baker MD, Fosarelli PD, Carpenter RO: Childhood fever: correlation of diagnosis with temperature response to acetaminophen, *Pediatrics* 80:315-318, 1987.
5. Baker MD, Avner JR, Bell LM: Failure of infant observation scales in detecting serious illness in

febrile, 4-8 week old infants, *Pediatrics* 85(6):1040-1043, 1990.

6. Baker R et al: Severity of disease correlated with fever reduction in febrile infants, *Pediatrics* 83(6):1016-1019, 1989.

7. Baraff LJ et al: Practice guidelines for the management of infants and children 0-36 months of age with fever without source, *Pediatrics* 92(1):1-12, 1993.

8. Baskin MN, O'Rourke EJ, Fleisher GR: Outpatient treatment of febrile infants 28-89 days of age with intramuscular administration of ceftriaxone, *J Pediatr* 120(1):22-27, 1992.

9. Bernardo LM et al: A comparison of aural and rectal temperature measurements in children with moderate and severe injuries, *J Emerg Nurs* 22(5):403-408, 1996.

10. Bonadio WA: Incidence of serious infections in afebrile neonates with a history of fever, *Pediatr Infect Dis J* 6:911-914, 1987.

11. Bonadio WA, Hegenbarth M, Zachariason M: Correlating reported fever in young infants with subsequent fever patterns and rate of serious bacterial infections, *Pediatr Infect Dis J* 9:158-160, 1990.

12. Bonadio WA, Romine K, Y Gyuro J: Relationship of fever magnitude to rate or serious bacterial infections in neonates, *J Pediatr* 733-734, May 1990.

13. Bonadio WA et al: Correlating infectious outcome with clinical parameters of 1130 consecutive febrile infants aged zero to eight weeks, *Pediatr Emerg Care* 9(2):84-86, 1993.

14. Brown RD et al: A probability nomogram to predict rectal temperature in children, *Clin Pediatr* 31(9):523-531, 1992.

15. Cheng TL, Partridge JC: Effect of bundling and high environmental temperature on neonatal body temperature, *Pediatrics* 92(2):238-240, 1993.

16. Erickson RS, Woo TM: Accuracy of infrared ear thermometry and traditional temperature methods in young children, *Heart Lung* 23(3):181, 1994.

17. Felter RA: Infectious disorders. In Barkin RM, ed: *Pediatric emergency medicine, concepts and clinical practice*, St Louis, 1992, Mosby.

18. Florida Emergency Medical Services for Children: Unpublished data, University of Florida Health Science Center, Jacksonville, Fla, 1988.

19. Freeman JM, Vining EP: Decision making and the child with febrile seizures, *Pediatr Rev* 13(8):298-304, 1992.

20. Gonzales Del Rey JA, Paul R: Seizures, febrile. In Barkin RM, ed: *Pediatric emergency medicine: concepts and clinical practice*, St Louis, 1992, Mosby.

21. Greenbaum EE et al: Recal thermometer-induced pneumoperitoneum in the newborn, *Pediatrics* 44:539-542, 1969.

22. Grover G et al: The effects of bundling on infant temperatures, *Pediatrics* 94(5):669-673, 1994.

23. Herzog LW, Coyne LJ: What is fever? Normal temperature in infants less than 3 months old, *Clin Pediatr* 32(3):142-145, 1993.

24. Isaacman DJ, Karaskic RB: Lack of effect of changing needles on contamination of blood cultures, *Pediatr Infect Dis J* 9(4):274-278, 1990.

25. Johnson KJ, Batia P, Bell EF: Infrared thermometry of newborn infants, *Pediatrics* 87:34-38, 1991.

26. Koziol-Melain J, Oman K, Edwards G: Ear temperatures: making research-based clinical decisions, *J Emerg Nurs* 22(1):77-79, 1996.

27. Kluger MJ: Fever: role of pyrogens and cryogens, *Physiol Rev* 71:93-127, 1991.

28. Mackowaik PA, Wasserman SS, Levine MM: A critical appraisal of 98.6° F, the upper limit of the normal body temperature, and other legacies of Carl Reinhold August Wunderlich, *JAMA* 268(12):1578-1580, 1992.

29. McCarthy PL: Controversies in pediatrics: what tests are indicated for the child under 2 with fever, *Pediatr Rev* 1(2):51-56, 1979.

30. McCarthy PL, Dolan TF: Hyperpyrexia in children—eight year emergency room experience, *Am J Dis Child* 130:849, 1976.

31. McCarthy PL, Jekel JF, Dolan TF: Temperature greater than or equal to 40°C in children less than 24 months of age: a prospective study, *Pediatrics* 59:663-668, 1977.

32. McCarthy PL et al: History and observation variables in assessing febrile children, *Pediatrics* 65(6):1090, 1980.

33. McCarthy PL et al: Observation scales to identify serious illness in febrile children, *Pediatrics* 70(5):802, 1982.

34. McClennan D, Giebnick GS: Perspectives on occult bacteremia in children, *J Pediatrics* 109:1-8, 1986.

35. McGowan JE et al: Bacteremia in febrile children seen in a "walk-in" pediatric clinic, *N Engl J Med* 288:1309-1312, 1973.

36. Offringa M et al: Seizures and fever: can we rule out meningitis on clinical grounds alone? *Clin Pediatr* 31:9, 514-522, 1992.

37. Powell KR: Evaluation and management of febrile infants younger than 60 days of age, *Pediatr Infect Dis J* 9(3):153-157, 1990.

38. Press S, Fawcett N: Association of temperature greater than 41.1°C with serious illness, *Clin Pediatr* 24:21, 1985.

39. Roddy SM, McBride MC: Seizure disorders. In Hoekelman RA, ed: *Primary pediatric care*, St. Louis, 1997, Mosby.

40. Romano MJ et al: Infrared tympanic thermometry in the pediatric intensive care unit, *Crit Care Med* 21(8):1181-1185, 1993.

41. Santer LJ, Stenklyft PH, Luten RC: *Handbook of common pediatric emergencies*, ed 2, Jacksonville, Fla, 1993, University of Florida Health Science Center.

42. Schuman AJ: The accuracy of infrared auditory canal

thermometry in infants and children, *Clin Pediatr* 32(6):347-354, 1993.

43. Selfridge J, Shea SS: The accuracy of the tympanic membrane thermometer in detecting fever in infants aged 3 months and younger in the emergency department setting, *J Emerg Nurs* 19(2):127-130, 1993.

44. Sharber J: A comparison of methods to reduce fever in young children, *J Emerg Nurs* 21(5):464, 1995.

45. Smiddy FG, Benson EA: Rectal perforation by thermometer, *Lancet* 2:805-806, 1969.

46. Soud T: The febrile child in the emergency department, *J Emerg Nurs* 19(4):355-358, 1993.

47. Styrt B, Sugarman B: Antipyresis and fever, *Arch Intern Med* 150:1589-1597, 1990.

48. Thomas V et al: National survey of pediatric fever management practices among emergency department nurses, *J Emerg Nurs* 20(6):505-509, 1994.

49. Torrey S et al: Temperature response to antipyretic therapy in children: relationship to occult bacteremia, *Am J Emerg Med* 3:190-192, 1985.

50. Vander Jagt EW: Fever. In Hoekelman RA, ed: *Primary pediatric care*, St Louis, 1997, Mosby.

51. Walson PD et al: Comparison of multidose ibuprofen and acetaminophen therapy in febrile children, *Am J Dis Child* 146:626-632, 1992.

52. Wasserman GM, White CB: Evaluation of the necessity for hospitalization of the febrile infant less than three months of age, *Pediatr Infect Dis J* 9(3):163-169, 1990.

53. Wong DL: *Whaley and Wong's essentials of pediatric nursing*, ed 5, St Louis, 1997, Mosby.

54. Wright PF et al: Patterns of illness in the highly febrile child: epidemiologic, clinical, and laboratory correlates, *Pediatrics* 67(5):694-700, 1981.

55. Yamamoto L et al: Relationship of bacteremia to antipyretic therapy in febrile children, *Pediatr Emerg Care* 3:223-227, 1987.

CHAPTER 27

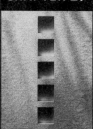

Environmental and Toxicologic Emergencies

Cheryl A. Tucker, Jay L. Schauben

Poisonings and Ingestions

EPIDEMIOLOGY

Over 250,000 drugs and commercial products are accessible to the average individual for ingestion.[26] With approximately 400 containers of potentially toxic substances entering the average home each year, it is no wonder that poisoning exposures account for nearly 10% of all emergency department visits and 5% to 10% of all medical admissions. In 1993 the Ameri-

---

Box 27-1   Substances Most Frequently Involved in Human Exposures

Cleaning substances
Analgesics
Cosmetics and personal care products
Cough and cold preparations
Plants
Bites/envenomations
Topicals
Pesticides (includes rodenticides)
Foreign bodies
Antimicrobials
Food products, food poisoning
Hydrocarbons
Sedatives/hypnotics/antipsychotics
Alcohols
Chemicals
Vitamins
Antidepressants

From Litovitz TL, Clark LR, and Soloway RA: *Am J Emerg Med* 12:546-584, 1994.

---

can Association of Poison Control Centers (AAPCC) reported over 1.7 million exposures to potentially toxic substances from 64 participating poison centers. Of these reported exposures, 90% occurred in the home, 86% were accidental, and 56% occurred in children under the age of 6 years. Extrapolating these data to encompass the entire United States population would predict a startling 4.3 million exposures each year. Fortunately, 45% of all poisoning exposures were classified as nontoxic and required no intervention. In general, poisoning exposures in children (75%) are unintentional in nature and therefore largely preventable with formalized public education (Box 27-1).[42]

NURSING HISTORY AND ASSESSMENT

The nursing history and assessment play an important role in the initial recognition of the poisoned child and in ongoing management. Data must be collected and interpreted rapidly to assess the toxic potential of the exposure. If the child's condition is unstable or has the potential to rapidly become unstable, emergency interventions are required.

The primary survey is the most important priority in the initial assessment and includes evaluation of the airway, breathing, and circulation. At the same time, caution must be used when moving a child to protect the cervical spine, particularly when a traumatic injury may have accompanied the exposure. The secondary survey includes a brief head-to-toe assessment to identify specific deviations from normal findings. A full neurologic survey is performed using recognized assessment tools such as the Glasgow Coma Scale (see Chapter 7, p. 137). Serial assessments using these scores are helpful and establish a progression of the child's clinical course.

After an ingestion, and whenever possible, the specific product container should be obtained. Similarities in brand names and the wide variety of active ingredients that could be involved leave too many possibilities for mismanagement if positive identification of the product is not obtained. Preexisting medical conditions, chronic medication use, substance abuse, or other items pertinent to the child's medical history are additional ingredients necessary for a complete patient assessment (Box 27-2).

TOXIC SYNDROMES

Over the years, clinicians have consistently grouped signs and symptoms of toxic ingestions as manifestations of a particular toxic exposure. Continuous patient assessment for the development of delayed symptoms or for these groups of symptoms (toxidromes) may lead to rapid identification of a specific toxin in the unknown exposure situation (Table 27-1). Patient history, physical examination, clinical symptoms, and laboratory results are all important when delineating a specific toxidrome. Recognition of the toxidrome alone may avert ordering an array of broad-spectrum, nonspecific toxicologic screens. Using the child's clinical symptoms when ordering specific toxicologic screens increases the probability of determining the toxin. One study actually compared the accuracy of the recognition of toxidromes in suspected overdose patients among nurses, physicians, and pharmacists. In this study, nurses achieved the highest percentage of correct toxidrome choices when compared to the drug screen results reported.[51]

NURSING INTERVENTIONS

EMERGENCY MANAGEMENT OF THE POISONED CHILD

Initial management of the emergently ill, poisoned child begins with the same procedures used for any patient requiring emergency care. Stabilization of the airway, breathing, and circulation (ABCs) always takes priority over other antidotal and decontamination interventions. Airway assessment for the gag or cough reflex, positioning the patient, clearing the airway via suction, and frequent monitoring of ventilatory function are essential. Depending on the source of the ingestion, the child may require ventilatory assistance with a bag-valve-mask device or maintenance of the airway with oral or nasopharyngeal devices. Supplemental oxygen is indicated for any child who is lethargic or obtunded and is universally used in the unstable child. Endotracheal intubation may be required to maintain a patent airway or to prevent the aspiration of gastric contents into the lungs. Assessment of oxygenation with arterial blood gas measurements or continuous monitoring via pulse oximeter should also be considered.

Intravenous access must be established rapidly, particularly when circulation is compromised or has the potential to become compromised rapidly. The child may be placed in the Trendelenburg position to improve venous return while being given intravenous (IV) fluids to correct hypovolemia.[66] The intrapulmonary (via endotracheal tube) and in-

Box 27-2	Essential Historical Data After an Exposure
Patient characteristics	Name, age, weight, sex, site where exposure occurred, medical history, current medications
Exposure characteristics	Substance, amount, route of exposure, how, when, why, presence of symptoms
	Positive identification of product (container obtained if possible)
	Associated trauma from exposure
	Chemicals or other products available in the environment
Management	Treatment rendered before arrival in emergency department
	Recognition of toxic syndrome

TABLE 27-1	Common Toxidromes		
TOXIN	VITAL SIGNS	MENTAL STATUS	OTHER
Anticholinergics	↑HR, ↑T	Delirium, hallucinations, lethargy to coma	Dry skin and mucous membranes, ↓ bowel sounds, urinary retention, flushed appearance, mydriasis
Beta blockers	↓BP, ↓HR	Confusion, dizziness	Cyanosis, seizures
Carbon monoxide	Varies from normal to cardiac arrest	May vary from lethargy to coma	Headache, dizziness, confusion, nausea, vomiting, electrocardiographic effects, seizures
Cyclic antidepressants	↑HR, ↓BP, ↑T	May vary from agitation, lethargy to coma	Confusion, mydriasis, dry mucous membranes, flushed, seizures, urinary retention, cardiac dysrhythmias
Iron	↓BP (late), ↑HR (late)	Normal unless ↓BP, lethargy	Nausea, vomiting, diarrhea, abdominal pain, hematemesis, acidosis, shock, seizures
Opioids	↓BP, ↓HR, ↓RR, ↓T	May vary from euphoria to coma	Miosis, absent bowel sounds, shallow respirations
Organophosphates	↓HR/↑HR, ↓BP/↑BP, ↓RR/↑RR	Sedation to coma	SLUDGE (Salivation, Lacrimation, Urination, Defecation, Gastrointestinal distress, Emesis), bronchorrhea, bronchoconstriction, weakness, muscle fasciculations, restlessness, seizures
Phenothiazines	↓BP, ↑HR; ↓T/↑T	Lethargy to coma	Dystonic reactions, ataxia, dizziness, tremor, seizures
Salicylates	↑T, ↑RR	Agitation to coma	Vomiting, tinnitus, confusion, diaphoresis, acidosis, shock
Sedative-hypnotics	↓RR, ↓T, ↓BP	Lethargy to coma	Ataxia, nystagmus, slurred speech
Sympathomimetics	↑HR, ↑BP, ↑T	Agitated, hyperactive	Tremors, sweating, seizures, cardiac dysrhythmias
Theophylline	↑HR, ↓BP, ↑RR, ↑T	Agitation to coma	Vomiting, diaphoresis, tremor, seizures

HR, Heart rate; BP, blood pressure; T, temperature; RR, respiratory rate.
Adapted from Goldfrank LR, et al: *Goldfrank's toxicologic emergencies*, Norwalk, CT, 1994, Appleton & Lange.

traosseous routes for drug administration may be used as alternatives if IV access cannot be established quickly. Vasopressors and/or inotropic agents may also be necessary to improve hemodynamic status.

If the child is unconscious or having a seizure, a rapid bedside assessment of blood glucose level is indicated before the administration of dextrose. Recent evidence suggests that the administration of glucose in the child with an altered mental status may not be as innocuous as previously believed. *Avoidance* of excessive glucose loads in patients at risk for cerebral ischemia (those with acute stroke, in impending cardiac arrest, with severe hypotension, or receiving cardiopulmonary resuscitation [CPR]) is now recommended.[10] The choice of therapy for seizure control often depends on the specific toxin involved. Higher than normal doses of anticonvulsant medication may be required to control toxin-induced seizures. In some circumstances, secondary therapeutic agents may be required to control seizures. For example, cyclic antidepressants require serum alkalinization to effectively control seizures and dysrhythmias; glucose is indicated when the child has overdosed on an oral hypoglycemic agent; and pyridoxine is indicated for an isoniazid overdose.

The child's status is often unstable and unpredictable after a toxic exposure. Therefore during the course of treatment the nurse must continuously reassess the child's airway, ventilatory status, hemodynamic and neurologic status, vital signs, and urinary output.

▌ EXTERNAL DECONTAMINATION

Various products available in the average home contain chemicals toxic to the skin or capable of dermal absorption. When a child has been exposed to a hazardous substance, the nurse must first don protective equipment, including gloves, a gown, and a protective mask. Immediate removal of the child's clothing followed by a complete and thorough washing of the skin with soap and water is imperative to terminate dermal damage. Flushing with warm water prevents inadvertent lowering of the child's body temperature. Special attention should be given to the eyes and other mucous membranes, as well as the hair, fingernails, and navel. "Neutralizing" an acid with a base and vice versa is not recommended because it may cause further thermal damage.

Ocular exposure to chemical substances requires immediate irrigation with copious amounts of water or saline solution. A minimum of 15 minutes' irrigation is recommended. The infant or toddler may be wrapped in a towel or blanket or may be placed on a restraining board to facilitate adequate irrigation of the eyes. Prolonged irrigation, approximately 30 minutes or longer for each eye, is indicated for exposures to caustic substances. Visual acuity should be assessed after all ocular exposures.

▌ GASTRIC DECONTAMINATION

SYRUP OF IPECAC

Ipecac syrup contains a mixture of the plant alkaloids emetine and cephaeline. Two distinct mechanisms of action are responsible for its emetic effect: direct irritation of the gastric mucosa and central stimulation of the brain's chemoreceptor trigger zone.[47] It has long been recognized as the emetic of choice for home management of the poisoned child, since most poisoning incidents in children are discovered within minutes of the ingestion.

The decision to induce vomiting is based on established criteria, which consider the toxic potential of the agent (both acute and delayed), the reliability of the historical data, and the patient's clinical status. If the child has ingested a nontoxic agent or a nontoxic amount of a potentially toxic agent, gastric emptying is not necessary. When induction of emesis is indicated, it is important to understand the characteristics of syrup of ipecac. The average recovery of drug from emesis is estimated at 28%, with a range of 0% to 78%,[30] and recovery is highly correlated with the administration time of ipecac after the ingestion.[50] Response to ipecac syrup varies with the time since ingestion, stomach contents, and individual receptiveness. Its emetic effects can persist for 45 minutes to 6 hours.[16]

Although ipecac syrup is effective in inducing emesis, its efficacy as a gastric decontamination procedure is questionable. The time delay encountered before the onset of emesis allows the ingested toxin to be partially absorbed in the gastrointestinal (GI) tract. In contrast, many drugs and toxic substances are rapidly adsorbed onto activated charcoal in the GI tract with very little lag time.[50]

A delay in the administration of activated charcoal can occur if gastric emptying with ipecac syrup has been initiated and continuing emesis occurs. Ipecac can also interfere with the retention of activated charcoal because of repeated emesis (up to 6 hours), potentially prolonging the time a child will need to remain in the emergency department.[37]

Emergency Department and nursing interventions. In general, the use of ipecac syrup is reserved for home management. Once the child arrives in the emergency department more definitive modes of therapy should be instituted. Some general information regarding the administration of ipecac follows.

Ipecac syrup administration is not recommended in children less than 6 months of age because of their immature airway protective reflexes. The dosing in older children or adults is adjusted by age (Table 27-2). Oral fluid administration after the administration of ipecac syrup augments the gastric emptying effect. A dose of 5 ml of water/kg body weight is recommended in infants and children, and 250 ml is recommended in older children or adults. Tepid water is preferred, since cold water reduces gastric emptying time.[65] Emesis usually occurs within 15 to 20 minutes of ipecac administration; however, if vomiting has not occurred within 30 minutes, the dose of ipecac can be repeated once. If the child becomes sleepy after repeated emesis, he or she should be placed on the left side to protect the airway in case of further emesis. The child who has received ipecac must be continuously monitored, and suction equipment must be readily available on arrival in the emergency department. Ipecac syrup administration is not without risks. Prolonged vomiting and diarrhea are not uncommon (Box 27-3).

GASTRIC LAVAGE

Lavage, as a means of gastric emptying, is indicated for the child who has ingested a potentially toxic substance and comes for treatment within a 1- to 2-hour time window. Although gastric lavage is widely used, recent studies have failed to show significant benefits

in patient outcome among acutely overdosed pediatric patients.[21,39,44] Nevertheless, the procedure is still performed as part of the overdose management protocol. Before the insertion of a lavage tube, the child's ability to protect the airway should be assessed. Endotracheal intubation is indicated if this ability is in question.

For practitioners still using gastric lavage, the indications for use include the following: (1) severe symptoms (seizures, cardiac disturbances, or respiratory depression [airway must be protected]); (2) ingestion of agents that decrease GI motility (anticholinergics, opioids) or cause pylorospasm (aspirin); (3) ingestion of solids rather than liquids; (4) moderate to severe potential for toxicity in a child coming for treatment less than 2 hours after ingestion; or (5) impending or potential loss of airway protective reflexes (as opposed to inducing vomiting using ipecac [airway must be protected]). Oral insertion of the gastric tube is desirable, since nasal insertion may injure the nasal mucosa or cause epistaxis.[22] Removal of partially dissolved tablet fragments, adherent masses of pills, or plant and mushroom parts may not be successful

TABLE 27-2	Ipecac Dosing
AGE	DOSE
Child 6 to 12 months	10 ml (2 tsp)
Child 1 to 5 years	15 ml (1 tbsp)
Over 5 years	30 ml (2 tbsp)
Additional dose	If no emesis in 30 minutes, repeat dose *once only*
Procedure	Administer with water (5 ml/kg or 250 ml in older children) Encourage fluids until emesis occurs Have the child sit up and stay active If child becomes sleepy, place on left side

Box 27-3 Ipecac Syrup: Contraindications and Adrenal Effects

Contraindications
Child less than 6 months of age
Ingestion of strong acid or alkali product
Comatose patient or one having seizures
Any patient whose condition is expected to rapidly deteriorate (i.e., ingestion of cyclic antidepressants or Lomotil)
Compromised gag reflex
Decreased level of consciousness
Evidence of significant vomiting before presentation
Ingestion of a foreign body
High-viscosity petroleum distillate ingestion or symptomatic hydrocarbon ingestion

Adverse effects
Protracted vomiting and diarrhea
Lethargy
Esophageal perforation in patients with history of Mallory-Weiss syndrome
Neuropathies and cardiomyopathies from chronic abuse of ipecac syrup in children with eating disorders

through a lavage tube. Agents known to cause gastric concretions, such as ferrous sulfate, meprobamate, glutethimide, and salicylates, may require prolonged lavage to dissolve or break up the mass of material. Continued deterioration or rising blood levels (for those agents whose levels are monitored) may indicate that a concretion exists[65] (Box 27-4).

Emergency Department and nursing interventions. To perform gastric lavage, the nurse must place the child in the left lateral Trendelenburg or swimmer's position. Immobilization with a backboard and straps or a large sheet may be necessary. A large-diameter orogastric lavage tube is used for the procedure (no. 24 to 28 French for the child less than 18 months old; no. 36 to 40 French for the child over 18 months to adult). Oral suction equipment must be readily available since vomiting usually occurs during the procedure. Because the tube is inserted orally, an oral airway or bite block may be required to prevent the child from biting and occluding the tube during the procedure (Fig. 27-1). Before lavage, the position

of the orogastric tube must be checked by (1) having the child speak (tube has not passed vocal cords); (2) pushing 50 ml of air through the tube while auscultating over the epigastrium for a rush of air; and/or (3) aspirating stomach contents through the syringe.

From 10 to 15 ml/kg of normal saline solution is administered in 50 ml increments to young children, and 200 to 250 ml increments of normal saline solution is given to older children. The use of a large syringe or commercially available lavage kit, with a receptacle for irrigation solution and one for gastric return, decreases contact with stomach contents. Gastric lavage should continue until the gastric return is clear; this requires approximately 500 ml in the child and 5 to 10 L in the older child. Occasionally the lavage tube becomes lodged against the stomach's mucosa during the procedure. Repositioning the tube will confirm that it is not clogged and that the return is clear. If activated charcoal and a cathartic are indicated, the lavage tube is then used as the vehicle for administration. On removal of the orogastric tube, suction equipment must be available, immediately, since vomiting frequently follows gastric lavage.

ACTIVATED CHARCOAL

Activated charcoal is the product of organic materials, such as wood and petroleum, that has been chemically treated and then heated to extremely high temperatures. This processing gives the black, gritty powder its large surface area and a tremendous adsorptive capac-

---

Box 27-4   Gastric Lavage

Indications
One to 2 hours after ingestion with moderate to severe toxicity potential
Agents that decrease GI motility or cause pylorospasm
Severely symptomatic patient

Contraindications
Nontoxic ingestion
Caustic or corrosive ingestions
Uncontrolled seizures
Significant dysrhythmias
Certain petroleum distillates
Ingestion of sharp object

Complications
Esophageal tears or perforation
Pulmonary aspiration, pulmonary hemorrhage, empyema
Tension pneumothorax
Endotracheal placement
Fluid and electrolyte imbalances if hypotonic solution (i.e., water) administered
Uncontrolled seizures—inability to insert tube orally

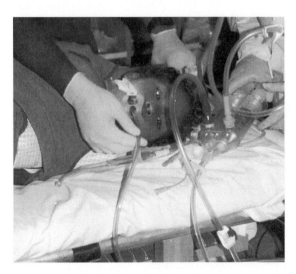

FIG. 27-1.   Gastric lavage procedure.

ity. Binding to the charcoal of potentially toxic substances in the GI tract prevents the systemic absorption of the toxin, lessening the potential for toxicity. Activated charcoal has been found to be superior in altering drug absorption when compared to ipecac syrup.[50]

Repetitive dosing with activated charcoal has also been shown to enhance the elimination of drugs by interfering with the enteroenteric recirculation, interfering with enterohepatic recirculation, and reducing the desorptive process (drugs unbinding from charcoal) of the drug.[71] The effect of high single and repetitive doses of charcoal on absorption and elimination of various drugs has been widely studied.[48,53,55] Its benefit in ingestions of large amounts of tablets, sustained-release products, or medications with prolonged elimination (phenobarbital, salicylate, theophylline, digoxin, carbamazepine) is substantial. Numerous studies to date have documented activated charcoal's ability to enhance the elimination of certain drugs that have already been absorbed into the systemic circulation, such as phenobarbital, theophylline, aminophylline, salicylates, and carbamazepine.[16,50,77] Its action is purported to be through a GI dialysis effect whereby the toxin is literally "pulled" from an area of higher concentration (blood) to an area of lower concentration (GI tract). This process results in acceleration of the drug's elimination in the feces. Not all substances bind equally to activated charcoal (Box 27-5).

Activated charcoal can be administered after ipecac-induced emesis, after gastric lavage, or as the sole intervention in an ingestion where gastric lavage would not be of benefit because of a delay in the patient coming for treatment. Initial or single doses of activated charcoal 1 to 2 g/kg are administered orally or via gastric tube. Multiple dose activated charcoal regimens are given at 1 g/kg initial dose, then 15 to 20 g (0.25 to 0.5 g/kg) every 4 to 6 hours.[31] It has become standard practice to concurrently administer a cathartic with activated charcoal to enhance elimination of the charcoal-toxin complex (see p. 629). Sorbitol has been found to improve the palatability of charcoal and is commonly added as the cathartic in charcoal suspensions. Flavorings such as cherry syrup, ice cream, milk, saccharin, sherbet, sorbitol, and sucrose have been used in the past to make charcoal more palatable. Numerous studies have found that some agents (ice cream, sherbet) decrease the absorptive capacity of charcoal, while others (chocolate syrup) have demonstrated contradictory results. Regardless of their impact on adsorption, palatability and acceptance in the pediatric patient were not significant (Box 27-6).[71]

Emergency Department and nursing interventions. Activated charcoal can be administered orally or via a nasogastric or orogastric tube. The dose is 1 to 2 g/kg per dose in young children and 50 to 100 g in older children; the multiple-dose regimen is 0.5 g/kg every 4 to 6 hours. Before administration, the abdomen must be auscultated for the presence of bowel sounds. When a multiple-dose regimen is used, bowel sounds must be auscultated before administering each dose. The solution tends to settle during shelf storage; therefore during preparation for administration, it must be vigorously shaken to resuspend the particles. Further dilution with 100 to 200 ml of water to create a black watery consistency also assists in resuspending settled particles and removes

---

Box 27-5   Agents Not Adsorbed by Activated Charcoal

- Alcohols: ethanol, methanol, ethylene glycol
- Boric acid
- Cyanide
- Heavy metals: arsenic, iron, lead, lithium, mercury
- Pesticides: DDT, malathion, N-methylcarbamate
- Petroleum distillates
- Strong acids or alkali

Box 27-6   Activated Charcoal

Contraindications
Caustic ingestions
Pure petroleum distillates or other hydrocarbon ingestions
Any agent not well adsorbed to charcoal that demonstrates a high risk for pulmonary aspiration

Adverse effects
Nausea, vomiting
Aspiration of charcoal and gastric contents
Diarrhea, constipation
Intestinal obstruction

residue from the container to ensure the optimal dose.[38] The watery consistency also improves the flow of the solution when administered through a orogastric or nasogastric tube.

When administered orally, acceptance of the solution can be a problem (Fig. 27-2). Some administration hints include using an opaque container with a fitted lid and straw to cover the appearance of the slurry; alternating the charcoal solution with sips of clear fluid; and adding ice to administer the charcoal solution as a cool liquid versus a lukewarm solution. The addition of flavorings is discouraged, since they may alter the adsorptive ability of the activated charcoal (Box 27-7).

If oral administration is unsuccessful, the solution may be administered via an orogastric tube, if one is already in place for gastric lavage, or a nasogastric tube. For either method, further dilution of the solution

may be required. A common side effect of administration via tube is stimulation of the gag reflex with resulting emesis. The use of a small-bore tube (i.e., Salem sump, Cantor tube, Duotube) introduced into the duodenum has been effective in limiting regurgitation.[67] Regardless of the method used, the airway must be protected from possible aspiration. Bedside suction must be available immediately during and following the procedure. In addition, the child must be in a position that allows easy rolling onto the side. After the activated charcoal is given, the tube should be flushed with normal saline solution to remove charcoal residue and ensure delivery of the appropriate dose of charcoal. Vomiting after administration may result from GI irritation.

CATHARTICS

Cathartics are used in conjunction with activated charcoal to expedite the transit of the toxin or toxin-charcoal complex. They serve to prevent constipation arising from charcoal administration and, to some degree, reduce the possibility of desorption, making

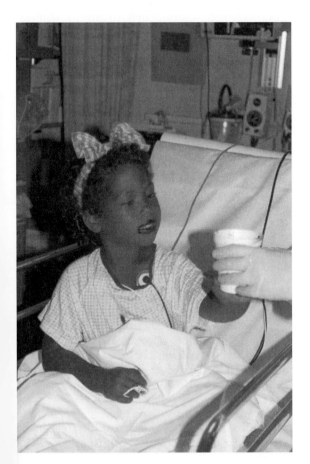

FIG. 27-2. Oral activated charcoal administration.

Box 27-7 Tips for Administering Activated Charcoal
• Dose 1 to 2 g/kg in children; 50 to 100 g in adults; multiple dose regimens 1 to 2 g/kg every 4 to 6 hours • Mix charcoal in 100 to 200 ml of water to a black, watery consistency • Auscultate for the presence of bowel sounds before administering each dose • If given orally, use an opaque container with a fitted lid and straw; cool the solution with ice to make it more palatable—alternate with sips of clear liquid • If oral administration is unsuccessful, further dilute the mixture and administer through a nasogastric tube or orogastric tube if one is already in place after gastric lavage • If sorbitol is administered, the 35% solution (not the 70% solution) must be used, or the 70% solution diluted to a 35% solution; it should not be given more often than every 12 hours

the drug available again for systemic absorption. The adverse effects from use in the child include excessive fluid loss through the gut, resulting in dehydration and electrolyte imbalances. For this reason, premixed solutions containing 70% sorbitol should be avoided, since hypernatremic dehydration can result. The recommended pediatric dose of sorbitol is 35%. If the 70% solution is all that is available, it must be diluted to a 35% solution. Caution should be used when administering any cathartic to children younger than 3 years of age. Cathartics are not recommended in children under 1 year of age. Repetitive cathartic dosing should be evaluated on a case-by-case basis; however, sorbitol should never be used more than once every 12 hours (Box 27-8).

Emergency Department and nursing interventions. As with activated charcoal, the abdomen must be auscultated for bowel sounds before giving a cathartic. After administration, the child's vital signs must be continuously monitored and the cardiac rate and rhythm evaluated. Documentation of intake and output is recommended.

If sorbitol is used, small children receive a more dilute solution than adults (35% versus 70%). When the 70% solution is all that is available, dilution to one-half strength is required before administration. Sorbitol is given orally or via nasogastric (NG) tube and is usually mixed with the charcoal solution. Cathartics are stopped once a charcoal stool appears.[54]

WHOLE BOWEL IRRIGATION

Recently, whole bowel irrigation has been advocated as a primary GI decontamination procedure after certain drug overdoses or poisonings. This procedure has been commonly used for bowel preparation before colonoscopy, barium enema, or bowel surgery. Golytely or Colyte is a polyethylene glycol (PEG) solution demonstrated to induce minimal water and electrolyte shifts because of its nonabsorbable nature. Large volumes can be safely given in pediatric patients who *do not* demonstrate a gastric obstruction or ileus.[77] Successful treatment of miniature battery ingestions in children initially proved this procedure's benefits. It is also suggested to be of value in the management of (1) ingestions of substances not well adsorbed by charcoal (i.e., iron, lithium), (2) massive ingestions of sustained-release preparations, (3) ingestions with concretion formation, or (4) patients who are "body packers" or "body stuffers" (have ingested wrapped or unwrapped medication in bulk).

Emergency Department and nursing interventions. In small children the PEG solution is administered at 25 ml/kg/hr; it is given at a rate of up to 2 L/hr for adolescents and adults. It is preferably administered by continuous infusion via NG tube for 4 to 6 hours, or until the rectal effluent is clear. Oral administration is generally not successful for children, since drinking large volumes of the fluid is required. The predominant adverse effect from this procedure is nausea and vomiting, which can be controlled by slowing the initial infusion rate and/or using antiemetics. A bedside commode close to the patient is required. This procedure is not recommended in the child with a decreased level of consciousness or one who is unable to protect the airway.

Box 27-8   Cathartics

Dosage
Magnesium sulfate, 250 mg/kg
Magnesium citrate, 5 ml/kg
Sorbitol, 1 g/kg (**35% solution**) (never administered more often than every 12 hours)

Contraindications
Dehydration
Preexisting diarrhea
Bowel obstruction or ileus
Avoid magnesium-containing cathartics in renal failure/congestive failure patients
Avoid sodium sulfate and sodium phosphate (Phospho-Soda) preparations in children

Adverse effects
Significant fluid loss or dehydration
Electrolyte depletion
Hypotension
Hypernatremia
Hyperosmolality
Hypermagnesemia (magnesium cathartics)
Abdominal distension (sorbitol)
Abdominal cramping
Vomiting

ALTERNATIVE METHODS OF ELIMINATION

The specific properties of a toxin make certain poisonings amenable to modalities that can potentially shorten the course of toxicity by enhancing the toxin's elimination. These modalities are often instituted based on the severity of symptoms and include forced diuresis, alkalinization of the urine, and extracorporeal drug removal.

Forced diuresis, which was advocated in the past, has since been abandoned because of associated significant side effects, including pulmonary and cerebral edema, and electrolyte and acid-base disturbances.

Alkalinization of the urine has proven effective for increasing the elimination of phenobarbital and salicylates.[58] It is performed by administering sodium bicarbonate intravenously to maintain a urine pH between 7.5 and 8.0, without allowing the serum pH to exceed 7.55. The result is an "ion-trapping" effect that enhances the elimination of specific pharmacokinetically amenable drugs. When this procedure is used, urine pH, serum electrolytes, and plasma pH must be monitored frequently. Hypokalemia and hypocalcemia are possible adverse effects. Acidification of the urine, although once used, is no longer advocated because of its significant adverse effects and questionable efficacy.

EXTRACORPOREAL DRUG REMOVAL TECHNIQUES

Extracorporeal drug removal techniques include peritoneal dialysis, hemodialysis, and hemoperfusion. Peritoneal dialysis has the benefit of being readily available and easily initiated, but its slow and inefficient (approximately 10% as effective as hemodialysis) removal of toxins across the peritoneal membrane does not often justify its use. In children, however, its use may be simpler and less hazardous than hemodialysis or hemoperfusion. Agents removed using peritoneal dialysis include barbiturates, bromides, phenytoin, ethanol, ethchlorvynol, ethylene glycol, inorganic mercury, isopropyl alcohol, lithium, methyprylon, quinidine, salicylate, and theophylline.[65]

Hemodialysis involves the use of a semipermeable membrane to separate diffusible from less diffusible or nondiffusible substances. This technique is usually reserved for use when the child has not responded to conservative medical treatment or for life-threatening situations when the child has a markedly elevated serum level of phenobarbital, salicylate, theophylline, methanol, ethylene glycol, or lithium.[5] The child's blood vessel size and small blood volume make hemodialysis very cumbersome. The procedure carries the risk for hemorrhage, infection, hypotension, air embolus, and nosocomial infections.

Hemoperfusion using charcoal-filled cartridges is also used to remove certain toxic compounds. Blood is directed through a column containing the adsorbent material. Affinity of the adsorbent for the toxin, rate of blood flow through the adsorbent, volume of distribution of the toxin, and its rate of equilibrium from peripheral tissues to blood determine the effectiveness of this technique.[56] During all of these procedures, blood chemistries, electrolytes, and vital signs must be closely monitored.

EXCHANGE TRANSFUSION

Exchange transfusion involves removing a given quantity of blood and replacing it with an equal amount of whole fresh blood. This technique is more successful with medications that are highly protein-bound. It may be of benefit when multidose activated charcoal cannot be given, the toxin is poorly adsorbed to activated charcoal, or the facility's access to pediatric hemodialysis or hemoperfusion is limited.[20]

ANTIDOTAL THERAPY

Only 30 to 40 antidotes exist for over 300,000 possible substances that a child can encounter.[64] Some of these antidotes involve conventional therapies; others are outdated and dangerous to the child.

The universal antidote—burned toast, magnesium oxide, and tannic acid—was recommended for years in many first aid courses. It is now known to be of no benefit for the management of the poisoned patient. Product labels frequently contain inappropriate, outdated antidotal therapies or misleading recommendations that can further harm the child, such as the administration of salt water to induce vomiting—with the inherent risk of hypernatremia—or using one's finger to induce vomiting by manipulation of the oropharynx. Acceptable antidotal therapies sometimes involve familiar medications used in unconventional ways. An example is the use of high doses of atropine for organophosphate toxicity. Regardless of the antidote used, general supportive care remains at the forefront of poisoning management in all children (Table 27-3).

TABLE 27-3	Common Antidotes Used in Children		
POISON	**ANTIDOTE**	**DOSAGE**	**COMMENTS**
Acetaminophen	N-Acetylcysteine (NAC)	Initial load: 140 mg/kg PO or via NG tube Maintenance: 70 mg/kg q4h for 17 doses	Dilute NAC to 5% with water, fruit juice, or soda; most effective if given within 16 hours of ingestion
Alcohols: methanol, ethylene glycol	Ethanol	Loading: 10 ml of 10% intravenous solution per kilogram of body weight Maintenance: 0.15 ml/kg/hr	Titrate to blood ethanol level of 100 to 150 mg/dl
Anticholinergic poisoning: antihistamines, certain mushrooms and plants	Physostigmine	0.03 mg/kg up to 0.5 mg IV over 2 minutes repeated to maximum dose of 2 mg if needed	May be useful if seizures or tachydysrhythmias present
Anticoagulants: coumadin, warfarin, or indandione rat poisons	Vitamin K	0.6 mg/kg subcutaneously (SQ) or slow IV (1 to 5 mg) 5 to 10 mg/day PO maintenance therapy	May cause flushing; decreased blood pressure
Benzodiazepines	Flumazenil (Romazicon)	0.2 mg over 30 seconds; if no response after 30 seconds, give 0.3 mg. If no response, give 0.5 mg over 30 seconds at 1-minute intervals up to total of 3 mg	Contraindicated in co-ingestion of tricyclic antidepressants or if taking benzodiazepines for seizure control
Beta-blocking agents, calcium channel–blocking agents	Glucagon	Initial: 0.1 mg/kg IV bolus (maximum 10 mg/dose given over 1 minute) Maintenance infusion: 0.05 to 0.1 mg/kg/hr	Titrate to response
Calcium channel blockers, fluorides, hydrofluoric acid	Calcium chloride/gluconate	Calcium chloride 10% 5 to 10 ml (0.1 to 0.2 ml/kg) or calcium gluconate 10% 10-20 ml (0.2 to 0.3 ml/kg) given slowly IV over 5 minutes Apply calcium gluconate gel 2.5% for dermal exposure	Requires continuous cardiac monitoring; SQ infiltration or arterial perfusion in severe cases of dermal exposure

	Common Antidotes Used in Children—cont'd		
TABLE 27-3			
POISON	**ANTIDOTE**	**DOSAGE**	**COMMENTS**
Cyclic antidepressants	Sodium bicarbonate	1 to 2 mEq/kg IV Titrate to response and arterial pH	Give if significant cardiac conduction delay or ventricular dysrhythmias
Digoxin, digitoxin, oleander, foxglove	Digoxin Immune Fab (Digibind)	Based on serum digoxin concentration and body weight; given intravenously	Approximately 65 mg of Fab binds 1 mg of digoxin
Heavy metals: arsenic, lead, organic/ inorganic mercury, gold	Dimercaptosuccinic acid (Chemet)	10 mg/kg PO q8h for 5 days, then 10 mg/kg PO q12h for 14 days	Given for blood lead levels more than 45 µg/day
Iron	Deferoxamine	90 mg/kg IM or IV to maximum of 1 g, q4-12h; not to exceed 6 g in 24 hours; IV slow infusion up to 15 mg/kg/hr	Given if serum iron >350 mg/dl or serum iron more than total iron capacity (TIBG); hypotension or shock
Opiates, possibly clonidine	Naloxone	0.1 mg/kg up to 1 to 2 mg IV, IM, via endotracheal tube, or sublingually; up to 8 mg in adolescent	May give continuous IV infusion
Organophosphate/ carbamate insecticides	Atropine	Initial dose, 0.05 to 1 mg/kg IV; usual dose 1 to 5 mg	Up to 5 mg IV q15min to dry secretions
Organophosphate insecticide	Pralidoxime	25 to 50 mg/kg IV over 2 minutes; repeat q8-12 hr if needed	Most effective when given within 24 hours after exposure; consider continuous IV infusion
Snake bite: Eastern or Texas coral snake	*Micrurus fulvius* antivenin	Three to five vials antivenin in 250 to 500 ml sodium chloride 0.9% continuous IV infusion over 4 to 6 hr	Hypersensitivity reactions are not dose related, may result in immediate anaphylactic reaction
Snake bite: rattlesnake, copperhead, or cottonmouth	Crotalidae polyvalent antivenin	Minimal envenomation: 5 to 8 vials antivenin Moderate envenomation: 8 to 12 vials antivenin Severe envenomation: 13 to 30+ vials of antivenin	Hypersensitivity reactions are not dose related, may result in immediate anaphylaxis

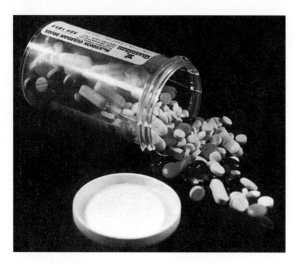

Fig. 27-3. Common household medications.

Common Poisonings in Children

Approximately 400 containers of potentially toxic substances enter the average home every year. Of these, the most common agents implicated in poison-ing exposures include products that contain alcohols, such as mouthwash, perfume, and hairspray, and medications such as acetaminophen, vitamins (chewable), and antihistamines/decongestants. An estimated 30 drugs are on hand in the average American home at any given time; it is therefore no surprise that approximately 40% of all ingestions in the United States involve medications[83] (Fig. 27-3).

Koren reviewed fatalities reported in children by the AAPCC from 1983 through 1989 and found that ingestion of a commercially available unit dose (one to two tablets, one tablespoon, or one teaspoon) in the toddler did not normally result in serious toxicity. However, a number of prescription medications proved to be profoundly dangerous in small amounts[36,48] (Table 27-4).

Obviously these are not the only medications that can be problematic. The local anesthetic benzocaine, present in such products as teething gels, first aid ointments, throat lozenges, hemorrhoid creams, or vaginal creams, may induce methemoglobinemia in the child. Children can also be more sensitive to certain drugs with regard to their hemodynamic depressant effects. Small amounts of imidazoline-derived sympathomimetic agents (as little as 2.5 ml), which are available over the counter as Visine, Afrin, Otrivin, or Clear Eyes, may cause bradycardia, hypotension, lethargy, and coma.[41]

TABLE 27-4	Potentially Fatal in a Single Dose
DRUG	**AVAILABLE SOURCE**
Antidiarrheal agents	Diphenoxylate with atropine (Lomotil), difenoxin (Motofen)
Camphor	Over-the-counter oils or liniments: Vicks Vaporub, Vicks Vapo-steam, Camphophenique
Chloroquine	Aralen (antimalarial, antiinflammatory)
Clonidine	Catapres
Ethchlorvynol	Placidyl
Glyburide, Glipizide	DiaBeta, Micronase, Glucotrol
Hydrocodone-based cough syrups	Hycodan, Tussionex
Lindane	Kwell
Lithium carbonate	Eskalith, Lithobid
Methyl salicylate	Oil of wintergreen, topical muscle liniments or ointments (Ben Gay, Icy Hot)
Phenothiazines	Thioridazine (Mellaril), chlorpromazine (Thorazine)
Propoxyphene	Darvon, Darvocet
Quinine	Over-the-counter preparations: antimalarial, skeletal muscle relaxant
Theophylline	Elixophyllin, Slo-bid, Theo-Dur
Tricyclics	Imipramine (Tofranil), desipramine (Norpramin)

A brief summary of the more common agents implicated in accidental poisonings follows. This is in no way intended to be a comprehensive review of the subject, but rather a quick reference to highlight the management of these exposures.

ACETAMINOPHEN

Acetaminophen is a popular analgesic and antipyretic. Available over the counter, acetaminophen comes in various forms such as tablets; caplets; combination products; pleasant tasting, chewable tablets; and flavored liquids. A reported 35,788 ingestions of a pediatric formulation of acetaminophen occurred in 1993.[42] Peak absorption of acetaminophen occurs approximately 4 hours after ingestion, and the drug is predominantly metabolized by the liver. Children may be more resistant to acetaminophen toxicity than adults.[60] Reasons for this difference are unclear, but they appear to be related to variations in the metabolic capacity of young children.[40] Nevertheless, acute ingestions of more than 140 mg/kg are considered toxic amounts.

The clinical presentation of acetaminophen toxicity may be divided into four stages. The first phase begins immediately after an acute toxic ingestion and may last up to 24 hours. Nausea, vomiting, anorexia, and diaphoresis may occur. However, many children remain asymptomatic during this phase. The second phase, lasting 24 to 72 hours, is marked by a latent period wherein the child becomes relatively asymptomatic. This may give the parent or nurse a false sense of security. During the third phase the child may experience right upper quadrant pain, elevation of liver enzyme and bilirubin levels, and prolongation of prothrombin time. Liver injury becomes evident 72 to 96 hours after ingestion in the untreated individual. In this third phase of acetaminophen poisoning, complications such as coagulation defects, jaundice, renal failure, and hepatic encephalopathy may appear. The fourth phase (recovery stage) begins approximately 5 days after ingestion. Liver enzyme levels will begin to return to normal in all but the most severe cases.

The optimal time to obtain an acetaminophen level is 4 hours after an acute ingestion, allowing for peak absorption of the drug. Once the level has been determined, it can be plotted on the Rumack-Matthew nomogram to determine the probability of toxic effects (Fig. 27-4). If the time of ingestion is unknown, the level should be measured immediately and again in 2 hours to assess the trend in plasma levels.

Emergency Department and nursing interventions. Since ipecac-induced emesis may delay the oral administration of the antidote, it is not recommended for acetaminophen ingestions. Large ingestions (≥140 mg/kg) treated within 2 hours of ingestion require gastric lavage, followed by the administration of activated charcoal to prevent further absorption of the drug. Although it has been speculated that charcoal administration may adversely affect the oral antidote's (*N*-acetylcysteine [NAC]) efficacy, limited clinical evidence exists to support this theory.[81] Some clinicians advocate gastric lavage to remove residual activated charcoal from the gut before NAC administration, whereas others stagger the dose of activated charcoal, giving it 1 to 2 hours after the NAC dose. By blunting the rise of toxic serum concentrations, early charcoal administration may prevent the need for subsequent antidote therapy.

NAC, the antidote for acetaminophen toxicity, is most effective if given within the first 8 hours after ingestion, although efficacy is purported to last up to 24 hours after ingestion. If, empirically, the amount ingested is considered toxic, antidotal therapy should be initiated until the serum acetaminophen level has been determined and further evaluation using the nomogram can be made. Initially a loading dose of NAC (140 mg/kg) is given orally or via nasogastric tube. Maintenance doses (70 mg/kg) are given orally every 4 hours for 17 additional doses if maintenance therapy is warranted by evaluation of the history or nomogram evaluation. When administered orally, NAC should be diluted 4:1 with cold orange or other fruit juice to increase acceptance and improve palatability; dilution with water is recommended for NG administration. If vomiting occurs within 1 hour of the NAC dose, the dose should be repeated.

ALCOHOLS

Alcohols were responsible for 46,594 exposures reported to poison centers in 1993.[42] The true incidence in children is difficult to determine, since many pharmaceutical and nonpharmaceutical products contain an alcohol as a main ingredient. Products containing *ethanol* are commonly found throughout the home in cough and cold preparations, perfumes, hair sprays, and mouthwashes. These products can produce varying degrees of CNS depression, depending on the concentration of ethanol in the product (range from 10% to 95%). Other alcohols (e.g., methanol, isopropyl, ethylene glycol) can produce symptoms much more severe than ethanol. *Isopropyl* (rubbing) alcohol

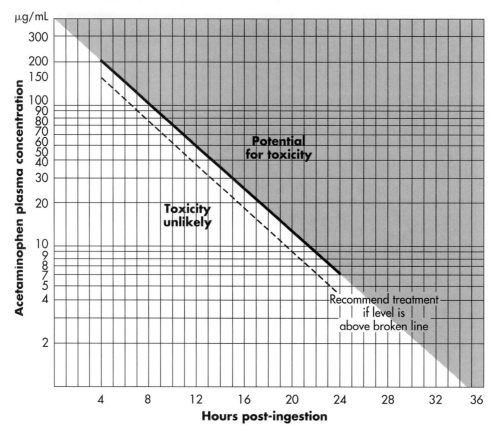

FIG. 27-4. Nomogram: plasma or serum acetaminophen concentration vs time after acetaminophen ingestion. (Used with permission from Rumack BM, Matthew M: Acetaminophen poisoning and toxicity, *Pediatrics* 55:871, 1975.)

is twice as potent a CNS depressant as ethanol and is metabolized in vivo to acetone. It may produce marked CNS depression, cardiovascular collapse, and severe GI irritation. *Methanol* (wood alcohol), found in gas-line antifreeze, solvents, or Sterno, is metabolized to formaldehyde and formic acid by the liver. These toxic metabolites are responsible for the severe metabolic acidosis and visual changes (haziness or "snowfield" appearance) characteristic of this exposure. Sweet-tasting *ethylene glycol,* found in antifreeze, brake fluid, and deicer, is metabolized to glycolaldehyde, glycolic acid, and oxalic acid, which can lead to significant metabolic acidosis, oxalate crystal formation, and, ultimately, renal dysfunction (Table 27-5).

Emergency Department and nursing interventions. Alcohols do not bind well to activated charcoal, and, since rapid CNS depression can develop, the use of ipecac syrup is not recommended. Ethanol

ingestion can cause profound hypoglycemia in children; measures to maintain normal glucose levels should be initiated. If the child is alert, a sugared beverage or sweet snack may be administered before arrival in the emergency department. Once the child arrives in the emergency department, IV dextrose administration must be considered. Interestingly, the antidotal treatment for methanol or ethylene glycol toxicity is an ethanol infusion (calculated to maintain a blood alcohol level of 100 to 150 mg/dl). Ethanol blocks the metabolism of methanol and ethylene glycol to their toxic metabolites. Therefore ethanol is the preferred substrate for alcohol dehydrogenase, the major pathway for alcohol metabolism. Hemodialysis is also used for severe isopropyl, methanol, and ethylene glycol exposures when severe acidosis, life-threatening complications, or significantly elevated blood levels (20 mg/dl methanol or ethylene glycol) exist.

TABLE 27-5	Alcohol Ingestions		
TYPES OF ALCOHOLS	**PRODUCTS CONTAINING ALCOHOL**	**CLINICAL PRESENTATION**	**EMERGENCY DEPARTMENT AND NURSING INTERVENTIONS***
Ethanol	• Cough and cold preparations • Perfumes • Hair spray • Mouthwash • Alcoholic beverages	• Varying degrees of central nervous system depression • Hypoglycemia • Seizures	• Stabilize the airway and breathing • Attach the child to a heart rate monitor • Obtain venous access • Obtain a bedside glucose level (ethanol ingestions) • Monitor serum electrolytes, glucose, and serum bicarbonate levels • Additional testing may include complete blood count, arterial blood gas levels, serum alcohol level, liver function tests, blood urea nitrogen, creatinine, and urinalysis • Strictly monitor intake and output • Continuously evaluate CNS status • Continuously evaluate respiratory and cardiovascular status • Administer IV dextrose for severe hypoglycemia (2 to 4 ml/kg of 25% dextrose in water) • For methanol and ethylene glycol ingestions, anticipate antidotal therapy of an ethanol infusion (to maintain a blood alcohol level of 100 to 150 mg/dl) • For severe ingestions, anticipate hemodialysis
Isopropyl	• Rubbing alcohol • Antiseptics • Cleaning agents	• Profound central nervous system depression • Respiratory depression • Cardiovascular collapse • Severe GI irritation	
Methanol	• Gas-line antifreeze • Solvents • Sterno • Windshield deicer	• Central nervous system depression • Severe metabolic acidosis • Visual changes (haziness or "snow-field" appearance) • Seizures	
Ethylene glycol	• Radiator antifreeze • Brake fluid • Windshield deicer	• Central nervous system depression • Severe metabolic acidosis • Renal dysfunction • Seizures	

*Syrup of ipecac is not recommended to treat alcohol ingestions because of the possibility of rapid central nervous system depression. Alcohols do not bind well to activated charcoal.

COUGH AND COLD PREPARATIONS

Over-the-counter cold medications are commonplace in the home. Of the 105,588 exposures reported by the AAPCC in 1993, a total of 72,540 victims were under the age of 6 years. Nationally, it was the fourth most common cause of poisoning.[42] Since upper respiratory infections and colds are so prevalent among children, parents tend to keep an adequate stock of these products in the home. They typically contain antihistamines, decongestants, and possibly ethanol or acetaminophen. Symptoms associated with the ingestion of decongestants such as phenylephrine phenylpropanolamine, and pseudoephedrine resemble the sympathomimetic toxic syndrome. Initially the child may be anxious, tachycardic, hypertensive, irritable, or complain of GI upset. Conversely, the antihistamines such as chlorpheniramine, diphenhydramine, and doxylamine are often responsible for sedative effects in the younger child. Older children may, paradoxically, have CNS stimulation. Symptoms associated with the ingestion of antihistamine and decongestant combination products include hyperactivity, tachycardia, ataxia, disorientation, hallucinations, tonic-clonic seizures, and respiratory depression. Another factor that may complicate the clinical picture is that many of these products also contain ethanol alcohol, further contributing to CNS depression. With combination products, it may be difficult to predict clinical symptomatology. Therefore the nurse must continually monitor the child for changes in clinical status and physiologic parameters.

Emergency Department and nursing interventions. With the wide variety of active ingredients potentially present in these exposures, each case should be assessed individually. First, the total dose of each ingredient should be determined to assess the potential for toxicity. Because liquid preparations are more quickly absorbed by the GI tract and many children with these ingestions do not arrive in the emergency department until 1 to 2 hours after the ingestion, the effectiveness of ipecac syrup or gastric lavage is questionable. However, GI decontamination should be considered for exposures involving very recent ingestions and the presence of significant anticholinergic effects. Treatment requires the prompt administration of activated charcoal for almost all of these exposures. The child must be continuously monitored for the development of additional signs and symptoms of toxicity for a minimum of 4 to 6 hours. Sustained-release products require additional observation because of their delayed absorption and prolonged action.

CYCLIC ANTIDEPRESSANTS

Cyclic antidepressants are commonly used medications for a variety of medical and psychiatric disorders. Amitriptyline (Elavil), doxepin (Sinequan), imipramine (Tofranil), and nortriptyline (Pamelor) are some of the more commonly used antidepressants. The toxicity of these drugs arises from their anticholinergic, sympatholytic, and quinidine-like effects. Anticholinergic effects include dry, flushed skin, dry mucous membranes, decreased bowel sounds, tachycardia, hypertension or hypotension, urinary retention, mydriasis, and agitation. More severe anticholinergic symptoms include hallucinations, seizures, and coma. The classic quinidine-like effects are demonstrated by myocardial depression and atrioventricular (AV) conduction delay. A QRS interval greater than 0.10 milliseconds correlates with more severe toxicity and the occurrence of seizures; an interval greater than 0.16 milliseconds correlates with seizures and ventricular dysrhythmias.

Clinically, the child may initially be alert and oriented. However, rapid progression to profound coma, seizures, or hypotension can occur without warning. Unfortunately, toxicity from these agents does not correlate well with the amount of drug ingested.

Emergency Department and nursing interventions. Aggressive management is warranted in this type of toxic exposure. Stabilization of the ABCs should be addressed immediately, with close monitoring of the cardiac rhythm and vital signs. The use of syrup of ipecac is contraindicated in cyclic antidepressant ingestions. Instead, gastric lavage is used with the subsequent administration of activated charcoal and a cathartic to limit systemic absorption. Alkalinization of the serum, considered to be antidotal by increasing protein binding of the drug, is indicated when vital signs are unstable, for ventricular dysrhythmias or seizures, or when the QRS interval is greater than 0.10 milliseconds. Either hyperventilation or the administration of a sodium bicarbonate (1 to 2 mEq/kg IV) bolus may be used to maintain an arterial pH in the 7.45 to 7.55 range. A minimum of 6 to 8 hours of observation after ingestion should be employed in the otherwise asymptomatic child. During this time the child must remain attached to a cardiac monitor and the nurse should continuously evaluate CNS status, vital signs, cardiac rhythm, and urinary output.

HYDROCARBONS

Hydrocarbon-containing products are commonly involved in accidental poisonings in the home. In 1993 a total of 25,373 exposures in children under the age of 6 years was reported by the AAPCC.[42] These products include mineral seal oil (found in furniture polish), gasoline, turpentine, kerosene, lighter-fluid, toluene, and mineral spirits. Often these agents are vehicles for more toxic substances, such as pesticides, camphor, or heavy metals. The potential for developing a chemical pneumonitis depends primarily on the viscosity and volatility of the product. Higher-viscosity hydrocarbons (mineral oil, automotive oils) are less irritating to mucous membranes and are not as likely to be aspirated into the lungs. Products with a low viscosity are more likely to enter the respiratory tract and subsequently cause a chemical pneumonitis. Most of these products are poorly absorbed by the GI tract or are highly filtered out by the liver and therefore are not a problem if left untreated.

Emergency Department and nursing interventions. The intentional induction of vomiting in a hydrocarbon ingestion is contraindicated, since vomiting increases the risk of aspiration. Signs of respiratory involvement, such as cough (continuing beyond the immediate exposure), dyspnea, or choking, may indicate aspiration of the chemical and an increased risk for the development of a chemical pneumonitis. Pulse oximetry, arterial blood gas levels, cardiac monitoring, baseline laboratory studies (complete blood count, electrolytes, creatinine, blood urea nitrogen), and single or serial chest x-rays are indicated with suspected pulmonary involvement.[50] The child should be observed over a period of 6 to 8 hours for the development of respiratory symptoms if significant ingestion or aspiration is suspected or known.

IRON

The availability of chewable vitamins with iron, iron supplements, and prenatal vitamins in the home probably fuels the continuing incidence of accidental iron ingestion. Children enjoy the sweet taste and familiar shapes of chewable vitamins, and the sugar coating and "candy-like" appearance of adult supplements prompts their ingestion. In 1992, six fatal iron poisonings were reported in children under the age of 2 years,[43] and three fatalities occurred in the same age group in 1993.[42] From 1983 through 1990, 16 children under 6 years of age died, making iron poisoning the leading cause of pediatric poisoning fatalities.[9] Ingestions of 20 mg of elemental iron/kg body weight normally result in only mild GI symptoms. A toxic ingestion occurs when more than 40 mg/kg is consumed.

Iron manifests direct corrosive effects on the gastric mucosa, as well as cellular toxicity in overdose quantities. The exact mechanism of cellular toxicity is still unknown. Subsequent to a toxic ingestion, vomiting, diarrhea, and hematemesis may occur, followed by a latent period of up to 12 hours during which the child shows improvement. Fever, hyperglycemia, bleeding, metabolic acidosis, and shock may appear after this phase. Later complications may include hepatic failure, seizures, and coma. Management is based on (1) obtaining an accurate history of the amount of iron ingested, (2) monitoring for associated clinical symptoms, and (3) using serum iron assessments.

Emergency Department and nursing Interventions. Treatment consists of initial decontamination using gastric lavage. An abdominal x-ray may be ordered to detect the presence of radiopaque tablets in the GI tract. Negative findings, however, do not always correlate with insignificant ingestions. Whole bowel irrigation is rapidly becoming the modality of choice to release iron from the GI tract, since activated charcoal does not bind iron.

The antidote for iron ingestions is deferoxamine, which is a chelating agent that removes iron from the tissues and free iron from the plasma. Intravenous administration of this antidote begins with up to 15 mg/kg/hour; the maximum daily dose is 6g.[31] With the use of deferoxamine, the urine may turn rose colored. Side effects include urticaria and hypotension, and these are more likely to occur when the drug is administered too rapidly.

Children with significant ingestions are monitored continuously. The gastric irritation produced by iron can lead to significant gastric hemorrhage, producing hypovolemia and shock. The nurse should continuously assess the child's vital signs, including blood pressure, and observe for the development of additional symptoms, including hematemesis, changes in CNS status, decreased urinary output, and/or signs of shock.

PLANTS

Plants were the fifth most common type of exposures reported to poison centers in 1993. Of 94,725 exposures, 72,773 occurred in children under the age of 6 years.[42] A wide variety of plants are commonly used for indoor decorating or outdoor landscaping. Many of these plants contain substances that can produce systemic toxicity, while others may produce local dermatitis, oral irritation, or mechanical injury. With some plants, only the stems, leaves, or flowers may individually contain a potentially toxic substance. Positive identification of the plant, determination of the part ingested, and estimation of the amount ingested are essential when assessing for the exposure's toxic potential.

Emergency Department and nursing interventions. In general, topical exposures should be thoroughly washed with soap and water. Some plants require specific agents to relieve the irritation or solubilize the offending ingredient. Ideally each plant should be positively identified before the initiation of treatment (Box 27-9).

Box 27-9 Harmful or Toxic Plants
Amaryllis
Angel's trumpet
Azalea
Boxwood
Caladium
Caroline jessamine
Castor bean
Century plant
Cherry laurel
Chinaberry
Daffodil
Deadly nightshade
Dumb cane
Elephant ear
Eucalyptus
Elderberry
English ivy
Foxglove
Holly
Hyacinth
Hydrangea
Japanese yew
Jerusalem cherry
Jimson weed
Juniper
Lantana
Ligustrum
Lily of the valley
Mandrake
Mistletoe
Morning glory
Mushrooms (wild)
Periwinkle
Pokeweed
Poison ivy, oak, or sumac
Poinsettia
Potato (leaves, green skin)
Purple queen
Rhododendron
Rhubarb
Tomato (stems, leaves)
Water hemlock
Wisteria
Yellow jessamine
Yew

PREVENTION OF POISONING EXPOSURES

Almost 60% of the 1.7 million exposures reported by the AAPCC in 1993 involved children under the age of 6 years. Obviously, this group represents the highest risks for unintentional poisonings. Parents commonly report a disruption in the family routine when an ingestion or exposure occurs, such as an ill parent, family tension, a guest in the home, vacation, or the parent's preoccupation with another child. Another common scenario is the parent being distracted while using a product (e.g., receives a phone call or visitor at the door), and neglecting to remove the product from the child's reach. Rooms that present the highest incidence of accidents are the kitchen, bathroom, and garage. For this reason these areas should be given special attention when "poison-proofing" a home.

With regard to the packaging of medications and other toxic substances, many parents possess a false sense of security with what are commonly referred to as "child-proof caps." These caps are actually only "child-resistant," slowing down the child's access to the container's contents. Therefore these items must be properly stored away from the child's reach. Safety latches for cabinets containing dangerous materials are recommended and will serve as a deterrent. Eventually, however, they will be mastered by every child after a certain age. Regardless, efforts at prevention should not stop. As children achieve developmental milestones, they become more mobile. Consequently, the risks in the environment increase as the child gains access to table tops, counters, closets, and drawers. Around 3 years of age, climbing becomes a new means of exploring and gaining access to dangerous items. Parents, or persons who care for children regularly, should continuously assess their environment and take active measures to "poison-proof" their home, based on the child's current and expected abilities.

Child abuse or neglect is occasionally suspected in poisoning exposures. Each situation must be evaluated for consistency of the events with the child's developmental abilities. Infants younger than 6 months of age are developmentally unable to gain purposeful access to toxic substances. Therefore suspicion should be raised for most poisoning exposures in these very young infants. Conversely, ingestions in children older than 6 years of age are usually intentional. These ingestions may be an attention-seeking behavior or a cry for help. Investigation into the motive behind the event and psychiatric counseling may be necessary.

Box 27-10 Tips for Poisoning Prevention

- Store medication out of the reach of children. Lock medicine-containing cabinets, and/or store all medications on high shelves in closets or cabinets. Keep purses out of children's reach if it is necessary to carry medication.
- Place chewable vitamins or pleasant-tasting children's medications out of reach. Children will ingest large amounts of these products.
- Avoid taking medication in front of children. They may imitate your behavior.
- Avoid combining several medications in one bottle for convenience.
- Use containers with child-resistant caps whenever possible.
- Never refer to medicine as candy. Explain to the child the reason for medication, and identify the appropriate people to give them medicine.
- Flush unused or old medicine down the toilet. Medicine tossed into the wastebasket is retrievable and a potential danger.
- Do not store household cleaning products and other potentially toxic substances under the kitchen or bathroom sink. Store these products on a high shelf or in a locked cabinet.
- Keep cleaning products, chemicals, and medications in their original containers. Do not transfer them to food or drink containers (soft drink bottles or cans, milk bottles, etc.).
- Keep a bottle of ipecac syrup available in the home for every child under the age of 5 years.
- Instruct children to *ask first* before eating or drinking any substance.
- Keep the emergency telephone number for the nearest poison information center by the phone. Inform relatives or babysitters of the availability of the phone number and ipecac syrup.
- Use caution when following product labels for first aid or emergency actions. These labels are often inaccurate, incomplete, or without warnings or product information.

Adapted from Weisman RS, Goldfrank LR: Prevention and the role of the poison center. In Goldfrank LR et al, eds: *Goldfrank's toxicologic emergencies,* ed 5, Norwalk, CT, 1994, Appleton & Lange.

DISCHARGE TEACHING

The emergency department nurse has an obligation to provide injury prevention advice to the parent or guardian before discharge from the department. Information should be printed, with verbal reinforcement on discharge. A review of emergency department records during one study revealed that only 1 in 10 children received injury prevention instructions at discharge.[18] By entering into the same potentially risky environment, the absence of active prevention education puts the child at risk for repeated poisoning accidents (Box 27-10).

POISON INFORMATION CENTERS

Since the inception of poison information centers in the early 1950s, directing the assessment, triage, and management of poisoned patients by telephone has become a routine event. These centers are staffed by nurses, pharmacists, and physicians who possess specialized knowledge and training in the management of the poisoned patient. The movement toward a centralized poison information system with standardized training and a dedicated staff has been much like that toward the utilization of a systems approach to emergency medical services around the country.[45] Nearly 72% of poison exposures can be treated at home with appropriate follow-up by the poison center, avoiding expensive emergency room visits.[42] During the early 1980s the AAPCC set standards for poison information center operation and outlined national accreditation criteria for these centers to ensure effective manpower, expertise, and resources.[78] Of the 64 poison centers reporting to the AAPCC in 1993, 36 are AAPCC certified as meeting the criteria set for regional centers (Fig. 27-5).

Nothing is more frightening to parents than realizing that their child has just become a poisoning victim. With the tremendous number and variety of products available in the average home, it is impossible to be informed about all of the potentially toxic substances in one's environment. A telephone call to the local poison center provides rapid, accurate information to the caller and quickly determines whether the victim needs medical attention. The information specialist can provide immediate relief to a panicked parent and reassurance by following up with a telephone call to ensure that no symptoms have developed. Having the telephone

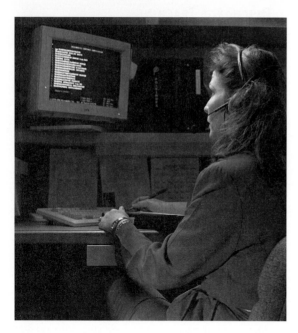

FIG. 27-5. Poison center—specialist in poison information.

number to the nearest poison center with other emergency numbers or attaching emergency telephone stickers to the telephone provides quick access in an emergency.

The poison center staff not only interacts with the general public, but also with healthcare professionals, providing direction for the evaluation and treatment of poisoning exposures. Intervention does not end with the initial call. Repeated follow-up contacts are performed for up to 24 hours to assess the status of the ongoing poison management. Although perceived as the main functional objective for a poison information center, answering telephone calls *is not* where the predominant cost-effectiveness or life-sparing abilities of these services reside. Since almost 90% of poison exposures are accidental, they can be prevented with public education and awareness of poison prevention. Poison centers have traditionally offered public education outreach programs in their regions with the goal of averting the occurrence of poisoning incidents on a grand scale and ultimately decreasing health care dollars spent.

| SECTION II | **Environmental Emergencies** |

∎ BITES AND STINGS

INSECT BITES

Etiology. In 1993 the AAPCC reported 60,516 bites and stings from ants, bees, wasps, hornets, caterpillars, mosquitos, and scorpions. Among the venomous insects, bees, wasps, and ants (Hymenoptera) were responsible for 16,186 human exposures.[42] Scorpion envenomations accounted for the third largest category of insect exposures in the 1993 AAPCC data. Caterpillars (Lepidoptera) are generally less toxic, but they can cause significant discomfort.

Frequently the offending insect is not observed in the act of biting, which would explain the 16,951 reported bites from an unknown insect or spider. Almost 3600 bites from black widow and brown recluse spiders took place in 1993, but no deaths were reported.[42] The black widow spider (*Latrodectus mactans*) can be quickly identified by its characteristic shiny black (sometimes brown), round body with a red hourglass marking on the underside. Children may be at greater risk from black widow bites due to stress from the intense pain and catecholamine release.[15] The brown recluse (*Loxosceles reclusa*) or "fiddle back" spider has a characteristic violin-shaped figure on the dorsum of the thorax. Local tissue necrosis results from envenomation with this spider. It is found most commonly in the Midwest, Southwest, and Pacific Northwest. Systemic reactions have occasionally been reported, characteristically manifesting hemolytic anemia with hemoglobinuria. The prevalence of specific insects and the incidence of stings or bites vary throughout geographic regions (Table 27-6).

Pathophysiology. Bees, wasps, and ant stings can produce various systemic effects, depending on individual sensitivity. The number of bites or stings may also determine the severity of symptoms in nonallergic individuals. Reactions may range from mild localized burning and itching to anaphylactic shock. Often the first exposure to a sting or bite results only in localized pain, mild redness, and edema. The danger exists on subsequent exposures where the individual becomes sensitized from previous antibody production (IgE antibody seen in allergic reactions).

TABLE 27-6	Common Insects Involved in Bites or Stings in the United States
ORDER	INSECTS
Hymenoptera	Honeybee, wasp, yellow jacket, hornet, fire ants
Aranea	Black widow, brown recluse
Lepidoptera	Puss caterpillar (woolly slug), flannel moth, io moth caterpillar, saddleback caterpillar, gypsy moth
Hemiptera (sucking bugs)	Assassin bugs, kissing bugs, bedbugs, giant waterbugs
Dipterans	Mosquitoes, biting midges ("no-seeums"), blackflies, sandflies, horse-flies
Scorpionida	Scorpions (bark scorpion, whip scorpion)

From Minton & Bechtel, 1989; Banner, 1989.

These antibodies cause basophils and mast cells to degranulate and release histamine and other substances. Symptoms consistent with an allergic reaction then appear. Wasp and bee venoms have been found to contain between 9 and 13 antigens, with some possessing potent allergic properties. It has been estimated that 4% of the general population show some degree of clinical allergy to insect venoms.[46]

Clinical presentation. Commonly, insect stings are inflicted on the head, neck, and extremities. Localized pain, edema, erythema, and wheal formation occur soon after the exposure. Multiple stings have produced vomiting, diarrhea, generalized edema, dyspnea, dizziness, muscle spasms, hypotension, cardiovascular collapse, and oliguria. Symptoms may be evident immediately or delayed more than 2 hours. Commonly, signs of systemic reaction appear within 30 minutes of the sting.[1] The honeybee has a barbed stinger containing a venom sac and often leaves the stinger in the wound after the attack (Table 27-7).

Emergency Department interventions. Interventions are based on symptoms, which may range from mild urticaria to fulminant anaphylaxis. In mild cases, antihistamine therapy with diphenhydramine 5 mg/kg/day, four times a day, can be given orally for pruritus. When the symptoms are more severe, diphenhydramine 1 mg/kg may be

administered every 6 to 8 hours via intravenous line or intramuscularly. For severe cases with signs of anaphylactic shock, epinephrine, volume therapy and the use of vasopressors are required (see discussion of anaphylaxis, p. 653).

Nursing care and evaluation. Children exhibiting mild signs are treated symptomatically. Children exhibiting moderate to severe symptoms should be cautiously monitored for the development of airway compromise or hemodynamic instability. These children require frequent vital signs, cardiac monitoring, and venous access. Children exhibiting signs of anaphylaxis require emergency stabilization of the ABCs (see discussion of anaphylaxis).

Once the child's condition is stabilized, the wound is cleaned and the stinger—if present—removed using a scraping motion. The use of tweezers may rupture the venom sack. Cold compresses can be applied to the wound(s), and antihistamine lotions or creams can be used. Baking soda paste or unseasoned meat tenderizer may be of benefit in the home setting. Oral analgesics and/or antihistamines may be necessary in some cases.

On discharge, the parent is told to observe the child closely for signs of infection within the next 24 to 72 hours. If warranted by severe allergy history, the patient, parent, and/or guardian is instructed in the use of an emergency insect bite kit and the need for a medical identification tag. Children who manifest a systemic reaction to a sting possess a 60% risk of life-threatening systemic reactions on reexposure.[72] The parent and child are instructed to avoid sudden movements around these insects; avoid perfumes, colognes, or hair sprays; and avoid dark-colored (brown, black, dark red) or loose fitting clothing with bright flowery patterns, which may attract insects. Children should wear shoes at all times when outdoors, shake out clothing and shoes before wearing, avoid outdoor areas where insects congregate (such as picnic sites), and avoid high-risk outdoor activities such as lawn mowing, hedge trimming, or emptying garbage cans.[1]

ANIMAL BITES

Etiology. Children experience bites from a variety of animals during the developing years. Animal bites account for approximately 1% of all emergency department visits, with the majority involving dogs, cats, humans, and rodents. Considering that 58% of families own a dog, the potential for this type of bite

TABLE 27-7	Common Signs and Symptoms After Venomous Insect Bites	
INSECT	**SIGNS AND SYMPTOMS**	**TREATMENT**
Honeybee, wasp, yellow jacket, hornet	Local swelling, redness and itching. Severe reactions: vomiting, diarrhea, urticaria, wheezing, dizziness, muscle spasms, hypotension, convulsions, collapse.	Remove stinger if present. Cleanse wound with antiseptic. Cold compress to area. Oral antihistamines and corticosteroids. Treat anaphylaxis as indicated.
Fire ants	Local reaction: reddened raised wheal leading to fluid-filled vesicle, pruritus, urticaria. Severe reaction: does not correlate with number of bites (<5 have caused severe anaphylactic reactions); symptoms same as honeybee, wasp, etc.	Local or systemic analgesics, antihistamines, steroids, antibiotics, baking soda paste. Anaphylactoid reactions: epinephrine, steroids, support respiratory and cardiovascular function.
Spiders		
Black widow	Severe pain in 15 to 60 minutes; increasing for 12 to 48 hours. Muscle rigidity in chest, back, shoulders, and abdomen. Dyspnea, nausea, vomiting, headache, sweating, paresthesias, hypertension.	Analgesics, diazepam, calcium gluconate 10% solution (0.1 ml/kg), muscle relaxants (i.e., methocarbamol) for muscle spasms. Antivenin for the young or old for uncontrolled hypertension or seizures.
Brown recluse	Bite often painless initially. Local pain and erythema 2 to 8 hours after the bite. Formation of bleb or blister, central induration and dark violet color next 48 to 72 hours. Area ulcerates and black eschar appears and eventually sloughs 2 to 5 weeks later. Systemic: headache, fever, nausea, vomiting, joint pain, rash, weakness, hemolytic anemia, disseminated intravascular coagulation, renal failure.	Ice compresses for short term, elevation and immobilization of bite site until pain resolves. Antibiotics, possible wound debridement, and skin grafting. Dapsone and steroids are controversial.
Caterpillars	Erythema, itching, swelling, and localized pain. Severe: nausea, headache, fever, vomiting, lymphadenopathy.	Application of tape to remove spines. Antipruritic creams/lotions. Analgesics for moderate pain.
Scorpions		
Non-*Centruroides*	Local pain and erythema, nausea, vomiting.	Wound cleansing; cool compresses; oral analgesics.
Whip scorpion	Secretes acetic and caprylic acid, which can be irritating to eyes or skin.	Prompt irrigation of eyes or skin.
Bark scorpion (*Centruroides exilicauda*)	Tachycardia, hypertension, vomiting, diarrhea, local hyperesthesia, muscle twitching, stridor, opisthotonus, roving eye movements, hyperactivity, visual defects.	Cool compresses, mild analgesics, supportive care; antivenin not approved by Food and Drug Administration.

is significant. In fact, dogs are responsible for 80% to 90% of mammalian bites, with cats accounting for only 10%.[24]

Localized infections account for more than 95% of complications from animal bites because of the variety of organisms that can be transmitted during the bite.[23] Rabies is a serious concern in children because of their desire for close contact with animals and the tendency to spend a good deal of time outdoors.[23]

Pathophysiology. Skin and soft tissue injuries are the first concern when evaluating animal bites. The variety of organisms that could be introduced into a wound increases a child's risk for infection. Over 40 organisms have been found in normal human mouth flora, including *Streptococcus, Staphylococcus aureus,* and *Eikenella corrodens.* Overall infection rates resulting from human bites vary from 15% to 50%, depending on the site. Dog bites are associated with a low incidence of infection (2% to 5%). *S. aureus, S. epidermidis,* and *Pasteurella multocida* are the organisms found most frequently. In contrast, cat bites result in a 30% to 50% rate of infection, with *P. multocida* the most prevalent organism implicated. Interestingly, a cat scratch will introduce the same organisms as a cat bite.

The most serious complication of an animal bite is the development of rabies, which should always be considered. Rabies is commonly carried in raccoons, foxes, bats, skunks, wolves, llamas, cattle, and unvaccinated domesticated dogs and cats. An unprovoked attack carries a higher risk of the rabies virus being transmitted, since unusual animal behavior may correlate with the animal's having rabies.[24] Skin penetration or contact with mucous membranes is necessary for transmission of the virus. The incubation period of the disease can range from 10 days to 8 months, although 1 to 2 months is average.[23]

Clinical presentation. Clinical presentation varies, depending on the severity of the bite, the source and location of the bite, and the length of time before seeking treatment. Wound evaluation includes an assessment of the severity of the injury as well as assessment for underlying injuries such as tendon or nerve damage. Cellulitis, erythema, swelling, and tenderness are seen in most animal bites. Fever and adenopathy may also be present. Other potential complications include closed-space infections, abscess formation, osteomyelitis, and septic arthritis. Wounds located on the hand or foot and puncture wounds have an increased incidence of

infection and require aggressive treatment. Wound infections normally surface within 3 to 5 days after the injury.

Emergency Department interventions. Treatment depends on the location, severity, and source of the bite. The wound is first cleaned and inspected for the degree of injury. Depending on findings, an x-ray of the injured area may be ordered to identify the presence of a foreign body or fracture. If the wound is infected, a culture is obtained. Suturing may be indicated, depending on the location and depth of the wounds, as well as the potential for wound infection. Facial wounds in particular are usually sutured for cosmetic reasons, and they have a low incidence of infection.

Antibiotic therapy is based on the source and location of the bite (high risk) and/or the organism(s) cultured. Tetanus prophylaxis is ordered based on immunization status. The rabies immunization series is initiated when the bite is considered high risk. Follow-up care is important to monitor for the development of an infection.

Nursing care and evaluation. On arrival in the emergency department the nurse must assess all wounds, evaluating the number of bites and the potential for underlying injuries. Wound management includes adequate cleansing of the wound(s). Irrigation under pressure and debridement may be necessary, as well as cleaning the wound with benzalkonium chloride, which kills the rabies virus. Scrubbing the wound with a brush should be avoided because it tends to increase the infection rate.[24] In more extensive wounds, local anesthesia may be employed before forceful irrigation. Copious amounts of normal saline solution are used to irrigate the wound. Antibiotics and immunizations should be anticipated.

Discharge instructions should include information on the importance of follow-up care (when and where), dressing application, and medication administration (antibiotics and/or where to obtain rabies prophylaxis). Parents should also be instructed to observe the wound(s) for signs of infection, which include fever, redness, tenderness, swelling, or drainage. The parent should be advised to restrict the child's access to unfamiliar animals in the future. Finally, local protocols must be followed based on city, county, or state requirements with regard to contacting animal control or the local health department for confinement of the animal if warranted.

SNAKEBITES

Etiology. Of the 72,637 bites and envenomations reported to the AAPCC in 1993, 4734 exposures involved the bite of a snake. Of these, 1150 were reported to involve venomous snakes, and almost 300 of these occurred in children under 17 years of age. In 1992 two deaths were recorded in adults, but none were reported in children.[43] No deaths were reported to poison centers in 1993.[42] The warmer months, between April and October, are the peak period for snakebites, since snakes are more active during this time. The most common snakebite in the United States is that of the copperhead snake.[28]

Two families of venomous snakes are indigenous to the United States. They are the pit vipers (Crotalidae) and the coral snakes (Elapidae). The pit vipers account for approximately 99% of all venomous snakebites in states reporting the highest incidence of snakebites (North Carolina, Arkansas, Texas, Missis-sippi, Arizona, and New Mexico) (Table 27-8). The majority of bites are to the extremities. The upper extremities are involved approximately two thirds of the time,[63] with 80% of bites on the finger and hand. The foot and ankle areas account for approximately 15% of snakebites.[74]

The Eastern and Western diamondback rattlesnakes are considered the more dangerous of the pit vipers because of their aggressiveness, their ability to inject a large amount of venom, and the hemotoxic activity of the venom. The coral snake's neurotoxic venom is thought to be more potent than that of the pit viper. The coral snake has a row of teeth instead of the fangs displayed by the pit viper and actually must "chew" to inject its venom.

Several characteristic features differentiate the pit vipers from nonvenomous snakes. The triangular-shaped head of the pit vipers contrasts to the oval or egg-shaped head of the nonvenomous snakes. Verti-

TABLE 27-8	Venomous Snakes of North America	
COMMON NAME	**NAME**	**AREA OF DISTRIBUTION**
Canebrake rattlesnake	*Crotalus horridus atricaudatus*	Southeastern states
Copperhead	*Agkistrodon contortrix*	Northeastern, Southeastern, Central, and Southwestern states
Cottonmouth	*Agkistrodon piscivorus*	Northeastern, Southeastern, Central, and Southwestern states
Eastern coral snake	*Micrurus fulvius fulvius*	Southeastern states
Eastern diamondback rattlesnake	*Crotalus adamanteus*	Southeastern states
Great Basin rattlesnake	*Crotalus viridus lutosus*	Central and Pacific states
Massasauga rattlesnake	*Sistrurus catenatus*	Central and Southwestern states
Mojave rattlesnake	*Crotalus scutulatus scutulatus*	Mojave Desert area in southern California and Southwestern states
Northern blacktailed rattlesnake	*Crotalus molossus molossus*	Southwestern states
Northern Pacific rattlesnake	*Crotalus viridis oreganus*	Pacific states
Pigmy rattlesnake	*Sistrurus miliaris*	Southeastern and Southwestern states
Prairie rattlesnake	*Crotalus viridis viridis*	Central and Southwestern states
Red diamondback rattlesnake	*Crotalus ruber ruber*	Southwestern and Pacific states
Sidewinder	*Crotalus cerastes*	Southwestern and Pacific states
Sonoran coral snake	*Micrurus euryxanthus*	Southwestern states
Southern Pacific rattlesnake	*Crotalus viridis helleri*	Pacific states
Texas coral snake	*Micrurus fulvius tenere*	Southwestern states
Timber rattlesnake	*Crotalus horridus horridus*	Northeastern and Central states
Western diamondback rattlesnake	*Crotalus atrox*	Southwestern and Pacific states

Adapted from Auerbach PS: *Wilderness medicine: management of wilderness and environmental emergencies,* ed 3, St Louis, 1995, Mosby.

cally elliptical pupils (similar to cat's eyes) differ from the round pupils of the nonvenomous snakes. However, the presence of an oval head or round pupils is not always indicative of strictly nonvenomous snakes. The coral snake possesses an oval head as well as round pupils. Other attributes of the pit vipers include the heat-sensitive pit (to detect its prey) located between the eye and nostril on the side of the head; two easily identifiable anterior fangs that fold posteriorly against the palate, readily available to advance forward to strike; the presence of a rattle on the tail; and a single row of ventral scales leading up to the anal plate.[28] The striking range of a snake is approximately one-half its length.

Pathophysiology. The presence of various protein and enzymatic components in the venom of the pit vipers is the basis for its extensive effects at the wound site and systemic effects on multiple organ systems. Locally the toxin causes increased vascular permeability, resulting in the extravasation of plasma, plasma proteins, and erythrocytes into the tissues.[79] Edema, hemorrhage, and tissue necrosis result. Venom may be carried through the lymphatic and blood systems, resulting in systemic effects, including microvascular damage to the endothelial cells and cellular plasma membranes.[79] The resultant extravasation of intravascular volume can lead to profound shock. Damage to plasma cellular membranes, coupled with the thrombin-like enzyme in crotalid venom, produces coagulopathies such as disseminated intravascular coagulation (DIC) and thrombocytopenia.[74] Uncontrollable hemorrhage can result.

Clinical presentation. The magnitude of clinical effects depends on the species and age of the snake, age and weight of the victim, location of bite, degree of envenomation, and promptness of care rendered. Massive tissue edema, shock, bleeding, and coagulation disturbances are the common effects of severe envenomation. In contrast, the coral snake's venom may cause little or no edema, necrosis, or pain. The venom is predominately neurotoxic, with symptoms appearing within 90 minutes or several hours.[62] Paresthesias and muscle fasciculations, flaccid paralysis, and respiratory failure may also develop.[61]

Approximately 30% of pit viper bites are dry bites and result in minimal local and systemic effects. The child may have one or two fang marks, immediate pain, and some local edema at the site. If actual envenomation occurred, progressive swelling will be evident within 5 minutes and may eventually involve the entire

extremity. Ecchymosis of the area varies and also depends on the degree of envenomation. Numbness and tingling around the mouth or face, weakness, nausea, vomiting, dizziness, and diaphoresis may also occur.[14]

Pit viper bites are classified according to severity of symptoms and are categorized as no envenomation and minimal, mild, moderate, or severe envenomation. Minimal envenomations demonstrate visible fang marks, pain, and localized swelling, without systemic signs of envenomation. Mild envenomation involves progressive swelling without systemic effects. Moderate envenomation involves marked swelling beyond the bite site, systemic signs as previously described, vital sign changes, and perhaps mild coagulation changes. Severe envenomation displays marked swelling, severe systemic symptoms, marked coagulopathy, and subcutaneous ecchymosis[63] (Fig. 27-6).

The incidence of coral snake envenomation is relatively low, with approximately 40% of all bites resulting in venom injection. The child bitten by a coral snake may exhibit little or no pain at the bite site. Bite marks may be difficult to visualize, since there are no fangs and swelling may be minimal. Early manifestations of envenomation involve paresthesias and muscle fasciculations at the site. Weakness or numbness may be evident within 90 minutes but may be delayed 12 hours or more. Other common symptoms

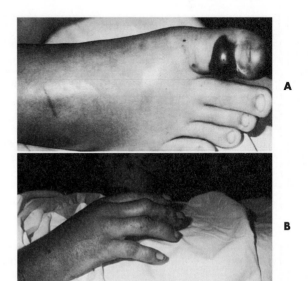

FIG. 27-6. **A,** Snake envenomation (moderate). **B,** Snake envenomation (mild).

include nausea, vomiting, dizziness, blurred vision, slurred speech, shortness of breath, and excessive salivation. Mild to moderate manifestations may eventually progress to paralysis and respiratory failure.

Emergency Department interventions. As with any emergency illness or injury, the ABCs must first be assessed and stabilized. Baseline laboratory values are obtained, including a complete blood count, serum electrolytes, serum creatinine, blood urea nitrogen, UA, prothrombin time, partial thromboplastin time, platelet count, fibrinogen level, and fibrin split products, as well as hold clot for type and cross match.[61] An electrocardiogram is indicated in all but minor cases. As symptoms progress, the administration of packed red blood cells, fresh-frozen plasma, and platelet replacement for coagulopathies may be required.

Serum antivenin administration is based on the suspected degree of envenomation and the source of the bite (Table 27-9). Early empiric administration of coral snake antivenin (Antivenin, *Micrurus fulvius* by Wyeth Laboratories) is advised in any bite where the suspicion for Elapidae envenomation is high. This is because of the difficulty in assessing envenomation because of the delay in symptomatology and the rapid progression of life-threatening symptoms once they become evident.

Nursing care and evaluation

Field care. Initial field management of the snakebite victim requires keeping the child warm and as calm as possible. Few snakebites cause immediate death; therefore prompt transport to the nearest health care facility is feasible. If the snake has been killed, it can be taken to the emergency department in a closed container for later identification. Direct handling of the snake is discouraged because of the presence of reflex activity, which can still enable the snake to envenomate anyone holding it. Immobilization of the extremity by splinting or with a sling, keeping the extremity at or below the level of the heart, and removal of any constrictive items (rings, watches, bracelets) is advised. The use of constrictive bands is extremely controversial. The possibility of increasing local tissue damage is one risk, as is applying the band too tightly so that all blood flow is occluded. It should be viewed as an adjunct in prehospital treatment until more definitive care at the emergency department is available.[11] Constricting bands should block lymphatic flow only. The proper procedure is to apply the band proximal to the bite site loosely with one to two fingerbreadths of room between the band and the skin surface. The application of ice is contraindicated because it may cause further tissue damage. Incision and suction in the field are not recommended

TABLE 27-9	Classification of Envenomation by the Pit Viper and Guidelines for Antivenin	
EXTENT OF ENVENOMATION	**SIGNS AND SYMPTOMS**	**ANTIVENIN GUIDELINES**
None	Fang marks present. No local swelling or systemic signs.	None
Minimal	Local swelling and pain. No systemic symptoms. No progression of signs.	None
Mild	Edema progresses slowly. Normal laboratory findings. No systemic effects.	0 to 5 vials
Moderate	Progression of swelling beyond bite site. Increase in pain and erythema. Perioral fasciculation, paresthesias, nausea, vomiting, or dizziness may occur. Minor laboratory changes.	5 to 10 vials
Severe	Rapid, progressive swelling; ecchymosis; petechiae, and necrosis. Systemic signs may include tachycardia, marked coagulopathy, shock, coma, renal failure, convulsions, hemolysis, or cardiac arrest.	10 to 40 vials

unless a significant delay in medical attention is expected, since the risk of infection or necrosis is significant and overzealous incision may cause additional injury. The use of a "Sawyer Extractor" may be of value in the first 30 to 60 minutes after a snakebite. It is applied directly over the incisions or fang punctures and acts as a suction device.[61]

Emergency Department interventions. Children coming to the emergency department with a positive history of a snakebite by a potentially venomous snake must be treated emergently. An initial evaluation of the ABCs is required, as is obtaining a complete set of baseline vital signs. The child must be continuously monitored for the development of systemic symptoms, with intake and output recorded. Intravenous access is obtained for the possible administration of fluids, blood components, and antivenin. Perfusion distal to the bite(s) must also be assessed, including color, skin temperature, capillary refill, and pulses. Compartment syndrome can develop after a venomous snakebite. It is most commonly associated with bites into the muscle fascia. Because of the presence of severe pain, cyanosis at the site, and massive edema with severe envenomations, the development of compartment syndrome may be difficult to detect.

The wound should be thoroughly examined and the child checked for the presence of other bite sites. Children often "freeze" from fear after the initial bite and may have more than one bite. If the bite is on an extremity, the circumference of the extremity must be measured to evaluate the progression of swelling, and the size is compared to the unaffected extremity. The extremity should be measured at the edge of edema in 4-inch increments proximally to the shoulder or groin. When the measuring tape is placed on the extremity, the skin should be marked on both sides of the tape so that the placement for subsequent measurements is in the exact same position. Measurements are taken every 15 minutes for the first 2 hours and then hourly. Tetanus prophylaxis is indicated, depending on immunization status. Standard wound cleansing is used. If the bite involves an extremity, the limb may be splinted in a functional position and kept at or below the level of the heart.

Antivenin. When antivenin administration is deemed necessary, two intravenous lines are recommended. One is for the antivenin and the other for fluid and medication therapy. Before administration, the skin is first tested for reactivity to identify children who are highly allergic to antivenin. Both serum sickness and anaphylaxis are serious side effects of antivenin administration, which is made from horse serum. With both skin testing and antivenin administration, emergency equipment and medications must be available to treat anaphylaxis. Skin testing involves the use of the test material supplied in the antivenin kit or reconstituted antivenin at a dilution

---

Box 27-11 Nursing Care of the Victim of a Venomous Snakebite

All children
- Stabilize the airway and breathing.
- Obtain a full set of baseline vital signs.
- Obtain vascular access and baseline laboratory studies.
- Attach the child to a cardiorespiratory monitor.
- Inspect and clean the wound; fully examine the child for the presence of other bites.
- Maintain strict intake and output.
- Continuously monitor the child for the development of systemic signs and symptoms.

Bites to an extremity
- Remove constricting clothing or items such as rings, watches, bracelets.
- Assess perfusion distal to the site; observe for the development of compartment syndrome.
- Splint the extremity and keep it at or below the level of the heart; do not apply ice.
- Serially measure the extremity in 4-inch increments, proximal to the site, every 15 minutes for 2 hours and then hourly.

Antivenin
- Prepare emergency equipment to treat the possible development of anaphylaxis.
- Perform skin testing based on package instructions.
- Gently mix the antivenin; do not shake the vial.
- Dilute the antivenin based on package instructions, the amount to be administered, and the size of the child (discuss with the ordering physician).
- Continuously monitor the child during the antivenin infusion.

of 1:10. The absence of a reaction does not guarantee that the child is not allergic to the antivenin; however, the majority of children with negative tests will tolerate the antivenin without acute adverse side effects.[74]

The antivenin is mixed by *gently* "rolling" the vial between the palms. Shaking or agitating the vial denatures the proteins in the antivenin. Children usually require more antivenin than adults.[28] Initially the antivenin is diluted according to package instructions, the size of the patient, and the amount of antivenin to be infused. The infusion is begun slowly (5 to 10 ml/kg/hr) and the child observed for approximately 10 minutes to see if an allergic response develops. If there is no reaction, the antivenin is administered over 1 to 2 hours.[74] When the child exhibits a positive response to skin testing yet has a severe envenomation requiring the use of the antivenin, premedication with diphenhydramine and cimetidine may be required. The use of corticosteroids is controversial. The child's condition must be monitored continuously throughout the antivenin infusion (Box 27-11).

▌ CLINICAL CONDITIONS

URTICARIA

Etiology. There are many causes of urticaria, including environmental vectors, drugs, food and food additives, diseases, insect bites, and stings (Box 27-12). At any given moment, up to 20% of the population can be afflicted with urticaria. Acute episodes are most common in children and in atopic individuals and are usually short-lived. Persons with chronic urticaria may have symptoms that last for more than 6 weeks. Frequently the etiology is not clearly determined.

Pathophysiology. Urticaria are believed to be induced by IgE antigen-antibody reactions.[68] These reactions cause basophil and mast cell mediators to be released, resulting in the characteristic vasodilation, erythema, and edema. The primary mediators purported to be responsible for this allergen-antibody reaction include histamine, bradykinin, and kallidin. Other substances also thought to be connected with this reaction are prostaglandins, leukotrienes, and plasmin. Several external factors appear to play a role in exacerbating urticaria, such as exertion, heat, and fever.[68]

Clinical presentation. The skin eruptions develop rapidly and are erythematous and pruritic. They usually manifest as a raised wheal with marked edema. The lesions are well-circumscribed, transitory, variable in size and pattern, and often have blanched centers.

Emergency Department interventions. No diagnostic tests are indicated for the acute, isolated urticarial reaction. The presence of systemic disease should always be considered in the differential diagnosis. Identification of the specific etiologic agents should be considered to prevent future occurrences. Antihistamines and epinephrine are the standard agents used in treating this condition. Episodes of mild urticaria generally respond well to antihistamines (histamine receptor blockers). Moderate cases of urticaria may require the addition of steroids. Treatment with epinephrine is reserved for severe and/or life-threatening reactions. The dose is 0.01 ml/kg/dose of the 1:1000 solution (maximum dose: 0.35 ml) given subcutaneously every 20 minutes as needed.

Most patients respond to low-dose, short-term therapy with steroids.[12] Steroids are given in conjunction with the administration of a histamine receptor (H_1) blocker such as diphenhydramine 5 mg/kg/24 hr every 6 hours orally, intramuscularly, or intravenously, or hydroxyzine 2 mg/kg/24 hr every 6 hours orally. Management of recurrent or persistent allergic urticaria should include the addition of H_2 blockers such as cimetidine 20 to 30 mg/kg/24 hr every 4 to 6 hours orally.[6]

Nursing care and evaluation. Severe reactions necessitate initial stabilization of the ABCs, as with any

---

Box 27-12	Common Etiologies of Urticaria

Contactants: moth scales, caterpillars, nettle plants, cat scratches
Drugs: antibiotics (penicillin) salicylates, narcotics
Foods and food additives: eggs, shellfish, nuts, fish
Inhalants: cat, horse
Infectious diseases: streptococcal pharyngitis, sinusitis, hepatitis, viral infection, mononucleosis
Insect bites and stings: bees, hymenoptera, fleas, mites
Neoplasms: leukemia, Hodgkin's disease
Trauma: mechanical, thermal (cold and heat), sun

life-threatening emergency. The child should be monitored for respiratory compromise with continuous vital sign assessment and cardiac monitoring. Intravenously administered medications are more rapidly effective in these circumstances. Antihistamines and epinephrine usually provide relief in acute episodes. Steroids may be indicated in more severe reactions or when response to initial therapeutic modalities is poor. Milder reactions warrant the use of oral medication, follow-up prescriptions, and discharge instructions, including methods for avoidance of the causative agents. Patients should be referred to their private physician for additional evaluation and follow-up.[59]

ANAPHYLAXIS/ANGIONEUROTIC EDEMA

Etiology. Anaphylaxis is a systemic allergic reaction immunologically mediated after exposure to an antigen. The antigen may be introduced orally, through inhalation, topically, or parenterally. Hypersensitivity to drugs, foods, or insect stings is common. Antibiotics, especially penicillin, are common causative agents. Genetic disposition appears to play a significant role in one's sensitivity to penicillin use and Hymenoptera stings (bee, wasp, yellow jacket, hornet, ants). Foods also known to induce this reaction include shellfish, nuts, eggs, fruits, vegetables, and milk. Other common etiologies include local anesthetics, diagnostic agents (radiographic contrast), narcotics, dust, animal dander, and pollen.

Pathophysiology. The anaphylactic reaction is mediated by IgE antibodies and caused by local and systemic release of endogenous vasoactive substances, such as histamine and leukotrienes. Anaphylaxis may also be produced by non-IgE-mediated mechanisms involving activation of the mast cells via anaphylatoxins. Initial sensitization to an offending agent causes antibody formation. Pathophysiologically, as part of the body's defense against these foreign agents, IgE antibodies bind to cell membranes of basophils and mast cells.[33] Subsequent exposures to the original sensitizing antigen set off events leading to the severe allergic reaction. In some rare instances these reactions may result from the initial exposure to the antigen.

In contrast to anaphylactic reactions, anaphylactoid reactions are not immunologically mediated. Certain agents may directly cause the degranulation of mast cells and basophils. Agents known to be associated with this include hyperosmolar solutions of mannitol, radiocontrast material, opiates, and vancomycin.[59]

Clinical presentation. Symptoms usually occur within 30 minutes of the exposure and range from simple urticaria to pruritus, bronchospasm, laryngeal edema, abdominal cramping, hypotension, or shock (Table 27-10).

Angioneurotic edema is an allergic disorder that usually occurs in the presence of urticaria. Areas involved include the lips, tongue, periorbital and perioral areas, dorsum of hands and feet, and scrotum. The mucous membranes of the larynx, bronchi, and gastrointestinal tract may be affected. Deeper layers of the skin are involved, causing a more diffuse swelling than the typical "hive" lesions. Localized subcutaneous edema of any body part may occur. Pronounced swelling of the airway can lead to stridor, hoarseness, dyspnea, and actual airway obstruction as a result of edema of the larynx. The symptoms may appear within several seconds of the exposure or up to several hours, and they may persist for 24 to 36 hours. Gastrointestinal involvement can manifest as acute abdominal pain with vomiting.

A form of hereditary angioedema appears to be much the same as anaphylaxis. In comparison to urticaria, the reaction occurs deeper in the dermis.[59] Occurrences may present spontaneously or be precipitated by trauma. Associated symptoms include prominent swelling in the face, lips, hands, and arms and edema of the tongue, uvula, oropharynx, and potentially the larynx. Edema of the GI tract may induce nausea, vomiting, and abdominal cramping.

TABLE 27-10	Signs and Symptoms of Anaphylactic Reaction	
SYSTEM	**SIGNS AND SYMPTOMS**
General	Weakness, malaise
Dermal	Urticaria, flushing, angioedema, pruritus, erythema
Respiratory	Stridor, hoarseness, cough, wheezing, chest tightness, tachypnea, rhinitis, cyanosis
Cardiovascular	Hypotension, tachycardia, shock, cardiac arrhythmias
Neurologic	Apprehension, syncope, seizures, coma
Gastrointestinal	Dysphagia, nausea, vomiting, diarrhea, abdominal pain

Pruritus is usually not associated with this disorder, nor does urticaria accompany its development. Epinephrine is not effective in treating hereditary angioedema.[84] Prophylaxis to prevent angioedema attacks with impeded androgens (stanozolol or danazol) has been successful.[59] Again, the most serious complication is edema of the larynx, which causes severe respiratory distress. Symptoms usually abate in 3 to 4 days.

Emergency Department interventions. Initial management depends on the severity of the response. An antihistamine such as diphenhydramine (1 mg/kg orally or IM) may be administered in combination with epinephrine (0.01 ml/kg of 1:1000 solution SQ) to treat mild symptoms. If symptoms are severe or rapidly progressing, intravenous access should be obtained to administer fluids and vasopressor therapy. If the child is hypotensive, volume replacement with 20 ml/kg of normal saline or lactated Ringer's solution is warranted, as well as intravenous epinephrine (0.01 mg/kg [1:10,000]/kg every 5 to 10 minutes, up to maximum of 0.1 mg). Intravenous epinephrine is also administered for bronchospasm. A continuous intravenous infusion of epinephrine may be required. It is administered at 0.1 µg/kg/min up to maximum 1.5 µg/kg/min. In severe cases, intravenous antihistamines may also be used. Commonly used histamine antagonists include diphenhydramine 1 mg/kg IV or IM or hydroxyzine hydrochloride 0.5 to 1 mg/kg IM or IV. Inhaled beta-agonist agents such as albuterol may be used for bronchospasm. Corticosteroids may be useful, but their effects may not be evident for 4 to 6 hours.[6] Baseline laboratory values may include complete blood count, serum electrolytes, clotting factors, and urinalysis; in severe cases, serial blood gas measurements are taken.

Nursing care and evaluation. Signs of anaphylaxis vary from mild symptoms to airway constriction and profound shock; therefore any child arriving with signs of anaphylaxis requires emergency management. The first priority of care is to establish or maintain a patent airway and provide oxygenation. Airway supplies, including a bag-valve-mask device and intubation equipment, and emergency drugs, including epinephrine, must be readily available. As the child's condition is being stabilized, evaluation for the presence of the offending agent should be made.

Frequent vital signs, cardiac monitoring, and pulse oximetry are required to monitor for the development of hypotension, dysrhythmias, or shock. If the child is maintaining a patent airway, the head of the bed is elevated to ensure optimum respiratory effort. If respiratory distress or shock is present, supplemental oxygen is indicated. Venous access is required to rapidly administer fluid and drug therapy. Epinephrine, used to treat both shock and bronchospasm, is not given if the heart rate is greater than 180 beats/min, nor is it effective in treating hereditary angioedema. Once the child's condition is stabilized, one should ensure that contact with the offending antigen has ceased.

Counseling should be provided for the child and parent to discuss the allergies and to ensure future avoidance of the exposure. Instructions should include the use of a home emergency kit for anaphylaxis and assistance in procuring a medical identification tag. Referral to an appropriate physician for evaluation of desensitization to specific allergens such as penicillin or bee venom may be indicated[59] (Box 27-13).

HYPOTHERMIA

Etiology. Hypothermia is defined as a core body temperature less than 35° C (95° F).[80] Commonly, it is thought of as a seasonal, geographically limited phenomenon. This, however, is not true, since hypothermia has been reported at various times throughout the year and from the entire country. Hypothermia is classified as both a symptom and a clinical disease. Primary hypothermia is caused by extreme exposure, near-drowning, subdural hematoma, or head or spinal cord injury. When death occurs from primary hypothermia, it is regarded as a violent or traumatic death and classified as accidental, homicidal, or suicidal in nature.[17] Secondary hypothermia results from complications of systemic disorders, including infection, carcinoma, endocrine/metabolic disorders intoxication, CNS disease, or vascular factors[6] (Box 27-14).

A number of predisposing factors contribute to the occurrence of hypothermia. Those components which decrease heat production (neonates delivered emergently, aging, endocrinologic failure, or insufficient nutrition), increase heat loss (poorly acclimated to cold, burns, dermatologic disorders, multiple pharmacologic and toxicologic agents, or ethanol), and impaired thermoregulation (central, peripheral, metabolic, pharmacologic, or toxicologic) contribute to the development of hypothermia. Neonates in particular are susceptible to hypothermia because of their large body surface area and low percentage of body fat. The subtle manner in which the child may present (poor feeding and/or lethargy) can further cloud the picture. Nonspecific symptoms such as hunger, nausea, chills, or dizziness are not readily associated with hypothermia.[17]

Box 27-13   Treatment of Anaphylaxis

1. Remove antigen, delay absorption
2. Establish and maintain the ABC's
   Airway: Position airway and administer 100% oxygen as indicated
   Breathing: Initiate BVM ventilation and intubate as necessary
   Circulation: Establish peripheral IV; volume expand as necessary with 20 ml/kg boluses of normal
       saline or lactated Ringer's solution
3. Epinephrine:
   Minor reaction or emergent treatment severe reaction: 0.01 ml/kg of 1:1,000 solution SQ or IM;
       repeat at 15 to 20 minute intervals
   Hypotension or airway obstruction: 0.01 mg/kg (which equals 0.1 ml/kg of 1:10,000 solution) IV
       or intraosseous (IO)
   Persistent hypotension: epinephrine drip 0.1 μ/kg/min titrated up to 1.5 μ/kg/min as necessary IV
       or IO
   Mix drip: $0.6 \times$ wt (kg) added to 5% dextrose in water to equal 100 ml; 1 ml/hour = 0.1 μ/kg/min
4. Corticosteroids:
   Methylprednisolone 1 mg/kg IV push every 4 hours as necessary; OR hydrocortisone 1.5 to 2 mg/kg
       IV push every 6 hours
5. Antihistamine: diphenhydramine 1-2 mg/kg IM or slow IV push; may repeat every 4 to 6 hours; alternatively cimetidine or ranitidine
6. Persistent hypotension: dopamine 5 to 20 μ/kg/min; norepinephrine 0.5 to 3 μ/kg/min
7. Persistent bronchospasm or airway obstruction: albuterol 2.5 mg/dose; terbutaline 1-2 mg/dose
8. Beta blocker-accentuated anaphylaxis: terbutaline 0.005 to 0.01 mg/kg SQ; isoproterenol drip 0.1
   to 1.5 μ/kg/min (mix as described above); glucagon 0.1 mg/kg (if less than 10 kg), 1 mg/dose if
   greater than 10 kgs, **slow** IV push, over 5 minutes

Compiled from Downs CE: Anaphylaxis. In Harwood-Nuss, A et al, ed: *The clinical practice of emergency medicine,* ed 2, Philadelphia, 1996, JB Lippincott; Zull, DN: Anaphylaxis. In Harwood-Nuss, A, et al, ed: *The clinical practice of emergency medicine,* ed 2, Philadelphia, 1996, JB Lippincott; Barone MA: *The Harriet Lane Handbook,* ed 14, 1996, St. Louis, Mosby.

Pathophysiology

Hypothermia. Normal core or deep body temperatures range from 36.4° to 37.5° C (97.5° to 99.5° F). A core temperature less than 35° C (95° F) is considered hypothermia. Normal exposure to a cold environment produces shivering, which in turn generates heat. Peripheral vasoconstriction results in an attempt to conserve heat. The sympathetic response produces an increased heart rate and a higher metabolic rate.[80] As the metabolic rate increases, both oxygen consumption and glucose utilization increase. Eventually glycogen stores are depleted and hypoglycemia and metabolic acidosis result. With core temperatures below 35° C (95° F), all major organ functions are affected, particularly the CNS, cardiovascular system, and respiratory system. In addition, cold-induced diuresis results from peripheral vasoconstriction and elevated blood volume and pressure. Complications arising from hypothermia in-

clude GI bleeding, acute renal failure, pancreatitis, coagulopathy, pulmonary edema, hypovolemia resulting from extracellular fluid shifts, and deep vein thrombosis.[6] With the presence of an underlying systemic disease process, the pathophysiologic cause is difficult to determine, since it depends on the prevailing etiology.

Frostbite. Frostbite results from prolonged exposure to subfreezing temperatures. The degree of tissue damage varies, depending on the duration of exposure, amount of protective clothing worn, wind chill factor, dampness of the environment, and ambient temperature. The endothelium, bone marrow, and nerve tissue are more prone to freezing than muscle, bone, or cartilage. When frostbite occurs, ice crystals form in the tissues, diminishing blood flow to the area. The result is a loss of cutaneous sensation. Next a vascular stasis phase follows, evidenced by blood vessel dilatation, spasticity, plasma leakage, stasis coagula-

---

Box 27-14   Causes of Hypothermia

Primary hypothermia
Environmental exposure
Near-drowning: Cold water immersion
Trauma   Head trauma
                 Spinal cord transection
Intoxication: Alcohol
                 Barbiturates
                 Carbon monoxide
                 Narcotics
                 Phenothiazines
                 Tricyclic antidepressants
                 General anesthetics

Secondary hypothermia
Infection: Bacterial meningitis
                 Encephalitis
                 Respiratory infection
                 Sepsis
Endocrine/metabolic
    disorders: Hypoglycemia
                 Hypothyroidism
                 Hypopituitarism
                 Diabetic ketoacidosis
                 Myxedema
                 Addison's disease
CNS dysfunction: Cerebrovascular accidents
                 CNS disease
Vascular disorders: Shock
                 Subarachnoid hemorrhage
                 Pulmonary embolism
Other: Burns
                 Protein-calorie malnutrition

---

tion, and shunting. In the late stage (ischemic phase), tissue ischemia leads to thrombosis or gangrene.[17]

Clinical presentation

Hypothermia.   In generalized hypothermia, presenting symptoms vary and depend on the presence of an underlying disease process or a pharmacologic agent that may predispose the child to hypothermia. Typically the hypothermic child presents with shivering, tachycardia, increased blood pressure, and increased respiratory rate. These are followed by signs of CNS involvement such as slurred speech or memory lapse. As the core temperature drops below 32° C (89.6° F), marked peripheral vasoconstriction, muscle rigidity, poor muscular coordination, and a depressed

level of consciousness are evident. Bradycardia, bradypnea, and a decline in respiratory depth are late findings. Symptoms associated with core temperatures less than 28° C (82.4° F) include rigidity, obtundation, myocardial irritability, decreased cardiac output, and dysrhythmias that progress to ventricular fibrillation and asystole. Ventricular fibrillation in pronounced hypothermia may be refractory to therapy until the core body temperature rises.[7]

Frostbite.   Areas most susceptible to frostbite are the extremities: fingers, hands, toes, feet, ears, and nose. Frostbite injuries are classified according to the degree of injury present after freezing and rewarming. First-degree injuries present with numbness, erythema, white or yellowish plaque, and edema in the absence of tissue loss. Second-degree injuries manifest as blisters filled with a clear or milky fluid with a erythematous, edematous area surrounding the blisters. Deeper tissue (subcutaneous) damage occurs in third-degree injuries with necrosis of the skin, ulceration, and edema often involving deeper blisters with purple, blood-containing fluid. Fourth-degree injuries involve the dermis and subcuticular tissues. Necrosis with gangrene may appear with this injury, which can include muscle and bone involvement.[7,17] (Table 27-11).

Emergency Department interventions.   As with all emergency situations, assessment of the ABCs is required. Laboratory evaluation should include arterial blood gases, complete blood count, electrolytes, blood urea nitrogen, creatinine, amylase, calcium, magnesium, creatinine phosphokinase, prothrombin time, partial thromboplastin time, and liver function studies. Fluid resuscitation with warmed IV solutions may be necessary because of the prevalence of dehydration in these patients. Diagnostic studies are initiated to determine the underlying cause of the hypothermia.

Ventricular fibrillation is treated with electrical defibrillation and drug therapy. Bretylium tosylate is preferred over lidocaine hydrochloride for hypothermia-related ventricular fibrillation. If the temperature is less than 30° C (86° F), an initial attempt at defibrillation can be made; however, the response to defibrillation is low. Attempts should not be pursued until the core temperature is a least 30° C.

Nursing care and evaluation

Hypothermia.   Hypothermia and frostbite are considered emergent conditions. Supplemental oxy-

TABLE 27-11	Phases of Frostbite Injury
DEGREE	**CLINICAL PRESENTATION**
First	Mottled skin, edema, erythema, white or yellowish plaque at injured area, burning and tingling, no tissue loss
Second	Blister formation (clear or milky fluid), paresthesia and anesthesia of area
Third	Deeper blisters (purple, blood-containing fluid), necrosis of skin with ulceration and edema, involvement of subcutaneous tissue
Fourth	Necrosis with gangrene, injury through the dermis, possible muscle and bone involvement

gen administration, intravenous access, cardiac monitoring, and pulse oximetry must be initiated. If the child requires cardiopulmonary resuscitation, it is approached with great caution. Although basic life support and the maintenance of a patent airway are essential, attempts at intubation can induce dysrhythmias. They therefore must be performed carefully while the child's heart rate and rhythm are constantly monitored. Resuscitative efforts must be continued until a core temperature of 32° C (89.6° F) is reached and further therapy is not successful.

Core temperature measurements must be checked frequently. An indwelling rectal or esophageal thermistor probe is ideal. In cases of mild hypothermia (core temperature > 32° C), passive external rewarming is performed with blankets. The temperature should not be raised more than 2° C/hr. If the core temperature is less than 32° C, more aggressive measures are required, including the use of warmed blankets, radiant heat sources such as water bottles, heating pads, and heating blankets. If the child's condition is unstable or if passive rewarming methods are unsuccessful and the child's temperature is less than 28° C, active core rewarming may be necessary. Heated, humidified oxygen can be administered, as well as warmed IV fluids, and GI irrigation with warmed fluids can be used. Other methods that may be indicated include peritoneal dialysis, extracorporeal rewarming, and diathermy. Once the core temperature reaches 32° to 34° C, warming measures can be terminated.

The victim of hypothermia must be constantly monitored for the development of dysrhythmias. Vi-

tal signs and urine output should be frequently evaluated.

Frostbite. In the frostbite victim, the nurse should cautiously handle the injured part while gently removing all clothing. The frostbitten area should not be rubbed. Superficial injuries may be warmed by covering with a clean, dry dressing. The more serious injuries should be rewarmed by immersing the affected part in cool or tepid water for 20 to 30 minutes.[17] Rewarming can be discontinued when the skin becomes pliable and erythematous at the most distal parts. The affected part is elevated, splinted, and sterile dressings applied. Tetanus prophylaxis, analgesics, and antibiotic therapy are administered as ordered.

The child should be assessed frequently, including vital signs, mental status, cardiac rhythm, and urine output. Tissue perfusion, sensation, and mobility of the extremity should be assessed regularly. If the child is to be discharged, the parent and child is instructed regarding home care and follow-up. Prevention must be stressed, including emphasis on the use of proper protective clothing.

INFECTIOUS DISORDERS
ROCKY MOUNTAIN SPOTTED FEVER

Etiology. Rocky Mountain spotted fever (RMSF) is the most common rickettsial illness in the United States.[35] Ticks act as vectors of rickettsial illnesses and transmit the infection to humans. The primary hosts of the ticks are warm-blooded animals such as dogs, rodents, or rabbits. In 1993 the AAPCC reported 2473 tick bites.

The incidence of RMSF appears to peak from April to September, presumably when ticks are most active. It has been reported in all the contiguous states except Maine. The incidence of the disease has actually decreased more than 10-fold in the mountain states,[25] while gradually increasing in the Southern and Eastern states. Two thirds of all cases of RMSF are reported in children.[21]

Pathophysiology. *Rickettsia rickettsii,* which is transmitted by ticks, is the organism responsible for RMSF. The principal vectors are the Eastern dog tick, Western wood tick, and Southwestern Lone Star tick.[70] Initially, the tick is small and difficult to detect. Once it is attached to the host and burrows into the skin to feed on blood, it becomes engorged. The spread of the organism to a human host occurs when an infected tick detaches from a primary host and feeds on a human. Transmission through conjunctival contact or through broken skin during the process of tick removal has also resulted in infection. The organism spreads through the vascular system and invades medial smooth muscle cells. Destruction of the vascular wall leads to an inflammatory response that results in thrombus formation and occlusion of the vessel lumen. This can lead to necrosis of peripheral structures such as the fingers, toes, ears, and scrotum.[25]

Clinical presentation. In children, 70% to 90% of RMSF patients report a history of tick bite. The incubation period ranges from 2 to 14 days.[13] Early symptoms are often nonspecific, typically consisting of sudden onset of headache, fever, and general malaise. Over the next several days, a red maculopapular rash appears on the extremities (wrists, hands, ankles, or feet), spreads to the entire body, and characteristically blanches when pressure is applied. The rash progresses to a petechial and purpuric eruption. More severe symptoms include meningismus, cerebral vasculitis, seizures, lethargy, confusion, and coma. Myocarditis, conduction abnormalities, dysrhythmias, pneumonitis, renal impairment, and vascular collapse may occur in severe cases. *Rickettsia*-induced vasculitis may induce small artery and vein occlusion and necrosis. Skin necrosis or gangrene of the extremities may indicate the presence of serious complications.[34]

Emergency Department interventions. Suspicion should be high for RMSF in endemic areas, especially if the patient has fever, headache, and myalgias lasting longer than 1 week. The classic rash and fever after the tick bite may be delayed for 3 to 4 days after the onset of illness. Early treatment with antibiotics is essential to prevent progression of the disease. Routine laboratory tests may provide some clues to the diagnosis. Electrolyte disturbances, thrombocytopenia, elevated bilirubin level, and liver function abnormalities may be observed. Immunofluorescent identification of the organism through biopsy of the skin rash has proven most helpful in early diagnosis.[25] Unfortunately, parents may not seek treatment for their child because of the similarity to and subsequent confusion with the measles rash. Indications for admission include (1) clinical evidence of toxicity, (2) encephalitis, (3) thrombocytopenia or alteration in clotting studies, and (4) hyponatremia.

Nursing care and evaluation. Nursing care depends on the severity of the symptoms. In cases where treatment has been delayed, the child may have sepsis and require emergency management. In less severe cases, where admission is indicated, intravenous access should be obtained for fluid and antibiotic administration.

It is not unusual for children to come to the emergency department with ticks embedded in the skin. Gloves and eye protection are required during tick removal. Ticks are removed with forceps by gentle, firmly applied upward traction. Care must be taken to remove the entire tick, including the head, and to prevent crushing it. Standard wound cleansing and care are then performed. Oral or parenteral antibiotic therapy is initiated as ordered.

When the child is discharged from the emergency setting, parents should be informed that the skin rash will resolve without further incident.[34] They should be instructed to follow the antibiotic regimen strictly and seek follow-up care if unusual symptoms develop. Discharge instructions should address the prevention of future bites, including the use of tick repellents. Clothes must be examined when the child has been in a tick-infested area.

LYME DISEASE

Etiology. Lyme disease is a tick-borne illness caused by the spirochete organism *Borrelia burgdorferi*. It is considered to be the most common tick-related illness in the continental United States and has been reported in 43 states.[57] However, its distribution is still predominantly regional, with most cases reported in the Northeast, upper Midwest and Pacific coastal regions.[57] The disease was originally reported in Lyme, Connecticut, in 1975 and has since increased steadily in occurrence. It is a multisystem disorder that involves dermatologic, cardiac, and neurologic complications.[25] A number of ticks have been implicated as vectors of the organism; however, the deer tick is the most frequently documented vector.

Pathophysiology. *B. burgdorferi* is initially introduced through the skin by the tick and becomes distributed throughout the body via the hematologic system. Invasion of the endothelial lining of blood vessels results in an inflammatory reaction.[21] The characteristic rash appears on the wrists, hands, ankles, and feet, then spreads to the rest of the body.[25] Eventually, most organ systems are involved and damaged by this diffuse vasculitis.[21]

Clinical presentation. The manifestations of Lyme disease are described in three stages. In *stage 1* a red annular skin lesion known as erythema chronicum migrans (ECM) appears between 2 and 32 days at the site of the tick bite. The lesion may expand to form multiple rings, called secondary lesions.[19] The lesions normally fade within a month. Fever, arthralgia, myalgia, headache, fatigue, stiff neck, lethargy, and lymphadenopathy are also associated with this stage.

In *stage 2,* more significant symptoms occur 2 to 12 weeks after the bite. Symptoms associated with this stage include neurologic manifestations, such as aseptic meningitis, encephalitis, cranial neuritis, and peripheral radiculoneuropathy, and cardiac manifestations, such as fluctuating atrioventricular heart block, myopericarditis, and left ventricular dysfunction.

Stage 3 is characterized by oligoarticular arthritis, which may develop several weeks to 2 years after the untreated tick bite. Swelling and pain in the larger joints is the typical manifestation. The child may suffer several brief, recurrent episodes. Chronic arthritis may linger in 10% of patients.[19]

Emergency Department interventions. Clinical evidence of Lyme disease and positive serologic testing are indications for treatment of the disease. If progression can be halted at stage I, the risk of the more serious symptoms in stages 2 and 3 can be avoided. Detection by immunofluorescence assay or enzyme-linked immunosorbent assay (ELISA) has been successful within weeks of the onset of Lyme disease.[57] Antibiotic therapy varies, depending on clinical presentation and progression of the disease. Early Lyme disease is treated with oral doxycycline, amoxicillin, or erythromycin. More serious symptoms such as Lyme carditis, neurologic manifestations, or Lyme arthritis require IV therapy with ceftriaxone or penicillin G.[57] Optimal doses and duration of therapy have not been established and should be individualized.

Nursing care and evaluation. As with any child, the ABCs must be assessed and stabilized on admission to the emergency department. The degree of care varies, depending on the stage of the disease and the symptoms present. If the disease is discovered early, supportive care may be all that is indicated. If the child is in a later stage of the disease, however, continuous monitoring of vital signs and assessment of hemodynamic and neurologic status are required. Rapid intravenous access may be ordered for fluid administration and prompt initiation of antibiotic therapy. Admission to the intensive care unit may be required to closely monitor the child's status and to continue appropriate therapy.

The child with an embedded tick requires removal of the tick with forceps by firmly applying gentle upward traction without crushing the tick. Universal precautions with an emphasis on glove and eye protection is indicated. Standard wound cleansing and care are required. If the child is to be discharged, instructions to the parent should include recognition of the early symptoms of Lyme disease and preventive techniques, such as how to use tick repellents and how to examine clothing twice daily when in tick-infested areas, especially during warm summer months. Diligence in making a habit of examining the child is important, since most tick bites are not noticed. Parents should also be instructed that the misuse of antibiotics prophylactically as a means to "prevent" the infection may introduce significant problems.[69]

REFERENCES

1. Adamski, DB: Assessment and treatment of allergic response to stinging insects, *J Emerg Nurs* 16:77-80, 1990.
2. Albertson TE et al: Superiority of activated charcoal alone compared with ipecac and activated charcoal in the treatment of acute toxic ingestion, *Ann Emerg Med* 18:56-59, 1989.
3. Auerbach PS, Geehr EC: *Management of wilderness and environmental emergencies,* St Louis, 1989, Mosby.
4. Banner W: Scorpion envenomation. In Auerbach PS, Geehr EC, eds: *Management of wilderness and environmental emergencies,* ed. 2, St Louis, 1989, Mosby.
5. Barkin RM, Kulig KW, Rumack BH: Poisoning and overdose management principles. In Barkin RM, Rosen P, eds: *Emergency pediatrics,* ed. 3, St Louis, 1990, Mosby.
6. Barkin RM, Rosen P: Anaphylaxis. In Barkin RM, Rosen P, eds: *Emergency pediatrics,* ed. 3, St Louis, 1990, Mosby.
7. Barkin RM, Rosen P: Dermatologic disorders. In Barkin RM, Rosen P, eds: *Emergency pediatrics,* ed. 3, St Louis, 1990, Mosby.
8. Barkin RM, Rosen P: Hypothermia. In Barkin RM, Rosen P, eds: *Emergency pediatrics,* ed. 3, St Louis, 1990, Mosby.
8a. Barone MA: *The Harriet Lane Handbook,* ed 14, St Louis, 1996, Mosby.
9. Berkovitch M et al: Recent increases in numbers and risk fatalities in young children ingesting iron preparations, *Veterinary Hum Toxicol* 36:53-55, 1994.
10. Browning RG et al: 50% dextrose: antidote or toxin? *Ann Emerg Med* 19:683-687, 1990.
11. Burgess JL et al: Effects of constriction bands on rattlesnake venom absorption: a pharmacokinetic study, *Ann Emerg Med* 21:1086-1093, 1992.
12. Christopher T: Urticaria. In Harwood-Nuss A et al,

eds: *The clinical practice of emergency medicine,* Philadelphia, 1991, JB Lippincott.

13. Crockett RK: Life-threatening rashes. In Harwood-Nuss A et al, eds: *The clinical practice of emergency medicine,* Philadelphia, 1991, JB Lippincott.

14. Cruz NS, Alvarez RG: Rattlesnake bite complications in 19 children, *Pediatr Emerg Care* 10:30-33, 1994.

15. Curry SC: Black widow spider envenomations. In Harwood-Nuss A et al, eds: *The clinical practice of emergency medicine,* Philadelphia, 1991, JB Lippincott.

16. Curtis RA, Barone J, Giacona N: Efficacy of ipecac and activated charcoal/cathartic, *Arch Inter Med* 144:48-52, 1984.

17. Danzl DF, Pozos RS, Hamlet MP: Accidental hypothermia. In Auerbach PS, Geehr ED, eds. *Management of wilderness and environmental emergencies,* ed. 2, St Louis, 1989, Mosby.

17a. Downs CE: Anaphylaxis. In Harwood-Nuss A et al, eds: *The clinical practice of emergency medicine,* ed 2, Philadelphia, 1996, JB Lippincott.

18. Dunn KA, et al: Injury prevention instruction in the emergency department, *Ann Emerg Med* 22:51-56, 1993.

19. Eichenfield AH, Athreya BH: Lyme disease: of ticks and titers, *J Pediatr* 114:328-333, 1989.

20. Fine JS: Pediatric principles. In Goldfrank, LR et al, eds: *Goldfrank's toxicologic emergencies,* ed 5, Norwalk, CT, 1994, Appleton & Lange.

21. Fleisher GR: Infectious disease emergencies. In Fleisher GR, Ludwin S, eds: *Textbook of pediatric emergency medicine,* ed 2, Baltimore, 1988, Williams & Wilkins.

22. Flomenbaum NE et al: General management of the poisoned or overdosed patient. In Goldfrank LR et al, eds: *Goldfrank's toxicologic emergencies,* ed 5, Norwalk, CT, 1994, Appleton & Lange.

23. Frenia ML, Lafin SM, Barone JA: Features and treatment of rabies, *Clin Pharm* 11:37-47, 1992.

24. Galloway RE: Mammalian bites, *J Emerg Med* 6:325-332, 1988.

25. Gentile DA: Tick-borne disease. In Auerbach PS, Geehr EC, eds: *Management of wilderness and environmental emergencies,* ed 2, St Louis, 1989, Mosby.

26. Goldfrank LR: General perspectives. In Goldfrank LR et al, eds: *Goldfrank's toxicologic emergencies,* ed 4, Norwalk, CT, 1990, Appleton & Lange.

27. Goldfrank LR et al: Vital signs and toxic syndromes. In Goldfrank, LR et al, eds: *Goldfrank's toxicologic emergencies,* ed 5, Norwalk, CT, 1994, Appleton & Lange.

28. Haddad LM, Podgorny G: Poisonous snakebite. In Haddad LM, Winchester JF eds: *Poisoning and drug overdose,* ed 2, Philadelphia, 1990, WB Saunders.

29. Harwood-Nuss A et al, eds: *The clinical practice of emergency medicine,* Philadelphia, 1991, JB Lippincott.

30. Joubert DW: Use of emetic, adsorbent, and cathartic agents in acute drug overdose, *J Emerg Nurs* 13:49-51, 1987.

31. Kearney TE: Activated charcoal. In Olson KR, ed: *Poisoning and drug overdose,* ed 2, Norwalk, CT, 1994, Appleton & Lange.

32. Kearney TE: Deferoxamine. In Olson KR, ed: *Poisoning and drug overdose,* ed 2, Norwalk, CT, 1994, Appleton & Lange.

33. Kelley MT: Anaphylaxis. In Grossman M, Dieckmann RA, eds: *Pediatric emergency medicine,* Philadelphia, 1991, JB Lippincott.

34. Kirkland KB et al: Rocky Mountain spotted fever complicated by gangrene: report of six cases and review, *Clin Infect Dis* 16:629-634, 1993.

35. Kohl S, Pickering L: Infectious diseases. In Behrman RE, Kliegman R, eds: *Nelson essentials of pediatrics,* Philadelphia, 1990, WB Saunders.

36. Koren G: Medications which can kill a toddler with one tablet or teaspoonful, *Clin Toxicol* 31:407-413, 1993.

37. Kornberg AE, Dolgin J: Pediatric ingestions: charcoal alone versus ipecac and charcoal, *Ann Emerg Med* 20:648-651, 1991.

38. Krenzelok EP, Lush RM: Container residue after the administration of aqueous activated charcoal products, *Am J Emerg Med* 9:144-146, 1991.

39. Kulig KW et al: Management of acutely poisoned patients without gastric emptying, *Ann Emerg Med* 14:562-567, 1985.

40. Lewis RK, Paloucek FP: Assessment and treatment of acetaminophen overdose, *Clin Pharm* 10:765-773, 1991.

41. Liebelt EL, Shannon MW: Small doses, big problems: a selected review of highly toxic common medications, *Pediatr Emerg Care* 9:292-297, 1993.

42. Litovitz TL, Clark LR, Soloway RA: 1993 annual report of the American Association of Poison Control Centers toxic exposure surveillance system, *Am J Emerg Med* 12:546-584, 1994.

43. Litovitz TL et al: 1992 annual report of the American Association of Poison Control Centers toxic exposure surveillance system, *Am J Emerg Med* 11:494-555, 1993.

44. Merigian KS et al: Prospective evaluation of gastric emptying in the self-poisoned patient, *Am J Emerg Med* 8:479-483, 1990.

45. Micik S: Emergency medical services and poison control, *Clin Toxicol* 12(3):309-317, 1978.

46. Minton SA, Bechtel HB: Arthropod envenomation and parasitism. In Auerbach PS, Geehr EC eds. *Management of wilderness and environmental emergencies,* ed 2, St Louis, 1989, Mosby.

47. Moran DM, Crouch DI, Finkle BS: Absorption of

ipecac alkaloids in emergency patients, *Ann Emerg Med* 13:43-45, 1984.

48. Morelli J: Pediatric poisonings: the 10 most toxic prescription drugs, *Am J Nurs* 93:27-29, 1993.

49. Neuvonen PJ, Olkkola KT: Oral activated charcoal in the treatment of intoxications: role of single and repeated doses, *Med Toxicol* 3:33-58, 1988.

50. Neuvonen PJ, Vartiainen M, Tokola O: Comparison of activated charcoal and ipecac syrup in prevention of drug absorption, *European J Clin Pharmacol* 24:557-562, 1983.

51. Nice A et al: Toxidrome recognition to improve efficiency of emergency urine drug screens, *Ann Emerg Med* 17:676-680, 1988.

52. Olson KR: Hydrocarbons. In Olson KR, ed: *Poisoning and drug overdose*, ed 2, Norwalk, CT, 1994, Appleton & Lange.

53. Park GD et al: Expanded role of charcoal therapy in the poisoned and overdosed patient, *Arch Intern Med* 146:969-973, 1986.

54. POISINDEX ® CCIS Substance Identification Computerized Database, Micromedex, Inc., Denver, CO.

55. Pond SM: Role of repeated oral doses of activated charcoal in clinical toxicology, *Med Toxicol* 1:3-11, 1986.

56. Pond SM: Techniques to enhance elimination of toxic compounds. In Goldfrank LR et al, eds: *Goldfrank's toxicologic emergencies*, ed 5, Norwalk, CT, 1994, Appleton & Lange.

57. Rahn DW, Malawista SE: Lyme disease: recommendations for diagnosis and treatment, *Ann Intern Med* 114:472-481, 1991.

58. Reed MD: Poisoning: general principles. In Blumer JL, ed: *A practical guide to pediatric intensive care*, ed 3, St Louis, 1990, Mosby.

59. Rosen FS: Urticaria, angioedema, and anaphylaxis, *Pediatr Rev* 13:387-390, 1992.

60. Rumack BH: Acetaminophen overdose in young children, *Am J Dis Child* 138:428-433, 1984.

61. Russell FE: Snake venom poisoning, *Veterinary Hum Toxicol* 33:584-586, 1991.

62. Russell FE: Identification and distribution of North American venomous snakes. In Russell FE, ed: *Snake venom poisoning*, Great Neck, NY, 1983, Scholum International, Inc.

63. Rydel JJ et al: Management considerations in copperhead envenomation, *J Emerg Nurs* 19:193-196, 1993.

64. Schauben JL, Frenia ML: Update on antidotal therapy, *J Pharm Pract* 6:63-73, 1993.

65. Schauben JL, Mofenson HC, Caraccio TR: Problems in the management of intoxications. In Luten RC ed. *Problems in pediatric emergency medicine*, New York, 1988, Churchill Livingstone.

66. Schauben JL, Spillane J: Poison emergencies, *US, Pharmacist* 16:37-57, 1991.

67. Schneider SM, Michelson EA: Enhanced activated charcoal delivery through small-bore tubing, *Veterinary Hum Toxicol* 35:503-505, 1993.

68. Sher T: Immunology and allergy. In Behrman BE, Kliegman R, eds: *Nelson essentials of pediatrics*, Philadelphia, 1990, WB Saunders.

69. Sigal LH: Current recommendations for the treatment of Lyme disease, *Drugs* 43:683-699, 1992.

70. Silvestri DL: Dermatologic problems in the intensive care unit. In Rippe, JM et al, eds: *Intensive care medicine*, ed 2, Boston, 1991, Little, Brown & Co.

71. Smilkstein MJ, Flomenbaum NE: Techniques used to prevent absorption of toxic compounds. In Goldfrank LR et al, eds: *Goldfrank's toxicologic emergencies*, ed 5, Norwalk, CT, 1994, Appleton & Lange.

72. Stafford CT, Moffitt JE, Yates AB: Insect sting anaphylaxis: referral is imperative, *Emerg Med* 24:230-234, 1992.

73. Sullivan JB Jr, Wingert WA: Reptile bites. In Auerbach PS, Geehr EC, eds: *Management of wilderness and environmental emergencies*, ed 2, St Louis, 1989, Mosby.

74. Sullivan JB: Snake envenomations. In Fuhrman BP, Zimmerman JJ, eds: *Pediatric critical care*, St Louis, 1992, Mosby.

75. Tenenbein M: Whole bowel irrigation as a gastrointestinal decontamination procedure after acute poisoning, *Med Toxicol* 3:77-84, 1988.

76. Reference deleted in proofs.

77. Tenenbein M, Cohen S, Sitar DS: Efficacy of ipecac-induced emesis, orogastric lavage, and activated charcoal for acute drug overdose, *Ann Emerg Med* 16:838-841, 1987.

78. Thompson DF et al: Evaluation of regional and nonregional poison centers, *New Engl J Med* 308:191-194, 1983.

79. Tully SA, Wingert WA: Venomous animal bites and stings. In Barkin RM, ed: *Pediatric emergency medicine: concepts in clinical practice*, St Louis, 1992, Mosby.

80. Varon J, Sadovnikoff N, Sternbach GL: Hypothermia, *Postgrad Med* 92:47-59, 1992.

81. Watson WA, McKinney PE: Activated charcoal and acetylcysteine absorption: issues in interpreting pharmacokinetic data, *DICP, Ann Pharmacotherapy* 25:1081-1084, 1991.

82. Weisman RS, Goldfrank LR: Prevention and the role of the poison center. In Goldfrank LR et al, eds: *Goldfrank's toxicologic emergencies*, ed 5, Norwalk, CT, 1994, Appleton & Lange.

83. Woolf AD, Lovejoy FH Jr: Epidemiology of drug overdose in children, *Drug Safety* 9:291-308, 1993.

84. Zull DN: Anaphylaxis. In Harwood-Nuss A et al, eds: *The clinical practice of emergency medicine*, ed 2, Philadelphia, 1996, JB Lippincott.

CHAPTER 28

Neonatal Topics

Syvil S. Burke

The term *neonates* includes all infants within the first 30 days of life. Neonates are seen in the emergency department for various reasons. Some are precipitously born in the department or on the way to the hospital. Others return to the hospital in the first month of life with chief complaints ranging from minor health problems to acute life-threatening illnesses.

Because neonates differ from older children and adults anatomically, physiologically, cognitively, and psychosocially, the approach to their care is different. Neonates depend on adults for their well-being. Their rudimentary methods of communication are often difficult for staff, and even parents, to interpret during the first month of life. In addition, the signs and symptoms of neonatal illness are subtle and can easily be overlooked or misinterpreted. Prompt identification and management of illness, however, can mean the difference between life and death, since immature body systems frequently cannot cope efficiently with illness. Rapid deterioration of neonates is common. Therefore all neonates must be promptly assessed and treated, then frequently evaluated for condition changes.

The onset of even minor neonatal illnesses or conditions, such as frequent crying or spitting up, can be frightening for parents. Concern about their infant's well-being commonly brings them to the emergency department for seemingly minor problems. Parents may also have difficulty recognizing the difference between normal variations and illness. By closely listening to parental concerns and thoroughly examining the infant, health care providers can differentiate between illness and normal variations. Educating parents about normal neonatal behavior and conditions is often reassuring.

This chapter focuses on neonatal anatomy and physiology, neonatal assessment, common parental concerns, and acute illnesses. Nursing care, management priorities, and discharge teaching are described. Neonatal resuscitation is discussed in Chapter 8.

NEONATAL ANATOMY AND PHYSIOLOGY

Throughout pregnancy, fetal body systems mature in preparation for extrauterine life. At birth, physiologic adjustments immediately occur to allow survival of the infant independent of the mother (see Chapter 11). Although most changes occur with the infant's first breaths, others, such as closure of the foramen ovale within the heart, may take hours, days, or months. Transitional physiology must be considered in the assessment and management of the neonate.

GROWTH AND METABOLISM

Neonates normally lose up to 10% of birth weight in the first few days of life as a result of loss of extracellular fluid (ECF), passage of meconium, and limited intake. Birth weight is regained by 8 to 12 days of age. Thereafter, normal neonatal weight gain of 0.5 to 1 ounce per day[8] is an important indicator of neonatal well-being (see Appendix D—Growth Charts).

The metabolic rate of neonates is higher than that of older children or adults, which contributes to greater heat and water losses and relatively increased oxygen, fluid, and nutrient requirements. The caloric requirements to meet metabolic demand and maintain growth in the newborn are approximately 55 kcal/kg/24 hr; however, by 1 week of age, 110 kcal/kg/24 hr is required.[41] Any stress, such as illness or hypothermia, can easily overwhelm the neonate's reserves; hypoxia, hypoglycemia, and fluid imbalances can occur rapidly.

PULMONARY SYSTEM

Newborns are normally endowed with adequate pulmonary structures to support oxygenation and ventilation. However, these structures are small and immature. Small conducting airways have relatively greater resistance to air flow; whenever any obstruction such as mucus or edema, occurs, the airway resistance is markedly increased. Since neonates are obligate nose breathers, nasal congestion can also interfere with ventilation.

The neonate has only 24 to 50 million alveoli as compared to the 300 to 400 million of the adult.[22,32] This generally provides enough surface area for gas exchange. However, whenever oxygen requirements increase, such as during illness or cold stress, the neonate is limited in the ability to increase gas exchange, and hypoxia develops rapidly. Neonates also have less pulmonary elastic and collagen tissue to maintain open alveoli at the end of expiration, increasing their susceptibility to atelectasis.

Since intercostal muscles are immature and ribs are horizontally oriented, the neonatal chest wall is limited in its ability to expand with inspiration. The diaphragm is the primary respiratory muscle in neonates and abdominal breathing is observed.

Because of their immature pulmonary systems, neonates can become rapidly fatigued and compromised whenever increased demands are placed on their respiratory system. Even relatively minor illnesses or conditions such as colds or hypothermia can produce respiratory distress in the neonate. Rapid progression to respiratory failure can then occur because of poor compensatory reserves.

CARDIAC SYSTEM

Newborns have a relatively high cardiac output (CO) that falls significantly within the first 2 weeks of life from approximately 400 to 200 ml/kg/min.[15] This high CO provides for increased neonatal metabolic requirements.

The neonatal myocardium is less compliant and has less contractile mass than the adult myocardium, limiting contractility and stroke volume (SV). The average neonatal SV is approximately 5 ml, as compared to 75 to 90 ml in the adolescent.[15,33] Because of limited contractility, SV cannot significantly increase during cardiovascular compromise such as hypovolemia. Therefore, to maintain CO, the neonate relies on increasing the heart rate (HR). Sustained bradycardia is an ominous sign in the neonate, indicating an inability to compensate.

Immaturity of the conduction system accounts for the frequency of cardiac dysrhythmias in the neonatal period. Stress or agitation can quickly cause a change in the HR or rhythm. Sensitivity to parasympathetic stimulation, such as suctioning or defecating, can create transient bradycardia or a pronounced sinus arrhythmia in the normal neonate.

NEUROLOGIC SYSTEM

All primary structures of the brain are present at birth, although the brain itself is only 25% of its mature adult weight.[15] Open sutures in the skull allow passage of the head through the birth canal and brain growth during infancy. The immaturity of the neurologic system is evidenced by the presence of infantile reflexes, uncoordinated movements, and cognitive limitations. Cranial nerves and spinal and protective reflexes are intact.

FLUIDS AND ELECTROLYTES

Neonates have proportionately more total body water and ECF than older children and adults. Total body water is approximately 75% in the neonate and 60% to 70% in the adult.[15] ECF comprises up to 40% of the newborn's total body water, compared to 20% in the adult.[44] The higher proportion of ECF predisposes neonates to more rapid loss of body fluids from normal mechanisms, including insensible and renal losses, as well as illnesses, such as vomiting and diarrhea. The neonate's higher metabolic rate, greater insensible and evaporative water losses from the large body surface area, and limited ability to concentrate urine contribute to a daily turnover of fluid of more than half the ECF volume, as compared to one-fifth in the adult. Normal urine excretion is approximately 2 ml/kg/hr.[15] Because of the relative inability to concentrate urine, the neonate cannot efficiently adjust to fluid imbalances.

HEMATOLOGIC AND IMMUNE SYSTEMS

Newborns have relatively high hematocrits and a predominance of fetal hemoglobin (Hb F). Compared to those of adults, neonatal red blood cells are more fragile and have a shorter life span. Over the first 2 to 3 months of life, the hematocrit and hemoglobin levels decrease to physiologically low levels, stimulating the bone marrow to increase red blood cell production.

Immaturity of the immune system, deficiency in immunoglobulin and polymorphonuclear leukocyte stores, and lack of previous exposure to antigens increase the neonate's susceptibility to infection. The neonate is also limited in the ability to synthesize new antibodies to protect against many viral and bacterial illnesses. Immature T-cell function additionally contributes to the neonate's susceptibility to viral infections.

Initial immunity is passively acquired from the mother. Immunoglobulins may be passed from the mother in utero (e.g., immunoglobulin G) or via breast milk (immunoglobulin A). In the first 3 to 5 months of life, passive immunity decreases while the production of immunoglobulins increases. During the transition, infants are particularly susceptible to serious bacterial and viral infections.

Gastrointestinal System

Enzyme deficiencies in the neonate limit the absorption of fats and the utilization of complex carbohydrates.[44] Young infants, therefore, cannot tolerate cow's milk or polysaccharides. Blood glucose levels are normally low in the newborn and, coupled with limited glycogen stores, predispose the neonate to hypoglycemia.

The neonatal liver is immature and cannot efficiently conjugate bilirubin. During the first several days of life, the increased production of bilirubin from the normal hemolysis of red blood cells can overwhelm the liver's ability to excrete bilirubin, resulting in physiologic jaundice.

Regurgitation or spitting up is normal in the neonate because of the relaxed cardiac sphincter and rapid peristalsis. Since neonatal salivary glands produce limited amounts of saliva, drooling is not common until the second to third month of life. Stool frequency may vary from several times a day to once every other day. Breast-fed babies usually have more frequent, looser bowel movements. Variation in stool patterns is common.

Thermoregulation

Neonates are particularly susceptible to cold stress caused by greater heat losses than in older children and limited ability to produce heat. The infant's proportionately larger body surface area (especially the head) allows a significant amount of heat loss. Heat production is limited by neonates' inability to shiver. Nonshivering thermogenesis, therefore, is the primary mechanism of heat production in the neonate. During this process, specialized neonatal brown fat is metabolized. Brown fat has a capacity for generating more metabolic activity and heat than regular fat tissue.[44] However, nonshivering thermogenesis increases oxygen and glucose consumption, which can quickly lead to hypoxia, lactic acidosis, hypoglycemia, pulmonary vasoconstriction, and right-to-left intracardiac shunting.[1,15]

❚ Neonatal Assessment

History

Initially a focused history of the chief complaint is obtained. Additional information about the prenatal, perinatal, and postnatal history is also important in identifying the infant's state of health and risk factors (Box 28-1). Parents know their infant better than any member of the emergency department staff. Listening to parental concerns not only provides clues to the infant's diagnosis, but also helps establish rapport and trust.

Physical Assessment

During the physical examination the neonate's limited energy must be conserved. Maintaining a normothermic environment and performing the assessment in an organized, efficient manner minimizes the amount of stress for the infant. Swaddling, holding, offering a pacifier, and soothing talk often calm the infant and facilitate accurate assessments.

Neonates present quite differently than older infants and children, exhibiting numerous normal variations (Table 28-1). Signs and symptoms of illness are often nonspecific.

Valuable information can be obtained using "hands-off" observation of the neonate. General appearance, respiratory status, and neurologic status can be assessed grossly by merely looking at the infant. The sequence of the physical examination generally proceeds in a toe-to-head fashion to avoid distressing the infant. Intrusive parts of the examination, such as rectal temperatures and otoscopy, should be performed last. Once the infant starts to cry, obtaining an accurate assessment of the heart, lungs, and abdomen is very difficult.

Following is a suggested approach to the neonatal physical examination. Changes in the sequence of the examination may be necessary, depending on the infant's behavior and presentation. The goal is to

Box 28-1	Birth History	
PRENATAL	**PERINATAL**	**POSTNATAL**
Did the mother receive prenatal care? Does the mother have any chronic illnesses, such as diabetes or a seizure disorder? Did the mother have any health problems during pregnancy, such as infections, toxemia, or premature labor? Did the mother take any prescribed or over-the-counter medications during pregnancy? Any smoking, alcohol, or drug use?	Was the birth "on time" or premature? How long was the labor? What kind of delivery was required—vaginal, cesarean section, or breech? Were there any problems during labor and delivery, such as placenta previa, excessive bleeding, decreased fetal heart rate, or meconium? What was the baby's birth weight?	Did the baby breathe immediately or require any resuscitation at birth? Any other problems at birth? Did the baby go to the regular nursery or to a special care or intensive care nursery? Did the baby have any problems during the first few days of life, such as jaundice, infections, or low blood sugar levels? Did the baby go home at the same time as the mother? Has the baby had any health problems at home? Any feeding problems, sleep disturbances, or irritability? Has the baby been gaining weight? Has the infant had any immunizations? What concerns do the parents have?

capture all pertinent information. A comprehensive discussion of physical assessment is found in Chapter 4.

General appearance. Initially the neonate is observed for level of consciousness, posture, activity, respiratory effort, skin color, behavior, facial expressions, nutritional status, and interaction with the environment. These observations are a good index of the neonate's overall state of health, as well as of the status of various body systems.

Skin. Changes in the skin color may or may not indicate serious illness. Transient peripheral or circumoral cyanosis and mottling of the extremities are normal responses to crying or a cold environment. However, cyanosis can also result from pulmonary, hematologic, central nervous system, or metabolic diseases, as well as from cardiac defects.[11] Pallor, severe jaundice, central cyanosis, and petechiae often reflect neonatal illness. Color changes must be evaluated in conjunction with other findings.

Various birthmarks may be present. These marks should be differentiated from bruises or rashes associated with illness or injury. For example, mongolian spots, which are bluish skin discolorations of the sacral, gluteal, and posterior thoracic areas often found on infants of African-American, Native American, or Mediterranean descent, are common birthmarks that can easily be mistaken for child abuse.

TABLE 28-1	Neonatal Assessment	
	COMMON NEONATAL VARIATIONS	**ABNORMAL FINDINGS**
Skin	Pink; peripheral or circumoral cyanosis may occur with crying or hypothermia	Central cyanosis; prolonged peripheral cyanosis; pallor
	Transient mottling in response to cold	Continuous mottling of extremities despite warming measures
	Jaundice between first and seventh days of life	Severe jaundice; persistent jaundice (>1 week of age); conjugated hyperbilirubinemia
	Newborn rashes, milia (distended sebaceous glands), birthmarks	Petechiae; bruises, especially soft tissue, except if associated with birth trauma
Chest and lungs	Quiet, easy respirations	Nasal flaring
	Abdominal breathing	Retractions
	Irregular (periodic) breathing	Stridor, crackles, wheezing
	Breast enlargement in newborns (may persist for several weeks); secretion of white milky substance (witch's milk)	Grunting respirations Apnea (>15 seconds' pause in respirations)
Heart	Murmurs caused by transitional physiology or innocent murmurs	Persistent heart murmurs associated with congenital heart defects (CHD)
	Transient bradycardia resulting from parasympathetic stimulation; sinus arrhythmia	Dysrhythmias such as prolonged bradycardia or supraventricular tachycardia (SVT)
Abdomen	Protuberent; poorly developed abdominal musculature	Intestinal masses Umbilical hernia
	Umbilical cord dries and falls off within 1 to 2 weeks	Purulent, odorous discharge from umbilicus
Genitourinary	Urinates in 24 hours after birth; normal urine output 1 to 2 ml/kg/hr	Decreased urination Hypospadias
	Female: pseudomenstruation (blood-tinged discharge) or white discharge	Yellow vaginal discharge Purulent drainage or bleeding of circumcision site
	Male: healing circumcision with small amount of dried yellow drainage	Undescended testicles; inguinal hernia
	Inability to retract foreskin of uncircumcised male	
	Testes palpable in scrotum or inguinal canal	
	Hydrocele	
Neurologic		
Level of consciousness (LOC)	Alert, looks around; focuses on people's faces	Does not focus; stares; does not follow bright objects
Posture	Flexed extremities	Limp, flaccid

TABLE 28-1	Neonatal Assessment—cont'd	
	COMMON NEONATAL VARIATIONS	**ABNORMAL FINDINGS**

Neurologic—cont'd

	COMMON NEONATAL VARIATIONS	ABNORMAL FINDINGS
Motor tone, movement	Resists extension of extremities	Poor muscle tone Seizure activity
	Moves all extremities spontaneously; quivering or transient tremors	Jitteriness from possible metabolic abnormalities or cocaine withdrawal
Activity	Vigorous response to intrusive procedures; consolable	Inconsolable; weak or no response to procedures
Cry	Vigorous cry	High-pitched or shrill cry; possible increased intracranial pressure (ICP)
Reflexes	See Table 28-2, p. 667	Weak or absent reflexes
Head	Proportionally larger than body as compared to adult	Enlarged head size per norms (hydrocephalus)
	Anterior fontanel closes between 9 and 18 months; posterior fontanel closes at birth or by 2 months of age	Bulging fontanel in the quiet infant indicates increased ICP Sunken fontanel indicates dehydration
	Molding, caput succedaneum (edema of scalp), cephalhematoma (bleeding into periosteum of bone); disappear in first few weeks	Craniosynostosis indicating premature closure of sutures
Eyes	Clear white sclera, positive red light reflex; pupils equal, round, and reactive to light; searching nystagmus	Red or jaundiced sclera; eye discharge Retinal hemorrhages or corneal abrasions
	Tears absent	
Ears	Small cartilaginous ear canals	No response to loud noises
Nose	Obligate nose breathers	Obstruction from mucus or choanal atresia
	Sneezing common	Thick, bloody nasal discharge without sneezing may indicate congenital syphilis
Mouth/throat	Minimal salivation	Thrush
	Strong, coordinated sucking	Cleft palate

Chest. Respiratory rate, effort, depth, rhythm, and breath sounds should be evaluated while the infant is at rest. Neonates commonly exhibit irregular breathing patterns, in which there are short pauses in respiration. Apnea, defined as breathing cessation for more than 15 seconds in the term neonate or 20 seconds in the premature infant, is considered pathologic.[27] Apnea associated with skin color changes and bradycardia requires prompt intervention.

Neonates are abdominal breathers, using the diaphragm as the primary muscle of respiration. Respirations can be counted by observing the rise and fall of the abdomen. Findings on auscultation can be misleading because transmission of breath sounds occurs easily across the neonate's thin chest wall. Therefore breath sounds should be evaluated in the axilla, in addition to the other lung fields.

Heart. Heart sounds, heart rate, and rhythm are best assessed in the quiet infant. Capillary refill is more accurately tested on the trunk, since perfusion to the extremities is vulnerable to other factors such as environmental temperature.

Neonatal HR is sensitive to a variety of factors, including crying, fever, parasympathetic stimulation such as stooling, and illness. Transient heart murmurs are common during the first few days of life. These functional murmurs usually disappear with closure of the ductus arteriosus and foramen ovale. Persistent murmurs, especially at the left sternal border or above the apical impulse, suggest a congenital heart defect (CHD).

Abdomen. The normal neonate's abdomen is soft, rounded, and protrudes slightly. Poorly developed abdominal musculature offers little protection to abdominal organs. The lower edge of the liver may be palpable 2 to 3 cm below the costal margin.

The umbilical cord dries and falls off within 1 to 2 weeks of age. Bleeding from the umbilicus is abnormal, except for a small amount of blood that may appear on the diaper or clothes when the cord falls off. Purulent, odorous drainage and erythema and swelling of the surrounding abdominal wall suggest a serious umbilical infection. Umbilical hernias are common and usually resolve without intervention.

Abdominal asymmetry, rigidity, distention, or visible masses require further evaluation. Palpable masses may indicate pyloric stenosis or intussusception. An enlarged liver is suggestive of congestive heart failure.

Genitourinary signs. Female neonates may normally excrete a white vaginal discharge. Occasionally a bloody discharge (pseudomenstruation) occurs in response to withdrawal from maternal hormones, as well as increased breast tissue and milky discharge from the breasts ("witch's milk").

In the newly circumcised male a small amount of bloody drainage may be observed. If the Plastibell procedure was used to remove the foreskin, the plastic ring remains on the penis for 5 to 8 days, when it separates and falls off, often accompanied by a small amount of bleeding.[44] Active bleeding, excessive swelling, and odorous purulent drainage are abnormal. In the uncircumcised male the foreskin often adheres closely to the glans penis and should not be forcibly retracted.

Neurologic status. Assessment of neurologic status includes level of response, musculoskeletal tone, and reflex responses. Much of the neurologic assessment occurs during other parts of the physical examination, for example, observation of muscle tone and response to stimuli. Alert neonates with intact vision are able to focus on and follow faces or bright objects. When disturbed, they react vigorously with a strong cry and increased movement, but they can usually be consoled by comforting measures such as holding and rocking. A change in the neonatal cry may represent changes in neurologic status. For example, a high-pitched or shrill cry can suggest increased intracranial pressure (ICP) or pain.

Healthy neonates maintain a flexed position and exhibit uncoordinated, spontaneous movements. Attempts at extending the extremities are met with active resistance. Neonates normally exhibit several immature as well as protective reflexes (Table 28-2). Weak or absent reflexes are abnormal, and the etiology should be identified as soon as possible.

Neonatal seizure activity is manifested differently than seizures in older infants and children. Although tonic-clonic movements may be seen, subtle seizures are more common. Seizures may be exhibited by staring spells, eye deviation, lip smacking, tongue thrusting, bicycling, and/or apnea.[5] Jitteriness, a seizure-like activity, is associated with such problems as cocaine withdrawal, hypoglycemia, and hypocalcemia.

Head. The posterior fontanel is often closed by compression of the head during delivery, but it may be palpable up to 2 months of age. The anterior fontanel, which is open, soft, and flat in the neonate, closes between 9 and 18 months of age. A bulging fontanel in the quiet upright infant suggests increased ICP. A sunken fontanel is associated with dehydration.

Increases in head size should be evaluated using a head circumference chart or the infant's personal growth chart, if available. However, this parameter is often deferred in the emergency department, since serial measurements are more meaningful. A head circumference measurement is indicated if increasing ICP is suspected.

Eyes, ears, nose, and throat. A normal neonatal eye examination shows bright and shiny corneas, clear white sclera, a positive red reflex, and briskly reactive pupils. Newborns can see objects within 12 inches and can follow a moving object or face. Tears may not be present with crying.

Neonatal tympanic membranes (TM) have similar landmarks, although they are more difficult to exam-

TABLE 28-2	Assessing Neonatal Reflexes	
REFLEX	**TESTING METHOD**	**NORMAL RESPONSE**
Babinski (plantar)	Stroke one side of the neonate's foot upward from the heel and across the ball of the foot.	Neonate hyperextends the toes, dorsiflexes the great toe, and fans the toes outward.
Blink (corneal)	Momentarily shine a bright light directly into the neonate's eyes.	Neonate blinks.
Crawl	Place the neonate prone on a flat surface.	Neonate attempts to crawl forward using the arms and legs.
Crossed extension	Position the neonate supine; extend one leg and stimulate the sole with a light pin prick or finger flick.	Neonate swiftly flexes and extends the opposite leg as though trying to push the stimulus away from the other foot.
Doll's eye	With the neonate supine, slowly turn the neonate's head to the left or right.	Neonate's eyes remain stationary.
Fencing (tonic neck)	With a swift motion, turn the neonate's head to either side.	Neonate extends the extremities on the side to which the head is turned and flexes the extremities on the opposite side.
Galant	Using a fingernail, gently stroke one side of the neonate's spinal column from the head to the buttocks.	Neonate's trunk curves toward the stimulated side.
Grasp	Palmar reflex: Place a finger in the neonate's palm.	Neonate grasps the finger.
	Plantar reflex: Place a finger against the base of the neonate's toe.	Neonate's toes curl downward and grasp the finger.
Moro	Suddenly but gently drop the neonate's head backward (relative to the trunk).	Neonate extends and abducts all extremities bilaterally and symmetrically; forms a C shape with the thumb and forefinger; and then adducts and flexes the extremities.
Pupillary (light)	Darken the room and shine a penlight directly into the neonate's eye for several seconds	Pupils constrict equally bilaterally.
Rooting	Touch a finger to the neonate's cheek or the corner of mouth. (The mother's nipple also should trigger this reflex.)	Neonate turns the head toward the stimulus, opens the mouth, and searches for the stimulus.
Startle	Make a loud noise near the neonate.	Neonate cries and abducts and flexes all extremities.
Stepping (automatic walking)	Hold the neonate in an upright position and touch one foot lightly to a flat surface (such as the bed).	Neonate makes walking motions with both feet.
Sucking	Place a finger in the neonate's mouth. (The mother's nipple should also trigger this reflex.)	Neonate sucks on the finger (or nipple) forcefully and rhythmically; sucking is coordinated with swallowing.

From Cantu D, Vaello L, Kenner C: Neonatal assessment. In Cohen S, Kenner C, Hollingsworth A, eds: *Maternal, neonatal, and women's health nursing,* Springhouse, 1991, Springhouse Corp.

Box 28-2	Normal Neonatal Vital Signs*
PARAMETER	NORMAL RANGES
Temperature	36.5° to 37° C (97.9° to 98.6° F)
Respiratory rate	30 to 60 breaths/min
HR	120 to 160 beats/min
Blood pressure	65 to 86/52 to 55* mm Hg Lower limit of normal systolic: 60 mm Hg

*Fiftieth percentile blood pressure range of boys and girls, birth to age 1 month.
From Chameides L, ed: *Textbook of pediatric advanced life support,* 1994, American Heart Association; Wong DL: *Whaley & Wong's essentials of pediatric nursing,* ed 5, St Louis, 1997, Mosby.

ine because of small, cartilaginous ear canals. Hearing is grossly tested by observing the neonate's reaction to sound. Normal responses include turning the head toward the sound or blinking the eyes. Loud noises often elicit the Moro reflex.

Nasal obstruction or deformities should be identified, since they can interfere with breathing or eating. The mouth and throat are most easily examined when the infant is crying. White patches on the mucosa that do not easily scrape off indicate thrush.

Vital signs. Resting HR and respiratory rate are most reliable and meaningful in the neonate (Box 28-2). Taking the infant's temperature and blood pressure usually induces crying; therefore these interventions should be reserved until the end of the examination. Tympanic thermometers are not recommended for neonates because correct placement within the ear canal is difficult. Also, accurate, reliable measurements are required to determine the presence of fever in the neonate.

Blood pressure is not a reliable indicator of serious illness in the neonate because of its variation with age and activity. Also, low blood pressure is a late sign of compromised circulation infants. A systolic blood pressure of less than 60 mm Hg in neonates is indicative of poor perfusion.

PARENT-INFANT RELATIONSHIP

An objective assessment of parent-infant interaction and attachment behaviors is important to identify high-risk social situations, which may impact the infant's physical health. In a healthy relationship the parent holds and comforts the infant, maintains eye contact with the infant, and provides appropriate auditory, visual, and tactile stimuli. Parents with poor attachment behaviors limit contact and communication with the infant, do not respond to the infant's cry, and are not attentive during the physical examination or feeding.[8,21] Observations of the parent-infant relationship are especially important in instances of suspected maltreatment.

ACUTE NEONATAL DISORDERS

SEPSIS

Etiology. Neonatal sepsis is a systemic illness caused by pathogens that invade the bloodstream. Signs and symptoms may be present at birth or develop in the first month of life. Because the neonate's immune system is immature, sepsis can rapidly progress to a life-threatening condition. The incidence of neonatal sepsis is estimated to be 1 to 10 cases per 1000 live births.[13]

Early sepsis, which occurs during the first 3 to 4 days of life, is associated with higher mortality and morbidity rates than later-onset sepsis. Bacteria acquired from the maternal genital tract either in utero or during delivery, including group B *Streptococcus, Escherichia coli* and other gram-negative rods, and *Listeria monocytogenes,* are the most common pathogens.[38]

After 3 to 4 days of age, sepsis is more often associated with focal disease, such as meningitis. Postnatally acquired organisms, such as staphylococci, *Pseudomonas aeruginosa,* other nosocomial organisms,[9] and various viruses or fungi, often cause late-onset sepsis. However, perinatally acquired organisms may also be involved.

Many factors increase the risk of neonatal sepsis. Perinatal risk factors include prematurity (<37 weeks gestation), low birth weight, prolonged rupture of the membranes, maternal infection, amniotic fluid abnormalities, multiple gestation, fetal distress or hypoxia, and obstetric or perinatal complications.[9] Postnatal susceptibility to infection is increased with neonatal intensive care admissions, invasive procedures, or artificial ventilation.

Pathophysiology. Early-onset sepsis is usually a multisystem fulminant illness presenting in the first 2 days of life. Pathogens are perinatally acquired by transplacental transfer, vaginal flora transmission after

Box 28-3   Signs and Symptoms of Neonatal Sepsis

Nonspecific
Temperature instability (hypothermia or hyperthermia)
Tachypnea
Feeding difficulties
Lethargy
Vomiting, diarrhea
Abdominal distention
Jaundice
Petechiae
Apnea spells

Shock
Tachycardia (early sign) → bradycardia (late sign)
Delayed capillary refill (<2 seconds)
Weak → absent peripheral pulses
Pallor, cyanosis, or mottling
Altered level of consciousness
Hypotension

Data from Burchfield DJ: Acute distress in the neonate and postnatal period. In Barkin RM, ed: *Pediatric emergency medicine*, St Louis, 1992, Mosby; Lott J: Assessment and management of immunologic dysfunction. In Kenner C, Brueggemeyer A, Gunderson L, eds: *Comprehensive neonatal nursing*, Philadelphia, 1993, Saunders.

Because the early signs and symptoms of neonatal sepsis are subtle and nonspecific, the diagnosis is considered in almost every neonate until proven otherwise. Without rapid recognition and treatment of sepsis, the risk of overwhelming infection and death is significantly increased.

The signs and symptoms of sepsis vary from subtle and nonspecific to profound shock (Box 28-3). Some neonates become ill rapidly, and others become ill over several days. Fever is generally an unreliable finding in the septic neonate. Most septic infants under 2 months of age are hypothermic.[36] Focal signs and symptoms are more common with late-onset sepsis. Tachypnea is a common finding in sepsis; however, signs of respiratory distress may indicate pulmonary pathology. Irritability, seizures, and a bulging fontanel suggest meningitis, which occurs more frequently in neonates than in other age groups.

Many other disorders mimic sepsis (Box 28-4). Certain endocrine, metabolic, and GI disorders may present with some of the typical GI symptoms observed in the septic infant, including vomiting, diarrhea, and abdominal distention. Other differential diagnoses include viral respiratory infections, neurologic disorders, child abuse, or congenital heart disease.

Emergency Department interventions

Diagnosis.   Because the presentation of neonatal sepsis is usually subtle, nonspecific, and potentially fulminant, diagnostic tests must be initiated expeditiously and followed by prompt antibiotic treatment. A complete septic workup, including urine, blood, and cerebrospinal fluid cultures, should be done on any infant with suspected sepsis before starting antibiotic therapy. Antibiotics administered before obtaining cultures alter bacterial culture results and possibly interfere with sensitivity testing. The lumbar puncture (LP) should be deferred if the infant displays significant respiratory or cardiovascular instability.[38]

A complete blood count with differential must be obtained and results evaluated according to age-appropriate norms. Neonatal sepsis may be associated with severe neutropenia, neutrophilia, or an increased ratio of immature to total granulocytes.[5,38] However, the white blood cell count and differential may be normal, especially in the early stage of the infection.

Other diagnostic tests include bedside and serum blood glucose determinations, urinalysis, and a chest x-ray. More detailed and specific tests may be necessary based on physical findings and clinical presentation.

rupture of the membranes, or aspiration of infected amniotic fluid. Sites of postnatal bacterial colonization include the skin, nasopharynx, oropharynx, conjunctiva, and umbilical cord.[13] Late-onset sepsis results from bacteria acquired perinatally with a delay in onset of symptoms, nosocomially from contaminated equipment or human contact, or through the umbilical cord, especially if hygiene is poor.

Neonates have limited ability to mount an immune response to pathogens. Mechanisms for localizing infection are immature, and production of gamma globulin does not occur until the second month of life.[44] Therefore neonates are vulnerable to fulminating, systemic infections that can rapidly progress to septic shock (see Chapter 6, Respiratory Failure and Shock).

Clinical presentation.   Parents often come to the emergency department with the complaint that their baby does not look right or is not acting normally.

Box 28-4   Differential Diagnosis of the Septic-Appearing Infant

Infectious diseases
    Bacterial sepsis
    Meningitis
    Urinary tract infection
    Virus infection
    Congenital syphilis
Cardiac diseases
    Congenital heart disease
    Paroxysmal atrial tachycardia
    Myocardial infarction
    Pericarditis
    Myocarditis
Endocrine disorders
    Congenital adrenal hyperplasia
Metabolic disorders
    Metabolic disorders
    Hyponatremia, hypernatremia
    Cystic fibrosis
    Inborn errors of metabolism
    Hypoglycemia
    Reye's syndrome
    Drug toxicity
Renal disorders
    Posterior urethral valves
Hematologic disorders
    Severe anemia
    Methemoglobinemia
Gastrointestinal (GI) disorders
    Gastroenteritis with dehydration
    Pyloric stenosis
    Intussusception
    Necrotizing enterocolitis
    Appendicitis, volvulus
Neurologic diseases
    Infant botulism
    Shunt obstruction, infection
    Child abuse—intracranial bleed

Adapted from Henretig S: Vomiting. In Fleisher G, Ludwig S, eds: *Textbook of pediatric emergency medicine*, ed 3, Baltimore, 1993, Williams & Wilkins.

Treatment.   Prompt treatment of neonatal sepsis is essential. As soon as the sepsis workup is complete, systemic antibiotics should be administered to neonates with suspected sepsis. Broad-spectrum antibiotics, including a combination of ampicillin with an aminoglycoside or third-generation cephalosporin such as ceftriaxone, are effective against the majority of neonatal infections. Once a definitive, causative agent is identified, antibiotics can be adjusted accordingly.[9] Admission to the hospital is warranted until sepsis is ruled out or the infection is adequately treated.

Nursing care and evaluation

Airway, breathing, and circulation (ABCs). Initial management of the potentially septic neonate requires stabilization of the ABCs. Emergency interventions include maintaining airway patency, oxygenation, ventilation, and perfusion. Continuous evaluation is necessary to identify early, nonspecific signs of sepsis, as well as to monitor responses to treatment and/or the progression of symptoms. Without prompt recognition and treatment, septic shock and death can result.

History and physical examination. A thorough history of the potentially septic neonate includes prenatal, perinatal, and postnatal information in order to identify risk factors for sepsis, such as prematurity and maternal infection. Treatment is often initiated in neonates with high-risk factors, even if they are asymptomatic. History of the chief complaint includes onset of signs and symptoms, exposure to infections, associated problems, and interventions initiated at home or by the primary health care provider. Obtaining information about the normal level of functioning before the onset of symptoms assists the nurse in evaluating the effect of the illness on the neonate.

A complete physical examination is important because of the neonate's tendency toward systemic, rather than focal, illness. Since symptoms are often nonspecific, other differential diagnoses must be ruled out by examination or diagnostic tests.

Diagnostic and therapeutic interventions. When obtaining blood specimens, it is prudent and less stressful to the neonate to simultaneously insert an intravenous (IV) catheter for fluid and medication administration. Urine for culture must be obtained by sterile catheterization or suprapubic tap, since bag urine specimens are not reliable. During the LP, close monitoring of the neonate for signs of respiratory compromise is required, since the position of the infant during the LP flexes the neck and increases the risk of airway obstruction. An oximeter can be used to monitor oxygenation during the procedure.

Medications should be administered as soon as possible after the cultures are obtained. Mixing medications with a small amount of fluid in a volumetric chamber and using an infusion pump prevents fluid overload, yet ensures timely infusion of the medication.

Family support and education. Parents of septic neonates are often frightened and worried. Ongoing reassurance that everything possible is being done, along with explanations of all procedures and test results, helps allay their fears. Identifying parental concerns and answering questions honestly helps develop rapport and a trusting relationship. The use of a breast pump should be offered to the nursing mother if her baby is unable to nurse.

Preparation for hospital admission includes the physical stabilization of the infant, documentation, and informing the parents of all pertinent admission information. Parents frequently want and should be allowed to stay with their hospitalized neonate.

HYPOGLYCEMIA

Etiology. Hypoglycemia is defined as a whole blood glucose concentration less than 30 mg/dl in the full-term newborn up to 3 days of age and less than 40 mg/dl in neonates more than 3 days of age. Neonatal hypoglycemia may result from a primary etiology or various other conditions. The numerous etiologic factors are categorized according to underlying pathology, including (1) decreased glycogen storage in the liver, (2) abnormal regulation of glucose metabolism, (3) hyperinsulinism, or (4) other factors that increase glucose utilization, such as sepsis (Box 28-5). Any illness or stressor in the neonate that increases glucose utilization can exhaust glycogen stores and lead to hypoglycemia. Endocrine disturbances such as hypopituitarism, hypothyroidism, and adrenal insufficiency can impair glucose production or availability, increasing the potential for hypoglycemia.

Pathophysiology. Neonates, especially those who are premature or small for gestational age, are particularly prone to hypoglycemia because of limited glycogen stores. The stress of birth, illness, or hypothermia frequently increases the neonate's glucose requirements beyond available supplies. Nonshivering thermogenesis, which produces heat for the cold neonate, rapidly utilizes glucose stores. Illnesses, such

as sepsis and respiratory distress, increase the metabolic rate and, in turn, glucose requirements.

Fetal hyperinsulinemia commonly occurs in response to high maternal glucose levels in diabetic mothers. After birth the high circulating insulin levels continue for several hours despite the withdrawal of maternal glucose supplies. Blood glucose levels drop precipitously, and hypoglycemia often develops in 2 to 4 hours. Insulin levels usually spontaneously return to normal within 6 to 12 hours.

Glycogen storage is a rare metabolic disorder that prevents hepatic glucose output. Hypoglycemia does not result from the lack of stored glycogen, but rather from the inability to use glycogen because of enzyme deficiencies.[10] Neonates with glycogen storage disease are completely dependent on exogenous glucose.

Clinical presentation. The signs and symptoms of hypoglycemia vary greatly. At the same low blood glucose level, some infants are asymptomatic, while others display many signs and symptoms, including lethargy, tremors, jitteriness, hypotonia, cyanosis, pallor, weak cry, poor feeding, and/or tachypnea. The hypoglycemic neonate can progress to seizures, coma, apnea, and cardiac arrest. Since signs and symptoms are often nonspecific, other diagnoses must be considered.

Box 28-5 Causes of Hypoglycemia in Infancy

Decreased glycogen storage
Prematurity
Small-for-gestational age infant

Hyperinsulinism
Infant of diabetic mother
Insulin-secreting tumor

Other factors that increase glucose utilization
Sepsis
Asphyxia
Cold stress

Metabolic
Galactosemia
Glycogen storage disease

Adapted from Burchfield DJ: Acute distress in the neonate and postnatal period. In Barkin RM, ed: *Pediatric emergency medicine*, St Louis, 1992, Mosby.

Emergency Department interventions

Diagnosis. When hypoglycemia is suspected, an immediate blood glucose level is obtained using one of the many available devices with glucose reagent strips. Laboratory confirmation of the serum glucose level must be obtained. However, treatment for suspected hypoglycemia should not be withheld awaiting laboratory reports.

Treatment. The treatment of choice for documented hypoglycemia is dextrose administration. The delivery method and rate are based on the presence or absence of symptoms and the clinical status of the infant. If vascular access cannot be attained quickly, glucagon 0.1 mg/kg/24 hr can be given intramuscularly to mobilize hepatic glycogen stores.[5]

Specific therapy should be initiated to alleviate any underlying cause of hypoglycemia, such as sepsis or metabolic disorders. Hypoglycemia associated with infants of diabetic mothers may require early feedings or occasionally parenteral dextrose until neonatal insulin levels return to normal.

Nursing care and evaluation.

After stabilizing the ABCs, subsequent interventions depend on the initial presentation of the neonate. A thorough history identifies risk factors for hypoglycemia as well as the presence of signs and symptoms. A complete physical examination and observation of the neonate confirm parental reports and identify signs that may not have been noticed by the parents. Neonates with risk factors or signs and symptoms that could be consistent with hypoglycemia should receive a rapid bedside glucose measurement, followed by a serum glucose level.

If the bedside glucose determination in an asymptomatic, clinically stable neonate indicates hypoglycemia, frequent oral feedings of glucose water or formula should be administered. If vascular access has been established, and glucose remains low despite oral feedings, parenteral dextrose is indicated.

A symptomatic or clinically unstable neonate with hypoglycemia requires immediate infusion of 3 to 5 ml/kg of a 10% dextrose solution (0.25 to 0.5 g/kg) over 1 to 2 minutes. This should be followed by a continuous infusion of 10% dextrose at 4 ml/kg/hr.[5] Blood glucose levels should be reevaluated after the bolus and every hour thereafter until they are stable. If results indicate hypoglycemia, the bolus should be repeated, and the dextrose infusion rate may be increased by 1 ml/hr.[5]

Because of the hyperosmolarity of dextrose solutions, concentrations greater than 10% should not be administered to the neonate. Therefore 25% or 50% solutions must be diluted with sterile water or normal saline solution before administration. In addition, IV line patency must be assured before administration, and the infusion must be given slowly to prevent sclerosing of the vein.

Additional nursing interventions include activities to reduce neonatal stress. Using warming devices or blankets and covering the neonate's head help prevent cold stress. Comforting measures, such as swaddling and pacifiers, can also reduce stress and conserve energy. Parents should be encouraged to assist in the care of their neonate.

HYPERBILIRUBINEMIA

Etiology. Neonatal jaundice is most commonly a manifestation of the normal transition the newborn undergoes after birth and rarely requires emergency intervention. The detection of jaundice is usually indicative of hyperbilirubinemia. Jaundice may, however, be a sign of an underlying problem and therefore must be evaluated (Box 28-6).

Unconjugated (indirect) hyperbilirubinemia may be caused by either a physiologic or a pathologic condition. Persistence of unconjugated hyperbiliru-

---

Box 28-6   Causes of Nonphysiologic Jaundice

Fetal-maternal blood group incompatibility
Breast milk jaundice
Sepsis
Polycythemia
Extravasation of blood (bruising, hematoma)
Abnormal red blood cells (spherocytosis, G-6-PD)
Inborn errors of metabolism (galactosemia, Gilbert's disease)
Hypothyroidism
Direct hyperbilirubinemia (biliary atresia, neonatal hepatitis, infections)

Adapted from Burchfield DJ: Acute distress in the neonate and postnatal period. In Barkin RM, ed: *Pediatric emergency medicine,* St Louis, 1992, Mosby.

binemia after the first week of life suggests a serious problem. Conjugated (direct) hyperbilirubinemia is usually pathologic.

Pathophysiology

Normal bilirubin metabolism. The hemoglobin released by the breakdown of red blood cells splits into heme and globin. The heme portion is converted to unconjugated (indirect) bilirubin. Because it is poorly soluble, unconjugated bilirubin binds to albumin for transport to the liver via the bloodstream. In the liver, glucuronyl transferase catalyzes the conjugation of bilirubin and glucuronic acid into a water-soluble substance.[44] The conjugated (direct) bilirubin is secreted into the bile and passes into the small intestine, where it can be excreted or unconjugated and reabsorbed. Any condition that increases the breakdown of red blood cells, such as hemolytic disorders, or decreases the conjugating capacity of the liver, bilirubin-albumin binding, or bowel excretion can lead to hyperbilirubinemia.

Physiologic jaundice. Normal bilirubin production in the neonate (6 to 8 mg/kg/day) is about twice that of an adult (3 to 4 mg/kg/day)[44] because the newborn has a higher concentration of circulating red blood cells with a shorter life span. As the red blood cells break down, increased amounts of bilirubin are produced. The neonatal liver, with its diminished supply of glucuronyl transferase, is initially unable to conjugate bilirubin efficiently. Therefore neonatal serum bilirubin levels are normally higher than the adult normal of <1 mg/dl. Most newborns reach peak bilirubin levels of less than 12 mg/dl by about the third day of life and then the level declines. Occasionally, infants with physiologic jaundice have indirect levels of bilirubin of >12 mg/dl. After 1 month of age, bilirubin levels should be less than 1 to 2 mg/dl.[20]

Breast milk jaundice. There are two mechanisms by which breast-feeding can increase the level of unconjugated bilirubin in the neonate. During the first week of life, breast-feeding may increase bilirubin levels because caloric insufficiency decreases liver transport and the excretion of bilirubin from the body.[23] Jaundice occurring in breast-fed babies after the first week of life is most likely caused by a decreased ability to conjugate bilirubin. The mechanism for this phenomena is controversial. It may involve hormonal, dietary, or enzymatic factors.[6]

Conjugated hyperbilirubinemia. The accumulation of conjugated or direct bilirubin may result from hepatocellular disease or an interruption in the transport system after bilirubin has been conjugated in the liver. The most common causes of conjugated hyperbilirubinemia are neonatal hepatitis and extrahepatic biliary atresia.[14] Biliary atresia is a mechanical obstruction to bile flow, resulting in hyperbilirubinemia. Dark urine and clay-colored stools may be present with hepatitis and biliary atresia.

Infections, especially gram-negative sepsis, may produce a mixed, conjugated and unconjugated hyperbilirubinemia in the neonate. Higher levels of unconjugated bilirubin result from the increased breakdown of red blood cells. Decreased hepatic excretion elevates the conjugated bilirubin.

Complications. The primary complication of high bilirubin levels is kernicterus (or bilirubin encephalopathy). Levels of unconjugated bilirubin greater than 20 to 25 mg/dl can be toxic to brain cells, leading to severe brain damage. Although this is rare, especially in healthy term babies, treatments such as phototherapy should be initiated early to prevent the increase in unconjugated bilirubin.

Clinical presentation. The clinical presentation of the neonate with unconjugated hyperbilirubinemia varies according to etiology and severity. Jaundice, the primary clinical manifestation, is not evident until the indirect bilirubin value exceeds 5 mg/dl. Progression of jaundice occurs from head to toe with increasing bilirubin levels.[6] Although progressive jaundice cannot be assessed in a single emergency room visit, dangerously high levels should be suspected in the infant whose entire body is yellow-orange.

Physiologic jaundice in the term baby usually peaks on the third day of life and declines by the fifth to seventh day. Jaundice occurring in the first 24 hours of life or persisting greater than a week in the full-term infant, is usually not pathologic (Table 28-3).

Signs and symptoms of underlying diseases may also be present. For example, the presence of lethargy, poor feeding, abdominal distention, or vomiting may be indicative of sepsis or GI causes of hyperbilirubinemia.

Emergency Department interventions

Diagnosis. The diagnosis and treatment of hyperbilirubinemia rely on serum levels of unconjugated (indirect) bilirubin. The upper limits of normal indi-

		BREAST-FEEDING ASSOCIATED		
	PHYSIOLOGIC JAUNDICE	JAUNDICE (EARLY ONSET)	BREAST MILK JAUNDICE (LATE ONSET)	HEMOLYTIC DISEASE
Cause	Immature hepatic function plus increased bilirubin load from red blood cell hemolysis	Poor milk intake related to fewer calories consumed by infant before mother's milk is well established; enterohepatic shunting	Possible factors in breast milk that prevent bilirubin conjugation Less frequent stooling	Blood antigen incompatibility causes hemolysis of large numbers of red blood cells Liver unable to conjugate and excrete excess bilirubin from hemolysis
Onset	After 24 hours (preterm infants, prolonged)	Second to fourth day	Fifth to seventh day	During first 24 hours (levels increase faster than 5 mg/dl/day)
Peak Duration	72 to 90 hours Declines on fifth to seventh day	Third to fifth day	Tenth to fifteenth day May remain jaundiced for 3 to 12 weeks	Variable
Therapy	Phototherapy if bilirubin levels increase significantly (rise in bilirubin greater than 5 mg/dl/day)	Frequent (10 to 12 times/day) breast-feeding Phototherapy for bilirubin 17 to 22 mg/dl in health term infants	Increase frequency of breast-feeding; use no supplementation such as glucose water Severe jaundice—temporary discontinuation of breast-feeding for up to 24 hours may be recommended if bilirubin levels decrease, breast-feeding can resume May include home phototherapy with uninterrupted breast-feeding	*Postnatal*—Phototherapy; if severe, exchange transfusion *Prenatal*—Transfusion (fetus) Prevent sensitization (Rh incompatibility) of Rh-negative mother with RhoGAM

From Wong DL: *Whaley & Wong's essentials of pediatric nursing,* ed 5, St Louis, 1997, Mosby.

rect bilirubin levels in full-term neonates are 13 mg/dl for bottle-fed and 15 mg/dl in breast-fed infants.[6] Previous serum bilirubin levels, if available, should be obtained and compared to present levels.

Depending on the clinical presentation, further studies may be indicated. A septic workup, complete blood count with differential and cultures, TORCH screen (toxoplasmosis, other (virus, bacteria, parasite), rubella, cytomegalovirus, herpes), and syphilis may identify an infectious etiology. Incompatible maternal and neonatal blood types, an elevated reticulocyte count, or a positive direct or indirect Coombs' test suggests a hemolytic process.[5] Clotting studies, ammonia, albumin, total protein, blood urea nitrogen (BUN), and creatinine levels may also provide helpful information.

Treatment. The primary goals of hyperbilirubinemia therapy are the prevention of kernicterus and the treatment of underlying pathology. Most neonates with an unconjugated bilirubin level greater than 15 mg/dl should receive phototherapy, which breaks down bilirubin in the skin into an excretable form. Home management with phototherapy lights or abundant sunshine is considered in many neonates, when close follow-up by a primary health care provider is available. Neonates with confirmed anemia or abnormal clotting studies may require blood transfusions. Inpatient admission is usually indicated for conjugated hyperbilirubinemia because the etiology is rarely identified in the emergency department.

Nursing care and evaluation. A complete history and physical examination is required to identify underlying etiologies and determine the severity of the illness. Certain factors, such as breast-feeding or prematurity, should alert the nurse to expect relatively higher bilirubin levels or a more prolonged course. Family history may increase the index of suspicion for problems such as red blood cell abnormalities. Results of the history, physical examination, and diagnostic workup dictate subsequent treatment.

Admission for phototherapy depends primarily on the level of indirect bilirubin. Other factors to consider include the rate of bilirubin rise (>5 mg/dl/day is excessive), gestational age, etiology, clinical status, proximity to follow-up care, availability of sunshine, and reliability of the caregivers. If the baby is discharged, instructions should be given concerning, home management (Box 28-7).

Controversy exists over whether breast milk hyperbilirubinemia is serious enough to warrant treatment. Hyperbilirubinemia is usually resolved if breast-feeding is briefly discontinued, but some feel that cessation of breast-feeding is unnecessary. If discontinuing breast-feeding for a couple of days is recommended, the emergency department nurse must evaluate both the mother's knowledge of breast pumping and the availability of appropriate equipment. A referral to a La Leche League or other breast-feeding resource may be helpful to promote continuation of breast-feeding. The parents should be

---

Box 28-7 Home Management of Hyperbilirubinemia

- Place the baby in a sunny area.
- Expose as much skin as possible to the sunlight, which provides a natural phototherapy.
- Make sure the baby stays warm.
- Breast-feed the baby more frequently to stimulate milk production. Increased intake by the baby stimulates the intestine so that bilirubin can be excreted.
- Report any change in signs and symptoms to a physician or return to the emergency department.
- Return for follow-up evaluation.

---

reassured that jaundice is only temporary and that breast milk is still beneficial for the infant.

COMMON COMPLAINTS

COLDS

Etiology. The common cold is a mild upper respiratory tract infection (URI) that is not life-threatening in the healthy neonate. However, parents frequently come to the emergency department for reassurance that their infant does not have a serious underlying disease.

Colds are primarily caused by rhinoviruses[28] but also by other viruses such as parainfluenza, adenovirus, and coronavirus.[42] Because there are over 200 different serotypes that can cause colds,[35] immunologically immature neonates are prone to frequent episodes. Prematurity, congenital disorders such as heart disease, and chronic illnesses such as bronchopulmonary dysplasia increase the susceptibility of the neonate to URIs, as well as increasing the severity of the illness.

Pathophysiology. The body responds to viral infection by initiating the inflammatory process. The resulting vasodilation, mucosal swelling, and secretion of nasal mucus account for the common cold symptoms. Nasal and pharyngeal irritation produce sneezing and coughing.

Clinical presentation. Colds present with a variety of symptoms that have a gradual onset. Nasal congestion and discharge are the major symptoms. Nasal discharge varies from watery to thick and usually changes consistency over the course of the illness. Sneezing is common. Coughing frequently occurs later in the course of the illness and is primarily caused by postnatal drip. Because infants are obligate nose breathers, mild signs of respiratory distress, such as tachypnea, and decreased feeding may occur because of nasal congestion. Fever is unusual in the neonate with a cold. Occasionally vomiting, especially after feedings, and diarrhea is present. Emesis usually contains large amounts of mucus. Cold symptoms generally resolve within 2 weeks.

Emergency Department interventions. There is no cure for the common cold. Antibiotics are not beneficial in treating viral illnesses. Supportive care is the recommended treatment. Neonates with cold symptoms require a complete examination to rule out underlying illnesses or congenital disorders. If fever is present, a complete septic workup is required to rule out sepsis.

Differential diagnoses that should be considered include otitis media, pneumonia, bronchiolitis, and sepsis. Frequent colds may raise suspicion of an underlying chronic illness.

Nursing care and evaluation. The history focuses on the current symptoms as well as baseline information related to when the infant last appeared well. Additional information should include alterations in normal activities such as sleep and feeding; past medical history; and medications or home remedies given. Cough medicines, acetaminophen, or even antibiotics are often given by caregivers without medical advice.

A complete physical assessment is required. Before the respiratory examination the nares of the congested infant are suctioned to relieve any nasal obstruction that may be affecting the respiratory status. Signs of upper and lower airway abnormalities should be identified, including signs of respiratory distress, such as retractions and nasal flaring. Tympanic membranes should be visualized by the physician or nurse practitioner, since otitis media commonly occurs as colds are resolving. Neonates with simple colds and no respiratory distress can safely be discharged home.

Parents should be instructed that nasal congestion may cause mild signs of respiratory distress and audible airway sounds such as "rattling" in the chest. With suctioning, however, these signs should disappear. Suctioning the infant before feeding allows the infant

---

Box 28-8 Discharge Instructions for the Common Cold in Neonates

- Use bulb syringe to carefully remove mucus from infant's nose, especially before feedings and sleep.
- If nasal discharge is thick, place 2 drops of salt water in each side of nose to loosen the mucus. Then suction out with bulb syringe. Commercial preparations can be used or a home recipe: dissolve ½ tablespoon salt in 4 ounces water.
- Use a cool mist or steam vaporizer pointed toward the baby to liquify secretions. Caution must be taken with steam vaporizers to prevent burns. Daily cleaning of the vaporizers is necessary to prevent bacterial growth. If a vaporizer is not available, take the baby into the bathroom with a hot shower running to create steam. Do not take the baby into the shower itself.
- Give the baby plenty of fluids to drink to help loosen secretions. Offer water between formula or breastmilk feedings.
- Keep the baby away from cigarette or other irritating smoke.
- If the baby develops a fever, the primary health care provider should be contacted. Acetaminophen should be given for fever *only* if recommended by your health care provider.
- Cough medicines or decongestant nose drops are not recommended in neonates.

---

to breath nasally, improving the ability to feed. Neonates with nasal congestion require frequent suctioning because they are unable to clear the nares by blowing their noses (Box 28-8).

CONSTIPATION

Etiology. Constipation is the regular passage of firm or hard stools unrelated to stool frequency.[8,44] Many parents view constipation as a serious problem and bring their baby to the emergency department with a chief complaint of irregular bowel movements or straining. Often what the parents describe is normal infant bowel habits. Sometimes, though, there are functional or pathologic causes.

Common causes of neonatal constipation include dietary changes, motility disorders, viral illnesses, and anal fissures. Life-threatening disorders such as mechanical obstruction and dehydration must also be considered.[25] Structural or congenital disorders of the anus, rectum, or colon, such as Hirschsprung's disease of anal displacement, can cause chronic constipation in the neonate (see Chapter 15, Gastrointestinal System, p. 337).

Pathophysiology. Digestive waste collects in the colon where sodium and water are reabsorbed. Distention of the rectum stimulates the defecation reflex, and fecal matter is expelled. This process is involuntary in the infant. Most newborns pass their first meconium stool in the first 48 hours of life.[13] Thereafter, normal neonatal stooling frequency ranges from one after every feeding to one every other day. Delayed passage of stools during the initial 48 hours of life may indicate structural or congenital problems.

Clinical presentation. Many parents misinterpret normal or colicky behavior as constipation. Neonates commonly strain, turn red in the face, and grunt with bowel movements despite the consistency of the stool. Colicky infants cry and draw up their legs. Parents frequently interpret this as abdominal pain from constipation, even when the bowel movements are soft.

Neonates with actual constipation have consistently hard, dry, and possibly blood-streaked bowel movements. Their abdomens may be firm and distended. They may have difficulty passing large, hard stool, especially if anal fissures are present. Pain may be manifested by crying and drawing up the legs. Differentiating between colic and constipation requires a complete history and physical examination, including inspection of the stool.

Emergency Department interventions. Infants with signs of constipation do not require an extensive diagnostic workup in the emergency department unless bowel obstruction is suspected. In this case, a surgical consultation is usually necessary. Diagnostic studies may include an abdominal flat plate, contrast studies, or ultrasound. For the constipated neonate, dietary changes can be instituted, with follow-up by the primary health care provider. More aggressive bowel management may be recommended for the uncomfortable infant with a large amount of stool impacted in the bowel.

Nursing care and evaluation. The history should include questions concerning usual bowel patterns, changes in bowel patterns, frequency of stools, and consistency. Changes in feeding should also be noted. These include dietary changes preceding the onset of constipation, the determination of whether the infant is bottle-fed or breast-fed, and if solids have been recently introduced.

Physical examination includes an abdominal and rectal examination. If possible, a stool sample is obtained and tested for occult blood. If the infant's stool is soft and the physical examination is negative, constipation does not exist, regardless of the reported stool infrequency.[25] If the infant is constipated, a fecal mass may be palpated in the lower left quadrant of the abdomen.

When a neonate is impacted with stool, treatment is often recommended to relieve discomfort. Digital rectal stimulation (with a thermometer, for example) can be attempted first. If this is not successful, a "chip" of a glycerin suppository is recommended. Enemas are a last resort and rarely used. If an enema is given, an isotonic solution should be used, since plain water can affect fluid and electrolyte balance in the neonate.[44]

If the neonate's bowel habits are normal, parental education and reassurance are necessary. Dietary changes are usually recommended for neonates with constipation. Increasing fluid intake, other than formula or milk, may prove beneficial. The infant's formula should be reviewed to detect overfeeding. Solid foods are not recommended in the neonatal period. Dark Karo syrup, 1 ounce per 8 ounce bottle of formula or water, may soften the stools. Parents should be advised to avoid suppositories and enemas at home. Some practitioners feel these practices can promote the formation of later behavioral problems regarding defecation. Follow-up care with a primary caregiver is recommended for all infants with constipation. If chronic or severe constipation is present, referral to a surgical or GI specialist may be indicated.

BLOODY STOOLS

Etiology. Neonatal blood loss from the GI tract can be alarming to parents. In the emergency department the health care provider must determine if blood in the stool arises from the GI tract or is secondary to local irritation.

There are numerous etiologies for bloody stools in the neonate. The most common cause is anorectal lesions, such as anal fissures. Swallowed maternal blood during delivery may pass into the stools of neonates younger than 7 days old.[13] Necrotizing enterocolitis (NEC), common in premature infants or full-term infants with birth asphyxia or cyanotic congenital heart disease, may cause lower GI bleeding.[29]

There have also been numerous case reports of bloody stools in exclusively breast-fed infants that have resolved when the nursing mother eliminated cow's milk protein from her diet, or breast milk was replaced by a casein hydrolysate formula or a soy protein–based formula.[39] Feeding neonates cow's milk instead of formula may also lead to intestinal blood loss and bloody stools.

The presence of bloody stools can be an emergency if associated with intestinal obstruction such as midgut volvulus secondary to malrotation.[3] Intussusception, another cause of bloody stools ("currant jelly"), is usually diagnosed in infants older than 1 month. Both conditions are surgical emergencies (see Chapter 15, Gastrointestinal System, p. 346-347).

Pathophysiology. The site of bleeding can sometimes be approximated by the quality of the stool. Melena, a black tarry stool, indicates bleeding proximal to the ileocecal valve. Gross blood usually arises from the lower intestinal tract. A small amount of blood streaked on the outside of the stool often indicates a localized lesion such as an anal fissure.

Clinical presentation. The majority of infants who come to the emergency department with bloody stools are hemodynamically stable. Neonates may have grossly bloody stools, streaks of visible blood in the stools, or tarry stools. Occult blood in the stool may be identified during further evaluation of the chief complaint.

Neonates with NEC often have abdominal distention, bilious vomiting, and lower GI bleeding. NEC does not usually require surgery unless signs of bowel perforation are present. Midgut volvulus presents with abdominal tenderness, bilious vomiting, and melena.[29]

Emergency Department interventions

Diagnosis. Stool should be examined for gross blood. If it is not readily apparent, a test for occult blood should be performed. Pathogens can be identified by stool culture. Depending on the severity and suspected etiology of the rectal bleeding, blood work may be ordered, including a complete blood count with differential. An elevated white blood cell count may be suggestive of an inflammatory response, and a decreased hemoglobin and hematocrit suggest anemia. Platelet counts and coagulation studies may be performed to rule out bleeding disorders.

Abdominal x-rays can identify obstructive causes of bloody stools and sometimes NEC. Additional radiologic studies such as an upper GI series and a barium enema may be performed for specific presentations.

Treatment. Treatment is based on the etiology of rectal bleeding. If an anal fissure is present, a stool softening regimen is prescribed (see the discussion of constipation). Frequent warm baths and petrolatum around the anus with diaper changes may promote comfort and healing. Treatment for NEC includes hospital admission and the administration of IV antibiotics, bowel rest, and hyperalimentation. If bowel perforation or obstruction is suspected, surgery is indicated.[29]

Nursing care and evaluation. A history of the onset, progression, amount, and quality of bleeding should be assessed. Specific amounts of blood should be requested, although they are often overestimated. Sometimes relating the size of blood spot on the diaper to a coin, such as a nickel or 50-cent piece is helpful. Parents should also describe the amount, color, and consistency of the stool.

If vomiting and abdominal distention are present with the bloody stool, there is a high index of suspicion for an obstruction. Hypoactive bowel sounds also suggest an obstruction. These infants require emergent management.

If the neonate's condition is hemodynamically stable and the infant does not exhibit signs of abdominal perforation or obstruction, a complete physical examination can be performed. This includes a visual examination of the anus to check for fissures.

Although the presence of bloody stools is not usually an emergency, parents may fear that the neonate has sustained a major blood loss. If an anal fissure is suspected, parents should be reassured that small amounts of bleeding may be expected. However, if an obstruction or perforation is suspected, parents require ongoing communication regarding the plan of care. Parents of these seriously ill neonates need support, understanding, and continuous updates as the nurse prepares the infant for surgery.

VOMITING

Etiology. Vomiting is an unexpected and unpleasant occurrence for any age group. When it occurs in the neonate, parents often seek medical attention for fear of dehydration or the possible onset of serious illness. Vomiting may be the primary complaint or may be associated with various other symptoms. Although it most frequently represents disturbances within the GI tract, it can also indicate disturbances in other areas of the body, including the central nervous system (e.g., head trauma), renal system (e.g., urinary tract infections), pulmonary system (e.g., pneumonia), and endocrine system (e.g., metabolic disorders). Vomiting caused by inborn errors of metabolism is sometimes mistakenly attributed to a GI tract obstruction or other etiology (Box 28-9).

A common variation of neonatal vomiting is physiologic regurgitation, or "spitting up." The immature lower esophageal sphincter allows stomach contents to reflux or regurgitate into the mouth. Gastroesophageal reflux is not forceful. Most infants continue to gain weight and outgrow reflux by 6 to 9 months of age.

Neonates whose onset of vomiting occurs in the first days of life should always be suspected of having a congenital GI anomaly that causes obstruction, such as intestinal atresia, malrotation with midgut volvulus, or Hirschsprung's disease.[16] Pyloric stenosis does not cause projectile vomiting until about 3 weeks of age.

Pathophysiology. The lower esophageal sphincter normally remains contracted to prevent food from refluxing back into the esophagus, opening only to allow food into the stomach. In neonates the underdeveloped muscle of this sphincter allows some reflux. Actual vomiting is mediated by two central nervous centers in the medulla. One center responds to stimuli from the pharynx, pleura, heart, GI tract, urogenital tract, and biliary tree.[30] The other triggers vomiting in response to metabolic disorders and certain drugs, such as ipecac.

The presence of bile in vomitus indicates a blockage distal to the ampulla of Vater (second portion of the duodenum). Absence of bile indicates that blockage, if present, is proximal to the ampulla of Vater.

Clinical presentation. The presentation of the infant with vomiting varies with the etiology. However, the quality of the emesis may offer clues to the pathology. For example, since gastric content alters the color of emesis, bright red vomitus indicates active bleeding above the stomach. Acute onset of

---

Box 28-9 Causes of Vomiting (Birth to 3 months)

Infectious
Viral gastroenteritis
Meningitis/encephalitis
Pneumonia/pertussis
Sepsis
UTI

Anatomic/congenital
Gastroesophageal reflux
Pyloric stenosis
Hernia
Hirschsprung's disease
Tracheoesophageal fistula
Intestinal stenosis
Malrotation with midgut volvulus
Esophageal web

Neurologic
Hydrocephalus
Cerebral edema
Intracranial tumor
Kernicterus

Metabolic
Congenital adrenal hyperplasia
Urea cycle defects
Organic acidemias
Amino acid metabolism defect
Hereditary fructose intolerance

Other
Milk allergy
Necrotizing enterocolitis

Adapted from Patterson MD: Vomiting. In Barkin RM, ed: *Pediatric emergency medicine*, St Louis, 1992, Mosby.

---

bilious vomiting in the neonate is presumed to be midgut volvulus, a surgical emergency, until proven otherwise.[40]

Dehydration is possible in any infant with vomiting. Signs and symptoms of dehydration often develop if the vomiting has been persistent and the intake minimal.

Emergency Department interventions. Diagnosis of the cause of vomiting is primarily based on the history and physical examination. Laboratory tests may include a complete blood count and differential, serum electrolytes and glucose, urinalysis, and others, depending on the presentation.

Abdominal x-rays and an upper GI series are commonly requested when obstructive lesions are suspected. If bilious vomiting is present, an emergency upper GI study is indicated.[34] Some physicians recommend ultrasound as the initial imaging approach to the infant who vomits. However, upper GI studies have been found to be sufficient and are less expensive.[12]

Surgical versus medical management is based on the diagnosis. If dehydration is present, parenteral or oral fluids are required based on the severity of symptoms.

Nursing care and evaluation. A detailed history can assist in the differentiation between the neonate with an emergency problem and one who is merely "spitting up." The history should include onset, duration, timing, quality, and amount of vomiting, along with any associated symptoms. Parents often need help in realistically defining the amount of vomitus. Comparison with common amounts, such as a teaspoon, tablespoon, or cup, is helpful. A description of the usual feeding pattern of the neonate is also an important part of the history. Past medical history may reveal risk factors for various etiologies of vomiting.

Observation of the infant's degree of illness is a valuable part of the physical examination. Some infants may "look sick," while others appear healthy. Gastroesophageal reflux is common in the neonate who appears well, with vomiting as the only complaint. The ill-appearing child may be lethargic, dehydrated, and/or have a serious underlying disorder. Fever, lethargy, or irritability may indicate an infectious process. Abdominal distention, high-pitched or absent bowel sounds, and visible peristalsis are signs of obstruction[17] (see Chapter 14, Fluid and Electrolyte Imbalances for specific signs and symptoms of dehydration).

Circulatory compromise is a possibility with some of the causes of vomiting (e.g., volvulus, intussusception, obstruction). If one of these conditions is suspected, vascular access is required to maintain hydration and/or administer fluid resuscitation. Abdominal decompression with a nasogastric tube may also be indicated. Infants suspected to have serious pathologic conditions are often admitted for further diagnostic evaluation, surgical intervention, or medical management.

Stable, well-hydrated infants with nonacute diagnoses who are tolerating fluids may be discharged from the emergency department. Discharge teaching should include information regarding vomiting in the neonate, frequency and types of oral fluids indicated (electrolyte solutions, formula), signs and symptoms of serious illness, and signs and symptoms of dehydration (Box 28-10). Parents must be given clear instructions about signs and symptoms of dehydration and when to call their primary care provider.

CRYING

Etiology. Crying is one of the few means by which a neonate can communicate. Infant crying is generally thought to signal an unmet need or distress. When parents are unable to identify the cause of their neonate's crying or when they are unable to console the infant, they may come to the emergency department.

One cause of crying in the infant is colic, which is discussed in the next section. Crying related to other conditions will be discussed in this section. There is a

---

Box 28-10   Discharge Teaching for Nonacute Causes of Vomiting in Neonates

- *Hydration:* Give the baby small, frequent amounts of clear fluids until vomiting stops. One half to 1 ounce every 15 to 30 minutes is a good starting point. Increase the amount of fluid slowly. Clear liquids (electrolyte solutions) are optimal to maintain adequate fluid and electrolyte balance. Avoid milk or formula until vomiting has stopped.
- *Recognition of signs of dehydration:* Keep track of the number and frequency of wet diapers. Notify the primary health care provider if there is less than half of the neonate's normal number of daily wet diapers or if the baby has not had a wet diaper every 6 to 8 hours. Report sunken fontanel, decreased activity, and dry mouth to the primary care provider
- *Caring for babies with reflux:* Position the baby with head elevated during and for a half hour after feedings. An infant seat is helpful for positioning.

certain degree of crying normally exhibited by infants during the first few months of life. Brazelton found that the number of times an infant cries each day peaks at about 6 to 8 weeks of age. Infant crying episodes did not occur uniformly throughout the day, but instead were clustered during the afternoon and evening.[2,4] Parents become concerned when they think their infant's crying is greater than what they anticipated.

Numerous medical conditions can cause inconsolable crying in infants. A 1-year study involving 56 infants brought to the Denver Children's Hospital Emergency Department for excessive crying identified many of these conditions, including GI disorders and metabolic disorders[31] (Box 28-11).

Clinical presentation. In the emergency department, neonates with a chief complaint of crying may cry inconsolably, cry sporadically, or not cry at all. Because of the brevity of the visit, health care providers rely heavily on the parent's description of the infant's behavior at home. The duration of crying before seeking medical attention can vary from 1 hour to several days.

Certain cries are associated with specific etiologies. For example, high-pitched cries are associated with pain, increased ICP, or drug withdrawal. A weak cry may be indicative of sepsis or neurologic disorders.

Emergency Department interventions. Diagnostic tests are based on the clinical findings. If a specific cause for crying is determined, treatment can be initiated accordingly. Colic is likely in infants with a negative physical examination and supportive history.

Nursing care and evaluation. A detailed history is necessary to determine the cause of persistent infant crying. Parents should be asked about the onset of crying, daily patterns, and any related events, such as recent immunizations, fever, or use of medications. The quality of the cry may be helpful in the diagnosis, as well as associated signs and symptoms.

A complete physical examination will help to identify signs of serious illness or injury. The Denver study found that the physical examination diagnosed the etiology of the crying in 41% of the cases. When the history and physical examination were combined, an additional 30% of the cases were diagnosed.[31]

The importance of examining the infant with the body undressed cannot be overemphasized. Fingers and toes should be examined for hair tourniquets. Bruises or burns on a neonate are highly suspicious of child abuse. The head should be evaluated for signs of

---

Box 28-11 Conditions Associated with Abrupt Onset of Unconsolable Crying in Young Infants

I. Discomfort caused by identifiable illness
A. Head and neck
  1. Meningitis*
  2. Skull fracture/subdural hematoma*
  3. Glaucoma
  4. Foreign body (especially eyelash) in eye†
  5. Corneal abrasion†
  6. Otitis media†
  7. Caffey's disease (infantile cortical hyperostosis)
  8. Battered child syndrome*
  9. Prenatal/perinatal cocaine exposure
B. Gastrointestinal
  1. Excess air because of improper feeding or burping technique
  2. Gastroenteritis†
  3. Intussusception*
  4. Anal fissure†
  5. Milk intolerance
C. Genitourinary
  1. Torsion of testis
  2. Incarcerated hernia*
  3. Urinary tract infections
D. Integument
  1. Open diaper pin
  2. Burn
  3. Strangulated finger, toe, penis (often because of an encircling hair)
E. Musculoskeletal
  1. Battered child syndrome*
  2. Extremity fracture (following a fall)
F. Toxic/metabolic
  1. Drugs: aspirin, antihistamines, atropinics, adrenergics, cocaine (including passive inhalation)*
  2. Metabolic acidosis, hypernatremia, hypocalcemia, hypoglycemia*
  3. Pertussis vaccine reactions
II. Colic—recurrent paroxysmal attacks of crying†

*Life-threatening causes.
† Common causes.
From Selbst S: The septic-appearing infant. In Fleisher G, Ludwig S, eds: *Textbook of pediatric emergency medicine*, ed 3, Baltimore, 1993, Williams & Wilkins.

trauma. The presence of retinal hemorrhages on fundoscopic examination is suggestive of shaken baby syndrome.[37] Since the infant cannot communicate verbally, emergency department health care providers must be alert to any physical signs of abuse, as well as evidence of poor parent-infant interaction.

Parental support is very important. Parents are often anxious and tired, particularly when they have been up with their crying baby for several nights. If the history and examination reveal a specific cause for crying, parental education regarding the specific condition is necessary. If the history is more suggestive of colic, specific approaches to the neonate are addressed in the next section.

COLIC

Etiology. The emergency nurse is likely to consider colic when faced with a frantic, sleep-deprived parent who has been dealing with prolonged periods of crying in an infant. Parents seek a cure, not only because they think their infant is in distress, but also because they need sleep.

The nature and cause of infantile colic are poorly understood. No universally accepted definition exists for colic, nor can consistent etiologies be identified. Most studies provide some evidence for either GI or non-GI causes (Box 28-12).

Although there is insufficient evidence to support the presence of a specific GI etiology, there are several theories. Dietary factors such as lactose intolerance, carbohydrate intolerance, and allergy to cow's milk have all been considered, as well as GI reflux and hormonal abnormalities. Most full-term infants cannot completely absorb the lactose in formula during the first several months of life. This results in increased gas production after feedings.[43] Starch, commonly found in cereal, is also not absorbed well by the young infant. In one study the prevalence of colic was found to be greater in a group of infants fed cereal within the first 3 months of life, compared to infants receiving no solids.[18]

Probably the most widely studied dietary theory for colic is that of cow's milk intolerance or allergy. The majority of studies have focused on the protein component of cow's milk rather than on lactose. Some evidence indicates that colic is associated with maternal consumption of cow's milk in breast-fed infants, although this is not supported by other studies.[19]

The literature suggesting non-GI etiologies for colic focuses on behavioral and interactive factors. According to this theory, there is no physical cause of

Box 28-12	Suggested Etiologies for Colic	
GI	**NON-GI**
Lactose intolerance	Crying variation
Carbohydrate malabsorption	Parental anxiety
Cow's milk allergy	Parent-infant interaction
Hormonal factors	

colic and the infant is not in pain or true distress. Instead, variations in normal crying and atypical parenting have been considered as major contributing factors. Maternal tension or poor parenting skills have been suggested; however, the behavioral and interactive data do not fully support non-GI causes.

Clinical presentation. Infant colic is most commonly characterized by excessive inconsolable crying; often occurring in the evenings; without an identifiable cause; and in an otherwise healthy infant between 2 weeks and 4 months of age. Physical signs such as pulling the legs up, tensing the abdomen, and passing flatus are frequently observed.

Criteria used to identify infants as colicky include 3 hours of crying per day for 3 days per week over a period of 3 weeks. Crying episodes usually start in the second to third week of life. The typical episode is described as crying that develops into an intense scream, as if the infant were in pain.

Emergency Department interventions. There is no cure for colic except time. Supportive treatment and parental support are the primary interventions until the infant outgrows the colic, which is usually by the fourth month of age.

Nursing care and evaluation. An organized approach to the history and physical examination helps rule out any physical cause of the crying (Fig. 28-1). When all other causes are excluded, the diagnosis of colic is usually made.

During the emergency department visit, parents should be taught strategies for decreasing the infant's crying. Some helpful approaches to decrease crying include rhythmic motion and positioning. Rocking the infant, taking the infant for a ride in a car, carrying the infant in a pack, and placing the infant in a swing often help, at least temporarily. Holding the infant in

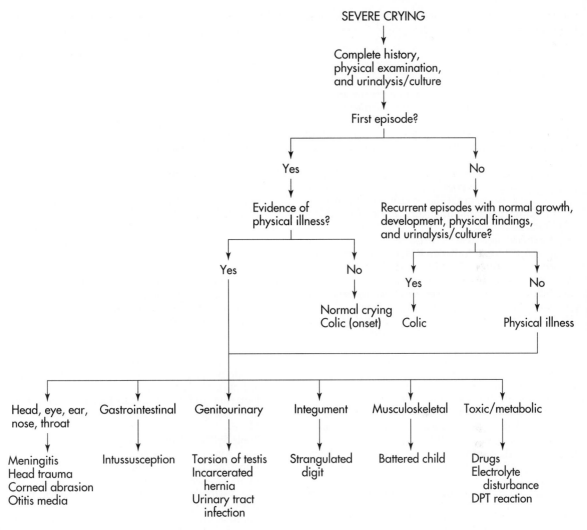

SEVERE CRYING

↓

Complete history,
physical examination,
and urinalysis/culture

↓

First episode?

- **Yes**
  - Evidence of physical illness?
    - **Yes**
    - **No**
      - Normal crying
      - Colic (onset)
- **No**
  - Recurrent episodes with normal growth, development, physical findings, and urinalysis/culture?
    - **Yes**
      - Colic
    - **No**
      - Physical illness

Head, eye, ear, nose, throat	Gastrointestinal	Genitourinary	Integument	Musculoskeletal	Toxic/metabolic
Meningitis Head trauma Corneal abrasion Otitis media	Intussusception	Torsion of testis Incarcerated hernia Urinary tract infection	Strangulated digit	Battered child	Drugs Electrolyte disturbance DPT reaction

FIG. 28-1. Approach to abrupt onset of severe crying in infancy. (From Henretig S: Crying and colic in early infancy. In Fleisher G, Ludwig S, eds: *Textbook of pediatric emergency medicine,* ed 3, Baltimore, 1993, Williams & Wilkins.)

the prone position on an arm is also frequently helpful. No medications are recommended for the infant with colic. Parents should be cautioned against using home cures, such as whiskey on the pacifier, since alcohol can be toxic to the neonate.

Parents frequently have difficulty coping with the colicky infant and often feel helpless and insecure. They should be encouraged to take time for themselves and to allow time to rest, so that they will have the energy to deal with the colicky periods. Reassurance that the parents are doing nothing wrong and

that this situation is time-limited is important. If other supportive services are needed, appropriate referrals must be made.

▮ SUMMARY

The care of neonates is highly specialized and challenging. Transitional and immature physiology contributes to the diseases typically seen in this age group and the differences in the manifestation of illness. The emergency department nurse must use astute observation skills and listen carefully to caregivers to identify subtle signs of neonatal illness.

REFERENCES

1. Aherne W, Hull D: Brown adipose tissue and heat production in the newborn infant, *J Pathol Bacteriol* 91:223, 1966.
2. Barr R, Kramer M, Bioisjoly C: Parental diary of infant cry and fuss behavior, *Arch Dis Child* 63:380–387, 1988.
3. Boyle J: Gastrointestinal bleeding. In Fleisher G, Ludwig S, eds: *Textbook of pediatric emergency medicine*, ed 2, Baltimore, 1988, Williams & Wilkins.
4. Brazelton T: Crying in infancy, *Pediatrics* 29:579–588, 1962.
5. Burchfield DJ: Acute distress in the neonate and postnatal period. In Barkin RM, ed: *Pediatric emergency medicine*, ed 2, St Louis, 1997, Mosby.
6. Cashore WJ: Hyperbilirubinemia. In Pomerance JJ, Richardson CJ, eds: *Neonatology for the clinician*, Norwalk, CT, 1993, Appleton & Lange.
7. Chameides L, Hazinski MF, eds: *Textbook of pediatric advanced life support*, Dallas, 1994, American Heart Association.
8. Chow MP et al: *Handbook of pediatric primary care*, New York, 1979, John Wiley & Sons.
9. Dashefsky B: Life threatening infections, *Pediatr Emerg Care* 7(4):244–253, 1991.
10. DiGiacomo J: Glucose homeostasis. In Merenstein G, Gardner S, eds: *Handbook of neonatal intensive care*, ed 2, St Louis, 1989, Mosby.
11. Driscoll JJ: Evaluation of the cyanotic newborn. Congenital heart disease, *Pediatr Clin North Am* 37(1):1–24, 1990.
12. Foley L et al: Evaluation of the vomiting infant, *Am J Dis Child* 143:660–661, 1989.
13. Gomella T: *Neonatology*, Norwalk, CT, 1992, Appleton & Lange.
14. Haber B, Lake A: Cholestatic jaundice in the newborn, *Clin Perinatol* 17(2):483–502, 1990.
15. Hazinski MF: Children are different. In Hazinski MF, ed: *Nursing care of the critically ill child*, ed 2, St Louis, 1992, Mosby.
16. Henretig F: Crying and colic in early infancy. In Fleisher G, Ludwig S, eds: *Textbook of pediatric emergency medicine*, ed 3, Baltimore, 1993, Williams & Wilkins.
17. Henretig F: Vomiting. In Fleisher G, Ludwig S, eds: *Textbook of pediatric emergency medicine*, ed 3, Baltimore, 1993, Williams & Wilkins.
18. Hide D, Guyer B: Prevalence of infant colic, *Arch Dis Child* 57:559–560, 1982.
19. Jakobsson I, Lindberg R: Cow's milk proteins cause infantile colic in breast-fed infants: a double blind crossover study, *Pediatrics* 71:268–271, 1983.
20. Johnson KB: *The Harriet Lane handbook*, St Louis, 1993, Mosby.
21. Lamper C: Facilitating attachment through well-baby care. In Hall JE, Weaver BR, eds: *Nursing of families in crisis*, Philadelphia 1974, JB Lippincott.
22. Langston C et al: Human lung growth in late gestation and the the neonate, *Am Rev Resp Dis* 129:607, 1984.
23. Lott J: Neonatal adaptation. In Cohen C, Kenner C, Hollingsworth A, eds: *Maternal, neonatal, and women's health nursing*, Springhouse, 1991, Springhouse Corp.
24. Lott J: Assessment and management of immunologic dysfunction. In Kenner C, Brueggemeyer A, Gunderson L, eds: *Comprehensive neonatal nursing*, Philadelphia, 1993, WB Saunders.
25. Ludwig S: Constipation. In Fleisher G, Ludwig S, eds: *Textbook of pediatric emergency medicine*, ed 3, Baltimore, 1993, Williams & Wilkins.
26. Reference deleted in proofs.
27. Martin GI: Infant apnea. In Pomerance JJ, Richardson CJ, eds: *Neonatology for the clinician*, Norwalk, CT, 1993, Appleton & Lange.
28. McMillan J et al: Rhinovirus infection associated with serious illness among pediatric patients, *Pediatr Infect Dis J* 12:321–324, 1992.
29. Ochsenschlager DW: Gastrointestinal bleeding. In Barkin RM, ed: *Pediatric emergency medicine*, ed 2, St Louis, 1997, Mosby.
30. Patterson MD: Vomiting. In Barkin RM, ed: *Pediatric emergency medicine*, ed 2, St Louis, 1997, Mosby.
31. Poole S: The infant with acute, unexplained, excessive crying, *Pediatrics* 88(3):450–455, 1991.
32. Robatham JL: Maturation of the respiratory system. In Shoemaker WC, Thompson WL, Holbrook PR, eds: *Textbook of critical care*, Philadelphia, 1988, WB Saunders.
33. Rudolph AM: The changes in circulation after birth, *Circulation* 41:343, 1970.
34. Rudolph C: Vomiting. In Grossman M, Diekmann R, eds: *Pediatric emergency medicine*, Philadelphia, 1991, JB Lippincott.
35. Santamaria JP, Abrunzo TJ: Ear, nose, and throat. In Barkin RM, ed: *Pediatric emergency medicine*, ed 2, St Louis, 1997, Mosby.
36. Selbst S: The septic-appearing infant. In Fleisher G, Ludwig S, eds: *Textbook of pediatric emergency medicine*, ed 3, Baltimore, 1993, Williams & Wilkins.
37. Singer J: A fatal case of colic, *Pediatr Emerg Care* 8:171–172, 1992.
38. Smith JB: Bacterial and fungal infections of the neonate. In Pomerance JJ, Richardson CJ, eds: *Neonatology for the clinician*, Norwalk, CT, 1993, Appleton & Lange.
39. Sullivan P: Cows' milk induced intestinal bleeding in infancy, *Arch Dis Infancy* 68:240–244, 1993.

40. Swischuk B: Acute-onset vomiting in a 15-day-old infant, *Pediatr Emerg Care* 8(6):359–360, 1992.

41. Vaughan VC, Litt IF: Growth and development. In Behrman RE, ed: *Nelson textbook of pediatrics,* ed 14, Philadelphia, 1992, WB Saunders.

42. Vogt HB: Rhinitis. In Bluestone CD, Stool WE, Scheetz MD, eds: *Pediatric otolaryngology,* Philadelphia, 1990, WB Saunders.

43. Walker-Smith J, Ford R, Phillips A: The spectrum of gastrointestinal allergies to food, *Ann Allergy* 53: 629–636, 1984.

44. Wong DL: *Whaley & Wong's essentials of pediatric nursing,* ed 5, St Louis, 1997, Mosby.

CHAPTER 29

Pain Assessment and Management

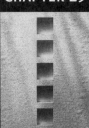

Lisa Marie Bernardo, Alice E. Conway

Pain is a common phenomenon confronted by emergency care professionals who treat ill and injured children. In the emergency department the routine assessment of pain can assist in identifying the severity of an illness or injury and in making the diagnosis. When the presence of pain is identified, pharmacologic and nonpharmacologic measures are initiated to minimize or alleviate the pain. After these interventions, evaluation is required to determine the treatment's effectiveness. This process guarantees the child's right to receive adequate pain control.

DEFINITION

The International Association for the Study of Pain (IASP) defines pain as "an unpleasant sensory and emotional experience associated with actual or potential tissue damage, or described in terms of such damage."[46] Most patients, unless severely ill or injured, are able to verbalize or describe the presence of pain, which is a subjective, personal experience. Infants, however, are unable to use language to describe pain; therefore the assessment of pain must rely on a suspicion of pain, and the presence of abnormal behavioral and physiologic parameters that might indicate pain. In infants, pain is defined as any perceived nociceptive (painful) input into the nervous system.[35]

PHYSIOLOGY OF PAIN

Nociception refers to the three types of noxious stimuli that excite pain receptors, including thermal, chemical, or mechanical energy. Any of these stimuli can impinge on the specialized nerve endings of A-delta and C-polymodal fibers, which carry the pain message.[35] Receptors preferentially sensitive to a noxious stimulus are called nociceptors. Prostaglandins at nociceptor sites sensitize nerve endings to perceive a nonpainful stimulus as painful.[36] Nociception, or nociceptor activity, is the initiating event in the perception of pain.[56]

TRANSMISSION OF PAIN

The perception of pain begins in the peripheral nervous system nociceptors, or pain receptors. The pain stimulus travels along two types of pain receptors: the A-delta fibers and the C-polymodal fibers. The A-delta fibers are myelinated, of small diameter, and mainly transmit mechanical and thermal pain. Because they are myelinated, the A-delta fibers transmit the painful stimulus quickly to the cortex, producing acute pain. The C-fibers are larger and unmyelinated. They transmit stimuli more slowly than the A-delta fibers, producing pain often characterized as an "ache," and account for the majority of chronic pain after an injury. The C-polymodal fibers respond to various stimuli, such as heat, pressure, chemicals, and inflammation[77] (Fig. 29-1).

Various chemical mediators affect impulse transmission and inhibition. Substance P is a neuropeptide that acts as a neurotransmitter in both the spinal cord and the periphery. It is slow to build up at the nerve site and does not dissipate immediately after the painful stimulus. This may account for the slow, chronic pain sometimes felt after the painful stimulus is removed.[26] Some pain mediators, including bradykinins, gamma-aminobutyric acid (GABA), endorphins, and norepinephrine, enhance the transmission of pain impulses at both the tissue and the central nervous system (CNS) levels,[76] thus increasing the child's pain. Endogenous opioids and serotonin modulate the transmission of painful stimuli, decreasing the experience of pain.

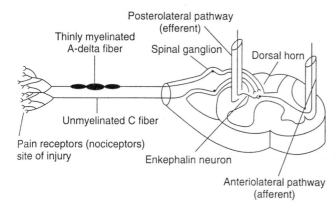

FIG. 29-1. Transduction, transmission, and modulation of pain. (From Betz C, Sowden L: *Mosby's pediatric nursing reference,* ed, 3, St Louis, 1996, Mosby.)

GATE THEORY

The gate control theory of pain proposed by Wall and Melzack[76] offers an explanatory and integrative theory about pain. In this theory a "gate" exists within the spinal cord. While this gate has not been identified anatomically, it accounts for the modification of ascending impulses by descending impulses. At the gate, both impulses are processed. If the ascending impulses are stronger than the descending ones, the gate opens, the impulse ascends to the brain, and pain is perceived. If descending impulses modulate the ascending ones, the gate remains closed and the effect is a decreased pain experience.[76]

PHYSIOLOGIC EFFECTS OF LONG-TERM AND SHORT-TERM PAIN

There are both short-term and long-term effects associated with pain. The short-term effects of acute pain include physiologic, hormonal, and metabolic changes. Pain stimulates the sympathetic nervous system, inducing increases in heart rate, blood pressure, respiratory rate, and muscle tension, as well as flushing, diaphoresis, palmar sweating, dilated pupils, and pallor. Hyperglycemia and decreased transcutaneous oxygen levels can also occur. If pain is repetitive or persists over time, sympathetic activation cannot be maintained, and physiologic parameters return to earlier levels. Consequently, physical signs of pain may decrease without a concomitant decrease in pain intensity.

The long-term effects of pain are well-known. School-aged children who experience chronic pain may gradually withdraw from their school and sports activities, leading to isolation and frustration.[42] Children with chronic pain do not sleep well, causing them to tire more easily, be more listless, and lose their ability to concentrate.[42] Thus persistent and/or unresolved pain experiences impact a child's ability to learn and interact socially and affect the child's perception of people and the world. In the neonate, painful experiences may have a permanent effect on neuronal architecture and memory (i.e., memory not accessible to conscious recall).[66]

PSYCHOSOCIAL ASPECTS OF PEDIATRIC PAIN

Pain is a multifaceted experience involving situational, behavioral, and emotional factors[39] (Fig. 29-2). It is mediated by the child's age and developmental level, health condition, emotional and cognitive states, personal concerns, family issues and attitudes, culture, and environment.[1] The child's pain may be affected by prior experiences with pain, advanced preparation for procedures, birth order, and gender.[19] Any of these variables can intervene to alter the experience of pain. For example, when a child is fearful and anxious, the pain experience may be more intense, particularly when the child hears other children (or adults) screaming or crying.[43] The presence of these variables helps to explain why some children respond to pain by lying very still and quiet while others are more vocal and active.

Behavioral expressions of pain are categorized as vocalizations, verbalizations, facial expressions, motor responses, and activity level[1] (Box 29-1). Verbal children are able to describe the unpleasantness and sensory attributes of pain, including its intensity, quality, location, and duration.[39-41] They are able to judge their current pain against pain they have already

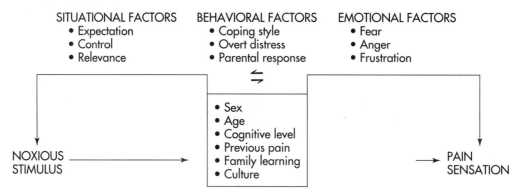

FIG. 29-2. McGrath's model of factors that affect pain. (From McGrath PA: Evaluating a child's pain, *J Pain Symptom Management* 4[4]:198-214, 1989.)

Box 29-1   Developmental Characteristics of Children's Responses to Pain

Young infants

Generalized body response of rigidity or thrashing, possibly with local reflex withdrawal of stimulated area

Loud crying

Facial expression of pain (brows lowered and drawn together, eyes tightly closed, mouth open and squarish)

Demonstrates no association between approaching stimulants and subsequent pain

Older infants

Localized body response with deliberate withdrawal of stimulated area

Loud crying

Facial expression of pain and/or anger (same facial characteristics as pain, but eyes may be open)

Physical resistance, especially pushing the stimulus away after it is applied

Young children

Loud crying, screaming

Verbal expressions of "Ow," "Ouch," or "It hurts"

Thrashing of arms and legs

Attempts to push stimulus away *before* it is applied

Uncooperative; needs physical restraint

Young children—cont'd

Requests termination of procedure

Clings to parent, nurse, or other significant person

Requests emotional support, such as hugs or other forms of physical comfort

May become restless and irritable with continuing pain

All these behaviors may be seen in anticipation of actual painful procedure

School-aged children

May see all behaviors of young child, especially *during* painful procedure but less in anticipatory period

Stalling behavior, such as "Wait a minute" or "I'm not ready"

Muscular rigidity, such as clenched fists, white knuckles, gritted teeth, contracted limbs, body stiffness, closed eyes, wrinkled forehead

Adolescents

Less vocal protest

Less motor activity

More verbal expressions, such as "It hurts" or "You're hurting me"

Increased muscle tension and body control

Data from Craig KD et al: Developmental changes in infant pain expression during immunization injections, *Soc Sci Med* 19(12):1331-1337, 1984; and Katz E. Kellerman J, Siegel S: Behavioral distress in children with cancer undergoing medical procedures: developmental considerations, *J Consult Clin Psychol* 48(3):356-365, 1980.

experienced and develop a vocabulary to describe pain, just as they develop a vocabulary to describe colors, shapes, and tastes.[39,40]

Nonverbal children, such as infants and young toddlers, are not able to provide a subjective report of pain. Consequently, the nurse must rely on behavioral responses, changes in physiologic parameters, parent report, and professional judgment. Even with this comprehensive assessment, it is sometimes impossible to differentiate pain from fear and anxiety. When a nurse suspects pain in the child, he or she should assess whether the child's injuries or illness would cause pain in someone else. If the answer is "yes," pain interventions should be initiated.

Children use strategies to help them cope with pain that vary with the child's age, developmental level, and previous pain experiences (Box 29-2).

| Box 29-2 | Coping Strategies Used by Infants, Children, and Adolescents |

Infants
Oral stimulation (sucking on hands, fingers, pacifier)
Crying
Lying in fetal position (promotes self-organization)

Toddlers
Oral stimulation
Hair twirling
Closing eyes/sleeping
Crying

Preschoolers
Rocking
Closing eyes/sleeping
Lying very still *or* being active

School-aged children
Being active *or* lying very still
Verbalizing one's pain
Telling jokes/watching television/playing video games
Sleeping

Adolescents
Verbalizing one's pain
Self-medication
Sleeping
Lying still

Asking the parent (or child) what helped the child deal with pain in the past may trigger inherent coping strategies. If these strategies are insufficient in the present situation, the nurse may try additional strategies to help the child cope.

INFLUENCES ON PEDIATRIC PAIN MANAGEMENT PRACTICES

Several factors influence the health care professional's ability to recognize and treat pain in children. Three of these factors are myths about pain, the use of placebos, and the prevention and anticipation of pain.

MYTHS ABOUT PAIN IN CHILDREN

A major myth among health care professionals is that infants do not experience pain because of neurologic immaturity.[14,15,19,61] It was erroneously believed that complete myelinization of the nerves is necessary for pain impulses to be transmitted. What is now suspected is that during the second trimester of gestation, the fetus has the anatomic and neurochemical abilities to experience discomfort.[6,14,22] Furthermore, complete myelinization is not necessary for pain impulses to be transmitted.[68]

Another facet to this myth is that infants and young children cannot verbalize or describe pain.[19] Therefore treatment for pain is withheld until a thorough examination distinctly identifies the presence of pain. While infants and young children cannot verbalize their pain, behaviors and vocalizations are indicative of how they feel.

Another myth is that children have no memory of pain.[19,61] Health care professionals erroneously assume that a short but painful procedure will be quickly forgotten. Studies have documented the persistence of behavioral changes, such as facial expression, body movements, and crying, in neonates after circumcision.[49] This implies the presence of memory and disputes the belief that young children do not remember pain.[6] Memory for circumstances leading to pain may be established by age 6 months, as evidenced by crying, resisting, and struggling before procedures.[73]

The administration of narcotics to children is an area of concern among health care professionals for two main reasons. One is the fear of narcotic addiction, and the second is the fear of respiratory depression.[19,61] For these reasons, narcotics are often withheld, even when the child has a condition(s) known to cause pain. In one study, only 62% of children with fractures were medicated with narcotic analgesics and only 53% of children with fractures and at risk for associated injuries were medicated.[24]

There is no evidence to suggest that infants or children who receive narcotics in the hospital become addicts after discharge[48] or are at increased risk of developing an addictive personality as an adult.[66] Therefore narcotics should never be withheld or limited for fear of addiction. In relation to respiratory depression, while narcotics would not be administered to a child with a severe head injury or hypovolemic shock, narcotics can be safely administered to children in severe pain. When narcotics are administered in the correct dosages with concomitant monitoring, they pose no more danger than the administration of any other medication.[19] Changes in physiologic measures, such as a decreasing heart and respiratory rate, can occur after the administration of opiates, but whether these changes result from opiate use or the relief of pain is arguable.[38]

Using Placebos to Assess Pediatric Pain

Although the pain experience varies from patient to patient, placebos have been found beneficial in some limited populations. However, the use of a placebo to assess the presence of pain in a child is never justified.[47] In fact, the use of placebos for this purpose in the child is considered unethical.[51] The result is that instead of being relieved of pain, the child continues to experience pain and learns to distrust health care professionals.[58]

Prevention and Anticipation of Pain

The best approach to pain management is to prevent the development of pain. Once pain is experienced, the routine administration of analgesics is recommended, rather than following an "as needed" schedule, since higher doses of analgesics may be required to alleviate pain than are needed to prevent pain.[60]

Another method of pain control is to tailor medications and administration routes to the child's needs. What works for some children may not work for others. For example, the intravenous (IV) route provides quick, effective pain relief for severe pain, while long-acting oral narcotics may be appropriate for prolonged pain.[60]

An often overlooked area of pain control in children is that of preparing them for painful procedures. Children of all ages will learn to mistrust health care

professionals if they are told a known painful procedure will be pain-free—or if they are given no preparation. The most effective approach is to (1) establish a relationship with the parents and the child; (2) use age-appropriate words and descriptions of the procedure; (3) assist the child during the procedure; and (4) comfort the child after the procedure.

The Nursing Process in Pain Management

The assessment of pain in infants, children, and adolescents involves a five-step process (Box 29-3). By following this process the emergency nurse can accurately determine the presence and degree of pain in the

---

Box 29-3   The Five-Step Process for Pain Assessment

1. Ask the child if he or she has pain.
   Use age-appropriate words (e.g., hurt).
   Consider cultural differences.
2. Administer a self-report measure to evaluate pain intensity.
   Keep pain rating scales readily available.
   If the child does not respond to one scale, try another one.
   Accept, and do not judge, the child's response.
3. Observe the child's behavior.
   Evaluate the child's verbalizations, vocalizations, body movements, facial expressions, and activity level.
   Determine if fear or anxiety is also present, which may also cause these behaviors.
4. Evaluate the child's physiologic measures (i.e., blood pressure, heart rate, respiratory rate).
   Record vital signs.
5. Ask the parent if he or she thinks the child has pain.
   Determine the parent's perception of the child's behaviors.
   Respect the parent's interpretation of the child's behavior and situation.
   Listen to the parent's suggestions on how to help relieve the child's pain.

child. When in doubt, child life specialists, pediatric or pain clinical nurse specialists, and other health care professionals can assist with the pain assessment (see the discussion of preparing children for painful treatments/procedures).

Step 1—Ask the Child

The first step in assessing pain is to ask the verbal child if he or she is experiencing pain. This step is sometimes overlooked because the nurse may believe the child does not understand what pain is or what pain means. Some nurses feel that asking about the presence of pain will lead a child to think that he or she should have pain. Yet if the nurse suspects pain, based on knowledge of the child's medical or nursing diagnoses and/or observation of the child's response to examinations and treatment, asking about the presence of pain only confirms what the nurse already suspects.

When asking the child if pain is present, a direct statement such as "Do you have pain?" can be used. Children under the age of 6 years, however, rarely know the meaning of the word *pain*.[19] Therefore it is necessary to identify words the child uses for pain, such as "hurt," "owie," or "boo-boo." Asking the child how he or she feels is another way to evaluate the presence of pain. Children can be very descriptive and may use words such as *burning, aching,* or *worst hurt I ever had*. It is also helpful to ask the child what he or she thinks is the cause of the pain, since young children may believe the pain is caused by an imagined misdeed or wrongdoing.[43]

The special needs child. Children with special needs, such as those with developmental delay, mental retardation, learning disabilities, or emotional disturbances, may require assistance when communicating the presence of pain. For example, the child with a hearing impairment may use a paper and pencil, a teletype writer, or sign language to communicate. The developmentally delayed or mentally retarded child may require the assistance of the parent or guardian—who recognizes emotional and behavioral signs of pain in the child—to communicate the presence of pain.

Pain denial. Occasionally children choose to deny pain, usually because of fear of receiving injections, fear of narcotic addiction, or avoidance of imagined undesirable events.[38] Young children who are fearful or in severe pain may deny pain because they are unable to recognize the relationship between the presence of pain and pain relief measures.[1] Denial of existing pain should be suspected when there is tissue damage (e.g., burns) that generally causes pain, when the child exhibits behavior or physiologic responses indicative of pain, or when the child moans.[38] Another situation where pain may be present but not expressed by the child is child maltreatment (physical or sexual).

Step 2—Administer a Self-report Measure

Self-report measures allow the child to describe the location or intensity of pain. The location of pain is assessed by pointing to the body location where the pain is experienced or by coloring or marking the location on a body outline drawing. The intensity of pain is measured by using a pain rating scale that assists in determining and tracking the intensity of pain as well as in evaluating the effectiveness of pain relief interventions.[38] Parents can be taught how to use these scales at home to continue to measure and subsequently treat the child's pain.

In children 4 years of age and older, effective self-report measures include the Oucher scale, the Poker Chip Tool, and the FACES Scale (Table 29-1). Older children, who understand the concepts of order and numbers (over the age of 6 to 7 years), can use the numeric rating scales, visual analog scales, and horizontal word-graphic rating scales.[60]

When pain is scored by the child, the emergency department nurse should not judge the child's score ("It doesn't really hurt that bad, does it?") because the child will tend to agree with the nurse.[11] In addition, the timing of the pain measurement and the interpretation of the results are important. Fear; anxiety; the need to void, vomit, or defecate; or the need for repositioning may all affect the child's perception and rating of pain.[11]

Some children are unwilling or unable to use a self-report measure. In these cases the parent or nurse can estimate the ratings. This proxy report must be used with caution, however, because only an estimate of the child's pain can be made based on deviations from normal behavior.

Step 3—Observe the Child's Behavior

Observations of behavior are the primary means of assessing the presence of pain in nonverbal children, but they can also be used to assess pain in verbal children.[1] Such observations can help the nurse to

TABLE 29-1	Pain Rating Scales for Children	

PAIN SCALE/ DESCRIPTION	INSTRUCTIONS	RECOMMENDED AGE
FACES Pain Rating Scale* (Nix, Clutter, and Wong, 1994; Wong and Baker, 1988): Consists of six cartoon faces ranging from smiling face for "no pain" to tearful face for "worst pain"	Explain to child that each face is for a person who feels happy because there is no pain (hurt) or sad because there is some or a lot of pain. Face 0 is very happy because there is no hurt. Face 1 hurts just a little bit. Face 2 hurts a little more. Face 3 hurts even more. Face 4 hurts a whole lot, but Face 5 hurts as much as you can imagine, although you don't have to be crying to feel this bad. Ask child to choose face that best describes own pain. Record the number under chosen face on pain assessment record.	Children as young as 3 years

    0   1   2   3   4   5

Oucher† (Beyer, 1989): Consists of six photographs of child's face representing "no hurt" to "biggest hurt you could ever have"; also includes a vertical scale with numbers from 0 to 100; scales for African-American and Hispanic children have been developed (Villarruel and Denyes, 1991) and validated (Beyer, Denyes, and Villarruel, 1992)	*Photographs:* Explain to child that face at bottom has "no hurt"; second picture, "just a little bit of hurt"; third picture, a "little bit more"; fourth picture, "even more hurt"; fifth picture, "pretty much hurt"; and last picture, "biggest hurt you could ever have." Ask child to choose face that best describes own pain. *Numbers:* Explain to child that 0 means you have "no hurt"; 0 to 29, "little hurts"; 30 to 69, "middle hurts"; 70 to 99, "big hurts"; and 100, "biggest hurt you could ever have." Ask child to choose any number between 0 and 100, not just numbers pictured on Oucher, that best describes own pain.	Children 3 to 13 years; use numeric scale if child can count to 100 by ones and identify larger of any two numbers (as in original instructions), or by 10s (Jordan-Marsh and others, 1994); otherwise use photographic scale

*Several variations of faces scales exist. Complimentary copies of Wong/Baker FACES Scale are available from Purdue Frederick Co., 100 Connecticut Ave., Norwalk, CT 06856; (203) 853-0123, ext. 4010.
†Oucher is available for a fee from Judith E. Beyer, PhD, RN, P.O. Box 47004, Aurora, CO 80047-0004.

TABLE 29-1	Pain Rating Scales for Children—cont'd	
PAIN SCALE/ DESCRIPTION	**INSTRUCTIONS**	**RECOMMENDED AGE**
Numeric Scale: Uses straight line with end points identified as "no pain" and "worst pain"; divisions along line are marked in units from 0 to 10 (high number may vary)	Explain to child that at one end of the line is a 0, which means that a person feels no pain (hurt). At the other end is a 10, which means the person feels the worst pain imaginable. The numbers 1 to 9 are for a very little pain to a whole lot of pain. Ask child to choose number that best describes own pain.	Children as young as 5 years, provided they can count and have some concept of numbers and their values of more or less

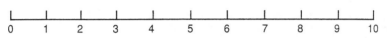

No pain .... Worst pain

0 1 2 3 4 5 6 7 8 9 10

Poker chip tool‡: Uses four red poker chips placed horizontally in front of child	Tell child, "These are pieces of hurt." Beginning at the chip nearest child's left side and ending at the one nearest child's right side, point to chips and say, "This [the first chip] is a little bit of hurt and this [the fourth chip] is the most hurt you could ever have." For a young child or for any child who does not comprehend the instructions, clarify by saying, "That means this [the first chip] is just a little hurt; this [the second chip] is a little more hurt; this [the third chip] is more hurt; and this [the fourth chip] is the most hurt you could ever have." Ask child, "How many pieces of hurt do you have right now?" Children without pain will say they don't have any. Clarify child's answer by words such as "Oh, you have a little hurt? Tell me about the hurt." Elicit descriptors, location, and cause. Ask the child, "What would you like me to do for you?" Record number of chips selected. *Spanish Instructions:* Follow English instructions, substituting the following words. Tell parent, if present: "Estas fichas son una manera de medir dolor. Usamos cuatro fichas." Say to child, "Estas son pedazos de dolor: una es un poquito de dolor y cuatro son el dolor maximo que tu puedes sentir. Cuantos pedazos de dolor tienes?"	Children as young as 4 to 4½ years, provided they can count and have some concept of numbers

‡Instructions for Poker Chip Tool and Word Graphic Rating Scale from Acute Pain Management Guideline Panel: *Acute pain management in infants, children, and adolescents: operative and medical procedures; quick reference guide for clinicians,* AHCPR Pub No 92-0020, Rockville, MD, 1992. Agency for Health Care Policy and Research, Public Health Service, US Department of Health and Human Services. Poker Chip Tool developed in 1975 by Nancy O. Hester, University of Colorado Health Sciences Center, Denver, CO. Spanish instructions from Jordan-Marsh M et al: *The Harbor-UCLA Medical Center Humor Project for Children,* Los Angeles, 1990, Harbor-UCLA Medical Center.

Continued.

TABLE 29-1 Pain Rating Scales for Children—cont'd

PAIN SCALE/ DESCRIPTION	INSTRUCTIONS	RECOMMENDED AGE
Word Graphic Rating Scale§ (Tesler, 1991): Uses descriptive words (may vary in other scales) to denote varying intensities of pain	Explain to child, "This is a line with words to describe how much pain you may have. This side of the line means no pain and over here the line means worst possible pain." (Point with your finger where "no pain" is, and run your finger along the line to "worst possible pain," as you say it.) "If you have no pain, you would mark like this." (Show example.) "If you have some pain, you would mark somewhere along the line, depending on how much pain you have." (Show example.) "The more pain you have, the closer to worst pain you would mark. The worst pain possible is marked like this." (Show example.) "Show me how much pain you have right now by marking with a straight, up-and-down line anywhere along the line to show how much pain you have right now." With a millimeter ruler, measure from the "no pain" end to the mark and record this measurement as the pain score.	Children as young as 5 years, although words may need explanation; words shown below were used with children ages 8 to 17 years

No pain	Little pain	Medium pain	Large pain	Worst possible pain

PAIN SCALE/ DESCRIPTION	INSTRUCTIONS	RECOMMENDED AGE
Visual Analogue Scale: Uses 10 cm horizontal line with end points marked "no pain" and "worst pain"	Ask child to place a mark on line that best describes amount of own pain. With a centimeter ruler, measure from the "no pain" end to the mark and record this measurement as the pain score.	Children as young as 4½ years; vertical or horizontal scale may be used (Walco and Ilowite, 1991)
Color Tool (Eland, 1993): Uses markers for child to construct own scale that is used with body outline	Present eight markers to child in a random order. Ask child, "Of these colors, which color is like . . . ?" (the event identified by the child as having hurt the most). Place the marker away from other markers. (Represents severe pain.) Ask child, "Which color is like a hurt, but not quite as much as . . .? (the event identified by the child as having hurt the most). Place the marker with the marker chosen to represent severe pain. Ask child, "Which color is like something that hurts just a little?" Place the marker with the other colors. Ask child, "Which color is like no hurt at all?" Show the four marker choices to child in order from the worst to the no-hurt color. Ask child to show on the body outlines where they hurt, using the markers they have chosen. After child has colored the hurts, ask if there are current hurts or hurts from the past. Ask if child knows why the area hurts if it is not clear to you why it does.	Children as young as 4 years, provided they know their colors, are not color blind, and are able to construct the scale if in pain

§Word Graphic Rating Scale is part of the Adolescent Pediatric Pain Tool and is available for a fee from Pediatric Pain Study, University of California, School of Nursing, Department of Family Health Care Nursing, San Francisco, CA 94143-0606; (415) 476-4040.
From Wong DL: *Whaley & Wong's Nursing care of infants and children*, ed 5, 1995, Mosby.

determine the presence of pain (see the discussion of psychosocial aspects of pediatric pain).

STEP 4—EVALUATE PHYSIOLOGIC MEASURES

The physiologic measures most often used to assess pain are heart rate, respiratory rate, blood pressure, and the presence of perspiration; all of these tend to increase in the presence of pain or anxiety. The use of these variables alone to identify pain is limited in the conscious child, since they are not specific for pain.[1] For example, the anxious or frightened child also experiences increased heart rate, respiratory rate, and blood pressure. Physiologic measures are useful in children who are chemically paralyzed and sedated.

STEP 5—ASK THE PARENT

If a parent or guardian is present, it is helpful to ask if he or she believes the child is in pain. Asking the parent, "Does your child have pain? How do you know?" will include the parent in the child's care and assist the emergency department nurse in validating the presence of pain. Often the parent is able to suggest interventions that help relieve a child's pain.

PHARMACOLOGIC INTERVENTIONS FOR PAIN RELIEF

Two types of pharmacologic agents are used to minimize or alleviate pain: analgesics and anesthetics. *Analgesics* reduce pain selectively without producing a loss of consciousness by (1) modulating the transmission of nociceptive signals to the brain (narcotics) or (2) inhibiting the metabolism of pain-producing substances in body tissues.[40] Analgesics used in the emergency department should ideally have a rapid onset and a short duration of effect. They should be easy to administer, provide effective analgesia, and have minimal side effects.[63]

Anesthetics reduce pain by removing all normal sensation, especially sensitivity to pain. A state of anesthesia may be produced by using an anesthetic substance, or through hypnotic suggestion. Anesthetic substances are classified as topical, local, regional, or general.

NONNARCOTIC ANALGESICS

Nonnarcotic analgesics include acetaminophen, aspirin and other salicylates, and nonsteroidal antiinflammatory drugs (NSAIDs)[32] (Table 29-2). Aspirin/salicylates and NSAIDs have analgesic, antipyretic, antiplatelet, and antiinflammatory actions.[32] In particular, aspirin and NSAIDs act on peripheral nerve endings at an injured site, producing analgesia by altering prostaglandin synthesis.[34] Prostaglandins may sensitize nociceptors to histamine and bradykinin, which are present in inflammation and lead to pain. When prostaglandin release is inhibited, it is believed that nerves are desensitized and the pain is reduced.

Acetaminophen. Acetaminophen is the most commonly administered analgesic and is as effective as aspirin with respect to analgesic and antipyretic properties.[32] It does not, however, have antiinflammatory properties.[34] Acetaminophen is metabolized in the liver and eliminated through the kidneys, with peak blood levels obtained 30 to 60 minutes after administration.[40] It can be given alone to children in mild to moderate pain or given with a narcotic to children in moderate pain. The usual dosage for acetaminophen is 15 mg/kg every 4 hours.[64] Preparations include drops, elixirs, suspensions, tablets, caplets, and suppositories. The child's familiarity with acetaminophen, such as its color and taste, may help with gaining his or her cooperation during its administration.

Salicylates. Aspirin was once the most commonly administered analgesic in children. Its use, however, has declined since its association with Reye's syndrome after viral illnesses, such as varicella. Salicylates are hydrolyzed to salicylic acid and metabolized primarily by the liver. They are ultimately excreted by the kidneys.[32] Aspirin can be administered for pain related to headache, myalgia, arthralgia, and sunburn. In sustained high doses, aspirin has an antiinflammatory effect that produces analgesia.[63,65]

Gastric irritation is a common side effect; therefore buffered or enteric-coated preparations are sometimes used. Offering food or milk, and encouraging fluid intake may also reduce the gastrointestinal symptoms. The analgesic dose of salicylates is 10 to 15 mg/kg/dose administered orally or rectally every 4 to 6 hours.[64]

Nonsteroidal antiinflammatory drugs. NSAIDs, such as ibuprofen, have more potent analgesic and antiinflammatory properties than aspirin or acetaminophen.[69] They are most often used for pain

TABLE 29-2	Nonnarcotic Analgesics			
MEDICATION	DOSE	ROUTE*	INDICATIONS	SIDE EFFECTS
Acetaminophen	15 mg/kg q4h	PO/PR	Mild to moderate pain (e.g., earache)	Uncommon; overdoses can cause renal and hepatic injury
Salicylates	10-15 mg/kg q4-6h	PO/PR	Mild pain; antiinflammatory (e.g., arthritis)	Gastric irritation; platelet dysfunction; exacerbation of asthma
NSAIDs (ibuprofen)	10 mg/kg q6h	PO	Mild pain (e.g., sprain/strain)	Gastric irritation; abdominal pain; inhibition of platelet functioning; renal and hepatic dysfunction

*PO, Orally; PR, rectally.

related to musculoskeletal, inflammatory, and rheumatoid conditions, as well as for dysmenorrhea, dental pain, and back pain.[32,36,63] NSAIDs are metabolized by the liver, excreted by the kidneys, and have a relatively slow onset of action. Common side effects include nausea, vomiting, or abdominal pain. The dose is 8 to 10 mg/kg every 6 hours administered orally.[64]

Ketorolac (Toradol) is a NSAID that can be administered orally or parenterally. It is approved for intramuscular (IM) use in children over 12 years of age weighing more than 50 kg who are in moderate to severe pain.[66] IV administration and use in infants and young children has not yet been approved.[66]

NARCOTIC ANALGESICS

Narcotics or opiates are used primarily in the treatment of acute, severe pain (e.g., fracture) and chronic pain during an acute episode (e.g., sickle cell crisis) (Table 29-3). Opioids are synthetic, such as meperidine or fentanyl, or naturally occurring, such as morphine and codeine.

It is believed that opiates mimic endogenous opiate peptides (called enkephalins) by binding to opioid receptors in the brain, brainstem, and spinal cord.[33] Narcotics therefore do not affect the painful stimulus, but instead alter a child's perception and interpretation of pain.[34]

Respiratory depression (caused by effects on the pontine and medullary centers) is the side effect of narcotics of most concern when administered to children. However, respiratory depression is usually dose related and readily reversed with naloxone. Healthy infants over the age of 3 months are no more sensitive to respiratory depression from opiate administration than are adults who achieve the same drug plasma levels.[77] Children at risk of respiratory depression include infants less than 3 months of age, particularly those who have a preexisting respiratory disorder or airway compromise, or children who have neurologic problems, such as increased intracranial pressure (ICP).[77] Because narcotics can mask worsening of a child's condition, they should be used with caution in children with substantial head, chest, or abdominal trauma and in children with significant CNS, cardiorespiratory, or abdominal disease or injury.[65]

Additional side effects include hypotension (due to local and CNS effects); urinary retention (due to smooth muscle contraction in the urinary tract); constipation; confusion; and dizziness.[34,63] Also, most children arriving in the emergency department have not fasted before narcotic administration; therefore the risk of emesis and aspiration is increased.

Emergency department nurses administering narcotic analgesics to children should understand the benefits and risks of their use and, if they are uncertain of a drug or dosage, should ask another nurse to double-check the medication. After administration of the drug the child is attached to a cardiorespiratory monitor and/or pulse oximeter. Narcotics should never be withheld from children in severe pain for fear of respiratory depression.

Routes of narcotic administration. Narcotics can be administered orally, nasally, sublingually, rec-

TABLE 29-3	Narcotic Analgesics			
MEDICATION	**DOSE**	**ROUTE***	**INDICATIONS**	**SIDE EFFECTS**
Morphine	0.1 to 0.2 mg/kg/ dose over 5 to 10 minutes (max dose 10 mg)	IV	Severe pain (burns)	Hypotension; respiratory depression
Fentanyl	0.5 to 3 µg/kg over 3 to 5 minutes 10 to 15 ug/kg	IV, IM, SL PO	Severe pain; treatment pain (closed reduction)	Respiratory depression; chest wall rigidity; apnea; bradycardia
Meperidine	1 to 2 mg/kg (max dose 100 mg)	IV, IM, PO, PR	Severe pain	Tachycardia; nervousness; tremors; disorientation; seizures
Codeine (usually administered with acetaminophen or NSAIDs)	0.5 to 1 mg/kg	PO	Moderate pain (minor burns)	Nausea, vomiting, constipation

*IV, Intravenous; IM, intramuscular; PO, oral; PR, rectal; SL, sublingual.

tally, intramuscularly, or intravenously. The *oral route* is preferred because it is noninvasive and many children will cooperate with administration. Orally administered narcotics may be mixed with a small amount of gelatin or taken with a drink of juice. The *sublingual route* can also be effective with medications such as fentanyl.

The *nasal route* is another popular route. Medications are absorbed more reliably through the nasal mucosa as compared to the oral route,[59] and the risk of gastric discomfort is eliminated. Another route gaining popularity is the *rectal route,* where a drug is injected into the rectum via a small feeding tube or a lubricated 1 ml syringe. This method is preferred in infants and toddlers who refuse oral medications.

The *intramuscular route* for narcotic administration may also be used in children. Intramuscular injections are painful, however, and the child equates the "shot" with pain, even if the medication is a narcotic.

For parenteral drug administration the *intravenous route* is preferred. It affords the most reliable and most controllable method for narcotic administration.[59]

Morphine. Morphine is the standard by which all other analgesics are compared and is the most extensively studied opiate in the pediatric population.[33] It is useful for children with fractures, burns, penetrating trauma, or sickle cell crisis.[63]

The dose of morphine is titrated until the desired analgesia is achieved, usually 0.1 to 0.2 mg/kg/dose IV, infused over 5 to 10 minutes (maximum dose is 10 mg).[63] The dose may be repeated every 3 to 4 hours.[63] A higher dose with a more frequent dosing schedule may be used in the child who does not achieve adequate pain relief or in children experiencing pain from chronic diseases, such as sickle cell disease or cancer.

Morphine has a histamine-releasing effect that can produce peripheral vasodilation and venous pooling.[33] When administered with a sedative, such as diazepam (or midazolam), or to a volume-depleted child, significant hypotension may result.[33] Although hypotension is an unwanted side effect, morphine should not be withheld from the injured child in severe pain who is awake, alert, and oriented; has stable vital signs; and has an IV line in place.[63]

Fentanyl. Fentanyl is 50 to 100 times more potent than morphine.[2] It is commonly used in the emergency department as an analgesic to relieve pain from injury, as well as to relieve pain during procedures such as closed reduction of fractures, extensive suturing, burn care, or wound cleaning.

Because histamine release is less than occurs with morphine administration, the risk of vasodilation producing hypotension is reduced.[33] Fentanyl is therefore the drug of choice for victims of trauma.[69] Side effects of fentanyl include respiratory depression, apnea, and bradycardia.

Fentanyl can be administered orally through lollipops, nasally, sublingually, or intravenously. When administered parenterally, it is rapid acting; however, its opiate effects quickly subside approximately 30 to 45 minutes after administration. The side effect of respiratory depression may last considerably longer.[13] Recommended IV doses range from 0.5 to 3 µg/kg.[13,65] To avoid respiratory depression the dose should be titrated in incremental doses until the desired anesthesia is achieved. Because fentanyl is rapid acting and because rapid administration can produce chest wall rigidity, fentanyl should be administered slowly over 3 to 5 minutes and the child continuously monitored for signs of respiratory depression[2,65] (see the discussion of conscious sedation, p. 699).

Meperidine. Meperidine is commonly administered for analgesia and is useful for procedures lasting longer than 30 minutes.[13] It is generally not used for controlling chronic pain because of the accumulation of its principal metabolite normeperidine. High levels of normeperidine can lead to nervousness, tremors, disorientation, and seizures,[64] and these effects cannot be reversed by the administration of naloxone.

The recommended dosage of meperidine is 1 to 2 mg/kg administered parenterally, orally, or rectally, with a maximum dose of 100 mg. Peak values may not be achieved for 90 minutes when the drug is administered IM and 120 minutes when administered rectally; the serum half-life is 3 to 4 hours.[13,63] Tachycardia is a common side effect.

Meperidine is frequently combined with narcotic potentiating agents such as hydroxyzine or promethazine, enhancing its sedative and analgesic effects. It is occasionally used in combination with phenergan and thorazine (DPT).

DPT. In the past the "DPT or lytic cocktail," a combination of IM demerol (2 mg/kg), phenergan (1 mg/kg), and thorazine (1 mg/kg), was used for its combined analgesic/sedative effect during suturing or fracture reduction. This combination of drugs offers no benefit over the administration of newer fast-acting narcotics and is associated with significant adverse side effects.[65] Phenothiazines (phenergan and thorazine) can produce profound hypotension, lower the seizure threshold, and cause dystonic reactions.[13] When com-

bined with meperidine, profound sedation and respiratory depression may result. For these reasons the Committee on Drugs of the American Academy of Pediatrics (AAP) has discouraged the use of the DPT cocktail in children.[4]

The onset of action after the IM administration of DPT is variable (approximately 20 to 30 minutes), and the effects can be prolonged (4.7 to 15 hours).[13,69] Therefore the child who has received this combination of drugs must be continuously evaluated and monitored until "fully aroused."

KETAMINE

Ketamine produces both analgesic and amnestic effects and is useful when performing short procedures such as suturing or burn debridement. Physiologically, ketamine produces a catatonic state of dissociative analgesia by blocking impulses between the cortical and limbic systems.

There are advantages and disadvantages to its use. The advantages are that it preserves carbon dioxide (CO_2) responsiveness, protects airway reflexes, and decreases airway reactivity and bronchospasm[30] (it has been used in the treatment of severe asthma; see Chapter 10, Respiratory System, p. 216). Disadvantages include increased heart rate, increased blood pressure, increased salivation, increased myocardial oxygen consumption, increased ICP and intraocular pressure,[13,30] and the risk of laryngospasm. Additionally, it can produce emergence phenomena such as hallucinations and nightmares, particularly when used in older children.

Dosage and administration. Ketamine can be administered orally, rectally, intravenously, or intramuscularly. The dosages vary, depending on the desired degree of sedation and the route of administration. When given parenterally, the onset of action is approximately 1 to 2 minutes. Parenteral doses range from 0.5 to 4 mg/kg. Doses of up to 5 to 10 mg/kg are occasionally given; however, these higher doses produce a deeply sedated child in a state of general anesthesia.[13] When given in conjunction with atropine, the increased salivation associated with ketamine administration is decreased.

Oral and rectal doses range from 6 to 10 mg/kg, and up to 30 minutes is required for onset of action. Because the solution contains benzyl alcohol, children may find the taste unacceptable. Masking the taste with a juice of choice may assist in gaining the child's cooperation.[72]

Emergency Department and nursing interventions. Ketamine produces a state of catatonic analgesia. This means the child's eyes will be open, yet there will be no response to verbal or painful stimulus. The child may exhibit random, purposeful movements. Parents observing the child in this state may become upset or frightened. Therefore they should be prepared for their child's reactions before ketamine is administered.

Because of the possibility of emergence phenomenon, lights should be kept dim (except for the procedure light) and noise at a minimum both during and after the procedure.

Nursing interventions for the child receiving ketamine are the same as those required for the child undergoing conscious sedation, although the insertion of an IV line is at the discretion of the treating physician.

CONSCIOUS SEDATION

Conscious sedation, as opposed to deep or unconscious sedation, is used when a child requires a short but relatively painful procedure such as a closed reduction of a fracture, extensive suturing of the face, burn debridement, wound care, or a dental procedure. It involves the use of a combination of sedatives (e.g., midazolam) and analgesics (e.g., fentanyl). Conscious sedation is defined as follows:

A medically controlled state of depressed consciousness that (1) allows protective reflexes to be maintained; (2) retains the patient's ability to maintain a patent airway independently and continuously; and (3) permits appropriate response by the patient to physical stimulation or verbal command, eg, "open your eyes.".[3]

Guidelines for the use of conscious sedation in the emergency department were established by the AAP.[3] Similarly, the American College of Emergency Physicians[5] has produced a policy statement regarding sedation and analgesia in children. Both groups mandate the attendance of a physician skilled in the administration of these medications, as well as a nurse whose sole purpose is to monitor the child throughout the procedure.

The advantage of conscious sedation is that the child's pain is adequately controlled. A disadvantage is that the procedure requires several emergency personnel, such as one physician to administer the medications, one nurse to monitor the patient, and another nurse or technician to assist with the procedure. Because personnel within the emergency department may be limited, additional health care professionals

such as anesthesia personnel, pediatric intensive care unit nurses, or pain control nurses may be asked to assist.

Emergency Department and nursing interventions. Before the procedure an IV line is inserted and the child is attached to a cardiorespiratory monitor, electronic blood pressure device, and pulse oximeter. If an end-expiratory CO_2 monitor is available, it should also be used. Airway equipment is required at the bedside, including a bag-valve-mask device, oxygen, suction, and intubation equipment. The choice of drugs is based on physician preference. Some institutions require the physician to obtain informed consent from the parent or guardian before the procedure (Box 29-4).

The drugs are administered by the physician, who titrates the dosage until the desired effects of pain relief

---

Box 29-4 Nursing Interventions for the Child Undergoing Conscious Sedation

Gather equipment:
Bag-valve-mask device
Oxygen mask and tubing
Suction catheters and large tonsil suction
Laryngoscope blade and handle appropriate for age
Endotracheal tube appropriate for age
Stylet

Attach child to monitors:
Cardiorespiratory monitor
Electronic blood pressure device
Pulse oximeter
End-expiratory CO_2 monitor (optional)

Obtain informed consent (physician).

Obtain drugs:
Naloxone
Analgesic (e.g., fentanyl)
Sedative (e.g., midazolam)

Continuously monitor and document:
Heart rate
Respiratory rate
Blood pressure
Oxygen saturation levels
Neurologic status

Remain with the child until fully aroused.

Box 29-5   Recommended Discharge Criteria for Conscious Sedation

- Cardiovascular function and airway patency are satisfactory and stable.
- The child is easily arousable, and protective reflexes are intact (child is able to swallow juice or eat a popsicle).
- The child can talk (as age appropriate).
- The child can sit up unaided (as age appropriate).
- If the child is incapable of the usually expected responses (e.g., very young or handicapped), the presedation level of responsiveness, or a level as close as possible to the normal level for that child, should be achieved.
- The child's state of hydration is adequate.

From American Academy of Pediatrics: Guidelines for monitoring and management of pediatric patients during and after sedation for diagnostic and therapeutic procedures, *Pediatrics* 89:1110-1115, 1992.

---

and sedation are achieved. The child usually remains awake or drowsy and ideally should be able to talk and answer questions. During the procedure the nurse should continuously monitor and record the child's vital signs, neurologic status, and oxygen saturation levels.

After the procedure the emergency department nurse must remain with the child and continue to monitor his or her condition until the effects of the medications have worn off. Before discharge, the child should have a patent airway and satisfactory cardiovascular function. In addition, the child should be awake and alert, able to sit unsupported, and able to drink juice or eat a popsicle. The verbal child should be able to talk (Box 29-5).

PATIENT-CONTROLLED ANALGESIA

Patient-controlled analgesia (PCA) involves the administration of narcotics through a specially designed IV pump that is controlled by the child. By pushing a button, the child can release a predetermined dose of narcotic (usually morphine) as needed. Alternatively, the narcotic of choice may be administered as a continuous infusion, with bolus administration for additional analgesia controlled by the child. Overdose is prevented by a "lockout" period between boluses.

Pediatric candidates for PCA include adolescents and older school-aged children; however, children as young as 5 or 6 years of age have used PCA successfully.[25] PCA can be initiated in the emergency department in children with sickle cell crisis, cancer pain, renal colic, or pain from other chronic illnesses.

SEDATIVES

Sedatives, such as midazolam, diazepam, and chloral hydrate, may be used alone or in conjunction with analgesics. While sedatives do not inhibit the child's perception of pain, they can block sensory input.[59] Sedatives are best used in conjunction with analgesics during painful procedures; however, the risk of respiratory depression is increased (Table 29-4).

Midazolam. Midazolam, a benzodiazepine, is a popular sedative administered to children not only for its anxiolytic effects, but because it produces amnesia as well. It is often the drug of choice when brief sedation is required, since it is rapid-acting and has a shorter half-life than diazepam.[13]

Midazolam can be administered orally, sublingually, nasally, rectally, and intramuscularly. When administered intravenously, it produces less venous irritation than diazepam because it is water-soluble. The dose varies, depending on the desired degree of sedation, route of administration, and use in conjunction with analgesics. Usual doses range from 0.05 to 0.2 mg/kg IV or IM, to 0.2 to 0.4 mg/kg orally or rectally. The parenteral solution is bitter, so before administration the child is instructed to swallow all of the medication at once, rather than sipping. Midazolam can also be mixed with sweet juice to disguise the taste. If the entire dose is not taken, however, the child may refuse to drink the remaining medication. When used in combination with analgesics, the risk of respiratory depression is increased. Respiratory arrest has been reported when midazolam was used in combination with fentanyl for sedation.[79]

Chloral hydrate. Chloral hydrate is one of the most commonly used sedatives in children. It is particularly popular before radiographic imaging. When used alone, the effects on the cardiovascular and respiratory systems are minimal. Because chloral hydrate has no analgesic effects, it is occasionally administered in combination with other sedatives or narcotics. When combined with these drugs, there is an increased risk of respiratory compromise.

TABLE 29-4	Sedatives Used in the Emergency Department		
MEDICATION	**DOSE***	**INDICATIONS**	**SIDE EFFECTS**
Midazolam	IV: 0.05 to 0.15 mg/kg IM: 0.2 mg/kg PO, IN, PR: 0.3 to 0.5 mg/kg	Used alone for sedation or with morphine, fentanyl, or demerol to produce muscle relaxation, amnesia, and sedation	Respiratory depression
Chloral hydrate	PR, PO: 50 to 75 mg/kg	Sedation	Prolonged sedation and hypoventilation (at high doses)
Diazepam	IV: 0.1 to 0.2 mg/kg PO, PR: 0.3 to 0.5 mg/kg	Sedation, antegrade amnesia	Respiratory depression

*IV, Intravenously; IM, intramuscularly; PO, orally; IN, nasally; PR, rectally.

Chloral hydrate can be administered orally or rectally in doses ranging from 50 to 75 mg/kg. Both irregular absorption and underdosing (doses less than 50 mg/kg) can prompt the administration of a second dose. The onset of action is approximately 20 to 30 minutes, with the serum half-life being 4 to 12 hours.

Diazepam. Diazepam is a benzodiazepine occasionally used for sedation in the pediatric population in the emergency department. Although it is a rapid-acting drug, its relatively long half-life and an increased risk of respiratory depression make it less popular than midazolam. Diazepam can be administered intravenously (which is painful), orally, or rectally in doses ranging from 0.1 to 0.2 mg/kg IV to 0.3 to 0.5 mg/kg orally or rectally.[69] Intramuscular administration is associated with severe pain and irregular absorption and is therefore not recommended.[13]

LOCAL ANESTHETICS

TAC, LAT, and TAS. Topical anesthetics include TAC (tetracaine, adrenaline, and cocaine), LAT (lidocaine, adrenaline, and tetracaine), and TAS (bipivacaine and norepinephrine). Topical anesthetics are as effective as lidocaine for most wounds on the face and scalp, but they are less effective for wounds on the extremities or trunk.[19a,23,64] Topical anesthetics should not be used in areas of the body where vasoconstriction is contraindicated, such as the fingers, nose, penis, pinna of the ears, or toes. Deaths have occurred in two children where TAC was absorbed through the mucous membranes—one na-

sally, the other when the solution was applied directly to a child's tongue.[23]

The dose for topical anesthetics is 3 to 5 ml applied directly to the wound using a cotton-tipped applicator or gauze pad.[62] Gloves are required when handling the solution, which must be applied by the nurse and held in place for 20 to 30 minutes by the nurse or parent. Care must be taken to prevent the solution from getting in the eyes or on the mucous membranes of the nose or mouth. When anesthetized, the area around the wound will blanch. The area may be tested with a needle prick; however, the child must be kept unaware of the presence of the needle.

EMLA. EMLA is a topical anesthetic containing pilocaine and lidocaine. It is used on intact skin before painful procedures such as venipuncture, lumbar punctures, and bone marrow aspirations. Because it must be applied at least 60 minutes before the procedure, its application in the emergency setting is limited. The use of EMLA in small, open wounds is currently being investigated. EMLA is not approved for use in infants less than 1 month of age because of its potential for pilocaine-induced methemoglobin and lidocaine toxicity. It should be used judiciously in infants older than 1 month of age with restrictions on the amount, area, and duration of cream application.[66]

Lidocaine. Injected anesthetics are used most often during suturing, but they can also be used to anesthetize an IV insertion site or the lumbar area before a lumbar puncture. Lidocaine is the most commonly used local anesthetic. For local infiltration the maximum dose is 3 to 5 mg/kg.[62] Individual doses are based on the concentration used: 1% solution, 0.5 ml/kg; 2% solution, 0.25 ml/kg. A combination of lidocaine and epinephrine can be administered when a vasoconstrictive effect is desired, with the dosage up to 7 mg/kg.[62] Because of its vasoconstrictive properties, lidocaine with epinephrine is not used on lacerations of the fingers, nose, penis, toes, or ears.

Lidocaine has a rapid onset of action and provides effective local anesthesia for approximately 30 to 45 minutes. Pain during injection is common. Many methods can be used to decrease this pain. They include injecting the lidocaine slowly using a small-gauge needle; rubbing the injection site before needle insertion and infiltration; buffering the solution with bicarbonate (10 parts [1%] lidocaine to 1 part sodium bicarbonate);[64] injecting the lidocaine in devitalized tissue or anesthetized areas; and waiting until the anesthetic effect has occurred before initiating the procedure.[64,66] Warming the solution may also be effective.

Nitrous oxide.   Nitrous oxide is sometimes used in the emergency department for children undergoing dental, orthopedic, or suturing procedures. When nitrous oxide is administered in a 50:50 ratio with oxygen, the effect is one of analgesia, not anesthesia. Therefore the child is awake and able to follow instructions.[62]

Candidates for nitrous oxide administration include alert, cooperative children. Children with an altered level of consciousness, respiratory distress, chest or facial trauma, abdominal distention, and prior intake of sedatives, narcotics, or alcohol should not receive nitrous oxide.[71] Any of these conditions may affect the child's level of consciousness, breathing, and subsequent ability to protect the airway.

Other contraindications to the use of nitrous oxide include children who have eaten within 2 hours of the procedure, in whom there is the potential for vomiting and aspiration. Furthermore, nitrous oxide must be administered by a physician who is skilled in its use, resuscitation equipment must be immediately available, and "capture equipment" is required to remove expired gases. The physician and nurse must remain with the patient during its use to observe for airway or respiratory compromise. As with conscious sedation, airway equipment, cardiorespiratory monitoring, and continuous observation are required.

Nitrous oxide can be administered by allowing the child to hold the oxygen mask to his or her nose. When adequate anesthesia has been achieved, the child usually drops the mask. Approximately 5 minutes of nitrous oxide inhalation is required to produce sedation and analgesia.[71]

REGIONAL ANESTHETICS

Regional (nerve) blocks are used for pain control during procedures such as extensive suturing or exploration for a foreign body.[71] Regional block sites include the axillary brachial plexus, wrist, digits, and ankle.[71] Contraindications for nerve blocks include infection at the needle puncture site, sepsis, bleeding disorders, use of anticoagulant therapy, compartment syndrome, or lymphadenopathy at the puncture site.[16] Lidocaine is used most often for regional blocks, with the dose being 5 mg/kg.[62] When a regional block is used, resuscitation equipment must be readily available in the event of an adverse reaction to the anesthetic. (Another type of regional anesthesia is the Bier block, which is reviewed in Chapter 23, Musculoskeletal and Soft Tissue Injuries, p. 559)

NONPHARMACOLOGIC INTERVENTIONS FOR PAIN RELIEF

When applied with pharmacologic interventions and individualized to meet the child's needs, nonpharmacologic interventions can modify the child's response to painful stimuli. Some nonpharmacologic interventions designed to help children cope with pain while in the emergency department include positioning and securing the child and using imagination training (IT). IT refers to self-directed behavioral interventions that use a selective focus to achieve a sense of control and an acceptance of an imagined reality.[12a] It includes techniques such as self-hypnosis, biofeedback, and guided imagery (Table 29-5).

POSITIONING AND SECURING

Simple measures, such as the application of ice,[17] heat, splints, or proper positioning, can minimize mild pain and/or prevent the exacerbation of pain in the child. For example, the pain associated with a fracture or sprain is often decreased when the extremity is splinted and/or elevated, and when ice is applied; the pain associated with an infiltrated IV line can be relieved with the application of a warm compress.

TABLE 29-5	Nonpharmacologic Techniques for Pain Reduction	
TECHNIQUE	**BENEFIT**	**LIMITATION**
Application of ice or heat	Helps to relieve pain by decreasing edema or relieving muscle tension	Short-term until definitive treatment is given
Massage	Loosens tight muscles; promotes comfort, especially when done in a slow, soothing manner	Works best with pharmacologic agents to relieve tension
Distraction and/or involvement	Requires no special training; works best for short-term procedures or treatments	May not be useful for long-term procedures
Relaxation and/or breathing	Requires no special training; works well with older children	May be difficult to use in uncooperative patients
Imagery	Requires no special training; useful in children with vivid imaginations	May not be useful if child/parent is not willing to participate
Therapeutic touch	Decreases anxiety and pain	Requires training; may be difficult to perform in busy emergency department
Hypnosis	Can work with hypersuggestible children	Requires training; may not be successful in busy emergency department
Biofeedback	Can work if child is familiar with procedure	Requires training
Positive self-talk/thought modeling/rehearsal	Does not require training; easy to implement; can reinforce positive behaviors	Requires verbal skills; may not be useful in emergency department environment

Assisting the child in finding a comfortable position is another intervention that can decrease the pain associated with an injury, illness, or procedure. The creative use of blankets, pillows, or towel rolls may help the child gain some pain relief, as may creative positioning on the stretcher (such as the side-lying position with legs drawn up for back pain). Sometimes simply allowing the parent to rock an infant or child who has been wrapped in a warm blanket decreases the anxiety associated with an emergency department visit and the perception of pain.

DISTRACTION AND/OR INVOLVEMENT

Distraction is a technique designed to focus a child's attention away from a procedure by having the child concentrate on a particular object, singing, counting, or storytelling.[7] Objects used for distraction can be kept in a "treasure chest" filled with toys such as dolls for demonstrating techniques, soap bubbles for blowing and counting, a magic wand with colored sparkles and shapes, and a soft ball to squeeze (i.e. "Squeeze the ball as hard as you can. Open your hand. Let's count until the ball regains its shape."). Other items such as a Slinky (for repetitive motion, which is very soothing); a soft, squeaking hammer (for pounding out frustration); story books; and stickers are appropriate for children. An additional item may be a "good luck" charm that has helped other children through this procedure.

Knowing the individual interests and developmental level of the child is an important consideration when choosing an effective distraction technique. Preschool children can be readily engaged in storytelling or singing. School-aged children may enjoy riddles and counting games. Adolescents in particular may enjoy listening to their favorite music on headsets.[63] Almost all children may enjoy viewing a videotape, such as a family-oriented or cartoon movie.

Engaging the child in the treatment process is also a distraction. By asking the child to participate in the procedure ("Please hold the Band-Aid for me"), the child regains some control of the situation and focuses on the task.

Emergency department treatment rooms that are "child friendly" can readily provide distractions. Wallpaper border patterns give the child something to focus on while being held by the parent or lying on the stretcher. Mobiles, kites, and other objects hanging from the ceiling allow the child to see something other than overhead lights and give the child something to talk about ("What color is the kite?").

RELAXATION AND/OR BREATHING

Deep breathing is a distraction method used to provide progressive relaxation and involves having the child concentrate on each breath by slowly inhaling and exhaling.[37] Blowing into a kazoo or party blower, blowing on a pinwheel, or creating soap bubbles can be used to initiate a deep, relaxing breathing pattern. Later the child can take the items home as a reward. Clenching or tightening and then relaxing various muscle groups is a relaxation technique that can be used with school-aged children and adolescents.

IMAGERY

Imagery is the concentrated focusing on images formed in the mind.[27] Imagining pleasant scenes is a helpful technique to facilitate relaxation in toddlers, preschool children, and older children.[55] With this technique the child is talked through the experience or relates a pleasant scenario, such as a picnic, holiday party, or other situation of the child's choosing. By describing an imagined situation the child relaxes, focusing on something other than the procedure or treatment.[12a]

Imagery requires the nurse or parent to describe the scenario and ask the child questions related to the imagined situation (e.g., "Let's imagine ourselves at the zoo. Who would you like to go with you? Which animal do you want to see first?"). Detailed stories provide the best distractions. Occasionally the child will take over the story, and the nurse or parent need only ask specific questions to guide the dialogue (e.g., "What color was that lion at the zoo? Was he a big one?").

THERAPEUTIC TOUCH

Therapeutic touch has been used since ancient times to facilitate healing and involves the conscious process of energy exchange through the practitioner's hands.[52] Therapeutic touch has been used to reduce anxiety in hospitalized patients[57] and stress in premature neonates.[20] Anecdotal reports have documented decreased pain and increased comfort in infants, children, and families.[21] While no studies using therapeutic touch in the emergency department have been published, this technique may be helpful to children and families requiring emergency treatment.

HYPNOSIS

Hypnosis is defined as an altered state of consciousness, where the mind focuses on one specific stimulus.[8] With hypnosis the child's own coping strategies are used while a painful or uncomfortable procedure is performed. Hypnosis techniques include checking readiness, induction, deepening techniques, trance maintenance, and de-induction/posthypnotic suggestions.[8]

Hypnosis works well in children, particularly preschool and school-aged children, because it capitalizes on their ability to fantasize. Children in these age ranges are also more vulnerable to suggestion.[31,53,54,81] When used with analgesics, hypnosis can be particularly effective.

BIOFEEDBACK

Biofeedback is another relaxation technique using either visual or auditory signals and then tightening and relaxing specific muscle groups. It can be used with older children and adolescents who are experiencing repeated procedures for chronic conditions, such as children with cancer. Therefore the emergency department nurse should inquire about what coping skills these children use to cope with painful procedures. For any child to successfully perform biofeedback, prior education regarding the technique and practice is required.

POSITIVE SELF-TALK AND THOUGHT STOPPING

Positive self-talk ("I can do it"), along with thought stopping, has been used for children undergoing repeated procedures.[82] Thought stopping consists of having the child say "stop" whenever he or she starts thinking of a feared procedure. This technique of positive self-statements, coupled with thought stopping, is effective for dealing with anticipatory distress and anxiety.

MODELING AND REHEARSAL

Modeling and rehearsal comprise another technique that can be used to enhance a child's coping ability for feared or repeated painful procedures.[28] The usual modeling technique has the child view a videotape of another child undergoing the same medical procedure where positive coping behaviors are observed. If such a videotape is not available, parents can be taught

specific coping behaviors that can be demonstrated to the child. The child can then practice or "rehearse" the specific coping strategies. This rehearsal reinforces positive behaviors. While this approach is not beneficial to the child requiring immediate interventions, it may be feasible for preoperative teaching or cast application.

▌EVALUATION OF PAIN RELIEF INTERVENTIONS

The evaluation of the pain relief interventions follows the five-step pain assessment process and is required for both pharmacologic and nonpharmacologic interventions. It begins with the emergency department nurse asking the verbal child how he or she is feeling and if the pain is still present. If a pain scale was used, the same scale should be readministered, preferably by the same emergency nurse. Changes in the child's behavior are observed and physiologic measures re-

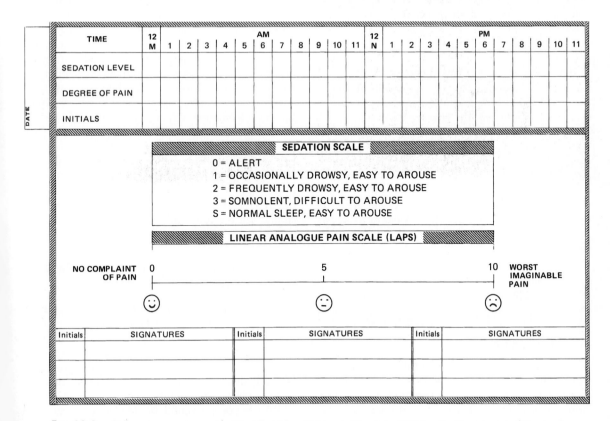

FIG. 29-3. Pain assessment record. (Modified from Children's Hospital of Pittsburgh, Department of Nursing.)

corded and compared to earlier values. The parent may be asked if any appreciable differences in the child are observed.

If no discernible changes are observed in the child's behavior after pharmacologic and nonpharmacologic pain relief measures, two considerations should be entertained. The first consideration is that the intervention(s) were inadequate; the second is that the child's behavior was not caused solely by pain.[38] The analgesic dose is then rechecked and the child assessed for other factors that may affect behavior, such as the absence of a parent, fear, or hunger. If continued pain is suspected, the nurse may consult with the physician and consider the administration of another dose of the same analgesic; administration of a different analgesic; and/or initiation of additional nonpharmacologic interventions.

Pain relief interventions are recorded on the emergency department record and/or pain flow sheet (if available) (Fig. 29-3). Recorded information includes results of pain scale measurements, observed pain-related behavior, pharmacologic and nonpharmacologic interventions, and their effectiveness.[38] The description, location, duration, radiation, and quality of the pain, as verbalized by the child, are also documented.

Before discharge from the emergency department, parents are encouraged to observe for signs of pain in their child and to administer prescription analgesics as ordered or to give over-the-counter medications such as acetaminophen. When parents are given prescriptions for over-the-counter medications, this action conveys the child's need for ongoing pain management.[64] A copy of the pain scale used in the emergency department can be given to the parent with instructions for use. Parents should be encouraged to follow-up with their health care provider or to return to the emergency department if the child's pain persists.

PREPARING CHILDREN FOR PAINFUL PROCEDURES OR TREATMENTS

While no one likes to tell a child that a procedure is potentially painful, it is unethical for the child not to receive advance preparation. A prepared child may be more cooperative and better able to cope with the procedure than one who has not been prepared. Even if the child does not cooperate during the procedure,

it is still in the child's best interest to know what will happen. Procedures initiated without adequate preparation deprive the child of the ability to anticipate, rehearse, and prepare for the procedure. Instead the child may feel helpless, angry, distrustful, and suspicious of health care providers.[19] Preparation for a procedure includes both procedural information (what will be done) and sensory information (what it may feel like).[80]

Before beginning the procedure, an age-appropriate explanation is offered, allowing the child to mobilize his or her coping skills.[19] School-aged children and adolescents can be told in advance what will happen, but toddlers and preschool children are told immediately before the procedure to avoid anticipatory anxiety. Next, the child is asked what he or she thinks will happen during the procedure ("Do you know what a cast is?"). The nurse can then clarify any misconceptions and answer any questions. Pictures, drawings, or dolls can help, as can allowing the child to touch the equipment (e.g., casting material).

Although preparing the child for a procedure can take 5 to 10 minutes (depending on the child's developmental level and previous pain experiences), that 10 minutes is better spent in allaying the child's fears than in struggling with the child during the procedure. Such an experience can be exasperating for the staff and devastating for the child and family.

Sometimes children ask, "Will it hurt?" A request for this information may be the child's way of asking for comfort and support.[51] The emergency department nurse should not lie to the child but can respond by describing the procedure and any anticipated sensations, such as cold or pinching. The nurse should also tell the child that everyone is different and that after the procedure the child should tell the nurse how it felt compared to other painful experiences.

SUPPORTING THE CHILD DURING PAINFUL PROCEDURES

During the procedure the nurse can use independent nursing interventions to help the child cope (Table 29-6). One method is to bring the child into the procedure using involvement techniques. This focuses the child's attention on one aspect of the procedure (see the discussion of nonpharmacologic interventions to relieve or minimize pain).

Whether or not a child should observe a procedure while it is being performed (e.g., suturing, wound cleaning, or IV insertion) depends on the child's

TABLE 29-6 | **Nursing Interventions to Promote Coping**

Infants

Provide containment, such as swaddling	Limits excessive movement and provides boundaries,[12b] which makes the infant feel safe.
Assist the infant with hand-to-mouth contact or nonnutritive sucking	Assists infants in coping with noxious stimuli. Neonates and infants have all of the necessary anatomic and neurochemical mechanisms to perceive pain.[6a]
Provide periods of rest between procedures and protect the infant from noise and bright lights	Helps to prevent overstimulation, behavioral disorganization, and fatigue.[23a]
Position infants 3 months of age and over on the parent's lap before or after procedures	Provides security and comfort.[45a]

Toddlers

Explain in simple, concrete words what the toddler will feel during the procedure just immediately before the procedure	Allows the child to anticipate what will happen.
Allow choices when possible (Do you want to drink juice or water after you drink your medicine?)	Helps to promote autonomy.
Encourage the toddler to hold the bandage, scream very loud, squeeze the parent's hand	Allows the toddler to express his or her pain and emotions in a safe manner that still allows for timely completion of the procedure.

Preschoolers

Allow the child to explore equipment and demonstrate how the equipment works	Helps to alleviate some of the child's fantasies associated with the procedure.
Using nonthreatening language, such as "fix" or "check"	Helps to prevent or minimize fears of body mutilation or pain.
Offer suggestions on how to master fear or pain; suggestions include "Hold my hand" or "say ouch if it hurts"	Promotes a sense of mastery and control.
Reinforce the child's coping by saying "You are such a big help"	Promotes self-esteem.

School-aged children

Allow enough time to ask questions; prompt the child who appears fearful but does not verbalize questions, saying, "Children your age who have this (procedure) often ask me about (common question). Do you have this question, too?"	Helps the child to express his or her thoughts. Helps the child to understand that others have had the same experience, too.
Tell the child how long a procedure will take	Allows the child to pace himself or herself through the procedure without becoming too restless or fidgety.

Adolescents

Encourage them to participate in the decision-making process related to procedures or treatments, whenever possible	Shows respect for the adolescent and promotes responsibility for one's health.
Encourage the verbalization of his or her feelings, and reaffirm the adolescent's normalcy	Promotes self-esteem.
Accept their questions and answer them honestly; respect their choice for a support person	Promotes self-esteem.

preferences and coping skills. The child given the option to watch or not to watch the procedure may feel a sense of control that can alleviate imagined fears. Telling the child to look away from a laceration or wound implies that the procedure is too horrible to watch.[39] Some wounds, however, may upset the child if they are made visible. Very young children, who fear a lack of body integrity, may also become more upset seeing a wound. Each situation is treated individually.

PARENTAL PRESENCE

Parental presence during procedures and treatments is a source of vigorous debate. One thought is that the child will feel betrayed if the parent remains in the room during a painful procedure because the child may perceive the parent as a participant in the pain-producing event. However, it is believed that from a child's point of view, more betrayal and anger may be felt if the parent leaves the room.[67] If the parent of a young child remains present, the child often cries and protests more during the procedure. Such behaviors may occur because the child feels safer and more comfortable in the parents' presence.[43] This freer expression of emotions is actually healthier than not expressing them.[67] The child whose parents are not present may inhibit pain behaviors because of fear of reprimand by the nurses or physicians.[43]

In support of parental presence during painful procedures is the fact that children look to their parents for comfort and support. If the parents are allowed to stay, they can distract and soothe the child during the procedure and model coping behaviors.[80] If the parents are unable to model effective coping behaviors and are distraught or distressed, the nurse can demonstrate such behaviors for the parents.[80] Keeping the parents informed and including them in decision-making will help them cope more effectively. The better the parents are able to cope, the more effective they will be in providing emotional support to their child.

DEBRIEFING CHILDREN AFTER PROCEDURES

After the procedure, pain or discomfort may be present. The child may also have anxieties related to what happened during the procedure. Praising the child for getting through the procedure and offering an appropriate reward (popsicle, sticker, drink of juice, etc.) helps allay these anxieties. Encouraging the child to ask questions, allowing the child to discuss thoughts

or feelings, and permitting the child to touch equipment validates the experience. Asking the child if any pain is present assists the emergency department nurse in determining the need for additional pain relief interventions.

PROFESSIONAL ISSUES ASSOCIATED WITH PAIN MANAGEMENT

The routine assessment, intervention, and evaluation of pain are a priority in pediatric emergency care. Children, like adults, experience pain, yet their responses vary based on numerous factors, including developmental level and coping abilities. To learn to identify and treat pain in children, emergency department nurses can attend (or develop) ongoing educational programs, such as seminars or lectures related to pediatric pain management.

From a hospital-wide perspective, nurses can and should serve on a hospital's interdisciplinary pain management team. If one is not available, emergency department nurses may help to organize one. Also, utilizing the expertise of pain consultants, when available, allows these individuals to share knowledge and make pain management recommendations.

Another means for assuring pediatric pain management in the emergency department is to make it a continuous quality improvement (CQI) indicator. CQI indicators can include yes/no measurements of documented pain assessment, analgesic administration, and evaluation after interventions. Other areas for quality improvement include nonpharmacologic options for pain management and evaluations of their effectiveness.

Finally, studies focusing on pain management practices or techniques that test and validate interventions and evaluate the nurse's role during procedures can be designed and implemented by emergency department nurses.[12] Examples of studies include the evaluation of pain rating scales in the pediatric emergency department population; the use of PCA in pediatric emergency department care; and the use of hypnosis and therapeutic touch in emergency care.

SUMMARY

Emergency department nurses play an important role in recognizing, assessing, and treating infants, children, and adolescents for pain. Knowing children's expressions of and responses to pain, as well as inherent coping strategies, allows the emergency department nurse to tailor pain management approaches to meet each child's needs. Incorporating the family into the child's treatment, as well as consulting with pediatric and pain specialists, assists the emergency department nurse to provide optimal pain management.

REFERENCES

1. Acute Pain Management Guideline Panel: *Acute pain management: operative or medical procedures and trauma. Clinical practice guideline,* AHCPR Pub. No. 92-0032. Rockville, MD, Feb 1992, Agency for Health Care Policy and Research, Public Health Service, US Department of Health and Human Services.
2. Algren JT, Algren CL: Sedation and analgesia for minor pediatric procedures, *Ped Emerg Care* 12(6): 435-441, 1996.
3. American Academy of Pediatrics: Guidelines for monitoring and management of pediatric patients during and after sedation for diagnostic and therapeutic procedures, *Pediatrics* 89(6):1110-1115, 1992.
4. American Academy of Pediatrics, Committee on Drugs: Reappraisal of lytic cocktail/Demerol, Phenergan, Thorazine (DPT) for sedation in children, *Pediatrics* 95:586-602, 1995.
5. American College of Emergency Physician: The use of pediatric sedation and analgesia, *Ann Emerg Med* 22(3):626-627, 1993.
6. Anand K, Hickey P: Pain and its effects on the human neonate and fetus, *N Engl J Med* 31(7):1321-1329, 1987.
6a. Anand K, McGrath P, eds: *Neonatal pain and distress,* Amsterdam; 1993, Elsevier.
7. Anderson C, Zeltzer L, Fanurik D: Procedural pain. In Schechter NI, Berde CB, Yaster M, eds: *Pain in infants, children and adolescents,* Baltimore, 1993, Williams & Wilkins.
8. Andolsek K, Novik B: Use of hypnosis with children, *J Fam Pract* 10(3):503-507, 1980.
9. Beyer JE: *The Oucher: a user's manual and technical report,* Denver, 1989, University of Colorado.
10. Beyer JE, Denyes MJ, Villarruel AM: The creation, validation and continuing development of the Oucher: a measure of pain intensity in children, *J Pediatr Nurs* 7(5):335-346, 1992.
11. Beyer JE, Wells N: The assessment of pain in children, *Pediatr Clin North Am* 36(4):837-854, 1989.
12. Brennan A: Caring for children during procedures: a review of the literature, *Contemp Pediatr* 12:22-36, 1995.
12a. Brown D: Imagination training: a tool with many uses, *Contemp Pediatr* 12:2, 22-36, 1995.
12b. Campos RG: Soothing pain-elicited distress in infants with swaddling and pacifiers. *Child Development,* 60:781-792, 1989.
13. Cote CJ: Sedation for the pediatric patient, *Pediatr Clin North Am* 41:1,21-58, 1994.
14. Craig K, Gronau R: Neonatal pain perception and behavioral measurement. In Anand K, McGrath PJ, eds: *Pain in neonates,* Amsterdam, 1993, Elsevier.
15. Cunningham N: Moral and ethical issues in clinical practice. In Anand K, McGrath PJ, eds: *Pain in neonates,* Amsterdam, 1993, Elsevier.
16. Dalens B: Peripheral nerve blockade in the management of postoperative pain in children. In Schechter NI, Berde CB, Yaster M, eds: *Pain in infants, children, and adolescents,* Baltimore, 1993, Williams & Wilkins.
17. Edgar L, Smith-Hanrahan C: Nonpharmacological pain management. In Watt-Watson J, Donovan M, eds: *Pain management: nursing perspective,* St Louis, 1992, Mosby.
18. Eland J: Children with pain. In Jackson OB, Saunders RB: *Child health nursing,* Philadelphia, 1993, JB Lippincott.
19. Eland JM, Anderson JE: The experience of pain in children. In Jacox AK, ed: *Pain: a source book for nurses and other health professionals,* Boston, 1977, Little, Brown.
19a. Ernst AA et al: LAT (lidocaine-adrenaline-tetracaine) versus TAC (tetracaine-adrenaline-cocaine) for topical anesthesia in face and scalp lacerations, *Am J Emerg Med* 13:2, 151-154, 1995.
20. Fedoruk RB: Transfer of the relaxation response: therapeutic touch as a method of reduction of stress in premature neonates. Unpublished doctoral dissertation, University of Maryland, 1984.
21. Finnerin D: Therapeutic touch for children and their families. In Borelli M, Heidt P, eds: *Therapeutic touch,* New York, 1981, Springer Publishing Co.
22. Fitzgerald M: Development of pain pathways and mechanisms. In Anand K, McGrath PJ, eds: *Pain in neonates,* Amsterdam, 1993, Elsevier.
23. Foley JJ: TAC: a controversial topical anesthetic for suture of skin lacerations, *J Emerg Nurs* 20:3,221-222, 1994.
23a. Franck L: Identification, management, and prevetion of pain in the neonate. In Kenner C, Brueggemeyer A, Gunderson L, eds: *Comprehensive neonatal nursing: a physiologic perspective,* Philadelphia, 1993, WB Saunders.
24. Friedland LR, Kulick RM: Emergency department analgesic use in pediatric trauma victims with fractures, *Ann Emerg Med* 23(2):203-207, 1994.
25. Gaukroger PB: Patient-controlled analgesia in children. In Schechter NI, Berde C, Yaster M, eds: *Pain

in infants, children, and adolescents, Baltimore, 1993, Williams & Wilkins.

26. Guyton AC: *Textbook of medical physiology,* ed 8, Philadelphia, 1991, WB Saunders.

27. Hockenberry M, Bologna-Vaughn S: Preparation for intrusive procedures using noninvasive techniques in children with cancer: state of the art versus new trends, *Cancer Nurs* 8:97-102, 1985.

28. Jay S et al: A comparative study of cognitive behavior therapy versus general anesthesia for painful medical procedures in children, *Pain* 62:39, 1995.

29. Jordan-Marsh M et al: Alternate Oucher from testing gender ethnicity and age variations, *Res Nurs Health* 17:111-118, 1994.

30. Keyes W: Sedative and analgesics. In Holbrook PR, ed: *Textbook of pediatric critical care,* Philadelphia, 1993, WB Saunders.

31. Kuttner L: Favorite stories: a hypnotic pain reduction technique for children in acute pain, *Am J Clin Hypnosis* 30:289-295.

32. Lau N: Pediatric pain management (part I), *J Pediatr Health Care* 6(2):87-92, 1992.

33. Lau N: Pediatric pain management (part II), *J Pediatr Health Care* 64(2):214-219, 1992.

34. LeBel-Schwartz A: Pain management in children. In Jellinek MS, Herzog DB, eds: *Psychiatric aspects of general hospital pediatrics,* Chicago, 1990, Year Book.

35. Loeser J: Pain education for health professionals. In Spross JA, Michel TH, Leuner JD, Conference Organizers: *Improving pain content in the curriculum.* Symposium conducted at the Faculty Pain Symposium of the Massachusetts General Hospital Institute of Health Professions, Boston, March 1992.

36. Maunuksela EL: Nonsteroidal anti-inflammatory drugs in pediatric pain management. In Schechter NL, Berde CB, Yaster M, eds: *Pain in infants, children and adolescents,* Baltimore, 1993, Williams & Wilkins.

37. McCaffery M, Beebe A: *Pain: clinical manual for nursing practice,* St Louis, 1989, Mosby.

38. McCaffery M, Wong DL: Nursing interventions for pain control in children. In Schechter NL, Berde CB, Yaster M, eds: *Pain in infants, children and adolescents,* Baltimore, 1993, Williams & Wilkins.

39. McGrath PA: Evaluating a child's pain, *J Pain Symptom Management* 4(4):198-214, 1989.

40. McGrath PA: *Pain in children: nature, assessment, and treatment,* New York, 1990, Guilford Press.

41. McGrath PA: Pain in the pediatric patient: practical aspects of assessment, *Pediatr Ann* 24:126-138, 1995.

42. McGrath PA: Psychological aspects of pain perception. In Schechter NL, Berde CB, Yaster M, eds: *Pain in infants, children and adolescents,* Baltimore, 1993, Williams & Wilkins.

43. McGrath PJ, Craig KD: Developmental and psychological factors in children's pain, *Pediatr Clin North Am* 36(4):823-836, 1989.

44. Melzack R, Wall P: Pain mechanism: a new theory, *Science* 150:971-979, 1965.

45. Melzack R, Wall P: Psychophysiology of pain, *Int Anesthesiol Clin* 8:3-34, 1970.

45a. Mercer R: Parent-infant attachment. In Sonstegard L, Kowalski K, Jennings B eds: *Women's health and childbearing, vol. II,* pp. 17-40, New York, 1987, Grune & Stratton.

46. Mersky H: Pain terms: a list with definitions and notes on usage. Recommended by the IASP subcommittee on taxonomy, *Pain* 6:249-252, 1979.

47. Miser AW: Management of pain associated with childhood cancer. In Schechter NL, Berde CB, Yaster M, eds: *Pain in infants, children and adolescents,* Baltimore, 1993, Williams & Wilkins.

48. Morrison R: Update on sickle cell disease; incidence of addition and choice of opioid in pain management, *Pediatr Nurs* 17(6):503, 1991.

49. Myron A, Maguire D: Pain perception in the neonate, implications for circumcision, *J Professional Nurs* 7:188-195.

50. Nix K, Clutter L, Wong DL: *The influence of the type of instructions in measuring pain intensity in young children using the* FACES *Pain Rating Scale,* unpublished manuscript, 1994.

51. Nolan K: Ethical issues in pediatric pain management. In Schechter NL, Berde CB, Yaster M, eds: *Pain in infants, children and adolescents,* Baltimore, 1993, Williams & Wilkins.

52. Nurse Healers—Professional Associates: *Therapeutic touch policy and procedure for health professionals,* New York, 1992, Nurse Healers—Professional Associates.

53. Olness, K: Hypnotherapy: a useful tool for the busy pediatrician, *Contemp Pediatr* pp 66-80, March, 1985.

54. Olness K, Gardner GG: Hypnotherapy: a useful tool for the busy pediatrician, *Contemp Pediatr* 66-80, March, 1985.

55. Ott MJ: Imagine the possibilities! Guided imagery with toddlers and preschoolers, *Pediatr Nurs* 22:34-38, 1996.

56. Purtillo K: *Pain in the critically ill,* Gaithersburg, MD, 1991, Aspen Publishers.

57. Quinn J: Therapeutic touch as energy exchange: replication and extension, *Nurs Sci Q* 20:79-87, 1989.

58. Rushton C: Placebo pain medications: ethical and legal issues, *Pediatr Nurs* 21:166-168, 1995.

59. Sacchetti A et al: Pediatric analgesia and sedation, *Ann Emerg Med* 23(2):237-250, 1994.

60. Schechter NL: Pain: acknowledging it, assessing it, treating it, *Contemp Pediatr* 4:16-46, 1987.

61. Schechter NL: The undertreatment of pain in chil-

dren: an overview, *Pediatr Clin North Am* 36(4): 781-794, 1989.

62. Selbst SM: Managing pain in the pediatric emergency department, *Pediatr Emerg Care* 5(1):56-63, 1989.

63. Selbst SM: Pain management in the emergency department. In Schechter NL, Berde CB, Yaster M, eds: *Pain in infants, children and adolescents,* Baltimore, 1993, Williams & Wilkins.

64. Selbst SM: Sedation and analgesia. In Fleisher G, Ludwig S, eds: *Textbook of pediatric emergency medicine,* ed 3, Baltimore, 1993, Williams & Wilkins.

65. Selbst SM, Henretig FM: The treatment of pain in the emergency department, *Pediatr Clin North Am* 48(1):131-136, 1989.

66. Strauss S, Lynn A, Spear R: Progress in pain control for very young infants *Contemp Pediatr* 12(5):80-100, 1995.

67. Sugarman M: Caring for children in hospitals. In Jellinek MS, Herzog DB, eds: *Psychiatric aspects of general hospital pediatrics,* Chicago, 1990, Year Book.

68. Swafford LI, Allen D: Pain relief in the pediatric patient, *Med Clin North Am* 48(1):131-136, 1968.

69. Terndrup TE: Pain control, analgesia, and sedation. In Barkin RM, ed: *Pediatric emergency medicine: concepts in clinical practice,* St Louis, 1992, Mosby.

70. Tesler M et al: The word-graphic rating scale as a measure of children's and adolescents' pain intensity, *Res Nurse Health* 14:361-371, 1991.

71. Thompson AE, Frader JE: Pain management in children. In Paris PM, Stewart RD, eds: *Pain management in emergency medicine,* Norwalk, CT, 1988, Appleton & Lange.

72. Tobias JD et al: Oral ketamine premedication to alleviate the distress of invasive procedures in pediatric oncology patients, *Pediatrics* 90(4):537-541, 1992.

73. Vaughan VC, Litt IF: Introduction. In Vaughan VC, Litt IF, eds: *Child and adolescent development: clinical implications,* Philadelphia, 1990, WB Saunders.

74. Villarruel AM, Denyes MJ: Pain assessment in children: theoretical and empirical validity, *Adv Nurs Sci* 14(2):32-41, 1991.

75. Walco GA, Ilowit NT: Vertical vs horizontal visual analog scales of pain intensity in children, *J Pain Symptom Management* 6(3):200, 1991.

76. Wall PD, Melzack R: *Textbook of pain,* New York, 1989, Churchill Livingstone.

77. Walters BL: Pain control in the emergency department. In Reisdorff EJ, Roberts MR, Wiegenstein JG, eds: *Pediatric emergency medicine,* Philadelphia, 1992, WB Saunders.

78. Wong D, Baker C: Pain in children: comparison of assessment scales, *Pediatr Nurs* 14(1):9-17, 1988.

79. Yaster M et al: Midazolam-fentanyl intravenous sedation in children: case report of respiratory arrest, *Pediatrics* 86:463-467, 1990.

80. Zeltzer LK, Anderson CT, Schechter NL: Pediatric pain: current status and new directions, *Curr Probl Pediatr* 20(8):411-486, 1990.

81. Zeltzer L, LeBaron S: Hypnosis and nonhypnotic techniques for reduction of pain and anxiety during painful procedures in children and adolescents with cancer, *J Pediatr* 101(6):1032-1035, 1982.

82. Zeltzer L, LeBaron S: The hypnotic treatment of children in pain. In Wolraich M, Routh D, eds: *Advances in developmental and behavioral pediatrics,* Greenwich, 1986, JAI Press.

CHAPTER 30

Children with Special Needs

Alison Schultz, Karen Chalanick

Children with special needs typically have congenital, hereditary, or acquired health conditions that actually or potentially interfere with normal growth and development.[6] Chronically ill and disabled children comprise a major portion of this population. Disabilities are conditions that functionally limit a person's abilities, such as walking, talking, or learning.[22] Serious chronic health conditions of childhood are defined as those lasting 3 months or more and affecting the child's functional ability in one or more areas.[12] The incidence of chronic conditions is about 1% of all live-born children. However, because advances in health care and medical technology have resulted in higher and longer-term survival rates, the population of children with special health care needs is increasing. The number of chronically ill or disabled children in the United States is estimated to be between 750,000 and 1,000,000.[4,15] About one-third cope with conditions of moderate severity or greater.[12]

Categories of chronic illness and disability that are commonly encountered in the emergency department (ED) include asthma, neurologic conditions, hematologic and oncologic conditions, cardiac conditions, and behavioral disorders.[17] The probability of one of these children coming to the ED with an illness or a complication of their underlying condition is relatively high. The incidence of the child arriving in the evening and requiring admission to the hospital is also high.[17]

NURSING HISTORY AND PHYSICAL EXAMINATION

HISTORY

The first step in the history is to identify the presence of the special health care condition, as many are "invisible." An important question to ask during the initial history is "does the child have a chronic or long-term illness or disability?" Most parents and some children readily answer this question, providing valuable information to guide further assessment.

The child's developmental status is another important component of the history. Information regarding developmental delays is valuable, not only as a clue to possible coexisting chronic conditions, but also in formulating strategies for developmentally appropriate approaches to the child.

In all but the most emergent situations, once it is known that a child has a chronic condition, detailed information about the child's home medical care should be elicited from the parents, including the time and dose of recently given medications and those that are due in the next few hours. Input from the child's primary or specialty health care provider, if possible, is invaluable.

PHYSICAL EXAMINATION

The physical examination proceeds based on the child's developmental level and follows the head-to-toe or toe-to-head format reviewed in Chapter 4. The developmental level and the child's abilities are determined based on findings obtained from the parents (and the child when possible) during the history. Not only do parents provide a wealth of information about a child's developmental level, but they also offer helpful hints for approaching and assessing the child.

Developmental abilities vary widely. It is important to note, however, that children with special needs do not necessarily have cognitive impairments or communication difficulties—although they may require the use of special equipment such as hearing aids, eyeglasses, or communication boards.

PSYCHOSOCIAL CONSIDERATIONS FOR CHILDREN WITH SPECIAL NEEDS

Children with special needs are more like their healthy and able-bodied peers than they are different. The child's developmental progression is often, however, affected by the psychologic burden of coping with a long-term illness or disability. Frequent and/or prolonged separations from parents related to hospitalizations threaten the development of trust, and the child's physical disabilities may threaten the development of autonomy. Socially, a child may be more whiny and clingy than usual for their age, or the child may appear advanced, perhaps in their knowledge of the disease and their ability to cope with procedures.

PSYCHOSOCIAL CONSIDERATIONS FOR FAMILIES

Children with special health care needs who require home management often become the center of their family's attention. The family's focus, however, is generally on the long-term nature of the illness or disability rather than on interventions for an acute illness or injury. Even parents of frequently hospitalized children have been found to poorly understand hospital policies and to be somewhat distrustful of health care professionals.[2] Parents report reluctance to be "too assertive" in their interactions with health care professionals for fear of being viewed negatively, leading to less optimal care for their child.[2]

Just as for previously well children who are hospitalized unexpectedly,[11] the family of the child with special needs may experience an acute sense of anxiety and feelings of loss of control when their child must be treated in the ED. In addition to losing their parental role and being confused and frightened by hospital routines, equipment, people, and procedures, separation of the parent and child in order to render emergency treatment may provoke extreme

---

Box 30-1 Psychosocial Considerations for Families of Children with Special Needs

- May experience an acute sense of anxiety
- May have feelings of a loss of parental control
- May view their child as "vulnerable"
- May fantasize or be unrealistic about the child's condition
- May experience grief or chronic sorrow
- May fear being too assertive, which they feel may impact negatively on the child's care

---

anxiety in both parent and child. Moreover, families are more likely to view their disabled or chronically ill children as "vulnerable,"[5] leading to overprotection (Box 30-1).

SPECIAL CONSIDERATIONS IN EMERGENCY NURSING CARE OF CHILDREN WITH SPECIAL NEEDS

Developmentally appropriate strategies, such as reducing separations from loved ones, facilitating play activities, encouraging verbalization of fears, and offering reassurance and understandable explanations, will assist the special needs child in coping with the stress of an ED visit. Parents cope more effectively with the stress of hospitalization when given more opportunities to assume normal parental role behaviors, such as comforting, feeding, or holding their child, as well as when given accurate information about their child's condition,[10,11] all of which can be facilitated while the child is in the ED.

MULTIDISCIPLINARY TEAMS

Children with complex medical needs are almost always discharged from tertiary medical centers, which have stringent criteria requiring the family to become experts in the child's care. Ideally these children are then followed by multidisciplinary teams from a tertiary medical center, as well as their health provider. Families who are providing complex health care for their child at home have usually developed a clear emergency plan that specifies which physician is responsible for decision-making regarding potential problems. Those families with little confidence in their decision-making skills or who have poor support systems are more likely to be referred to the ED for evaluation after speaking with their physician.

HOME HEALTH CARE

Caretaker fatigue and a loss of objectivity are real problems for families who are caring for children with complex illnesses at home. Children whose needs are continuous, such as those on continual ventilator support, require almost constant attention by qualified personnel. Other children, such as those with gastrostomy tubes or indwelling central lines, or children with continuous oxygen therapy may require frequent visits by a home health nurse to evaluate the child's status, administer medications, or provide support to the parents. Although these services may be indicated, they are not always available— particularly when a family requires respite care. Insufficient numbers of qualified home care nurses, a paucity of respite care facilities, and inadequate funding may require a family to bear the burden of a child's care with little or no home care support. Regardless of the availability of services, a family who has missed several nights of sleep because of a lack of home nursing support or an exacerbated illness loses their ability to accurately assess, and cope with, the child's condition. Although hospitals are not the most appropriate places to provide relief to families when their home care plan has fallen apart, there is often no other place for these families to turn. If the overall goal of providing safe care at home is not being met, the immediate solution may be admission to the hospital.

"DO NOT RESUSCITATE" ORDERS

Occasionally the family of a disabled child with a certain prognosis of early death or for whom treatment means imposing undue pain and suffering has decided on limited interventions or a "do not resuscitate" (DNR) order for their child. State laws and regulations and hospital policies vary in terms of how such decisions and advance directives are to be handled, and nurses must be knowledgeable about these in order to act swiftly when the need arises (see Chapter 2, Legal and Ethical Considerations).

CHILDREN WITH COMMUNICATION OR SENSORY DEFICITS

DEVELOPMENTALLY DELAYED CHILDREN

Etiology. Developmental delays can occur in any developmental sphere; for the purposes of this section, "developmental delays" will be equated with "mental retardation" (MR). According to the American Association on Mental Retardation,

Mental retardation refers to substantial limitations in present functioning. It is characterized by significantly subaverage intellectual functioning existing concurrently with related limitations in two or more of the following applicable adaptive skills: communications, self-care, home living, social skills, community use, self-direction, health and safety, functional academics, leisure, and work. Mental retardation manifests before age 18.[1]

MR has many causes and is found in frequent or uniform association with many other conditions (Box 30-2). Because of advances in both the understanding of MR and in the technology that supports diagnostic

---

Box 30-2 Causes of Mental Retardation
• Hereditary disorders (e.g., Tay-Sachs disease, Hurler syndrome, neurofibromatosis, tuberous sclerosis)
• Alterations in embryonic development (e.g., chromosomal changes, prenatal influences)
• Pregnancy-related problems (e.g., placental insufficiency)
• Perinatal problems (e.g., prematurity, birth asphyxia)
• Sequela from childhood diseases/injuries (e.g., encephalitis, meningitis, asphyxia from near-drowning)
• Environmental/behavioral problems (e.g., deprivation, parental neurosis, psychosis, childhood neurosis, psychosis)
• Unknown causes

Modified from Crocker AC: The causes of mental retardation, *Pediatr Ann* 18:623, 1989.

investigation, it is now possible in many cases to determine the cause of a particular child's MR and/or the condition with which it is associated.

Pathophysiology. The pathophysiology for MR varies with the cause. For example, chromosomal variations generally lead to a direct disruption in normal brain growth and organization, while fetal malnutrition results in inadequate support for normal prenatal brain growth and development. Perinatal stresses usually lead to an insult to the brain such as hemorrhage or anoxia, affecting both existing brain structure and subsequent development.

Clinical presentation. Children with MR, even if unassociated with another disabling condition such as cerebral palsy, may have delays in psychomotor skills, speech and language, and/or functional independence. Infants often do not exhibit signs of delay until several months of age, when motor milestones begin to be missed or primitive reflexes do not fade. Later, standardized testing reveals subaverage intellectual functioning along with the need for assistance in activities of daily living, and the MR diagnosis is confirmed.

As a general rule, more severely affected individuals with MR usually have a greater degree of retardation in communication and adaptive skills and are more likely to have shorter attention spans and exhibit impulsive, aggressive, or even self-injurious behaviors.[8] Children who are less affected sometimes behave in a manner somewhat like children who have attention deficit disorder; that is, they may be impulsive, overactive, and tend to act out their frustrations. Children with multiple disabilities may have additional frustrations. For example, children who have a short attention span, difficulty with impulse control, and a mobility impairment are especially frustrated as they attempt gains in the psychomotor arena.

Emergency Department interventions. Children with MR are brought to the ED for all of the same problems as children with typical developmental patterns. Assessing the chief complaint and constructing a plan of care must take into account the child's developmental variance. This information is best obtained from the parents or home caregivers. Additionally, the child's primary pediatrician or nurse-practitioner can be consulted. Treatment of the child depends on the chief complaint presenting signs, and symptoms and suspected underlying etiology.

Nursing care and evaluation. Delivering care to a child with MR is fundamentally different from the typical situation only in terms of the child's ability to understand and participate in the experience in an age-appropriate manner (Box 30-3). All other differences result from pathophysiology related to the condition(s) that accompany the MR. Assessment for these problems is performed in the same manner as for other children. Treatment of the child's illness or injury requires all of the usual attention to detail as for other children, plus special attention to safety.

Decreasing stress is an important goal of nursing care. Children with MR often have a poor concept of time and become very fearful and agitated when separated from familiar caregivers or family for even brief periods. A family member should stay with the child whenever possible. Security objects can also be kept close to the child. It is best to minimize the number of health care providers who must interact with the child and family. Including the parents in as many aspects of the child's assessment and treatment

---

Box 30-3 Nursing Care Approaches to the Mentally Retarded Child

- Allow the parents to participate in the child's care whenever possible.
- Allow a family member and/or a security object to remain with the child whenever possible.
- Provide developmentally appropriate explanations and preparation for procedures. Assume the child can understand what is being said.
- Give "permission" for regressive behaviors.
- Use the child's name or nickname consistently.
- Learn the child's words or signs for essential functions and feelings.
- Present only one thought, question, or instruction at a time.
- Allow the child to use communication aids.
- Ensure the child's safety (e.g., never leave alone, keep side rails/crib sides up at all times, and use restraints as necessary).
- Offer positive reinforcement (verbal, touch, stickers, etc.).

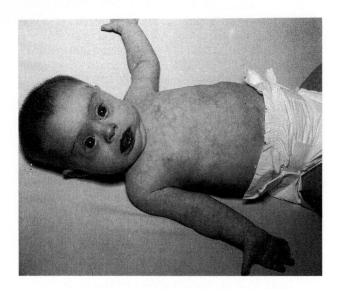

FIG. 30-1. A child with Down syndrome has characteristic features. (From Wong DL: *Whaley & Wong's essentials of pediatric nursing,* ed 5, St Louis, 1997, Mosby.)

as possible and keeping them informed helps reduce their stress. Reducing parental stress diminishes the child's stress.

Communicating effectively with children with MR requires patience and skill. Often the child's receptive language skills exceed his or her expressive skills. The nurse should assume that children with MR can understand what is being said, even if they cannot respond or act on it. Consistently using the child's name or nickname and listening to the child conveys caring and respect. The child's words or signs for essential functions and feelings such as pain, hunger, and elimination should be identified. Use of communication aids the parents have brought along, such as eyeglasses, hearing aids, or communication boards, should be encouraged.

DOWN SYNDROME (TRISOMY 21)

Etiology. Down syndrome (DS) is an autosomal chromosome abnormality in which the affected individual has 47 chromosomes rather than the usual 46, with the additional chromosome being a number 21. DS is the most common human malformation-mental retardation syndrome, occurring at a rate of about 1 to 1.2 per 1000 live births. The probability of a pregnancy resulting in a child with DS increases with maternal age, but in the United States, most are born to younger mothers, since the birth rate is so much higher among younger women. The incidence of DS

does not differ significantly among members of different races, ethnic groups, or socioeconomic classes.[16] Since these children have a characteristic appearance and because chromosome analysis is definitive, DS is usually diagnosed in infancy (Fig. 30-1).

In most cases the additional chromosome 21 has resulted from accidental nondisjunction during division of the germ cell. The specific cause or causes of DS are as yet unclear. It is known that in 95% of cases the germ cell with the extra chromosome is maternal.[16]

Pathophysiology. In DS, the additional chromosome 21 is usually found in all cell lines, since it was introduced into the zygote through fertilization. Thus there is the potential for effects in many of the major body systems and organs, for example, the central nervous system (brain development/mental retardation), cardiac system (congenital cardiac anomalies), skin (characteristic dermatoglyphics), craniofacial areas (abnormalities, including microcephaly and flat occiput), and gastrointestinal system (higher incidence of duodenal and esophageal atresia). Individual patients do not have all possible sequelae, however, and the severity varies among affected individuals (Box 30-4).

Clinical presentation

Growth abnormalities. Infants with DS frequently have delayed growth. Older children, adoles-

> ### Box 30-4   Pathophysiologic Conditions Associated with Down Syndrome
>
> Mental retardation (usually mild)
> Muscular hypotonia
> Delayed growth
> Conditions that may be associated with DS
>   Congenital heart defects
>   Gastrointestinal malformations (e.g.,
>   duodenal atresia, tracheoesophageal
>   fistula, Hirschsprung's disease, Meckel's
>   diverticulum)
>   Hearing problems
>   Leukemia
>   Dental problems
>   Respiratory problems (e.g., tracheal
>   hypoplasia/stenosis, obstructive sleep
>   apnea, gastroesophageal reflux, primary
>   pulmonary hypertension)
>   Emotional problems
>   Genitourinary problems
>   Immunologic deficiencies
>   Reproductive problems
> Conditions more common in older children,
>   adolescents, and adults
>   Atlantoaxial subluxation
>   Cataracts
>   Thyroid conditions
>   Obesity
>   Seizures
>
> Modified from Cooley W, Graham JM: Down syndrome—an update and review for the primary pediatrician, *Clin Pediatr* 30(4):233-253, 1991.

cents, and adults with DS more commonly have problems with obesity.

Infections.   Immunologic defects, in conjunction with anatomic differences, render children with DS more susceptible to infection. Upper and lower respiratory infections account for the majority of ED visits. Pneumonia can be a serious problem for a child with DS, particularly those with cardiac anomalies or primary pulmonary pathology.

The eustachian tube is often short in children with DS, and this, coupled with increased nasal secretions and inadequate drainage, predisposes these children to serous and acute otitis media. Complicating the

evaluation is the fact that the external ear is often abnormally shaped and the external ear canal is very narrow. The frequency of ear infections may be partially at fault for the high incidence of hearing loss in this population.

Surgical complications.   Infants with DS and associated cardiac and/or gastrointestinal defects usually undergo surgical correction during infancy. They may therefore come to the ED with any of the postsurgical complications associated with cardiothoracic or gastrointestinal surgery. Most common among these are wound infections and dehiscence. Recovery of infants with DS may be more prolonged than that of others because of their predisposition to infection and failure to thrive.

Atlantoaxial instability.   Approximately 15% of children with DS have atlantoaxial instability.[18] To screen for this condition a cervical x-ray is taken at 3 and 12 years of age. If the x-ray is abnormal, the child should refrain from participating in certain sports such as tumbling, gymnastics, and diving.[18] If a child with DS has neurologic signs that are consistent with cervical cord compression, such as lower limb spasticity, torticollis, progressive weakness, or loss of bowel or bladder control, atlantoaxial instability should be suspected.

Leukemia.   Approximately 1% of children with DS develop leukemia; most are affected between 1 and 4 years of age. Fifty percent develop acute megakaryoblastic leukemia (AMKL). Newborns with DS frequently develop a transient AMKL, which is often discovered on the complete blood count (CBC) and differential completed during a routine sepsis workup. Although this condition usually disappears around 3 months of age, there is a higher risk for developing true AMKL later in life.

Emergency Department interventions.   ED interventions depend on presenting signs and symptoms of illness or injury and the likelihood of an underlying pathology. In the young child with DS and signs of pneumonia, mycoplasma may be the infectious agent.[13] For this reason, not only are the usual laboratory and radiologic tests for pneumonia performed, but additionally a cold agglutinin blood test or specific titer for mycoplasma is done. Appropriate inpatient or outpatient antibiotic treatment is instituted, as indicated.

Ear infections are treated aggressively after investigation of chronicity and previous treatment. The child is then referred back to the primary care provider for follow-up. Care by a specialist is often indicated.

Atlantoaxial instability must be considered in the Down syndrome child with neurologic signs. Although only a small percentage of these children have atlantoaxial instability, situations producing forceful injuries to the head and neck (particularly motor vehicle crashes) can precipitate overt symptoms of cervical cord compression. These children are immobilized and evaluated for cervical spine compression. Lateral x-rays of the upper cervical spine in neutral, flexion, and extension are obtained. A computed tomography (CT) scan and magnetic resonance imaging (MRI) will provide more accurate and detailed information.

Nursing care and evaluation. Children with DS are often thought of as cute, cuddly, happy youngsters with developmental delay. In fact, children with DS have a wide range of abilities and personalities, as do all children, and therefore must be approached as the unique individuals they are. Because many children with DS have hearing and speech difficulties, communication may be difficult and parents' assistance is valuable. As always, developmentally appropriate strategies for effective communication and anxiety reduction must be employed.

Safety is of particular concern for these children because, although they are developmentally delayed, mobility impairment is unlikely. Children and adolescents with DS should therefore never be left unattended while in the ED.

CHILDREN WHO ARE DEPENDENT ON MEDICAL TECHNOLOGY

"Technology-dependent" describes a small subset in the population of chronically ill children. Technology dependence is defined as "the need for both a medical device to compensate for the loss of a vital body function and substantial and ongoing nursing care to avert death or further disability".[20]

The technologically dependent child can present a major challenge to the ED staff. Home equipment may be unfamiliar to the ED nurse, and the presence of a parent who has been extensively

trained to perform home care can create a situation in which the nurse feels unprepared to provide optimal care.

OXYGEN DEPENDENCE

Etiology. The most common pediatric conditions for which home oxygen therapy is used include bronchopulmonary dysplasia (BPD), cystic fibrosis, and cardiac disease. However, there are many other indications for long-term oxygen supplementation. Home oxygen therapy is considered for two broad categories of children.[19] The first group has serious disease, but the prospect of improvement, and perhaps recovery, exists. The treatment goal is eventual weaning from the oxygen while carefully monitoring the child's growth, development, stamina, and cardiopulmonary status. The infant with BPD is an example of reversible pulmonary disease. The second group has end-stage pulmonary (e.g., severe cystic fibrosis) or cardiac disease. Home oxygen is used to improve the child's quality of life.

Clinical presentation. The type of oxygen delivery system used at home is determined by several factors, including whether the child requires continuous or intermittent oxygen, a portable or stationary system, and high or low liter flow or concentration of oxygen.

Home oxygen may be delivered by various methods. It is usually delivered by nasal cannulas, tracheostomy masks, oxygen tents, or ventilators. Face masks and nasal catheters are not well tolerated by most children who use oxygen regularly at home.

Children with chronic lung disease commonly have signs and symptoms of respiratory distress. They are more likely than healthy children to develop significant pulmonary compromise in response to respiratory infections. Other common causes of respiratory distress in children on home oxygen include bronchoconstriction, equipment failure, and progression of the chronic pulmonary disease. End-stage, terminal disease is characterized by increasing oxygen requirements and progressive respiratory compromise. The child may have DNR orders, or the issue may need to be considered if it appears that respiratory arrest is imminent (see Chapter 2, Legal and Ethical Considerations, pp. 35-37).

Emergency Department and nursing interventions. On initial presentation of the child on home oxygen therapy, the ED nurse must first determine the child's baseline pulmonary function. Parents or home nurses can provide information concerning the child's usual oxygen saturation, respiratory rate and effort, and color, as well as a history of the child's responses to past interventions (Box 30-5). Other systems should also be assessed, particularly the cardiac system for signs of right-sided heart failure. Ongoing evaluations compare the child's current status to initial assessment findings. Decisions to discharge or admit rely on the child's current health status in comparison to the parent's and/or child's primary or specialty health care provider's description of baseline.

Nursing interventions depend on the chief complaint and clinical condition. If equipment failure has occurred, the child may require a temporary increase in oxygen to ensure rapid recovery. When the equipment is functioning well, other causes of deterioration are sought and the appropriate interventions begun.

TRACHEOSTOMY TUBES

Etiology. A tracheostomy is a surgically created opening in the trachea at the level of the cricoid cartilage. A plastic or metal tube is inserted to keep the stoma patent, allowing air movement in and out of the lungs (Fig. 30-2 and Table 30-1). Children require tracheostomy tubes for various medical reasons. The most common indications are a congenital upper airway obstruction; acquired upper airway obstruction as a result of trauma or foreign bodies; complications from long-term endotracheal intubation; and the need for a comfortable, stable airway for long-term ventilation.

Clinical presentation. Children with tracheostomy tubes have various illnesses or injuries that may or may not be directly related to the tracheostomy. The most common presentations in the ED that are directly related to the tracheostomy include obstruction of the tracheal opening by a mucus plug, increased airway secretions, or a foreign body. Another reason for presentation is accidental decannulation of the stoma.

Clinical presentation depends on the degree of airway obstruction. Mild obstructions are associated with minimal respiratory distress. Severe obstructions are associated with tachypnea, cyanosis, decreased breath sounds, and severe retractions.

Emergency Department and nursing interventions. On arrival in the ED the child's general condition is assessed. If the child arrives with a complaint that is unrelated to the tracheostomy, such as a laceration to the finger, routine triage protocols may be followed. If a segregated or well-child waiting area cannot be provided, however, the child may be placed in a private room, away from children with respiratory illnesses.

The child with severe respiratory distress or with signs of respiratory failure is treated emergently. Tracheostomy-related causes of respiratory distress (e.g., occlusion or decannulation) must be differentiated from other causes (e.g., infection or bronchoconstriction).

To best evaluate the child's condition, historical information relating to the child's baseline status is

---

Box 30-5 Nursing History and Physical Examination for the Child with Home Respiratory Technology

History

What is the child's normal respiratory pattern, and how does the current status differ?

What interventions have been tried at home, and what was the child's response?

Does the child's respiratory status vary during the day and evening, and has this changed?

Have any other associated signs and symptoms been observed (e.g., fever, vomiting, diarrhea, color changes)?

Has the child been exposed to any known illnesses?

Is oxygen required? If so, how much and when?

Have oxygen requirements increased? If so, how much?

Physical examination

Assess airway patency.

Assess breathing/ventilation (respiratory effort, breath sounds, skin color).

Assess circulation (pulses, capillary refill).

Assess neurologic status (level of consciousness, activity level, motor tone).

Evaluate vital signs.

Assess oxygen delivery system (if used):

  Adequate amount of oxygen in the tank

  Connections at the child and the oxygen source

  Percentage of oxygen delivered

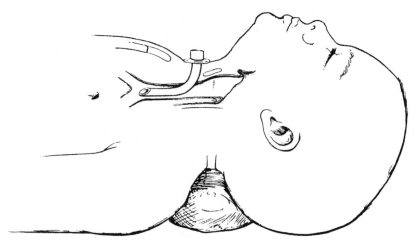

FIG. 30-2. A plastic or metal tube is inserted through a surgical incision at the level of the cricoid cartilage. (From Rowe MI et al, eds: *Essentials of pediatric surgery*, St Louis, 1995, Mosby.)

TABLE 30-1	Tracheostomy Tubes Commonly Used in Pediatrics	
	SINGLE CANNULA, PLASTIC/SILICONE, PEDIATRIC AND NEONATAL TUBES	**DOUBLE CANNULA, PLASTIC/SILICONE TUBES**
Usual age group	Premature infants, newborns, young children	Older children, adolescents, and adults
Distinguishing features	Wide variety of diameters and lengths that accommodate very small tracheas	Large outer diameter precludes use in infants, young children
	Anatomically designed to fit the curve of small children's tracheas	Available with or without fenestration (hole in outer cannula that allows for easier vocalization when inner cannula is not in use)
		Low profile cannula available (protrudes less), but does not attach to ventilator or bag-valve device
		Decannulation plugs available that occlude the trachea and allow for breathing through the upper airways
Materials	Soft, flexible materials	Made of a more rigid plastic
Cuffs	Not available with cuffs	Available with or without
Care and cleaning	Easy for home care providers to change and care for	Inner cannula may be easily removed to clean or check for mucus
	Must remove entire tube if concerned about mucus occlusion	Standard inner cannula must be in place for mechanical ventilation and BVM ventilation

obtained from the parent, as well as information concerning interventions attempted by the parents before arrival in the ED. The physical examination includes evaluation of the patency of the tracheostomy (e.g., the ability to pass a suction catheter through the tube and the ability to provide effective manual ventilation) and evaluation of the child's ventilatory status. If the tube is occluded or dislodged, it is removed and replaced with a new one.

When replacement of a tracheostomy tube is indicated, suction equipment, oxygen equipment, a bag-valve-mask device, and a new cannula the same size as the previously used one, or one size smaller, must be available. If the situation is an emergency and a tracheostomy tube is not available or the child cannot be ventilated, an endotracheal tube may be placed in the stoma. It must not, however, be inserted beyond the carina. To insert a tracheostomy tube, the child is placed supine with the head and neck extended. Oxygen can be administered both to the nose and mouth and to the stoma. The new tracheostomy tube is then inserted posteriorly and then caudally, following the course of the tracheal fistula. The tube is securely tied around the child's neck, and placement is confirmed with an improvement in the child's ventilatory status and by chest x-ray (Fig. 30-3). Cloth ties, such as umbilical cord tape, are most commonly used to secure the tube. Ties should be snug around the neck but still allow one finger to be inserted underneath. Other methods that may be used, depending on regional preferences and safety considerations, include Velcro fasteners and stainless steel beaded chains.

General considerations for the child with a tracheostomy. Tracheostomies bypass the body's natural humidification and filtering devices located in the nose and pharynx. Therefore humidification of the airways is provided, especially for children with small, single cannula tubes that can easily become occluded with dried secretions. The air compressor that runs home humidification systems is not easily portable and is not usually brought to the ED. Tracheostomy collars with humidification and oxygen (if necessary) should be provided while the child is in the ED (Fig. 30-4). A small and easy-to-use humidification device is the heat-moisture exchanger or artificial nose, which attaches to the outer diameter of the tracheostomy tube. A felt or gauze filter traps exhaled moisture and heat, which can then be used to humidify subsequent inspired breaths. Most artificial noses are disposable and should be discarded when the filter becomes saturated. They should be checked regularly for blockage by expectorated secretions.

Since the amount of air passing through the vocal cords is dramatically reduced by a tracheostomy, the child's ability to make sound is diminished. Speech is possible, however, if any air is leaking around the tracheostomy tube and up through the vocal cords. The esophagus is not altered, so there is no inherent reason why a child with a tracheostomy cannot eat. Many infants and young children do, however, develop feeding problems.

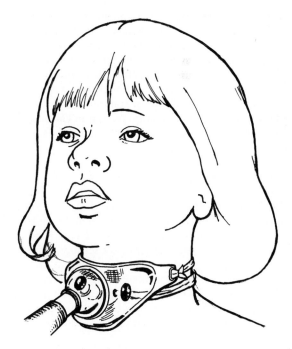

FIG. 30-4. Tracheostomy collars are used to deliver humidification and/or oxygen to the child with a tracheostomy.

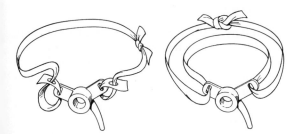

FIG. 30-3. Two methods of securing tracheostomy tubes around a child's neck.

MECHANICAL VENTILATORS

Etiology. The number of children who require ventilator assistance at home, either continuously or intermittently, has increased dramatically in the past 10 years. The most successful home ventilator management is achieved in patients whose day-to-day cardiopulmonary status is stable, even though they are unable to provide the ventilatory effort needed to support life.[9] Chronic ventilator assistance is most commonly required in children with severe BPD, neuromuscular disorders that affect the strength and effectiveness of respiratory movements, and congenital anomalies that either directly or iatrogenically cause chronic respiratory failure. Head or spinal cord injury may also result in chronic respiratory failure.

Clinical presentation. When the ventilator-assisted child comes to the ED with respiratory distress, various causes must be considered. Problems may include illnesses, such as respiratory tract infections or bronchoconstriction; aspiration; tracheostomy problems, such as plugging or extubation; or mechanical ventilator dysfunction.

The type of ventilator, the amount of ventilatory support, and the intensity of home care required are determined by the child's medical condition. Portable home ventilators have been streamlined for ease of use outside the hospital. Most are relatively compact, easy to operate, and run on various power sources. Since home ventilators are not designed to support critically ill children, a ventilator capable of delivering ventilation in different modes may be necessary if the child becomes acutely ill. The most common type of home ventilator is a positive pressure ventilator. Chronically ventilated children usually have tracheostomies.

Emergency Department and nursing interventions

Assessment. On arrival in the ED the home-ventilated child's usual state of health and ventilator settings are identified by history and compared to current clinical status and ventilator settings. If home nursing support has been used, significant clinical information is usually documented in a notebook. The past several days of nurse's notes, if available, can help to accurately assess the child's condition and determine the cause of the current problem.

Interventions. If the child is in moderate to severe respiratory distress, or if mechanical problems are suspected, the ventilator should be immediately disconnected, bag-valve-tracheostomy ventilation with 100% oxygen initiated, and tube placement checked. If the upper airway is clear, bag-valve-mask ventilation can be used as long as the stoma or tracheostomy is occluded. The ventilator can then be carefully checked and problems corrected if necessary. If the machine is functioning well and respiratory distress is evident, pathologic causes should be sought and treated.

Trouble-shooting for the ventilator. The ventilator settings, power source, connections, peak inspiratory pressure, alarm settings, and humidification source are checked. Home ventilators remain plugged into an electrical outlet whenever possible. Other sources of power include an internal battery that lasts less than an hour and an external battery that lasts about 8 hours. An alarm sounds when the internal battery is almost depleted. The ventilator's *humidification source* is often disconnected during transport to the ED; this should be checked and replaced, if necessary, to prevent drying of secretions.

Peak inspiratory pressure (PIP) reflects the amount of airway pressure that is required to inflate the lungs when a preset volume is delivered. It may vary from breath to breath. A leak in the system lowers the PIP, and an occlusion in the system increases the PIP.

Pressure alarms reflect deviations from the safe airway pressure range for the child. Activation of the high pressure alarm may indicate an obstruction somewhere in the system or increased resistance in the lungs. Activation of the low pressure alarm may indicate a leak in the system or the delivery of an inadequate volume. Alarms should never be set outside the range for the child's safety. The usual high pressure alarm setting is 45 to 50 cm H_2O; the usual low pressure alarm setting is 10 to 15 cm H_2O (Table 30-2).

GASTROSTOMY TUBES

Etiology. A gastrostomy is an external opening from the stomach to the abdomen. Gastrostomies can be used for prolonged gastric decompression but are most commonly used for the long-term feeding of infants and children who, for various reasons, cannot consume adequate amounts of nutrients by mouth (Box 30-6).

Clinical presentation. Children with gastrostomy dysfunction may come to the ED with a dis-

TABLE 30-2	Home Ventilator Settings	
SETTING	**CHARACTERISTICS OF THE SETTING**
Three modes	Assist control (AC) (volume ventilation with pre-set volume)
	Synchronized intermittent mandatory ventilation (SIMV) (intermittent volume ventilation with preset volume)
	SIMV with pressure limit control (intermittent *pressure* ventilation—child receives variable volumes as condition changes)
Breath rate	The higher the rate, the less likely spontaneous breaths will occur
Tidal volume	The amount of gas needed to inflate the lungs; based on the child's weight (10 to 15 ml/kg is average); adjusted as the child grows
Inspiratory time	Usually between 0.6 and 1.0 seconds
Pressure limit (maximum amount of airway pressure delivered with each inspiration)	Set in pressure-limited mode
	Usual home pressure limit is 26 to 30 cm H_2O
Positive end expiratory pressure (PEEP) (amount of pressure required to keep lungs from collapsing after expiration)	At home, PEEP usually does not exceed 5 cm H_2O
Oxygen	Usually 40% is maximum used in home setting; not all children require oxygen

---

Box 30-6 Common Indications for the Placement and Use of a Gastrostomy Tube

Poor oral-motor function as a result of CNS damage

Infants who were initially gavage fed and lack sucking skills

Esophageal atresia

Oral and esophageal burns

Infants and children who require high calorie diets and are unable to orally consume sufficient calories

From Paarlberg J, Balint J: Gastrostomy tubes: practical guidelines for home care, *Pediatr Nurs* March/April:99-102, 1985.

---

lodged tube or gastrointestinal symptoms. When a child with a gastrostomy develops vomiting or abdominal distention, tube dysfunction must be considered, as well as gastroenteritis, absorption problems, or other gastrointestinal disorders. It should be noted that children who have had a fundoplication* are unable to vomit.

Emergency Department and nursing interventions. Gastrostomy tube malfunctions are occasionally the chief complaint on arrival in the ED. Because problems such as accidental dislodgement or blockage are not life-threatening emergencies, they are ideally handled outside the ED by the family themselves, the pediatrician, or the specialist. However, if the physician is unavailable or the problem cannot be corrected at home, the child may be brought to the ED. When the child arrives, the nursing history and physical examination focus on problems that may be related to the gastrostomy tube, the gastrointestinal tract, or other associated findings (Box 30-7 and Table 30-3).

Types of gastrostomy tubes. There are two main types of pediatric gastrostomies. The type of gastrostomy and tubing is selected based on the individual needs of the child and the surgeon's personal prefer-

*A fundoplication is a surgical procedure in which the fundus of the stomach is wrapped around the distal esophagus to prevent gastroesophageal reflux.

Box 30-7   Assessment of Gastrostomy Tube Function

Inspect the gastrostomy tube and stoma; note drainage, leakage, and condition of skin around tube
Establish patency of tube by gently flushing
Inspect for abdominal distention
Palpate abdomen; note any rigidity or pain
Inspect any emesis or diarrhea for amount, consistency, color, blood, mucus, guaiac stool

---

ence. The most common gastrostomy requires that a tube remain in place at all times. The second type uses the wall of the stomach to make a kind of permanent tunnel. The tube is inserted when it is time to feed the child.

Indwelling tubes must have a mechanism to maintain placement in the stomach. The Malecot and Pezzar tubes have ends that mushroom out and expand after the tube is inserted into the stomach. Foley catheters, MIC tubes, and Flow-Thru tubes have a small balloon at the tip of the tube. After the tube is inserted into the stomach, the balloon is inflated with water to keep it from coming out.

When the wall of the stomach is made into a

TABLE 30-3	Potential Problems Related to Gastrostomy Tubes
PROBLEM	**INTERVENTIONS**
Blocked tube	Gently milk tube to dislodge blockage
	Try to draw back plunger of syringe to facilitate movement of fluid in tube
	Change tube if necessary
Vomiting and/or diarrhea	If child is otherwise healthy, may indicate that tube has slipped from position
	Gently pull back on tube to assess tube postion
	Assess parent's technique in administration of feeding; rapid feedings may cause vomiting
Abdominal cramping	Assess parent's technique in administration of feeding; feedings that are too cold or given too fast may cause cramping
Leaking around tube	Gently pull back on tube to make sure the inner balloon is snug against the wall of the abdomen
	Change tube as indicated
	If g-button is leaking, the antireflux valve may be stuck in the open position; gently insert the obturator or a small suction catheter into the button until it moves the button back into the closed position
Bleeding/drainage around tube	Minimal amount of bleeding may follow a tube change
	Assess parent's method for securing tube; make sure tube is not being pulled too taut
	Some drainage is normal; apply clean dressing around stoma and change dressing frequently
Accidental dislodgement	Not an emergency, but tube should be reinserted within 1 to 2 hours if possible
	Try to reinsert the tube
	If unable to reinsert, cover site with gauze until tube can be reinserted by specialist

From Paarlberg J, Balint J: Gastrostomy tubes: practical guidelines for home care, *Pediatr Nurs* March/April: 99-102, 1985.

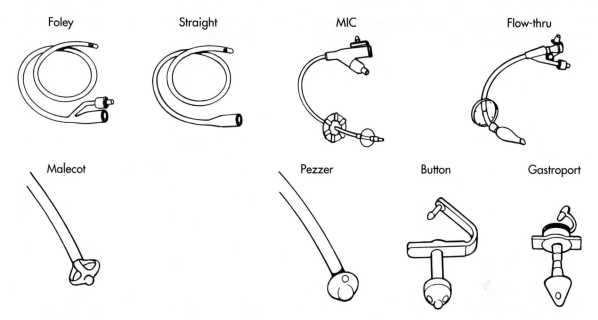

FIG. 30-5. Types of gastrostomy tubes. (From University of Colorado Health Sciences Center, School of Nursing: *Home gastrostomy care for infants and young children,* Lawrence, KS, 1990, Learner Managed Design, Inc.)

permanent tunnel (the Janeway procedure), commonly used tubes include Foley catheters and straight catheters. These types of tubes are inserted into the stoma for feeding and removed when the feeding is complete.[21]

The gastrostomy feeding button has become popular in children for whom long-term enteral feedings are expected. It is a skin-level feeding device that lies flat on the abdomen. A mushroom-like tip expands in the stomach and keeps the tube in place. For feedings, a special adapter is attached to the button and connected to the appropriate feeding tube. The benefits of the gastrostomy button in children include appearance, decreased chance for accidental dislodgement, and increased comfort and mobility.[7] A button can only be inserted after a traditional gastrostomy has been performed and the site is well established (usually after 6 to 12 weeks) (Fig. 30-5).

▮SUMMARY

In summary, the care of children with special needs can be challenging. However, when the child's special needs and communication impairments are approached as areas that require a modified approach to care—but do not change the child's intrinsic value—

the ED visit can be immensely rewarding for the child, the family, and the staff.

REFERENCES

1. American Association on Mental Retardation: *Mental retardation: definition, classification, and systems of supports,* ed 9, Washington DC, 1992, American Association on Mental Retardation.
2. Burke SO et al: Hazardous secrets and reluctantly taking charge: parenting a child with repeated hospitalizations, *Image J Nurs Scholarship* 23:39-45, 1991.
3. Cooley WC, Graham JM Jr: Common syndromes and management issues for primary care physicians. Down syndrome—an update and review for the primary pediatrician, *Clin Pediatr* 30(4):233-253, 1991.
4. Gale CA: Inadequacy of health care for the nation's chronically ill children, *J Pediatr Health Care* 3(1): 20-27, 1989.
5. Green M, Solnit A: Reactions to the threatened loss of a child: a vulnerable child syndrome, *Pediatrics* 34:58-66, 1964.
6. Haley K, ed: *Emergency nursing pediatric course manual,* Chicago, 1993, Emergency Nurses Association.
7. Huth M, O'Brien M: The gastrostomy feeding button, *Pediatr Nurs* 13(4):241-245, 1987.

8. Kenny TJ, Nitz K: Mental retardation. In Hoekelman RA, ed: *Primary pediatric care,* ed 2, St Louis, 1997, Mosby.

9. Lucas J: Ventilator care at home. In Golish J, Sleeper G, O'Ryan J, eds: *Home respiratory care,* Norwalk, CT, 1988, Appleton & Lange.

10. Melnyk BM: Coping with unplanned childhood hospitalization: effects of informational interventions on mothers and children, *Nurs Res* 43(1):50-55, 1994.

11. Miles MS et al: Maternal and paternal stress reactions when a child is hospitalized in a pediatric intensive care unit, *Issues Comprehensive Pediatr Nurs* 7:333-342, 1984.

12. Newacheck PW, Taylor WR: Childhood chronic illness: prevalence, severity and impact, *Am J Public Health* 82(3):364-371, 1992.

13. Orliek SL, Walker MS, Kuhls TL: Severe mycoplasma pneumonia in young children with Down syndrome, *Clin Pediatr* 31(7):409-412, 1992.

14. Paarlberg J, Balint J: Gastrostomy tubes: practical guidelines for home care, *Pediatr Nurs* March/April:99-102, 1985.

15. Perrin JM, MacLean WE Jr: Biomedical and psychosocial dimensions of chronic illness in childhood. In Kavoly P, ed: *Handbook of child health assessment: biosocial perspectives,* New York, 1988, John Wiley.

16. Pueschel SM: The child with Down syndrome. In Levine MD, Carey WB, Crocker AC, ed: *Developmental-behavioral pediatrics,* ed 2, Philadelphia, 1992, WB Saunders.

17. Reynolds S et al: Children with chronic conditions in a pediatric emergency department, *Pediatr Emerg Care* 12(3):166, 1996.

18. Rogers PT: Down syndrome: managing the child and family. In Hoekelman RA et al, ed: *Primary pediatric care,* ed 3, St Louis, 1997, Mosby.

19. Sewell E, Holsclaw P, Schidlow D, McGeady S, Berger B, Kolb S: The use of oxygen for children in their homes. Philadelphia Pediatric Pulmonary Center, Maternal and Children Training Grant #MCJ-009-021-05-01, 1987.

20. *Technology-dependent children: hospital v. home care—a technical memorandum,* OTA-TM-H-38, Washington, DC, 1987, Government Printing Office.

21. University of Colorado Health Sciences Center, School of Nursing: *Home gastrostomy care for infants and young children,* Lawrence, KS, 1990, Learner Managed Design, Inc.

22. Wong DL: *Whaley & Wong's essentials of pediatric nursing,* ed 5, St Louis, 1997, Mosby.

CHAPTER 31

Psychosocial and Behavioral Problems

Melinda Sciera

Pediatric psychosocial and behavioral problems are best dealt with by primary care physicians and professionals skilled in behavioral evaluation. Occasionally, however, the child comes to the emergency department with a complication of his or her disorder, such as a drug overdose or suicidal tendencies, that requires emergency management. Others come to the emergency department because parents or teachers are unable to control or cope with the child's behavior at home or school. Sometimes access to inpatient or acute mental health care is available only through the emergency department.

NURSING HISTORY AND ASSESSMENT

The components of the nursing history and assessment depend on the child's or parents' chief complaint and presenting signs and symptoms. In some cases, particularly those where substance abuse or sexual promiscuity are suspected, it may be best to obtain separate histories from the parent and child. Each viewpoint helps clarify the current problem and direct appropriate interventions. Observation of the family's behavior and interactions during the examination reflects their ability to respond to the child in distress. (Specific information regarding the history and physical examination is offered within each subsequent topic) (Box 31-1).

ADOLESCENT ISSUES

Adolescents deserve special mention because they have unique developmental needs. Risk-taking behaviors, "magical thinking," and a sense of invulnerability all render the adolescent susceptible to traumatic injuries as well as various behavioral disorders.

Sexual experimentation is common among adoles-

Box 31-1 Psychosocial Database

Chief complaint
What is the parent/caregivers' chief concern?

Family composition/dynamics
Who lives in the home, and how does the child react to those living in the home?
Is there any history of mental illness or substance abuse in the family?

Relationship with peers
What is the child's relationship with their peers and members of the opposite sex?

Personal history
Have there been previous behavioral or psychiatric problems?
How has the child adapted to prior psychosocial crises?
Is the child sexually active?
What are the child's habits (e.g., smoking, use of alcohol or drugs)?
What are the child's usual activities outside of school?
How is the child's school performance?

Future plans
What are the child's immediate plans?
Is there suicidal ideation or intent?

Compiled from Adams and Fras, 1988; Hofman and Greydanus, 1989; Wong, 1997.

---

cents as they seek to establish an "adult identity," establish independence, improve self-esteem, and satisfy a need for love and intimacy.[22] By the age of 16 years, 29% of boys and 17% of girls report having had sexual intercourse. These percentages increase dramatically by the age of 18 years, where 65% of boys and 51% of girls report having had sexual intercourse.[39] Approximately 50% of adolescents report not having used contraceptives with their first sexual experience, with younger adolescents less likely than older adolescents to use protection.[28]

APPROACH TO THE ADOLESCENT

The approach to the adolescent in the emergency department is individualized based on their developmental needs.[27] Parental involvement, the content of the questions, the language used, and the style and pace of the interview are all affected by the child's developmental level.

When interviewing an adolescent, the timing, location, and content of the interview are important considerations. In the triage or registration area the adolescent may find it difficult to express the true reason for a visit, particularly if the area is open or visible to others. In this situation the phenomenon of an "imaginary audience" may cause the adolescent to feel as if he or she is on a stage, with all the world watching and judging his or her feelings and actions.[16] They may be embarrassed about their problems or worried about "getting in trouble" with parents or other authority figures. Additionally, "hidden agendas" such as an unwanted pregnancy may be overlooked or not discussed at all.

During the treatment of adolescents, privacy is maintained and modesty respected. Wide variations in growth and development between early and late adolescence means that physiologic, psychologic, and cognitive maturation do not always correlate. Therefore the physically large child who is in early adolescence will likely experience the same degree of anxiety over the suturing of a facial laceration as his or her smaller classmates of the same age.

▌ ATTENTION DEFICIT ▌ HYPERACTIVITY DISORDER

ETIOLOGY

Attention deficit hyperactivity disorder (ADHD) refers to a constellation of behaviors found in school-aged children. It is characterized by developmentally inappropriate problems of inattention, impulsivity, and hyperactivity.[3] The cause of ADHD has not been established; however, the etiology is thought to be of neurologic origin. Although brain damage or brain injury (trauma, infection, central nervous system [CNS] disease) can be associated with ADHD, biologic factors such as prematurity, perinatal asphyxia, or neurologic disorders are thought to be the most common predisposing conditions that produce ADHD.[11] Other factors that correlate with the presence of ADHD include maternal cigarette and alcohol use during pregnancy and genetic factors.[7] Relatives of children with attention deficit disorder (ADD), with or without hyperactivity, have been found to be seven times more likely to be affected than relatives of normal children.[7]

Estimates of the prevalence of this disorder range from 3% to 20% of elementary school children, occurring up to 10 times more often in boys than girls.[13,15] It is estimated that these symptoms persist in as many as 50% to 80% of children with ADHD as they move into adolescence.[56]

PATHOPHYSIOLOGY

Because the etiology of ADHD has not been established, the pathophysiology is not well understood. Disordered pathways between prefrontal and limbic structure, mediated by dopamine and noradrenergic systems, are a suggested cause.[4]

CLINICAL PRESENTATION

Each child with ADHD manifests a different constellation of symptoms, including attention difficulties, impulsivity, and hyperactivity. These behaviors vary in their level of severity. Attention difficulties may result in an inability to complete tasks, poor organizational skills, or high distractibility. Impulsivity manifests as difficulty with self-control, resulting in emotional outbursts and temper tantrums. Lack of self-control may also be seen in stealing, lying, and other acting-out behavior.[26] Hyperactivity is characterized by aimless, non-goal-directed behaviors that range from excessive gross motor activity to subtle fidgeting behaviors. Hyperactivity tends to be worse in group situations, making it difficult to observe during one-to-one medical or psychiatric interviews. The severity of ADHD symptoms is evidenced by the degree of impairment of functioning at home, at school, and with peers (Box 31-2).

EMERGENCY DEPARTMENT INTERVENTIONS

The comprehensive workup required for the diagnosis of ADHD is not appropriate in the emergency department setting. Signs and symptoms consistent with ADHD that are observed in undiagnosed children are documented and communicated to the child's primary care provider. Physical causes for hyperactive behavior, such as the use of asthma medications, should also be considered. Medications administered to treat ADHD include CNS stimulants such as methylphenidate hydrochloride (Ritalin), dextroamphetamine (Dexedrine), or pemoline (Cylert). Methylphenidate hydrochloride is by far the most commonly prescribed medication used to treat ADHD.[53] Dosages are adjusted based on the child's response but generally range from 0.3 to 1.0 mg/kg two to three times a day for school-aged children and 0.3 to 0.5 mg/kg two to three times a day for preschoolers. The primary side effects of the stimulant medications include growth suppression, appetite suppression, and sleep disturbance.

Clonidine 0.1 to 0.2 mg/day has also been used successfully as an alternative to the stimulants in the management of ADHD.[31] The major side effect of clonidine is transient somnolence. Because clonidine is an antihypertensive medication, the child's blood pressure is also monitored.[14]

NURSING CARE AND EVALUATION

Children with ADHD arrive in the emergency department for a variety of reasons. Although children with ADHD rarely present with acute conditions that are directly related to the disorder, exceptions involve consequences of the disorder such as the adolescent who has ingested a toxic substance or one who is exhibiting suicidal tendencies.

Nursing interventions for the child with ADHD include providing for the child's safety, keeping environmental stimuli to a minimum, and assisting with the examination. The child may be disruptive to others and/or damage hospital property. To keep stimulation to a minimum, brief, yet specific explanations of procedures and clearly stated expectations for behavior are beneficial. Limiting the number of care providers with whom the child and family must interact also helps. Age-appropriate diversional activities may maintain the child's attention and cooperation. Parental input on successful behavioral management strategies used at home or school can be invaluable.

▌CONDUCT DISORDERS

ETIOLOGY

A conduct disorder is characterized by a "repetitive and persistent pattern of behavior (lasting at least 6 months), that violates the basic rights of others or age-appropriate societal rules."[3] The etiology of conduct disorders is complex and not completely understood. Problematic behaviors include stealing, running away, lying, setting fires, truancy, vandalism, destruction of others' property, rape, fights involving weapons, or cruelty to animals. Such delinquent behavior is approximately five times more common in boys, and boys are more likely to inflict violent behavior on others.[26] Aggressive or violent acts often result in incarceration of the child (Box 31-3).

PATHOPHYSIOLOGY

Although the pathophysiology leading to a conduct disorder is unknown, some suggested etiologies include biochemical abnormalities of the CNS, such as decreased levels of serotonin and dopamine β-hydroxylase[9,47] and excessive testosterone levels in males,[38] both of which have been documented is aggressive behavior. Other factors, such as CNS injury or parental psychopathology have also been implicated.

CLINICAL PRESENTATION

Children with conduct disorders may come to the emergency department with anger, hostility, and/or anxiety. Physiologic signs of *anxiety,* which often precede aggressive and violent behavior, include increased heart rate and respiratory rate, sweating, dry

---

Box 31-3   DSM-IV Diagnostic Criteria for Conduct Disorder

Presence of at least three of the following criteria in the past 12 months, with at least one criterion present in the past 6 months:

- Aggression to people and animals
- Destruction of property
- Deceitfulness or theft
- Serious violations of rules (e.g., staying out late at night despite parental rules, running away from home, truant from school) or prohibitions, beginning before age 13 years

Modified from American Psychiatric Association: *Diagnostic and statistical manual of mental disorders,* ed 4, Washington, DC, 1992, American Psychiatric Press.

---

mouth, nausea, and palpitations. Other symptoms include feelings of tension, talk with increased pitch and volume, difficulty with attention span, or hyperactivity with pacing, hand tremors, and wringing of the hands.[40]

The *angry child* may demonstrate an increased tone of voice and facial expressions, including flaring nostrils, a flushed face, and tight lips.[46] Deliberate pacing, clenched fists, crossed arms, and hands resting on the hips are additional signs of anger. The child may also be demanding and sarcastic.

Hostile children are more often adolescents. They may be aggressive and demonstrate a lack of impulse control. They have difficulty controlling their voices and may be verbally abusive. Restlessness and agitation are often observed. Other symptoms include homicidal or suicidal ideation.

EMERGENCY DEPARTMENT INTERVENTIONS

The goals for managing aggressive and disruptive children in the emergency department include (1) ensuring the safety of the child, staff, and family; (2) ruling out possible underlying medical conditions that may be contributing to behavior; and (3) making appropriate referrals for individual and/or family counseling.[26] Disposition of the child, whether it be admission, incarceration, or discharge, usually requires the input of social workers, psychiatric health care providers, and/or law enforcement officers.

NURSING CARE AND EVALUATION

The child with a conduct disorder may endanger himself or herself, staff, visitors, or other patients. Nursing care is therefore aimed primarily at providing a safe environment for the child.

The most effective method of controlling potentially volatile situations is early recognition of signs of hostile and aggressive behavior, including anxiety and anger. Early recognition allows time to defuse or control the situation before it escalates. The child displaying a high level of anxiety or anger is not left unattended. Environmental stimuli are reduced, and verbal interactions are limited to short, simple sentences.[48] If the child is angry, interventions are best provided on a one-on-one basis using a calm, clear but firm voice.[48] Limits are set in terms of appropriate behavior and language.

Hostile children require immediate intervention. These children are kept in a quiet, secure area where stimuli are reduced. The hostile child is never approached by a single staff member in a secluded area. When these children are approached, an "escape route" is maintained for both the nurse and the child, and a safe distance (at least 3 feet) is maintained from the child. When communicating with the child the nurse maintains eye contact, speaks firmly, and calmly conveys expectations for the child's immediate behavior. The consequences of negative behavior are also conveyed. Verbalization is kept to a minimum, and arguing is avoided.

Objects in the immediate environment that could be potential weapons, including call light cords, jewelry, and stethoscopes, are identified and removed. External control provided by the use of restraints may help a child feel safe and regain personal control.[26] The child in physical restraints is supervised at all times by emergency department staff or a parent/caregiver. Institutional policies regarding the use of restraints, frequency of release (for hygiene and range of motion exercises), and documentation is followed. Once medical or toxicologic causes of out-of-control behavior are ruled out, pharmacologic restraints may be necessary. Benzodiazepines, such as lorazepam, or antipsychotics, such as haloperidol or chlorpromazine, may be administered to control acute agitation.

▌ DEPRESSION AND SUICIDE

Depression and suicidal behavior are major contributing factors to the morbidity and mortality of children and adolescents. The relationship between depression and suicide is by no means straightforward. While the two problems overlap, they are not synonymous.[3] As in adults, depressed children are not necessarily suicidal, and many who are suicidal are not depressed.

DEPRESSION

Etiology. Childhood depression includes a number of affective disorders, or disturbances in mood/affect, which vary in severity and duration.[55] The cause of depression in children and adolescents is unknown. Although many factors have been associated with an increased incidence of childhood depression, the single most important risk factor seems to be the affliction of at least one parent with an affective disorder. Depression in the child is therefore thought to be both genetic and caused by the inability of the parent to provide effective and appropriate parenting.

The rate of occurrence of depression depends on the child's age. Rates among prepubertal children vary, depending on the source of sample data, from 0.3% (in preschoolers) to 2% of all prepubertal children.[55] Incidence in the adolescent population is difficult to quantify because of the lack of a generally agreed-upon definition of depression and the varying nature of populations studied. However, estimates range from 20% to 33%.[26]

Pathophysiology. The pathophysiology of depression is unclear; however, the strong association of depression with genetics has led to much research related to neurotransmitters and biogenic amines. These studies have suggested abnormalities in noradrenergic and serotonergic neurotransmission.[8]

Clinical presentation. The clinical manifestations of depression vary with developmental stage, Box 31-4 describes characteristics of depression in children of all ages.

Emergency Department interventions. When the depressed child or the child suspected to be depressed arrives in the emergency department, the first goal of care is to identify suicide potential by direct questioning of the child and/or parents. The child or adolescent who admits to suicidal ideation requires psychiatric consultation.

Emergency department treatment requires providing for the safe disposition of the child (e.g., admission or discharge with outpatient mental health follow-up care). Although antidepressants may be required for treatment of the disorder, these drugs are not pre-

---

Box 31-4   Factors Associated with Depression

Past history:
Illnesses, especially chronic conditions[5]
Physical abuse[32]
Genetic factors, especially parent with affective disorder[10]
School problems, including learning disabilities[26]
ADHD[26]

Clinical manifestations:
Decreased initiative and responsiveness to stimulation; apathy
Sadness, dejection, gloominess
Decreased attachment or social withdrawal
Irritability, self-criticism, mood swings, cries easily
Weight loss, loss of appetite
Somatic complaints
Academic problems
Changes in sleep behavior

---

scribed in the emergency department because follow-up cannot be assured and the positive effects of the drug may decrease the probability the family will pursue ongoing care.[26]

Nursing care and evaluation. When the depressed child or the child suspected to be depressed arrives in the emergency department, an evaluation of suicide potential is made. If suicide potential is high, the child is triaged emergently and placed in an area visible to staff. A safe environment is provided by removing objects that may be used to inflict self-injury. A caregiver or parent should remain with the child (also see the discussion of nursing care and evaluation in suicide attempts).

SUICIDE ATTEMPTS

Etiology. Suicide is rare in young children. Although school-aged children express suicidal ideation, cognitive immaturity probably prevents planning and executing a lethal attempt.[50] Suicide attempts increase with age, however, and the sharpest increase occurs after 16 years of age.[50] In children between the ages of 10 and 19 years, suicide accounts for 10% of all deaths.[19] Suicide is the second leading cause of death in adolescents between 15 and 19 years of age.[52]

Pathophysiology. Many factors are associated with suicidal behavior in children and adolescents. Suicide attempts may be precipitated by acute stress, including interpersonal loss (the death of a friend or relative), a disciplinary or legal crisis (being reported for cheating or truancy at school or being arrested), peer humiliation, or the threatened or actual break-up with a boyfriend or girlfriend.[50] Specific risk factors that suggest a child is at risk for completed suicide or for reattempts at suicide include a constellation of behaviors, including (1) previous suicide attempts; (2) early sexual behavior; (3) substance abuse; (4) trouble in school and with law enforcement; and (5) depression[17] (Box 31-5).

Adolescent females are more likely to attempt suicide using nonlethal methods (especially pills). Adolescent males tend to choose more lethal means, such as firearms and hanging. Males are therefore approximately four to five times as likely to commit "successful" suicide.

Clinical presentation. The presentation of the child after a suicide attempt depends on the type and lethality of the method used, as well as the time elapsed since the event. In adolescents, drug overdoses are the most common emergency department presentation. Ingestions usually involve prescription drugs found within the household or common over-the-counter medications such as acetaminophen or ibuprofen. Other methods include wrist slashing, lethal weapons, hangings, or car crashes. The child's condition on arrival in the emergency department may range from awake and alert to comatose. Combative behavior may be displayed, especially if alcohol or drugs were involved.

Pediatric suicidal behavior is most commonly an impulsive attempt to obtain attention or signal the need for help, without any attempt to cause serious injury or death (suicidal gesture). After a suicidal gesture, adolescents frequently inform friends or family members, which results in a "rescue" from harm. Occasionally, severely depressed adolescents are intent on killing themselves and conceal their plans from everyone. Social isolation appears to be the most significant distinguishing factor characteristic of "successful" vs "unsuccessful" suicides.[58]

Emergency Department interventions. When the child who has attempted suicide arrives in the emergency department, initial interventions first address stabilization of the airway, breathing, and circulation (ABCs) and the treatment of life-threatening conditions. Once physiologic stability has been achieved, evaluation of the suicide attempt begins. Three dimensions are considered in the evaluation of the suicide attempt, including (1) medical lethality, (2) suicidal intent, and (3) strengths and supports available to the youth.[26] Disposition of the child depends on the child's medical condition, emotional stability, and suicidal intent as well as the family's ability to monitor the child at home. If the potential for a repeat attempt is high, the child is admitted and one-to-one nurse care arranged. Discharge of the child who has attempted suicide is only considered when the risk for a repeat attempt is low and only into a situation in which the family is willing and able to monitor the child's behavior. Specific follow-up care must be assured (Box 31-6).

Nursing care and evaluation. The child who has attempted suicide is triaged emergently. Because suicide attempts are not always obvious on presentation to the emergency department, any child or adolescent who has "accidental" or otherwise "unintentional" injuries, especially if high risk factors are present, is questioned directly for the possibility of suicidal intent.

Box 31-5   Risk Factors for Suicidal Behavior

Psychiatric illness
  Mood disorders, including depression
  Conduct disorders
  Psychosis
  Family history of mood disorders and
    suicide
Substance abuse
Past suicide attempts
Chronic physical illnesses, such as seizure disorders
Environmental factors
  History of abuse or neglect
  Parental discord or absence
  Suicide of friend or admired figure
  Multiple stressors
  Availability of firearms

Adapted from Barnett TM: Psychiatric and behavioral disorders. In Barkin RM, ed: *Pediatric emergency medicine: concepts and clinical practice,* St Louis, 1992, Mosby.

After assessment and stabilization of the ABCs, the child or adolescent requires close observation of both physiologic parameters and mood. Placing the child in an area that allows privacy but is still visible to staff facilitates observation. The child's environment is assessed and consideration given to the potential lethality of equipment and supplies such as monitor lead wires, scissors, electrical outlets, windows, and other objects that might be used in a repeat attempt. Physical restraints may be necessary to protect the child from further self-inflicted harm.

Barriers to providing empathetic care to suicidal youngsters and their families include (1) ambivalence regarding the seriousness of the attempt; (2) negative attitudes toward the treatment of this type of emergency in a medical setting; (3) high levels of distress arising from forcing the patient to perform such unpleasant activities as drinking charcoal; and (4) feelings toward the parents of the patient, such as blame for the suicide attempt and anger for interrupting work with questions regarding their child's care.[45] By recognizing these barriers, nurses can provide more comprehensive and compassionate care to the child who has attempted suicide.

Parents and family members also require support and understanding. A useful therapeutic intervention for the family is to encourage them to verbalize their feelings. Families of suicidal children may benefit from a referral to family counseling.

If the child is to be discharged, the parents are consulted. If they feel competent to care for the child at home, they are provided with a list of warning signs of depression or suicidal behavior. The parents are also provided with follow-up care recommendations (Box 31-7).

Box 31-6 Assessing Childhood and Adolescent Suicidal Intent

Circumstances of suicide attempt
  Nature of suicide attempt (pills vs violent means)
  Use of multiple methods
  Method used to extreme (all vs some pills ingested)
  Suicide note written
  Secrecy of attempt (attempt concealed vs revealed)
  Premeditation (impulsive vs long-planned attempt)
  History of prior attempts
Child self-report
  Premeditation of attempt
  Anticipation of death
  Desire for death
  Attempt to conceal attempt
  Nature of precipitating stresses
Child mental status
  Orientation/cognitive intactness
  Presence/absence of psychosis
  Manner of relating to physician
  Current suicidality
    Response to being saved/being unsuccessful in attempt
    Active plan for another attempt
    Readiness to discuss stresses
    Readiness to accept external and family support
Nature of orientation toward future

From Hodas GR, Sargent J: Psychiatric emergencies. In Fleisher G, Ludwig S, eds: *Textbook of pediatric emergency medicine,* ed 3, Philadelphia, 1993, Williams & Wilkins.

Box 31-7 Prevention of Childhood and Adolescent Suicide: Warning Signs for Parents

Withdrawal (from peers, parents, siblings)
Somatic complaints
Irritability
Crying
Diminished school performance
Sad or anxious appearance
Significant loss (rejection by peer group, breakup of romance, poor grades, failure to achieve important goal)
Major event or change within family
Casual mention of suicide or being "better off dead"
Explicit suicide threat
Minor, seemingly unimportant suicide "gestures"
Apparent "accidents"
Other unusual behavior patterns—housebound behavior, breaking curfew, running away, drug or alcohol abuse, bizarre or antisocial actions

From Hodas GR, Sargent J: Psychiatric emergencies. In Fleisher G, Ludwig S, eds: *Textbook of pediatric emergency medicine,* ed 3, Philadelphia, 1993, Williams & Wilkins.

EATING DISORDERS

ETIOLOGY

Eating disorders such as anorexia nervosa and bulimia nervosa are characterized by persistent concerns with one's body shape and size. Eating disorders most commonly occur in white upper middle-class female adolescents, with the peak age of onset being 14 to 18 years of age. While there is continuing debate over specific defining criteria for anorexia nervosa and bulimia nervosa, many experts suggest that they are actually a continuum of disorders.[37] In general, bulimia nervosa is characterized by binge eating followed by self-induced vomiting and/or the use of cathartics. Anorexia nervosa is characterized by refusal to maintain body weight because of intense fear of becoming fat, even though the child may be underweight[3] (Boxes 31-8 and 31-9).

Theories regarding the etiology of eating disorders reflect their complexity and suggest an interaction between familial (genetic and sociocultural), individual (neurochemical and developmental), social, and cultural factors.[37] The incidence of anorexia nervosa has increased approximately 500% in the past three decades.[43] The current incidence of anorexia among females is 0.5% to 1%, and the incidence of bulimia is 1% to 3%.[35] Bulimia tends to start later in adolescence than anorexia.

PATHOPHYSIOLOGY

Treatable medical conditions are present in one third to one half of all patients with eating disorders;[20] however, physical complications of these disorders can involve nearly every organ system. Life-threatening complications result from disturbances in fluid and electrolyte balance, the gastrointestinal system, the cardiopulmonary system, and the CNS, which are described in Table 31-1. Other complications include endocrine dysfunction, with alterations in hypothalamic and pituitary function. Amenorrhea is common and results primarily from malnutrition. Most patients report irregular or absent menstrual periods at weights less than 15% below ideal body weight.[57] Evidence of relative hypothyroidism, with dry skin, hair loss, hypothermia, and hyporeflexia, may also be seen.[54] Thermoregulatory dysfunction is common and results in lowered body temperature and inability to respond to changes in environmental temperature.[20]

Bone marrow suppression, secondary to malnutrition, can lead to leukopenia, anemia, and, rarely, thrombocytopenia. White blood cell counts in the range of 2500 to 4000 cells/mm^3 are not uncommon, with both relative neutropenia and lymphopenia, as well as hemoglobin values of 10.5 to 12.5 g/dl.[44]

Box 31-8   DSM-IV Diagnostic Criteria for Anorexia Nervosa

- Refusal to maintain body weight over a minimal normal weight for age and height (e.g., weight loss resulting in body weight 15% below that expected or failure to gain weight as expected during period of growth, resulting in weight 15% below that expected)
- Intense fear of gaining weight or becoming fat, even though underweight
- Disturbance in perception of one's body weight, size, or shape (e.g., self-perception of being "fat" when in fact emaciated or perception of "fat thighs" when underweight)
- In females, absence of at least three consecutive menstrual cycles when otherwise expected to occur (primary or secondary amenorrhea)

Adapted from American Psychiatric Association: *Diagnostic and statistical manual of mental disorders*, ed 4, Washington, D.C., 1992, American Psychiatric Press.

Box 31-9   DSM-IV Diagnostic Criteria for Bulimia Nervosa

- Recurrent episodes of binge eating (rapid consumption of large amount of food in brief period of time)
- Feeling of lack of control over eating behavior during binge episodes
- Self-induced vomiting, use of laxatives or diuretics, strict dieting or fasting, or vigorous exercise to prevent weight gain
- Minimum average of two binge eating episodes a week for at least 3 months
- Persistent overconcern with body shape and weight

Adapted from American Psychiatric Association: *Diagnostic and statistical manual of mental disorders*, ed 4, Washington, D.C., 1992, American Psychiatric Press.

TABLE 31-1	Complications of Eating Disorders	
CATEGORY	**COMPLICATIONS**	**ETIOLOGY**
Fluid and electrolyte disturbances	Abnormal serum levels of sodium, potassium, chloride, bicarbonate, blood urea nitrogen	Vomiting Use of diuretics Diarrhea from laxatives Restricted fluid intake
	Dehydration	Diarrhea related to laxative use
	Hypochloremic metabolic alkalosis	
Gastrointestinal disorders	Decreased cardiac sphincter tone leading to spontaneous vomiting without need for mechanical stimulation and gastroesophageal reflux	Vomiting
	Mallory-Weiss tear (esophageal rupture)	
Cardiopulmonary disorders	Decreased heart size and cardiac mass	Malnutrition
	Pericardial effusion	Fluid/electrolyte imbalance
	Electrocardiographic abnormalities	Electrolye imbalance; use of syrup of ipecac
	Subcutaneous emphysema; pneumomediastinum	Vomiting
Neurologic disturbances	Seizures (rare)	Electrolyte imbalance
	Muscle weakness	Malnutrition/weight loss

CLINICAL PRESENTATION

The clinical presentation of the child with an eating disorder varies, depending on the severity, nature, and duration of the problem. Vital sign alterations, such as slow heart rate (under 60 beats/min), low blood pressure, postural hypotension, and subnormal temperature (less than 36°F), commonly result from decreased metabolism, diminished cardiac output, and thermoregulatory dysfunction. The recurrent vomiting associated with bulimia may be associated with the erosion of tooth enamel and/or dryness or irritation of the oral mucosa from the acid pH of regurgitated stomach contents.[1] Self-induced vomiting may also result in scars or calluses on the knuckles (Russell's sign), as well as purpura or petechiae on the face or subconjunctival hemorrhage caused by increased intrathoracic pressure. The gag reflex may also be diminished. Other common signs and symptoms of an eating disorder includes fatigue, dizziness/fainting, swollen extremities, constipation, missed or irregular menses, and a sad facial expression. Dermatologic manifestations of malnutrition include (1) growth of fine lanugo-like hair on the face, back, arms, or legs; (2) loss of subcutaneous fat; (3) pedal or pretibial edema; (3) orange discoloration of the skin secondary to increased ingestion of yellow (low-calorie) vegetables; (4) brittle hair and nails; and (5) dry, cold, scaly skin.[20]

EMERGENCY DEPARTMENT INTERVENTIONS

The first priority of care for the child with a suspected or known eating disorder is to evaluate the child's physiologic status and to treat life-threatening disorders. The degree of diagnostic testing and the extent of treatment depend on the child's history and clinical presentation. Baseline diagnostic testing to determine the severity of nutritional deficits and electrolyte disturbances includes a complete blood count (CBC), serum electrolyte levels, urinalysis, and an electrocardiogram (ECG). Additional testing, such as magnetic resonance imaging (MRI), computerized tomography (CT) scans, or an upper or lower gastrointestinal series, may be required to rule out an organic cause for weight loss, such as malignancies, inflammatory bowel disease, or malabsorption disorders.

Fluid and electrolyte imbalances are treated with intravenous fluid and electrolyte therapy (see Chapter 14, Fluid and Electrolyte Disorders). Pharmacologic management of complications of the eating disorder may or may not be useful. For example, inotropic or chronotropic agents are not effective when, as in the case of an eating disorder, bradycardia represents compensation for a hypometabolic state.[34]

The course of treatment and disposition of the child require evaluation of the history, physical examination, and diagnostic testing as well as the child's emotional status. Severe emotional or physiologic disturbances indicate the need for hospital admission. If a child is to be discharged, the family and child are referred for multidisciplinary interventions, including medical, behavioral, individual psychiatric, and family therapy.

NURSING CARE AND EVALUATION

Adolescents with eating disorders may come to the emergency department before diagnosis with related or unrelated complaints. More commonly, however, they come after diagnosis with severe weight loss and complications of the disorder. The child with a suspected or known eating disorder who arrives with signs of dehydration or shock, bradycardia, or hypothermia is triaged emergently.

If the child's condition is undiagnosed, suspicion of an eating disorder is initially aroused when the adolescent is found to have severe weight loss, an electrolyte imbalance secondary to vomiting or the use of laxatives or diuretics, or ketonuria related to starvation. Behavioral characteristics associated with an eating disorder may be identified during the history-taking process or in general conversation with the child or parent[37] (Table 31-2).

When a eating disorder is suspected, a detailed

TABLE 31-2	Behavioral Characteristics of Anorexia and Bulimia Nervosa	
CHARACTERISTICS	**ANOREXIA NERVOSA**	**BULIMIA NERVOSA**
Drive for thinness	Feels fat when thin	Seeks to avoid obesity
Body image	Distorted, severely; preoccupation with weight	Distorted to varying degrees; preoccupation with weight
Self-concept deficit	Low self-esteem; lack of trust	Low self-esteem; lack of trust
Food-related behaviors	Food rituals	Chaotic eating patterns
	Rigid eating patterns	Binges (composed of large amounts of food in a short period of time) when feeling bored, angry, depressed, lonely
	Calorically dense foods avoided	
	Sudden increase in cooking, diet books, calories	
		Fad diets—vomits, fasts, exercises after meals
		Ingests laxatives, diuretics, ipecac to promote weight loss
Individual personality characteristics	Perfectionistic	Impulsive
	Obsessive	Mood swings
Miscellaneous behaviors	Repetitive, frequent exercise	Wears baggy clothes to hide weight loss
	Co-addictions possible	Repetitive, frequent exercise
	Wears baggy clothes	Co-addictions possible
	Social withdrawal	Social withdrawal
	Decreased school performance or increased effort to maintain performance	

From Connolly C, Corbett-Dick P: *J School Health* 60(8):403, 1990.

weight history is obtained. Eating behaviors, including patterns of binge eating, restriction of intake, and purging, are explored. Information regarding the child's relationships with parents and peers, school performance, sexual activity, and substance abuse is also important. Parental input regarding the child's eating behaviors and demeanor is also useful.

The physical examination involves obtaining a weight measurement and a full set of vital signs, including oral temperature, respiratory rate, orthostatic blood pressure, and apical pulse measured in lying, sitting, and standing positions. While the practitioner is performing the physical examination, the child is observed for physiologic manifestations of malnutrition, repetitive vomiting, and laxative and/or diuretic use. Although these children are often hypothermic, warming measures, such as a hypothermia units, are contraindicated because the hypothermia is a result of low caloric intake. Emergency nursing interventions, in addition to stabilization of the ABCs, include frequent monitoring of the child for changes in cardiovascular and neurologic status and keeping the family updated regarding the plan of care. If the child is not admitted to the hospital, referral for long-term follow-up care is essential.

▌SUBSTANCE ABUSE

Substance abuse is a problem of increasing significance for society. Children and adolescents are not immune and are at particularly high risk for associated problems. Experimentation at a young age can interfere with normal psychosocial development, lead to more serious substance abuse, and disrupt school performance and social relationships with family and friends.[21] In early adolescence, tobacco and alcohol are the most commonly abused substances.[42] Among older adolescents, the degree of substance abuse rises but is likely to be underestimated, since surveys do not reach school dropouts, a group that tends to be involved in heavier drug use.

Substance abuse problems that precipitate an emergency department visit range from acute intoxication, withdrawal, and associated unintentional trauma (e.g., motor vehicle crashes, falls, near-drowning) to life-threatening medical complications. Behavioral changes and parental desire for drug testing may also bring the substance-abusing adolescent to the emergency department.[18]

PATHOPHYSIOLOGY AND CLINICAL PRESENTATION

CNS stimulants

Amphetamines. Amphetamines are CNS stimulants that are generally taken orally, but may be used intravenously or subcutaneously (called "skin popping"). Mild doses produce increased energy, euphoria, dilated pupils, flushed skin, and decreased ability to sleep. Increased doses produce restlessness, irritability, tremors, hyperreflexia, diaphoresis, and body temperature elevation. Severe side effects include cardiovascular toxicity and CNS toxicity. Cardiovascular toxicity produces hypertension and dysrhythmias. Severe hypertension can lead to encephalopathy or intracerebral hemorrhage. Common dysrhythmias include sinus tachycardia, atrial tachycardia, and ventricular tachycardia. CNS toxicity may be evidenced by agitation, hyperactivity, seizures, hemorrhage, or stroke.[23] Acute toxicity can produce paranoid symptoms and result in spontaneous violence.[24]

Cocaine. Cocaine is a CNS stimulant that is generally snorted or smoked but may also be injected. Because it is readily absorbed through the mucous membranes, effects are felt within minutes. CNS stimulation results in euphoria and a sense of well-being. With long-term use, autonomic stimulation can produce hypertension and tachycardia. Excessive stimulation of the CNS and autonomic nervous system is responsible for most toxic manifestations.[23] Dysrhythmias associated with cocaine use include sinus tachycardia, ventricular fibrillation, atrial tachycardia and fibrillation, ventricular tachycardia, and asystole.[41] Myocardial infarction, aortic dissection, and pulmonary edema represent severe adverse sequelae. Neurologic complications include headache, subarachnoid hemorrhage, stroke, and seizures. Other severe complications include renal infarction, hepatotoxicity, and rhabdomyolysis (muscle necrosis).

Sedatives/hypnotics.

The sedative/hypnotic group of drugs includes barbiturates, methaqualone, alcohol, and benzodiazepines. Effects include sedation or somnolence as well as "mellowness" when awake. Overdose, especially of the barbiturates and similar compounds, can be fatal, as can the combined use of benzodiazepines and alcohol.[24]

Alcohol. Ethanol alcohol is an intoxicating agent that is absorbed into the bloodstream largely via the intestinal tract and, to a smaller extent, through the stomach. The rate of absorption is affected by many factors, including the rate of ingestion of the alcohol, the rate of gastric emptying (i.e., the presence of food in the stomach), and the age, sex, and size of the child.

The most notable acute manifestations of alcohol ingestion are the effects on the CNS, which include slurred speech, gait disturbances, dulled reflexes, and personality changes such as belligerence, irritability, euphoria, and lack of social inhibition. When the blood alcohol level rises rapidly, memory blackouts may occur. Severe CNS effects include sedation, coma, and/or seizures. An alcohol overdose can result in death (also see Chapter 27, Environmental and Toxicologic Emergencies).

Hallucinogens. Hallucinogens include lysergic acid diethylamide (LSD), phencyclidine (angel dust), mescaline, and marijuana. Intoxication varies from mild stimulation, euphoria, enhanced senses, and increased energy to hallucinations, altered sensorium, and disorientation.[24]

Phencyclidine. Phencyclidine (PCP) was originally developed as an anesthetic agent with analgesic and depressant properties. Other effects include sympathomimetic and CNS stimulation. PCP can be used orally or nasally, or it can be mixed with marijuana or tobacco and smoked.[23] Disorientation, slurred speech, ataxia, muscle rigidity, and myoclonic jerks may result from acute intoxication. Nystagmus is a characteristic physical finding. Psychologic manifestations such as paranoia, auditory hallucinations, and violent behavior are the most obvious adverse reactions associated with drug use. Adverse physical findings can include hypertension, diaphoresis, tremors, tachycardia, respiratory depression, dysrhythmias, coma, or seizures.

Marijuana (Cannabis). Marijuana is a plant substance that is generally smoked but occasionally eaten. Intoxication results in a euphoric sedation with a heightening of the senses, including hunger. Tachycardia or sensory effects may precipitate a panic or anxiety attack at the onset of use, characterized by palpitations, hyperventilation, apprehension, and the feeling of imminent death.[51] Pleasurable but sometimes frightening sensory stimuli can occur, including streaks or trails of light following the movement of objects across the field of vision. Toxic delirium from marijuana use is rare.

Opioids. Opioids or narcotics are a group of drugs that include morphine, heroin, codeine, and methadone. Drug use results in sedation, analgesia, and euphoria. While heroin and other narcotics are not frequently a drug of choice for adolescents, oral narcotics may be used in combination with other drugs. The major effects of opioids include CNS depression and decreased gastric motility. Flushed and itchy skin can also occur. Overdoses of narcotics can rapidly produce respiratory depression or arrest, coma, and bradycardia. Narcotic antagonists such as naloxone are used to reverse adverse affects.

Inhalants and volatile substances. Inhalants such as glue, toluene, and other hydrocarbons produce euphoric effects that can be sought by children as young as in grade school. These substances are inexpensive and tend to be readily available.[36] Toxicity may result in asphyxia or hypoxemia, with respiratory depression and hypoventilation. CNS effects can include hallucinations, ataxia, confusion, seizures, and coma. Cardiac depression may result in dysrhythmias or cardiovascular collapse.[23]

EMERGENCY DEPARTMENT AND NURSING INTERVENTIONS

The child who is suspected of substance abuse is triaged emergently on arrival in the emergency department. Initial interventions require assessment and stabilization of the ABCs, obtaining a full set of vital signs, and attaching the child to a heart rate monitor and pulse oximeter. A thorough history is obtained, including information from paramedics and/or family and friends to determine the nature of the ingestion[23] (see also Chapter 27, Environmental and Toxicologic Emergencies).

Diagnostic testing includes obtaining blood for toxicologic and metabolic studies. Toxicology screening tests performed on blood or urine specimens are sometimes limited in the types of agents measured. They can, however, be helpful in confirming suspicions regarding a particular ingested substance. As with all patients who present acutely with a decreased level of consciousness, determination of blood glucose level by the rapid finger-stick/reagent strip method is performed. If the source of the ingestion is unknown, and intravenous access has been established, the universal antidotes dextrose and naloxone (Narcan) may be ordered.

Nursing care requires constant bedside management of the child with frequent assessments for signs of respiratory depression, compromised airway, cardiovascular instability (hypotension, hypertension, bradycardia, dysryhthmias), and neurologic compro nise. Temperature management may be required if he child is hyperthermic or hypothermic. All intake nd output are monitored. A calm, quiet atmosphere s provided, and the child and family are continuously eassured.

RUNAWAY/HOMELESS CHILDREN AND ADOLESCENTS

lightly more than 1 million adolescents run away rom home each year. They may be motivated to leave nome for various reasons, including physical and/or exual abuse, severe family discord, conflicts in school or in social relationships, economic hardship within he family, early pregnancy, and personal or family drug/alcohol abuse.[33]

Homeless youth frequently come to the emer- gency department seeking medical care as well as helter. Inadequate environmental and nutritional conditions may predispose them to health problems requiring acute intervention. Some exchange sexual ctivity for money, food, shelter, or drugs (referred o as "survival sex"). These behaviors result in sexu- lly transmitted diseases or pregnancy. While it is not uncommon for an adolescent to come to the emer- gency department without a parent or other care- giver, a safe destination at discharge should be en- ured. Social services may be enlisted to assist with he child's discharge.

SUMMARY

Children and adolescents come to the emergency department with a variety of behavioral, psychosocial, nd/or psychiatric disorders. The basis for these disorders may be a combination of biopsychosocial actors. Evaluation and management require an un- lerstanding of child and adolescent development and pplication of this knowledge using a family-centered pproach.

REFERENCES

1. Abrams RA, Ruff JC: Oral signs and symptoms in the diagnosis of bulimia, *JADA* 113:761-764, 1986.
2. Adams P, Fras I: *Beginning child psychiatry*, New York, 1988, Brunner/Mazel.
3. American Psychiatric Association: *Diagnostic and statistical manual of mental disorders*, ed 4, Wash- ington, DC, 1992, American Psychiatric Associa- tion.
4. Anthony BJ, Phillips S: Attention deficit hyperactiv- ity disorder. In McAnarney ER et al, eds: *Textbook of Adolescent Medicine*, Philadelphia, 1992, WB Saunders.
5. Austin J: Assessment of coping mechanisms used by parents and children with chronic illness; *MCN* 15:98-102, 1990.
6. Barnett TM. Psychiatric and behavioral disorders. In Barkin RM, ed: *Pediatric emergency medicine: con- cepts and clinical practice*, St Louis, 1992, Mosby.
7. Biederman J et al: Family-genetic and psychosocial risk factors in DSM-III attention deficit disorder, *Child Adolesc Psychiatry* 29:526, 1990.
8. Brent DA: Depression and suicide in children and adolescents, *Pediatr Rev* 14(10):380-388, 1993.
9. Brown GL et al: Aggression, suicide and serotonin: relationships to CSF amine levels, *Am J Psychiatry* 139:741, 1982.
10. Carlson GA, Cantwell DP: Suicidal behavior and depression in children and adolescents, *J Am Acad Child Adolesc Psychiatry* 21:4, 361-368, 1982.
11. Clunn P: Disruptive behavior disorders of early childhood. In Clunn P, ed: *Child psychiatric nursing*, Philadelphia, 1991, Mosby.
12. Connolly C, Corbett-Dick P: Eating disorders: a framework for school nursing initiatives, *J School Health* 60(8):401-405, 1990.
13. Copeland L, Wolraich M: Disorders of behavioral development: attention deficit hyperactivity disor- der. In Wolraich ML, ed: *The practical assessment and management of children with disorders of development and learning*, Chicago, 1987, Year Book.
14. Culbert TP, Banez GA, Reiff MI: Children who have attentional disorders: interventions, *Pediatr Rev* 15(1):5-14, 1994.
15. Dulcan MK: Attention deficit disorder: evaluation and treatment, *Pediatr Ann* 14:383-398, 1985.
16. Elkind D: Understanding the young adolescent, *Adolescence* 55:126, 1978.
17. Ensminger MD: Adolescent sexual behavior as it relates to other transition behaviors in youth. In Hoffert SL, Hayes CD, eds: *Risking the future: adolescent sexuality, pregnancy and childbearing*, Washington, DC, 1987, National Academy of Sci- ences.
18. Felter R, Izsak E, Lawrence HS: Emergency depart- ment management of the intoxicated adolescent, *Pediatr Clin North Am* 34:399-421, 1987.
19. Fingerhut LA, Kleinman JC: *Trends and current status in childhood mortality, United States, 1900-85, Vital and Health Statistics*, Series 3, No.2 (DHHS Publication No. PHS 89-1410), Hyattsville, MD, 1989, National Center for Health Statistics.
20. Fisher M: Medical complications of anorexia and bulimia nervosa, *Adolesc Med* 3(3):487-502, 1992.
21. Gans JE, Blyth DA, Elster AB: *America's adolescents: how healthy are they? Profiles of Adolescent Health Series* Vol 1, Chicago, 1990, American Medical Association.

22. Grace E, Strasburger V: Normal sexuality. In McAnarney ER et al, eds: *Textbook of adolescent medicine,* Philadelphia, 1992, WB Saunders.

23. Graham CJ: Emergency care of the substance-abusing adolescent, *Adolesc Med* 4(1):167-180, 1993.

24. Halikas J: Substance abuse in children and adolescents. In Garfinkel B, Carlson G, Weller E, eds: *Psychiatric disorders in children and adolescents,* Philadelphia, 1990, WB Saunders.

25. Hayes CD, ed: *Risking the future: adolescent sexuality, pregnancy and childbearing,* Washington, DC, 1987, National Academy Press.

26. Hodas GR, Sargent J: Psychiatric emergencies. In Fleisher G, Ludwig S, eds: *Textbook of pediatric emergency medicine,* ed 3, Philadelphia, 1993, Williams & Wilkins.

27. Hodgman CH, Jack MS: Interviewing. In McAnarney ER et al, eds: *Textbook of adolescent medicine,* Philadelphia, 1992, WB Saunders.

28. Hofferth SL, Hayes CD: *Risking the future: adolescent sexuality, pregnancy, and childbearing,* vol 2, Washington, DC, 1987, National Academy Press.

29. Hofman AD, Greydanus DE: Principles of psychosocial evaluation and counseling. In *Adolescent medicine,* ed 2, Norwalk, CT, 1989, Appleton & Lange.

30. Joffe A: Too little, too much: eating disorders in adolescents, *Contemp Pediatr* 7(3):114-135, 1990.

31. Johnson KB, ed: *The Harriet Lane handbook: a manual for pediatric house officers,* ed 13, St Louis, 1993, Mosby.

32. Kazdin A et al: Depressive symptoms among physically abused and psychiatrically disturbed children, *J Abnormal Psychol* 94:298-307, 1985.

33. Kennedy M: Homeless and runaway youth mental health issues: no access to the system, *J Adolesc Health Care* 12:576-579, 1991.

34. Kreipe RE, Harris JP: Myocardial impairment resulting from eating disorders, *Pediatr Ann* 21(11):760-68, 1992.

35. Lavelle JM: Adolescent emergencies. In Fleisher G, Ludwig S, eds: *Textbook of pediatric emergency medicine,* ed 3, Philadelphia, 1993, Williams & Wilkins.

36. Linden CH: Volatile substances of abuse, *Emergency Med Clin North Am* 8:559-577, 1990.

37. Love CC, Seaton H: Eating disorders: highlights of nursing assessment and therapeutics, *Nurs Clin North Am* 26(3):677-697, 1991.

38. Mattson A: Psychoendocrine aspects of male delinquency and aggression. In Lewis DO, ed: *Vulnerabilities to delinquency,* New York, 1981, Spectrum Publications.

39. Moore KA: *Facts at a glance,* Washington, DC, 1988, Child Trends, Inc.

40. Muscari ME: The "acting-out" adolescent: identification and management, *Pediatr Nurs* 18(4):362-366, 1992.

41. Nanji AA, Filipenko JD: Asystole and ventricular fibrillation associated with cocaine intoxication, *Chest* 85:132-133, 1984.

42. National Institute on Drug Abuse (NIDA): *National household survey on drug abuse: population estimates 1988* (DHHS Publication No. ADM 89 1636), Washington, DC, 1989, US Government Printing Office.

43. Nussbaum MP: Nutritional conditions: anorexia nervosa. In McAnarney ER et al, eds: *Textbook of adolescent medicine,* Philadelphia, 1992, WB Saunders.

44. Palla B, Litt IF: Medical complications of eating disorders in adolescents, *Pediatrics* 81:613-623, 1988.

45. Piacentini J: Evaluating adolescent suicide attempters: what emergency nurses need to know, *J Emerg Nurs* 19:465-466, 1993.

46. Pond V: The angry adolescent, *J Psychosocial Nurs* 26(12):15-17, 1988.

47. Rogeness GA et al: Clinical characteristics of emotionally disturbed boys with very low activities of dopamine-beta-hydroxylase, *J Am Acad Child Adolesc Psychiatry* 23:203, 1984.

48. Schulz JN, Dark SL: *Manual of psychiatric nursing care plans,* ed 2 Boston, 1986, Little, Brown.

49. Shaffer D, Fisher P: The epidemiology of suicide in children and young adolescents, *J Am Acad Child Psychiatry* 20:545-565, 1981.

50. Shaffer D, Hicks R: Suicide and suicidal behaviors. In McAnarney ER et al, eds: *Textbook of adolescent medicine,* Philadelphia, 1992, WB Saunders.

51. Sheehy SB: *Emergency nursing principles and practice,* ed 3, St Louis, 1992, Mosby.

52. Simmons K: Adolescent suicide: second leading death cause, *JAMA* 257:3329, 1987.

53. Smitherman CH: A drug to ease attention deficit disorder, *MCN* 15:362-365, 1990.

54. Weiner H: The physiology of eating disorders, *Int J Eating Dis* 4:347-388, 1985.

55. Weller E, Weller R: Depressive disorders in children and adolescents. In Garfinkel B, Carlson G, Weller E, eds: *Psychiatric disorders in children and adolescents,* Philadelphia, 1990, WB Saunders.

56. Wender PH: Attention-deficit hyperactivity disorder in adolescents and adults. In Garfinkel B, Carlson G, Weller E, eds: *Psychiatric disorders in children and adolescents,* Philadelphia, 1990, WB Saunders.

57. Wentz AC: Body weight and amenorrhea, *Obstet Gynecol* 56:482-487, 1980.

58. Wong DL: *Whaley & Wong's essentials of pediatric nursing,* ed 5, St Louis, 1997, Mosby.

Comparison of EMS Data Collection Recommendations

COMMON DATAPOINTS	EMSC	ACS	JCAHO
Hospital identifier #	♦	♦	
Hospital patient # (medical rec. #)		♦	♦
Date of Admission	♦	♦	♦
Time of Admission		♦	♦
Type of Admission			♦
Discharge Date	♦	♦	♦
Discharge Time			♦
Live/Died	♦	♦	
Diagnosis at Discharge/ICD-9	♦	♦1	♦
Discharge Disposition	♦	♦	♦
Date of Birth (Age)	♦	♦2	♦
Sex	♦	♦	♦
Race/Ethnic origin	♦	♦	
Patients ZIP code of residence	♦	♦	
Insurance/Payor code	♦	♦	
Mode of Transport from injury scene			♦
Ambulance I.D.	♦		
Ambulance run report present			♦3
Date & Time: ED Disposition			♦
ED Disposition			♦
Transferring Hosp. ID#/(to, from or not)		♦	
Mechanism of Injury	♦		
E-code	♦	♦	
E-code site		♦	
Attending MD identifier		♦	
Vital Signs (RR, HR, Temp)	♦	♦4	♦
LOS ICU	♦		
OR Procedure Codes		♦5	♦

♦ Necessary data requested
1 ACS data set includes Abbreviated Injury Scale (AIS).
2 ACS lists "+ flag if estimate".
3 JACHO includes EMS scene arrival date/time, departure date/time, and ED arrival date and time.
4 ACS Vital signs on arrival in ER: Systolic BP, Pulse, Respiratory Rate, GSC, Intubated (yes/no).
5 ACS list in OR: ICD-9 procedure code, date, time and surgeon identifier for each operation.
Reprinted, with permission, from Seidel, J.S., and Henderson, D.P. (1991). *EMSC: A Report to the Nation.* Arlington, VA: National Center for Education in Maternal Child Health.

ALABAMA

State Contact
Steve Haynes, Director of Training, EMS
(334) 613-5383

ALASKA

(ENH-1) Alaska EMSC
Sharron Lobaugh, MEd, MS, Project Coordinator
(907) 465-3027

ARIZONA

(ENH-II) Arizona EMSC
Daniel W. Spaite, MD, Principal Investigator
(602) 626-6312

ARKANSAS

State Contact
Debra H. Fiser, MD, Chairman,
Department of Pediatrics
(501) 320-5262

(R-II) Quality & Cost Containment-Peds. Intensive Care
John Tilford, PhD, Project Director
(501) 320-3340

CALIFORNIA

State Contact
Ernestine Crowder, EMSC Project Coordinator
(916) 322-4336, ext. 341

(RC) National EMSC Resource Alliance (NERA)
Deborah P. Henderson, PhD, RN
James S. Seidel, MD, PhD
Project Co-Directors
(310) 328-0720

(R) Prehospital Pediatric Intubation and Patient Outcome
Marianne Gausche, MD, Project Director
(310) 222-3508

COLORADO

State Contact
David Miller, EMSC Project Director
(303) 692-2995

CONNECTICUT

(IMP-I) Connecticut EMSC
Cheryl Berglund, MPH
(860) 509-7978

DELAWARE

State Contact
Steve Blessing, Office of Paramedic Administrator
(302) 739-6637

DISTRICT OF COLUMBIA

State Contact
Mary J. Berkeley, Director, Special Projects
(202) 994-3921

(RC) EMSC National Resource Center (NRC)
Jane Ball, RN, DrPH, Project Director
(202) 884-4927

(TI-I) EMSC in Managed Care
Michele Solloway, PhD
(202) 530-2307

*Contact NERA for additional information on current EMSC grants and/or EMSC State contact people.
Key I = First Year; II = Second Year; III = Third Year; CE = Continuing Education grant; ENH = Enhancement grant;
IMP = Implementation grant; PL = Planning grant; R = Research grant; RC = Resource Center; TI = Targeted Issue

FLORIDA

State Contact
Lou Romig, MD, Pediatric Emergency Specialist
(305) 666-6511 Ext. 3588

GEORGIA

(ENH-I) Georgia EMSC
Chuck McLean, Project Coordinator
(404) 656-4800

HAWAII

(ENH-I) Hawaii EMSC
Donna Maiava, Project Coordinator
(808) 733-9210

IDAHO

State Contact
Dia Gainor, Director, EMS Bureau
(208) 334-4000

ILLINOIS

*(CE-I) EMSC Regions Leadership Conference:
   Injury Prevention*
Ron W. Lee, MD, MBA
(708) 327-2556

(IMP-I) Illinois EMSC
Linda Gutfeld, RN, BSN, EMSC Manager
(708) 327-3672

INDIANA

(IMP-I) Indiana EMSC
Tres Scherer, MD, Chairman, EMSC Advisory
   Committee
(317) 274-5437

IOWA

(IMP-I) Iowa EMSC
Katrina Altenhofen, EMT-P, Project Coordinator
(515) 242-6285

KANSAS

(PL) Kansas EMSC
Joe Moreland, Planning & Information Systems
   Coordinator
(913) 296-1399

KENTUCKY

State Contact
Coy Harris, NREMT-P
(502) 866-2121

(IMP-I) Kentucky EMSC
Susan Pollack, MD, Project Director
(606) 257-6749

LOUISIANA

(ENH-I) Louisiana EMSC
Beth Toups, Project Administrator
(504) 342-4881

MAINE

State Contact
Patrick Cote, RN, EMT-P, Project Director
(207) 622-7566

MARIANA ISLANDS

(IMP-I) Mariana Islands EMSC
Tom Manglona, EMT-P
011-670-235-9110

MARYLAND

State Contact
Cynthia Wright-Johnson, EMSC Administrator
(410) 706-3178

*(R-III) Injury Prevention in an Urban Pediatric
   Clinic*
Andrea Gielen, ScD
(410) 955-2397

MASSACHUSETTS

(CE-I) Medical Care of Children During Disaster
Richard V. Aghababian, MD
(508) 624-5431

(ENH-I) Massachusetts EMSC
Janet Berkenfield, Project Director
(617) 624-5431

MICHIGAN

(ENH-III) Michigan's Pediatric Emergency Dev't System
Robin Shivley, Project Coordinator
(517) 335-8559

(ENH-I) Michigan EMSC
Stephen Boyer, Project Director
(517) 335-8518

MINNESOTA

(ENH-I) Minnesota EMSC
Susan Ager, Project Director
(612) 282-3863

MISSISSIPPI

State Contact
Wade Spruill, Director, EMS
(601) 987-3880

MISSOURI

State Contact
Stephen Hise, EMSC Project Coordinator
(573) 751-6356

MONTANA

State Contact
Ken Threet, Training Coordinator, EMS Bureau
(406) 444-3895

(IMP-II) Montana EMSC
Drew Dawson, Project Director
(406) 444-3895

NEBRASKA

(PL) Nebraska EMSC
Debbie Kuhn, Coordinator
(402) 471-2158

NEVADA

State Contact
Jan Franklin, Children's Foundation, Nevada EMSC
(702) 380-1010

NEW HAMPSHIRE

(TI-I) Children with Special Health Care Needs
Janet Houston, MHA, Project Director
(603) 650-1813

NEW JERSEY

State Contact
Joyce Ordun, RN, MS
(609) 588-3633

NEW MEXICO

State Contact
Connie Monahan, Program Manager
(505) 272-5063

NEW YORK

State Contact
Ed Wronski, EMS Director
(518) 474-2219

(TI-III) NYC EMSC Project: TRIPP
George Foltin, MD, Project Director
(212) 562-4470

NORTH CAROLINA

State Contact
Bob Bailey
(919) 733-2285

(ENH-II) North Carolina EMSC
Karen Frush, MD, Project Director
(919) 733-2285

NORTH DAKOTA

(PL) North Dakota EMSC
Jack Geller, MD, PhD
(701) 777-3848

OHIO

(ENH-I) Ohio EMSC
Cyndi Young, Project Coordinator
(614) 466-9459

OKLAHOMA

(TI-II) Child Care Health & Safety
Paul Marmen, BS, EMT, Project Coordinator
(405) 271-3307

OREGON

State Contact
Gregg Landers, EMT-P, Acting Chief
(503) 731-4011

(R-III) Pediatric Prehospital Critical Care Skills Retention
Eustacia Su, MD, Project Director
(503) 494-7500

PENNSYLVANIA

(IMP-III) Pennsylvania EMSC
Jim Abromotis, Project Coordinator
(717) 730-9000

(R-II) Applying Biomed, Epidemiology to Injury Prediction
Flaura Winston, MD, Project Director
(215) 590-5208

(R-III) Cost-Effective ED Screening-UTI in Febrile Children
Kathy N. Shaw, MD
(215) 590-1944

PUERTO RICO

State Contact
Amaury Hernandez, EMSC Project Coordinator
(809) 781-1066

RHODE ISLAND

(TI-I) A Model for the Coordination of EMSC with Special Health Care Needs
Gary Kleinman, NREMT-P, Project Coordinator
(401) 444-8210

SOUTH CAROLINA

(IMP-III) South Carolina EMSC
Susan Collins, Project Coordinator
(803) 737-7204

SOUTH DAKOTA

(ENH-I) South Dakota EMSC
David Boer, BS, NREMT-P, Project Coordinator
(605) 357-1371

(CE-II) EMSC Regional Conference
Stephen Karl, MD
(605) 357-1371

TENNESSEE

(IMP-III) Tennessee EMSC
Rhonda Phillippi, RN, Project Coordinator
(615) 343-1506

(R-II) Emergency Mental Health Services for Children
Charles Glisson, PhD, Project Director
(615) 974-6481

TEXAS

State Contact
Gay Knight, Program Administrator
(512) 834-6700

(TI-II) A Model for KTU
Robert Wiebe, MD, and Joseph Weinberg, MD, Project Directors
(214) 640-6116

(TI-II) Improving Primary Care Physician Education & Involvement
Karin McCloskey, MD, Project Director
(214) 640-5854

UTAH

State Contact
Lisa Carlson, RN, MS
(801) 538-6720

(RC) National EMSC Data Analysis Research Center (NEDARC)
Mike Dean, MD, Principal Investigator
Pat Nechodom, Project Director
(801) 581-6410

UTAH (CONTINUED)

(TI-II) EMSC for Children with Special Health Care Needs
Breck Rushton, RN, BSN
(801) 538-6719

(R-II) Epidemiology and Cost of EMSC
Anthony Suruda, MD, Project Director
(801) 581-3841

VERMONT

(ENH-II) Vermont EMSC
Patrick Malone, EMT-P, Special Project Director
(802) 863-7310

VIRGIN ISLANDS

(IMP-I) Virgin Islands EMSC
Jerry Stein, EMS Coordinator
(809) 773-1311 ext. 3054

VIRGINIA

(PL) Virginia EMSC
Amy Hatten, EMSC Project Coordinator
(804) 828-6932

WASHINGTON

State Contact
Kathy Williams, MS
(360) 705-6738

WEST VIRGINIA

(IMP-I) West Virginia EMSC
Patty Hawkins, EMSC Coordinator
(304) 366-8764

WISCONSIN

(ENH-II) Wisconsin EMSC
David Burke, EMSC Project
(608) 265-8161

(TI-I) Project UJIMA: Youth Violence Intervention/ Prevention
Jenifer Wincek, RN, MPH, Contact Person
(414) 266-3064

WYOMING

(IMP-II) Wyoming EMSC
Carol Zorna, Project Coordinator
(307) 777-7955

Summary of Recommendations of the Committee on Pediatric Emergency Medical Services

The following recommendations are from EMERGENCY MEDICAL SERVICES FOR CHILDREN, by the Institute of Medicine Committee on Pediatric Emergency Medical Services, Jane S. Durch and Kathleen N. Lohr, editors, Division of Health Care Services, Institute of Medicine. (National Academy Press, Washington, DC, 1993).

The committee recommends that:

EDUCATION AND TRAINING

- States and localities develop and sustain programs to provide to the general public of all ages adequate and age-appropriate levels of education and training in safety and prevention, in first aid and cardiopulmonary resuscitation, and in when and how to use the emergency medical services system appropriately for children. It recommends further that:
  - the content of such programs reflect the particular needs of each community;
  - the content of such programs reflect the special medical, developmental, and social needs of children;
  - parents and other adults who are responsible for the care and education of children (e.g., day-care workers, teachers, coaches) receive highest priority in such programs; and
  - adolescents also be a high priority in this endeavor.
- States and localities develop and maintain specific guidelines or criteria to ensure basic consistency and quality of educational programs across communities and populations reached, including specific content elements that those education programs should cover.
- Organizations that accredit training programs for prehospital care providers require that the curricula for EMT-Basic, EMT-Intermediate, and EMT-Paramedic provide training in pediatric basic life support; in the medical, developmental, and social needs of all children; and in caring for children with special health care needs.

- Accreditation organizations require that curricula for EMT-Paramedic programs include training in advanced life support for children.
- Appropriate accrediting organizations require that the primary curricula for all health care professionals include training in basic resuscitation skills and the use of the emergency medical services system. These curricula must give specific attention to the unique medical, developmental, and social needs of children.
- Appropriate accrediting organizations ensure that graduate nursing programs in emergency, pediatric, and family practice nursing include training in emergency care for children, including advanced resuscitation.

The Accreditation Council for Graduate Medical Education ensure that residency programs for emergency medicine, family medicine, pediatrics, and surgery include training in emergency care for children, including advanced resuscitation.

PUTTING ESSENTIAL TOOLS IN PLACE

- All state regulatory agencies with jurisdiction over hospitals and emergency medical services systems require that hospital emergency departments and emergency response and transport vehicles have available and maintain equipment and supplies appropriate for the emergency care of children.
- All state regulatory agencies with jurisdiction over hospitals and emergency medical services systems address the issues of categorization and regionalization in overseeing the development of EMS-C and its integration into state and regional EMS systems.

COMMUNICATIONS AND 9-1-1 SYSTEMS

- All states ensure that 9-1-1 systems are implemented. The 9-1-1 system must be universally accessible and effectively linked to the emergency medical services system. Communities with 9-1-1 systems in place should move toward enhanced

9-1-1 capabilities. Communities with no 9-1-1 system should move directly to an enhanced 9-1-1 system.

Planning, Evaluation, and Research

- States and other relevant bodies adopt requirements that ICD-9-CM E-codes be reported for all injury diagnoses for hospital and emergency department discharges.
- States implement a program to collect, analyze, and report data on emergency medical services; those data should include all of the elements of a national uniform data set and describe the nature of emergency medical services provided to children.
- Mechanisms be developed to link all data on a specific case, where those data are generated by separate parts of the emergency medical services system.
- The federal center responsible for emergency medical services for children develop guidelines for a national uniform data set on emergency medical services for children.
- Research in emergency medical services for children be expanded and that priority attention be given to seven areas: clinical aspects of emergencies and emergency care; indices of severity of injury and, especially, severity of illness; patient outcomes and outcome measures; costs; system organization, configuration, and operation; effective approaches to education and training,

including retraining and skill retention; and prevention.

Federal and State Agencies and Funding

- Congress direct the Secretary of the Department of Health and Human Services to establish a federal center or office to conduct, oversee, and coordinate activities related to planning and evaluation, research, and technical assistance in emergency medical services for children.
- Congress direct the Secretary to establish a national advisory council for this center; members should include representatives of relevant federal agencies, state and local governments, the health care community, and the public at large.
- States establish a lead agency to identify specific needs in emergency medical services for children and to address the mechanisms appropriate to meeting those needs.
- State advisory councils be established for these agencies; members should include representatives of relevant state and local agencies, the health care community, and the public at large.
- Congress appropriate $30 million each year for five years—a total of $150 million over the period—to support activities of the federal center and the state agencies related to emergency medical services for children.

BOYS: BIRTH TO 36 MONTHS
PHYSICAL GROWTH
NCHS PERCENTILES*

NAME _____ RECORD # _____

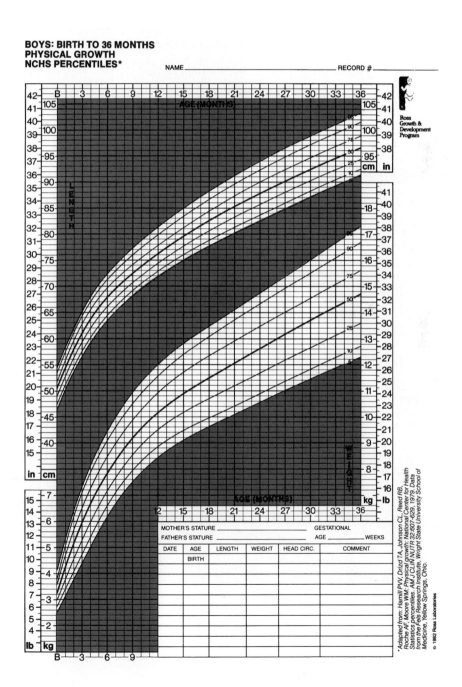

*Adapted from: Hamill PVV, Drizd TA, Johnson CL, Reed RB,
Roche AF, Moore WM: Physical growth: National Center for Health
Statistics percentiles. AM J CLIN NUTR 32:607-629, 1979. Data
from the Fels Research Institute, Wright State University School of
Medicine, Yellow Springs, Ohio.
© 1982 Ross Laboratories

Ross
Growth &
Development
Program

DATE	AGE	LENGTH	WEIGHT	HEAD CIRC.	COMMENT
	BIRTH				

MOTHER'S STATURE _____ GESTATIONAL
FATHER'S STATURE _____ AGE _____ WEEKS

BOYS: 2 TO 18 YEARS
PHYSICAL GROWTH
NCHS PERCENTILES*

NAME _____ RECORD # _____

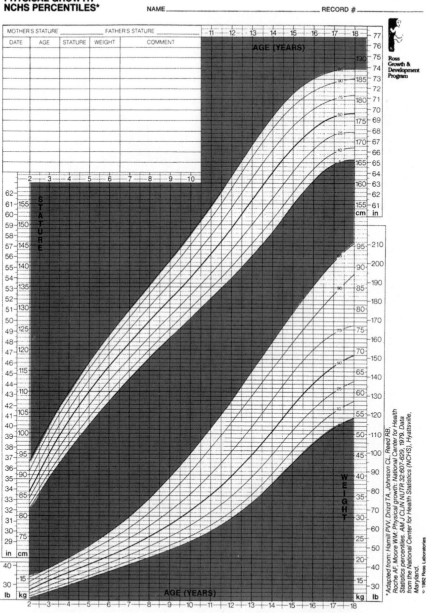

*Adapted from: Hamill PVV, Drizd TA, Johnson CL, Reed RB, Roche AF, Moore WM. Physical growth: National Center for Health Statistics percentiles. AM J CLIN NUTR 32:607-629, 1979. Data from the National Center for Health Statistics (NCHS), Hyattsville, Maryland.

© 1982 Ross Laboratories

Ross
Growth &
Development
Program

GIRLS: BIRTH TO 36 MONTHS
PHYSICAL GROWTH
NCHS PERCENTILES*

NAME_____   RECORD #_____

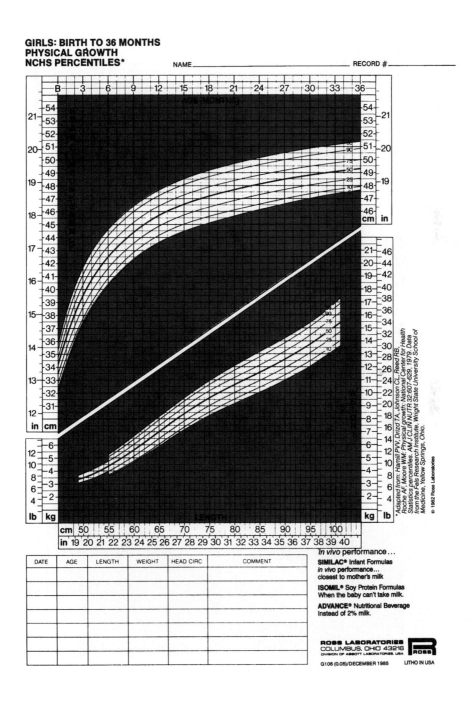

DATE	AGE	LENGTH	WEIGHT	HEAD CIRC	COMMENT

*Adapted from: Hamill PVV, Drizd TA, Johnson CL, Reed RB, Roche AF, Moore WM: Physical growth: National Center for Health Statistics percentiles. AM J CLIN NUTR 32:607-629, 1979. Data from the Fels Research Institute, Wright State University School of Medicine, Yellow Springs, Ohio.

© 1982 Ross Laboratories

in vivo performance...
SIMILAC® Infant Formulas
in vivo performance...
closest to mother's milk.

ISOMIL® Soy Protein Formulas
When the baby can't take milk.

ADVANCE® Nutritional Beverage
Instead of 2% milk.

ROSS LABORATORIES
COLUMBUS, OHIO 43216
DIVISION OF ABBOTT LABORATORIES, USA

G106 (0.05)/DECEMBER 1985   LITHO IN USA

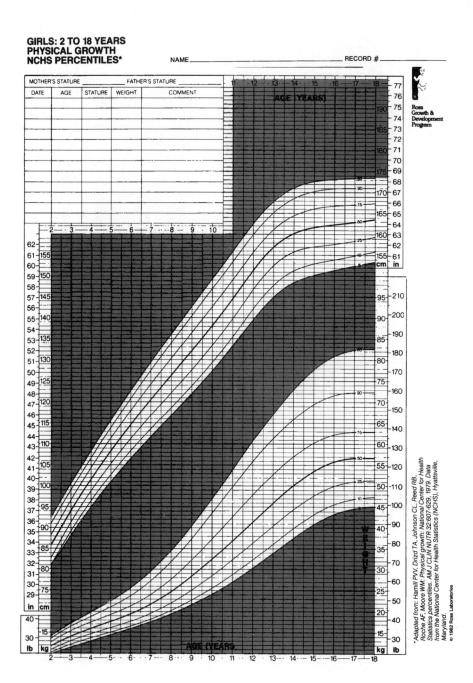

GIRLS: 2 TO 18 YEARS
PHYSICAL GROWTH
NCHS PERCENTILES*

NAME_____ RECORD #_____

Index

A

AAP; *see* American Academy of Pediatrics
Abbreviated Injury Scale, 494-495
ABCs of assessment
  coma, 140
  status epilepticus, 129-130
  triage, 99, 493-494
Abdomen
  acute, 349
  breathing assessment, 196, 197
  cardiovascular assessment, 235-236
  circumferential burn, 583
  free air in, 531
  physical examination, 85, 335
    intussusception, 347
    neonatal, 664
  tenderness, 85
  trauma, 527-535, 536
    multiple injury management, 507-508
  x-ray in iron poisoning, 639
Abdominal breathing by neonate, 661
Abdominal distention
  Hirschsprung's disease, 354
  thoracoabdominal injuries, 534
Abdominal muscle, 64
Abdominal pain, 338-339
  appendicitis, 348
  assessment, 85, 334-335
  Henoch-Schönlein purpura, 388
  intussusception, 346-347
  malrotation of bowel with volvulus, 350
  pelvic inflammatory disease, 369
  sickle cell anemia, 406
  urban *versus* rural prehospital calls, 4
Abdominal thrusts in foreign body airway obstruction, 152-153
Abrasion, 4, 561
Abscess
  peritonsillar, 469
  retropharyngeal, 469
Absence seizure, 271, 273
Absolute neutrophil count, 400
Abstract thinking, 56
Abuse
  child, 586-605
    definitions, 586-587
    documentation, 133
    emergency department intervention, 595
    failure to thrive, 602-604
    fractures, 556-557
    legal issues, 597-598

Abuse—cont'd
  child—cont'd
    Munchausen syndrome by proxy, 601-602
    muscular dystrophy *versus,* 311
    nursing care and evaluation, 595-597
    nursing history, 588-589
    physical assessment, 591-592
    poisoning as, 640
    policies and protocols, 19
    psychosocial assessment, 589-591
    as reportable incidence, 29
    shaken baby syndrome, 515, 602
    status epilepticus, 131, 133
    sexual, 587, 598-601
      clinical manifestations, 591
      gonococcal pharyngitis, 469
      pelvic inflammatory disease, 372
      policies and protocols, 19
      as reportable incidence, 29
  substance, 737-739
Accessory muscle use in asthma, 212, 213
Accidental Death and Disability: The Neglected Disease of Modern Society, 2
Accreditation in regionalizing care, 14
Acetabular pelvic fracture, 548
Acetaminophen
  body temperature reduction, 609, 617, 618
  migraine headache, 270
  pain management, 695, 696
  poisoning, 632, 634, 635
Acetazolamide, 273
Acetic acid, 460
N-Acetylcysteine, 632, 635
Acetylsalicylic acid, 299
Acid burn injury, 582
Acid-base balance, 109-110, 326-327
  disorders, 125, 327-330
  respiratory failure and, 109-110
Acidemia in near-drowning, 222
Acid-fast stain
  meningitis, 279
  tuberculosis, 211
Acidosis
  metabolic, 125, 327
    diabetic ketoacidosis, 477
    hypercyanotic spell, 252
    hyperkalemia, 322, 323, 324
    sodium bicarbonate for, 162
    oxygen-hemoglobin saturation curve, 109

Acidosis—cont'd
  respiratory, 110, 328-329
  status epilepticus, 128
Acquired immunity, 394, 395
Acquired immunodeficiency syndrome, 396-400
Acrocyanosis
  cardiovascular assessment, 235
  neonatal, 170
ACT; *see* Auditory canal thermometer
ACTH; *see* Adrenocorticotropic hormone
Activated charcoal, 627-629
  acetaminophen poisoning, 635
  cough and cold preparation poisoning, 638
  cyclic antidepressant poisoning, 638
Active transport, 313
Activity level during physical examination, 75
Acupuncture, 39
Acute chest syndrome, 405, 406
Acute glomerulonephritis, 378-380
Acute megakaryoblastic leukemia, 717
Acute otitis media, 460-461
Acute renal failure, 382-385
Acute respiratory distress syndrome, 145
Acyanotic congenital heart defects, 237-241
Acyclovir, 430
ADD; *see* Attention deficit disorder
A-delta fiber, 686
Adenohypophysis, 473
Adenoids, 64, 467
Adenosine
  pediatric resuscitation, 163
  supraventricular tachycardia, 160, 260
Adenovirus
  conjunctivitis, 454
  gastroenteritis, 341
  pericarditis, 254
  pneumonia, 203
ADH; *see* Antidiuretic hormone
ADHD; *see* Attention deficit hyperactivity disorder
Adhesive tape
  Broselow resuscitation, 153, 154, 155
  neonatal intubation, 170
Admission documentation in litigation risk management, 34
Adolescent
  chest pain, 258-259

Adolescent—cont'd
common injuries, 63, 490
coping strategies, 689, 706
gaining cooperation of, 74
growth and development, 56-58, 59
headache, 269
interviewing, 71, 72, 728
normal values
blood volume, 67
respiratory rate, 198
urine output, 366
pain responses, 688
pelvic inflammatory disease, 369, 372
psychosocial and behavioral problems, 727-728
seizure etiology, 271
suicide, 731-733
triage assessment, 82
vision testing, 81
Adrenal cortex, 473
Adrenal insufficiency, 483-486
Adrenal medulla, 473
Adrenaline
for local anesthesia, 701
release of, 475
Adrenergic response in congestive heart failure, 250
Adrenocorticotropic hormone, 473, 484
Advanced Cardiac Life Support Course, 10
Advanced directives, 37
Advanced life support, 153-164
airway and ventilation, 154-157
circulation, 158-159
defibrillation and cardioversion, 160-161
dysrhythmia management, 159-160
equipment, 153-154, 155
hypovolemia management, 159
intubation, 157-158
neonatal, 164-175
airway, 168
breathing, 169-170, 171
circulation, 170-173
equipment, 165-166
fluids and medications, 173-175
meconium aspiration, 175-176
obstetric history, 167
prehospital transport, 166-167
preterm deliveries, 176
stimulation and temperature control, 167-168
team responsibilities, 165
tension pneumothorax, 176
resuscitation drugs, 161-164
sequence of resuscitation activities, 153
team member responsibilities, 153
Advanced Pediatric Life Support course, 12
Advocates for children, 21

Aerolized therapy
bronchiolitis, 207
cystic fibrosis, 226
Aerosol inhalation injury, 579
African-American population
pityriasis rosea, 433
sickle cell anemia, 403
umbilical hernias, 85
Afterload, 233-234
cardiogenic shock, 118
pulmonary stenosis, 241-242
AG; see Anion gap
Age
body fluid composition, 314
circulating blood volume, 502
common injuries, 490
juvenile rheumatoid arthritis, 298
Agitation, shock and, 116
AGN; see Acute glomerulonephritis
AI; see Adrenal insufficiency
AIDS; see Acquired immunodeficiency syndrome
Air enema, 347
Air transport, neonatal, 166
Airway
advanced life support, 154-157, 168
anaphylaxis, 652
anatomy and physiology, 66-67, 193, 194, 195
basic life support, 149, 150, 152
burn injury, 574, 582
comatose child, 136-138, 140
inhalation injury, 580
meningitis, 281
neonatal sepsis, 670
Pediatric Trauma Score, 9
poisoning, 623
respiratory distress, 199
seizure, 272, 273
shock, 122
sickle cell crisis, 407, 408
status epilepticus, 129, 130
trauma management
of head and neck, 522
multiple injury, 493, 497-500
treatment protocols, 5
triage assessment, 94, 96, 98, 99
Airway obstruction
anaphylaxis, 652
angioneurotic edema, 652
asthma, 212
bacterial tracheitis, 202-203
basic life support, 149
breath sounds, 198
bronchiolitis, 206
chemical ingestion, 583
epiglottitis, 201-202
foreign body, 151-153, 217-219
inhalation injury, 579
juvenile rheumatoid arthritis, 299-300
multiple trauma management, 497-500

Airway obstruction—cont'd
nursing care, 203
respiratory failure, 108
triage assessment, 98
viral croup, 200-201
AIS; see Abbreviated Injury Scale
Akinetic seizure, 273
Albumin
glomerulonephritis, 380, 381
hypocalcemia, 482-483
for volume resuscitation, 123, 575
Albuterol
asthma, 213, 214
bronchiolitis, 207
hyperkalemia, 323, 324
pertussis, 209
Alcohol
abuse, 737-738
poisoning, 632, 634, 635-637
Aldactone; see Spironolactone
Aldosterone, 473
adrenal insufficiency, 483, 484
body fluid regulation, 314
Alertness in asthma assessment, 213
Alkali burn injury, 582
Alkaline disk battery
in ears and nose, 462
ingestion, 360, 361
Alkaline solutions, 124
Alkalosis, 321, 328
Allen picture card examination, 454
Allergy
anaphylaxis, 651
angioneurotic edema, 651-652
basophils, 392
conjunctivitis, 454
dermatitis
atopic, 442-443
contact, 444-446
diarrhea, 337
insect stings, 642-643
latex, 287
penicillin, 280
triage assessment, 96
Alpha receptors
pediatric shock therapy, 124
sympathetic and parasympathetic nervous system stimulation, 115
Alternate pathway in septic shock, 120
AL-TEs; see Apparent life-threatening events
Alveolar ventilation, 109-110
Alveoli
anatomy and physiology, 193
neonatal, 661
Amcinonide, 445
Amebiasis, 356, 357
American Academy of Pediatrics
conscious sedation, 699
ground and air transport, 5
immunization recommendation, 87
neonatal resuscitation, 167
paramedic education, 4

American Academy of Pediatrics—cont'd
  Pediatric Advanced Life Support course, 12
American Association of Poison Control Centers, 628, 641
American College of Emergency Physicians, 699
American College of Surgeons, 16
American Heart Association
  cardiopulmonary resuscitation and first aid education, 16
  defibrillation and cardioversion safety, 161
  neonatal resuscitation, 167
  pediatric emergency training of physicians, 10-12
American Nurses Association, 35, 36
American Red Cross, 16
Amiloride, 226
Aminocaproic acid, 411
Aminoglycoside, 670
Aminomethane, 125, 145
Aminophylline, 215, 216
Amitriptyline
  migraine headache prophylaxis, 270
  poisoning, 638
AMKL; see Acute megakaryoblastic leukemia
Amnesia, 514
Amoxicillin
  acute otitis media, 461
  Lyme disease, 657
  sinusitis, 467
  urinary tract infection, 375
Amoxicillin-clavulanate
  pneumonia, 206
  urinary tract infection, 375
Amphetamines, 737
Ampicillin
  meningitis, 279
  neonatal sepsis, 670
  osteomyelitis, 295
  pneumonia, 206
  septic arthritis, 296
  Shigella gastroenteritis, 342
Amrinone, 124, 125
Anal stage of toddler development, 47-49
Analgesics, 695
  burn injury, 576
  head and neck injury, 525
  intussusception, 347
  laceration repair, 562
  migraine headache, 270
  narcotic, 696-698
  nonnarcotic, 695-696
  patient-controlled, 700
  septic arthritis, 297
Anaphylactic shock, 114
Anaphylactoid purpura, 387
Anaphylaxis, 651-652, 653
  antivenin administration, 650

ANC; see Absolute neutrophil count
Ancylostoma ceylanicum, 358
Ancylostoma duodenale, 358
Anectine; see Succinylcholine
Anemia, 401-403, 404, 405
  anorexia and bulimia nervosa, 734
  infective endocarditis, 253
  juvenile rheumatoid arthritis, 299
  sickle cell, 403-408
    limp and, 293
    palpable spleen, 85
    sickled cells of, 392
Anesthesia, 695
  Bier block, 558, 559
  local, 701-702
  rapid sequence induction, 111, 130, 499
  regional, 702
  status epilepticus, 130, 131
Anesthesia ventilation bag, 154-157, 502
  neonatal, 169
Angel dust, 738
Anger
  in child, 730
  family in crisis, 179
Angioneurotic edema, 651-652, 653
Angiotensin I, 314
Angiotensin II, 314
Angiotensin-aldosterone system, 115
Angiotensin-converting enzyme inhibitors, 119
Animal bite, 643-645
Anion gap, 326, 327
Anisocoria, 521, 536
Ankle
  bones of, 548
  fracture, 547, 556
Anlagen, 418-419
Anorexia nervosa, 734-737
Ant sting, 642, 644
  anaphylactic reaction, 651
Anterior chamber, 80-81
Antibiotics
  acute otitis media, 461
  animal bite, 645
  bacterial meningitis, 279-280
  bacterial tracheitis, 203
  bronchopulmonary dysplasia, 227
  conjunctivitis and, 455
  cystic fibrosis, 225-226
  diarrhea, 336
  disseminated intravascular coagulation, 413
  epiglottitis, 202
  impetigo, 434
  increased intracranial pressure, 141
  infective endocarditis, 253
  Lyme disease, 657
  muscular dystrophy respiratory infection, 311
  neonatal sepsis, 670
  osteomyelitis, 294, 295

Antibiotics—cont'd
  pelvic inflammatory disease, 372, 373
  pericarditis, 254
  pharyngitis, 470
  pneumonia, 206
  preorbital and orbital cellulitis, 457
  Rocky Mountain spotted fever, 656
  septic arthritis, 296
  septic shock, 121
  sinusitis, 467
  urinary tract infection, 375
Anticholinergics
  asthma, 215, 216
  poisoning, 624, 632
Anticipatory grief, 182
Anticoagulant poisoning, 632
Anticonvulsants
  head and neck injury, 525
  near-drowning, 222
  status epilepticus, 131, 132
  sudden withdrawal, 128
Antidepressant poisoning, 624, 633, 638
Antidiarrheal agent poisoning, 634
Antidiuretic hormone, 473
  body fluid regulation, 313-314
  diabetes insipidus, 481
  shock and, 115
Antidotal therapy, 631-633
Antidumping law, 24
Antiemetics in migraine headache, 270
Antiepileptic therapy, 272, 274
Antifungals, 439-440
Antihistamines
  anaphylaxis, 652, 653
  chickenpox, 430
  insect bites, 643
  poisoning, 632, 634
  urticaria, 450, 650
Antiprotease therapy, 226
Antipyretics, 609, 617, 618
Antirheumatic drug, 299, 300
Antiseborrheic shampoo, 446
Antistreptolysin-O antibody test, 255-256
Antivenin, 633, 648, 649-650
Anus, child abuse and, 591-592, 600-601
Anxiety
  conduct disorders, 729-730
  muscular dystrophy, 311, 312
  as obstacles to patient care, 71
  parental, 59-60
  separation, 46, 47, 49
  stranger, 46, 47
AOM; see Acute otitis media
Aorta
  coarctation of, 242-243
  patent ductus arteriosus, 238, 239
  transposition of great arteries, 244
Aortic stenosis, 243-244

Aortic valve
  hypoplastic left heart syndrome, 248
  rheumatic fever, 255
Apgar score, 168
APLS; *see* Advanced Pediatric Life Support
Apnea, 228-230, 665
Apparent life-threatening events, 228-330
Appearance
  child abuse, 591
  general survey, 77, 78
  neonatal assessment, 663
  preschooler, 51
  toddler, 48
Appendicitis, 333, 348-350
  limp and, 292
Arachnoid mater
  anatomy and physiology, 266, 511, 512
  meningitis, 277
Arbovirus, 281
ARF; *see* Acute renal failure
Arginine vasopressin, 314
Aristocort; *see* Triamcinolone acetonide
Arm
  coarctation of aorta and, 243
  trauma, 549-555
    nursing care and evaluation, 556-559
Arsenic poisoning, 633
ART; *see* Automated reagin test
Arterial blood gases
  asthma, 212
  congenital heart defects, 249
  near-drowning, 221
  normal values, 109, 326
  pediatric anatomic and physiologic differences, 66
  respiratory failure, 110
Arterial carbon dioxide tension
  head and neck injury, 523
  increased intracranial pressure, 141, 143
  normal values, 109, 326
Arterial hemoglobin saturation
  oxygen transport, 108-109
  pulse oximetry, 105
  sickle cell crisis, 407
  triage assessment, 105
Arterial oxygen partial pressure, 108
Arthritis
  cricoarytenoid, 297, 299
  Henoch-Schönlein purpura, 388
  juvenile rheumatoid, 297-301
  limp and, 292
  Lyme disease and, 657
  septic, 295-297
Arthropod-borne virus in encephalitis, 281
AS; *see* Aortic stenosis
Ascariasis, 357, 359
Ascites, 380

ASD; *see* Atrial septal defect
Aseptic meningitis, 277-283
Asian population, 183
Asphyxia, traumatic, 492, 530
Aspiration
  bone marrow
    intraosseous access, 504-505
    septic arthritis, 296
  foreign body, 217-219
  meconium, 175-176
  suprapubic bladder, 376
Aspirin, 695
  hemophilia and, 410
  juvenile rheumatoid arthritis, 300
Assault, sexual, 587, 595, 600
Assent of child, 28
Assessment; *see also* Physical examination
  across the room, 95-97
  head-to-toe
    comatose child, 139-140
    trauma management, 492, 506-508
  triage, 90-91
Asthma, 211-217
  atopic dermatitis, 442-443
  chronic sinusitis, 466
  foreign body aspiration *versus,* 218
Asystolic arrest, 160, 163
Atelectasis
  bronchiolitis, 206
  foreign body aspiration, 217
Ativan; *see* Lorazepam
Atlantoaxial instability, 717, 718
Atlas, cervical spine, 516-517
Atonic seizure, 273
Atonic/astatic syndrome, 283
Atopic dermatitis, 442-444, 445
Atrial fibrillation, 260-261
Atrial flutter, 260, 261
Atrial septal defect, 239-240
  total anomalous pulmonary venous return, 247
  tricuspid atresia, 246
Atrioventricular block, 260
Atrioventricular canal defect, 241
Atrium, pulmonary stenosis and, 242
Atrophy, 424
Atropine
  as antidote, 633
  intubation, 158
  pediatric resuscitation, 162, 163
  rapid sequence induction, 112, 499
  symptomatic bradycardia, 159-160
Atrovent; *see* Ipratropium bromide
Attachment, 668
Attention deficit disorder, 728
Attention deficit hyperactivity disorder, 728-729
Attenuation, 599
Auditory canal, 458
  inflammation, 458-460
Auditory canal thermometer, 616

Augmentin; *see* Amoxicillin-clavulanate
Auscultation
  abdominal, 85, 335
    activated charcoal administration, 628
    multiple trauma management, 507
  breath sounds, 196-198, 236-237
    asthma, 213
    multiple trauma management, 501
    pneumonia, 204
  heart sounds, 236-237
    atrial septal defect, 240
Automated reagin test, 369
Automatic walking reflex, 667
Automotive oil poisoning, 638
Autonomic nervous system
  cardiovascular function, 113
  pediatric anatomic and physiologic differences, 64, 68
  shock and, 113-114, 115
Autonomy, 47-49
Autopsy, 186
Autoregulation
  cardiovascular function, 114-115
  intracranial pressure, 142
Autosomal dominant inherited disorder, 408
Autosomal recessive inherited disorder
  cystic fibrosis, 223
  sickle cell anemia, 403
Autotransfusion, 544
Aveeno; *see* Oatmeal bath
AVPU score, 102, 505, 521
Avulsion, 561
  pelvic fracture, 548
  urban *versus* rural prehospital calls, 4
Axillary temperature, 616
AZT; *see* Zidovudine

B

B cell, 394, 395
Babinski reflex, 64, 68, 667
Baby No-neck collar, 522
Bacille Calmette-Guérin vaccine, 211
Back blows for foreign body airway obstruction, 151-153
Back in multiple trauma management, 508
Back pain, 4
Bacteremia
  fever and, 612
  neutropenia with fever, 400
  osteomyelitis, 293, 294
Bacterial infection
  acute otitis media, 460, 461
  conjunctivitis, 454, 455, 456
  cutaneous, 434-437
  diarrhea, 337
  epiglottitis, 201-202
  gastroenteritis, 339-340
  pericarditis, 254
  pneumonia, 204, 205, 206

Bacterial infection—cont'd
  sinusitis, 466-467
  tracheitis, 201, 202-203
Bacterial meningitis, 277-283
Bactroban; see Mupirocin
Bag-valve-mask ventilation
  advanced life support, 154
  neonatal, 169, 171
  respiratory failure, 111
  status epilepticus, 130
  trauma management
    head and neck, 522
    multiple injury, 498, 502
Balanitis, 448
Balloon valvuloplasty, 249
Barbiturate coma, 145
Barbiturates
  erythema multiforme and, 448
  head and neck injury, 525, 526
  increased intracranial pressure, 143-144
  urticaria and, 450
Barium enema, 347
Barium swallow, 353
Barking cough, 200, 202
Baroreceptors, 114
Barrel chest, 84
  bronchopulmonary dysplasia, 227
Bascular access, 130
Basic life support, 149-153
  equipment and supplies, 11
  hypothermia, 655
Basic needs neglect, 587
Basilar skull fracture, 516
Basophils, 391, 392, 394
  insect stings, 643
  urticaria, 650
Bathtub scald injury, 565, 571
Battered child syndrome, 586
Battery
  in ears and nose, 462
  ingestion, 360, 361
Battle's sign, 507
Bed rest
  rheumatic fever, 256
  toxic or transient synovitis, 302
Bee sting, 642, 643, 644
  anaphylactic reaction, 651
  urticaria, 450
Beef tapeworm, 359
Behavior
  anorexia and bulimia nervosa, 736
  child abuse, 589, 590
  family in crisis, 179
  headaches, 269
  increased intracranial pressure, 136
  pain
    assessment, 691-695
    expressions of, 687-689
  risk-taking, 57-58, 63
Behavior disorders, 727-739
  adolescent issues, 727-728

Behavior disorders—cont'd
  attention deficit hyperactivity disorder, 728-729
  conduct disorders, 729-730
  depression and suicide, 730-733
  eating disorders, 734-737
  history and assessment, 727
  Legg-Perthes disease, 303
  runaways/homelessness, 739
  substance abuse, 737-739
Bell-clapper deformity, 377, 378
Beneficence, 35, 36
Benzathine penicillin
  rheumatic fever, 256
  syphilis, 370
Benzocaine poisoning, 634
Benzodiazepines
  hyponatremia, 319
  poisoning, 632
  status epilepticus, 131
Best eye opening in Glasgow Coma Scale, 137
Beta blocker poisoning, 624, 632
Beta receptors
  pediatric shock therapy, 124
  sympathetic and parasympathetic nervous system stimulation, 115
Beta-agonists
  asthma, 213, 214
  bronchopulmonary dysplasia, 227
Beta-endorphins, 120
Beta-hemolytic streptococci
  cellulitis, 435
  epiglottitis, 201
  glomerulonephritis, 379
  impetigo, 434
  pharyngitis, 469
  rheumatic fever, 255-256
  scarlet fever, 430, 431
  tracheitis, 202
Beta-hydroxylase, 729
Betamethasone dipropionate, 445
Bicarbonate
  diabetic ketoacidosis, 478
  metabolic acidosis, 327
  metabolic alkalosis, 328
Bicarbonate radical
  normal values, 109, 326
  respiratory failure, 110
Bicarbonate-carbonic acid system, 326-327
Bicycle helmet safety, 487
Bier block, 558, 559
Bile
  gallbladder storage, 334
  in neonatal vomitus, 679
Bilirubin
  in neonate, 662
  obstructive jaundice, 344
Biofeedback, 703, 704
Birth
  herpes simplex virus type 2 transmission, 343

Birth—cont'd
  neonatal care following, 167-168
  preterm, 176
  resuscitation after; see Neonatal resuscitation
  trauma, 78
Birth history, 663
  cardiovascular assessment, 234
  neurologic assessment, 268
Birth weight
  cardiovascular assessment, 234
  cerebral palsy seizures and, 284
  neonate loss of, 660
Birthmark, 86, 663
Bites
  animal, 643-645
  as child abuse, 593
  insect, 642-643, 644
  snakebite, 646-650
Black widow spider bite, 642, 644
Blackbird Preschool Vision Screening System, 454
Bladder, 364
Bleeding; see Hemorrhage
Blepharitis, 80
Blindness, erythema multiforme and, 449
Blink reflex, 80, 667
Blister in hypothermia, 654
Block
  atrioventricular, 260
  Bier, 558, 559
  heart, 262-263
    symptomatic bradycardia, 160
  nerve, 702
Blood
  anatomy and physiology, 65, 390-395
  disorders, 401-415
    anemia, 401-403, 404, 405
    disseminated intravascular coagulation, 411-413
    hemophilia, 408-411
    idiopathic thrombocytopenic purpura, 413-415
    sickle cell anemia, 403-408
  history and physical examination, 395-396
  neonatal, 661-662
Blood culture
  neutropenia with fever, 401
  osteomyelitis, 294
  pneumonia, 205
Blood flow
  cerebral, 513
  left-to-right shunting, 237
  patent ductus arteriosus, 239
Blood glucose
  diabetic ketoacidosis, 478
  hypoglycemia, 472, 475, 671
  neonatal, 662, 671
  shock, 125
  status epilepticus, 131

Blood loss
hypovolemic shock, 117
surgical thoracotomy, 535
Blood pressure
cardiovascular assessment, 236
coarctation of aorta and, 243
criteria for transport to pediatric
critical care center, 7
dehydration, 100, 319
hypothermia, 654
increased; see Hypotension
multiple trauma management, 506
neonatal, 668
normal values, 103, 116, 668
pain assessment, 695
pediatric anatomic and physiologic
differences, 67
Pediatric Trauma Score, 9
pericardial tamponade, 530
pericarditis, 254
shock, 114, 116
septic, 121
triage assessment, 94, 104
Blood transfusion
disseminated intravascular coagulation, 413
hemolytic-uremic syndrome, 387
hypovolemic cardiopulmonary arrest, 159
idiopathic thrombocytopenic purpura, 414
for Jehovah's Witness, 32, 33
poisoning, 631
shock, 123
sickle cell crisis, 407
thoracic injury, 544
Blood urea nitrogen
dehydration, 316
diabetic ketoacidosis, 478
glomerulonephritis, 381
hemolytic-uremic syndrome, 387
Blood volume
cardiovascular compensatory response, 114, 116
Frank-Starling law, 114
normal findings, 502
pediatric anatomic and physiologic
differences, 67
shock and, 111, 114, 116
Bloody diarrhea
hemolytic-uremic syndrome, 386
Hirschsprung's disease, 354
Bloody stool, 338
neonatal, 677-678
Blowout ocular fracture, 537
BLS; see Basic life support
Blunt thoracoabdominal trauma, 527
Blunted sensorium, 221
Board restraint, 463
Body fluid; see Fluid
Body image of adolescent, 56, 57, 58
Body proportion, 63

Body surface area
burn injury assessment, 566
fluid therapy requirements, 317, 575
pediatric anatomic and physiologic
differences, 63
Body temperature
anorexia and bulimia nervosa, 735
fluid therapy determination, 317
grunting respirations, 100
immunologic or hematologic assessment, 396
increased intracranial pressure, 145
meningitis, 281
methods for obtaining, 616
neonatal, 167-168, 662, 668
normal values, 606
pelvic inflammatory disease, 372
pyloric stenosis, 353
regulation of, 607-608, 662
status epilepticus, 131
trauma management, 506
triage assessment, 94, 103, 104
Body weight
average daily water losses, 314
at birth
cardiovascular assessment, 234
cerebral palsy seizures and, 284
neonate loss of, 660
color-coding of resuscitation equipment, 155
failure to thrive, 602
fluid therapy requirements, 575
neonatal intubation equipment, 170
pediatric anatomic and physiologic
differences, 61-63
Bohr effect, 116
Bolus therapy
dehydration, 316
hyponatremia, 319
intussusception, 347
shock
cardiogenic, 119
hypovolemic, 118
septic, 121
status epilepticus, 130
Bonding, 668
Bone; see also Musculoskeletal system
infection, 291-295
palpation, 291
red blood cell production in, 390,
392
Bone marrow
intraosseous access, 504-505
osteomyelitis, 293
red blood cell production in, 390,
392
Bone scan
Legg-Perthes disease, 303
osteomyelitis, 294
Bordetella pertussis, 208
Borrelia burgdorferi, 656
Bowel; see Intestine

Bowel elimination
Hirschsprung's disease, 353
neonatal, 662, 677
Bowel sounds, 85
activated charcoal administration, 628
multiple trauma management, 507
Bowing fracture, 542
BP; see Blood pressure
BPD; see Bronchopulmonary dysplasia
Braces in muscular dystrophy, 311
Bradycardia
cardiac output and, 101, 104
cardiovascular assessment, 236
epinephrine dosages, 162, 163
hypoxic, 147
intubation and, 157, 169, 499
neonatal, 661
symptomatic, 159-160
Bradydysrhythmia, 259
Bradykinin
pain and, 686
urticaria, 650
Brain; see also Neurologic system
anatomy and physiology, 64, 266,
512
neonatal, 661
blood flow, 513
cerebral palsy and, 283
edema, 142, 513
encephalopathy and, 282
herniation, 134, 135
increased intracranial pressure
and, 142, 513-514
hyperemia, 513
near-drowning and, 220, 221-222
trauma; see Head and neck trauma
Brain death, ethical considerations, 37
Brainstem
anatomy and physiology, 266, 267,
512
compression, 134
reflexes in assessment of, 134
Breast
examination, 83
neonatal, 364, 664
Breast milk jaundice, 673, 674, 675
Breath sounds
assessment, 84, 196-198
endotracheal tube placement evaluation, 158
multiple trauma management, 501
triage assessment, 99
Breathing
adventitious breath sounds, 197,
198
basic life support, 149, 152
burn injury, 574
central nervous system control, 194
comatose child, 138, 140
meningitis, 281
neonatal, 661

Breathing—cont'd
neonatal resuscitation, 169-170, 171
neonatal sepsis, 670
pain management, 703, 704
pediatric anatomic and physiologic
differences, 67
rescue, 149
respiratory distress, 199
seizure, 272, 273
sickle cell anemia, 408
status epilepticus, 130
trauma management, 493, 500-502
triage assessment, 94, 96, 98-100
Bretylium
pediatric resuscitation, 163
ventricular tachycardia, 262
Broad-spectrum antibiotics
acute otitis media, 461
bacterial meningitis, 279-280
bacterial tracheitis, 203
bronchopulmonary dysplasia, 227
disseminated intravascular coagulation, 413
increased intracranial pressure, 141
neonatal sepsis, 670
pericarditis, 254
Bronchiolitis, 206-208
Bronchodilators
asthma, 216
bronchiolitis, 207
bronchopulmonary dysplasia, 227
cystic fibrosis, 225
Bronchopulmonary dysplasia, 226-
228, 718
Bronchoscopy, 218
Broselow resuscitation tape, 19, 153,
154, 155
Brown fat, 607, 662
Brown recluse spider bite, 642, 644
Brudzinski's sign, 278
Bruising
child abuse, 592-593
color changes in, 593
hemophilia, 409
idiopathic thrombocytopenic pur-
pura, 414
BSA; see Body surface area
Buckle fracture, 542
Buck's traction, 303
Buddy taping, 555
Bulimia nervosa, 734-737
Bulla, 420, 422
impetigo, 434
Bumetanide, 251
Bumex; see Bumetanide
BUN; see Blood urea nitrogen
Burn center referral criteria, 572
Burn injury, 564-585
chemical, 582-583
child abuse, 565, 593-594
circumferential, 583-584
classification, 565-571

Burn injury—cont'd
criteria for transport to pediatric
critical care center, 8
electrical, 581-582
emergency department preparation, 573
emergency management, 572
field care, 572-573
hypovolemic shock, 117
inhalation, 579-581
nursing care and evaluation, 573-
578
prevention, 564-565
triage criteria, 571-572
Burned toast as universal antidote, 631
Butalbital, 270
Buttock bruising from child abuse, 592
Button tube, 725
BVM; see Bag-valve-mask

C
Caffeine, 270
Calamine lotion, 430
Calcaneus fracture, 547
Calcium
balance disorders, 323-326
burn injury, 575
hypercalcemia, 325
hypocalcemia, 324-325, 482, 483
shock, 125
Calcium channel blocker poisoning, 632
Calcium chloride
as antidote, 632
hypocalcemia, 125
pediatric resuscitation, 162, 163
Calcium gluconate
as antidote, 632
hypocalcemia, 325
hypocalcemia seizure, 483
renal failure, 384
Calicivirus, 341
Caloric intake
cystic fibrosis, 225
neonatal, 660
Caloric reflex test, 521-522
Camphor poisoning, 634
Campylobacter
diarrhea, 336
gastroenteritis, 340, 341
Candidiasis
diaper dermatitis, 441
oral, 440
septic shock, 119
stomatitis, 343
Cannabis, 738
Capillary leak syndrome, 120, 122
Capillary refill
criteria for transport to pediatric
critical care center, 7
extremities in assessment of, 235

Capillary refill—cont'd
neonatal
normal, 666
sepsis, 669
shock, 116
triage assessment, 94, 101
Capoten; see Captopril
Captopril, 251
Caput succedaneum, 78
Car accident, 490-491
Children's Trauma Tool, 10
Car seat
as EMS equipment, 11
in injury prevention, 489
Carbamate insecticide poisoning, 633
Carbamazepine
antiepileptic therapy, 273
poisoning, 628
Carbenicillin, 295
Carbicarb, 125, 327
Carbon dioxide
cystic fibrosis, 226
endotracheal tube placement evaluation, 158
respiratory alkalosis, 328
respiratory failure and, 107-108,
109
Carbon dioxide partial pressure
asthma, 213
metabolic alkalosis, 328
respiratory acidosis, 328
Carbon monoxide poisoning, 579,
580, 624
Carbonic acid, 110
Carboxyhemoglobin in inhalation injury, 580
Cardiac catheterization, 249
Cardiac output, 233-234
calculation, 115
congestive heart failure, 250
intrinsic autoregulation, 114
neonatal, 661
pediatric anatomic and physiologic
differences, 67
shock, 114-115
cardiogenic, 118
hemorrhagic, 117
septic, 121
Cardiac sounds
assessment, 84, 236-237
neonatal, 666
atrial septal defect, 240
Cardiac tamponade, 503
juvenile rheumatoid arthritis, 301
Cardiogenic shock, 114, 118-119
Cardiopulmonary arrest
epidemiology, 147
hypovolemic, 159
near-drowning, 220
respiratory failure and shock leading
to, 107
urban versus rural prehospital calls, 4

Cardiopulmonary resuscitation; *see also*
  Resuscitation
  cessation guidelines, 37
  community education, 16
  continuous quality improvement pro-
    grams and, 16
  drowning survival rates and, 148
  hypothermia, 655
Cardiovascular disease, 237-263
  acquired, 252-255
  anorexia and bulimia nervosa, 735
  apnea and, 228
  chest pain, 258-259
  congenital heart defects, 237-238
    acyanotic with left-to-right
      shunting, 238-241
    cyanotic with right-to-left
      shunting, 244-248
    obstructive, 241-244
  congestive heart failure, 250-251,
    252
  dysrhythmias, 259-263
  grunting respirations, 100
  hypercyanotic episode, 252
  Kawasaki disease, 256
  nursing intervention, 256-258
  rheumatic fever, 255-256
Cardiovascular system, 233-265
  AIDS manifestations, 399
  anatomy and physiology, 66-67,
    233-234
    neonatal, 661
  disease; *see* Cardiovascular disease
  frequency of injury, 527
  hemorrhagic shock classifica-
    tion, 503
  history and physical assessment, 84,
    234-237
    neonatal, 664
  hyperkalemia, 323
  intrinsic autoregulation, 114, 116
Cardioversion
  advanced life support, 160-161
  atrial flutter, 260
  supraventricular tachycardia, 160,
    260
  ventricular tachycardia, 160, 262
Caregiver; *see* Parent
Casting, 558, 559
Catarrhal stage of pertussis, 208
Catatonic analgesia, 699
Catecholamines, 473
Categorization in regionalizing
  care, 14
Caterpillar bite, 642, 644
Cathartics, 628, 629-630
Catheterization
  cardiac, 249
  cerebral shunting, 276
  esophageal foreign body re-
    moval, 361, 362
  intracranial pressure monitor-
    ing, 144, 145

Catheterization—cont'd
  intubation, 158
  umbilical, 171-173
  for urine collection, 376
CAVCD; *see* Complete atrioventricular
  canal defect
Cefaclor, 375
Cefazolin
  cellulitis, 435
  osteomyelitis, 295
Cefotaxime
  epiglottitis, 202
  meningitis, 279
Cefoxitin, 373
Ceftriaxone
  acute otitis media, 461
  epiglottitis, 202
  Lyme disease, 657
  meningitis, 279
  neonatal sepsis, 670
  preorbital and orbital cellulitis, 457
  Shigella gastroenteritis, 342
  syphilis, 370
Cefuroxime, 202
Celiac artery, 334
Cell-mediated immunity, 394
Cellular metabolism; *see* Metabolism
Cellulitis, 435
  periorbital and orbital, 455-457
Central apnea, 228-229
Central cyanosis
  neonatal, 170
  tricuspid atresia, 246
Central dispatch, 4
Central downward cerebral herniation, 135
Central nervous system
  apnea and, 228
  control of breathing, 194
  hemorrhagic shock classifica-
    tion, 503
  hypoglycemia and, 474
  hypothermia and, 653
  narcotic analgesics and, 696
  Pediatric Trauma Score, 9
  respiratory failure and, 108
  stimulants, 737-738
Central venous access
  burn injury, 576
  multiple trauma management, 504
  resuscitation, 158-159
Central venous pressure in shock, 122
Cephalexin
  impetigo, 434
  preorbital and orbital cellulitis, 457
  urinary tract infection, 375
Cephalohematoma, 78
Cephalosporin
  bacterial tracheitis, 203
  epiglottitis, 202
  neonatal sepsis, 670
  pneumonia, 206
  preorbital and orbital cellulitis, 457

Cephalosporin—cont'd
  scarlet fever, 431
  urticaria and, 450
Cephalothin, 295
Cerebellum
  anatomy and physiology, 266, 267,
    512
  herniation, 514
Cerebral blood flow, 513
Cerebral cortex
  coma and, 134
  febrile seizure and, 610
Cerebral edema, 142, 513
Cerebral herniation, 134, 135, 142,
  513-514
Cerebral hyperemia, 513
Cerebral palsy, 283-285
  head examination and, 78
Cerebral perfusion pressure
  calculation, 513
  monitoring, 144
Cerebral resuscitation in near-
  drowning, 221-222
Cerebrospinal fluid, 266
  hydrocephalus, 275
  meningitis, 277, 279
  ventricular drainage of, 144, 507,
    520
Cerebrum, 266, 267, 512
Certification of emergency medical ser-
  vice providers, 4-5
Cerumen removal, 458
Cervical collar, 500, 501
Cervical spine
  immobilization, 500, 501
    before basic life support, 149, 150
    head and neck injury, 522, 524
    juvenile rheumatoid arthritis
      and, 299
    near-drowning injury, 219, 221
    physical examination, 80, 83
    trauma; *see* Head and neck trauma
Cervical spine collar, 522
Cervicitis, child abuse and, 600
CF; *see* Cystic fibrosis
Charcoal, activated, 627-629
CHDs; *see* Congenital heart defects
Chemet; *see* Dimercaptosuccinic acid
Chemical injury, 582-583
Chemoreceptors, 108
Chemotherapy, 97
Chest
  cardiovascular assessment, 235-236
  circumferential burn, 583
  flail, 529
  neonatal intubation placement, 169
  observation for breathing assess-
    ment, 99, 196, 197
    during basic life support, 149
  paddle placement, 161
  physical examination, 83-84
    neonatal, 664, 665
  protrusion or depression, 84

Chest—cont'd
  trauma, 527-530, 531-535, 536
    multiple injury management, 507
Chest circumference, 83
Chest compression
  basic life support, 150-151
  multiple trauma management, 503-504
  neonatal, 170-171
Chest pain, 254, 258-259
Chest physiotherapy, 225
Chest thrusts for foreign body airway obstruction, 151-153
Chest tube
  sizes of, 502
  thoracoabdominal injuries, 534-535
Chest wall
  anatomy and physiology, 193-194
  inflammation, 259
  neonatal, 661
  palpation, 237
Chest x-ray
  asthma, 212
  bronchiolitis, 207
  bronchopulmonary dysplasia, 227
  congenital heart defects, 249
  congestive heart failure, 250
  cystic fibrosis, 225
  endotracheal tube placement evaluation, 158
  foreign body aspiration, 218
  inhalation injury, 580
  myocarditis, 254
  near-drowning, 220-221
  pericarditis, 254
  pneumonia, 204
  respiratory failure, 110
  septic shock, 121
  tension pneumothorax, 176
  tuberculosis, 210
CHF; see Congestive heart failure
Chiari II malformation, 275
Chickenpox, 425, 429-430
Chief complaint
  interviewing and, 72
  triage assessment, 96
Child
  anatomic and physiologic differences, 61-68
    cardiovascular system, 67
    metabolism and fluid and electrolyte balance, 63-66
    neurologic system, 67-68
    physical growth, 61-63, 64
    pulmonary system, 66-67
    thermoregulation, 68
  assent given by, 28
  coping strategies, 58-59
  crisis intervention, 181
  death of, 182-186
  growth and development, 43-58, 59; See also Growth and development

Child—cont'd
  interviewing, 71, 72
  parental involvement, 59-61
  special needs, 712-726; see also Special needs child
  terminally ill, 35-37
Child abuse, 586-605
  bite marks, 593
  bruising, 592-593
  burns, 565-566, 593-594
  characteristics and risk factors, 587-588
  definitions, 586-587
  documentation, 133
  emergency department intervention, 595
  failure to thrive, 602-604
  fractures, 556-557, 594-595
  head injury, 595
  legal issues, 597-598
  Munchausen syndrome by proxy, 601-602
  muscular dystrophy versus, 311
  nursing care and evaluation, 595-597
  nursing history, 588-589
  physical assessment, 591-592
  poisoning as, 640
  policies and protocols, 19
  prevention, 604
  psychosocial assessment, 589-591
  as reportable incidence, 29
  shaken baby syndrome, 515, 602
  status epilepticus, 131, 133
Child Protective Services, 597
Child-life programs, 18-19
Children's Trauma Tool, 9, 10
Chiropractics, 39
Chlamydia
  child abuse and, 600
  infection in newborn, 82
  ophthalmia neonatorum, 454
  pelvic inflammatory disease, 369
  pneumonia, 203
  as sexually transmitted disease, 368, 370
Chloramphenicol
  bacterial tracheitis, 203
  meningitis, 280
Chloride
  body fluid balance, 315
  pyloric stenosis, 353
Chloroquine poisoning, 634
Chlorothiazide, 251
Chlorpheniramine poisoning, 637
Chondromalacia of patella, 292
Choral hydrate, 700-701
Christmas disease, 408
Chronic illness, 97
Chronic renal failure, 382-385
Chvostek's sign, 325, 483
CIE; see Counterimmune electrophoresis

Cigarette smoking, 461
Cimetidine, 651
Ciprofloxacin, 226
Circulation
  advanced life support, 158-159
  basic life support, 149-151, 152
  burn injury, 574
  comatose child, 138-139, 140
  fetal, 233, 234
  gastrointestinal, 334
  meningitis, 281
  neonatal resuscitation, 170-173
  neonatal sepsis, 670
  renal, 365
  in respiratory distress, 199
  shock, 122-123
  sickle cell crisis, 407, 408
  status epilepticus, 130
  trauma management
    head and neck injury, 523
    multiple injury, 497, 502-505
  triage assessment, 94, 96, 100-101
Circumcision assessment, 666
Circumferential burn injury, 583-584
CISD; see Critical incident stress debriefing
CISM; see Critical incident stress management
Clavicular fracture, 549-550
Clavicular retractions, 197
Clean catch urine collection, 376
Clindamycin
  bacterial tracheitis, 203
  pelvic inflammatory disease, 373
Clobetasol propionate, 445
Clonazepam, 273
Clonidine
  attention deficit hyperactivity disorder, 729
  poisoning, 633, 634
Clostridium tetani, 508
Clotrimazole, 440
Clotting factor
  disseminated intravascular coagulation, 411, 412
  hemophilia, 408, 411
  snakebite, 647
Clotting studies in suspected child abuse, 595
Cloxacillin, 434
Clubbing of digit, 235, 236
CNS; see Central nervous system
CO; see Cardiac output
CO_2; see Carbon dioxide
COA; see Coarctation of aorta
Coagulation; see Clotting
Coalition building, 21
Coarctation of aorta, 242-243
COBRA; see Consolidation Omnibus Budget Reconciliation Act
Cocaine
  abuse, 737
  local anesthesia, 701

Codeine, 697
  abuse, 738
  extremity injury, 557
  migraine headache, 270
  upper respiratory infection, 199
Cognitive development
  adolescent, 56-58
  cerebral palsy, 283
  infant, 44-46
  Piaget's theory, 44
  preschooler, 50-52, 53
  school-age child, 54, 55
  toddler, 48, 49
Cognitive function, 268
Cold; see Common cold
Cold agglutinins, 205
Cold calorics in coma, 134-136
Cold preparation poisoning, 634, 637-638
Cold sore, 343
Cold stress, neonatal, 168
Colic, 682-683
Colistin, 226
Collagen, 307
Collar, cervical, 500, 501
Colle's fracture, 552, 553
Colloids
  burn injury, 575
  hypovolemic cardiopulmonary arrest, 159
  shock, 122, 123
Colon; see Large intestine
Color Tool for pain assessment, 694
Color-coding of resuscitation
  equipment, 155
Colyte, 630
Coma, 133-141
  barbiturate, 145
  diffuse axonal injury, 514
  hepatic, 356
  nonketotic hyperosmolar, 478
Comminuted fracture, 542
Common cold, 82, 198-199
  neonatal, 675-676
Common fears; see Fears
Communicable disease, 420-434
  fifth disease, 431-432
  hand-foot-mouth disease, 433-434
  pityriasis rosea, 432-433
  roseola infantum, 432
  rubella, 429
  rubeola, 420-428
  scarlet fever, 430-431
  varicella, 429-430
Communicating hydrocephalus, 275
Communication
  cerebral palsy, 285
  crisis intervention, 179-180
  family with abused child, 595-596
  infant, 46
  litigation prevention, 30-31
  mental retardation, 716
  preschooler, 52, 53

Communication—cont'd
  school-age child, 54
  toddler, 49
  tracheostomy and, 721
Community education, 15-16
Compartment syndrome, 559-560
  humerus fractures, 551
  metatarsal fractures, 548
  snakebite, 649
Compartmental pressure measurement, 560
Compazine; see Prochlorperazine
Complaints, 33
Complement system, 391, 395
  septic shock, 120
Complete atrioventricular canal defect, 241
Complete blood count
  bronchiolitis, 207
  child abuse, 595
  juvenile rheumatoid arthritis, 299
  neonatal sepsis, 669
  rheumatic fever, 255
Compound skull fracture, 516
Compression fracture, 542
Computed tomography
  abdominal injury, 532, 533
  encephalopathy, 282
  hydrocephalus, 276
  increased intracranial pressure, 141
  meningitis, 279
  preorbital and orbital cellulitis, 456
  seizure, 272
  sinusitis, 467
Concha, 464
Concrete thinking
  adolescent, 56, 57
  school-age child, 54, 55
Concussion, 514
Conduct disorders, 729-730
Conduction in body temperature regulation, 607
Condylomata acuminata, 600
Confirmation in regionalizing care, 14
Congenital adrenal hyperplasia, 484, 485
Congenital aganglionic
  megacolon, 353-355
Congenital disorder
  child abuse and, 588
  incarcerated hernias, 351-352
  malrotation of bowel with volvulus, 350
  syphilis, 368
Congenital heart defects, 237-250
  acyanotic with left-to-right
    shunting, 238-241
  cyanotic with right-to-left
    shunting, 244-248
  diagnostic testing, 249
  obstructive, 241-244
  treatment, 250
Congenital rubella syndrome, 429

Congestive heart failure, 250-251, 252
  anemia, 402, 403
  cardiogenic shock, 119
  chest x-ray, 249
  complete atrioventricular canal defect, 241
  patent ductus arteriosus, 239
  tachypnea, 236
Conjugated hyperbilirubinemia, 673
Conjunctiva
  examination, 80
  trauma, 537
Conjunctivitis, 80, 448, 454-455
Connective tissue disorder, 307
Conscious sedation, 699-700
Consent for treatment, 27-29
Consolidation Omnibus Budget Reconciliation Act, 24-27
  triaging out of emergency departments, 92
Constipation, 337-338
  Hirschsprung's disease, 354
  myelomeningocele, 286, 287
  neonatal, 676-677
Constrictive band for snakebite, 648-649
Contact dermatitis, 444-446
Continuous quality improvement
  EMSC, 16, 17
  nurses' role, 21
  pain management, 708
Contractility, 234
  intrinsic autoregulation, 114
Contrecoup injury, 514
Contusion
  cerebral, 514
  pulmonary, 528, 529
  soft tissue, 561
  urban versus rural prehospital calls, 4
Convalescent stage of pertussis, 208, 209
Convection in body temperature regulation, 607
Cooperation during physical
  examination, 73-74, 75, 76-77
Coping strategies, 58-59, 689
  painful procedures, 706-708
Copperhead snake bite, 633, 646
Coral snake bite, 633, 646, 647-648
Cordran; see Flurandrenolide
Cornea
  anatomy, 453
  conjunctivitis and, 454-455
  examination, 80
  trauma, 537
Corneal reflex
  coma, 136
  head and neck injury, 521
  neonatal assessment, 667
Coronary sinus atrial septal defect, 239
Cort-Dome; see Hydrocortisone
Cortex
  adrenal, 473

Cortex—cont'd
  cerebral
    coma and, 134
    febrile seizure and, 610
  renal, 364-365
Corticospinal pathways, 68
Corticosteroids
  anaphylaxis, 652, 653
  asthma, 213-216
  bronchopulmonary dysplasia, 227
  glomerulonephritis, 381
  hemophilia, 411
  juvenile rheumatoid arthritis, 299, 300
  pertussis, 209
Corticotropin-releasing factor, 484
Cortisol, 483, 484
Costochondritis, 259
Cottonmouth snake bite, 633, 646
Cough
  asthma, 212
  bacterial tracheitis, 201, 202
  cystic fibrosis, 224
  epiglottitis, 201
  pertussis, 209
  as pulmonary protection, 195
  viral croup, 200, 201
  whooping, 208-209, 210
Cough preparations
  poisoning, 634, 637-638
  upper respiratory infection, 199
Coumadin poisoning, 632
Counterimmune electrophoresis, 205
Coup injury, 514
Court cases in suspected child abuse, 597-598
Court orders, 32
Cow's milk, colic and, 682
Coxsackievirus
  encephalitis, 281
  hand-foot-mouth disease, 433
  myocarditis, 254
  stomatitis, 343
CP; see Cerebral palsy
CPK; see Creatine phosphokinase
C-polymodal fiber, 686
CPP; see Cerebral perfusion pressure
CPR; see Cardiopulmonary resuscitation
CQI; see Continuous quality improvement
Crackles
  bronchopulmonary dysplasia, 227
  pneumonia, 204
  respiratory assessment, 197, 198
Cradle cap, 446
CRAMS Scale, 8
Cranial nerves
  head and neck injury, 521-522
  meningitis, 277, 278
Cranial sutures, 266
  examination, 77-78, 79

Cranial sutures—cont'd
  pediatric anatomic and physiologic differences, 64, 67
  premature closure of, 78
Craniosynostosis, 78
Cranium, 266, 512
Crawl reflex, 667
C-reactive protein, 255
Creatine phosphokinase, 311
Creatinine, 315-316
CRF; see Chronic renal failure; Corticotropin-releasing factor
Cribriform plate, 464
Cricoarytenoid arthritis, 297, 299
Cricoid, 195
  endotracheal intubation, 498, 499
Cricothyroidotomy, 499, 500
Crisis, defined, 178
Crisis intervention, 178-192
  communication, 179-180
  critical incident stress management, 186-188
  death of child, 182-186
  homicide and violence, 189-191
  initial interview, 180
  resuscitation, 181
  signs and symptoms, 179
  sudden infant death syndrome, 188-189, 190
  violent behavior, 181-182
Crisis management, 178
Critical incident stress debriefing, 187
Critical incident stress management, 186-188
Crossed extension reflex, 667
Crotalidae polyvalent antivenin, 633
Croup, 200-201
Crush injury of hand, 555
Crust, 420, 423
Crying
  in febrile child, 611
  gastrointestinal examination, 335
  neonatal, 662, 665, 680-682
  during physical examination, 75, 662
  as symptom of pain, 102
  triage assessment, 102, 103
Cryoprecipitate, 413
Cryptosporidiosis, 357
Crystalloids
  hypovolemic cardiopulmonary arrest, 159
  increased intracranial pressure, 139
  shock, 122, 123
CSF; see Cerebrospinal fluid
Cuboid fracture, 547
Cuffed tube, 157
Cullin's sign, 530
Cultural factors, 61
  febrile child, 614, 617
  gastroenteritis, 340
  grieving process, 183
  neonatal sepsis, 669

Cultural factors—cont'd
  neutropenia with fever, 401
  osteomyelitis, 294
  pelvic inflammatory disease, 369
  pertussis, 209
  pneumonia, 205
  septic shock, 121
  sexual abuse, 595, 600
  sickle cell anemia, 403
  sinusitis, 467
  treatment rooms, 18
  urinary tract infection, 374-375
Cuneiform fracture, 547
Cushing's triad, 143
Custody disputes, 598
Cut-downs, 504
Cuticle, 419
CVP; see Central venous pressure
Cyanosis
  congenital heart disease, 235
  criteria for transport to pediatric critical care center, 7
  neonatal, 170, 663
  respiratory distress and failure, 100, 110, 196, 501
  tricuspid atresia, 246
Cyanotic congenital heart defects, 238, 244-248
Cyclic antidepressant poisoning, 624, 633, 638
Cyclocort; see Amcinonide
Cylert; see Pemoline
Cyproheptadine, 270
Cyst, 420, 422
Cystic fibrosis, 223-226
Cystitis, 374
Cytokines, 120
Cytotoxic cerebral edema, 142
Cytotoxic T cell, 394, 395

D

Dactylitis, 406
Dance's sign, 347
Dandy-Walker syndrome, 275
Data collection
  abused child, 596-597
  for continuous quality improvement programs, 16
  EMS, 9-10
  murdered child, 189
DDAVP; see 1-Desamino, 8-D-arginine vasopressin
Death
  acquired immunodeficiency syndrome, 396
  burn injury, 564
  child abuse, 586
  child's right to die, 37
  continuous quality improvement programs and, 16
  crisis intervention, 182-186
  diabetic ketoacidosis, 477

Death—cont'd
  drownings, 219
  homicidal, 189
  hypothermia, 652-653
  injury prevention and, 15
  poisoning, 634
  support of family, 19-20
  thoracoabdominal injury, 527
Debriefing, 187
Decaderm; *see* Dexamethasone
Decadron; *see* Dexamethasone
Decerebrate posturing, 134, 138
Decision making, ethical, 34-35
Decongestants
  poisoning, 634
  upper respiratory infection, 199
Decontamination, gastric, 625-630
Decorticate posturing, 134, 138
Decubitus ulcer, 284
Deductive reasoning in school-age
  child, 54
Deep partial-thickness burn, 567, 568,
  570
Deep tendon reflex in spinal cord injury, 134
Defecation; *see* Bowel elimination
Deferoxamine, 633, 639
Defibrillation
  advanced life support, 160-161
  emergency medical technician classi-
    fication, 3
  near-drowning, 221
  ventricular fibrillation, 160
Deftazidime, 295
Dehydration, 315-318
  criteria for transport to pediatric
    critical care center, 8
  diabetes insipidus, 481
  diabetic ketoacidosis, 477, 478
  diarrhea, 337
  gastroenteritis, 340
  hypernatremic, 320, 321
  hyponatremic, 318, 319
  hypovolemic shock, 117
  intussusception, 347
  pyloric stenosis, 352-353
  renal failure, 384
  signs and symptoms, 100
  triage assessment, 100
  vomiting, 680
Delivery
  herpes simplex virus type 2 transmis-
    sion, 343
  neonatal care following, 167-168
  preterm, 176
  resuscitation after; *see* Neonatal resus-
    citation
  trauma, 78
Delta virus, 345
Demerol, 698
  burn injury, 576
Dens process, 516-517
Denver Eye Screening Test, 454

Deoxyribonucleic acid, 397
Department of Children's Ser-
  vices, 597
Department of Health and Human
  Services, 20-21
Department of Social Services, 597
Department of Transportation, 21
Depressed skull fracture, 516
Depression, 730-731
Dermatitis, 440-446
  atopic, 442-444, 445
  contact, 444-446
  diaper, 441-442
  seborrheic, 446
Dermis
  anatomy and physiology, 418
  burn injury, 418
Dermovate; *see* Clobetasol propionate
1-Desamino, 8-D-arginine vaso-
  pressin, 482
Designation in regionalizing care, 14
Desipramine poisoning, 634
Desonide, 445
DesOwen; *see* Desonide
Desoximetasone, 445
Developmental stages; *see* Growth and
  development
Developmentally delayed child, 714-
  716
Dexamethasone
  increased intracranial pressure, 143
  meningitis, 279
  potency guide, 445
Dexedrine; *see* Dextroamphetamine
Dextran, 123
Dextroamphetamine, 729
Dextromethorphan, 199
Dextrose
  diabetic ketoacidosis, 480
  hypoglycemia, 475
    neonatal, 672
  neonatal resuscitation, 166
DFA; *see* Direct fluorescent antibody
DI; *see* Diabetes insipidus
Diabetes insipidus, 481-482
  increased intracranial pressure, 145
Diabetic ketoacidosis, 477-480
Diagnostic peritoneal lavage, 508,
  532-533
Diaper dermatitis, 440, 441-442
Diaper rash in urinary tract infec-
  tion, 374
Diaphragm
  abdominal breathing in neonate, 661
  anatomy and physiology, 193-194
  frequency of injury, 527
Diaphyseal fracture, 542
Diarrhea, 336-337
  cystic fibrosis, 224, 225
  gastrostomy tube, 724
  Hirschsprung's disease, 354

Diarrhea—cont'd
  hypovolemic shock, 117
Diary, headache, 270
Diazepam, 697, 701
  head and neck injury, 525, 526
  rapid sequence induction, 113
  status epilepticus, 131, 132
Dichloroacetate, 125, 327
Dicloxacillin, 434
Didanosine, 397-398
Diencephalon, 139
Diet
  diarrhea, 337
  neonatal colic, 682
  triage assessment, 96
Difenoxin poisoning, 634
Diffuse axonal injury, 514
Diffusion, 108, 313
Digiband; *see* Digoxin immune fab
Digit, clubbing, 235, 236
Digitalis, 250
Digoxin
  congestive heart failure, 251
  myocarditis, 255
  supraventricular tachycardia, 260
  toxicity, 252, 633
Digoxin immune fab, 633
Dilantin; *see* Phenytoin
Dilute urine in diabetes insipidus, 481,
  482
Dimercaptosuccinic acid, 633
Diphenhydramine
  anaphylaxis, 652, 653
  insect bites, 643
  poisoning, 637
  urticaria, 651
Diphenoxylate with atropine poison-
  ing, 634
Diphyllobothrium latum, 359
Diplegia, spastic, 283
Diprosone; *see* Bethamethasone
Dipylidium caninum, 359, 360
Direct current cardioversion, 260, 262
Direct fluorescent antibody, 207
Disability, 96, 99
  comatose child, 139
  respiratory distress, 199
  school-age child fear of, 54
  status epilepticus, 130
  trauma management, 494, 505-506
  triage assessment, 94, 99, 101-102
Discharge
  nasal
    assessment, 465
    breath sounds and, 84
    head trauma and, 82
    neonatal upper respiratory infec-
      tion, 676
    sinusitis, 466
  ocular, 80
  vaginal
    newborn, 364
    sexual abuse, 600

Discharge teaching
  animal bite, 645
  asthma, 216-217
  burn injury, 577, 578
  documentation of for litigation risk
    management, 34
  fractures, 559
  headache, 270
  seizures, 274, 275
  tuberculosis, 211
  viral croup, 201
Discomfort in triage assessment, 99,
  102-103
Dislocation in cerebral palsy, 284
Dispatch in prehospital care, 4
Disseminated intravascular
  coagulation, 411-413
  meningococcal meningitis, 279
  snakebite, 647
Distraction in pain management, 703-
  704
Distributive shock, 113, 114
Diuresis
  forced in poisoning, 631
  hypovolemic shock, 117
Diuretics
  bronchopulmonary dysplasia, 227
  congenital heart defects, 250
  congestive heart failure, 251
  head and neck injury, 525
  hyperkalemia, 323, 324
  increased intracranial pressure, 141,
    143, 524
  metabolic alkalosis, 328
  near-drowning, 222
Diving reflex, 219
DKA; see Diabetic ketoacidosis
DNA; see Deoxyribonucleic acid
DNR; see Do not resuscitate
Do not resuscitate, 714
Dobutamine
  myocarditis, 255
  pediatric resuscitation, 163
  shock, 124
Documentation
  child abuse, 133, 596-597
  conscious sedation, 699
  litigation risk management, 34
  murdered child, 189
  pediatric trauma team responsibil-
    ity, 496
  poisoning, 625
  status epilepticus, 133
Dog bite, 643-645
Doll's eyes
  coma, 134
  head and neck trauma, 522
  neonatal assessment, 667
Dopamine
  conduct disorders, 729
  myocarditis, 255
  pediatric resuscitation, 163
  shock, 124

Dopaminergic receptors, 115
Down syndrome, 716-718
  Hirschsprung's disease in, 354
Doxepin poisoning, 638
Doxycycline
  chlamydia, 370
  Lyme disease, 657
  pelvic inflammatory disease, 373
Doxylamine poisoning, 637
D-penicillinase, 300
DPL; see Diagnostic peritoneal lavage
DPT, 698
Drainage, cerebrospinal fluid, 144,
  507
Drooling
  airway obstruction, 98
  epiglottitis, 202
Drowning, 219-223
  primary hypothermia, 653
  survival rates, 148
Drugs
  abuse, 737-739
  diarrhea and, 337
  dosages, 5, 19
  metabolism and excretion, 65-66
  overdoses, 732
  resuscitation, 161-164
    neonatal, 173-175
  triage assessment, 96, 97
  urticaria, 650
Dry drowning, 219
Duchenne's muscular dystrophy, 310-
  312
Duodenum, 332
Dura mater, 266, 511, 512
Dwarf tapeworm, 359, 360
Dysphagia in airway obstruction, 98
Dysplasia,
  bronchopulmonary, 226-228, 718
Dyspnea
  asthma, 213
  pericarditis, 254
Dysrhythmia, 259-263
  advanced life support, 159-160
  electrical burn injury, 581, 582
  hypothermia, 654, 655
  neonatal, 661
Dystrophin, 310
Dystrophy, Duchenne's
  muscular, 310-312

E

Ear, 457-463
  AIDS manifestations, 398
  anatomy and physiology, 64, 457-
    458
  disorders, 458-463
    acute otitis media, 460-461
    foreign bodies in, 462-463
    otitis externa, 458-460
  history, 458

Ear—cont'd
  physical examination, 80, 81, 82,
    458, 459
    neonatal, 665, 666
Ear drum, 457, 458
Early septic shock, 121
Eating disorders, 734-737
Ecchymosis, 420
  snakebite, 647
Echocardiography
  congenital heart defects, 249
  congestive heart failure, 251
  Kawasaki disease, 256
  myocarditis, 254-255
  pericarditis, 254
  septic shock, 121
Echovirus, 281
ED; see Emergency department
EDAP; see Emergency department approved for pediatrics
Edema
  angioneurotic, 651-652, 653
  bronchopulmonary dysplasia, 227
  cerebral, 513
    increased intracranial pres-
      sure, 142
  eyelid, 80
  glomerulonephritis, 380, 381
  snakebite, 647
  urticaria, 650
Education
  burn injury prevention, 564
  emergency department
    personnel, 10-13, 19
  Emergency Medical Services For
    Children recommendations, 747
  interfacility transport personnel, 14-
    15
  nurses, 21
  pediatric triage, 90
  prehospital providers, 4-5
  public, 15-16
  safety, 61, 62-63
  trauma management, 492, 496-497
EEG; see Electroencephalography
Effortless tachypnea
  hypoplastic left heart syndrome, 248
  transposition of great arteries, 245
Egocentricity in toddler, 49
Eisenmenger's syndrome, 240
Elavil; see Amitriptyline
Elbow
  fracture, 556
  nursemaid's, 552-554
Electrical burn injury, 581-582
Electrical outlets in pediatric emergency
  departments, 18
Electrocardiography
  congenital heart defects, 249
  congestive heart failure, 250
  hyperkalemia, 323
  hypocalcemia, 483
  hypokalemia, 322

Electrocardiography—cont'd
in intubation, 157
myocarditis, 254
near-drowning, 220-221
pericarditis, 254
septic shock, 121
snakebite, 648
Electroencephalography
encephalopathy, 282
increased intracranial pressure, 141
seizure, 272
Electrolyte balance, 314-315; see also
Fluid and electrolyte balance
Electrolyte imbalance; see Fluid and
electrolyte imbalance
Electromechanical dissociation, 160
Elimination
bowel
Hirschsprung's disease, 353
neonatal, 662, 677
urinary, 364
Elimite; see Permethrin
ELISA; see Enzyme-linked immunosorbent assay
Emancipated minor, 29
EMD; see Electromechanical dissociation
Emergency department
caring for children in adult
facilities, 19-20
continuous quality improvement, 16
ideal, 17-19
personnel education, 10-13
promotion of injury prevention, 15
triaging out of, 92
Emergency department approved for
pediatrics, 16-17
criteria for transport to, 7-8
rural population transport to, 14
urban population transport to, 13
Emergency Medical and Injury Prevention Systems for Children, 20
Emergency medical service, 1
access to, 15-16
activation during field resuscitation, 149, 151, 152
categorization of providers, 3
data collection recommendations,
741
education of providers, 4-5, 492
state contacts, 742-746
Emergency medical service systems,
1-2, 3
Emergency medical services for
children, 1-23
adult emergency departments
and, 19-20
components of, 3
continuous quality improvement, 16, 17
data and research, 9-10
development of, 2-3, 4
emergency departments approved for
pediatrics, 16-17

Emergency medical services for
children—cont'd
emergency medical services
systems, 1-2, 3
equipment, 9, 11
funding, 20-21
hospital care, 10-13, 14
emergency department
education, 10-13
intensive care/specialized
care, 13, 14
rehabilitation, 13
ideal pediatric emergency
departments, 17-19
nurses' role in, 21
prehospital care, 3-6
dispatch in, 4
field treatment protocols, 5
identification in, 3-4
provider education in, 4-5
public education and EMS
access, 15-16
regional development, 13-15
scoring systems, 6-9
transport systems, 5-6, 7-8
Emergency Medical Services For Children recommendations, 747-748
Emergency medical technician, 2, 3
Emergency Nurse Pediatric
Course, 12, 497
Emergency Nursing Advanced Pediatric
Management, 13
Emetics, 625
EMIPSC; see Emergency Medical and
Injury Prevention Systems for Children
EMLA, 701
Emotional abuse, 587, 590
EMS; see Emergency medical service
EMSC; see Emergency medical services
for children
EMSS; see Emergency medical service
systems
EMT; see Emergency medical techni-
cian
EN-APM; see Emergency Nursing Ad-
vanced Pediatric Management
Encephalitis, 281-283
Encephalopathy, 142, 282
Endocarditis, 253
Endocrine system, 472-486
adrenal insufficiency, 483-486
anatomy and physiology, 472, 473
diabetes insipidus, 481-482
diabetic ketoacidosis, 477-480
hypocalcemia, 482-483
hypoglycemia, 472-477
hypothermia, 653
Endorphins
pain and, 686
septic shock, 120
Endoscopy, 361, 362
Endothelial cells
hemolytic-uremic syndrome, 386

Endothelial cells—cont'd
septic shock, 120
Endotracheal intubation, 157-158
bacterial tracheitis, 203
epiglottitis, 202
multiple trauma management, 498-
499
near-drowning, 221
neonatal, 169-170, 171
meconium staining, 176
poisoning, 623
resuscitation drug delivery, 161,
173-174
tube size in, 499
viral croup, 200
End-stage renal disease, 385
Enema
intussusception, 347
myelomeningocele, 287
neonatal constipation, 677
Enkephalins, 696
Enophthalmus, 452-453
ENPC; see Emergency Nurse Pediatric
Course
Entamoeba histolytica, 356, 357
Enteric bacteria, 119
Enterobiasis, 358, 359
Enterocolitis, 354
Enterovirus
hand-foot-mouth disease, 433
pericarditis, 254
Enuresis in diabetes insipidus, 481
Environmental emergencies, 642-657
anaphylaxis and angioneurotic
edema, 651-652, 653
bites and stings, 642-650
animal, 643-645
insect, 642-643, 644
snakebite, 646-650
hypothermia, 652-655
Lyme disease, 656-657
Rocky Mountain spotted fever, 655-
656
urticaria, 650-651
Environmental factors
care of child in adult emergency departments, 19
congenital heart defects, 237
Lyme disease, 656
nosebleed, 465
as obstacles to patient care, 71
pharyngitis, 469
primary hypothermia, 653
Rocky Mountain spotted fever, 655
suicidal behavior, 732
triage assessment, 103
Enzyme-linked immunosorbent assay
bronchiolitis, 207
HIV infection, 397
Lyme disease, 657
Enzymes
neonatal, 662
pediatric anatomic and physiologic
differences, 64

Eosinophilia, 209
Eosinophils, 392, 393, 394
Epidermal appendages, 418-419
Epidermis
  anatomy and physiology, 417, 418
  burn injury, 567, 568, 570
Epidural hematoma, 514-515
Epidural space, 511
Epiglottal reflex, 195
Epiglottitis, 201-202
Epilepsy Foundation of America, 274
Epinephrine
  anaphylaxis, 652, 653
  asthma, 214
  asystolic arrest, 160
  resuscitation
    neonatal, 166, 174
    pediatric, 161-162, 163
  shock, 124
  symptomatic bradycardia, 159
  urticaria, 450, 650
  ventricular fibrillation, 160
  viral croup, 200
Epinephrine administration kit, 450
Epiphyseal fracture, 542
Epiphysis
  anatomy and physiology, 290
  osteomyelitis, 293
  septic arthritis, 296
  slipped capital femoral, 303-306,
    307, 308
  limp and, 292
Epispadias, 367
Epistaxis, 465-467
Epithelial cells, intestinal, 332-333
Equipment
  in adult emergency departments, 19
  conscious sedation, 699
  EMS, 9, 11
  interfacility transport, 14-15
  intubation, 111, 157-158
  resuscitation, 153-154, 155
    neonatal, 165-166
  spinal immobilization, 500
  trauma, 495-496
  triage, 91
Ergotamines, 270
Erikson's psychosocial developmental
    theory, 44
  adolescent, 56, 57-58
  infant, 44, 45
  preschooler, 49, 51
  school-age child, 52, 55
  toddler, 47-49
Erosion, 424
Erysipelas, 435
Erythema chronicum migrans, 657
Erythema infectiosum, 426, 431-432
Erythema multiforme, 448-450
Erythrocyte, 390-391; see also Red
  blood cells
Erythrocyte sedimentation rate
  arthritis
    juvenile rheumatoid, 299

Erythrocyte sedimentation rate—cont'd
  arthritis—cont'd
    septic, 296
  infective endocarditis, 253
  Kawasaki disease, 256
  osteomyelitis, 294
  pelvic inflammatory disease, 372
  rheumatic fever, 255
  toxic or transient synovitis, 301
Erythromycin
  Campylobacter gastroenteritis, 341
  chlamydia, 370
  impetigo, 434
  Lyme disease, 657
  pertussis, 209
  pneumonia, 206
  rheumatic fever, 256
  scarlet fever, 431
Erythropoietin, 390
Escharotomy, 583-584
Escherichia coli
  meningitis, 277
  neonatal sepsis, 668
  urinary tract infection, 372
Esophageal pacing
  atrial flutter, 260
  supraventricular tachycardia, 260
  symptomatic bradycardia, 160
Esophagus
  anatomy and physiology, 332, 333
  foreign body lodged in, 360-361
ESR; see Erythrocyte sedimentation rate
Estrogen, 473
Ethambutol, 211
Ethanol
  as antidote, 632, 636
  poisoning, 635, 637
Ethchlorvynol poisoning, 634
Ethical considerations, 34-41
  alternative health care practices, 38-
    41
  beneficence and nonmaleficence, 35,
    36
  brain death, 37
  child's right to die, 37
  decision making, 34-35
  justice, 35
  organ donation, 37-38
  respect for persons, 35
  terminal illness, 35-37
Ethnic factors; see Cultural factors
Ethosuximide, 273
Ethylene glycol poisoning, 632, 636
Eustachian tube
  acute otitis media and, 460-461
  anatomy, 64, 457
Evaporation in body temperature regulation, 607
Evidence collection
  abused child, 596-597
  murdered child, 189
Ewing's sarcoma, 292
Exanthems
  assessment, 87

Exanthems—cont'd
  infectious, 420-434
    fifth disease, 431-432
    hand-foot-mouth disease, 433-434
    pityriasis rosea, 432-433
    roseola infantum, 432
    rubella, 429
    rubeola, 420-428
    scarlet fever, 430-431
    varicella, 429-430
Exchange transfusion, 631
Excoriation, 420, 423
Excretion of drugs and toxins, 65-66
Exercise
  cardiovascular assessment, 234, 235
  Legg-Perthes disease, 303
  pulmonary stenosis, 242
Exocrine gland dysfunction in cystic fibrosis, 224
Exophthalmos, 452
Expiration, 197; see also Breathing
Expiratory stridor in viral croup, 200
Expiratory wheezing
  asthma, 212
  bronchiolitis, 207
Exposure
  status epilepticus, 130
  trauma management, 494, 506
  triage assessment, 103
Express consent, 28
External auditory canal, 458-460
Extracellular fluid, 313, 314
  diabetic ketoacidosis, 477
  electrolyte balance, 314-315
  hyperkalemia, 322
  hypernatremia, 320
  hypokalemia, 321-322
  hyponatremia, 318
  neonatal, 661
  pediatric anatomic and physiologic
    differences, 63
Extremities
  blood pressure technique, 236
    coarctation of aorta, 243
  cardiovascular assessment, 235, 236
  circumferential burn, 583, 584
  coarctation of aorta and, 243
  fracture, 542-544
    nursing care and evaluation, 556-
      559
  intraosseous access, 159
  osteomyelitis of, 293
  physical examination, 86
  septic arthritis, 296
  snakebite, 649
  trauma, 542-544, 549-555
    multiple injury, 508
    nursing care and evaluation, 556-
      559
  triage assessment, 92, 103
Eye, 452-457
  AIDS manifestations, 398
  anatomy and physiology, 64, 452,
    453

Eye—cont'd
assessment, 78-81, 452-454
neonatal, 665, 666
chemical exposure, 625
coma and, 134, 138
dehydration, 100
disorders, 454-457
erythema multiforme and, 448-449, 450
head and neck injury assessment, 521-522
hydrocephalus and, 275
hypertonic *versus* hypotonic dehydration, 319
juvenile rheumatoid arthritis, 301
juvenile rheumatoid arthritis and, 297-298, 300
oculocephalic reflex, 134
trauma, 536-538
Eyeball, 95-97, 452
Eyelid
edema, 80
sunken, 80
trauma, 536

F

FAB; *see* Fluorescent antibody testing
Face
examination, 78, 79
laceration repair, 562
FACES Scale, 691, 692
Factor replacement, 410, 411
Failure to thrive
AIDS, 397
child abuse, 602-604
cystic fibrosis, 224
Falls, 491
cerebral palsy, 284
Children's Trauma Tool, 10
muscular dystrophy, 310, 311
window, 489
Family
adolescent relationship with, 56, 57, 58
in crisis, 178-186, 188-191
communication, 179-180
death of child, 182-186
homicide and violence, 189-191
initial interview, 180
resuscitation, 181
signs and symptoms, 179
sudden infant death syndrome, 188-189, 190
violent behavior, 181-182
physical comfort of in emergency departments, 17-18
presence in treatment rooms, 19
of special needs child, 713
status epilepticus and, 131-132
Family history
apnea, 229
cardiovascular assessment, 234

Family history—cont'd
Legg-Perthes disease, 302
neurologic assessment, 268
Fantasy; *see* Magical thinking
Farm machinery injury, 491-492
Fasciotomy, 584
Fat, brown, 607, 662
FBA; *see* Foreign body aspiration
FBAO; *see* Foreign body airway obstruction
Fears
adolescent, 57, 58
infant, 45, 46
preschooler, 51, 52
school-age child, 54, 55
toddler, 48, 49
Febrile child; *see* Fever
Febrile seizure, 128, 609-610
roseola infantum, 432
Federal government, EMSC support, 20
Feedings
acute otitis media, 461
congestive heart failure, 250
ventricular septal defect, 241
Felbamate, 273
Feldenkrais, 39
Female genitalia
anatomy, 364, 365
physical assessment, 367
neonatal, 664, 666
sexual abuse, 599-600
Femoral epiphysis, slipped capital, 292, 303-306, 307, 308
Femoral head, osteochondrosis of, 302
Femur
fracture, 544-545, 556
intraosseous access, 504
red blood cell production in, 392
Fencing reflex, 268, 667
Fentanyl, 697-698
extremity injury, 557
midazolam and, 700
Ferrous sulfate poisoning, 626
Fetal hemoglobin, 391
Fetus
cardiovascular development, 233, 234
rubella and, 429
Fever, 606-621
bacterial tracheitis, 201, 202
bronchiolitis, 206-207
clinical presentation, 610-613
defined, 606-607
emergency department intervention, 614-615
epiglottitis, 201
etiology, 607
fluid therapy determination, 317
grunting respirations, 100
increased intracranial pressure, 145
Kawasaki disease, 256
measles, 428

Fever—cont'd
meningitis, 279, 281
neonatal sepsis, 669
neutropenia with, 400-401
nursing care and evaluation, 615-619
osteomyelitis, 293
pathophysiology, 607-610
pelvic inflammatory disease, 372
Rocky Mountain spotted fever, 656
roseola infantum, 432
seizures, 128, 431, 609-610
supraventricular tachycardia, 260
toxic or transient synovitis, 301
triage assessment, 94, 103, 104
viral croup, 201
Fiberoptic catheter, 144, 145
Fibrillation
atrial, 260-261
ventricular, 262
advanced life support, 160
electrical burn injury, 581
hypothermia, 654, 655
near-drowning, 220
Fibula fracture, 545-546, 547
Field treatment; *see also* Prehospital care
burn injury, 572-573
protocols, 5
resuscitation etiology, 147
snakebite, 648-649
Field triage; *see* Triage
Fifth disease, 426, 431-432
Finger
position for chest compression, 151
in neonate, 171
trauma, 555, 556
Finger sweep for foreign body removal, 218
Fingernail, 419
loss of in crush injury, 555
Fingerprinting in hypotonic dehydration, 319
Fiorinal, 270
Fire ant bite, 644
Firearm injury, 516
First aid
community education, 5, 16
prehospital provider training, 5
First responder, 3
First-degree burn, 567, 570
Fish tapeworm, 359
Fissure, 424
Flail chest, 529
Flame injury, 566
Fleets enema, 287
Flow-Thru tube, 724, 725
Flucinolone acetonide, 445
Fluid
loss
daily, 314
hypovolemic shock, 117
shift
burn injury, 574-575
hypovolemic shock, 117-118

Fluid and electrolyte balance
  anatomy and physiology, 63-66,
    313-315
  encephalopathy, 282
  neonatal, 661
Fluid and electrolyte imbalance
  acid-base disorders, 326-329
  anorexia and bulimia nervosa, 735,
    736
  burn injury, 575
  calcium balance disorders, 323-326
  dehydration, 315-318
  diabetic ketoacidosis, 477
  hyperkalemia, 322-323, 324
  hypernatremia, 320-321
  hypokalemia, 321-322
  hyponatremia, 318-319, 320
  nursing care, 329-330
  renal failure, 383-384
  shock, 125
Fluid and electrolyte therapy; see Fluid
  therapy
Fluid restriction in increased intracranial pressure, 143
Fluid therapy
  anaphylaxis, 652
  asthma, 216
  burn injury, 574-578
  comatose child, 138-139
  dehydration, 316
  diabetes insipidus, 482
  diabetic ketoacidosis, 479
  disseminated intravascular coagula-
    tion, 413
  febrile child, 618
  gastroenteritis, 340
  hyponatremia, 319, 320
  hypovolemic cardiopulmonary ar-
    rest, 159
  increased intracranial pressure, 143
  intussusception, 347
  maintenance calculation, 317
  malrotation of bowel with
    volvulus, 350-351
  meningitis, 279
  near-drowning, 222
  neonatal resuscitation, 166, 173-175
  renal failure, 385
  shock, 122
    cardiogenic, 119
    hypovolemic, 118
    septic, 121
  sickle cell crisis, 407
  status epilepticus, 130
  trauma management
    head and neck, 523
    multiple injury, 505
Flumazenil, 632
Fluocinonide, 445
Fluonid; see Flucinolone acetonide
Fluorescent antibody testing, 209
Fluoride poisoning, 632
Flurandrenolide, 445

Flutter, atrial, 260, 261
Folate deficiency, 285
Foley catheter
  esophageal foreign body re-
    moval, 361, 362
  gastrostomy tube, 725
Folic acid deficiency in anemia, 402
Follicle-stimulating hormone, 473
Follow-up information after transfer, 15
Fontanels, 266
  anatomy, 68, 511
  dehydration, 100, 319
  examination, 78, 79, 666
  hydrocephalus, 275
  triage assessment, 94, 102
Food
  anaphylactic reaction, 651
  aspiration, 217
  hypoglycemia treatment, 475
  urticaria, 450, 650
Foot
  assessment in lower extremity frac-
    ture, 543
  bones of, 548
  fracture of, 547-548, 556
Foramen ovale, 242
Forced diuresis, 631
Forceps, McGill, 157
Forearm fracture, 551-552, 553, 556
Foreign body
  in ears and nose, 462-463
  ingestion, 360-362
Foreign body airway obstruction, 151-
  153, 198, 217-219
Foreign body aspiration, 217-219
Formal operations stage of development, 56, 57
Fourth-degree burn, 571
Foxglove poisoning, 633
Fracture
  blowout ocular, 537
  cerebral palsy, 284
  child abuse, 594-595
  Legg-Perthes disease, 302
  limp and, 292
  lower extremity, 542-544
  nursing care and evaluation, 556-559
  open, 560-561
  osteogenesis imperfecta, 308, 309,
    310
  Pediatric Trauma Score, 9
  rib, 529, 594-595
  skull, 516, 595
  triage assessment, 103
  types and patterns, 542
  upper extremity, 549-552, 554-555
  urban versus rural prehospital calls, 4
Frank-Starling law, 233
Fresh frozen plasma
  disseminated intravascular coagula-
    tion, 413
  hemolytic-uremic syndrome, 387

Freud's psychosexual developmental
  theory, 44
  adolescent, 57
  infant, 45
  preschooler, 50, 51
  school-age child, 55
  toddler, 47-49
Friction rub
  juvenile rheumatoid arthritis, 297
  pericarditis, 254
Frostbite, 654, 655
Fruity breath, 477
FSH; see Follicle-stimulating hormone
FTT; see Failure to thrive
Full-thickness burn, 567, 570, 571,
  583
Funding, 20-21, 748
Fundoplication, 723
Funeral arrangements, 183
Fungal infection
  cutaneous, 437-440
  meningitis, 279
  otitis externa, 459
Funnel chest, 84
Furosemide
  bronchopulmonary dysplasia, 227
  congestive heart failure, 251
  glomerulonephritis, 381
  head and neck injury, 525
  hypercalcemia, 325
  hyperkalemia, 323, 324
  hyponatremia, 319
  increased intracranial pressure, 141,
    143, 524
  myocarditis, 255
  renal failure, 383, 384

G

GABA; see Gamma-aminobutyric acid
Gabapentin, 273
GAβHS; see Group A beta-hemolytic
  streptococci
Gag reflex
  bulimia nervosa, 735
  coma, 136
Gait in lower extremity fracture, 543
Galant reflex, 667
Galeazzi fracture, 552, 553
Gallbladder, 334
Gamma-aminobutyric acid, 686
Gangrene in hypothermia, 654
Gas exchange, 108, 193
Gas inhalation injury, 579
Gasoline poisoning, 638
Gastoport tube, 725
Gastric decompression, neonatal, 169
Gastric decontamination, 625-630
Gastric emptying, 332
Gastric lavage for poisoning, 626-627,
  635
Gastroenteritis, 339-340, 341-343
Gastroesophageal reflux, 332

Gastrografin enema, 287
Gastrointestinal system, 332-363
  AIDS manifestations, 399
  anatomy and physiology, 64, 332-
    334
  cystic fibrosis and, 224, 225
  disorders, 339-362
    anorexia and bulimia nervosa, 735
    apnea and, 228
    appendicitis, 348-350
    foreign body ingestion, 360-362
    gastroenteritis, 339-340, 341-343
    hemorrhage, 338
    Hirschsprung's disease, 353-355
    incarcerated hernia, 351-352
    inconsolable crying, 681
    intestinal parasites, 356-360
    intussusception, 346-347
    liver transplantation for, 355-356
    malrotation of bowel with
      volvulus, 350-351
    pyloric stenosis, 352-353
    stomatitis, 340-344
    viral hepatitis, 344-346
  history and assessment, 334-335
  neonatal, 662
  signs and symptoms, 335-339
    abdominal pain, 338-339
    constipation, 337-338
    diarrhea, 336-337
    rectal bleeding, 338
    vomiting, 335-336
  trauma, 527, 531
Gastrostomy tube, 722-725
Gate theory, 687
GBS; see Group B streptococci
GCS; see Glasgow Coma Scale
Gender
  juvenile rheumatoid arthritis, 298
  pyloric stenosis, 352
  urinary tract infection, 373
Gene therapy for hemophilia, 411
General appearance
  child abuse, 591
  general survey, 77, 78
  neonatal assessment, 663
  preschooler, 51
  toddler, 48
General survey, 77-79, 80
Generalized seizure, 271, 272, 273
Genetic factors
  anaphylaxis, 651
  congenital heart defects, 237
  cystic fibrosis, 223-224
  febrile seizure, 609
  pyloric stenosis, 352
Genital herpes, 368
Genital stage of adolescent development, 57
Genitalia
  anatomy and physiology, 364, 365
  child abuse, 591-592, 599-600
  multiple trauma management, 508

Genitalia—cont'd
  physical assessment, 85, 366-367
  neonatal, 664, 666
Genitourinary system, 364-389
  anatomy and physiology, 64, 364-
    365, 366
  disorders, 367-388
    acute glomerulonephritis, 378-
      380
    hemolytic-uremic syndrome, 386-
      387
    Henoch-Schönlein purpura, 387-
      388
    inconsolable crying, 681
    nephrotic syndrome, 380-382
    pelvic inflammatory disease, 369-
      372, 373
    renal failure, 382-385
    renal transplantation for, 385-
      386
    sexually transmitted disease, 367-
      369, 370-371
    testicular torsion, 377-378
    urinary tract infection, 372-375
    vesicoureteral reflux, 375-377
  history and physical
    examination, 85-86, 365-366
    neonatal, 664
  trauma, 527
Gentamicin
  osteomyelitis, 295
  pelvic inflammatory disease, 373
  pneumonia, 206
German measles, 429
GH; see Growth hormone
Ghon complex, 210
Giardia lamblia, 356-359
Glasgow Coma Scale, 134, 137, 139,
  494
  drowning survival rates and, 148
  field triage, 6
  head and neck injury, 520
  multiple trauma management, 505-
    506
  neurologic triage assessment, 102
GLIAS; see Glycerol 30%-sodium ascorbate 20%
Glipizide poisoning, 634
Glomerular filtration rate, 365
  calculation of, 365
  chronic renal failure, 382
  metabolic alkalosis, 328
Glomerulonephritis, 378-380
Glottic opening in endotracheal intubation, 498
Gloving, 400
Glucagon, 473
  anaphylaxis, 653
  as antidote, 632
  glucose regulation, 474
  hypoglycemia, 475-476
Glucocorticoids, 473, 485-486
Gluconate, 483

Glucose
  altered mental status, 624-625
  diabetic ketoacidosis, 478
  hyperkalemia, 323, 324
  hypoglycemia, 472, 475, 671
  increased intracranial pressure, 141
  meningitis, 279
  neonatal, 662, 671
  regulation of, 472-474
  for resuscitation, 162-164, 174-175
  shock, 125
  status epilepticus, 128, 131
Glucuronyl transferase, 673
Glue, 738
Glutethimide poisoning, 626
Glyburide poisoning, 634
Glycerin suppository, 677
Glycerol 30%-sodium ascorbate 20%,
  145
Glycogen storage, 472-474
  neonatal hypoglycemia and, 671
Glycogenolysis, 474
Gluconeogenesis, 474
Goalpost technique, 173
Gold compound for juvenile rheuma-
  toid arthritis, 300
Gold poisoning, 633
Golytely, 630
Gonadotropins, 473
Gonococcal pharyngitis, 469
Gonorrhea, 368, 369, 371
Gowning, 207
Gram stain in meningitis, 279
Gram-negative organisms, 668
  gastroenteritis, 341-343
  septic shock, 119, 121
Gram-positive organisms, 121
  septic shock, 119
Granulocytes, 391, 394
Grasp reflex, 667
Greenstick fracture, 542, 549, 550
Grief, 182-186
  murdered child, 189
Griseofulvin, 439
Ground transport, 5, 166
Group A beta-hemolytic streptococci
  cellulitis, 435
  epiglottitis, 201
  glomerulonephritis, 379
  impetigo, 434
  osteomyelitis, 293
  pharyngitis, 469
  rheumatic fever, 255-256
  scarlet fever, 430, 431
  tracheitis, 202
Group B streptococci
  meningitis, 277
  neonatal sepsis, 668
  osteomyelitis, 293
  pneumonia, 203
  septic shock, 119
Growth and development, 43-58, 59
  adolescent, 56-58, 59

Growth and development—cont'd
  developmentally delayed child, 714-716
  growth charts, 749-752
  growth parameters, 74-75
  infant, 44-47
  mental retardation, 716-717
  neonatal, 660
  neurologic assessment, 268
  pediatric anatomic and physiologic differences, 61-63, 64
  preschooler, 49-52, 53, 54
  school-age child, 52-56
  toddler, 47-49, 50
Growth charts, 74, 749-752
Growth hormone, 473
Growth parameters, 74-75
Growth plate, 86
  anatomy and physiology, 290
  fracture, 541-542
    ankle, 547
    knee, 547
  Legg-Perthes disease, 306
  septic arthritis, 296
Grunting respirations
  criteria for transport to pediatric critical care center, 7
  pneumonia, 204
  respiratory distress, 196
  triage assessment, 100
Guaifenesin, 410-411
Guardian; see Parent
Guidelines for Air and Ground Transport of Neonatal and Pediatric Patients, 5

H
H technique, 173
Haddon Matrix, 487, 488
Haemophilus influenzae
  acute otitis media, 460
  cellulitis, 435
    preorbital and orbital, 455, 457
  conjunctivitis, 454
  meningitis, 277
  osteomyelitis, 293
  pneumonia, 203
  septic arthritis, 296
  septic shock, 119
  sinusitis, 466
Haemophilus influenzae type B
  epiglottitis, 201
  meningitis, 277, 280
  septic arthritis, 296
  tracheitis, 202
Hair, 418-419
  pubic, 85-86
Halcinonide, 445
Hallucinogens, 738
Halog; see Halcinonide
Hand
  anorexia and bulimia nervosa, 735

Hand—cont'd
  posterior view, 554
  trauma, 555, 556
Hand-foot syndrome in sickle cell anemia, 406
Hand-foot-mouth disease, 427, 433-434
Handgun injury, 189
Handwashing
  AIDS, 400
  impetigo, 434
  neutropenia with fever, 401
Hard palate, 468
HCO_3; see Bicarbonate radical
Head
  heat loss and, 68
  multiple trauma management, 506-507
  pediatric anatomic and physiologic differences, 64
  physical examination, 77-78, 79, 80
  neonatal, 666
Head and neck trauma, 511-527
  attention deficit hyperactivity disorder, 728
  cerebral palsy, 284
  cervical spine immobilization, 500, 501
  cervical spine injury, 516-519
  child abuse, 595
  Children's Trauma Tool, 10
  closed head injury, 514-516
  emergency department intervention, 519
  hemophilia, 410
  increased intracranial pressure, 141
  multiple trauma
    management, 505-506
  nasal discharge, 82
  near-drowning, 219, 221
  neurologic assessment, 505-506
  nursing intervention and evaluation, 520-527
  skull fracture, 516
  urban versus rural prehospital calls, 4
Head circumference
  hydrocephalus, 275
  measuring of, 78
  neonate, 77
Head lice, 447-448
Headache, 267-270
  Rocky Mountain spotted fever, 656
Head-tilt chin-lift position
  basic life support, 149, 150
  respiratory failure, 111
Head-to-toe assessment
  comatose child, 139-140
  trauma management, 492, 506-508
Health maintenance organizations, 27
Hearing assessment, 81, 458
Hearing loss, 280
Heart, 233-265
  AIDS manifestations, 399

Heart—cont'd
  anatomy and physiology, 66-67, 233-234
    neonatal, 661
  disease; see Heart disease
  frequency of injury, 527
  hemorrhagic shock classification, 503
  history and physical assessment, 84, 234-237
    neonatal, 664
  hyperkalemia, 323
  intrinsic autoregulation, 114, 116
Heart attack; see Cardiopulmonary arrest
Heart block, 262-263
  symptomatic bradycardia, 160
Heart disease, 237-263
  acquired, 252-255
  anorexia and bulimia nervosa, 735
  chest pain, 258-259
  congenital heart defects, 237-238
    acyanotic with left-to-right shunting, 238-241
    cyanotic with right-to-left shunting, 244-248
    obstructive, 241-244
  congestive heart failure, 250-251, 252
  dysrhythmias, 259-263
  grunting respirations, 100
  hypercyanotic episode, 252
  Kawasaki disease, 256
  nursing intervention, 256-258
  rheumatic fever, 255-256
Heart murmur
  aortic stenosis, 244
  assessment, 84, 236-237
    neonatal, 664, 666
  atrial septal defect, 240
  coarctation of aorta and, 243
  complete atrioventricular canal defect, 241
  pulmonary stenosis, 242
  ventricular septal defect, 240
Heart rate
  anemia, 402
  anorexia and bulimia nervosa, 735
  Apgar score, 168
  cardiac output and, 114-115, 233
  neonatal, 661, 666, 668
    assessment, 170
    chest compression, 171
    intubation, 169
  normal, 103
  pain assessment, 695
  pediatric anatomic and physiologic differences, 67
  supraventricular tachycardia, 259
  symptomatic bradycardia, 159
  triage assessment, 103-104
  ventricular septal defect, 241
Heart sounds, 84, 236-237
  atrial septal defect, 240

Heart sounds—cont'd
  neonatal, 666
Heart valve
  hypoplastic left heart syndrome, 248
  rheumatic fever, 255
Heat application for pain management, 703
Heat loss
  neonatal, 662
  through head, 68
Heavy metal poisoning, 633
Heel fracture, 547
Heimlich maneuver, 152
Helium-oxygen mixture for viral croup, 200-201
Helper T cell, 394, 397
Hemarthrosis, 409
Hematocrit
  anemia, 405
  congenital heart defects, 249
  dehydration, 315-316
  neonatal, 661
  pediatric anatomic and physiologic differences, 65
Hematogenous osteomyelitis, 293, 294
Hematologic system; see also Blood
  anatomy and physiology, 65, 390-395
  disorders, 401-415
    anemia, 401-403, 404, 405
    disseminated intravascular coagulation, 411-413
    hemophilia, 408-411
    idiopathic thrombocytopenic purpura, 413-415
    sickle cell anemia, 403-408
  history and physical examination, 395-396
  neonatal, 661-662
Hematoma, 514-515
Hematuria
  infective endocarditis, 253
  renal failure, 383
Hemiplegia, spastic, 283
Hemodialysis for poisoning, 631, 636
Hemoglobin, 391
  anemia, 405
  anorexia and bulimia nervosa, 734
  bilirubin metabolism, 673
  congenital heart defects, 249
  cyanosis and, 196
  neonatal, 661
Hemolytic-uremic syndrome, 386-387
Hemoperfusion for poisoning, 631
Hemophilia, 408-411
  limp and, 292-293
Hemoptysis, 225, 226
Hemorrhage
  anemia, 403
  criteria for transport to pediatric critical care center, 7
  disseminated intravascular coagulation, 412

Hemorrhage—cont'd
  epistaxis, 465-467
  femur fractures, 544-545
  gastrointestinal, 338
  hemophilia, 408-411
  idiopathic thrombocytopenic purpura, 413-414
  increased intracranial pressure, 142
  intracranial, 514-516
  rectal, 338
  snakebite, 647
  subjunctival, 80
  tube thoracostomy, 502
Hemorrhagic shock, 117
  multiple trauma management, 503
Hemothorax, 502, 527, 529
Henoch-Schönlein purpura, 387-388
Heparin, 413
Hepatic artery, 334
Hepatic coma, 356
Hepatic enzymes, 64
Hepatic system
  acetaminophen poisoning, 635
  AIDS manifestations, 399
  anatomy and physiology, 64, 334
    neonatal, 662
  palpation, 85, 237
  roundworm migration to, 359
  transplantation, 355-356
  trauma, 530-531
    frequency, 527
    referred pain in, 507
  viral hepatitis, 344-346
Hepatitis, 344-346
Herald patch, 432, 433
Herbalism, 39
Hereditary factors; see Genetic factors
Hereditary spherocytosis, 402
Hernia
  cerebral, 134, 135, 513-514
  incarcerated, 351-352
  traumatic diaphragmatic, 530
  umbilical, 85
Heroine, 738
Herpangina, 343
Herpes simplex virus
  child abuse and, 600
  encephalitis, 281, 282
  genital herpes, 368
  stomatitis, 343
Hetastarch, 123
Hip
  Legg-Perthes disease, 303, 304-305
  septic arthritis, 296
  toxic or transient synovitis, 301
HIPs; see Hospital insurance plans
Hirschsprung's disease, 353-355
Histamine
  anaphylactic reaction, 651
  insect stings, 643
  urticaria, 450, 650
Histamine blockers, 651
Histoacryl Blue, 562
Histocytes, 392

History, 70-72
  apnea, 229
  burn injury, 574
  cardiovascular, 234-237
  child abuse, 588-589
  comatose child, 140-141
  crisis intervention, 180
  cystic fibrosis, 226
  febrile child, 612, 613
  gastrointestinal, 334-335
  genitourinary, 365-366
  head and neck trauma, 520
  hematologic and immune system, 395-396
  Legg-Perthes disease, 302
  musculoskeletal, 290, 291
  neonatal, 662
  neonatal resuscitation, 167
  neonatal sepsis, 670
  neurologic, 266-267, 268
  obstetric, 167
  pelvic inflammatory disease, 372
  poisoning, 623
  respiratory assessment, 110, 195
  special needs child, 712
  status epilepticus, 129
  trauma management, 492, 506
  triage, 95
HIV; see Human immunodeficiency virus infection
Hives, 450-451
HLHS; see Hypoplastic left heart syndrome
HMOs; see Health maintenance organizations
Hoarseness in viral croup, 200
Home care
  apnea monitoring, 229-230
  mechanical ventilators, 722, 723
  oxygen dependence, 718-719
  special needs child, 714
Homelessness, 739
Homeopathy, 40
Homicide of child, 189-191
Hookworm, 358
Hormones; see Endocrine system
Hornet sting, 644, 651
Hospital agreements, 14
Hospital care, 10-13, 14
  emergency room education, 10-13
  intensive care/specialized care, 13, 14
  rehabilitation, 13
Hospital insurance plans, 27
Host factors in pneumonia, 204
Hostile child, 730
House fire, 564-565, 579
HR; see Heart rate
HSV; see Herpes simplex virus
Human bite, 645
Human herpesvirus 6, 432
Human immunodeficiency virus infection, 396-400, 409
Human parvovirus B19, 431

Human plasma for volume resuscitation, 123
Humerus fracture, 550-551, 556
Humoral immunity, 395
HUS; *see* Hemolytic-uremic syndrome
Hydration; *see* Fluid therapy
Hydrocarbon
    abuse, 738
    poisoning, 638-639
Hydrocephalus, 274-277
    head examination, 78
    increased intracranial pressure, 142
    myelomeningocele, 285
Hydrocodone-based cough syrup poisoning, 634
Hydrocortisone
    adrenal insufficiency, 485
    potency guide, 445
Hydrocortisone cream, 441-442
Hydrocortisone valerate, 445
Hydrofluoric acid poisoning, 632
Hydrogen ion concentration, 326; *see also* pH
    respiratory failure, 110
    respiratory sensitivity to, 107-108
Hydroxyethyl starch, 123
Hydroxylase, 729
Hydroxymethyl, 125
Hydroxyurea, 408
Hydroxyzine
    sickle cell anemia, 406
    urticaria, 450, 651
Hymen, 86, 367
    in child abuse, 599-600
Hymenolepis nana, 359
Hyperactivity
    attention deficit hyperactivity disorder, 728, 729
    Legg-Perthes disease, 303
Hyperbilirubinemia, 672-675
Hypercalcemia, 325-326
Hypercyanotic episode, 244, 252
Hyperdynamic state, 121
Hyperemia, cerebral, 513
Hyperglycemia, 477, 478
    pain and, 687
    pediatric resuscitation, 164
Hyperkalemia, 322-323, 324
    burn injury, 575
    renal failure, 383-384, 385
Hyperkinetic cerebral palsy, 283
Hyperlipidemia, 381
Hypernatremia, 319, 320-321
Hyperpigmentation, 484
Hyperplasia, 484, 485
Hypersensitivity reaction, 450
Hypertension
    coarctation of aorta and, 243
    renal failure, 383
Hyperthermia
    increased intracranial pressure, 145
    status epilepticus, 131
    triage assessment, 94, 105

Hypertonic dehydration, 315, 320-321
    diabetes insipidus, 481
Hyperventilation
    cyclic antidepressant poisoning, 638
    head and neck injury, 523
    increased intracranial pressure, 141, 143
    respiratory alkalosis, 328
Hyphema, 537
Hypnosis, 703
Hypnotics
    abuse, 737
    intubation, 158
    poisoning, 624
Hypoalbuminemia
    burn injury, 575
    glomerulonephritis, 380, 381
Hypocalcemia, 324-325, 482-483
    renal failure, 384
    shock, 125
Hypoglycemia, 472-477
    adrenal insufficiency, 484, 485
    cardiovascular disorder and, 257
    ethanol ingestion, 636
    neonatal, 671-672
    pertussis, 209
    resuscitation
        neonatal, 174-175
        pediatric, 164
    shock, 125
    status epilepticus, 128, 131
Hypokalemia, 321-322
Hypomagnesemia, 483
Hyponatremia, 318-319, 320
    renal failure, 383, 384
    viral hepatitis, 346
Hypopharynx, 467, 468
Hypopituitarism, 484
Hypoplastic left heart syndrome, 248
Hypoproteinuria, 381
Hypospadias, 367
Hypotension
    coma, 136
    criteria for transport to pediatric critical care center, 7
    disseminated intravascular coagulation, 413
    narcotic analgesics and, 696
    pericardial tamponade, 530
    shock, 116
    tension pneumothorax, 528-529
Hypothalamic-pituitary-adrenal axis, 483, 484
Hypothalamus
    body temperature regulation, 607
    cardiovascular function, 113
Hypothermia, 652-655
    increased intracranial pressure, 145
    meningitis, 281
    near-drowning, 219, 220, 222, 223
    oxygen-hemoglobin saturation curve, 109
    pyloric stenosis, 353

Hypothermia—cont'd
    trauma management
        head and neck, 524
        multiple injury, 506
        triage assessment, 94, 104-105
Hypotonic dehydration, 315
Hypoventilation
    muscular dystrophy, 310, 311
    respiratory failure, 110
Hypovolemia
    advanced life support, 159
    burn injury, 574, 575
    nosebleed, 465
Hypovolemic shock, 114, 117-118
    burn injury, 574
Hypoxemia, 227, 228
Hypoxia
    asthma, 212, 216
    bronchopulmonary dysplasia, 227
    respiratory failure, 147
    status epilepticus, 128

I

Iatrogenic adrenal insufficiency, 484
Ibuprofen, 696
    body temperature reduction, 609, 617, 618
    hemophilia and, 410
    juvenile rheumatoid arthritis, 300
Ice application for pain management, 702, 703
ICP; *see* Intracranial pressure
Identification in prehospital care, 3-4
Identity *versus* role confusion in adolescent development, 56, 57-58
Idiopathic thrombocytopenic purpura, 413-415
Ilium, 332
Imagery for pain management, 703, 704
Imaginary audience, 728
Imagination training, 702
Imidazoline poisoning, 634
Imipramine poisoning, 634, 638
Immobilization
    cervical spine, 500, 501
        before basic life support, 149, 150
    septic arthritis, 297
    snakebite, 648
Immune globulin
    idiopathic thrombocytopenic purpura, 414
    varicella-zoster, 430
    viral hepatitis, 345, 346
Immune system
    anatomy and physiology, 65, 390-395
    disorders, 396-401
        acquired immunodeficiency syndrome, 396-400
        neutropenia with fever, 400-401
    history and physical examination, 395-396

Immune system—cont'd
low-grade fever and, 609
neonatal, 661-662, 662
Immunity, 394-395
neonatal, 662
Immunization, 87
bacille Calmette-Guérin, 211
pneumococcal, 206
triage assessment, 96
tuberculosis prevention, 211
varicella, 429
Immunocompromised child
acquired immunodeficiency
syndrome, 396-400
differential diagnosis, 397
neutropenia with fever, 400-401
septic shock, 119
stomatitis, 344
triage assessment, 97
Immunofluorescence, 657
Immunoglobulin E
anaphylactic reaction, 651
insect stings, 642
urticaria, 650
Immunoglobulin G, 65
Immunoglobulins, 395
neonatal, 662
Impacted fracture, 542
Impetigo, 434-435
Implied consent, 28, 29
in Verbal response, Glasgow Coma
Scale, 137
Incarcerated hernia, 351-352
Incest, 587
Incident reports, 33
India ink, 279
Indomethacin
hemophilia and, 410
juvenile rheumatoid arthritis, 300
Industry versus inferiority in school-age
child development, 52, 55
Infant
approach, 46-47, 76
basic life support, 152
bronchopulmonary dysplasia, 226-
228
chest compression, 150, 151
common fears, 45, 46
common injuries, 62, 490
congenital heart disease, 235
coping strategies, 689, 706
endotracheal tube size, 158
febrile
clinical presentation, 610-612
triage assessment, 104
foreign body airway
obstruction, 151-152
gaining cooperation of, 73-74
general survey, 75
growth and development, 44-47
hematologic and immune system, 65
increased intracranial pressure, 136,
142-143

Infant—cont'd
normal values
arterial blood gases, 109
blood volume, 67
urine output, 366
vital signs, 103, 198
pain responses, 688
reflexes, 268
seizure etiology, 271
sleep position, 188
temperature control in, 608
triage assessment, 82, 102
urinary tract infection, 374, 375
vision testing, 81
Infant car seat, 11, 489
Infantile spasm, 271, 272
Infarction in sickle cell anemia, 405
Infection
animal bites, 645
apnea and, 228
bacterial; see Bacterial infection
bone, 291-295
fever caused by, 608-609
fungal
cutaneous, 437-440
meningitis, 279
otitis externa, 459
genital tract, 367-372, 373
hypothermia, 653
increased intracranial pressure,
142
lower respiratory, 203-211
bronchiolitis, 206-208
muscular dystrophy, 310, 311
pertussis, 208-209, 210
pneumonia, 203-206
tuberculosis, 209-211
Lyme disease, 656-657
mental retardation and, 717
muscular dystrophy and, 310
neutropenia with fever, 400
oral cavity, 340-344
parasitic
cutaneous, 446-448
diarrhea, 337
eosinophil attachment to, 392
intestinal, 356-360
Rocky Mountain spotted fever, 655-
656
shunt, 275-276
sickle cell anemia and, 405, 406,
407, 408
upper respiratory
bacterial tracheitis, 202-203
common cold, 198-199
epiglottitis, 201-202
neonatal, 675
viral croup, 200-201
urinary tract, 372-375
in myelomeningocele, 286-287
vesicoureteral reflux, 375
urticaria, 650
viral; see Viral infection
Infection control, 207

Infectious exanthems, 420-434
fifth disease, 431-432
hand-foot-mouth disease, 433-434
pityriasis rosea, 432-433
roseola infantum, 432
rubella, 429
rubeola, 420-428
scarlet fever, 430-431
varicella, 429-430
Infective endocarditis, 253
Inferior mesenteric artery, 334
Infiltrates in bacterial tracheitis, 203
Inflammation
amebiasis, 356
appendicitis, 348
arthritis, 296, 297
asthma, 211-217
bacterial pneumonia, 204
bronchiolitis, 206
chest wall, 259
cystic fibrosis, 224
encephalitis, 282
endocarditis, 253
meningitis, 277
myocarditis, 254
ocular, 454
pertussis, 208
rheumatic fever, 255-256
septic shock, 120
Influenza, 203
Influenza vaccine, 206
Informed consent, 27, 28, 29
Ingestion; see also Poisoning
chemicals, 582-583
foreign body, 360-362
urban versus rural prehospital
calls, 4
Inguinal hernia, 351
INH; see Isoniazid
Inhalants
abuse, 738
urticaria, 650
Inhalation injury, 579-581
Initiative versus guilt in preschooler de-
velopment, 49, 51
Injury; see Trauma
Injury Severity Score, 6, 8, 495
Innate immunity, 394, 395
Inner ear, 457
Inotropic agents, 251, 255
Insect as foreign body, 462
Insect bites, 642-643, 644
Insecticide poisoning, 633
Inspiration; see Breathing
Institute of Medicine report, 20-21
Insulin, 473
diabetic ketoacidosis, 477, 479-480
glucose regulation, 474
Insurance companies, 27
Intake and output
bronchopulmonary dysplasia, 227
encephalopathy, 282
near-drowning, 222
Integumentary system; see Skin

Intellectual development
  adolescent, 56-58
  infant, 44-46
  preschooler, 50-52, 53
  school-age child, 54, 55
  toddler, 48, 49
Intensive care, 13, 14
Intentional injury, 489-490
Intercostal retraction, 84, 99, 196, 197
Interfacility transport, 14-15
Interleukin-1, 120, 121
Interstate agreements, 15
Interview, 70-72; *see also* History
  adolescent, 728
  of child abuse victim, 589
Intestinal parasites, 356-360
Intestine
  anatomy and physiology, 332-333
  incarcerated hernia, 351
  intussusception, 346-347
  irrigation in poisoning, 630
  malrotation with volvulus, 350-351
  obstruction
    abdominal examination, 85
    Hirschsprung's disease, 353-354
    intussusception, 346, 347
    malrotation of bowel with volvulus
      and, 350
    neonatal bloody stools, 678
  trauma, 531
Intraabdominal trauma, 527-535, 536
Intracellular fluid, 313, 314
  diabetic ketoacidosis, 477
  electrolyte balance, 314-315
  hyperkalemia, 322
  hypernatremia, 320
  hypokalemia, 321-322
  hyponatremia, 318
Intracranial hemorrhage
  hemophilia, 409
  idiopathic thrombocytopenic pur-
    pura, 414
  from trauma, 514-516
Intracranial pressure
  cerebrospinal fluid reabsorption
    and, 266
  increased, 141-145
    clinical manifestations, 136
    comatose child, 136, 138-139
    encephalopathy, 282
    head and neck injury, 513-514,
      519, 523-524
    hydrocephalus, 275, 276
    meningitis, 279
    multiple trauma management, 505
  monitoring, 144-145
  normal, 142
  pediatric anatomic and physiologic
    differences, 68
Intracranial volume, 513
Intraosseous access
  multiple trauma management, 504-
    505

Intraosseous access—cont'd
  resuscitation, 158-159
  status epilepticus, 130
Intrastate agreements, 15
Intrathoracic trauma, 527-535, 536
Intravenous access
  poisoning, 623
  resuscitation, 158
  status epilepticus, 130
Intubation
  advanced life support, 157-158
    neonatal, 169-170, 171
  bacterial tracheitis, 203
  epiglottitis, 202
  poisoning, 623
  preterm infant, 176
  rapid sequence induction, 111
  respiratory failure, 111
  status epilepticus, 129, 130
  trauma management
    head and neck, 522-523
    multiple injury, 498-499
  tube size in, 499
  viral croup, 200
Intussusception, 346-347
  neonatal, 678
Involvement for pain
  management, 703-704
IO; *see* Intraosseous
Ionized calcium, 482
Ipecac syrup, 625-626
Ipratropium bromide, 215
Iris, 80-81, 453
Iron poisoning, 624, 633, 639
Irrigation
  animal bite, 645
  chemical burn, 583
  ear, 458, 462
  rectal, 354-355
  whole bowel, 630
Irritability
  intussusception, 347
  as red flag, 102
Irritant contact dermatitis, 444-446
Islands of Langerhans, 473
Isolation
  impetigo, 434
  neutropenia with fever, 401
  triage assessment, 97
Isoniazid, 211
Isopropyl alcohol poisoning, 635-636,
  637
Isoproterenol
  anaphylaxis, 653
  shock, 124, 125
  symptomatic bradycardia, 160
Isotonic dehydration, 315, 316-317
Isotonic solutions, 119, 122
ISS; *see* Injury Severity Score
IT; *see* Imagination training
Itching; *see* Pruritus
ITP; *see* Idiopathic thrombocytopenic
  purpura
IV; *see* Intravenous

J
Janeway procedure, 725
Jaundice
  neonatal, 672-675
  viral hepatitis, 344
Jaw-thrust position
  basic life support, 149, 150
  multiple trauma management, 498
  respiratory failure, 111
Jehovah's Witness, 32, 33
Jejunum, 332
Joint
  arthritis
    juvenile rheumatoid, 297
    septic, 295, 296, 297
  cerebral palsy, 283
  hemophilia, 409
  Henoch-Schönlein purpura, 388
  Lyme disease, 657
  palpation, 291, 297
Joint Commission on Accreditation of
  Healthcare Organizations, 16
JRA; *see* Juvenile rheumatoid arthritis
Justice, 35
Juvenile Dependency Court, 598
Juvenile rheumatoid arthritis, 292,
  297-301

K
Kallidin, 650
Kawasaki disease, 256
Kayexalate, 323, 324
Kehr's sign, 530
Keloid, 423
Kenalog; *see* Triamcinolone acetonide
Kerions, 438
Kernicterus, 673
Kernig's sign, 278
Kerosene poisoning, 638
Ketamine
  asthma, 216
  pain management, 698-699
  rapid sequence induction, 112
Ketoacidosis, diabetic, 477-480
Ketorolac, 696
Kidney
  in acid-base balance, 326
  AIDS manifestations, 399
  anatomy and physiology, 63, 64, 65,
    364-365
  disorders, 378-386
    acute glomerulonephritis, 378-
      380
    nephrotic syndrome, 380-382
    renal failure, 382-385
    renal transplantation for, 385-386
  hemorrhagic shock classifica-
    tion, 503
  Henoch-Schönlein purpura, 388
  shock and, 115
  trauma, 527, 531
  urinary tract infection ascending
    to, 374

Killer T cell, 394
Knee
    Osgood-Schlatter disease, 306
    septic arthritis of hip and, 296
    trauma, 546-547
    urban *versus* rural prehospital calls, 4
Knee-chest position, 252
Knuckle, 735
Koplik's spots, 420
Kupffer's cells, 392
Kussmaul respirations, 477
Kwell; *see* Lindane

L

Labia
    anatomy, 364, 365
    physical assessment, 367
        in child abuse, 599
Labor, Consolidated Omnibus Budget
    Reconciliation Act and, 24
Laceration
    cerebral, 516
    soft tissue, 561-562
    urban *versus* rural prehospital
        calls, 4
Lactated Ringer's solution
    anaphylaxis, 652
    burn injury, 575
    diabetic ketoacidosis, 479
    hypovolemic shock, 118
    Parkland formula, 575
    status epilepticus, 130
Lactic acidosis, 128
Lactose, 682
Lamotrigine, 273
Language development
    adolescent, 56-58
    infant, 44-46
    preschooler, 50-52, 53
    school-age child, 54, 55
    toddler, 48, 49
Language used by nurse, 53
Lap-belt complex, 531
Large intestine
    anatomy and physiology, 333
    intussusception, 346-347
    irrigation, 630
    trauma, 531
Laryngoscope blade for intuba-
    tion, 157, 170
Laryngotracheobronchitis, 200-201
Larynx, 195
    edema in hereditary angioedema,
        652
    inhalation injury, 580
Lasix; *see* Furosemide
Latency stage in school-age child devel-
    opment, 55
Latex agglutination, 205
Latex allergy, 287
Latex precautions, 287
Latrodectus mactans, 642

Lavage
    gastric, 626-627
    peritoneal, 508, 535
Lead poisoning, 633
Left-to-right shunt, 237-238
    atrial septal defect, 239-240
    complete atrioventricular canal de-
        fect, 241
    nursing intervention, 257
    patent ductus arteriosus, 238-239
    ventricular septal defect, 240-241
Leg
    blood pressure in, 236
        coarctation of aorta, 243
    fracture, 542-544
        nursing care and evaluation, 556-
            559
    intraosseous access, 159
    osteomyelitis of, 293
    septic arthritis, 296
Legal considerations, 24-34
    child abuse, 597-598
    consent for treatment, 27-29
    legislative and reimbursement
        issues, 24-27
    medical negligence/malpractice,
        30-31
    refusal of care, 32-33
    reportable incidents, 29-30, 597
    risk management, 33-34
    telephone advice, 31-32
Legg-Calvé-Perthes disease, 302-303,
    304-305
Legislation
    EMSC funding, 20
    legal considerations, 24-27
Lens, 452, 453
LES; *see* Lower esophageal sphincter
Lethargy, 133
    algorithm for chief complaint of, 94
    diabetes insipidus, 481
    intussusception, 347
    shock, 116
Leukemia, 717
Leukocyte, polymorphonuclear
    neonatal, 662
    septic shock, 120
Leukocytosis, 299
Leukopenia, 734
Leukotrienes, 651
Level of consciousness, 133
    coma assessment, 134
    immunologic or hematologic assess-
        ment, 396
    increased intracranial pressure, 143
    near-drowning, 220, 221
    neonatal assessment, 664
    neurologic examination, 267
    triage assessment, 94
LH; *see* Luteinizing hormone
Liaison nurse, 496
Lice, 447-448
Lichenification, 420, 423, 443

Lidex; *see* Fluocinonide
Lidocaine, 701-702
    pediatric resuscitation, 163
    rapid sequence induction, 112
    ventricular tachycardia, 262
Life-threatening neurologic
    emergencies, 128-146
    coma, 133-141
    increased intracranial pressure, 141-
        145
    status epilepticus, 128-133
Lighter-fluid poisoning, 638
Limp, 290, 292-293
    Legg-Perthes disease, 303
    lower extremity trauma, 542-544
    toxic or transient synovitis, 301
Lindane
    pediculosis, 448
    poisoning, 634
    scabies, 447
    toxicity, 448
Linear skull fracture, 516
Lipids, 380
Lipoid pneumonia, 217
Listening
    active, 595-596
    child abuse and, 595-596
    during interview, 71
Listeria monocytogenes
    meningitis, 277
    neonatal sepsis, 668
    septic shock, 119
Literature review on public educa-
    tion, 16
Lithium carbonate poisoning, 634
Litigation
    prevention, 30-31
    risk management, 33-34
Live insect as foreign body, 462
Liver
    acetaminophen poisoning, 635
    AIDS manifestations, 399
    anatomy and physiology, 64, 334
        neonatal, 662
    palpation, 85, 237
    roundworm migration to, 359
    transplantation, 355-356
    trauma, 530-531
        frequency, 527
        referred pain in, 507
    viral hepatitis, 344-346
Liver enzymes, 64
Liver transplantation, 355-356
Living will, 37
Lobar consolidation in
    pneumonia, 204-205
Local anesthesia, 701-702
Local pediatric center, 14
Longitudinal fracture, 542
Loop diuretics, 323, 324
Loop of Henle, 365
Lorazepam
    head and neck injury, 525, 526

Lorazepam—cont'd
  status epilepticus, 131, 132
Lotrimin; see Clotrimazole
Lower esophageal sphincter, 64, 332
Lower extremity
  blood pressure in, 236
    coarctation of aorta, 243
  fracture, 542-544
    nursing care and evaluation, 556-559
  intraosseous access, 159
  osteomyelitis of, 293
  septic arthritis, 296
Lower respiratory infection, 203-211
  bronchiolitis, 206-208
  pertussis, 208-209, 210
  pneumonia, 203-206
  tuberculosis, 209-211
Loxosceles reclusa, 642
LP; see Lumbar puncture
LPC; see Local pediatric center
LSD; see Lysergic acid diethylamide
Lumbar puncture
  encephalopathy, 282
  febrile child, 617-618
  increased intracranial pressure, 141
  meningitis, 279, 281
  neonatal sepsis, 670
  preorbital and orbital cellulitis, 456
Lund and Browder chart, 566, 568
Lung; see also Respiratory system
  AIDS manifestations, 398
  anatomy and physiology, 66-67, 194-195
  anorexia and bulimia nervosa, 735
  bronchopulmonary dysplasia, 227
  juvenile rheumatoid arthritis, 297, 299, 301
  muscular dystrophy, 310-311
  neonatal, 661, 664
  roundworm migration to, 359
  trauma
    contusion, 528, 529
    frequency of injury, 527
    hemothorax, 529
    pneumothorax, 528-529
  venous congestion, 250
Luteinizing hormone, 473
Lyme disease, 656-657
Lymphangitis in cellulitis, 435
Lymphatic system, 195
Lymphocyte monoclonal antibody, 386
Lymphocytes, 393, 394
Lymphopenia, 734
Lysergic acid diethylamide, 738

M

Macrophages, 392, 394
  acquired immunodeficiency syndrome and, 397
  septic shock, 120

Macule, 420, 421
Magical thinking, 49, 50
Magnesium
  burn injury, 575
  hypercalcemia, 326
  hypocalcemia, 483
Magnesium citrate, 630
Magnesium oxide as universal antidote, 631
Magnesium sulfate
  asthma, 216
  as cathartic, 630
Magnetic resonance imaging
  hydrocephalus, 276
  seizure, 272
Malassezia furfur, 437, 438
Male genitalia
  anatomy, 364
  physical assessment, 367
    neonatal, 664, 666
Malecot tube, 724, 725
Malpractice, 30-31, 33-34
Malrotation of bowel with volvulus, 350
Maltreatment; see Child abuse
Mannitol
  head and neck injury, 525
  increased intracranial pressure, 141, 143, 524
  renal failure, 383
Marijuana, 738
Mask
  neonatal intubation, 149
  rescue breathing, 149
  respiratory syncytial virus control, 207
  resuscitation bag, 157
Massage for pain management, 703
Mast cell, 643, 650
Maternal and Child Health Bureau
  funding of EMS systems, 20
  Institute of Medicine report, 20-21
  paramedic education, 4-5
Maternal factors
  neonatal hypoglycemia, 671, 672
  neonatal resuscitation, 167
Mature minor, 29
McGill forceps, 157
McGrath model, 688
MCHB; see Maternal and Child Health Bureau
MCHC; see Mean corpuscular hemoglobin concentration
MCNS; see Minimal change nephrotic syndrome
MCV; see Mean corpuscular volume
MD; see Muscular dystrophy
Mean corpuscular hemoglobin concentration, 405
Mean corpuscular volume, 405
Measles, 420-428
  encephalitis, 281
  German, 429

Meatus, 464
Mechanical ventilation
  bronchopulmonary dysplasia, 227
  cystic fibrosis, 226
  dependence on, 722, 723
  increased intracranial pressure, 143
  near-drowning, 221
Meconium
  aspiration, 175-176
  failure to pass in Hirschsprung's disease, 354
Medical negligence, 30-31
Medical screening examination, 24, 27
Medication; see also Drugs
  dosages, 5, 19
  triage assessment, 96, 97
Medication nurse in pediatric trauma team, 496
Medulla, 139
Melanocyte-stimulating hormone, 473
Melena, 678
Memory B cell, 394
Memory T cell, 394, 395
Meninges, 266, 511, 512
Meningitis, 277-281
  criteria for transport to pediatric critical care center, 8
  tuberculosis, 210, 211
Meningococcal meningitis, 278-279
Meningoencephalitis, 281
Menstruation
  last date of in triage history, 97
  pelvic inflammatory disease and, 369
Mental retardation, 714-716
  cerebral palsy, 284
Mental status
  criteria for transport to pediatric critical care center, 7
  dehydration, 100
  encephalopathy, 282
  head and neck injury, 520
  hemolytic-uremic syndrome, 387
  hypertonic versus hypotonic dehydration, 319
  meningitis, 281
  renal failure, 384, 385
  respiratory distress, 199
  shock, 125
  sickle cell anemia, 408
  trauma management, 494, 505-506, 507
  triage assessment, 99, 100-101
Menteggia's fracture, 552, 553
Meperidine, 697, 698
  extremity injury, 557
  migraine headache, 270
  sickle cell anemia, 406
Meprobamate poisoning, 626
Mercury poisoning, 633
Mescaline, 738
Mesenteric artery, 334, 350
Metabolic acidemia, 222

Metabolic acidosis, 125, 327
  diabetic ketoacidosis, 477
  hypercyanotic spell, 252
  hyperkalemia, 322, 323, 324
  sodium bicarbonate for, 162
Metabolic alkalosis, 328
Metabolism, 313, 314
  apnea and, 228
  bilirubin, 673
  of drugs and toxins, 65-66
  hepatic, 334
  hypothermia, 653, 654
  neonatal, 660
  pediatric anatomic and physiologic
    differences, 63-66
  shock and, 115-116
Metacarpal fracture, 555
Metaphyseal fracture, 542
Metatarsal fracture, 548
Metered-dose inhaler, 214, 215
Methadone abuse, 738
Methanol poisoning, 632, 636, 637
Methicillin-resistant organism, 280
Methyl salicylate poisoning, 634
Methylphenidate hydrochloride, 729
Methylprednisolone
  anaphylaxis, 653
  asthma, 215
  head and neck injury, 525, 526
  increased intracranial pressure, 143
  potency guide, 445
  renal transplantation rejection, 386
Methylxanthines, 215
Metoclopramide, 270
Metolazone, 251
Metronidazole, 371
Mexican American population, 183
MGCS; see Modified Glasgow Coma
  Scale
Micatin; see Miconazole
MICN; see Mobile intensive care nurse
Miconazole, 440
Microsporum, 437, 439
Micrurus fulvius antivenin, 633
Midazolam, 700, 701
  head and neck injury, 524, 525
  rapid sequence induction, 113
Middle ear
  anatomy, 457
  inflammation, 460
Migraine headache, 269
Miliary tuberculosis, 210, 211
Miller blade, 170
Mind/body/spirit balance, 40
Mineral sea oil poisoning, 638
Mineral spirits poisoning, 638
Mineralocorticoids, 485-486
Minimal change nephrotic syn-
  drome, 380
Minor, emancipated and mature, 29
Mite, 446
Mitral valve
  hypoplastic left heart syndrome, 248

Mitral valve—cont'd
  rheumatic fever, 255
Mobile intensive care nurse, 3
Mobility in myelomeningocele, 285
Mobitz type I heart block, 262
Mobitz type II heart block, 262
Modeling, 705
Modified Glasgow Coma Scale, 520-
  521
Modified Parkland formula, 575
MODS; see Multiple organ dysfunction
  syndrome
Moisturizing treatment for atopic der-
  matitis, 443
Mongolian spots, 663
Monitoring
  apnea, 229-230
  conscious sedation, 699
  intracranial pressure, 144-145
  intubation, 158
  triage, 103-105
Monoclonal antibodies, 121
Monocytes, 392, 393, 394
Monro-Kellie principle, 142
Moraxella
  preorbital and orbital cellulitis,
    455
  sinusitis, 466
Morbidity, injury prevention and, 15
Moro reflex, 68, 268, 667
Morphine, 697
  abuse, 738
  burn injury, 576
  congestive heart failure, 251
  extremity injury, 557
  head and neck injury, 524, 525
  hypercyanotic spell, 252
  intussusception, 347
  sickle cell anemia, 406
Mortality; see Death
Mosquito, 281
Motor development
  adolescent, 57-58
  infant, 45, 46
  preschooler, 51-52
  school-age child, 55
  toddler, 48
Motor function
  comatose child, 134
  Glasgow Coma Scale, 134, 137
  head and neck trauma assessment,
    522
  neonatal assessment, 665
Motor vehicle accident, 490-491
  blunt intestinal injury, 531
  Children's Trauma Tool, 10
Mourning, 182-183
Mouth
  anatomy, 64, 468
  infection or ulceration, 340-344
  neonate suctioning, 168
  physical examination, 80, 82-83
    neonatal, 665

MSH; see Melanocyte-stimulating hor-
  mone
MSP; see Munchausen syndrome by
  proxy
Mucociliary escalator mechanism, 195
Mucocutaneous lymph node syn-
  drome, 256
Mucous membrane
  angioneurotic edema, 651
  dehydration, 100, 319
Mucus secretions in cystic fibro-
  sis, 223, 224
Multi-drug resistant organisms, 211
Multiple organ dysfunction syn-
  drome, 121
Multiple trauma management; see
  Trauma
Multisystem disorders
  hemolytic-uremic syndrome, 386-
    387
  Henoch-Schönlein purpura, 387-
    388
Mumps, 425
Munchausen syndrome by proxy, 601-
  602
Mupirocin, 434
Murmur; see Heart murmur
Muscle contraction in tension head-
  ache, 269, 270
Muscle relaxants, 111, 113
Muscle tone
  cerebral palsy, 283
  triage assessment, 94
Muscle weakness
  hypokalemia, 322
  muscular dystrophy, 310, 311
Muscular dystrophy, 310-312
Musculoskeletal system, 290-312
  AIDS manifestations, 399
  anatomy and physiology, 65, 290
  disorders, 291-312
    Duchenne's muscular
      dystrophy, 310-312
    inconsolable crying, 681
    juvenile rheumatoid arthritis, 297-
      301
    Legg-Perthes disease, 302-303,
      304-305
    Osgood-Schlatter disease, 306-
      307
    osteogenesis imperfecta, 307-310
    osteomyelitis, 291-295
    respiratory failure and, 108
    septic arthritis, 295-297
    slipped capital femoral
      epiphysis, 303-306, 307, 308
    toxic or transient synovitis, 301-
      302
  history, 290, 291
  physical examination, 290, 291,
    292-293
  trauma, 540-561
    compartment syndrome, 559-560

Musculoskeletal system—cont'd
    trauma—cont'd
        growth plate, 541-542
        lower extremity, 542-549
        nursing care and evaluation, 556-559
        open fracture, 560-561
        upper extremity, 549-555
Myalgia, Rocky Mountain spotted fever and, 656
Mycobacterium catarrhalis, 202
Mycobacterium tuberculosis
    pneumonia, 203
    tuberculosis, 209
Mycoplasma
    erythema multiforme, 448
    pneumonia, 203, 204
Myelomeningocele, 285-287
Myocarditis, 254
Myocardium
    cardiogenic shock, 114, 118
    neonatal, 661
    pediatric anatomic and physiologic differences, 67
Myoclonic seizure, 273
Myoglobinuria, 580

N

NAC; *see* N-Acetylcysteine
Nafcillin
    bacterial tracheitis, 203
    cellulitis, 435
        preorbital and orbital, 457
    osteomyelitis, 295
    pneumonia, 206
Nail, 419
    loss of in crush injury, 555
    tinea, 437
Naloxone
    as antidote, 633
    resuscitation
        neonatal, 166, 174
        pediatric, 162, 163
Naproxen, 300
Narcan, 121
Narcotics, 690, 696-698
    abuse, 738
    addiction, 690
    migraine headache, 270
    sickle cell anemia, 406, 407
Nasal congestion, 82
Nasal decongestants, 199
Nasal discharge
    assessment, 465
    breath sounds and, 84
    head trauma and, 82
    neonatal upper respiratory infection, 676
    sinusitis, 466
Nasal flaring, 7
Nasal obstruction, neonatal, 668
Nasal washing, 207

Nasogastric tube
    increased intracranial pressure, 141
    multiple trauma management, 498
    rapid sequence induction, 111
    status epilepticus, 130
Nasopharyngeal airway, 498
Nasopharynx, 464, 467, 468
Nasotracheal intubation, 157, 523
National EMSC Data and Research Center, 10
National Highway Traffic Safety Administration, 21
    on databases, 10
    funding of EMS systems, 20
National Hydrocephalus Foundation, 277
National Pediatric Trauma Registry, 8-9
National standards for emergency medical technician training, 5
Native American population, 183
Natural killer cell, 394
Navicular fracture, 547
Near-drowning, 219-223
    primary hypothermia, 653
    survival rates, 148
Nebulized albuterol, 214, 323, 324
Nebulized ipratropium bromide, 215
NEC; *see* Necrotizing enterocolitis
Necator americanus, 358
Neck; *see also* Cervical spine
    physical examination, 80, 83
    trauma; *see* Head and neck trauma
    urban *versus* rural prehospital calls, 4
Neck x-ray
    epiglottitis, 202
    viral croup, 200
Necrotizing enterocolitis, 678
NEDARC; *see* National EMSC Data and Research Center
Needle
    intraosseous access, 159, 504-505
    umbilical catheterization, 173
Needle containers, 18
Needle cricothyroidotomy, 499, 500
Needle decompression, 534
Needle thoracostomy, 502
Negativism of toddler, 47
Neglect, 587
    clinical manifestations, 590
    in poisoning, 640
    policies and protocols, 19
    as reportable incidence, 29
Negligence, 30-31
Neisseria gonorrhoeae, 371
    child abuse and, 600
    conjunctivitis, 454
    ophthalmia neonatorum, 454
Neisseria meningitidis
    meningitis, 277, 280
    septic shock, 119
Nembutal sodium, 525
Neomycin, 460

Neonatal resuscitation, 164-175
    airway, 168
    breathing, 169-170, 171
    circulation, 170-173
    equipment, 165-166
    fluids and medications, 173-175
    meconium aspiration, 175-176
    prehospital transport, 166-167
    preterm deliveries, 176
    stimulation and temperature control, 167-168
    team responsibilities, 165
Neonate
    AIDS, 397
    anatomy and physiology, 660-662
    assessment, 662-668
    bloody stools, 677-680
    cardiovascular system, 233
    care of after birth, 167-168
    colic, 682-683
    common cold, 675-676
    conjunctivitis, 454-455
    constipation, 676-677
    crying, 680-682
    defined, 660
    febrile, 104
    head of, 77-78, 79
    hematologic and immune system, 65
    hydrocephalus, 275
    hyperbilirubinemia, 672-675
    hypoglycemia, 671-672
    hypothermia, 653
    hypoxemia, 228
    normal values
        arterial blood gases, 109
        blood pressure, 116
        blood volume, 67
        vital signs, 103
    obstetric history, 167
    resuscitation; *see* Neonatal resuscitation
    seizure etiology, 271
    sepsis, 668-671
    tension pneumothorax, 176
    urinary tract infection, 374, 375
    visual acuity, 452
    volvulus, 350
    vomiting, 679-680
Neoplasm, 292
Nephron, 365, 366
Nephrotic syndrome, 380-382
Nerve block, 702
Neural tube defect, 285
Neurogenic shock, 114, 523
Neurohypophysis, 473
Neurologic status
    criteria for transport to pediatric critical care center, 7
    dehydration, 100, 319
    encephalopathy, 282
    head and neck injury, 520
    hemolytic-uremic syndrome, 387
    meningitis, 281

Neurologic status—cont'd
    poisoning, 624
    renal failure, 384, 385
    respiratory distress, 199
    shock, 125
    sickle cell anemia, 408
    trauma management, 494, 505-506,
        507
    triage assessment, 99, 100-101
Neurologic system, 266-289
    AIDS and, 397, 398
    anatomy and physiology, 64, 67-68,
        266, 267
    apnea and, 228
    cardiovascular regulation, 114
    control of breathing, 194
    disorders, 277-287
        anorexia and bulimia nervosa, 735
        cerebral palsy, 283-285
        encephalitis, 281-283
        meningitis, 277-281
        myelomeningocele, 285-287
    hemorrhagic shock classifica-
        tion, 503
    hypoglycemia and, 474
    hypothermia and, 653
    life-threatening emergencies, 128-
        146
        coma, 133-141
        increased intracranial
            pressure, 141-145
        status epilepticus, 128-133
    Lyme disease and, 657
    narcotic analgesics and, 696
    neonatal, 661, 664-665
    nursing history and assessment, 266-
        267, 268
    Pediatric Trauma Score, 9
    respiratory failure and, 108
    signs and symptoms, 267-277
        headache, 267-270
        hydrocephalus, 274-277
        seizures, 270-274, 275
    stimulants, 737-738
Neuromuscular assessment in head and
    neck injury, 520
Neuromuscular blockers for intuba-
    tion, 158
Neutropenia
    anorexia and bulimia nervosa, 734
    with fever, 400-401
Neutrophil count, 400
Neutrophils, 391-392, 393, 394
    meningitis, 279
    septic arthritis, 296
Newborn; see Neonate
Nifedipine, 270
Nightstick fracture, 552, 553
Nikolsky's sign, 436
9-1-1 systems, 4
    education and access, 16
    Emergency Medical Services For
        Children recommendations, 747-
        748

Nipride; see Sodium nitroprusside
Nitrofurantoin, 375
Nitroglycerin, 119
Nitroprusside
    cardiogenic shock, 119
    congestive heart failure, 251
    myocarditis, 255
Nitrous oxide, 702
Nix; see Permethrin
Nociception, 686
Nodule, 421
Noncommunicating hydroceph-
    alus, 275
Nonketotic hyperosmolar coma, 478
Nonmaleficence, 35, 36
Nonnarcotic analgesics, 695-696
Non-shivering thermogenesis, 68, 607
Nonsteroidal antiinflammatory
    drugs, 695-696
    juvenile rheumatoid arthritis, 299,
        300
    toxic or transient synovitis, 302
Nonurgent care, 92
Norcuron; see Vecuronium
Norepinephrine
    pain and, 686
    shock, 124-125
Normal saline
    anaphylaxis, 652
    diabetic ketoacidosis, 479
    gastric lavage, 627
    hypercalcemia, 325
    hypovolemic shock, 118
    status epilepticus, 130
Nortriptyline poisoning, 638
Norwalk virus, 339, 340
Nose, 463-467
    AIDS manifestations, 398
    anatomy and physiology, 64, 463-
        464
    congestion, 82
    discharge
        assessment, 465
        breath sounds and, 84
        head trauma and, 82
        neonatal upper respiratory infec-
            tion, 676
        sinusitis, 466
    disorders, 465-467
    history, 464-465
    neonatal
        obstruction, 668
        physical examination, 665
        suctioning, 168
    physical examination, 80, 81-82,
        465-466
Nosebleed, 465-467
NPTR; see National Pediatric Trauma
    Registry
Nurse
    advanced life support responsibili-
        ties, 153
    child abuse cases and
        prevention, 588-589, 596, 604

Nurse—cont'd
    considerations in choosing lan-
        guage, 53
    critical incident stress
        management, 186-188
    death of child, 184-186
    emergency medical service for chil-
        dren, 21
    injury prevention, 61, 62-63, 487
    malpractice suits against, 30-31
    pediatric emergency training for, 12-
        13
    pediatric trauma team, 496
    triage, 90
Nursemaid's elbow, 552-554
Nutracort; see Hydrocortisone
Nuts, 450
Nystatin, 440

O
Oatmeal bath, 430
Object permanence, 46
Oblique fracture, 542
OBRA; see Omnibus Budget Reconcili-
    ation Act
Observation
    cardiovascular assessment, 235-236
    musculoskeletal assessment, 291
    pain assessment, 691-695
    respiratory assessment, 196-198
Obstetric history, 167
Obstruction
    airway; see Airway obstruction
    apnea, 228
    appendicitis, 348
    cardiovascular defects, 238, 241-244
    nasal, 668
    pyloric stenosis, 352
Obstructive jaundice, 344
Obstructive shock, 111-113, 114
Occiput, cervical spine immobilization
    and, 522, 524
Oculocephalic reflex, 134
Oculovestibular response
    coma, 134-136
    head and neck injury, 521-522
Odontoid process, 516-517
OES; see Oral electrolyte solution
OI; see Osteogenesis imperfecta
Oleander poisoning, 633
Omnibus Budget Reconciliation
    Act, 27
Opalescent dentin, 309
Open book deformity, 549
Open fracture, 560-561
Open wound, 9
Ophthalmia neonatorum, 454
Opiate antagonists, 121
Opiates
    pain management, 696
    poisoning, 633
Opioids
    abuse, 738

Opioids—cont'd
poisoning, 624
Optic nerve, 452
Oral airway, 498
Oral candidiasis, 440
Oral cavity
anatomy, 64, 468
infection or ulceration, 340-344
neonate suctioning, 168
physical examination, 80, 82-83
neonatal, 665
Oral electrolyte solution, 317, 318
Oral rehydration, 317
diabetic ketoacidosis, 479
fever, 618
Oral stage of infant development, 45
Orbital cellulitis, 455-457
Organ donation, 37-38, 185-186
Organophosphate poisoning, 624, 633
Orientation of new personnel, 30
Orogastric tube
gastric lavage, 627
neonatal insertion, 169
Oropharyngeal airway, 11
Oropharynx, 467, 468
Orotracheal intubation, 523
Osgood-Schlatter disease, 292, 306-307
Osmolality, 314
diabetes insipidus, 481
mannitol administration, 143, 524
normal, 314
Osmosis, 313
Osteoblasts, 308
Osteochondrosis of femoral head, 302
Osteogenesis imperfecta, 307-310
Osteogenic sarcoma, 292
Osteomyelitis, 291-295
Osteopenia, 307
Osteoporosis, 307
Ostium secundum defect, 239
Otic medication drop instillation, 460
Otitis externa, 458-460
Otitis media, 460-461
Otomycosis, 459
Oucher Scale, 691, 692
Ovary, 473
Oxygen challenge test, 249
Oxygen partial pressure
chemoreceptor stimulation, 108
congenital heart defects, 249
near-drowning, 221
normal values, 109, 326
oxygen transport, 108-109
sickle cell crisis, 407
Oxygen saturation
asthma, 213
pulse oximetry, 105
total anomalous pulmonary venous
return, 247
triage assessment, 105
Oxygen therapy
asthma, 216
bronchopulmonary dysplasia, 227

Oxygen therapy—cont'd
cardiovascular disorder, 257
congestive heart failure, 251
cystic fibrosis, 226
dependence on, 718-719
head and neck injury, 522
hypercyanotic spell, 252
inhalation injury, 580
metabolic acidosis, 125
multiple trauma management, 501
pertussis, 209
poisoning, 623
rapid sequence induction, 111
respiratory failure, 111
with resuscitation bags, 154-157
shock, 122
sickle cell crisis, 407
status epilepticus, 129-130
symptomatic bradycardia, 159
symptomatic supraventricular tachycardia, 160
tracheostomy tube replacement, 721
viral croup, 200-201
Oxygen toxicity, 226
Oxygen transport, 108-109
anemia, 402
cellular metabolism and, 115
respiratory failure and, 108-109
septic shock, 120
Oxygen-hemoglobin saturation
curve, 108-109
Oxytocin, 473

P

P wave, 323
Pacing, 160, 260
Packed red blood cells
hemolytic-uremic syndrome, 387
hypovolemic cardiopulmonary arrest, 159
idiopathic thrombocytopenic purpura, 414
sickle cell crisis, 407
Paco₂; see Arterial carbon dioxide tension
Paddle placement in defibrillation and
cardioversion, 161
Pain
abdominal; see Abdominal pain
assessment, 690-695, 705
chest, 258-259
compartment syndrome, 560
defined, 686
denial, 56, 691
headache, 269
Henoch-Schönlein purpura, 388
Legg-Perthes disease, 306
lidocaine injection, 702
muscular dystrophy, 311, 312
myths, 689-690
otitis externa, 460
physiology, 686-687
prevention and anticipation, 690

Pain—cont'd
psychosocial aspects, 687-689
referred, 339
hepatic injury, 507
septic arthritis of hip, 296
sickle cell anemia, 405-406, 408
testicular torsion, 377
toxic or transient synovitis, 301
triage assessment, 99, 102-103
urban *versus* rural prehospital calls, 4
Pain management
anesthesia, 701-702
biofeedback, 704
burn injury, 576
conscious sedation, 699-700
distraction and involvement, 703-
704
in dying patient, 35, 36
evaluation, 705-706
fractures, 557-558
headache, 270
imagery and hypnosis, 704
intussusception, 347
juvenile rheumatoid arthritis
and, 300
ketamine, 698-699
modeling and rehearsal, 705
narcotics, 696-698
nonnarcotic analgesics, 695-696
during painful procedures, 706-708
patient-controlled analgesia, 700
positioning and securing, 702-703
positive self-talk and thought
stopping, 705
professional issues, 708
relaxation and breathing, 704
sedatives, 700-701
sickle cell anemia, 406, 407, 408
therapeutic touch, 704
Palate, 468
Palatine tonsil, 468
Palm method in burn assessment, 566
Palmar grasp, 268
Palpation
abdominal, 85, 335
intussusception, 347
articular, 291
bone, 291
cardiovascular, 237
fracture, 556
liver and spleen, 85
neck, 83
rectal, 86
septic arthritis, 297
PALS; see Pediatric Advanced Life Support course
Palsy, cerebral, 283-285
Pamelor; see Nortriptyline
Pancreas
anatomy and physiology, 334
trauma, 527
Pancreatic enzyme replacement, 225
Pao₂; see Oxygen partial pressure
Papule, 420, 421

Paradoxic irritability, 102
Parainfluenza
    pneumonia, 203
    viral croup, 200
Paralysis in myelomeningocele, 286
Paramedic, 3, 4
Paranasal sinus, 464
Parasitic infection
    cutaneous, 446-448
    diarrhea, 337
    eosinophil attachment to, 392
    intestinal, 356-360
Parasympathetic nervous system, 114
Parathyroid gland, 473
Parathyroid hormone, 473
    hypocalcemia, 324, 482-483
Parenchyma, renal failure and, 383
Parent
    of abused child
        behavior, 589-591
        communication, 595-596
        history, 589
        support of family, 596
    cerebral palsy and, 285
    death of child, 38
    general appearance, 77, 78
    interviewing, 71-72
    involvement of during emergency de-
        partment visit, 59-61, 73
    notification of emergency, 28-29,
        180
    presence during procedures, 60-61,
        497, 708, 715-716
    relieving infant anxiety, 46-47
Parental attachment, 44, 668
Parkland formula, 575
Paroxysmal stage of pertussis, 208-209
Partial seizure, 271, 272, 273
Partial thromboplastin time
    child abuse, 595
    hemophilia, 409, 410
Partially treated meningitis, 277
Partial-thickness burn, 567-568, 570
PASGs; see Pneumatic antishock
    garments
Patch, 421
Patella, 292
Patent ductus arteriosus, 238-239
Pathologic fracture, 542
Patient advocacy, 21
Patient care obstacles, 70, 71
Patient complaints, 33
Patient positioning; see Positioning
Patient Self-Determination Act, 37
Patient transfer form, 25-26
Patient-controlled analgesia, 700
PCA; see Patient-controlled analgesia
PCP; see Phencyclidine hydrochloride;
    Pneumocystis carinii pneumonia
PCR; see Polymerase chain reaction
PDA; see Patent ductus arteriosus
PdLNs; see Pediatric liaison nurses
Peak expiratory flow rate in
    asthma, 212-213

Peak inspiratory pressure in mechanical
    ventilation, 722
Pedestrian struck, 491
    Children's Trauma Tool, 10
    criteria for transport to pediatric
        critical care center, 7
    prevention, 489
Pediatric Advanced Life Support
    course, 12
Pediatric cart, 10, 12
Pediatric critical care center
    standards for, 17
    transport
        criteria for, 7-8
        of rural population, 14
        of urban population, 13
Pediatric emergency departments, 17-
    19; see also Emergency department
Pediatric Emergency Nursing Educa-
    tion Program, 13
Pediatric Emergency Nursing Manual,
    12
Pediatric Glasgow Coma Scale, 137
    multiple trauma
        management, 505-506
    neurologic triage assessment, 102
Pediatric liaison nurses, 16, 17
Pediatric scoring instruments, 8-9
Pediatric Trauma Score, 8-9, 494, 495
Pediculosis capitis, 447-448
Peer group, 52, 56, 57, 58
PEFR; see Peak expiratory flow rate
Pelvic examination, 369
Pelvic inflammatory disease, 369-372,
    373
    limp and, 292
Pelvis
    fracture, 548-549
    multiple trauma management, 508
Pemoline, 729
PENEP; see Pediatric Emergency Nurs-
    ing Education Program
Penetrating trauma
    Children's Trauma Tool, 10
    thoracoabdominal, 527-528
Penicillin
    allergy, 280
    anaphylactic reaction, 651
    cellulitis, 435
    erythema multiforme and, 448
    pharyngitis, 470
    scarlet fever, 431
    sickle cell anemia infection prophy-
        laxis, 406
    urticaria and, 450
Penicillin G
    Lyme disease, 657
    meningitis, 279
Penis, 364, 367
Penobarbital, 525
Pentothal; see Thiopental
Percussion
    abdominal, 335
    skull, 78

Perforation of appendix, 348, 349
Periactin; see Cyproheptadine
Pericardial tamponade, 529-530
Pericardiocentesis, 535, 536
Pericarditis, 254, 297, 299, 301
Periorbital cellulitis, 455-457
Periosteum, 65
Peripheral cyanosis
    neonatal, 170
    respiratory assessment, 196
Peripheral pulses
    shock, 116
    triage assessment, 94
Peristaltic waves, 352
Peritoneal dialysis, 631
Peritoneal lavage
    diagnostic, 508
    thoracoabdominal injuries, 535
Peritonsillar abscess, 469
Permethrin, 447, 448
Perspiration in pain assessment, 695
Pertussis, 208-209, 210
Petechia, 420
    idiopathic thrombocytopenic pur-
        pura, 413, 414
    meningitis, 279, 280
    scarlet fever, 431
    septic shock, 121
    triage assessment, 103
Pezzer tube, 724, 725
pH, 326
    alkalization of urine for poison-
        ing, 631
    diabetic ketoacidosis, 480
    hypokalemia, 322
    metabolic acidosis, 327
    metabolic alkalosis, 328
    normal values, 109, 326
    respiratory acidosis, 328
    respiratory alkalosis, 328
Phagocyte, 195
Phalangeal fracture, 555
Phallic stage of preschooler develop-
    ment, 50, 51
Pharyngeal tonsils, 467
Pharyngitis, 469-470
    epiglottitis, 201
    rheumatic fever and, 255
Pharynx
    AIDS manifestations, 398
    anatomy and physiology, 64, 467-
        468
    assessment, 83, 468
        neonatal, 64, 666-667
Phenazopyridine, 375
Phencyclidine hydrochloride, 738
Phenergan, 698
Phenobarbital
    antiepileptic therapy, 273
    head and neck injury, 525
    poisoning
        activated charcoal and, 628
        urine alkalization in, 631
    status epilepticus, 131, 132

Phenothiazine poisoning, 624, 634
Phenylbutazone, 410
Phenylephrine poisoning, 637
Phenylpropanolamine poisoning, 637
Phenytoin
    antiepileptic therapy, 273
    erythema multiforme and, 448
    head and neck injury, 525, 526
    status epilepticus, 131, 132
    urticaria and, 450
    ventricular tachycardia, 262
PHI; see Prehospital Index
Philadelphia collar, 522
Phosphate, 326
Photographs in suspected child
    abuse, 597
Phototherapy for hyperbilirubine-
    mia, 674, 675
Physeal fracture, 541-542
Physical abuse, 586-587
Physical comfort in emergency
    departments, 17-18
Physical development; see Growth and
    development
Physical disability, 54
Physical examination, 72-87
    abdomen, 85
    approaches
        adolescent, 77
        infant, 46-47, 76
        preschooler, 52, 54, 76
        school-age child, 54-56, 77
        toddler, 49, 50, 76
    cardiovascular, 234-237
    chest, 83-84
    child abuse, 591-595
    cutaneous, 86-87
    documentation for litigation risk
        management, 34
    ear, 81, 82
    extremities, 86
    eye, 78-81
    gaining child's cooperation, 73-74,
        75, 76-77
    gastrointestinal, 335
    general survey, 77-79, 80
    genitourinary, 85-86, 366-367
    growth parameters, 74-75
    head, 77-78, 79, 80
    hematologic and immune sys-
        tem, 396
    mouth, 82-83
    musculoskeletal, 290, 291, 292-293
    nasal, 81-82
    neck, 83
    neonatal, 662-668
    neonatal sepsis, 670
    neurologic, 267, 268
    parental involvement, 73
    psychosocial considerations, 713
    rectal, 86
    respiratory, 195-198
    rewarding child after, 73
    special needs child, 712

Physical examination—cont'd
    status epilepticus, 131
    triage, 97-103
        airway, 98, 99
        breathing, 98-100
        circulation, 100-101
        discomfort/pain, 102-103
        exposure/environment, 103
        neurologic status, 101-102
    well child care recommendations, 87
Physician
    advanced life support responsibili-
        ties, 153
    pediatric emergency training for, 10-
        12
    telephone orders from, 32
Physiologic jaundice, 673, 674
Physostigmine, 632
Pia mater
    anatomy, 511-513, 512
    meningitis, 277
Piaget's theory of cognitive develop-
    ment, 44
    adolescent, 56, 57
    infant, 44, 45
    preschooler, 50, 51
    school-age child, 54, 55
    toddler, 48, 49
PID; see Pelvic inflammatory disease
Pigeon chest, 84
Pigmentation in adrenal insuffi-
    ciency, 484
Pilocaine, 701
Pinna
    assessment, 458, 459
    manipulation of during tympanic
        membrane examination, 81
Pinworm, 358, 359
    child abuse and, 600
PIP; see Peak inspiratory pressure
Pit viper snake bite, 646, 647, 648
Pituitary gland, 473
Pityriasis rosea, 427, 432-433
Pityrosporum, 437
Placing response, 268
Plant poisoning, 639, 640
Plantar reflex, 667
Plaque, 421
Plasma cell, 394
Plasma for volume resuscitation, 123
Plasma protein fraction, 123
Plasmanate; see Plasma protein fraction
Plastibell procedure, 666
Platelet count
    child abuse, 595
    hemolytic-uremic syndrome, 387
    idiopathic thrombocytopenic pur-
        pura, 414
    normal, 394
Platelets
    anatomy and physiology, 391, 392-
        394
    disseminated intravascular coagula-
        tion, 412, 413

Platelets—cont'd
    hemolytic-uremic syndrome, 386,
        387
    idiopathic thrombocytopenic pur-
        pura, 413, 414
    septic shock, 120
Play area in emergency depart-
    ment, 18, 19
Play in toddler physical examina-
    tion, 49, 74, 75
Pleural cavity
    hemothorax, 529
    pneumothorax, 528
Pleural effusion
    juvenile rheumatoid arthritis, 297,
        301
    pneumonia, 205
Pneumatic antishock garments, 123,
    505
Pneumococcal vaccine, 206
Pneumocystis carinii pneumonia, 399
Pneumonia, 203-206
    lipoid, 217
    muscular dystrophy, 310-311
    pertussis, 208
    Pneumocystis carinii, 399
Pneumonitis in juvenile rheumatoid ar-
    thritis, 297
Pneumoperitoneum, 531
Pneumothorax, 502, 528-530
    from blunt trauma, 528
    cystic fibrosis, 225, 226
    frequency of injury, 527
    needle decompression in, 534
    neonatal resuscitation, 176
Poison ivy, 446
Poisoning, 622-641
    acetaminophen, 635, 636
    alcohol, 635-637
    antidotal therapy, 631-633
    carbon monoxide, 579, 580
    cough and cold preparations, 637-
        638
    cyclic antidepressants, 638
    epidemiology, 622
    exchange transfusion, 631
    external documentation, 625
    extracorporeal drug removal, 631
    gastric decontamination, 625-630
    history and assessment, 622-623
    hydrocarbons, 638-639
    iron, 639
    nursing intervention, 623-625
    plants, 639, 640
    poison information centers, 641-642
    prevention, 640-641
    primary hypothermia, 653
    salt, 321
Poker Chip Tool, 691, 693
Policies and procedures
    care of child in adult emergency de-
        partments, 19
    litigation prevention, 30
Polycythemia, 249

Polydipsia, 481
Polyethylene glycol, 630
Polymerase chain reaction
  HIV infection, 397
  pertussis, 209
Polymorphonuclear leukocyte
  neonatal, 662
  septic shock, 120
Polymorphonuclear neutrophils, 279, 391
Polymyxin B sulfate, 460
Polyuria, 481
Pons, 139
Pork tapeworm, 359
Portal system, 334
Portal vein, 334
Positioning
  airway obstruction, 98
    foreign body, 151-152
  cerebral palsy, 284, 2885
  gastric lavage, 626
  head and neck injury, 522
  hypercyanotic spell, 252
  increased intracranial pressure, 145
  neonatal intubation, 169
  oral examination, 83
  pain management, 702-703
  respiratory failure, 111
Positive end-expiratory pressure
  in mechanical ventilation, 722
  near-drowning, 221
Positive pressure ventilation
  neonatal, 169
  tension pneumothorax, 176
Positive self-talk, 703, 705
Posture
  neonatal assessment, 664
  pediatric anatomic and physiologic differences, 64
Potassium
  body fluid balance, 315
  burn injury, 575
  dehydration, 316
  diabetic ketoacidosis, 477, 479
  hyperkalemia, 322, 323
  hypokalemia, 321, 322
  pyloric stenosis, 353
  shock, 125
Pralidoxime, 633
Prednisolone, 215
Prednisone
  asthma, 215
  glomerulonephritis, 381
  Henoch-Schönlein purpura, 388
  juvenile rheumatoid arthritis, 300
Pregnancy
  emancipated minor and, 29
  fifth disease, 431, 432
  rubella and, 429
Prehn's sign, 377
Prehospital care, 1, 3-6, 493-494
  advanced life support, 153
  burn injury, 572-573

Prehospital care—cont'd
  continuous quality improvement, 16
  dispatch in, 4
  field treatment protocols, 5
  identification in, 3-4
  neonatal transport, 166-167
  nurses' role, 21
  protocols, 5
  provider education in, 4-5
  resuscitation etiology, 147
  snakebite, 648-649
  survival rates, 147-148
Prehospital Index, 8
Preload, 114, 233
Premature infant
  apnea, 228
  bronchopulmonary dysplasia, 226
Preoperational thinking, 50, 51, 54, 55
Prerenal acute renal failure, 382, 383, 384
Preschooler
  approach to, 52, 54, 76
  common fears, 51, 52
  common injuries, 62
  coping strategies, 689, 706
  gaining cooperation of, 74
  general survey, 77
  growth and development, 49-52, 53, 54
  interviewing, 72
  laceration repair, 562
  normal vital signs, 103, 198
  triage assessment, 82
  vision testing, 81
Pressure alarm in mechanical ventilation, 722
Pressure sore in cerebral palsy, 284
Preterm deliveries, 176
Priapism in sickle cell crisis, 407
Primary survey, 493-494, 497
Privacy
  adolescent treatment, 728
  in pediatric emergency departments, 18
  triage, 89
Procainamide, 262
Procardia; see Nifedipine
Prochlorperazine, 270
Proerythroblast, 391
Progesterone, 473
Projectile vomiting, 352
Prolactin, 473
Prone position for sleeping infant, 188
Prophylaxis
  meningitis, 280, 281
  migraine headache, 270
  sickle cell anemia infection, 406
  tetanus, 508-509
    animal bite, 645
    burn injury, 576
    snakebite, 649
Propoxyphene poisoning, 634

Propranolol
  hypercyanotic spell, 252
  migraine headache prophylaxis, 270
  ventricular tachycardia, 262
Proptosis, 452
Prostacyclin, 386
Prostaglandins
  body temperature regulation, 608
  cardiovascular disorder, 257, 258
  pain reception, 686
Protein
  glomerulonephritis, 380, 381
  meningitis, 279
Prothrombin time
  child abuse, 595
  hemophilia, 409, 410
Provider education, 4-5
Proximal tubule, renal, 365
Pruritus
  atopic dermatitis, 444
  chickenpox, 430
PS; see Pulmonary stenosis
Pseudoephedrine poisoning, 637
Pseudomenstruation, 664, 666
Pseudomonas
  cystic fibrosis, 223, 225, 226
  neonatal sepsis, 668
  osteomyelitis, 293
  otitis externa, 459
  septic shock, 119
Psychosexual development, 44
Psychosocial development
  adolescent, 56, 57-58
  Erikson's theory, 44
  infant, 44, 45-46
  preschooler, 49-50, 51-52
  school-age child, 52-54, 55
  toddler, 47-49
Psychosocial factors
  headache, 270
  increased intracranial pressure, 141
  neurologic assessment, 268
  pain, 687-689
  special needs child, 713
Psychosocial problems, 727-739
  adolescent issues, 727-728
  attention deficit hyperactivity disorder, 728-729
  conduct disorders, 729-730
  depression and suicide, 730-733
  eating disorders, 734-737
  history and assessment, 727
  runaways/homelessness, 739
  substance abuse, 737-739
PT; see Prothrombin time
PTH; see Parathyroid hormone
PTS; see Pediatric Trauma Score
PTT; see Partial thromboplastin time
Pubic diastasis fracture, 549
Pubic hair, 85-86
Pubic lice, 447, 448
Public education, 15-16
  burn injury prevention, 564

Publications; *see* Literature review
Pulmonary artery
  patent ductus arteriosus, 238, 239
  transposition of great arteries, 244
Pulmonary balloon valvuloplasty, 249
Pulmonary blood flow
  atrial septal defect, 240
  complete atrioventricular canal defect, 241
  patent ductus arteriosus, 239
  pulmonary stenosis, 242
  tetralogy of Fallot, 244
  total anomalous pulmonary venous return, 247, 248
  truncus arteriosus, 245
  ventricular septal defect, 240
Pulmonary edema, 227
Pulmonary stenosis, 241-242
  tetralogy of Fallot, 244
  truncus arteriosus, 245
Pulmonary system, 194-195
  AIDS manifestations, 398
  anatomy and physiology, 66-67, 194-195
  anorexia and bulimia nervosa, 735
  bronchopulmonary dysplasia, 227
  juvenile rheumatoid arthritis, 297, 299, 301
  muscular dystrophy, 310-311
  neonatal, 661, 664
  roundworm migration to, 359
  trauma
    contusion, 528, 529
    frequency of injury, 527
    hemothorax, 529
    pneumothorax, 528-529
    venous congestion, 250
Pulmonary vascular resistance
  total anomalous pulmonary venous return, 247
  truncus arteriosus, 245, 246
  ventricular septal defect, 240
Pulse
  criteria for transport to pediatric critical care center, 7
  prehospital assessment, 149-150
  triage assessment, 94
Pulse oximetry
  asthma, 216
  limitations, 198
  respiratory assessment, 198
  status epilepticus, 130
  triage assessment, 105
Pulseless arrest, epinephrine dosages, 162, 163
Pulsus paradoxus, 254
Puncture wound, 561
  osteomyelitis, 293
Pupil
  anatomy, 452
  coma and, 134, 138
  examination, 80
  increased intracranial pressure, 143

Pupil—cont'd
  near-drowning, 220
  trauma management, 536
    multiple injury, 507
  venomous *versus* nonvenomous snake, 646-647
Pupillary reflex, 667
Purpura, 420
  Henoch-Schönlein, 387-388
  idiopathic thrombocytopenic, 413-415
  meningitis, 279, 280
Purpura fulminans, 411
Purulent discharge
  pelvic inflammatory disease, 369
  sinusitis, 466
Pustule, 420, 422
Pyelonephritis, 374
Pyloric sphincter, 332
Pyloric stenosis, 352-353
Pylorus, 332
Pyrazinamide, 211
Pyrethrin, 448
Pyrogen, 608

Q

QRS complex
  cyclic antidepressant poisoning, 638
  electromechanical dissociation and, 160
  hyperkalemia, 323
Quadriplegia, spastic, 283, 284
Quality improvement, 16, 17, 21
Quinine poisoning, 634

R

Rabies, 645
Raccoon's eyes, 507
Radial fracture, 551-552
Radial nerve, humerus fracture and, 551
Radiation in body temperature regulation, 607
Radio communication in field triage, 6
Radiography; *see* X-ray
Rales
  bronchopulmonary dysplasia, 227
  pneumonia, 204
  respiratory assessment, 197, 198
Ramenofsky's six components of emergency care, 2-3
Range of motion exercise in Legg-Perthes disease, 303
Range of motion in cerebral palsy, 283
Rape, 587, 595, 600
Rapid antigen detection
  bronchiolitis, 207
  pneumonia, 205
Rapid sequence induction intubation, 111

Rapid sequence induction intubation—cont'd
  multiple trauma management, 499
  status epilepticus, 130
Rash
  assessment, 87
  chickenpox, 430
  Henoch-Schönlein purpura, 388
  Lyme disease, 656-657
  meningitis, 279, 280
  Rocky Mountain spotted fever, 656
  syphilis, 368
  triage assessment, 103
Rashkind atrial septostomy, 249
Rattlesnake bite, 633, 646
Reactive airway disease, 211-230
Receptors, pain, 686
Recessive disorder
  cystic fibrosis, 223
  hemophilia, 408
  muscular dystrophy, 310
  osteogenesis imperfecta, 309
  sickle cell anemia, 403
Recording nurse, 496
Rectal irrigation in Hirschsprung's disease, 354-355
Rectal temperature, 616
  antipyretic guidelines, 618
  in febrile child, 607
  mean values, 606
  triage assessment, 104
Rectum
  anatomy and physiology, 333
  hemorrhage, 338
  physical examination, 86
Red blood cells
  anatomy and physiology, 65, 390-391, 392
  neonatal, 661
  anemia and, 401-402
  packed
    hemolytic-uremic syndrome, 387
    hypovolemic cardiopulmonary arrest, 159
    idiopathic thrombocytopenic purpura, 414
    sickle cell crisis, 407
REDAP; *see* Rural emergency department approved for pediatrics
Referred pain, 339
  hepatic injury, 507
  septic arthritis of hip, 296
Reflexes
  Apgar score, 168
  coma, 134-136
  diving, 219
  near-drowning, 220
  neonatal, 268, 665, 666, 667
  neurologic assessment, 267, 268
  pediatric anatomic and physiologic differences, 64, 68
  as pulmonary protection, 195
Reflexology, 39

Reflux
  gastroesophageal, 332
  vesicoureteral, 375-377
Refractory septic shock, 121
Refusal of care, 32-33
Regional anesthesia, 702
Regional development, 13-15
Reglan; see Metoclopramide
Regression, 49, 58-59
Regurgitation, neonatal, 662, 679
Rehabilitation, 13
Rehearsal in pain management, 703,
  705
Reimbursement, 15, 24-27
Relaxation in pain management, 703,
  704
Religious factors
  organ donation, 37
  refusal of care, 32, 33
Remodeling, 302
Renal cortex, 364-365
Renal failure, 382-385
Renal system
  in acid-base balance, 326
  AIDS manifestations, 399
  anatomy and physiology, 63, 64, 65,
    364-365
  disorders, 378-386
    acute glomerulonephritis, 378-
      380
    nephrotic syndrome, 380-382
    renal failure, 382-385
    renal transplantation for, 385-386
  hemorrhagic shock classifica-
    tion, 503
  Henoch-Schönlein purpura, 388
  shock and, 115
  trauma, 527, 531
Renal transplantation, 385-386
Renin-angiotensin-aldosterone sys-
  tem, 115, 314
Reportable incidents, 29-30, 597
Reproductive system, 64
Rescue breathing, 149, 152
Research
  Emergency Medical Services For
    Children recommendations, 748
  EMS, 9-10
  nurses' role, 21
  public education, 16
Respect for persons, 35
Respiration; see Breathing
Respiratory acidosis, 110, 328-329
Respiratory center, 107-108
Respiratory disorders, 198-232
  abdominal pain and, 339
  anorexia and bulimia nervosa
    and, 735
  apnea, 228-230
  asthma, 211-230
  bronchopulmonary dysplasia, 226-
    228
  cystic fibrosis, 223-226

Respiratory disorders—cont'd
  foreign body aspiration, 217-219
  lower respiratory infection, 203-211
    bronchiolitis, 206-208
    muscular dystrophy, 310, 311
    pertussis, 208-209, 210
    pneumonia, 203-206
    tuberculosis, 209-211
  near-drowning, 219-223
  respiratory failure and, 108
  upper respiratory infection
    bacterial tracheitis, 202-203
    common cold, 198-199
    epiglottitis, 201-202
    neonatal, 675
    sinusitis and, 466
    viral croup, 200-201
Respiratory distress
  assessment, 84
  bacterial tracheitis, 202
  cerebral palsy, 284
  cystic fibrosis, 226
  esophageal foreign body, 360, 361
  glomerulonephritis, 381
  juvenile rheumatoid arthritis, 299,
    301
  multiple trauma management, 498,
    501
  nursing care, 198, 199
  pneumonia, 204
  respiratory failure versus, 110
  signs and symptoms, 99-100, 196-
    198
  triage assessment, 99-100
  urban versus rural prehospital calls, 4
Respiratory effort, 84
Respiratory failure, 107-111, 112, 113
  assessment, 84
  cardiopulmonary arrest, 147, 148
  clinical presentation, 110
  emergency department interven-
    tion, 110
  etiology, 107, 108
  hypoxia-induced, 147
  nursing care and evaluation, 111
  pathophysiology, 107-110
  potential versus actual, 148
  prehospital survival rates, 148
  rapid sequence induction, 111
  signs and symptoms, 196-198
  trauma management
    multiple injury, 498, 501
    thoracoabdominal injuries, 534
Respiratory rate
  Apgar score, 168
  asthma, 213
  criteria for transport to pediatric
    critical care center, 7
  hypoplastic left heart syndrome, 248
  hypothermia, 654
  multiple trauma management, 506
  neonatal, 665, 668
  normal, 103, 198

Respiratory rate—cont'd
  pain assessment, 695
  respiratory assessment, 198
  triage assessment, 103-104
Respiratory syncytial virus
  bronchiolitis, 206-207
  bronchopulmonary dysplasia, 227
  pneumonia, 203
Respiratory system, 193-232
  in acid-base balance, 326
  AIDS manifestations, 398
  anatomy and physiology, 66-67,
    193-195
  depression of with narcotics, 696
  disorders; see Respiratory disorders
  hemorrhagic shock classifica-
    tion, 503
  inhalation injury, 579-580
  juvenile rheumatoid arthritis, 297,
    299, 301
  muscular dystrophy, 310-311
  neonatal, 661
  nursing history and assessment, 195-
    198
  roundworm migration to, 359
  trauma
    contusion, 528, 529
    hemothorax, 529
    pneumothorax, 528-529
Responsiveness in basic life support, 149
Restraint, 463
Resuscitation, 147-177
  advanced life support, 153-164
    airway and ventilation, 154-157
    circulation, 158-159
    defibrillation and
      cardioversion, 160-161
    dysrhythmia management, 159-
      160
    equipment, 153-154, 155
    hypovolemia management, 159
    intubation, 157-158
    pediatric resuscitation drugs, 161-
      164
    sequence of resuscitation activi-
      ties, 153
    team member responsibilities, 153
  basic life support, 149-153
  cardiopulmonary arrest epidemiol-
    ogy, 147
  crisis intervention, 181
  do not resuscitate orders, 714
  family presence during, 181
  field treatment and priority of
    care, 147
  hypothermia, 655
  near-drowning, 220, 221-222
  neonatal, 164-175
    airway, 168
    breathing, 169-170, 171
    circulation, 170-173
    equipment, 165-166

Resuscitation—cont'd
  neonatal—cont'd
    fluids and medications, 173-175
    meconium aspiration, 175-176
    obstetric history, 167
    prehospital transport, 166-167
    preterm deliveries, 176
    stimulation and temperature
      control, 167-168
    team responsibilities, 165
    tension pneumothorax, 176
  outcome following, 147-148
  recognition of prearrest
    condition, 148-149
  sudden infant death syndrome, 189
  of terminally ill child, 35
Resuscitation bag, 154, 156, 169
Reticular activating system, 134
Reticulocytes, 405
Reticulum cell, 392
Retina, 452, 453
Retractions
  asthma, 212
  respiratory distress, 84, 99, 196,
    197
Retropharyngeal abscess, 469
Revised Trauma Score for Children, 9,
  494
Rewarding after physical examina-
  tion, 73
Reye syndrome, 282
RhDNase, 226
Rheumatic fever, 255-256
Rheumatoid arthritis, juvenile, 292,
  297-301
Rhinology and Paranasal Subcommittee
  of American Academy of Otolaryn-
  gology, 467
Rhinovirus, 198
Rhonchi, 197
Rib
  examination, 84
  fracture, 529
    child abuse and, 594-595
    frequency of, 527
  red blood cell production in, 392
Ribavirin, 207
Ribonucleic acid, 397
Rickettsial illness, 655-656
Rid; see Pyrethrin
Rifampin
  meningitis prophylaxis, 280, 281
  tuberculosis, 211
Right-to-left shunt, 238, 244-248,
  257-258
Risk management programs, 33-34
Risk-taking behavior, 57-58, 63
Ritalin; see Methylphenidate hydrochlo-
  ride
RMSF; see Rocky Mountain spotted
  fever
RNA; see Ribonucleic acid
Robert Wood Johnson Foundation, 2

Rocky Mountain spotted fever, 655-
  656
Romazicon; see Flumazenil
Rooting reflex, 268, 667
Roseola infantum, 427, 432
Rotavirus, 339, 341
Roundworm, 359
RR; see Respiratory rate
RSI; see Rapid sequence induction intu-
  bation
RSV; see Respiratory syncytial virus
Rubbing alcohol poisoning, 635-636
Rubella, 425, 429
Rubeola, 420-428, 425
Rule of nines, 566, 567
Rumack-Matthew nomogram, 635,
  636
Runaways, 739
Rural emergency department approved
  for pediatrics, 14
Rural population
  chief complaints for prehospital
    calls, 4
  EMSC transport system, 14
  triage scoring systems, 6
Russell's sign, 735

S
Safety
  bicycle, 487
  cerebral palsy, 284
  defibrillation and cardioversion, 161
  education, 61, 62-63
  in pediatric emergency depart-
    ments, 18
Safety seat, 11, 489
Salicylates
  pain management, 695, 696
  poisoning, 624
    activated charcoal and, 628
    gastric lavage, 626
    juvenile rheumatoid arthritis, 300
    urine alkalization in, 631
  rheumatic fever, 256
Salmonella
  diarrhea, 336
  gastroenteritis, 340, 342
  osteomyelitis, 293
Salt poisoning, 321
Salter-Harris classification, 542
Sao₂; see Arterial hemoglobin saturation
Sarcoma, 292
Sarcoptes scabiei, 446
Sawyer Extractor, 649
SBE; see Subacute bacterial endocarditis
Scabies, 446-447
Scald injury, 565, 566, 570, 571
Scalded skin syndrome, 435-437
Scale, 19, 423
Scalp
  anatomy, 511
  fungal infection, 437-440

Scalp—cont'd
  seborrheic dermatitis, 446
Scar, 423
Scarlet fever, 426, 430-431
School-age child
  approach to, 54-56
  cardiopulmonary resuscitation and
    first aid education, 16
  common injuries, 63, 490
  coping strategies, 689, 706
  gaining cooperation of, 74
  growth and development, 52-56
  interviewing, 72
  laceration repair, 562
  normal vital signs, 103, 198
  pain responses, 688
  triage assessment, 82
  vision testing, 81
SCIWORA; see Spinal cord injury with-
  out radiographic abnormalities
Sclera, 80, 452
Scoliosis, 293
Scoring systems in field triage, 6-9,
  494-495
Scorpion envenomation, 642, 644
Screening
  Consolidated Omnibus Budget Rec-
    onciliation Act, 24
  Omnibus Budget Reconciliation
    Act, 27
  pediatric emergency care, 16, 17
Scrotum, 364, 367
Seafood urticaria, 450
Seat belts, 489, 490, 491, 531
Sebaceous gland, 419
Seborrheic dermatitis, 446
Sebum, 419
Secondary survey, 496, 506
Second-degree burn, 567-568, 570
Secretions
  bacterial tracheitis, 202
  comatose child, 138
  cystic fibrosis, 223, 224
  nasal
    assessment, 465
    breath sounds and, 84
    head trauma and, 82
    neonatal upper respiratory infec-
      tion, 676
    sinusitis, 466
  ocular, 80
  pertussis, 209
  vaginal
    newborn, 364
    sexual abuse, 600
Sedation
  conscious, 699-700
  manual reduction of incarcerated
    hernia, 351-352
  near-drowning, 222
Sedatives, 700-701
  abuse, 737
  head and neck injury, 524, 525

Sedatives—cont'd
  intubation, 158
  poisoning, 624
  rapid sequence induction, 112-113
Seesaw respirations, 84
Seizure, 270-274, 275
  cerebral palsy, 284
  febrile, 128, 432, 609-610
  head and neck injury, 526
  hypernatremia, 321
  hypocalcemia, 483
  hyponatremic, 319
  increased intracranial pressure, 143
  meningitis, 278, 281
  neonatal, 666
  renal failure, 383
  status epilepticus, 128-133
  urban *versus* rural prehospital calls, 4
Selenium sulfide shampoo, 439
Self-inflating resuscitation bag, 154,
    156, 502
Sellick maneuver, 222, 499
Selsun Blue; *see* Antiseborrheic sham-
    poo
Semicoma, 133
Sensorimotor stage of develop-
    ment, 44, 45, 48, 49
Sensory function, 522
Separation anxiety, 46, 49
Sepsis
  defined, 120
  disseminated intravascular coagula-
      tion, 411
  neonatal, 668-671
  neutropenia with fever, 400
Sepsis syndrome, 120-121
Septic arthritis, 295-297
Septic shock, 114, 119-121
  bacterial meningitis, 279
  neonatal, 669
  osteomyelitis, 295
  septic arthritis, 297
Septicemia, 294
Septum
  anatomy, 464
  assessment, 465
  atrial septal defect, 239
  complete atrioventricular canal de-
      fect, 241
  transposition of great arteries, 245
Sequestration crisis in sickle cell ane-
    mia, 405, 406
Serotonin, 729
Serum albumin
  glomerulonephritis, 381
  hypocalcemia, 482-483
Serum bicarbonate, 478
Serum calcium, 324-325, 482, 483
Serum carboxyhemoglobin, 580
Serum creatinine, 316
Serum electrolytes, 66, 316
Serum glutamic oxaloacetic transami-
    nase, 531

Serum glutamic pyruvic transami-
    nase, 531
Serum osmolality
  diabetes insipidus, 481
  mannitol administration, 143, 524
  normal, 314
Serum pH
  in alkalization of urine for poison-
      ing, 631
  diabetic ketoacidosis, 480
Serum potassium
  dehydration, 316
  diabetic ketoacidosis, 477
  hyperkalemia, 322, 323
  hypokalemia, 321, 322
Serum sodium
  dehydration, 315, 316
  diabetes insipidus, 482
  hypernatremia, 320, 321
  hyponatremia, 318
  meningitis, 279
Set point, hypothalamic, 608
Setting sun sign, 275
Severity Index for Acute Pediatric Ill-
    ness, 9
Sex hormones, 473
Sex roles in preschooler develop-
    ment, 50
Sexual abuse, 587, 598-601
  clinical manifestations, 591
  gonococcal pharyngitis, 469
  pelvic inflammatory disease, 372
  policies and protocols, 19
  as reportable incidence, 29
Sexual assault, acute, 587, 595, 600
Sexual history, 372
Sexually transmitted disease, 367-369,
    370-371
  child abuse and, 600
  ophthalmia neonatorum, 454
SGOT; *see* Serum glutamic oxaloacetic
    transaminase
SGPT; *see* Serum glutamic pyruvic
    transaminase
Shaken baby syndrome, 131, 515, 602
Shampoo
  antiseborrheic, 446
  pediculosis, 448
  tinea versicolor, 439
Sheet restraint, 463
Shigella
  diarrhea, 336
  gastroenteritis, 340, 342
Shock, 111-116
  adrenal insufficiency, 485
  anaphylaxis, 652
  anemia, 402, 403
  cardiogenic, 114, 118-119
  cardiopulmonary arrest, 148-149
  dehydration, 100
  encephalopathy, 282-283
  glomerulonephritis, 381
  hypovolemic, 114, 117-118, 574

Shock—cont'd
  multiple trauma management, 503
  nursing care and evaluation, 122-
      126
  pediatric anatomic and physiologic
      differences, 67
  septic, 114, 119-121
    bacterial meningitis, 279
    neonatal, 669
    osteomyelitis, 295
    septic arthritis, 297
  sickle cell crisis, 407, 408
  snakebite, 647
  trauma management, 493-494
Shotgun wound, 189
Shunt
  cerebral, 275-277, 286
  left-to-right, 237-238
    atrial septal defect, 239-240
    complete atrioventricular canal de-
        fect, 241
    nursing intervention, 257
    patent ductus arteriosus, 238-239
    ventricular septal defect, 240-
        241
  right-to-left, 238, 244-248, 257-
      258
SIADH; *see* Syndrome of inappropriate
    antidiuretic hormone
Sibilant wheezing, 197
Sibling death, 184, 185
Sickle cell anemia, 403-408
  limp and, 293
  palpable spleen, 85
  sickled cells of, 392
SIDS; *see* Sudden infant death syn-
    drome
Silent lung, 212
Sinequan; *see* Doxepin
Sinus venosus defect, 239
Sinus x-ray, 467
Sinuses, 463-467
Sinusitis, 466-467
Skeletal system; *see* Musculoskeletal sys-
    tem
Skin, 417-451
  adrenal insufficiency and, 484
  AIDS manifestations, 398
  anatomy and physiology, 417-419
  animal bites and, 645
  anorexia and bulimia nervosa, 735
  cardiogenic shock, 118
  criteria for transport to pediatric
      critical care center, 7
  dehydration, 100, 319
  disorders; *see* Skin disorders
  hemorrhagic shock classifica-
      tion, 503
  history and assessment, 86-87, 419-
      420, 421-422, 423-424
  neonatal, 663, 664
  lesion; *see* Skin lesion
  shock, 116

Skin color
  Apgar score, 168
  asthma, 213
  cardiovascular assessment, 235
  compartment syndrome, 560
  in febrile child, 611
  hypertonic *versus* hypotonic dehydration, 319
  respiratory assessment, 196
  triage assessment, 94
Skin disorder
  inconsolable crying, 681
  parasitic infestation, 446-448
Skin disorders
  bacterial infection, 434-437
  dermatitis, 440-446
  erythema multiforme, 448-450
  fungal infection, 437-440
  infectious exanthems, 420-434
    fifth disease, 431-432
    hand-foot-mouth disease, 433-434
    pityriasis rosea, 432-433
    roseola infantum, 432
    rubella, 429
    rubeola, 420-428
    scarlet fever, 430-431
    varicella, 429-430
Skin lesion, 421-424
  assessment, 87
  chickenpox, 430
  Henoch-Schönlein purpura, 388
  Lyme disease, 656-657
  meningitis, 279, 280
  Rocky Mountain spotted fever, 656
  syphilis, 368
  triage assessment, 103
Skin testing before antivenin administration, 650
Skull, 511, 512
  fracture, 516
    child abuse, 595
  neonatal, 266
Sleep
  cerebral palsy, 284
  disturbance after emergency department visit, 49
  infant positioning, 188
Sleep apnea, 228
Sling and swathe, 551
Slipped capital femoral epiphysis, 292, 303-306, 307, 308
Small intestine
  anatomy and physiology, 332-333
  intussusception, 346-347
Smith's fracture, 552, 553
Smoke detector, 565
Smoke inhalation, 579
Smoking, 461
Snakebite, 633, 646-650
Snellen symbol chart, 454
Snuffbox tenderness, 555
Sodium
  body fluid balance, 315

Sodium—cont'd
  burn injury, 575
  deficit calculations, 320
  dehydration, 315, 316
  diabetes insipidus, 482
  hypernatremia, 320, 321
  hyponatremia, 318, 319
  meningitis, 279
  pyloric stenosis, 353
Sodium bicarbonate, 633
  alkalization of urine for poisoning, 631
  cyclic antidepressant poisoning, 638
  hyperkalemia, 323, 324
  metabolic acidosis, 125, 327
  near-drowning, 222
  renal failure, 384
  resuscitation, 162, 163, 166, 174
Sodium carbonate, 327
Sodium chloride, 223
Sodium nitroprusside, 251, 255
Sodium polystyrene sulfonate, 323, 324, 383
Soft palate, 468
Soft tissue trauma, 561-563
Solu-Medrol; *see* Methylprednisolone
Somatic pain, 339
Somatostatin, 473
Sonorous wheezing, 197
Sorbitol, 628, 630
Sore throat, 469-470
  epiglottitis, 201
  rheumatic fever and, 255
Southeast Asian population, 183
Spasm
  hypocalcemia, 483
  infantile, 271, 272
Spastic diplegia, 283
Spastic hemiplegia, 283
Spastic quadriplegia, 283, 284
Special needs child, 712-726
  developmentally delayed, 714-716
  do not resuscitate orders, 714
  Down syndrome, 716-718
  history and physical examination, 712-713
  home health care, 714
  multidisciplinary teams, 713-714
  pain assessment, 691
  technology-dependent, 718-725
    gastrostomy tubes, 722-725
    mechanical ventilators, 722, 723
    oxygen dependent, 718-719
    tracheostomy tubes, 719-721
Specialized care, 13, 14
Specific gravity
  dehydration, 316
  diabetes insipidus, 145
  renal failure, 383
Spectinomycin, 370
Speech
  Glasgow Coma Scale, 137
  tracheostomy and, 721

Spherocytosis, hereditary, 402
Spider bite, 642, 644
Spina bifida, 78, 285-287
Spina Bifida Association of America, 287
Spinal cord injury, 134
Spinal cord injury without radiographic abnormalities, 519
Spine
  immobilization, 500, 501
    before basic life support, 149, 150
  juvenile rheumatoid arthritis and, 299
  near-drowning injury, 219, 221
Spiral fracture, 542
  child abuse, 595
  femur, 545
Spirometry, 212-213
Spironolactone, 251
Spitting up, 336, 662, 679
Spleen
  palpation, 85
  pediatric anatomic and physiologic differences, 64
  sickle cell anemia and, 405
  trauma, 527, 530, 531
Splenic sequestration, 405, 406
Splinting
  fracture, 558
    clavicular, 550
    femur, 557
    humerus, 551
  juvenile rheumatoid arthritis, 300-301
Sponging to reduce fever, 617
Sprain, 292
Sputum examination
  muscular dystrophy respiratory infection, 311
  pneumonia, 205
  tuberculosis, 210
SSSS; *see* Staphylococcal scalded skin syndrome
ST segment
  hypocalcemia, 483
  near-drowning, 221
Staff
  critical incident stress management, 186-188
  death of child, 184-186
  for triage, 89-90
Staphylococcal scalded skin syndrome, 435-437
Staphylococcus aureus
  cellulitis, 435
    preorbital and orbital, 455
  conjunctivitis, 454
  impetigo, 434
  infective endocarditis, 253
  osteomyelitis, 293
  septic arthritis, 296
  septic shock, 119
  tracheitis, 202

Startle reflex, 667
State contacts, 742-746
Status epilepticus, 8, 128-133
Statute of limitations, 31
STD; *see* Sexually transmitted disease
Stenosis
    aortic, 243-244
    pulmonary, 241-242
        tetralogy of Fallot, 244
        truncus arteriosus, 245
    pyloric, 352-353
Stepping reflex, 667
Sterile technique, 172
Sternum
    depression, 84
    examination, 84
    protrusion, 84
    red blood cell production in, 392
    resuscitation compression, 150-151,
        171
Steroids
    asthma, 214-215
    atopic dermatitis, 443-444, 445
    conjunctivitis and, 455
    head and neck injury, 525, 526
    idiopathic thrombocytopenic pur-
        pura, 414
    increased intracranial pressure, 141,
        143
    meningitis, 279
    septic shock, 121
    urticaria, 650, 651
    viral croup, 200
Stevens-Johnson syndrome, 448-450
Stillbirth, 307, 308
Stimulation, neonatal, 167-168
Stings, 642-643
    anaphylactic reaction, 651
Stomach, 332
Stomatitis, 340-344, 448
Stool
    bloody, 338
    cystic fibrosis, 225
    Hirschsprung's disease, 354
    intussusception, 346, 347
    neonatal, 662, 677-678
    pyloric stenosis, 352
Stool examination
    amebiasis, 356
    gastroenteritis, 340
    giardiasis, 359
    neonatal bloody stool, 678
Strabismus, 452
Strain, 292
Stranger anxiety, 46, 47
Strangulated hernia, 351
Streptococci
    acute otitis media, 460
    conjunctivitis, 454
    group A
        cellulitis, 435
        epiglottitis, 201
        glomerulonephritis, 379

Streptococci—cont'd
    group A—cont'd
        impetigo, 434
        osteomyelitis, 293
        pharyngitis, 469
        rheumatic fever, 255-256
        scarlet fever, 430, 431
        tracheitis, 202
    group B
        meningitis, 277
        neonatal sepsis, 668
        osteomyelitis, 293
        pneumonia, 203
        septic shock, 119
    infective endocarditis, 253
    meningitis, 277
    nephritogenic, 378
    pneumonia, 203, 204
    preorbital and orbital cellulitis, 455
    septic shock, 119
    sinusitis, 466
    tracheitis, 202
Streptomycin, 211
Stress
    child abuse and, 596
    critical incident stress
        management, 186-188
    defined, 178
    events that influence, 179
    parental, 59-60
    school-age child response to, 54-55
    tension headache, 269, 270
    toddler response to, 49
Stress fracture, 542
Stridor
    airway obstruction, 98
    bacterial tracheitis, 201, 202
    epiglottitis, 201
    respiratory assessment, 197, 198
    viral croup, 200, 201
Stridor at rest
    criteria for transport to pediatric
        critical care center, 7
    viral croup, 200
String test, 359
Stroke volume, 233-234
    anemia, 402
    in cardiac output, 115
    neonatal, 661
    pediatric anatomic and physiologic
        differences, 67
Stupor, 133
Stylet for neonatal intubation, 170
Subacute bacterial endocarditis, 253
Subarachnoid hemorrhage, 515-516
Subarachnoid screw, 144
Subarachnoid space, 277
Subcutaneous tissue, 418
    burn injury, 571
    hypothermia, 654
Subdural hematoma, 515
Subdural space, 266, 511
Subjunctival hemorrhage, 80

Sublimaze; *see* Fentanyl
Sublingual narcotic administra-
    tion, 697
Substance abuse, 737-739
Substance P, 686
Succinylcholine, 113
Sucking reflex, 268, 667
Suctioning
    basic life support, 149
    comatose child, 138
    gastric lavage, 626
    intubation, 157, 158, 170
    near-drowning, 222
    neonatal, 168
    neonatal resuscitation, 166
    pertussis, 209
Sudden infant death syndrome, 4, 188-
    189, 190
Sugar-tong splint, 551
Suicide, 730-733
Sulfate, 326
Sulfisoxazole, 375
Sulfonamide
    erythema multiforme, 448
    urticaria, 450
Sumatriptan succinate, 270
Sunburn, 567, 570
Superficial burn, 567, 570
Superficial partial-thickness burn, 567,
    568, 570
Superior mesenteric artery
    gastrointestinal calculation, 334
    malrotation of bowel with volvulus
        and, 350
Supplies
    in adult emergency departments, 19
    EMS, 9, 11
    neonatal resuscitation, 166
    triage, 91
Support group in death of child, 183
Suppressor T cell, 394-395
Supraclavicular retraction, 84, 99, 196,
    197
Supracondylar fracture, 551
Supraglottitis, 201-202
Suprapubic bladder aspiration, 376
Suprasternal retraction, 84, 99, 196,
    197
Supraventricular tachycardia, 259-260
    advanced life support, 160
    cardiogenic shock, 118, 119
Surgery, mental retardation and, 717
Surgical debridement in osteomyeli-
    tis, 294
Surrogate consent, 28
Sutures, cranial, 266
    examination, 77-78, 79
    pediatric anatomic and physiologic
        differences, 64, 67
    premature closure of, 78
Suturing, 562
SV; *see* Stroke volume
SVT; *see* Supraventricular tachycardia

Sweat, cystic fibrosis and, 223
Sweat chloride test, 225
Sweat gland, 418, 419
Swimmer's ear, 458
Swimmer's position, 626
Swischuk line, 518, 519
Sympathetic nervous system, 67, 114
Sympathomimetics
  poisoning, 624
  shock, 124-125
Symptomatic bradycardia, 159-160
Symptomatic supraventricular tachycardia, 160
Synacort; see Hydrocortisone
Synalar; see Flucinolone acetonide
Synchronized cardioversion, 160-161, 260
Syncope, 242
Syndrome of inappropriate antidiuretic hormone, 318
  encephalopathy, 282
  increased intracranial pressure, 145
  meningitis, 277-278, 279
Synovial membrane, 301
Synovitis, 292, 301-302
Syphilis, 368, 370
  child abuse and, 600
Syrup of Ipecac, 625-626
Systolic blood pressure
  criteria for transport to pediatric critical care center, 7
  Pediatric Trauma Score, 9
  pericarditis, 254

T

T cell, 394
  cell-mediated immunity, 394-395
  human immunodeficiency virus and, 397
  neonatal, 662
  pediatric anatomic and physiologic differences, 65
T wave
  hyperkalemia, 323
  hypocalcemia, 483
  near-drowning, 221
TA; see Truncus arteriosus
TAC, 701
Tachycardia
  anemia, 402
  cardiac output and, 104, 114-115
  cardiovascular assessment, 236
  hypothermia, 654
  shock, 114-115, 116
  supraventricular, 259-260
    cardiogenic shock, 118, 119
    symptomatic, 160
  tension pneumothorax, 528-529
  ventricular, 261-262
    advanced life support, 160
Tachydysrhythmia, 259

Tachypnea
  asthma, 212
  congestive heart failure, 236
  effortless
    hypoplastic left heart syndrome, 248
    transposition of great arteries, 245
  neonatal sepsis, 669
  shock, 116
  tension pneumothorax, 528-529
  ventricular septal defect, 241
Tactile neonatal stimulation, 168
Taenia saginata, 359
Taenia solium, 359
Talus fracture, 547
Tamponade
  cardiac, 503
    juvenile rheumatoid arthritis, 301
  pericardial, 529-530
Tannic acid, 631
Tapeworm, 359-360
TAPVR; see Total anomalous pulmonary venous return
Target lesion, 448
TB; see Tuberculosis
TBSA; see Total body surface area
Team responsibilities
  advanced life support, 153
    neonatal, 165
  pediatric trauma, 496
Technology-dependent child, 718-725
  gastrostomy tubes, 722-725
  mechanical ventilators, 722, 723
  oxygen dependent, 718-719
  tracheostomy tubes, 719-721
Teeth, 309
Telephone
  central dispatch assessment, 4
  legal considerations of telephone advice, 31-32
  parental consent, 29
  private physician orders from, 32
Telogen, 418-419
Temovate; see Clobetasol propionate
Temperature; see Body temperature
Temporal lobe
  herniation, 514
  unilateral displacement, 135
Tension headache, 269, 270
Tension pneumothorax, 502, 528-530
  needle decompression in, 534
  neonatal resuscitation, 176
Terbutaline
  anaphylaxis, 653
  asthma, 214
Terminal illness, ethical decisions, 35-37
Testes, 86, 473, 664
Testicle, 364
Testicular torsion, 377-378
Testosterone, 473
TET spell, 252
  tetralogy of Fallot, 244

Tetanus, 508-509
  animal bite, 645
  burn injury, 576
  snakebite, 649
Tetany, 483
Tetracaine, 701
Tetracycline, 370
Tetralogy of Fallot, 244
TGA; see Transposition of great arteries
Thalamus, 267
THAM; see Aminomethane
Theophylline
  asthma, 216
  bronchopulmonary dysplasia, 227
  poisoning, 624, 628, 634
Therapeutic touch, 39, 703, 704
Thermal inhalation injury, 579
Thermogenesis, non-shivering, 68
Thermometer, tympanic, 104
Thermoregulation, 607, 662
  neonatal, 662
  pediatric anatomic and physiologic differences, 68
Thiopental, 112
Third-degree burn, 567, 570, 571
Third-generation cephalosporin
  bacterial tracheitis, 203
  epiglottitis, 202
  neonatal sepsis, 670
Third-spacing of fluids, 574
Thirst mechanism, 313
Thoracentesis
  juvenile rheumatoid arthritis, 299
  tension pneumothorax, 176
Thoracoabdominal trauma, 527-535, 536
Thoracostomy, 502, 534
Thorazine, 698
Thought modeling, 703
Thought stopping, 705
Thrills, 237
Throat
  AIDS manifestations, 398
  anatomy and physiology, 64, 467-468
  assessment, 83, 468
    neonatal, 64, 666-667
  pharyngitis, 469-470
Thrombocytes; see Platelets
Thrombocytopenia, 394
  anorexia and bulimia nervosa, 734
Thrush, 440
Thumb for neonatal chest compression, 171
Thyrocalcitonin, 473
Thyroid gland, 473
Thyroid hormones, 473
Thyroid-stimulating hormone, 473
TI; see Triage Index
Tibia
  fracture, 545-546, 547
  intraosseous access, 159, 504
  Osgood-Schlatter disease, 306

Tibia—cont'd
  red blood cell production in, 392
Tick
  encephalitis, 281
  Lyme disease, 656
  removal, 656, 657
  Rocky Mountain spotted fever, 655
Tidal volume, 194
  in mechanical ventilation, 722
  neonatal, 169
  self-inflating resuscitation bag, 154, 502
Tinactin; see Tolnaftate
Tinea, 437-440
Tissue perfusion in shock, 118, 125
Toast as universal antidote, 631
Tobramycin, 226
Toddler
  approach to, 49, 50, 76
  common fears, 48, 49
  common injuries, 62, 490
  coping strategies, 689, 706
  fever presentation, 612
  gaining cooperation of, 74, 75
  general survey, 75-77
  growth and development, 47-49, 50
  laceration repair, 562
  normal respiratory rate, 198
  pain responses, 688
  triage assessment, 82
  vision testing, 81
Toddler's fracture, 546
Toe fracture, 547, 556
Toenail, 419
Tofranil; see Imipramine
Toilet training, 47
Tolmetin, 300
Tolnaftate, 440
Toluene
  abuse, 738
  poisoning, 638
Tongue, 468
  as airway obstruction, 149, 195, 497
  assessment, 82
  scarlet fever, 431
Tongue depressor, 83
Tonic neck reflex, 268, 667
Tonic seizure, 273
Tonic-clonic seizure, 128, 129, 272, 273
Tonicity, term, 314
Tonsil, 64, 467
Tonsillar pillars, 468
Topicort; see Desoximetasone
Topicort LP; see Desoximetasone
Toradol; see Ketorolac
Torsion, testicular, 377-378
Torus fracture, 542
Total anomalous pulmonary venous return, 246-248
Total body surface area in burn injury assessment, 566
Toxic synovitis, 292, 301-302

Toxicity, 622-641
  acetaminophen, 635, 636
  alcohol, 635-637
  antidotal therapy, 631-633
  bacterial tracheitis, 201
  carbon monoxide, 579, 580
  cough and cold preparations, 637-638
  cyclic antidepressants, 638
  digoxin, 252
  epidemiology, 622
  epiglottitis, 201
  exchange transfusion, 631
  external documentation, 625
  extracorporeal drug removal, 631
  gastric decontamination, 625-630
  history and assessment, 622-623
  hydrocarbons, 638-639
  iron, 639
  lindane, 448
  nursing intervention, 623-625
  osteomyelitis, 293
  oxygen, 226
  plants, 639, 640
  poison information centers, 641-642
  prevention, 640-641
  primary hypothermia, 653
  salicylate, 300
  salt, 321
  vitamin D, 325-326
Toxidromes, 623, 624
Toxins
  cellulitis, 435, 436
  metabolism and excretion, 65-66
  pertussis, 208
  snakebite, 647
Toys, 19
Trachea, 195
  airway obstruction, 497
  endotracheal intubation, 498
Tracheitis, 201, 202-203
Tracheostomy tube, 719-721
Traction, 303, 306
Traction splint, 557
Tractor accident, 491-492
Training; see Education
Transfers
  checklist, 15
  Consolidated Omnibus Budget Reconciliation Act and, 24, 25-26
  continuous quality improvement programs and, 16
  documentation of for litigation risk management, 34
  hospital agreements, 14
  Omnibus Budget Reconciliation Act and, 27
  patient transfer form, 25-26
Transfusion; see Blood transfusion
Transient synovitis, 301-302
Transillumination
  sinusitis, 467
  tension pneumothorax, 176

Transit disorders, 336
Transplantation
  liver, 355-356
  renal, 385-386
Transport, 5-6, 7-8
  to burn care center, 577
  of family after death of child, 184, 186
  neonatal, 166-167
  to pediatric critical care center, 7-8, 492-494
  regional development of training and equipment, 14-15
  urban versus rural population, 13, 14
Transport monitor, 11
Transport provider training, 14-15
Transposition of great arteries, 244-245
Transthoracic pacing, 160
Transverse fracture, 542
Trauma, 487-510, 511-539, 530-531
  access to care, 492-494
  basic life support following, 149
  birth, 78
  cellulitis following, 435
  Children's Trauma Tool, 10
  criteria for transport to pediatric critical care center, 7
  by developmental stage, 62-63
  etiology and mechanisms, 489-492
  frequency, 527
  handgun, 189
  head and neck; see Head and neck trauma
  hemophilia and, 409, 410
  increased intracranial pressure, 141
  intentional verus unintentional, 489-490
  limp and, 292
  musculoskeletal, 540-561
    compartment syndrome, 559-560
    growth plates, 541-542
    lower extremity, 542-549
    nursing care and evaluation, 556-559
    open fracture, 560-561
    triage assessment, 92, 103
    upper extremity, 549-555
  nosebleed, 465
  nursing care, 496-509
    airway, 497-500
    breathing, 500-502
    cervical spine immobilization, 500, 501
    circulation, 502-505
    disability, 505-506
    exposure and body temperature control, 506
    head-to-toe assessment, 506-508
    parental presence, 497
    primary and secondary surveys, 497, 506
    tetanus, 508-509

Trauma—cont'd
nursing care—cont'd
vital signs and history, 506
ocular, 536-538
pediatric trauma area/
equipment, 495-496
prehospital care, 492
prevention, 61, 62-63, 487-489
nurses' role, 21
prehospital care, 2, 3-4
public education, 15
seizing child, 130
referred pain in, 507
scoring systems, 6-9, 494-495
soft tissue, 561-563
spinal cord, 134
thoracoabdominal, 527-535, 536
abdominal injury, 530-531
anatomy and physiology, 528
emergency department
intervention, 531-533
nursing care and evaluation, 533-
535, 536
thoracic injury, 528-530
Trauma Score, 6, 495
Trauma Triage Rule, 8
Traumatic asphyxia, 492, 530
Traumatic brain injury; see Head and
neck trauma
Traumatic diaphragmatic hernia, 530
Treatment rooms, 18, 19
Trendelenburg position, 626
Treponema pallidum, 368
Triage, 89-106
ABCDEs of, 99
assessment, 90-91
burn injury, 571-572
criteria, 93, 94, 95
examination, 95-105
across the room assessment,
95-97
history, 96, 97
physical assessment, 97-103
vital signs/monitoring, 103-105
fever, 615-616
intervention, 91-92
out of emergency department, 92
scoring systems, 6-9
settings for, 89
staffing, 89-90
transport systems, 5-6, 7-8
triage nurse, 90
Triage decision, 95
Triage desk, 19
Triage Index, 6
Triage-Revised Trauma Score, 8
Triamcinolone acetonide, 445
Trichomonas, 368, 371
Trichophyton, 437, 438, 439
Tricuspid atresia, 246, 247
Tricyclic poisoning, 634
Tridesilon; see Desonide
Trimethoprim-sulfamethoxazole
meningitis, 280

Trimethoprim-sulfamethoxazole—
cont'd
Pneumocystis carinii pneumonia pre-
vention in AIDS, 399
Shigella gastroenteritis, 342
urinary tract infection, 375
Yersinia gastroenteritis, 343
Tripod position
airway obstruction, 98
criteria for transport to pediatric
critical care center, 7
Tris, 125
Trisomy 21, 716-718
Tromethamine
increased intracranial pressure, 145
metabolic acidosis, 327
Trousseau's sign, 325, 483
T-RTS; see Triage-Revised Trauma
Score
Truncus arteriosus, 245-246
Trust versus mistrust in infants, 44, 45
TS; see Trauma Score
TSH; see Thyroid-stimulating hormone
TTR; see Trauma Triage Rule
Tube
gastric lavage, 626
gastrostomy, 723-724, 725
tracheostomy, 720
Tuberculosis, 209-211, 279
Tuberous sclerosis, 271
Tubule, renal, 365
necrosis in renal failure, 365
Tumor, 422
Tumor necrosis factor, 120, 121
Turbinates, 464
Turner's sign, 530
Turpentine poisoning, 638
Tympanic membrane
anatomy, 457, 458
assessment, 81, 458, 459
neonatal, 666-667
upper respiratory infection, 676
Tympanic thermometer, 104
Tympanometry in acute otitis media,
461

U

Ulcer, 420, 424
decubitus, 284
oral cavity, 340-344
Ulna fracture, 551
Ultrasound
appendicitis, 349
pyloric stenosis, 353
Umbilical catheterization, 171-173
Umbilical cord assessment, 664, 666
Umbilical hernia, 85
Uncal herniation, 134, 135, 514
Unconjugated
hyperbilirubinemia, 672-673
Unconscious patient
foreign body airway
obstruction, 152-153

Unconscious patient—cont'd
prehospital pulse assessment, 150
Uniform Anatomical Gift Act of 1968,
37-38
Unintentional injury, 489
United States Department of Health
and Human Services, 20-21
Universal precautions, 400
Upper respiratory infection
bacterial tracheitis, 202-203
common cold, 198-199
epiglottitis, 201-202
neonatal, 675
sinusitis and, 466
viral croup, 200-201
Urban population
chief complaints for prehospital
calls, 4
EMSC transport system, 13
Ureter, 364
vesicoureteral reflux, 375
Urethra
anatomy, 364
vesicoureteral reflux, 375
Urgent care, 92
URI; see Upper respiratory infection
Urinalysis
dehydration, 316
febrile child, 614, 617
glomerulonephritis, 379, 380-381
renal failure, 383
urinary tract infection, 374
Urinary elimination, 364
Urinary frequency in urinary tract infection, 374
Urinary system; see Genitourinary system
Urinary tract infection, 372-375
myelomeningocele, 286-287
vesicoureteral reflux, 375
Urine
alkalinization of for poisoning, 631
dilute in diabetes insipidus, 481, 482
vesicoureteral reflux, 375
Urine culture
febrile child, 614, 617
methods of collection, 49, 375, 376
urinary tract infection, 374-375
Urine output
burn injury, 576
cardiovascular disorders, 258
dehydration, 100
glomerulonephritis, 381
increased intracranial pressure, 141
neonatal, 661
normal values, 366
renal failure, 383
shock, 116, 125
septic, 121
Urine pH in alkalization of urine for
poisoning, 631
Urticaria, 450-451, 650-651
UTI; see Urinary tract infection
Uveitis, 297-298, 300
Uvula, 468

V

Vaccine, 87
  bacille Calmette-Guérin, 211
  pneumococcal, 206
  triage assessment, 96
  tuberculosis prevention, 211
  varicella, 429
Vaginal discharge
  newborn, 364
  sexual abuse, 600
Valium; see Diazepam
Valproic acid, 273
Valvular aortic stenosis, 243-244
Valvuloplasty, 249
Vancomycin, 280
Varicella, 425, 429-430
  encephalitis, 281
  pericarditis, 254
Varicella-zoster immune globulin, 430
Vascular access
  comatose child, 138
  meningitis, 281
  multiple trauma management, 504
Vascular resistance
  cardiogenic shock, 118
  pulmonary
    total anomalous pulmonary venous
      return, 247
    truncus arteriosus, 245, 246
    ventricular septal defect, 240
Vascular system, Rocky Mountain spotted fever and, 656
Vasogenic cerebral edema, 142
Vasoocclusive crisis in sickle cell anemia, 403, 406, 407
Vasopressin
  body fluid regulation, 314
  diabetes insipidus, 481
  shock and, 115
Vecuronium, 113, 525
Veganism, 40
Vegetarianism, 40
Venomous snake bite, 646-650
Venous access
  adrenal insufficiency, 485
  anaphylaxis, 652
  cerebral palsy, 284-285
  cystic fibrosis, 226
  electrolyte disturbance acid-base bal-
    ance, 329
  right-to-left shunting, 258
Ventilation, 194
  advanced life support, 154-157
  bag-valve-mask
    advanced life support, 154
    neonatal, 169, 171
    respiratory failure, 111
    status epilepticus, 130
    trauma management, 498, 502,
      522
  mechanical
    bronchopulmonary dysplasia, 227
    cystic fibrosis, 226

Ventilation—cont'd
  mechanical—cont'd
    dependence on, 722, 723
    increased intracranial pres-
      sure, 143
    near-drowning, 221
  positive pressure, 169
  respiratory control, 107-108
Ventilation to pulmonary blood flow
  ratio, 108
Ventricular drain, 144
Ventricular fibrillation, 262
  advanced life support, 160
  electrical burn injury, 581
  hypothermia, 654, 655
  near-drowning, 220
Ventricular septal defect
  coarctation of aorta and, 243
  transposition of great arteries, 245
  tricuspid atresia, 246
Ventricular tachycardia, 261-262
  advanced life support, 160
Ventriculoperitoneal shunt, 275, 276,
  286
Verapamil, 160, 260
Verification in regionalizing care, 14
Versed, 576
Vertebra
  anatomy, 517-518
  red blood cell production in, 392
  trauma, 518-519
Vesicle, 420, 422
Vesicoureteral reflux, 375-377
Violence
  against child, 189-191
  in emergency department, 181-182
Viral hepatitis, 344-346
Viral infection
  acute otitis media, 460
  as asthma trigger, 212
  conjunctivitis, 454, 455
  croup, 200-201
  diarrhea, 337
  encephalitis, 281-283
  gastroenteritis, 340
  meningitis, 279
    encephalitis versus, 282
  myocarditis, 254
  pharyngitis, 469-470
  pneumonia, 204, 205, 206
Viral shedding, 207
Visceral pain, 338
Visual acuity, 452
  assessment, 78-79, 81, 454
    juvenile rheumatoid arthritis, 301
    traumatic eye injury, 538
  pediatric anatomic and physiologic
    differences, 64
Visual Analog Scale, 694
Vital signs
  anorexia and bulimia nervosa, 735
  cardiovascular assessment, 236, 258
  coma, 136, 139

Vital signs—cont'd
  criteria for transport to pediatric
    critical care center, 7
  head and neck trauma, 520
  increased intracranial pressure, 143
  neonatal, 668
  normal, 103
  poisoning, 624
  respiratory assessment, 198
  trauma management, 506
  triage, 103-105
Vitamin B_{12} deficiency in anemia, 402
Vitamin D
  deficiency, 324
  hypercalcemia, 324, 325-326
  hypocalcemia, 482-483
  toxicity, 325-326
Vitamin K
  as antidote, 632
  viral hepatitis, 344
Vitamin poisoning, 634
Vitamin therapy, 40
Vocal cord in endotracheal intubation, 498
Voiding, 364
Volume expanders; see Fluid therapy
Volume resuscitation; see Fluid therapy
Volvulus, 350-351
Vomiting, 335-336
  appendicitis, 348
  bulimia nervosa, 735
  chemical ingestion, 583
  gastroenteritis, 340
  gastrostomy tube, 724
  with headache, 269, 270
  hypovolemic shock, 117
  induction in poisoning, 625
  intussusception, 347
  malrotation of bowel with volvu-
    lus, 350
  in metabolic alkalosis, 328
  neonatal, 679-680
  pertussis, 209
  pyloric stenosis, 352
  upper respiratory infection, 676
Von Willebrand's disease, 408
V:Q ratio; see Ventilation to pulmonary
  blood flow ratio
VSD; see Ventricular septal defect
VUR; see Vesicoureteral reflux
VZIG; see Varicella-zoster immune
  globulin

W

Waddells' triad, 491
Waiting area, 89
Warfarin poisoning, 632
Warming measures in near-
  drowning, 223
Washing, nasal, 207
Wasp sting, 642, 643, 644
Water deprivation test, 482

Water temperature in pediatric emergency departments, 18
Waterhouse-Friderichsen syndrome, 485
Waters view, 467
Weight; *see* Body weight
Weight loss
  dehydration, 100, 117, 315
  diabetes insipidus, 482
  hypovolemic shock, 117
  pyloric stenosis, 352
Well child care, 87
Westcort; *see* Hydrocortisone valerate
Western blot assay, 397
Wet drowning, 219
Wheal, 420, 421
Wheezing
  asthma, 212
  bronchiolitis, 207
  pneumonia, 204
  respiratory assessment, 197, 198
White blood cell count
  anemia, 405
  anorexia and bulimia nervosa, 734
  febrile child, 614
  hemolytic-uremic syndrome, 387
  Henoch-Schönlein purpura, 388
  neonatal bloody stool, 678
  pelvic inflammatory disease, 372

White blood cell count—cont'd
  pertussis, 209
  pneumonia, 205
  toxic or transient synovitis, 301
White blood cells
  anatomy and physiology, 391-392,
    393, 394
  in meningitis, 279
Whole bowel irrigation, 630
Whooping cough, 208-209, 210
Window fall, 489
Witch's milk, 666
Wood alcohol poisoning, 636
Wood's light examination, 438
Word Graphic Rating Scale, 694
Wound, Pediatric Trauma Score, 9
Wound care
  animal bite, 645
  burn injury, 576-577
  snakebite, 645
Wrist fracture, 554-555, 556

X

X-linked recessive disorder
  hemophilia, 408
  muscular dystrophy, 310
X-ray
  cervical spine injury, 519

X-ray—cont'd
  chest; *see* Chest x-ray
  child abuse, 595
  foreign body ingestion, 360, 361,
    362
  fracture, 556, 557
    clavicular, 550
    limp and, 544
    toddler's fracture, 546
  iron poisoning, 639
  Legg-Perthes disease, 306, 308
  septic arthritis, 296
  sinusitis, 467
  thoracic injury, 544

Y

Yale scale, 610, 611
Yellow jacket sting, 644
  anaphylactic reaction, 651
Yersinia, 342-343

Z

Zaroxolyn; *see* Metolazone
ZDV; *see* Zidovudine
Zidovudine, 397-398